Quick Guide to Bivar

Level of measurement of dependent variable	Group Comparisons: Number of groups (the independent variable)				Correlational analyses (To examine relationship strength)
	2 Groups		3+ Groups		
	Independent Groups Tests	Dependent Groups Tests	Independent Groups Tests	Dependent Groups Tests	
Nominal (Categorical)	χ^2 p. 401 (or Fisher's exact test) p. 402	McNemar's test p. 402	χ^2 p. 401	Cochran's Q	Phi coefficient (dichotomous) or Cramér's V (not restricted to dichotomous) p. 403
Ordinal (Rank)	Mann-Whitney Test p. 396	Wilcoxon signed ranks test p. 396	Kruskal-Wallis H test p. 400	Friedman's test p. 400	Spearman's rho (or Kendall's tau) pp. 403
Interval or Ratio (Continuous)*	Independent group t test pp. 394-395	Paired t test p. 396	ANOVA pp. 396-399	RM-ANOVA pp. 400	Pearson's r p. 402
	Multifactor ANOVA for 2+ independent variables p. 398				
	RM-ANOVA for 2+ groups x 2+ measurements over time p. 424				

*For distributions that are markedly nonnormal or samples that are small, the nonparametric tests in the row above (for ordinal measures) may be needed.

Polit and Beck's
NURSING RESEARCH
Generating and Assessing Evidence for Nursing Practice

Twelfth Edition

Jane Flanagan, PhD, RN, ANP-BC, AHN-B, FNI, FNAP, FAAN
Associate Professor
William F. Connell School of Nursing
Chestnut Hill, Massachusetts

Cheryl Tatano Beck, DNSc, CNM, FAAN
Distinguished Professor
School of Nursing
University of Connecticut
Storrs, Connecticut

Wolters Kluwer

Philadelphia • Baltimore • New York • London
Buenos Aires • Hong Kong • Sydney • Tokyo

Vice President and Publisher: Julie K. Stegman
Director of Nursing Education and Practice Content: Jamie Blum
Senior Acquisitions Editor: Joyce Berendes
Director of Product Development: Jennifer K. Forestieri
Senior Development Editor: Jacquelyn Saunders
Editorial Coordinator: Janet Jayne
Marketing Manager: Wendy Mears
Editorial Assistant: Sara Thul
Design Coordinators: Stephen Druding, Leslie Caruso
Art Director, Illustration: Jennifer Clements
Production Project Manager: Matthew West
Manufacturing Coordinator: Margie Orzech-Zeranko
Prepress Vendor: TNQ Tech

Twelfth Edition

Copyright © 2025 Wolters Kluwer.

Copyright © 2021 Wolters Kluwer. Copyright © 2017 Wolters Kluwer. Copyright © 2012 Wolters Kluwer Health | Lippincott Williams & Wilkins. Copyright © 2008, 2004, 1999 by Lippincott Williams & Wilkins. Copyright © 1995, 1991, 1987, 1983, 1978 by J. B. Lippincott Company.

All rights reserved. This book is protected by copyright. No part of this book may be reproduced or transmitted in any form or by any means, including as photocopies or scanned-in or other electronic copies, or utilized by any information storage and retrieval system without written permission from the copyright owner, except for brief quotations embodied in critical articles and reviews. Materials appearing in this book prepared by individuals as part of their official duties as US government employees are not covered by the abovementioned copyright. To request permission, please contact Wolters Kluwer at Two Commerce Square, 2001 Market Street, Philadelphia, PA 19103, via email at permissions@lww.com, or via our website at shop.lww.com (products and services).

9 8 7 6 5 4 3 2 1

Printed in Mexico

Library of Congress Cataloging-in-Publication Data

ISBN-13: 978-1-975223-80-9

Cataloging in Publication data available on request from publisher.

This work is provided "as is," and the publisher disclaims any and all warranties, express or implied, including any warranties as to accuracy, comprehensiveness, or currency of the content of this work.

This work is no substitute for individual patient assessment based upon healthcare professionals' examination of each patient and consideration of, among other things, age, weight, gender, current or prior medical conditions, medication history, laboratory data, and other factors unique to the patient. The publisher does not provide medical advice or guidance, and this work is merely a reference tool. Healthcare professionals, and not the publisher, are solely responsible for the use of this work including all medical judgments and for any resulting diagnosis and treatments.

Given continuous, rapid advances in medical science and health information, independent professional verification of medical diagnoses, indications, appropriate pharmaceutical selections and dosages, and treatment options should be made, and healthcare professionals should consult a variety of sources. When prescribing medication, healthcare professionals are advised to consult the product information sheet (the manufacturer's package insert) accompanying each drug to verify, among other things, conditions of use, warnings, and side effects and identify any changes in dosage schedule or contraindications, particularly if the medication to be administered is new, infrequently used, or has a narrow therapeutic range. To the maximum extent permitted under applicable law, no responsibility is assumed by the publisher for any injury and/or damage to persons or property, as a matter of products liability, negligence law or otherwise, or from any reference to or use by any person of this work.

shop.lww.com

TO

The memory of Denise F. Polit

1946–2021

From Denise's son:

Denise Polit was, above all, a force of nature. She was brilliant and kind, giving and strong, and passionate to the point of danger. She tasked herself with constant improvement so that she could lift up others. She would agonize for hours over a sentence, trying to find the perfect way to help others understand a difficult concept. As you read these pages, I hope that you can catch a glimpse of the passion she had for this material, for the desire she had to make a difference to those who dedicated themselves to trying to learn a difficult subject. She cared, deeply, about the book you're about to read, and I hope that, like myself and so many others, you will find that her passion and dedication will help guide you and make you a better version of yourself.

Denise is survived by her stepdaughters Norah, Lauren, and Alaine and their wonderful families, as well as by her son Alex, who still hopes that, one day, he will be worthy of all that she did for him.

Respectfully,
N. Alexander O'Hara

Acknowledgments

We must start this 12th edition of the book by acknowledging the tremendous loss of Dr. Denise Polit—not only for her family but also for the discipline of nursing. Dr. Polit was not a nurse, but how extremely fortunate our discipline has been to have had her devote her career to supporting the learning, knowledge, and professional development of nurses, specifically in the field of nursing research. Since Denise wrote the first edition of this book in 1978, there has been no other individual who we believe has had more of an impact on the development of generations of nurses in regard to nursing research than Dr. Denise Polit. Denise would often call this book "her baby," which she tenderly cared for throughout each of the first 11 editions. She will be deeply missed!

This 12th edition, like the previous 11 editions, depended on the contributions of dozens of people. Many faculty and students who used the text have made invaluable suggestions for its improvement, and to all of you who have, we are very grateful. In addition to all those who assisted us over the past 40 plus years with the earlier editions, the following individuals deserve special mention.

We would like to acknowledge the comments of reviewers of the previous edition of this book, anonymous to us initially, whose feedback influenced our revisions. We would like to thank Dr. Carrie Morgan Eaton at the University of Connecticut who provided regular feedback and updates to computer-assisted qualitative data analysis software.

We also extend our thanks to those who helped to turn the manuscript into a finished product. The staff at Wolters Kluwer has been of great assistance to us over the years. We are indebted to Joyce Berendes, Jacquelyn Saunders, Janet Jayne, Wendy Mears, Matthew West, and all the others behind the scenes for their fine contributions.

Finally, we thank our family and friends. Our husbands Richard Nangle and Chuck and children Curt and Lisa have become accustomed to our demanding schedules, but we recognize that their support involves a lot of patience and many sacrifices.

Reviewers

Kelley M. Anderson, PhD, FNP, CHFN-K
Associate Professor
Department of Professional Nursing Practice
Georgetown University
Washington, District of Columbia

Debra Bacharz, PhD, MSN, RN
Professor of Nursing
Leach College of Nursing
University of St. Francis
Joliet, Illinois

Kimberly Balko, PhD, RN
Assistant Professor
Department of Nursing
SUNY Empire State College
Saratoga Springs, New York

Susan A. Bonis, PhD, RN
Assistant Clinical Professor
College of Nursing
University of Wisconsin—Milwaukee
Milwaukee, Wisconsin

Barbara Brewer, PhD, RN, MALS, MBA
Associate Professor
College of Nursing
The University of Arizona
Tucson, Arizona

Kathleen A. Fagan, PhD, RN, APN
Associate Professor
Graduate Nursing
School of Nursing
Felician University
Lodi, New Jersey

Tracia Forman, PhD, RN-BC, CNE
Assistant Professor
Department of Nursing
University of Texas Rio Grande Valley
Brownsville, Texas

LaDawna R. Goering, DNP, APN, ANP-BC
Assistant Professor
Department of Nursing
Northern Illinois University
DeKalb, Illinois

Ashlyn Johnson, DNP, FNP-BC
Assistant Professor of Nursing
MSN Program (FNP & PMHNP Tracks)
Mount Marty College
Yankton, South Dakota

Rebecca Witten Jones, PhD, RN, MSN, NP-C, CNL
Clinical Assistant Professor
Dr. Susan L. D\avis, RN, & Richard J. Henley
  College of Nursing
Sacred Heart University
Fairfield, Connecticut

Kara Misto, PhD, RN
Assistant Professor
School of Nursing
Rhode Island College
Providence, Rhode Island

Stephen J. Stapleton, PhD, MS, RN, CEN, FAEN
Associate Professor
Mennonite College of Nursing
Illinois State University
Normal, Illinois

Debbie Stayer, PhD, RN-BC, CCRN-K
Assistant Professor
Department of Nursing
Bloomsburg University
Bloomsburg, Pennsylvania

Kathleen Thompson, PhD, RN, CNE
Clinical Professor
Department of Nursing
University of Tennessee, Knoxville
Knoxville, Tennessee

Ann Tritak, EdD, RN
Associate Dean
Department of Graduate Nursing
Felician University
Lodi, New Jersey

Shelly Wells, PhD, MBA, MS, APRN-CNS
Division Chair and Professor
Division of Nursing
Northwestern Oklahoma State University
Alva, Oklahoma

Kelli D. Whittington, PhD, RN, CNE
Chair, Division of Nursing
McKendree University
Lebanon, Illinois

Preface

Research methodology is a dynamic enterprise. Even after 11 editions of this book, we have continued to draw new material and inspiration from ground-breaking advances in research methods and in nurse researchers' use of those methods. It is thrilling to share many of those developments in this new edition. We expect that many of the new methodologic and technological enhancements will be translated into powerful evidence for nursing practice. We are pleased that that this 12th edition has built on the foundation of the previous versions We have retained many features that made this book a classic textbook and resource, including its focus on research as a support for evidence-based nursing; but as with other editions, we have introduced important information that we hope will help to shape the future of nursing research.

NEW TO THIS EDITION

New and Added Content

Throughout the book, we have included up-to-date information on methodologic innovations that have arisen in nursing, medicine, and the social sciences during the past 4 to 5 years. These changes reflect the 2022–2026 NINR Strategic Plan and the AACN Essentials. The many additions and changes are too numerous to describe here, so here are just two examples. In Chapter 2 we included a discussion regarding the importance of original research in the practice setting. We have added information about the role of the PhD-prepared nurse in developing new knowledge and working in collaboration with DNP-prepared nurses who will implement this knowledge in care settings. In Chapter 25 there is an expanded and updated CAQDAS computer software for managing qualitative data. Also added is a large section on secondary qualitative data analysis. Braun and Clarke's reflexive thematic analysis and Kyngas et al.'s qualitative content analysis method have also been added to this chapter.

Every chapter has an online supplement (and some chapters in this edition have two supplements), which gave us the opportunity to add a considerable amount of new material.

Here is a complete list of the supplements for the 33 chapters of the textbook:

1. The History of Nursing Research
2. A. Evaluating Clinical Practice Guidelines—AGREE II
   B. Evidence-Based Practice in an Organizational Context
3. Deductive and Inductive Reasoning
4. Complex Relationships and Hypotheses
5. A. Finding Evidence for a Clinical Query
   B. Literature Review Summary Tables
6. Prominent Conceptual Models of Nursing Used by Nurse Researchers, and a Guide to Middle-Range Theories
7. Historical Background on Unethical Research Conduct
8. Research Control
9. Randomization Strategies
10. A. Selected Experimental and Quasi-Experimental Designs: Diagrams, Uses, and Drawbacks/Validity Threats
    B. Plausibility Assessments and Other Strategies When Randomization is Not Possible

11. Other Specific Types of Research
12. Statistical Process Control
13. Sample Recruitment and Retention
14. Other Types of Structured Self-Reports
15. Cross-Cultural Validity and the Adaptation/Translation of Measures
16. Overview of Item Response Theory
17. SPSS Analysis of Descriptive Statistics
18. SPSS Analysis of Inferential Statistics
19. SPSS Analysis and Multivariate Statistics
20. Some Preliminary Steps in Quantitative Analysis Using SPSS
21. Clinical Significance Assessment with the Jacobson–Truax Approach
22. Historical Nursing Research and Other Types of Qualitative Inquiry
23. Models of Generalizability in Qualitative Research
24. Additional Types of Unstructured Self-Reports
25. Transcribing Qualitative Data
26. Whittemore and Colleagues' Framework of Quality Criteria in Qualitative Research
27. Transforming Quantitative and Qualitative Data
28. Complex Intervention Development: Additional Resources
29. Examples of Various Pilot and Feasibility Objectives
30. A. Publication Bias in Systematic Reviews
    B. Supplementary Resources for Qualitative Evidence Synthesis
31. The RE-AIM Framework
32. A. Tips for Publishing Reports on Pilot Intervention Studies
    B. Impact Factor and Publication Information for Selected Nursing Journals
33. Proposals for Pilot Intervention Studies

Another feature of this edition concerns readers' access to references we cited. To the extent possible, the studies we have chosen as examples of research methods are published as open-access articles. These studies are identified in the reference list at the end of each chapter.

We hope that our many revisions will help users of this book to maximize their learning experience.

ORGANIZATION OF THE TEXT

The content of this edition is organized into six main parts.

- **Part 1—Foundations of Nursing Research and Evidence-Based Practice** introduces fundamental concepts in nursing research. Chapter 1 briefly summarizes the history and future of nursing research, discusses the philosophical underpinnings of qualitative research versus quantitative research, and describes the major purposes of nursing research. In this chapter, nursing research is discussed in light of the Institute of Medicine 2020–2030 report, The National Institute of Nursing Research Strategic Plan (2020–2026), the AANC Essentials, and the 2021 Magnet Application Manual. Chapter 2 offers guidance on using research to support evidence-based practice. Chapter 3 introduces readers to key research terms and presents an overview of steps in the research process for both qualitative and quantitative studies.

- **Part 2—Conceptualizing and Planning a Study to Generate Evidence for Nursing** further sets the stage for learning about the research process by discussing issues relating to a study's conceptualization: the formulation of research questions and hypotheses (Chapter 4), the review of relevant research (Chapter 5), the development of theoretical and conceptual contexts (Chapter 6), and the fostering of ethically acceptable approaches in doing research (Chapter 7). Chapter 8 provides an overview of important issues that researchers must attend to during the planning of any study.

- **Part 3—Designing and Conducting Quantitative Studies to Generate Evidence for Nursing** presents material on undertaking quantitative nursing studies. Chapter 9 describes fundamental principles of quantitative research design, and Chapter 10 focuses on methods to enhance the rigor of a quantitative study, including mechanisms of research control. Chapter 11 examines research with different and distinct purposes, such as noninferiority trials, realist evaluations, surveys, and outcomes research. Chapter 12 is devoted to methods used in quality improvement and improvement science. Chapter 13 presents strategies for sampling study participants in quantitative research. Chapter 14 describes structured data collection methods that yield quantitative information. Chapter 15 discusses the concept of measurement and then focuses on methods of assessing the quality of formal measuring instruments. We describe methods to assess the properties of point-in-time measurements (reliability and validity) and longitudinal measurements—that is, change scores (reliability of change scores and responsiveness). Chapter 16 presents material on how to develop high-quality self-report instruments. Chapters 17–19 present an overview of univariate, bivariate, and multivariate statistical analyses, respectively. Chapter 20 describes the development of an overall analytic strategy for quantitative studies, including material on handling missing data. Chapter 21 discusses the issue of interpreting results and making inferences about clinical significance.

- **Part 4—Designing and Conducting Qualitative Studies to Generate Evidence for Nursing** presents material on undertaking qualitative nursing studies. Chapter 22 is devoted to research designs and approaches for qualitative studies, including information on critical theory, feminist, and participatory action research. Chapter 23 discusses strategies for sampling study participants in qualitative inquiries. Chapter 24 describes methods of gathering unstructured self-report and observational data for qualitative studies. Chapter 25 discusses methods of analyzing qualitative data, with specific information on grounded theory, phenomenologic, and ethnographic analyses. Greater guidance on coding qualitative data has been added to this edition. Chapter 26 elaborates on methods qualitative researchers can use to enhance (and assess) integrity and trustworthiness throughout their inquiries.

- **Part 5—Designing and Conducting Mixed Methods Studies to Generate Evidence for Nursing** presents material on mixed methods nursing studies. Chapter 27 discusses a broad range of issues, including asking mixed methods questions, designing a study to address the questions, sampling participants in mixed methods research, and analyzing and integrating qualitative and quantitative data. Chapter 28 presents information about using mixed methods approaches in the development of complex nursing interventions. In Chapter 29, we provide suggestions for designing and conducting pilot studies and using data from the pilots to make decisions about "next steps."

- **Part 6—Building an Evidence Base for Nursing Practice** provides additional information on linking research and clinical practice. Chapter 30 offers an overview of methods of conducting systematic reviews that support EBP. In this chapter, we provide guidance on conducting the integrative review, meta-analyses (and an evaluation of confidence in the evidence using the GRADE system), metasyntheses, qualitative evidence syntheses using meta-aggregation, and mixed studies reviews. Chapter 31 offers cutting-edge advice on strategies to enhance the *applicability* of practice-based evidence to clinical decisions for individuals and subgroups. Chapter 32 discusses the dissemination of evidence—how to prepare a research report (including theses and dissertations) and how to publish research findings. The concluding chapter (Chapter 33) offers suggestions on developing research proposals to obtain financial support; it includes information about developing a proposal for a pilot intervention study.

KEY FEATURES

This textbook was designed to be helpful to those who are learning how to do research, to those who are learning to appraise research reports critically, and to use research findings in practice. Many of the features successfully used in previous editions have been retained in this 12th edition. Among the basic principles that helped to shape this and earlier editions of this book are (1) an unswerving conviction that the development of research skills is critical to the nursing profession, (2) a fundamental belief that research is intellectually and professionally rewarding, and (3) a steadfast opinion that learning about research methods does not need to be intimidating nor dull. Consistent with these principles, we have tried to present the fundamentals of research methods in a way that both facilitates understanding and arouses curiosity and interest. Key features of our approach include the following:

- **Research examples** Each chapter concludes with one or two actual research examples designed to highlight methodologic features described in the chapter and to sharpen the reader's critical thinking skills. In addition, many research examples are used throughout the book to illustrate key points and to stimulate ideas for a study. Many examples used in this edition are published as open-access articles that can be used for further learning and classroom discussion.
- **Specific practical tips on doing research** The textbook is filled with practical suggestions on how to translate the abstract notions of research methods into realistic strategies for conducting research. Every chapter includes several tips for applying the chapter's lessons to real-life situations. These tips are an acknowledgment that there is often a gap between what gets taught in research methods textbooks and what a researcher needs to know to conduct a study.
- **Critical appraisal guidelines** Almost all chapters include guidelines for conducting a critical appraisal of various aspects of a research report.
- **A comprehensive index** We have crafted an exceptionally thorough index. We know that our book is used as a reference book as well as a textbook, and we recognize how crucial it is to access needed information efficiently.
- **Aids to student learning** This book includes several additional features designed to enhance and reinforce learning, including the following: succinct, bulleted summaries at the end of each chapter; tables and figures that provide examples and graphic materials in support of the text discussion; and a detailed glossary.
- **Clear, user-friendly style** Our writing style is designed to be easily digestible and nonintimidating. Concepts are introduced carefully and systematically, difficult ideas are presented clearly, and readers are assumed to have no prior exposure to technical terms.

A Note About Language Used In This Book

Wolters Kluwer recognizes that people have a diverse range of identities, and we are committed to using inclusive and nonbiased language in our content. In line with the principles of nursing, we strive not to define people by their diagnoses, but to recognize their personhood first and foremost, using as much as possible the language diverse groups use to define themselves and including only information that is relevant to nursing care.

We strive to better address the unique perspectives, complex challenges, and lived experiences of diverse populations traditionally underrepresented in health literature. When describing or referencing populations discussed in research studies, we will adhere to the identities presented in those studies to maintain fidelity to the evidence presented by the study investigators. We follow best practices of language set forth by the *Publication Manual of the American Psychological Association, 7th edition*, but acknowledge that language evolves rapidly, and we will update the language used in future editions of this book as necessary.

A COMPREHENSIVE PACKAGE FOR TEACHING AND LEARNING

To further facilitate teaching and learning, a carefully designed ancillary package has been developed to assist faculty and students.

Resources for Instructors

Tools to assist you with teaching your course are available upon adoption of this text at http://thepoint.lww.com/Flanagan12e.

- An **e-Book** gives you access to the book's full text and images online.
- The **Test Generator** lets you put together exclusive new tests from a bank containing more than 790 questions to help you in assessing your students' understanding of the material.
- **PowerPoint Presentations** summarizing key points in each chapter provide an easy way for you to integrate the textbook with your students' classroom experience, either via slide shows or handouts. Multiple-choice and true/false questions are integrated into the presentations to promote class participation and allow you to use i-clicker technology.
- An **Image Bank** of all the images in the book allows you to use these illustrations in your PowerPoint slides or as you see fit in your course.
- Other helpful resources include **Answers to Application Exercises** and **Strategies for Effective Teaching**.

Contact your sales representative for more details and ordering information.

A COMPREHENSIVE, DIGITAL, INTEGRATED COURSE SOLUTION: *LIPPINCOTT® COURSEPOINT*

Lippincott® CoursePoint is an integrated, digital curriculum solution for nursing education that provides a completely interactive experience geared to help students understand, retain, and apply their course knowledge and be prepared for practice. The time-tested, easy-to-use and trusted solution includes engaging learning tools, case studies, and in-depth reporting to meet students where they are in their learning, combined with the most trusted nursing education content on the market to help prepare students for practice. This easy-to-use digital learning solution of Lippincott® CoursePoint, combined with unmatched support, gives instructors and students everything they need for course and curriculum success!

Lippincott® CoursePoint includes:

- Engaging course content provides a variety of learning tools to engage students of all learning styles.
- Adaptive and personalized learning helps students learn the critical thinking and clinical judgment skills needed to help them become practice-ready nurses.
- Unparalleled reporting provides in-depth dashboards with several data points to track student progress and help identify strengths and weaknesses.
- Unmatched support includes training coaches, product trainers, and nursing education consultants to help educators and students implement CoursePoint with ease.

It is our hope that the content, style, and organization of *Nursing Research,* 12th Edition continue to meet the needs of a broad spectrum of nursing students and nurse researchers. We also hope that the book will help to foster enthusiasm for the kinds of discoveries that research can produce and for the knowledge that will help support an evidence-based nursing practice.

About the Authors

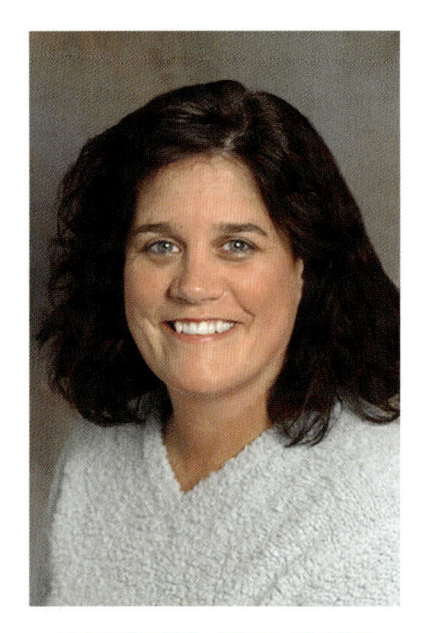

JANE FLANAGAN
PhD, RN, ANP-BC, AHN-B, FNI, FNAP, FAAN

Jane Flanagan is an Associate Professor and department chairperson at the William F. Connell School of Nursing, Boston College. Jane is a certified nurse practitioner and holds appointments as a nurse scientist at the Massachusetts General Hospital (MGH) Yvonne Munn Center for Nursing Research and as an associate clinical scientist at the Phyllis Cantor Center at the Dana-Farber Cancer Institute. Jane serves on the Board of Directors at the Sherrill House in Boston and as an advisor to the Board at Fox Hill Village in Westwood, MA.

Jane is the editor of the *International Journal of Nursing Knowledge* and *Visions,* the official journal of the Society of Rogerian Scholars in *Advances in Nursing Science*. Jane also serves on the editorial board for the *International Journal for Human Caring*. She is an appointed fellow in NANDA-I, the National Academy of Practice, and the American Academy of Nursing. She is the immediate past president of the Eastern Nursing Research Society (ENRS). Jane's funded research using mixed methods is focused on strategies to improve the experience of older adults—especially dementia caregivers and those with chronic health conditions.

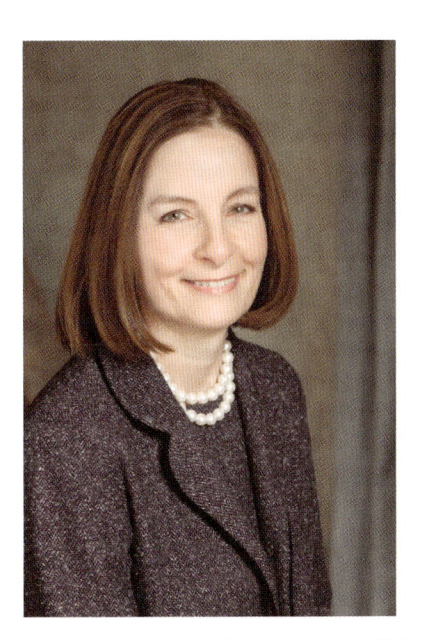

CHERYL TATANO BECK
DNSc, CNM, FAAN

Dr. Beck is a Distinguished Professor at the University of Connecticut, School of Nursing. She also has a joint appointment in the Department of Obstetrics and Gynecology at the School of Medicine. She received her master's degree in maternal-newborn nursing and her certificate in nurse-midwifery from Yale University. Her Doctor of Nursing Science degree is from Boston University. She is a fellow in the American Academy of Nursing and is inducted into the Sigma Theta Tau International Nurse Researcher Hall of Fame and Sigma XI, the Scientific Research Honor Society. She was awarded the Marcé Medal by the International Marcé Society for Perinatal Mental Health for the significant contributions of her research program. She has received numerous other awards such as the Association of Women's Health, Obstetric and Neonatal Nursing's Distinguished Professional Service Award, the Distinguished Alumna Award from Yale University, and Eastern Nursing Research Society's Distinguished Researcher Award.

Over the past 40 years, Cheryl has focused her research efforts on developing a research program on postpartum mood and anxiety disorders. Her Postpartum Depression Screening Scale is based on her series of qualitative studies. She has published over 195 journal articles. In addition to coauthoring award-winning research methods textbooks with Denise Polit, Cheryl coauthored with Dr. Jeanne Watson Driscoll *Postpartum Mood and Anxiety Disorders: A Clinician's Guide*, which received the *2006 American Journal of Nursing Book of the Year Award*. Other books Cheryl has written include *Traumatic Childbirth, Developing a Program of Research in Nursing, Secondary Qualitative Data Analysis in the Health and Social Sciences*, and *Introduction to Phenomenology: Focus on Methodology*.

Contents

PART 1 FOUNDATIONS OF NURSING RESEARCH AND EVIDENCE-BASED PRACTICE 1
Chapter 1 Introduction to Nursing Research in an Evidence-Based Practice Environment 2
Chapter 2 Evidence-Based Nursing: Translating Research Evidence Into Practice 21
Chapter 3 Key Concepts and Steps in Qualitative and Quantitative Research 42

PART 2 CONCEPTUALIZING AND PLANNING A STUDY TO
GENERATE EVIDENCE FOR NURSING 64
Chapter 4 Research Problems, Research Questions, and Hypotheses 65
Chapter 5 Literature Reviews: Finding and Critically Appraising Evidence 83
Chapter 6 Theoretical Frameworks 113
Chapter 7 Ethics in Nursing Research 130
Chapter 8 Planning a Nursing Study 152

PART 3 DESIGNING AND CONDUCTING QUANTITATIVE STUDIES TO
GENERATE EVIDENCE FOR NURSING 174
Chapter 9 Quantitative Research Design 175
Chapter 10 Rigor and Validity in Quantitative Research 205
Chapter 11 Specific Types of Quantitative Research 224
Chapter 12 Quality Improvement and Improvement Science 239
Chapter 13 Sampling in Quantitative Research 257
Chapter 14 Data Collection in Quantitative Research 275
Chapter 15 Measurement and Data Quality 307
Chapter 16 Developing and Testing Self-Report Scales 338
Chapter 17 Descriptive Statistics 362
Chapter 18 Inferential Statistics 380
Chapter 19 Multivariate Statistics 406
Chapter 20 Processes of Quantitative Data Analysis 428
Chapter 21 Clinical Significance and Interpretation of Quantitative Results 441

PART 4 DESIGNING AND CONDUCTING QUALITATIVE STUDIES TO GENERATE EVIDENCE FOR NURSING 461

Chapter 22 Qualitative Research Design and Approaches 462
Chapter 23 Sampling in Qualitative Research 487
Chapter 24 Data Collection in Qualitative Research 499
Chapter 25 Qualitative Data Analysis 522
Chapter 26 Trustworthiness and Rigor in Qualitative Research 551

PART 5 DESIGNING AND CONDUCTING MIXED METHODS STUDIES TO GENERATE EVIDENCE FOR NURSING 568

Chapter 27 Basics of Mixed Methods Research 569
Chapter 28 Developing Complex Nursing Interventions Using Mixed Methods Research 595
Chapter 29 Feasibility and Pilot Studies of Interventions Using Mixed Methods 614

PART 6 BUILDING AN EVIDENCE BASE FOR NURSING PRACTICE 635

Chapter 30 Systematic Reviews of Research Evidence 636
Chapter 31 Applicability, Generalizability, and Relevance: Toward Practice-Based Evidence 677
Chapter 32 Disseminating Evidence: Reporting Research Findings 705
Chapter 33 Writing Proposals to Generate Evidence 730

Appendix: Statistical Tables 749
Glossary 755
Index 787

Part 1

FOUNDATIONS OF NURSING RESEARCH AND EVIDENCE-BASED PRACTICE

Chapter 1 Introduction to Nursing Research in an Evidence-Based Practice Environment
Chapter 2 Evidence-Based Nursing: Translating Research Evidence Into Practice
Chapter 3 Key Concepts and Steps in Qualitative and Quantitative Research

1

Introduction to Nursing Research in an Evidence-Based Practice Environment

Learning Objectives

1. Describe the importance of nursing research to clinical practice.
2. Recognize the historical trends and future directions of nursing research.
3. Identify the sources of evidence for nursing practice.
4. Outline the two paradigms of nursing research and the research methods associated with them.
5. Describe the difference between basic and applied nursing research.

NURSING RESEARCH IN PERSPECTIVE

Many factors have contributed to a heightened awareness of the need for nurses at all levels to recognize their role in designing, creating opportunities for, implementing, and disseminating knowledge for practice. While technical skill acquisition and competency remain essential to nursing academic and practice settings alike, there is a greater appreciation of the need for nurses to develop, translate, and implement the most trustworthy and sound evidence for practice. **Evidence-based practice (EBP)** is a process that considers not only the best evidence, but also patient preferences and circumstances, social determinants of health, and nurses' clinical judgment, to make informed patient care decisions. Given the nursing focus on health, healing and holism, the best evidence that guides nursing practice is informed by nurses and others with whom they collaborate.

What Is Nursing Research?

Research inquiry relies on a variety of methods to answer questions or solve problems. Nurses are increasingly engaged in research intended to improve patient care. **Nursing research** is designed to generate evidence about issues of importance to the delivery and outcomes of patient care and as a result, may include work focused on the nursing profession, practice, education, and administration. In this book, we emphasize **clinical nursing research** aimed at guiding nursing practice that improves the health and quality of life of the patients, families/supports, and communities nurses serve.

Nursing research has experienced remarkable growth in the past few decades, providing nurses with a growing evidence base on which to practice. Yet many questions persist, and mechanisms for incorporating research innovations into nursing practice still are in development.

Examples of Nursing Research Questions
- What are the impact and effectiveness of telehealth-delivered psychoeducational and behavioral interventions among persons with dementia and their caregivers? (Saragih, et al., 2022)
- What is the effect of a web-based self-care program for patients with primary hypertension on cardiovascular risk-factors, self-efficacy, and self-care behaviors? (Chen et al., 2022)

The Importance of Research in Nursing

Findings from rigorous research provide evidence for informing nurses' decisions. Nurses have come to accept the desirability of incorporating research evidence into their actions, if the evidence shows that the actions are clinically appropriate and result in positive patient outcomes.

In some countries, research plays an important role in nursing credentialing and status. For example, the American Nurses Credentialing Center—an arm of the American Nurses Association and a prestigious credentialing organization in the United States—developed a Magnet Recognition Program to acknowledge healthcare organizations that provide high-quality nursing care. The 2023 Magnet application manual incorporates a perspective that recognizes global issues in nursing and healthcare. In addition to the 2017 revisions that strengthen evidence-based requirements, the 2021 manual calls for an example with supporting evidence of a clinical nurse who implemented a new or revised EBP practice within the organization (ANCC, 2023; Graystone, 2017). Applicants must now submit at least three nursing studies reflecting varied types of scholarship: Magnet hospitals must not only be involved in implementing EBP but also in the creation of original nursing research and the dissemination the new knowledge generated. Although it can be challenging to make direct correlations, there is evidence to suggest that Magnet hospitals with their focus on research and EBP may lead to some improved patient outcomes. For example, Aamodt et al. (2021) found that in patients with Parkinson disease, Magnet hospitals had lower rates of mortality and several nurse-sensitive outcomes than those admitted to non-Magnet hospitals, even when differences in other hospital characteristics were taken into account. Also Dierkes et al. (2021) reported that hospitals with Magnet status had 30% lower odds of value-based purchasing penalties suggesting they had fewer hospital readmissions and hospital-acquired conditions in relation to non-Magnet hospitals.

The primary focus of the literature on hospital-based research nurse scientists prepared with a PhD and advanced practice nurses prepared as DNPs is about describing the role in practice. Future work will likely be focused on the impact of the nurse scientist generating original research and the DNP implementing the findings into practice with a focus on the impact on patient care outcomes.

Example of Evidence-Based Practice
The Fall TIPS Program (Dykes et al. (2020); Dykes & Hurley (2021) aimed at reducing the risk of falls in hospitalized patients is now routinely practiced nationwide in hospitals and other patient care facilities such as nursing home settings, but prior to its early development, there were no evidence-based options for preventing falls in the hospital settings despite the known risks to patients and extensive costs of care. Expanded adoption of this nurse-led program reflects mounting evidence that the Fall Tips Program prevents falls in hospitalized patients.

The Consumer–Producer Continuum in Nursing Research

Most nurses are likely to engage in research activities along a continuum of participation. At one end are consumers of nursing research, who read research reports or research summaries to keep up-to-date on findings that might affect their practice. EBP depends on well-informed research consumers.

At the other end of the continuum are producers of nursing research: nurses who conduct research. At one time, most nurse researchers were academics who taught in nursing schools, but research is increasingly being conducted by clinical nurses who seek solutions to recurring problems in patient care.

Between these end points on the continuum lie a variety of research activities that are undertaken by nurses. Even if you never personally carry out a study, you may (1) contribute to an idea for a clinical study; (2) gather information for a study; (3) advise clients about participating in research; (4) seek answers to a clinical problem by searching for and appraising research evidence; or (5) discuss the implications of a study in a **journal club** in your practice setting, which involves meetings (in groups or online) to discuss research articles. Understanding research can improve the depth and breadth of every nurse's professional practice.

> **TIP** The Cochrane Collaboration, an important organization for EBP, offers an online journal club resource with podcasts, slides, and discussion questions (https://www.cochranelibrary.com/cdsr/journal-club). Journal clubs, including virtual ones, may help to create an environment of lifelong learning, foster a commitment to EBP, and stimulate nursing research (Rosen & Ryan, 2019).

Nursing Research in Historical Perspective

Table 1.1 summarizes some of the key events in the historical evolution of nursing research.

Florence Nightingale is credited as the first nursing researcher. Her most well-known research contribution involved an analysis of factors affecting soldier mortality and morbidity during the Crimean War (1853–1856). Based on skillful analyses, she was successful in effecting changes in nursing care—and, more generally, in public health. After Nightingale's work, research was absent from the nursing literature until the early 1900s, but most early studies concerned nurses' education rather than patient care.

In the 1950s, research by nurses began to accelerate. For example, the American Nurses' Foundation, which is devoted to the promotion of nursing research, was founded. The surge in the number of studies conducted in the 1950s created the need for a new journal; *Nursing Research* came into being in 1952. As shown in Table 1.1, dissemination opportunities in professional journals grew steadily thereafter.

In the 1960s, nursing leaders expressed concern about the shortage of research on practice issues. Professional nursing organizations, such as the Western Interstate Council for Higher Education in Nursing, established research priorities, and practice-oriented research on various clinical topics began to emerge in the literature.

During the 1970s, improvements in client care became a more visible research priority, and guidance on assessing research for application in practice settings emerged. Also, nursing research expanded internationally. For example, the Workgroup of European Nurse Researchers was established in 1978 to develop greater communication and opportunities for partnerships among 25 European National Nurses Associations.

In the United States, the National Center for Nursing Research (NCNR) at the National Institutes of Health (NIH) was established in 1986. Several forces outside of nursing also helped to shape the nursing research landscape in the 1980s. A group from the McMaster Medical School in Canada designed a clinical learning strategy that was called evidence-based medicine (EBM). EBM, which promulgated the view that research findings were superior to the opinions of authorities as a basis for clinical decisions, constituted a profound shift for medical education and practice, and has had a major effect on all healthcare professions.

Nursing research was strengthened and given more visibility when NCNR was promoted to full institute status within the NIH. In 1993, the **National Institute of Nursing Research (NINR)** was established, helping to put nursing research more into the mainstream of health research. Funding opportunities for nursing research expanded in other countries as well.

Current and Future Directions for Nursing Research

Nursing research continues to develop at a rapid pace and will undoubtedly flourish throughout the 21st century. Broadly speaking, the priority for future nursing research will be the promotion of excellence in nursing science. Toward this end, nurse researchers and practicing nurses will be sharpening their research skills and using those skills to address emerging issues of importance

TABLE 1.1 • Historical Landmarks in Nursing Research

YEAR	EVENT
1859	Nightingale's Notes on Nursing is published.
1900	*American Journal of Nursing* begins publication.
1923	Columbia University establishes first doctoral program for nurses.
	Goldmark Report with recommendations for nursing education is published.
1936	Sigma Theta Tau awards first nursing research grant in the United States.
1948	Brown publishes report on inadequacies of nursing education.
1952	The journal *Nursing Research* begins publication.
1955	Inception of the American Nurses' Foundation to sponsor nursing research.
1957	Establishment of nursing research center at Walter Reed Army Institute of Research.
1963	*International Journal of Nursing Studies* begins publication.
1965	American Nurses' Association (ANA) sponsors nursing research conferences.
1969	*Canadian Journal of Nursing Research* begins publication.
1972	ANA establishes a Commission on Research and Council of Nurse Researchers.
1976	Stetler and Marram publish guidelines on assessing research for use in practice.
	Journal of Advanced Nursing begins publication.
1982	Conduct and Utilization of Research in Nursing (CURN) project publishes report.
1983	*Annual Review of Nursing Research* begins publication.
1985	ANA Cabinet on Nursing Research establishes research priorities.
1986	National Center for Nursing Research (NCNR) is established within U.S. National Institutes of Health.
1988	Conference on Research Priorities is convened by NCNR.
1989	The U.S. Agency for Health Care Policy and Research (AHCPR) is established.
1993	NCNR becomes a full institute, the National Institute of Nursing Research (NINR).
	The Cochrane Collaboration is established.
	Magnet Recognition Program makes first awards.
1995	Joanna Briggs Institute, an EBP collaborative, is established in Australia.
1997	Canadian Health Services Research Foundation is established with federal funding.
1998	The European Academy of Nursing Science (EANS) is launched.
1999	AHCPR is renamed Agency for Healthcare Research and Quality (AHRQ).

TABLE 1.1 • Historical Landmarks in Nursing Research (Continued)

YEAR	EVENT
2000	NINR's annual funding exceeds $100 million. The Canadian Institute of Health Research is launched. Council for the Advancement of Nursing Science (CANS) is established.
2005	The Quality & Safety Education for Nurses (QSEN) initiative is inaugurated.
2006	NINR issues strategic plan for 2006–2010.
2010	The Institute of Medicine publishes a report, *The Future of Nursing*, that includes research priorities and recommendations for lifelong learning.
2011	NINR celebrates 25th anniversary and issues a new strategic plan.
2016	NINR issues *The NINR Strategic Plan: Advancing Science, Improving Lives*.
2019	NINR budget exceeds $145 million.
2022	NINR issues the 2022–2026 Strategic Plan with this mission: to lead nursing research to solve pressing health challenges and inform practice and policy-optimizing health and advancing health equity into the future.

to the profession and its clientele. Among the trends we foresee for the early 21st century are the following:

- *Strengthening of **interprofessional collaboration** through team science.* Collaboration of nurses with researchers in related fields has expanded in the 21st century as researchers address fundamental healthcare problems with each member bringing their own disciplinary perspective to the design and implementation of the research. In turn, such collaborative efforts could lead to nurse researchers playing a more prominent role in national and international healthcare policies. One major recommendation in the Institute of Medicine's (IOM) influential 2010 report, *The Future of Nursing*, reiterated and expanded upon in the 2021 report, *The Future of Nursing 2020–2030: Charting a Path to Achieve Health Equity* (Wakefield et al., 2021), was that nurses should be full partners with physicians and other healthcare professionals in redesigning healthcare with the goal of achieving health equity for all.
- *A new emphasis on health equity.* Along with the IOM, the NINIR Strategic Plan 2020–2026 calls for emphasis on health equity. NINR has embraced research focused on health equity, social determinants of health, population and community health prevention and health promotion, systems, and models of care (NINR, 2020).
- *Continued focus on EBP.* Encouragement for nurses to engage in evidence-based patient care and lifelong learning is sure to continue. In turn, improvements will be needed both in the quality of studies and in nurses' skills in locating, understanding, critically appraising, and using relevant study results. Relatedly, there is an emerging interest in **translational research**, which involves research on how findings from studies can best be translated into practice.
- *Continued emphasis on research synthesis with an appreciation of the **systematic and narrative reviews**.* Research syntheses that integrate research evidence across studies are the cornerstone of EBP. However, all types of reviews are critical to EBP. A systematic review is important because it uses a well-defined process to integrate research findings on a narrowly defined research question and includes a rating appraisal of the evidence. Clinical practice guidelines

typically rely on such systematic reviews. We offer some guidance on how to create, as well as how to appraise, research syntheses in this book. Narrative reviews are equally important to nursing science as they provide perspective, highlight gaps in what is known, result in a deep understanding and a critique of the topic while often sparking the need for original research (Flanagan, 2022).

- *Expanded local research and quality improvement efforts in healthcare settings.* Projects designed to solve local problems are increasing. This trend will be reinforced as more nurses earn terminal degrees in nursing (DNP, PhD) and as hospitals apply for (and are recertified for) Magnet status in the United States and in other countries. Mechanisms need to be developed to ensure that evidence from these projects becomes available to others facing similar problems.
- *Increased emphasis on patient-centeredness.* **Patient centeredness** has become a central concern in healthcare, as well as in research. In the United States, the Patient-Centered Outcomes Research Institute funds research focused on assisting communities, patients, and their caregivers to make well-informed healthcare decisions with an enhanced commitment to diversity, equity, and inclusion. Efforts are increasing to ensure that research is relevant to patients and that patients play a role in setting research priorities. **Comparative effectiveness research**, which involves direct comparisons of alternative treatments, has emerged as an important tool for patient-centered research.
- *Relatedly, greater interest in the* **applicability** *of research.* More attention is being paid to figuring out how study results can be applied to individual patients or groups of patients. A limitation of the current EBP model is that standard strategies offer evidence on average effects of healthcare interventions under ideal circumstances. Ideas are emerging about how best to enhance the applicability of research in real-world settings.
- *Growing interest in defining and ascertaining* **clinical significance**. Research findings increasingly must meet the test of being clinically significant, and patients have taken center-stage in efforts to define clinical significance.
- *Focusing on what nurses are likely to be studying in the future.* Although there is rich diversity in research interests—as we will illustrate throughout this book in the research examples—research priorities have been articulated by several nursing organizations, including NINR, Sigma Theta Tau International, and other nursing organizations throughout the world. Change is a given as nursing must keep up with the trends that influence research agendas, but with a focus on the person, care partner, and community nursing is able to be nimble and respond to the demands.

SOURCES OF EVIDENCE FOR NURSING PRACTICE

Nurses make clinical decisions based on knowledge from many sources, including coursework, textbooks, and their own personal and clinical experiences. Because evidence is constantly evolving, learning about best practice nursing will persist throughout your career.

Some of what you have learned is based on systematic research, but some is not. What are the sources of evidence for nursing practice? Until recently, knowledge primarily was handed down from one generation to the next based on experience, trial and error, tradition, and expert opinion. A brief discussion of some alternative sources of evidence shows how research-based information is different.

Tradition and Authority

Decisions are sometimes based on custom or tradition. Certain "truths" are accepted as given, and such "knowledge" is so much a part of a common heritage that few seek validation. Some nursing interventions are based on custom and "unit culture" rather than on sound evidence. Indeed, one analysis suggested that some "sacred cows" (ineffective traditional habits) persisted even in a healthcare center recognized as a leader in EBP (Hanrahan et al., 2015).

Another common source of information is an authority, a person with specialized expertise. Reliance on authorities (such as faculty or textbook authors) is unavoidable but imperfect: authorities are not infallible, particularly if their expertise is based primarily on personal experience or out-of-date materials.

Clinical Experience and Trial and Error

Clinical experience is a functional source of knowledge and plays an important role in EBP. Yet personal clinical experience has some limitations as a knowledge source because each nurse's experience is too narrow to be generally useful. Moreover, the same objective event is often perceived differently by different nurses.

Trial and error involve trying alternatives successively until a solution to a problem is found. Trial and error may offer a practical means of securing knowledge, but the method tends to be haphazard and solutions may be idiosyncratic.

Logical Reasoning

Solutions to some problems are developed by logical reasoning, which combines experience, the intellect, and formal systems of thought. **Inductive reasoning** involves developing generalizations from specific observations. For example, a nurse may observe the anxious behavior of (specific) hospitalized children and conclude that (in general) children's separation from their parents is stressful. **Deductive reasoning** involves developing specific predictions from general principles. For example, if we assume that separation anxiety occurs in hospitalized children (in general), then we might predict that (specific) children in a hospital whose parents do not room-in will manifest symptoms of stress. Both types of reasoning are useful for understanding phenomena, and both play a role in research. Logical reasoning by itself, however, is limited because the validity of reasoning depends on the accuracy of the initial premises.

Assembled Information

In making clinical decisions, healthcare professionals rely on information that has been assembled for various purposes. For example, local, national, and international *benchmarking data* provide information on such issues as infection rates or the rates of various procedures (e.g., cesarean births) and can facilitate evaluations of clinical practices. Cost data—information on the costs associated with certain procedures, policies, or practices—are sometimes used as a factor in clinical decision-making. *Quality improvement and risk data*, such as medication error reports, can be used to assess the need for practice changes. Such sources are useful, but they do not provide a mechanism for making clinical decisions or guiding improvements.

Disciplined Research

Research conducted in a disciplined framework is the best method of acquiring knowledge. Nursing research combines logical reasoning with other features to create evidence that, although fallible, tends to be especially reliable. Carefully synthesized findings from rigorous research are especially valuable. The current emphasis on EBP requires nurses to base their clinical practice to the greatest extent possible on research-based findings rather than on tradition, authority, intuition, or personal experience—although nursing will always remain a rich blend of art and science.

PARADIGMS AND METHODS FOR NURSING RESEARCH

A **paradigm** is a world view, a general perspective on the complexities of the world. Paradigms for human inquiry are often characterized in terms of the ways in which they respond to basic philosophical questions, such as, "What is the nature of reality?" and "What is the relationship between the inquirer and those being studied?"

Disciplined inquiry in nursing has been conducted mainly within two broad paradigms, *positivism* and *constructivism*. This section describes these two paradigms and outlines the research methods associated with them. In later chapters, we describe the transformative paradigm that underpins critical theory research (Chapter 22) and a pragmatism paradigm that underlies mixed methods research (Chapter 27).

The Positivist Paradigm

The paradigm that dominated healthcare research for decades is called **positivism** (or *logical positivism*). Positivism is rooted in 19th century thought, guided by such philosophers as Newton and Locke. Positivism reflects a broader cultural phenomenon (*modernism*) that emphasizes the rational and the scientific.

A fundamental assumption of positivists is that there is a reality *out there* that can be studied and known. (An **assumption** is a basic principle that is believed to be true without proof.) Adherents of positivism assume that nature is basically ordered and regular and that reality exists independent of human observation (Table 1.2). The related assumption of **determinism** refers to the positivists' belief that phenomena are not haphazard but rather have antecedent causes. If a person has a cerebrovascular accident, a positivist assumes that there must be a reason that can be potentially identified. Within this

TABLE 1.2 • Major Assumptions of the Positivist and Constructivist Paradigms

PHILOSOPHICAL QUESTION	POSITIVIST PARADIGM ASSUMPTION	CONSTRUCTIVIST PARADIGM ASSUMPTION
What is the nature of reality?	Reality exists; there is a real world driven by real natural causes	Reality is multiple and subjective, mentally constructed by individuals
In what way is the researcher related to those being researched?	The researcher is independent from those being researched; findings are not influenced by the researcher	The researcher interacts with those being researched; findings are the creation of the interactive process
What is the role of values in the inquiry?	Values and biases are to be held in check; objectivity is sought	Subjectivity and values are inevitable and desirable
What are the best methods for obtaining evidence?	Deductive processes → hypothesis testing	Inductive processes → hypothesis generation
	Emphasis on discrete, specific concepts	Emphasis on entirety of a phenomenon, holistic
	Focus on the objective and quantifiable	Focus on the subjective and nonquantifiable
	Outsider knowledge—researcher is external, separate	Insider knowledge—researcher is part of the process
	Fixed, prespecified design	Flexible, emergent design
	Controls over context	Context-bound
	Large, representative samples	Small, information-rich samples
	Measured (quantitative) information	Narrative (unstructured) information
	Statistical analysis	Qualitative analysis
	Seeks generalizations	Seeks in-depth understanding

paradigm, much research activity is aimed at understanding the underlying causes of phenomena.

Positivists value objectivity and attempt to hold personal beliefs and biases in check. The positivists' scientific approach involves using orderly procedures with tight controls of the research situation to test hunches about the phenomena being studied.

Strict positivist thinking has been challenged, and few researchers adhere to the tenets of pure positivism. In the **post positivist paradigm**, there is a belief in reality and a desire to understand it, but post positivists recognize the impossibility of total objectivity. They do, however, see objectivity as a goal and strive to be as neutral as possible. Post positivists also recognize the obstacles to knowing reality with certainty and therefore seek *probabilistic* evidence—i.e., learning what the true state of a phenomenon *probably* is. This modified positivist position remains a dominant force in healthcare research. For the sake of simplicity, we refer to it as positivism.

The Constructivist Paradigm

The **constructivist paradigm** (also called the *naturalistic paradigm*) began as a countermovement to positivism with writers such as Weber and Kant. Just as positivism reflects the cultural phenomenon of modernism that burgeoned after the industrial revolution, naturalism is an outgrowth of the cultural transformation called postmodernism. Postmodern thinking emphasizes the value of deconstruction, taking apart old ideas and structures, and reconstruction, putting ideas and structures together in new ways. The constructivist paradigm represents a major alternative system for conducting disciplined research in nursing. Table 1.2 compares the major assumptions of the positivist and constructivist paradigms.

For the naturalistic inquirer, reality is not a fixed entity but rather is a construction of the people participating in the research; reality exists within a context, and many constructions are possible. Naturalists thus take the position of relativism: if there are multiple interpretations of reality that exist in people's minds, then there is no process by which the ultimate truth or falsity of the constructions can be determined.

The constructivist paradigm assumes that knowledge is maximized when the distance between the researcher and those under study is minimized. The voices and interpretations of study participants are crucial to understanding the phenomenon of interest. Findings in a constructivist inquiry are the product of the interaction between the inquirer and the participants.

Paradigms and Methods: Quantitative and Qualitative Research

Research methods are the techniques researchers use to structure a study and to gather and analyze information relevant to the research question. The two alternative paradigms correspond to different approaches to developing evidence. A key methodologic distinction is between **quantitative research**, which is most closely allied with positivism, and **qualitative research**, which is associated with constructivist inquiry—although positivists sometimes undertake qualitative studies and constructivist researchers sometimes collect quantitative information. This section provides an overview of the methods associated with the two paradigms.

The Scientific Method and Quantitative Research

The traditional **scientific method** refers to a set of orderly, disciplined procedures used to acquire information. Quantitative researchers use deductive reasoning to generate predictions that are tested in the real world. They typically move in a systematic fashion from the definition of a problem and the selection of concepts on which to focus, to the solution of the problem. By **systematic**, we mean that the investigator progresses logically through a series of steps, according to a prespecified plan of action.

Quantitative researchers use various control strategies. **Control** involves imposing conditions on the research situation so that biases are minimized and validity is maximized. Control mechanisms are discussed at length later in this book.

Quantitative researchers gather **empirical evidence**—evidence that is rooted in objective reality and gathered through the senses (e.g., through sight or hearing). Observations of the presence or absence of skin inflammation, patients' agitation, or infant birth weight are all examples of empirical observations. Reliance on empirical evidence means that findings are grounded in reality rather than in researchers' personal beliefs.

Evidence for a study in the positivist paradigm is gathered according to an established plan, using structured methods to collect needed information. Usually the information gathered is **quantitative**—that is, numeric information that is obtained through a formal *measurement* and is analyzed statistically.

A traditional scientific study strives to go beyond the specifics of a research situation. For example, quantitative researchers are typically not as focused on understanding why a particular person has a stroke as in understanding what factors generally influence its occurrence in people. The degree to which research findings can be generalized to individuals other than those who participated in a study is called **generalizability**.

The scientific method has enjoyed considerable stature as a method of inquiry and has been used productively by nurse researchers studying a wide range of nursing problems. This approach cannot, however, solve all nursing problems. One important limitation—common to both quantitative and qualitative research—is that research cannot be used to answer moral or ethical questions. Many intriguing questions about humans fall into this area—questions such as whether euthanasia should be practiced or abortion should be legal.

The traditional research approach also must address measurement challenges. To study a phenomenon, quantitative researchers try to measure it using numeric values that express quantity. For example, if the phenomenon of interest is patient stress, researchers would want to assess if patients' stress is high or low. Physiologic phenomena like blood pressure can be measured with great accuracy and precision, but measuring psychological phenomena (e.g., stress, resilience, depression) is challenging.

Another issue is that nursing research focuses on humans, who are inherently complex and diverse. Quantitative studies typically concentrate on relatively few concepts (e.g., weight gain, fatigue, pain). Complexities tend to be controlled and, if possible, eliminated, rather than studied directly, and this narrowness of focus can sometimes obscure insights. Quantitative research within the positivist paradigm has been accused of an inflexibility of vision that fails to capture the full breadth of human experience.

Constructivist Methods and Qualitative Research

Researchers in constructivist traditions emphasize the inherent complexity of humans, their ability to shape and create their own experiences, and the idea that truth is a composite of realities. Constructivist studies focus on understanding the human experience as it is lived, usually through the collection and analysis of qualitative materials that are narrative and subjective.

Researchers who criticize the scientific method believe that it is overly reductionist—that is, it reduces human experience to the few concepts under investigation, and those concepts are defined in advance by the researcher rather than emerging from the perspective of those under study. Constructivist researchers tend to emphasize the dynamic and holistic aspects of human life and attempt to capture those aspects in their entirety.

Researchers use flexible, evolving procedures to capitalize on findings that emerge during the study. Constructivist inquiry often takes place in the **field** (i.e., in naturalistic settings), sometimes over an extended time period. In constructivist research, the collection of information and its analysis typically progress concurrently; as researchers sift through information, they gain insights, new questions emerge for them, and they seek further evidence to amplify or confirm the insights. Through an inductive process, researchers integrate information to develop a theory or description that helps illuminate the phenomenon of interest.

Constructivist studies yield rich, in-depth information that can elucidate varied dimensions of a complicated phenomenon. Findings from qualitative research are typically grounded in the real-life experiences of people with first-hand knowledge of a phenomenon.

Nevertheless, the approach has several limitations. Human beings are used directly as the instrument through which information is gathered, and humans are extremely intelligent and sensitive—but fallible—tools. The subjectivity that enriches the analytic insights of skillful researchers can yield trivial and obvious "findings" among less competent ones.

Another potential limitation involves the subjectivity of constructivist inquiry, which sometimes raises concerns about the idiosyncratic nature of the conclusions. Would two constructivist researchers studying the same phenomenon in similar settings arrive at similar conclusions? The situation is further complicated by the fact that most constructivist studies involve a small group of participants. Thus, the generalizability of findings from constructivist inquiries is sometimes a potential concern.

Multiple Paradigms and Nursing Research

Paradigms should be viewed as lenses that help to sharpen our focus on phenomena, not as blinders that limit intellectual curiosity. Nursing knowledge would be thin if there were not a rich array of methods available within the two paradigms—methods that are often complementary in their strengths and limitations. We believe that intellectual pluralism is advantageous.

We have emphasized differences between the two paradigms and associated methods so that distinctions would be easy to understand. Subsequent chapters of this book elaborate further on differences in terminology, methods, and research products. It is equally important to note, however, that the two main paradigms have many features in common, only some of which are mentioned here:

- *Ultimate goals.* The aim of disciplined research, regardless of paradigm, is to answer questions and solve problems. Both quantitative and qualitative researchers seek to capture the truth about an aspect of the world in which they are interested, and both groups can make meaningful contributions to evidence for nursing practice.
- *External evidence.* Although the word *empiricism* has come to be associated with the classic scientific method, researchers in both traditions gather and analyze evidence empirically, that is, through their senses.
- *Reliance on human cooperation.* Human cooperation is essential in both qualitative and quantitative research. To understand people's circumstances and experiences, researchers must persuade them to participate in the investigation *and* to speak and act candidly.
- *Ethical constraints.* Research with human beings is guided by ethical principles that sometimes are at odds with research goals. Ethical dilemmas sometimes confront researchers, regardless of paradigm or method.
- *Fallibility of disciplined research.* Virtually all studies have limitations. Every research question can be addressed in many ways, and inevitably there are tradeoffs. The fallibility of any single study makes it important to understand and critically appraise researchers' methodologic decisions when evaluating evidence quality.

Thus, researchers using traditional scientific or constructivist methods face many similar challenges despite philosophic and methodologic differences. The selection of an appropriate method depends on researchers' personal philosophy and on the research question. If a researcher asks, "What are the effects of cryotherapy on nausea and oral mucositis in patients undergoing chemotherapy?" the researcher needs to study effects by carefully measuring patient outcomes. On the other hand, if a researcher asks, "What is the process by which parents learn to cope with the death of a child?" the researcher would be hard pressed to quantify such a process. Personal world views of researchers help to shape their questions.

In reading about the alternative paradigms for nursing research, you likely were more attracted to one of the two paradigms. It is important, however, to learn about both approaches to disciplined inquiry and to recognize their respective strengths and limitations. In this textbook, we describe methods associated with both qualitative and quantitative research to assist you in becoming methodologically bilingual. This is especially important because large numbers of nurse researchers are now undertaking **mixed methods research** that involves the collection and analysis of both qualitative and quantitative data (Chapters 27–29).

THE PURPOSES OF NURSING RESEARCH

The general purpose of nursing research is to answer questions and solve problems of relevance to nursing. Specific purposes can be classified in various ways. For example, a distinction sometimes is made between basic and applied research. **Basic research** is undertaken to discover general principles of human behavior and biophysiologic processes. Some basic research (*bench research*) is performed in laboratory settings and focuses on the molecular and cellular mechanisms that underlie disease. **Applied research** is aimed at examining how basic principles can be used to solve practice problems. Nurse researchers undertake both types of research.

Another way to classify research purposes concerns the extent to which studies provide explanatory information. Specific study goals can range along a descriptive/explanatory continuum, but a fundamental distinction is between studies whose primary intent is to describe phenomena and those that are **cause-probing**—that is, designed to illuminate the underlying causes of phenomena. The descriptive/explanatory continuum includes studies whose purposes are identification, description, exploration, prediction/control, and explanation of health-related phenomena. For each purpose, various types of questions are addressed—some more amenable to qualitative than to quantitative inquiry, and vice versa. Table 1.3 gives examples of questions asked for these purposes.

TABLE 1.3 • Research Purposes and Questions on the Description/Explanation Continuum

PURPOSE	TYPES OF QUESTIONS: QUANTITATIVE RESEARCH	TYPES OF QUESTIONS: QUALITATIVE RESEARCH
Identification		What is this phenomenon? What is its name?
Description	How prevalent is the phenomenon? How often does the phenomenon occur? How intense is the phenomenon?	What are the dimensions or characteristics of the phenomenon? What is important about the phenomenon?
Exploration	What factors are related to the phenomenon? What are the antecedents of the phenomenon?	What is the full nature of the phenomenon? What is really going on here? How is the phenomenon experienced? What is the process by which the phenomenon evolves?
Explanation	What is the underlying cause of the phenomenon? Does the theory explain the phenomenon?	How does the phenomenon work? What does the phenomenon mean? How did the phenomenon occur?
Prediction	If phenomenon X occurs, will phenomenon Y follow? What will happen if we modify a phenomenon or introduce an intervention?	—
Control	Can the occurrence of the phenomenon be prevented or controlled?	—

In both nursing and medicine, researchers have written several books to facilitate EBP, and these books categorize studies in terms of the types of information needed by clinicians (Guyatt et al., 2015; Melnyk & Fineout-Overholt, 2022). These writers focus on several types of clinical purposes: Therapy/intervention; Diagnosis/assessment; Prognosis; Etiology (causation)/prevention of harm; Description; and Meaning/process.

Therapy/Intervention

Therapy/intervention questions are addressed by healthcare researchers who want to learn about the effects of specific actions, products, or processes. Typically, researchers addressing this type of question are evaluating whether a new treatment or a practice change has beneficial effects.

The name "Therapy" for this category originates from promoters of EBP in medicine who focused on studies of the effects of "therapeutic" medical interventions, such as new drugs or surgical procedures. However, this category should be thought of more broadly to include research on the effects of alternative ways of doing things, usually with the intent of testing strategies for making improvements. Therapy questions are foundational for evidence-based decision-making. Evidence for changes to nursing practice, nursing education, and nursing administration comes from studies that have specifically tested the effects of intervening in a particular way. Table 1.4 provides some examples of studies in which nurse researchers addressed diverse Therapy/intervention questions. If such questions are answered in a rigorous fashion, the evidence might suggest a practice change or the implementation of an institutional innovation.

Studies in this category range from evaluations of highly specific treatments (e.g., comparing two types of cooling blankets for febrile patients) to assessments of complex multisession interventions designed to change behaviors (e.g., nurse-led health promotion programs). **Intervention research** is essential for EBP, and nurses are increasingly engaging in this type of research. Research addressing Therapy questions is inherently cause-probing: the researcher wants to know if a certain intervention will cause improved outcomes.

TABLE 1.4 • Examples of Therapy/Intervention Questions

THERAPY/INTERVENTION QUESTION	AREA OF FOCUS
Does an education intervention improve teenagers' knowledge and behaviors relating to contraception? (Pivatti et al., 2019)	Nursing practice
Do muscle relaxation or nature sounds reduce fatigue in patients with heart failure? (Seifi et al., 2018)	Nursing practice
Does a nurse-led phone follow-up education program reduce cardiovascular risk among patients with cardiovascular disease? (Zhou et al., 2018)	Nursing practice
Does a simulation-based palliative care communication skill workshop improve self-perception of skills in expressing empathy and discussing spiritual issues among healthcare workers and students? (Brown et al., 2018)	Interprofessional education
Does simulation improve the ability of first year nursing students to learn vital signs? (Eyikara & Baykara, 2018)	Nursing education
Does a bundle of interventions to support nurses' engagement in evidence-based practice (EBP) increase their knowledge, attitudes, and use of library resources? (Carter et al., 2018)	Nursing administration

Diagnosis/Assessment

A burgeoning number of nursing studies concern the rigorous development and evaluation of formal instruments to screen, diagnose, and assess patients and to measure important clinical outcomes—that is, they address **Diagnosis/assessment questions**. High-quality instruments with documented accuracy are essential for both clinical practice and research. Typically, the question being addressed is "Does this new instrument yield reliable and valid information about an outcome, situation, or condition of importance to nursing?" Studies addressing Diagnosis questions are not cause-probing.

Example of a Study Aimed at Diagnosis/Assessment
Banister et al. (2022) examined the nursing assessment and documentation recorded in the electronic health records of patients admitted over 1 month during the height of the COVID-19. Using a nursing assessment framework, they captured the clinical decision-making, nursing diagnoses, and key social determinant of health.

Prognosis

Researchers who ask **Prognosis questions** strive to understand the outcomes that are associated with a disease or a health problem (i.e., its consequences), to estimate the probability the outcomes will occur, and to predict the types of people for whom the outcomes are most likely. Such studies facilitate the development of long-term care plans for patients and can suggest the need for appropriate interventions. For example, Prognosis studies provide valuable information for guiding patients to make lifestyle choices or to be vigilant for key symptoms. Prognosis questions are typically cause-probing; the researcher wants to know if, for example, a certain disease or behavior causes subsequent adverse outcomes.

Example of a Study Aimed at Prognosis
Lazard et al. (2020) studied a peer-to-peer app aimed at promoting social support in young cancer survivors to determine their preferences for such a tool.

Etiology (Causation)/Prevention of Harm

Nurses encounter patients who face potentially harmful exposures as a result of environmental agents or because of personal behaviors or characteristics. Providing information to patients about such harms and how best to avoid them depends on the availability of accurate evidence about factors that contribute to health risks. For example, there would be no smoking cessation programs if research had not provided strong evidence that smoking cigarettes causes or contributes to a wide range of health problems. Thus, identifying factors that affect or cause illness, mortality, or morbidity is an important purpose of many nursing studies. **Etiology questions** are inherently cause-probing—the purpose is to understand factors that cause health problems.

Example of a Study Aimed at Identifying and Preventing Harm
Wang et al. (2023) conducted a randomized clinical control trial to compare a midwife-led weight management program to a control group. Findings indicated that the nurse midwife-led weight management program encouraged appropriate gestational weight gain, health literacy, and improved the experience of antenatal care.

Description

Description questions are not in a category typically identified in EBP-related classification schemes, but so many nursing studies have a descriptive purpose that we include it here. Examples of phenomena that nurse researchers have described include patients' pain, physical function, confusion, and levels of depression. Quantitative description focuses on the prevalence, size, intensity, and measurable attributes of phenomena. Qualitative researchers, by contrast, describe the dimensions or the evolution of phenomena.

Example of a Quantitative Study Aimed at Description
Schoenfisch et al. (2019) did a study to describe hospital nursing staff's use of lift or transfer devices. They found that only 40% of the nurses used equipment for at least half of lifts/transfers.

Example of a Qualitative Study Aimed at Description
Dickins et al. (2021) undertook a study among low-income midlife and older women to describe the patterns of healthcare use, facilitators, barriers, and opportunities to optimize primary/preventive care engagement.

Meaning/Process

Designing effective interventions, motivating people to comply with treatments and health promotion activities, and providing sensitive advice to patients are among the many healthcare activities that can benefit from understanding clients' perspectives. Research that provides evidence about what health and illness mean to clients, what barriers to positive health practices they face, and what processes they experience in a transition through a healthcare crisis are important to evidence-based nursing practice. Studies that address **Meaning/process questions** are seldom focused on identifying the underlying causes of phenomena but might offer important clues.

Example of a Study Aimed at Understanding Meaning/Process
Mattson and coresearchers (2024) studied the process by which women use self-management of opioid recovery through pregnancy and early parenting.

Study Purposes and Evidence-Based Practice

Studies that address therapy/intervention questions provide the most direct evidence for EBP. If we want to know, for example, whether wedge-shaped foam cushions are more effective in preventing heel pressure ulcers than standard foam pillows, we would need to look for rigorous studies that have addressed this therapy question. However, other questions also play a role in improving the quality of nursing care, albeit in different ways.

Table 1.5 presents examples of different types of questions relating to cigarette smoking, using the study purpose categories we just described. Only one of these questions is directly actionable—the Therapy question. If there is strong evidence that nurse-led smoking cessation programs are effective in reducing smoking among young adults, we might consider initiating such a program in our own community.

If the other questions in Table 1.5 were answered in rigorous studies, the evidence could also play a role in guiding efforts to improve nursing practice—but not as directly. Answers to some of these questions might help target those most in need of an intervention. For example,

TABLE 1.5 • Different Categories of Questions Related to Cigarette Smoking

TYPE OF QUESTION	EXAMPLE OF A RELATED RESEARCH QUESTION ON CIGARETTE SMOKING
Therapy/intervention	Does a nurse-led smoking cessation program for young adults reduce smoking?
Diagnosis/assessment	Is our Smoking Susceptibility Index a valid and reliable measure of propensity to initiate smoking in teenagers?
Prognosis	Is a diagnosis of smoking-related lung cancer associated with increased risk of suicidal ideation?
Etiology (causation)/prevention of harm	Does being poor increase the risk that a person will smoke cigarettes?
Description	What percentage of high school students smoke 1+ packs of cigarettes/week, and what percentage of smokers have tried to quit?
Meaning/process	What is it like for long-term smokers to attempt and fail at quitting?

based on studies addressing the Diagnosis question, we could launch a prevention effort aimed at teenagers with high scores on the evidence-based Smoking Susceptibility Index, or results from an Etiology study might lead us to offer a smoking-cessation initiative in low-income neighborhoods. Evidence from the Prognosis question might prompt us to develop a strong program of emotional support for patients with lung cancer. We might be motivated to implement an intervention for high school students if we knew that rates of smoking were high (the Description question). And, if we knew that a high percentage of smokers in our community had been unsuccessful in efforts to quit, we might design an intervention with that information in mind. The stories from long-term smokers who failed to quit despite efforts to do so (the Meaning question) could lead us to involve them in the design of an intervention for hardened smokers.

Nurse researchers are making strides in addressing all types of questions about important health problems—but evidence regarding what "works" to address problems comes from studies focused on Therapy questions. Evidence about the scope of a problem, factors affecting the problem, the consequences of the problem, and the meaning of the problem can, however, play a crucial role in efforts to design better interventions, to aim our resources at those in greatest need, and to provide appropriate guidance to clients in everyday practice.

ASSISTANCE FOR USERS OF NURSING RESEARCH

This book is designed primarily to help you develop skills for conducting research, but in an environment that stresses EBP, it is extremely important to hone your skills in reading, evaluating, and using nursing studies. We provide specific guidance to consumers in most chapters by including guidelines for critically appraising aspects of a study covered in the chapter. The questions in Box 1.1 are designed to assist you in using the information in this chapter in an overall preliminary assessment of a research report.

RESEARCH EXAMPLES

Each chapter of this book presents brief descriptions of studies conducted by nurse researchers, focusing on aspects emphasized in the chapter. Read the full journal articles to learn more about the methods and results of these studies.

Research Example of a Quantitative Study

Study: Psychosocial predictors of adverse outcomes in rural heart failure (HF) caregivers (Grant et al., 2021).

Study purpose: The purpose of the study was to examine whether social support, problem solving, and family function predicted depressive symptoms,

---

BOX 1.1 Questions for a Preliminary Overview of a Research Report

1. How relevant is the research question in this study to the actual practice of nursing? Does the study focus on a topic that is a priority area for nursing research?
2. Was the research quantitative or qualitative?
3. What was the underlying purpose (or purposes) of the study—identification, description, exploration, explanation, or prediction and control? Does the purpose correspond to an EBP focus such as therapy/intervention, diagnosis/assessment, prognosis, etiology (causation)/prevention of harm, description, or meaning/process?
4. Is this study fundamentally cause-probing?
5. What might be some clinical implications of this research? To what type of people and settings is the research most relevant? If the findings are valid, how might I use the results of this study in my clinical work?

caregiving-related life changes, self-care, and caregiver burden in rural HF caregivers and (2) to compare the findings related to these variables to those in urban caregivers.

Study methods: The sample was recruited using multiple strategies including social media and face-to-face strategies. There was a total sample of 540 (rural = 114, urban = 426) participants who completed online surveys that captured demographic information and measures related to social support, problem-solving, self-care, family functioning, depressive symptoms, caregiver burden, and life changes. A secondary analysis was conducted to compare the two groups.

Key findings: Rural caregivers experienced significantly less social support, had fewer problem-solving skills and more family functioning challenges, and had greater depressive symptoms and more subjective burden than the urban participants. There were no significant differences in caregiver self-care or perceived life changes between the two groups.

Conclusions: Grant and colleagues concluded that social support and problem solving have significant effects on depressive symptoms in rural HF caregivers. Problem solving and family function also affect caregiver burden, while social support and family functioning influence caregiver life changes.

Research Example of a Qualitative Study

Study: Perspectives of Maternal Mortality Among Women Who Live in Indiana (Renbarger et al., 2023).

Study purpose: The purpose of this descriptive qualitative study was to explore the perspectives of women in the lay public in Indiana on the topic of maternal mortality.

Study methods: Twenty women were recruited from Facebook groups aimed at women with children. Researchers used semi-structured phone interviews and asked participants to describe their understanding of maternal mortality and their related experiences.

Key findings: Analysis of the interviews revealed three main themes: (1) Women are not worried about mortality until they experience pregnancy complications, (2) Women have limited information on maternal mortality, and (3) Women often feel dismissed during maternity care.

Conclusions: Nurses and other clinicians need to increase their efforts to effectively communicate about maternal morbidity and to follow evidence-based guidelines for respectful maternity care.

SUMMARY POINTS

- **Nursing research** is systematic inquiry undertaken to develop evidence on problems of importance to nurses. Nurses are adopting an **evidence-based practice (EBP)** that incorporates research findings into their clinical decisions.
- Nurses can participate in a range of research-related activities that span a continuum from being consumers of research (those who read and evaluate studies) to being producers of research (those who design and undertake studies). Engagement with research often occurs in practice settings through participation in a **journal club**.
- Nursing research began with Florence Nightingale but developed slowly until its rapid acceleration in the 1950s. Since the 1980s, the focus has been on **clinical nursing research**—that is, on problems relating to clinical practice.
- The **National Institute of Nursing Research (NINR)**, established at the U.S. National Institutes of Health in 1993, affirms the stature of nursing research in the United States.
- Contemporary issues in nursing research include the growth of EBP, expansion of local research and quality improvement efforts, research synthesis through **systematic reviews**, **interprofessional** studies, **patient-centeredness** in both clinical care and in research, interest in the **applicability** of research to individual patients or groups, interest in precision healthcare and symptom science, and efforts to measure the **clinical significance** of research results.
- Disciplined research stands in contrast to other knowledge sources for nursing practice, such as tradition, authority, personal experience, trial and error, and logical reasoning.

- Nursing research is conducted mainly within one of two broad **paradigms**—world views with underlying **assumptions** about reality: the positivist and the constructivist paradigms.
- In the **positivist paradigm**, it is assumed that there is an objective reality and that natural phenomena are orderly. The assumption of **determinism** is the belief that phenomena result from prior causes and are not haphazard.
- In the **constructivist** (naturalistic) **paradigm**, it is assumed that reality is not fixed, but it is a construction of human minds; "truth" is a composite of multiple constructions of reality.
- The positivist paradigm is associated with **quantitative research**—the collection and analysis of numeric information. Quantitative research is typically conducted within the traditional **scientific method**, which is a systematic, controlled process. Quantitative researchers gather and analyze **empirical evidence** (evidence collected through the human senses) and strive for **generalizability** of their findings.
- Researchers within the constructivist paradigm emphasize understanding the human experience as it is lived through the collection and analysis of subjective, narrative materials using flexible procedures that evolve in the **field**; this paradigm is associated with **qualitative research**.
- **Basic research** is designed to extend the knowledge base for the sake of knowledge itself. **Applied research** focuses on discovering solutions to immediate problems.
- A fundamental distinction, especially relevant in quantitative research, is between studies whose primary intent is to describe phenomena and those that are **cause-probing**—i.e., designed to illuminate underlying causes of phenomena. Specific research purposes on the description/explanation continuum include identification, description, exploration, prediction/control, and explanation.
- Nursing studies can be classified in terms of several EBP-related aims: **Therapy/intervention**; **Diagnosis/assessment**; **Prognosis**; **Etiology** (causation)/prevention of **harm**; **Description**; and **Meaning/process**. Rigorous answers to Therapy questions are foundational for EBP.

REFERENCES CITED IN CHAPTER 1

2023 Magnet® Application Manual. American Nurses Credentialing Center; 2023.

Aamodt, W. W., Travers, J., Thibault, D., & Willis, A. W. (2021). Hospital magnet status associates with inpatient safety in parkinson disease. *Journal of Neuroscience Nursing*, 53(3), 116–122. https://doi.org/10.1097/JNN.0000000000000582

Banister, G., Carroll, D. L., Dickins, K., Flanagan, J., Jones, D., Looby, S. E., & Cahill, J. E. (2022). Nurse-sensitive indicators during COVID-19. *International Journal of Nursing Knowledge*, 33(3), 234–244. https://doi.org/10.1111/2047-3095.12372

Brown, C., Back, A., Ford, D., Kross, E., Downey, L., Shannon, S., Curtis, J. R., Engelberg, R. A., & Engelberg, R. (2018). Self-assessment scores improve after simulation-based palliative care communication skill workshops. *American Journal of Hospice & Palliative Care*, 35(1), 45–51.

Carter, E., Rivera, R., Gallagher, K., & Cato, K. (2018). Targeted interventions to advance a culture of inquiry at a large, multicampus hospital among nurses. *Journal of Nursing Administration*, 48(1), 18–24.

Chen, T. Y., Kao, C. W., Cheng, S. M., & Chang, Y. C. (2022). A web-based self-care program to promote healthy lifestyles and control blood pressure in patients with primary hypertension: A randomized controlled trial. *Journal of Nursing Scholarship*, 54(6), 678–691. https://doi.org/10.1111/jnu.12792

Dickins, K. A., Malley, A., Bartels, S. J., Baggett, T. P., & Looby, S. E. (2021). Barriers, facilitators, and opportunities to optimize care engagement in a diverse sample of older low-income women: A qualitative study. *Geriatric Nursing*, 42(5), 965–976. https://doi.org/10.1016/j.gerinurse.2021.06.015

Dierkes, A. M., Riman, K., Daus, M., Germack, H. D., & Lasater, K. B. (2021). The Association of Hospital Magnet® status and pay-for-performance penalties. *Policy Politics & Nursing Practice*, 22(4), 245–252. https://doi.org/10.1177/15271544211053854

Dykes, P. C., Burns, Z., Adelman, J., Benneyan, J., Bogaisky, M., Carter, E., Ergai, A., Lindros, M. E., Lipsitz, S. R., Scanlan, M., Shaykevich, S., & Bates, D. W. (2020). Evaluation of a patient-centered fall-prevention tool kit to reduce falls and injuries: A nonrandomized controlled trial. *JAMA Network Open*, 3(11), e2025889. https://doi.org/10.1001/jamanetworkopen.2020.25889

Dykes, P. C., & Hurley, A. C. (2021). Patient-centered fall prevention. *Nursing Management*, 52(3), 51–54. https://doi.org/10.1097/01.NUMA.0000733668.39637.ba

Eyikara, E., & Baykara, Z. (2018). Effect of simulation on the ability of first year nursing students to learn vital signs. *Nurse Education Today*, 60, 101–106.

Flanagan, J. (2022). The lost art of the narrative review. *International Journal of Nursing Knowledge*, 33(2), 83. https://doi.org/10.1111/2047-3095.12368

Grant, J. S., Graven, L. J., Schluck, G., & Abbott, L. (2021). Psychosocial predictors of adverse outcomes in rural heart failure caregivers. *Rural Remote Health*, *21*(3), 6497. https://doi.org/10.22605/RRH6497

Graystone, R. (2017). The 2019 Magnet® application manual: Nursing excellence standards evolving with practice. *Journal of Nursing Administration*, *47*(11), 527–528.

Guyatt, G., Rennie, D., Meade, M., & Cook, D. (2015). *Users' guide to the medical literature: Essentials of evidence-based clinical practice* (3rd ed.). McGraw Hill.

Hanrahan, K., Wagner, M., Matthews, G., Stewart, S., Dawson, C., Greiner, J., Pottinger, J., Vernon-Levett, P., Herold, D., Hottel, R., Cullen, L., Tucker, S., & Williamson, A. (2015). Sacred cow gone to pasture: A systematic evaluation and integration of evidence-based practice. *Worldviews on Evidence-Based Nursing*, *12*(1), 3–11. https://doi.org/10.1111/wvn.12072

Lazard, A. J., Saffer, A. J., Horrell, L., Benedict, C., & Love, B. (2020). Peer-to-peer connections: Perceptions of a social support app designed for young adults with cancer. *Psychooncology*, *29*(1), 173–181. https://doi.org/10.1002/pon.5220

Mattson, N. M., Ohlendorf, J. M., & Haglund, K. (2024). Grounded theory approach to understand self-management of opioid recovery though pregnancy and early parenting. *JOGNN*, *53*(1), 34–45.

Melnyk, B. M., & Fineout-Overholt, E. (2022). *Evidence-based practice in nursing and healthcare: A guide to best practice* (4th ed.). Lippincott Williams & Wilkins.

National Institute of Nursing Research. (2020). *The national institute of nursing research 2022–2026 strategic plan*. NINR.

Pivatti, A., Osis, M., & de Moraes Lopes, M. H. B. (2019). The use of educational strategies for promotion of knowledge, attitudes and contraceptive practice among teenagers: A randomized clinical trial. *Nurse Education Today*, *72*, 18–26.

Renbarger, K. M., Place, J. M., Twibell, R., Trainor, K., & McIntire, E. (2023). Perspectives of maternal mortality among women who live in Indiana. *Journal of Obstetric Gynecologic, & Neonatal Nursing*, *52*(1), 62–71. https://doi.org/10.1016/j.jogn.2022.09.006

Rosen, J., & Ryan, M. (2019). A virtual nursing journal club: Bridging the gap between research evidence and clinical practice. *Journal of Nursing Administration*, *49*(12), 610–616. https://doi.org/10.1097/NNA.0000000000000824

Saragih, I. D., Tonapa, S. I., Porta, C. M., & Lee, B. O. (2022). Effects of telehealth intervention for people with dementia and their carers: A systematic review and meta-analysis of randomized controlled studies. *Journal of Nursing Scholarship*, *54*(6), 704–719. https://doi.org/10.1111/jnu.12797

Schoenfisch, A., Kucera, K., Lipscomb, H., McIlvaine, J., Becherer, L., James, T., & Avent, S. (2019). Use of assistive devices to lift/transfer, and reposition hospital patients. *Nursing Research*, *68*(1), 3–12.

Seifi, L., Najafi Ghezeljeh, T., & Haghani, H. (2018). Comparison of the effects of Benson muscle relaxation and nature sounds on the fatigue in patients with heart failure: A randomized controlled clinical trial. *Holistic Nursing Practice*, *32*(1), 27–34.

Wakefield, M., Williams, D. R., & Le Menestrel, S. (2021). *The future of nursing 2020-2030: Charting a path to achieve health equity*. National Academy of Sciences.

Wang, X., Zhu, C., Liu, H., Sun, L., Zhu, W., & Gu, C. (2023). The effects of a midwife-led weight management program for pregnant women: A randomized controlled trial. *International Journal of Nursing Studies*, *137*, 104387. https://doi.org/10.1016/j.ijnurstu.2022.104387

Zhou, Y., Liao, J., Feng, F., Ji, M., Zhao, C., & Wang, X. (2018). Effects of a nurse-led phone follow-up education program based on the self-efficacy among patients with cardiovascular disease. *Journal of Cardiovascular Nursing*, *33*(1), E15–E23.

2 | Evidence-Based Nursing: Translating Research Evidence Into Practice

Learning Objectives

1. Define evidence-based practice and its importance to nursing.
2. Identify various types of reviews conducted to synthesize research findings.
3. Describe the pros and cons of clinical guidelines.
4. Describe the common features of the various models of evidence-based practice.

INTRODUCTION

Evidence-based practice (EBP) has been a major force in the health professions for the past few decades. In nursing, many organizations and initiatives have promoted EBP. For example, EBP has been named as one of the six core competencies in the Quality and Safety Education for Nurses initiative (Tracy & Barnsteiner, 2021).

This book will help you to develop skills to generate, and to evaluate, research evidence for nursing practice. Before we delve into the "how-tos" of research, we discuss key aspects of EBP to clarify the key role that research plays in EBP.

BACKGROUND OF EVIDENCE-BASED NURSING PRACTICE

This section provides a context for understanding evidence-based nursing practice and closely related concepts.

Definition of Evidence-Based Practice

Dozens of definitions of EBP have been proposed. Here is the one offered by Melnyk and Fineout-Overholt (2019) in their textbook on EBP: "A paradigm and lifelong problem-solving approach to clinical decision making that involves the conscientious use of the best available evidence (including a systematic search for and critical appraisal of the most relevant evidence to answer a clinical question) with one's own clinical expertise and patient values and preferences to improve outcomes for individuals, communities, and systems" (p. 753). This definition, like many others, declares that EBP is a *decision-making* (or *problem-solving*) *process*. Most definitions also include the idea that EBP is built on a "three-legged stool," each "leg" of which is essential to the process: *best evidence, clinical expertise*, and *patient preferences and values*. Figure 2.1 depicts these concepts.

> **TIP** Huo et al. (2022) conducted a concept analysis of evidence-based practice (EBP). They identified 11 core elements related to the process. They propose that EBP is a transformative process involving dynamic capabilities informing leadership and educators alike in the implementation of EBP aimed at improving patient care outcomes.

Best Evidence

A basic feature of EBP as a clinical problem-solving strategy is that it de-emphasizes decisions

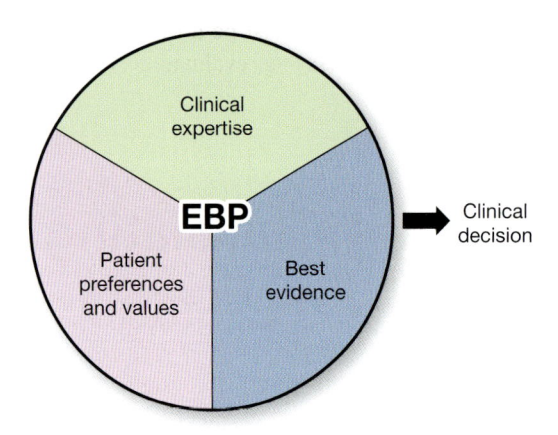

FIGURE 2.1 Evidence-based practice components.

based on tradition or expert opinions. The emphasis is on identifying and evaluating the best available research evidence as a tool for solving problems.

> **TIP** The consequences of *not* using research evidence can be devastating. For example, from 1956 through the 1980s, Dr. Benjamin Spock—who was considered an expert on the care of infants—published a top-selling book, *Baby and Child Care.* Spock advised putting babies on their stomachs to sleep. In their systematic review, Gilbert et al. (2005) wrote, "Advice to put infants to sleep on the front for nearly half a century was contrary to evidence from 1970 that this was likely to be harmful" (p. 874). They estimated that if medical advice had been guided by research evidence, over 60,000 infant deaths might have been prevented.

There continues to be debate about what qualifies as "*best*" evidence. Numerous organizations and authors have created *evidence hierarchies* that rank evidence sources according to the degree to which they provide unbiased evidence to guide clinical decisions. We discuss evidence hierarchies in more detail later in this chapter. Evidence, however, whether "best" or not, is never by itself a sufficient basis for clinical decision-making.

Patient Values and Preferences

Patient-centered care has been defined by the Institute of Medicine (2001) as "providing care that is respectful of and responsive to individual patient preferences, needs and values, and ensuring that patient values *guide* all clinical decisions." Patient-centered care is an important feature of EBP.

"Patient preferences" encompass several concepts, including patient preferences for type of treatment; preferences for being involved in decision-making; patients' social or cultural values; preferences about involving family members in healthcare decisions; patients' priorities regarding quality-of-life issues; and their spiritual or religious values. Decisions also require understanding patients' circumstances, such as the resources at their disposal. Nurses thus need the skills to elicit and understand patient preferences—and to communicate information about "best evidence" to patients.

Clinical Expertise and Experiential Evidence

Decision-making in clinical practice ultimately relies on clinicians' expertise, which is an amalgam of academic knowledge gained during training and continuing education, experiences with patient care, and interdisciplinary sharing of new knowledge. David Sackett, the pioneer of evidence-based medicine, strongly advocated for the importance of clinical expertise in making decisions because even very strong research evidence may not be appropriate or applicable for individual patients.

Newhouse (2007) stressed the importance of *experiential evidence*, which is internal evidence from local monitoring or evidence-gathering efforts, such as quality improvement projects. Clinical expertise and experiential evidence, combined with patient preferences, guide how "best evidence" can be used to make healthcare decisions.

Evidence-Based Practice and Related Concepts

During the 1980s, concern about research utilization began to emerge. **Research utilization (RU)** is the use of findings from a study in a practical application. In RU, the emphasis is on translating new knowledge into real-world applications. EBP is a broader concept than RU because it integrates research findings with other factors, as just noted. Also, whereas RU begins with the research itself

(How can I put this new knowledge to use in my clinical setting?), the start-point in EBP typically is a clinical question (What does the evidence suggest is the best approach to solving this clinical problem?).

During the 1980s and 1990s, RU projects were undertaken by numerous hospitals and nursing organizations. These projects were institutional attempts to implement changes in nursing practice based on research findings. During the 1990s, however, the call for research utilization was superseded by the push for EBP.

The EBP movement originated in the fields of medicine and epidemiology during the 1990s. British epidemiologist Archie Cochrane criticized healthcare practitioners for failing to incorporate research evidence into their decision-making. His work led to the establishment of the **Cochrane Collaboration**, an international partnership with centers established in 43 countries. The Collaboration prepares and disseminates reviews of research evidence and has a goal of making Cochrane "the home of evidence" relating to healthcare decision-making.

> **TIP** The Cochrane Collaboration publishes systematic reviews, protocols, and editorials: https://www.cochranelibrary.com/browse-by-review-group. Cochrane Reviews provide the most recent systematic reviews by topic. For example, Wilfling et al. (2023) reviewed the evidence of nonpharmacological interventions for sleep disturbances in people with dementia. The findings are also presented in plain language format so that they are accessible to the general public.

Also during the 1990s, a group from McMaster Medical School in Canada (led by Dr. David Sackett) developed a clinical learning strategy, which they called *evidence-based medicine*. The evidence-based medicine movement has shifted to a broader conception of using best evidence by all healthcare practitioners (not just physicians) in a multidisciplinary team. EBP is considered a major shift for healthcare education and practice. In the EBP environment, a skillful clinician can no longer rely on a repository of memorized information but rather must be a lifelong learner who is adept in accessing, evaluating, and using new evidence.

> **TIP** A debate has emerged concerning whether the term "evidence-based practice" should be replaced with "*evidence-informed practice*" (EIP). Those who advocate for EIP have argued that the word "based" suggests a stance in which patient preferences are not sufficiently considered in clinical decisions (e.g., Glasziou, 2005). Yet, as noted by Melnyk and Newhouse (2014), all current models of EBP incorporate clinicians' expertise and patients' preferences. They argued that "Changing terms now...will only create confusion at a critical time where progress is being made in accelerating EBP" (p. 348). We concur and use the term EBP throughout this book.

Knowledge translation (KT) is a related term that is often associated with efforts to enhance systematic change in clinical practice. The term was coined by the Canadian Institutes of Health Research (CIHR), which defined KT as "the exchange, synthesis, and ethically-sound application of knowledge—within a complex system of interactions among researchers and users—to accelerate the capture of the benefits of research for Canadians through improved health, more effective services and products, and a strengthened healthcare system" (CIHR, 2004). The World Health Organization (WHO) (2005) adapted the CIHR's definition and defined KT as "the synthesis, exchange, and application of knowledge by relevant stakeholders to accelerate the benefits of global and local innovation in strengthening health systems and improving people's health." Institutional projects aimed at KT often use methods and models that are similar to organizational EBP projects.

Translational research has emerged as a discipline devoted to developing methods to promote KT and the use of evidence. Translational science involves the study of interventions, implementation processes, and contextual factors that affect the uptake of new evidence in healthcare practice (Titler, 2014). In nursing, the need for translational research was an important impetus for the development of the Doctor of Nursing Practice degree. We discuss translational research in Chapter 11.

EBP can be undertaken by individual nurses working with patients or as a project taken on by a team within a healthcare organization. Organizational EBP projects share certain features with **quality improvement (QI)** efforts. We describe methodologic strategies for quality improvement in Chapter 12.

> **TIP** EBP is widely endorsed in nursing, but its adoption often faces many challenges. Some of the obstacles include nurses' lack of research appraisal skills; their misperceptions about EBP; heavy patient loads and lack of time; nurses' and administrators' resistance to change; and lack of autonomy about practice decisions. Factors that facilitate EBP include strong organizational support; the availability of EBP mentors and resources; collaboration among healthcare professionals; and participation in journal clubs (Gardner et al., 2016; Newhouse & Spring 2010).

RESOURCES FOR EVIDENCE-BASED PRACTICE IN NURSING

Although EBP can present challenges to nurses, resources to support EBP are increasingly available. We offer some guidance and urge you to explore other ideas with your colleagues, mentors, and health information experts.

Preprocessed and Preappraised Evidence

Searching for best evidence requires skill, especially because of the accelerating pace of evidence production. Thousands of studies of relevance to nurses are published each month in professional journals. These **primary studies** are not preappraised for quality or clinical utility.

Fortunately, finding evidence useful for practice is often facilitated by the availability of evidence sources that are preprocessed (synthesized) and sometimes pre appraised. DiCenso et al. (2009) have created a "6S" hierarchy of evidence sources, which is intended as a guide to evidence retrieval. The 6S hierarchy, typically shown as a pyramid, places five types of preprocessed evidence at the top, and individual studies at the bottom. The hierarchy is intended to help you see how to proceed with an evidence search. A clinician seeking evidence would start at the top of the hierarchy and work downward if appropriate evidence was lacking at a given level. Table 2.1 shows the **6S hierarchy** and provides examples at each level. In this section, we describe each evidence source, starting at the bottom of the hierarchy because higher levels build on the ones that precede them.

> **TIP** The 6S hierarchy does not imply a gradient of evidence in terms of *quality*, but rather in terms of ease in retrieving relevant evidence to address a clinical question. At all levels, the evidence should be assessed for quality and relevance.

Level 6 in the 6S Hierarchy: Single Studies

Reports describing a single original study are at the base of the 6S hierarchy because single studies are not ready for immediate use in making EBP decisions. At a minimum, individual primary studies need to be critically appraised for their rigor and their relevance to clinical problems. Clinicians searching for best evidence for a clinical query would start with a single study *only* if evidence from higher levels was unavailable or was judged to be flawed. We describe the major source of research reports (journal articles) in Chapter 3 and provide guidance in searching for studies in Chapter 5.

Level 5 in the 6S Hierarchy: Synopses of Single Studies

A synopsis of a study provides a brief overview of the research, often with sufficient detail to understand the evidence. As noted by DiCenso et al. (2009), a synopsis offers three advantages over the original report: (1) the brevity of the synopsis makes it more readily accessible to practitioners; (2) the study was likely chosen for abstraction because an expert believed the study was important; and (3) the synopsis is sometimes accompanied by commentary about the clinical utility

TABLE 2.1 • The "6S" Hierarchy of Evidence Sources[a]

EVIDENCE SOURCE	DESCRIPTION/EXAMPLES	EXAMPLES OF RESOURCES
1. Systems ↓	• Computerized decision support systems	• In some electronic health records systems
2. Summaries ↓	• Evidence-based clinical practice guidelines • Online EBP summary resources	• U.S. National Guidelines Clearinghouse • Registered Nurses Association of Ontario Best Practices • EBSCO Nursing Reference Center; JBI COnNECT+; UpToDate
3. Synopses of syntheses ↓	• Synopses published in evidence-based abstraction journals or compiled by organizations	• *Evidence-Based Nursing* • DARE Database of Reviews of Evidence • The Centre for Reviews and Dissemination (CRD)
4. Syntheses ↓	• Systematic reviews • Rapid reviews	• Joanna Briggs Institute Database • Cochrane Database • AHRQ Evidence Reports • *BMC Systematic Reviews*
5. Synopses of studies ↓	• Brief summaries of single studies, often with commentary on clinical applicability	• *Evidence-Based Nursing* • *ACP Journal Club*
6. Single original studies	• Not preprocessed, primary studies published in journals	• PubMed (MEDLINE) • CINAHL

AHRQ, Agency for Healthcare Research and Quality; EBP, evidence-based practice.

[a]The "6S" hierarchy depicting the efficiency of evidence retrieval for different sources was proposed by DiCenso et al., 2009.

of the evidence (i.e., preappraised). Several evidence-based journals include synopses of original studies, including *Evidence-Based Nursing, Evidence-Based Midwifery, ACP Journal Club,* and *The Online Journal of Knowledge Synthesis for Nursing.*

Level 4 in the 6S Hierarchy: Syntheses

EBP relies on meticulous integration and synthesis of research evidence on a topic. The importance of such syntheses has given rise to many different types of research review (Grant & Booth, 2009), but the most familiar type of synthesis is the systematic review. A systematic review is not a literature review, which is described further in Chapter 5. A systematic review is a methodical, scholarly inquiry that follows many of the same steps as those for primary studies. It yields a summary of the current best evidence at the time the review was written. Chapter 30 offers guidance on conducting and critically appraising systematic reviews and describes a few other types of synthesis, such as *scoping reviews, realist reviews*, and *umbrella reviews*.

Systematic reviewers sometimes integrate findings from quantitative studies using statistical methods, in what is called a **meta-analysis**. Meta-analysts treat the findings from a study as one piece of information. The findings from multiple studies on the same topic are combined and analyzed statistically. Instead of individual people being the **unit of analysis** (the basic entity of a statistical analysis) as in most primary studies, meta-analysts use findings from individual studies as the unit of analysis. Meta-analysis is an objective method of integrating a body of findings and of observing patterns that might otherwise have gone undetected.

> **Example of a Meta-Analysis**
> Meng and colleagues (2022) conducted a systematic review and meta-analysis of the effectiveness of coaching on lifestyle modification and hypertension. In their analysis of 12 randomized controlled trials, they found that health coaching reduces blood pressure, improves dietary behaviors, and increases self-efficacy among patients with high blood pressure. The most common and effective health coaching was delivered by nurses via telephone. They conclude that there is a need for policies to implement these interventions into practice.

Systematic reviews of qualitative studies often take the form of metasyntheses, which are rich resources for EBP (Beck, 2009). A **metasynthesis**, which involves integrating qualitative research findings on a topic, is less about reducing information and more about amplifying and interpreting it. For certain qualitative questions, an approach to systematic synthesis called **meta-aggregation** may be appropriate, as we describe in Chapter 30. Strategies have also been developed for **systematic mixed studies review** (also called *mixed research syntheses*), which are efforts to integrate and synthesize both quantitative and qualitative evidence on a topic (Heyvaert et al., 2017; Sandelowski et al., 2013).

> **Example of a Mixed Studies Review**
> Beck and Vo (2020) conducted a mixed studies review on fathers' stress related to their infants' NICU hospitalization. They synthesized a total of 21 studies: 10 were quantitative and 11 were qualitative.

Many systematic reviews are published in professional research journals that can be accessed using standard literature search procedures; others are available in dedicated databases. A major example is the Cochrane Database of Systematic Reviews, which contains thousands of systematic reviews. Most Cochrane reviews involve meta-analyses, and most of them relate to healthcare interventions—but the Cochrane Collaboration now also includes qualitative evidence syntheses. Cochrane reviews are done with great rigor and have the advantage of being checked and updated regularly.

Rapid reviews have become increasingly important for health policy decisions and in under-resourced countries facing critical health problems that require immediate intervention (Tricco, et al., 2022). This type of review exploded with the emergence of COVID-19 as the world sought evidence about how to diagnose and treat this deadly disease. These streamlined reviews are less rigorous than systematic reviews but are typically completed in weeks rather than months or years. Rapid reviews are described in Chapter 30.

> **TIP** Many resources are available for finding systematic reviews. For example, the Joanna Briggs Institute in Australia (http://joannabriggs.org/) and the Centre for Reviews and Dissemination at the University of York in England (http://www.york.ac.uk/inst/crd/index.htm) produce useful systematic reviews.

Level 3 in the 6S Hierarchy: Synopses of Syntheses

Synopses of systematic reviews make rigorously integrated evidence even more handy for practitioners seeking answers to clinical queries. Many abstract journals mentioned in connection with Level 5 synopses of studies (e.g., *Evidence-Based Nursing, Evidence-Based Midwifery*) also include synopses of selected systematic reviews.

Level 2 in the 6S Hierarchy: Summaries

For some clinical questions, best evidence may be conveniently available in "Summaries," which include online EBP summary resources and clinical practice guidelines.

Dozens of evidence-based, point-of-care (PoC) resources for healthcare professionals have become available. These web-based resources are designed to provide rapidly accessible evidence-based information (and, sometimes, guidance) that is periodically updated. Nickum and colleagues (2022) created a rubric to evaluate PoC summary resources for nurses. The rubric considered the content, coverage of nursing-based topics, transparency of the evidence, user perception, and customization of the PoC for supporting nursing practice. They reported that no PoC resource met all five criteria. However, for nursing, they found Lippincott's Advisor had the highest coverage of diagnoses, while ClinicalKey for Nursing had strong content focused on nursing interventions and outcomes. Kwag and colleagues (2016), who focused on evidence summaries for physicians, also came to the conclusion that UpToDate and BMJ Best Practice were two of the best and most reliable resources out of the 23 they evaluated.

Evidence-based **clinical practice guidelines**, like systematic reviews, represent efforts to distill a large body of evidence into a manageable form, but guidelines differ from reviews in a number of respects. First, clinical practice guidelines, which are usually based on systematic reviews, give specific recommendations for evidence-based decision-making. Second, guidelines attempt to address all issues relevant to a clinical decision, including balancing benefits and risks. Third, systematic reviews are evidence-driven—that is, they are undertaken when a body of evidence has been produced and needs to be synthesized. Guidelines, by contrast, are developed to guide clinical practice—even when available evidence is limited or of unexceptional quality (Straus et al., 2018). Fourth, systematic reviews are done by researchers, but guideline development typically involves the consensus of a group of researchers, experts, and clinicians. For this reason, guidelines based on the same evidence may result in different recommendations. Differences across guidelines sometimes reflect genuine contextual factors—for example, guidelines that are appropriate in the United States may be unsuitable in India.

It can be challenging to find clinical practice guidelines because there is no single guideline repository. One approach is to search for guidelines in comprehensive guideline databases. For example, in the United States, nursing and other healthcare guidelines are maintained by the National Guideline Clearinghouse (www.guideline.gov), and similar databases are available in other countries. An important nursing guideline resource comes from the Registered Nurses Association of Ontario (www.rnao.org/bestpractices).

In addition to looking for guidelines in national clearinghouses and in the websites of professional organizations, you can search bibliographic databases such as MEDLINE or EMBASE. Search terms such as the following can be used: *practice guideline, clinical practice guideline*, *best practice guideline*, *evidence-based guideline*, and *consensus statement*. Be aware, though, that a standard search for guidelines in bibliographic databases will yield many references—but often a frustrating mixture of citations to not only the actual guidelines, but also to commentaries, anecdotes, implementation studies, and so on.

Example of a Nursing Clinical Practice Guideline
In 2022, the Registered Nurses Association of Ontario (RNAO) published the second edition of a best practice guideline called "*Promoting smoking reduction and cessation with indigenous peoples of reproductive age and their communities.*" The guideline is intended for use "by nurses and other members of the interprofessional healthcare team to enhance the quality of their practice pertaining to the assessment and management of adult asthma."

There are many topics for which practice guidelines still need to be developed, but the opposite problem is also true: the dramatic increase in the number of guidelines means that there are sometimes multiple guidelines on the same topic. Worse yet, because of variations in the rigor of guideline development and in interpretations of the evidence, different guidelines sometimes offer different and even conflicting recommendations. Thus, those who wish to adopt clinical practice guidelines to address a clinical problem are urged to critically appraise them to identify ones that are based on the strongest and most up-to-date evidence, have been meticulously developed, are user-friendly, and are appropriate for local use.

Several guideline appraisal instruments are available, but the one that has gained the broadest support is the Appraisal of Guidelines Research and Evaluation Instrument, now in its second version

(Brouwers et al., 2010). This tool has been translated into many languages and has been endorsed by the WHO. A shorter and simpler tool for evaluating guideline quality is called the iCAHE Guideline Quality Checklist (Grimmer et al., 2014). A "mini-checklist" for assessing guideline quality for daily practice use has also been proposed (Siebenhofer et al., 2016).

TIP The U.S. Agency for Healthcare Research and Quality offers "guideline syntheses" that provide systematic comparisons of agreement and disagreement among selected guidelines on the same topic (https://www.guidelines.gov/syntheses/index).

One final issue is that guidelines change more slowly than original research or syntheses. If a high-quality guideline is not recent, it is advisable to determine whether more up-to-date evidence would alter (or strengthen) the guideline's recommendations. It has been recommended that, to avoid obsolescence, guidelines should be reassessed every 3 years.

TIP In addition to clinical guidelines, evidence-based **care bundles** are being developed. The concept of care bundles, developed by the Institute for Healthcare Initiatives (www.ihi.org), refers to a set of interventions to treat or prevent a specific cluster of symptoms. There is evidence that a bundle of strategies produces better outcomes than a single intervention.

Level 1 in the 6S Hierarchy: Systems

In a perfect world, evidence-based clinical information systems would link rigorous, up-to-date evidence (e.g., from summaries or syntheses) about a problem with information about a *particular* patient from the patient's electronic health record. Clinicians would then, with best evidence in hand, incorporate their own expertise and patient preferences in arriving at a course of action. Although few current systems match this ideal, some computerized decision support systems have been developed for particular problems, including decisional support tools available on laptops and smartphones.

We can expect progress on such systems in the years ahead.

Example of a Clinical Decision Support Systems
Gengo e Silva and colleagues (2018) described an electronic decision support system in a Brazilian hospital that links nursing diagnoses, outcomes, and interventions performed by nurses caring for medical and surgical patients.

Evidence Hierarchies and Level of Evidence Scales

The EBP movement has led to a proliferation of different **evidence hierarchies,** which are intended to show a ranking of evidence sources in terms of their risk of bias. (These are distinct from the 6S hierarchy discussed in the previous section, which rank evidence sources in terms of the ease and efficiency of finding answers to clinical questions.) Evidence hierarchies are often presented as pyramids, with the highest-ranking sources—those presumed to have the least bias for making inferences about the effects of an intervention—at the top.

The hierarchies form **level of evidence (LOE) scales** that rank order types of evidence. Level I evidence usually is considered the best (least biased) type of evidence, and almost all leveling schemes put systematic reviews at the top level. Some LOE scales have only three levels, while others have 10 or more levels.

Figure 2.2 shows our eight-level evidence hierarchy for Therapy/intervention questions. This hierarchy ranks sources of evidence with respect to the *readiness* of an intervention to be put to use in practice. In our scheme, the Level I evidence source is a systematic review of a type of study called a *randomized controlled trial* (RCT), which is the "gold standard" type of study for Therapy questions. An individual RCT is a Level II evidence source in our hierarchy. Going down the "rungs" of the evidence hierarchy for Therapy questions results in evidence with a higher risk of bias in answering questions about "what works." For example, Level III evidence comes from a type of study called quasiexperiments (the terms in Figure 2.2 are explained later in the book). Of course, there continue to be

Pyramid: Polit-Beck Evidence Hierarchy

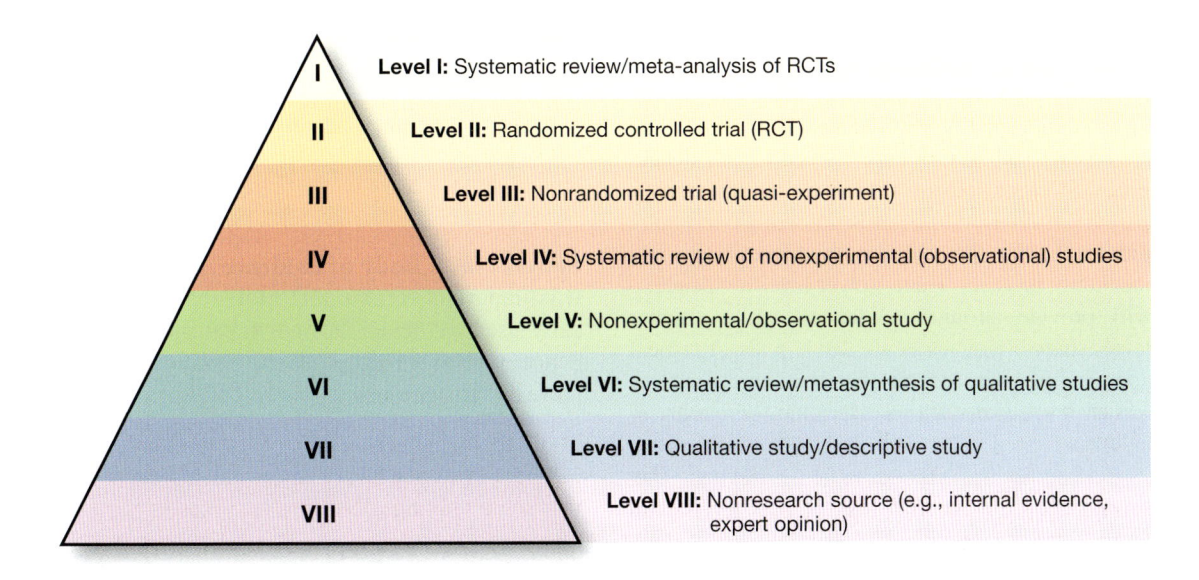

- **Level I:** Systematic review/meta-analysis of RCTs
- **Level II:** Randomized controlled trial (RCT)
- **Level III:** Nonrandomized trial (quasi-experiment)
- **Level IV:** Systematic review of nonexperimental (observational) studies
- **Level V:** Nonexperimental/observational study
- **Level VI:** Systematic review/metasynthesis of qualitative studies
- **Level VII:** Qualitative study/descriptive study
- **Level VIII:** Nonresearch source (e.g., internal evidence, expert opinion)

FIGURE 2.2 Polit–Beck evidence hierarchy/levels of evidence scale for therapy questions.

clinical practice questions for which there is relatively little research evidence. In such situations, nursing practice must rely on other sources, including internal evidence from pathophysiologic data, local projects, and expert opinion (Level VIII). As Straus et al. (2018) have noted, one benefit of the EBP movement is that a new research agenda can emerge when clinical questions arise for which there is no satisfactory evidence.

Hierarchies and Level of Evidence Scales: Some Caveats

Although evidence hierarchies are intended as an EBP resource, considerable confusion exists regarding LOE scales. The fact that there are dozens from which to choose exacerbates this confusion.

One important issue that needs to be acknowledged is that different types of questions require different hierarchies. For example, an evidence hierarchy for prognosis questions differs from the hierarchy for therapy questions. The concept of evidence hierarchies arose in medicine to inform decisions about medical interventions—thus, early evidence hierarchies explicitly ranked evidence for Therapy/intervention questions. Few currently published hierarchies make this point clear, the major exceptions being the LOE hierarchies created by the Oxford Centre for Evidence-Based Medicine (http://www.cebm.net/ocebm-levels-of-evidence/) and the Joanna Briggs Institute (http://joannabriggs.org/jbi-approach.html). We also provide LOE scales in this book for different types of questions (see Chapter 9). As we noted in Chapter 1, evidence for non-Therapy questions can play a role in EBP, but such evidence does not directly support practice changes.

TIP As an example, if we wanted to know whether drinking alcohol during pregnancy puts females at higher risk of a miscarriage (an etiology question), we would not find "best evidence" from a systematic review of RCTs. Pregnant females would never be assigned at random to a "drinking" vs. non-drinking condition to assess whether miscarriage rates are higher in the drinking group.

A second issue is that LOE scales have been used for different purposes. Some writers suggest that LOE scales are similar to the 6S hierarchy—the highest level offers the best starting place in a search for evidence. Others, however, use evidence hierarchies to "level" or grade evidence sources, implying that higher levels provide better quality evidence. As pointed out by Levin (2014), an evidence hierarchy "is not meant to provide a quality rating for evidence retrieved in the search for an answer" (p. 6). The Oxford Centre for Evidence-Based Medicine concurs: the levels in their scheme are "NOT intended to provide you with a definitive judgment about the quality of evidence. There will inevitably be cases where 'lower level' evidence… will provide stronger evidence than a 'higher level' study" (Howick et al., 2011, p. 2). A critical appraisal of each study or evidence source, regardless of level, is needed to determine the *quality of evidence*.

Related to this second issue is the fact that some LOE scales conflate risk of bias levels with terms implying quality. For example, in Melnyk and Fineout-Overholt's (2019) evidence hierarchy (Box 1.3), Level II is defined as *well-designed* RCTs.

Another word of caution: evidence hierarchies need to be sufficiently detailed to include the full range of possible evidence sources. Users of LOE scales often must "read between the lines" and use some judgment. For example, in our hierarchy, if a systematic review included both RCTs *and* nonrandomized trials, we would still consider this Level I evidence. However, if a systematic review included several nonrandomized trials but no RCTs, we might consider this to be evidence somewhere between Levels I and II. As another example, in the Melnyk and Fineout-Overholt (2019) hierarchy, there is no level specified for RCTs that are not especially "well-designed."

As noted by Levin (2014), those who wish to use an LOE scale must choose one that matches their needs from the many that exist, keeping in mind that "leveling" a study based on the chosen scale is not a substitute for a critical appraisal of the evidence.

> **TIP** Evidence hierarchies and LOE scales are rather firmly entrenched in the EBP literature, but they are not without controversy. Concern was expressed initially by critics who felt that qualitative evidence was being undervalued. For example, for therapy questions, qualitative studies are typically near the bottom of the hierarchy. Another criticism of these ranking systems is that they focus exclusively on the risk of certain types of bias, rather than on biases that might undermine the applicability of evidence in real-world settings (e.g., Goodman, 2014). We discuss this important concern about EBP in Chapter 31.

Systems for a Body of Evidence

It is important to note that LOE scales are typically used to "level" an individual piece of evidence, such as a single study. Other systems exist, however, for grading an entire body of evidence with regard to the *strength of evidence*. By far the most widely used system is the Grading of Recommendations Assessment, Development, and Evaluation (GRADE) system (Guyatt et al., 2008). The GRADE system involves two components—grading the quality of an overall body of evidence and ranking the strength of recommendations based on that evidence. GRADE is used with increasing frequency in systematic reviews and in the development of clinical practice guidelines. We discuss GRADE at some length in Chapter 30.

Models for Evidence-Based Practice

Models of EBP are important resources for designing and implementing EBP projects in practice settings. Some models focus on the use of research from the perspective of individual clinicians (e.g., the Stetler Model), but most focus on institutional EBP efforts (e.g., the Iowa Model). Another way to categorize existing models is to distinguish process-oriented models (e.g., the Iowa Model) and models that are explicitly mentor models, such as the ARCC-E (Advanced Research and Clinical Practice Through Close Collaboration in Education) model.

The many worthy EBP models are too numerous to list comprehensively, but a few are shown in Box 2.1. Melnyk and Fineout-Overholt (2019) provide a good synthesis of several EBP models, and Schaffer and colleagues (2013) identify features to consider in selecting a model to plan an EBP project. Although each model offers different perspectives on translating research findings

> **BOX 2.1** Selected Models for Evidence-Based Practice
>
> - ACE Star Model of Knowledge Transformation (Stevens, 2012)
> - Advancing Research and Clinical Practice Through Close Collaboration in Education (ARCC-E) Model (Melnyk & Fineout-Overholt, 2019)
> - Diffusion of Innovations Model (Rogers, 1995)
> - Iowa Model of Evidence-Based Practice to Promote Quality Care (Buckwalter et al., 2017; Titler et al., 2001)
> - Johns Hopkins Nursing EBP Model (Dearholt & Dang, 2012)
> - Promoting Action on Research Implementation in Health Services (PARiHS) Model (Harvey & Kitson, 2016; Rycroft-Malone et al., 2013)
> - Stetler Model of Research Utilization (Stetler, 2010)

into practice, several steps and procedures are similar across the models. Figure 2.3 shows a diagram of one prominent EBP model, the revised **Iowa Model** of EBP (Buckwalter et al., 2017).

Example of Using an Evidence-Based Practice Model

Sage-Rockoff and colleagues (2018) used the Iowa Model in their EBP project designed to improve thermoregulation for trauma patients in the emergency department.

INDIVIDUAL AND ORGANIZATIONAL EVIDENCE-BASED PRACTICE

Individual nurses make many decisions and convey important healthcare information and advice to patients, and so they have ample opportunity to put research into practice. Here are three clinical scenarios that provide examples of such opportunities:

- Clinical Scenario 1. You work in an allergy clinic and notice how difficult it is for many children to undergo allergy scratch tests. You wonder if an interactive distraction intervention would help reduce children's anxiety when they are being tested.
- Clinical Scenario 2. You work in a rehabilitation hospital, and one of your older patients, who had total hip replacement, tells you she is planning a long airplane trip to visit her daughter after rehabilitation treatments are completed. You know that a long plane ride will increase her risk of deep vein thrombosis and wonder if compression stockings are an effective in-flight treatment for her. You decide to look for the best evidence to answer this question.
- Clinical Scenario 3. You are caring for a hospitalized cardiac patient who tells you that he has sleep apnea. He confides in you that he is reluctant to undergo continuous positive airway pressure (CPAP) treatment because he worries it will hinder intimacy with his wife. You wonder if there is any evidence about what it is like to experience CPAP treatment so that you can better address your patient's concerns.

In these and thousands of other clinical situations, research evidence can be put to good use to improve the quality of nursing care. Thus, individual nurses need to have the skills to personally search for, appraise, and apply evidence in their practice.

For some clinical scenarios that trigger an EBP effort, individual nurses have sufficient autonomy to implement research-informed actions on their own (e.g., answering patients' questions about experiences with CPAP). In other situations, however, decisions are best made among a team of nurses (or with an interprofessional team) working together to solve a common clinical problem. Institutional EBP efforts typically result in a formal policy or protocol affecting the practice of many nurses and other staff.

Many of the steps in institutional EBP projects are the same as those we describe in the next

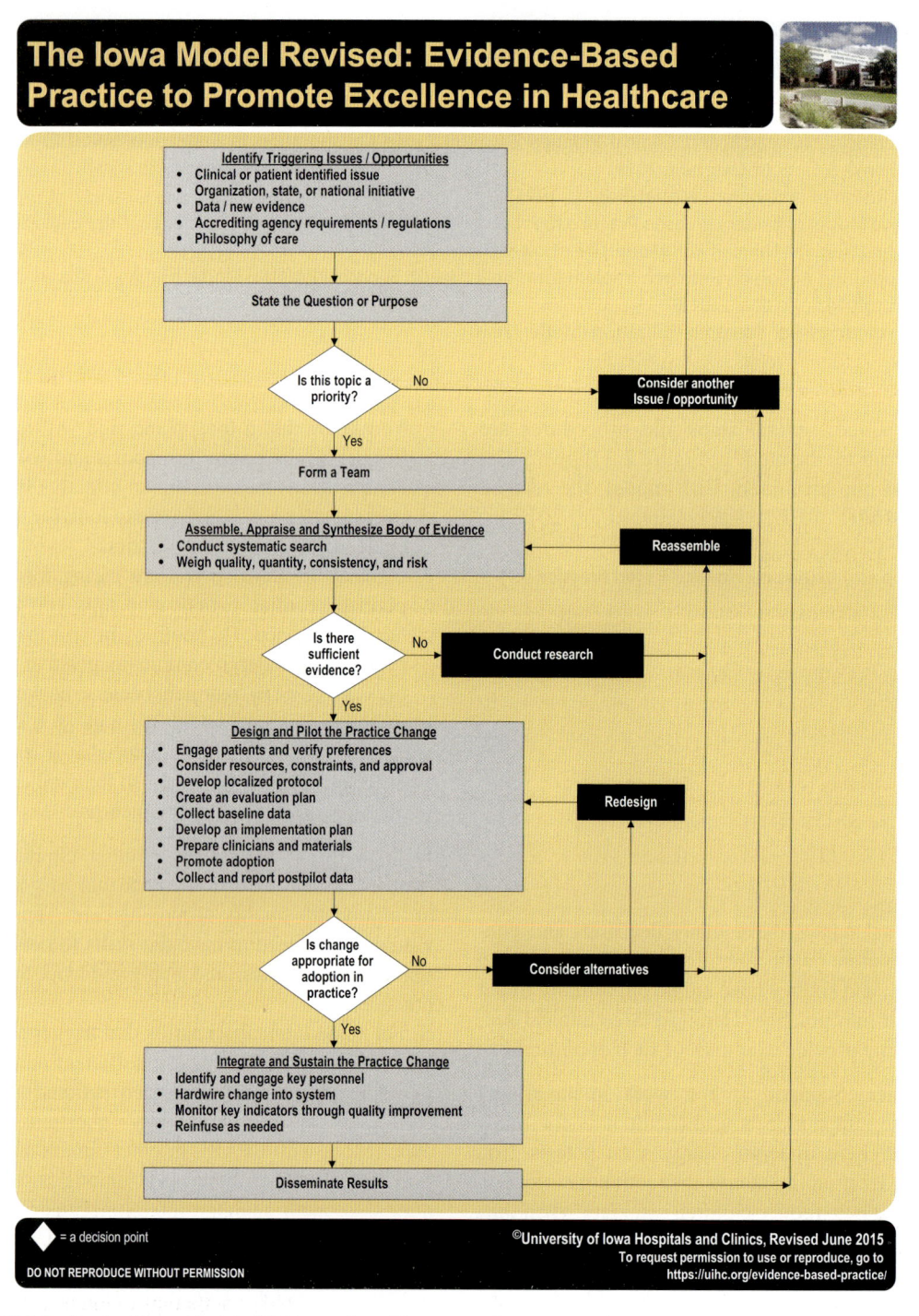

FIGURE 2.3 (Revised Iowa Model of Evidence-Based Practice to Promote Quality Care Iowa Model Collaborative. (2017). Iowa model of evidence-based practice: revisions and validation. *Worldviews on Evidence-Based Nursing, 14*(3), 175–182. doi:10.1111/wvn.12223. Used/reprinted with permission from the University of Iowa Hospitals and Clinics, copyright 2015. For permission to use or reproduce, please contact the University of Iowa Hospitals and Clinics at 319-384-9098.)

section, but additional issues are of relevance at the organizational level. For example, as shown in the Iowa Model (Figure 2.3), some of the activities include assessing whether the question is an organizational priority, forming a team, and conducting a formal evaluation.

MAJOR STEPS IN EVIDENCE-BASED PRACTICE

In this section, we provide an overview of how research evidence can be put to use in clinical settings. In describing the basic steps in the EBP process, we use a mnemonic device (the 5 As) that we have adapted from several sources (e.g., Guyatt et al., 2015; EBP blogs by nurse educator Cathy Thompson [https://nursingeducationexpert.com]).

- Step 1: **Ask**—Ask a well-worded clinical question that can be answered with research evidence;
- Step 2: **Acquire**—Search for and retrieve the best evidence to answer the clinical question;
- Step 3: **Appraise**—Critically appraise the evidence for validity and applicability to the problem and situation;
- Step 4: **Apply**—After integrating the evidence with clinical expertise, patient preferences, and local context, apply it to clinical practice; and
- Step 5: **Assess**—Evaluate the outcome of the practice change.

The EBP process cannot be undertaken in a vacuum, however. A precondition for the entire undertaking is to have an openness to change and a desire to provide the best possible care, based on evidence showing benefits to patient outcomes. Melnyk and Fineout-Overholt (2019) call this Step 0: Cultivating a spirit of inquiry. Johnston and Fineout-Overholt (2005) noted that "getting from zero to one" involves having nurses be reflective about their clinical practice. An additional step after Step 5 is to disseminate information about the EBP project.

Step 1: Ask a Well-Worded Clinical Question

A crucial first step in EBP involves converting information needs into well-worded clinical questions that can be answered with research evidence. Where do the questions come from? Some EBP models distinguish two types of "triggers" for an EBP undertaking: (1) *problem-focused triggers*—a clinical practice problem in need of solution, or (2) *knowledge-focused triggers*—readings in the research literature. Problem-focused triggers may arise in the normal course of clinical practice and include both patient-identified and clinician-identified issues. The Iowa Model (Figure 2.3) includes examples of both types of triggers in the top box.

EBP experts distinguish between background and foreground questions. *Background questions* are foundational questions about a clinical issue, for example: What is cancer cachexia (progressive body wasting), and what is its pathophysiology? Answers to such background questions are typically found in textbooks. *Foreground questions,* by contrast, are those that can be answered based on current research evidence on diagnosing, assessing, or treating patients, or on understanding the meaning or prognosis of their health problems. For example, we may wonder, is a fish oil–enhanced nutritional supplement effective in stabilizing weight in patients with advanced cancer? The answer to such a Therapy question may provide direction on how to address the needs of patients with cachexia. In other words, foreground questions seek the specific information needed to make clinical decisions.

Most guidance for EBP uses the acronyms PIO and PICO to help practitioners develop well-worded questions. In the PICO form, the clinical question is worded to identify four components:

1. P: the *Population* or *patients* (What are key characteristics of the patients or people?)
2. I: the *Intervention*, *influence*, or *exposure* (What is the intervention or therapy of interest? Or what is a potentially harmful or beneficial influence?)

3. C: an explicit *Comparison* to the "I" component (With what is the intervention or influence being compared?)
4. O: the *Outcome* (What is the outcome or consequence in which we are interested?)

Applying this scheme to our question about cachexia, our *population* (P) is cancer patients with cachexia; the *intervention* (I) is fish oil–enhanced nutritional supplements; and the *outcome* (O) is weight stabilization. In this question, the *comparison* is not formally stated, but the implied "C" is the *absence* of fish oil–enhanced supplements—the question is in a PIO format. However, when there is an explicit comparison of interest, the full PICO question is required. For example, we might be interested in learning whether fish oil–enhanced supplements (I) are better than melatonin (C) in stabilizing weight (O) in patients with cancer (P).

For questions that can best be answered with qualitative information (e.g., about the meaning of an experience or health problem), two components are most relevant:

1. the *population* (What are the characteristics of the patients or clients?) and
2. the *situation* (What conditions, experiences, or circumstances are we interested in understanding?)

For example, suppose our question was "What is it like to suffer from cachexia?" In this case, the question calls for rich qualitative information; the *population* is patients with advanced cancer, and the *situation* is the experience of cachexia.

In addition to the basic PICO components, other components may be used in an evidence search. For example, some EBP experts suggest adding a "T" component (PICOT) to designate a time frame. For example, take the following question: Among caregivers of people with dementia (P), what is the effect of participation in a caregiver intervention (I), compared with not participating in the intervention (C) on quality of life (O) 6 months after enrollment (T)? Other experts, however, consider the time frame as part of the outcome: e.g., quality of life 6 months after enrollment (O). Still others prefer to search for the PICO elements without filtering out evidence from studies that used a different period of follow-up, such as 4 months after enrollment.

TIP The Cochrane Collaboration has launched a PICO project—a *Strategy to 2020* initiative—to annotate its systematic reviews with PICO component identification to facilitate retrieval efforts.

Table 2.2 offers question templates for asking well-framed clinical foreground questions for specific types of questions. The right-hand column includes questions with an explicit comparison (PICO questions), while the middle column does not (PIO). The questions are categorized in a manner similar to that discussed in Chapter 1 (EBP purposes), as featured in Table 1.3. Note that although there are some differences in components across question types, there is always a P component.

Step 2: Acquire Research Evidence

By asking clinical questions in a well-worded form, you should be able to search the research literature for the information you need. Using the templates in Table 2.2, the information inserted into the blanks constitutes *keywords* for undertaking an electronic search.

Earlier in this chapter, we described resources to facilitate an efficient search for evidence. As shown in the 6S hierarchy (Table 2.1), there is a range of preappraised evidence sources that can help you acquire evidence regarding your question. Starting with preappraised evidence might lead you to a quick answer—and potentially to a better answer than would be possible if you had to start at the bottom rung with individual studies. Researchers who prepare systematic reviews and synopses usually have excellent research skills and use established standards to evaluate the evidence. Thus, when preprocessed evidence is available to answer a clinical question, you may not need to look any farther, unless the review is not recent or is of poor quality. When high-quality preprocessed evidence cannot be located or is old, you will need to look for best evidence in primary studies, using strategies we describe in Chapter 5.

TABLE 2.2 • Question Templates for Selected Clinical Foreground Questions: PIO and PICO

TYPE OF QUESTION	PIO QUESTION TEMPLATE (QUESTIONS WITHOUT AN EXPLICIT COMPARISON)	PICO QUESTION TEMPLATE (QUESTIONS WITH AN EXPLICIT COMPARISON)
Therapy/ treatment/ intervention	In _____ (**P**opulation), what is the effect of _____ (**I**ntervention) on _____ (**O**utcome)?	In _____ (**P**opulation), what is the effect of _____ (**I**ntervention), in comparison to _____ (**C**omparative/alternative intervention), on _____ (**O**utcome)?
Diagnosis/ assessment	For _____ (**P**opulation), does _____ (**I**dentifying tool/procedure) yield accurate and appropriate diagnostic/assessment information about _____ (**O**utcome)?	For _____ (**P**opulation), does _____ (**I**dentifying tool/procedure) yield more accurate or more appropriate diagnostic/assessment information than _____ (**C**omparative tool/procedure) about _____ (**O**utcome)?
Prognosis	In _____ (**P**opulation), does _____ (**I**nfluence/exposure to disease or condition) increase the risk of _____ (**O**utcome)?	In _____ (**P**opulation), does _____ (**I**nfluence/exposure to disease or condition), relative to _____ (**C**omparative disease/condition OR absence of the disease/condition) increase the risk of _____ (**O**utcome)?
Etiology/ harm	In _____ (**P**opulation), does _____ (**I**nfluence/exposure/characteristic) increase the risk of _____ (**O**utcome)?	In _____ (**P**opulation), does _____ (**I**nfluence/exposure/characteristic) compared to _____ (**C**omparative influence/exposure OR lack of influence or exposure) increase the risk of _____ (**O**utcome)?
Description (prevalence/ incidence)	In _____ (**P**opulation), how prevalent is _____ (**O**utcome)?	*Explicit comparisons are not typical, except to compare different populations*
Meaning or process	What is it like for _____ (**P**opulation) to experience (condition, illness, circumstance)? OR What is the process by which _____ (**P**opulation) cope with, adapt to, or live with (condition, illness, circumstance)?	*Explicit comparisons are not typical in these types of questions*

> **TIP** In Chapter 5, we describe the free internet resource, PubMed, which offers a special tool for those seeking evidence for clinical decisions. Another important database, CINAHL, allows users to restrict a search with an "EBP" limiter.

Step 3: Appraise the Evidence

The evidence acquired in Step 2 of the EBP process should be appraised before taking clinical action. Critical appraisal for EBP may involve several types of assessments. Various criteria have been proposed for EBP appraisals, including the following:

1. *Quality:* To what extent is the evidence valid—that is, how serious is the risk of bias?
2. *Magnitude:* How large is the effect of the intervention or influence (I) on the outcome (O) in the population of interest (P)? Are the effects clinically significant?
3. *Quantity:* How much evidence is there? How many studies have been conducted, and did those studies involve a large number of study participants?
4. *Consistency:* How consistent are the findings across various studies?
5. *Applicability:* To what extent is the evidence relevant to my clinical situation and patients?

Evidence Quality

The first appraisal issue is the extent to which the findings in a research report are valid. That is, were the study methods sufficiently rigorous that the evidence has a low risk of bias? Melnyk and Fineout-Overholt (2019) propose the following formula: LOE (e.g., Figure 2.2) + quality of evidence = strength of evidence. Thus, in coming to a conclusion about the quality of the evidence, it is insufficient to simply "level" the evidence using an LOE scale—it must also be appraised. We offer guidance on appraising the quality of evidence from primary studies throughout this book, and Chapter 5 includes an appraisal worksheet.

If there are several primary studies and no existing systematic review, you would need to draw conclusions about the body of evidence taken as a whole. The previously mentioned GRADE system (Guyatt et al., 2008) is being used increasingly to summarize evidence quality for a body of evidence in systematic reviews (Chapter 30).

Magnitude of Effects

The appraisal criterion relating to magnitude considers how powerful the effects of an intervention or influence are. Estimating the magnitude of the effect for quantitative findings is especially important when an intervention is costly or when there are potentially negative side effects. If, for example, there is good evidence that an intervention is only marginally effective in improving a health problem, it is important to consider other factors (e.g., evidence regarding its effects on quality of life). There are various ways to quantify the magnitude of effects, such as an *effect size index* that we describe later in this book.

The magnitude of effects also has a bearing on *clinical significance*. We discuss how to assess the clinical significance of study findings in Chapter 21.

Quantity and Consistency of Evidence

A rigorously conducted primary study of a RCT offers especially strong evidence about the effect of an intervention on an outcome of interest. But *multiple* RCTs are better than a single study. Moreover, large-scale studies (such as multisite studies) with a large number of study participants are especially desirable.

If there are multiple studies that address your clinical query, however, the strength of the evidence is likely to be diminished if there are inconsistent results across studies. In the GRADE system, inconsistency of results leads to a lower quality-of-evidence grade. When the results of different studies do not corroborate each other, it is likely that further research will have an impact on confidence about an intervention's effect.

Applicability

It is also important to appraise the evidence in terms of its relevance for the clinical situation at hand—that is, for *your* patient in a specific clinical setting. Best practice evidence can most readily be applied to an individual patient in your care if they are similar to people in the study or studies under review. Would your patient have qualified for participation in the study—or is there some factor such as age, illness severity, or comorbidity that would have excluded the patient? Practitioners must reach conclusions about the applicability of research evidence, but researchers also bear some responsibility for enhancing the applicability of their work. As we discuss in Chapter 31, concerns about the fact that "best evidence" is usually about "average" patients from restricted populations has made the issue of applicability increasingly salient.

TIP An appraisal of evidence for use in your practice may involve additional factors. In particular, costs are likely to be an important consideration. Some interventions are expensive, and so the amount of resources needed to put best evidence into practice would need to be factored into any decision. Of course, the cost of *not* taking action is also important.

Actions Based on Evidence Appraisals

Appraisals of the evidence may lead you to different courses of action. You may reach this point and conclude that the evidence is not sufficiently sound, or that the likely effect is too small, or that the cost of applying the evidence is too high. The evidence may suggest that "usual care" is the best strategy—or it may lead you to pose an alternative clinical query. You may also consider the possibility of undertaking your own study to add to the body of evidence relating to your original clinical question. If, however, the initial appraisal of evidence suggests a promising clinical action, then you can proceed to the next step.

Step 4: Apply the Evidence

As the definition for EBP implies, research evidence needs to be integrated with your own clinical expertise and knowledge of your clinical setting. You may be aware of factors that would make implementation of the evidence, no matter how sound or promising, inadvisable. Patient preferences and values are also important. A discussion with the patient may reveal negative attitudes toward a potentially beneficial course of action, contraindications (e.g., comorbidities), or possible impediments (e.g., lack of health insurance).

Armed with rigorous evidence, your own clinical know-how, and information about your patient's circumstances, you can use the resulting information to make an evidence-based decision or provide research-informed advice. Although the steps in the process, as just described, may seem complicated, in reality the process can be efficient—*if* there is an adequate evidence base and especially if it has been skillfully preprocessed. EBP is most challenging when findings from research are contradictory, inconclusive, or "thin"—that is to say, when better quality evidence is needed.

One final issue is the importance of integrating evidence from qualitative research, which can provide rich insights into how patients experience a problem, or about barriers to complying with treatment. A new intervention with strong potential benefits may fail to achieve desired outcomes if it is not implemented with sensitivity and understanding of patients' perspectives. As Morse (2005) so aptly noted, evidence from an RCT may tell you whether a pill is effective, but qualitative research can help you understand why patients may not swallow the pill.

Step 5: Assess the Outcomes of the Practice Change

One last step in many EBP efforts concerns evaluating the outcomes of the practice change. Did you achieve the desired outcomes? Were patients satisfied with the results?

Straus et al. (2018) remind us that part of the ongoing evaluation involves how well you are performing EBP. They offer self-evaluation questions that relate to the EBP steps, such as asking answerable questions (Am I asking any clinical questions at all? Am I asking well-formulated question?) and acquiring external evidence (Do I know the best sources of current evidence? Am I becoming more efficient in my searching?).

TIP Every nurse can play a role in using research evidence. Here are some strategies:
- *Read widely and critically.* Professionally accountable nurses keep abreast of important research developments relating to their specialty by reading professional journals.
- *Attend professional conferences.* Conference attendees have opportunities to meet researchers and to explore practice implications of new research.
- *Insist on evidence that a procedure is effective.* Every time nurses or nursing students are told about a standard nursing procedure, they have a right to ask: Why? Nurses need to develop expectations that the clinical decisions they make are based on sound, evidence-based rationales.
- *Become involved in a journal club.* Many organizations that employ nurses sponsor journal clubs that review studies with potential relevance to practice.
- *Pursue and participate in EBP projects.* Several studies have found that nurses who are involved in research activities (e.g., an EBP project or data collection activities) develop more positive attitudes toward research and better research skills.

RESEARCH EXAMPLE

Thousands of EBP projects are underway in practice settings. Many that have been described in the nursing literature offer information about planning and implementing such an endeavor.

Study: Implementation of the MEDFRAT to promote quality care and decrease falls in community hospital emergency rooms (McCarty et al., 2018).

Purpose: An interprofessional team undertook an EBP implementation project at a large healthcare delivery system with 12 emergency departments (EDs). The focus of the project was to decrease falls in community hospital EDs.

Framework: The project used the Iowa Model as its guiding framework. The EBP team identified a problem-focused trigger—the inconsistent use of fall-risk assessments and variation in falls in the EDs.

Approach: The project team assembled relevant literature to identify an appropriate assessment tool for use in EDs. The team selected the Memorial Emergency Department Fall-Risk Assessment Tool (MEDFRAT) because it was simple to use (only six questions) and had been validated for use in EDs (i.e., it had evidence-based utility). The tool creates two risk-stratification levels, and each has suggested fall-risk prevention interventions. For example, possible interventions included hourly rounding, bed in low position, bedside alarms, and locating patients into view of the nurses' station. Information systems staff built the MEDFRAT into the electronic medical record. The team then created and implemented a 1-hour education session about falls for nurses in the EDs. The EDs in the project were visited over a 4-month period, with 60 nurses attending the sessions. The participating nurses offered feedback and further suggestions. Several nurses mentioned the lack of bedside alarms, and so portable alarms were ordered. Another suggestion concerned the use of different colored grip socks to identify patients at high risk of a fall. Overall, the nurses' reactions to MEDFRAT were unanimously positive.

Evaluation: The MEDFRAT has been implemented in all 12 EDs in the system. Baseline levels of falls in the ED over a 4-year period ranged from 0 (in EDs with under 10 beds) to 76 in the ED with the most beds. Data regarding the effectiveness of the intervention were not available when the report was written, but short-term outcomes and longer-term outcomes (decrease in ED falls) are being monitored.

Conclusions: The authors of the report concluded that the Iowa Model was a useful framework. They were optimistic about the outcomes and about using the Iowa Model to implement other evidence-based nursing interventions in their setting.

SUMMARY POINTS

- **Evidence-based practice (EBP)** is the conscientious integration of current best evidence and other factors in making clinical decisions. The three main components of EBP are (1) best research evidence; (2) your own clinical experience and knowledge; and (3) patient preferences, values, and circumstances.

- Two underpinnings of the EBP movement are the **Cochrane Collaboration** (which is based on the work of British epidemiologist Archie Cochrane) and the clinical learning strategy called *evidence-based medicine* developed at the McMaster Medical School.
- **Research utilization (RU)** and EBP are overlapping concepts that concern efforts to use research as a basis for clinical decisions, but RU *starts* with a research-based innovation that gets evaluated for possible use in practice.
- **Knowledge translation (KT)** is a term used primarily about system-wide efforts to enhance systematic change in clinical practice or policies. **Translational research** is a discipline devoted to developing methods to promote KT and the use of evidence.
- Resources to support EBP are growing at a phenomenal pace. Preprocessed (synthesized) and preappraised evidence is especially useful and efficient in addressing clinical queries. The **6S hierarchy** of preappraised evidence offers a guide for efficient evidence searches. This hierarchy includes (6) systems at the pinnacle; (5) summaries; (4) synopses of syntheses; (3) syntheses; (2) synopses of single studies; and (1) individual primary studies, which are not preappraised, at the base.
- Systematic reviews (Syntheses) have been considered the cornerstone of EBP. **Systematic reviews** are rigorous integrations of research evidence from multiple studies on a topic. Systematic reviews can involve either narrative approaches to integration (including **meta-synthesis** and **meta-aggregation** of qualitative studies) or quantitative methods (**meta-analysis**) that integrate findings statistically by using individual studies as the **unit of analysis.** The emergence of **rapid reviews** reflects the need for less rigorous, but more timely, syntheses of evidence.
- Evidence-based **clinical practice guidelines** are a major example of preappraised evidence in the "Summaries" category of the 6S hierarchy. These guidelines combine a synthesis and appraisal of research evidence from a systematic review with specific recommendations for clinical decision-making. Clinical practice guidelines should be carefully and systematically appraised, for example, using the Appraisal of Guidelines Research and Evaluation (*AGREE II*) instrument.
- The EBP movement has given rise to a proliferation of **evidence hierarchies** that provide a preliminary guidepost for finding "best" evidence—evidence with the lowest risk of bias. Evidence hierarchies reflect **LOE scales** that rank order types of evidence source. Most published LOE scales are appropriate only for Therapy/intervention questions. In LOEs for Therapy questions, systematic reviews of RCTs are considered Level I sources. However, at every level, the quality of the evidence must be appraised: Strength of evidence = level + quality.
- Many models of EBP have been developed, including models that provide a framework for individual clinicians (e.g., the **Stetler model**) and others for organizations or teams of clinicians (e.g., the **Iowa Model** of Evidence-Based Practice to Promote Quality Care).
- Although organizational projects include additional steps, the most basic steps in EBP for both individuals and team are as follows (the 5 As): *Ask* a well-worded clinical question; *Acquire* the best evidence to answer the question; *Appraise* and synthesize the evidence; *Apply* the evidence, after integrating it with patient preferences and clinical expertise; and *Assess* the effects of the practice change.
- A widely used scheme for asking well-worded clinical questions involves four primary components, an acronym for which is **PICO**: Population or patients (P), Intervention or influence (I), Comparison (C), and Outcome (O).
  - An appraisal of the evidence involves such considerations as the quality of the evidence, in terms of the risk of bias; the magnitude of the effects and their clinical importance; the quantity of evidence; the consistency of evidence across studies; and the applicability of the evidence to particular settings and patients.

STUDY ACTIVITIES

REFERENCES CITED IN CHAPTER 2

Beck, C. (2009). Metasynthesis: A goldmine for evidence-based practice. *AORN Journal*, *90*(5), 701–710.

Beck, C. T. & Vo, T. (2020). Fathers' stress related to their infants' NICU hospitalization: A mixed research synthesis, *Archives of Psychiatric Nursing*, *34*(2), 75–84. https://doi.org/10.1016/j.apnu.2020.02.001

Brouwers, M., Kho, M., Browman, G., Burgers, J., Cluzeau, F., Feder, G., Graham, I. D., Grimshaw, J, Hanna, SE, Littlejohns, P, Makarski, J, Zitzelsberger, L, Fervers, B., & for the AGREE Next Steps Consortium. (2010). Agree II: Advancing guideline development, reporting and evaluation in health care. *Canadian Medical Association Journal*, *182*(18), E839–E842.

Buckwalter, K. C., Cullen, L., Hanrahan, K., Kleiber, C., McCarthy, A. M., Rakel, B, Steelman, V, Tripp-Reimer, T., & Tucker, S; Iowa Model Collaborative. (2017). Iowa model of evidence-based practice: Revisions and validation. *Worldviews on Evidence-Based Nursing*, *14*(3), 175–182.

Car In Hat Ra. (2004). *Knowledge translation strategy 2004–2009: Innovation in action*. Canadian Institutes of Health Research.

Dang, D., Dearholt, S., Bissett, K., Ascenzi, J., & Whalen, M. (Eds.). (2012). *Johns Hopkins nursing evidence-based practice: Model and guidelines*. Sigma Theta Tau International.

DiCenso, A., Bayley, L., & Haynes, B. (2009). Accessing preappraised evidence: Fine-tuning the 5S model into a 6S model. *Evidence-Based Nursing*, *12*(4), 99–101.

Gardner, K., Kanaskie, M., Knehans, A., Salisbury, S., Doheny, K., & Schirm, V. (2016). Implementing and sustaining evidence based practice through a nursing journal club. *Applied Nursing Research*, *31*, 139–145.

Gengo e Silva, R., Dos Santos Diogo, R., da Cruz, D., Ortiz, D., Ortiz, D., Peres, H., & Moorhead, S. (2018). Linkages of nursing diagnoses, outcomes, and interventions performed by nurses caring for medical and surgical patients using a decision support system. *International Journal of Nursing Knowledge*, *29*(4), 269–275.

Gilbert, R., Salanti, G., Harden, M., & See, S. (2005). Infant sleeping position and the sudden infant death syndrome: Systematic review of observational studies and historical review of recommendations from 1940 to 2002. *International Journal of Epidemiology*, *34*(4), 874–887.

Glasziou, P. (2005). Evidence-based medicine: Does it make a difference? Make it evidence informed with a little wisdom. *British Medical Journal*, *330*(7482), 92–94.

Goodman, C. S. (2014). *Hta 101: Introduction to health technology assessment*. National Information Center on Health Services Research and Health Care Technology.

Grant, M., & Booth, A. (2009). A typology of reviews: An analysis of 14 review types and associated methodologies. *Health Information and Libraries Journal*, *26*(2), 91–108.

Grimmer, K., Dizon, J., Milanese, S., King, E., Beaton, K., Thorpe, O., Lizarondo, L., Luker, J,. Machotka, Z., Kumar, S. (2014). Efficient clinical evaluation of guideline quality: Development and testing of a new tool. *BMC Medical Research Methodology*, *14*, 63.

Guyatt, G., Oxman, A., Vist, G., Kunz, R., Falck-Ytter, Y., Alonso-Coello, P., Schünemann, HJ, & GRADE Working Group (2008). Grade: An emerging consensus on rating quality of evidence and strength of recommendations. *BMJ*, *336*(7650), 924–926.

Guyatt, G., Rennie, D., Meade, M., & Cook, D. (2015). *Users' guide to the medical literature: Essentials of evidence-based clinical practice* (3rd ed.). McGraw Hill.

Harvey, G., & Kitson, A. (2016). PARIHS revisited: From heuristic to integrated framework for the successful implementation of knowledge into practice. *Implementation Science*, *11*, 33.

Heyvaert, M., Hannes, K., & Onghena, P. (2017). *Using mixed methods research synthesis for literature reviews*. Sage Publications.

Howick, J., Chalmers, I., Glasziou, P., Greenhalgh, T., Heneghan, C., Liberati, A., … Thornton, H. (2011).*The 2011 Oxford CEBM levels of evidence: Introductory document*. Centre for Evidence-Based Medicine.

Huo, M., Zhao, B., Li, Y., & Li, J. (2022). Evidence-based practice dynamic capabilities: A concept derivation and analysis. *Annals of Translational Medicine*, *10*(1), 22. https://doi.org/10.21037/atm-21-6506

Institute of Medicine. (2001). *Crossing the quality chasm: A new health care system for the 21st century*. National Academic Press.

Johnston, L., & Fineout-Overholt, E. (2005). Teaching EBP: "Getting from zero to one." moving from recognizing and admitting uncertainties to asking searchable, answerable questions. *Worldviews on Evidence-Based Nursing*, *2*, 98–102.

Kwag, K. H., Gonzalez-Lorenzo, M., Banzi, R., Bonovas, S., & Moja, L. (2016). Providing doctors with high-quality information: An updated evaluation of web-based point-of-care information summaries. *Journal of Medical Internet Research*, *18*(1), e15.

Levin, R. F. (2014). Levels, grades, and strength of evidence: "What's it all about, Alfie?". *Research and Theory for Nursing Practice*, *28*(1), 5–8.

McCarty, C., Woehrle, T., Waring, S., Taran, A., & Kitch, L. (2018). Implementation of the MEDFRAT to promote quality care and decrease falls in community hospital emergency rooms. *Journal of Emergency Nursing*, *44*(3), 280–284.

Melnyk, B. M., & Fineout-Overholt, E. (2019). *Evidence-based practice in nursing and health care* (4th ed.). Lippincott Williams & Wilkins.

Melnyk, B. M., & Newhouse, R. (2014). Evidence-based practice versus evidence-informed practice: A debate that could stall forward momentum in improving health care quality, safety, patient outcomes, and costs. *Worldviews on Evidence-Based Nursing, 11*, 347–349.

Meng, F., Jiang, Y., Yu, P., Song, Y., Zhou, L., Xu, Y., & Zhou, Y. (2023). Effect of health coaching on blood pressure control and behavioral modification among patients with hypertension: A systematic review and meta-analysis of randomized controlled trials. *International Journal of Nursing Studies, 138*, 104406. Advance online publicationhttps://doi.org/10.1016/j.ijnurstu.2022.104406.

Morse, J. M. (2005). Beyond the clinical trial: Expanding criteria for evidence. *Qualitative Health Research, 15*(1), 3–4.

Newhouse, R. P. (2007). Diffusing confusion among evidence-based practice, quality improvement, and research. *Journal of Nursing Administration, 37*(10), 432–435.

Newhouse, R. P., & Spring, B. (2010). Interdisciplinary evidence-based practice: Moving from silos to synergy. *Nursing Outlook, 58*(6), 309–317.

Nickum, A., Johnson-Barlow, E., Raszewski, R., & Rafferty, R. (2022). Focus on nursing point-of-care tools: Application of a new evaluation rubric. *Journal of the Medical Library Association: JMLA, 110*(3), 358–364. https://doi.org/10.5195/jmla.2022.1257

Registered Nurses' Association of Ontario (2017). *Adult asthma care: Promoting control of asthma* (2nd ed.). Retrieved from http://rnao.ca/bpg/guidelines/adult-asthma-care

Rogers, E. M. (1995). *Diffusion of innovations* (4th ed.). Free Press.

Rycroft-Malone, J., Seers, K., Chandler, J., Hawkes, C., Crichton, N., Allen, C., Bullock, I, Strunin, L, Strunin, L. (2013). The role of evidence, context, and facilitation in an implementation trial: Implications for the development of the PARIHS framework. *Implementation Science, 8*, 28.

Sandelowski, M., Voils, C. I., Crandell, J. L., & Leeman, J. (2013). Synthesizing qualitative and quantitative research findings. In Beck, , (Ed.). *Routledge international handbook of qualitative nursing research* (pp. 347–356). Routledge.

Saqe-Rockoff, A., Schubert, F., Ciardiello, A., & Douglas, E. (2018). Improving thermoregulation for trauma patients in the emergency department: An evidence-based practice project. *Journal of Trauma Nursing, 25*(1), 14–20.

Schaffer, M. A., Sandau, K., & Diedrick, L. (2013). Evidence-based practice models for organizational change: Overview and practical applications. *Journal of Advanced Nursing, 69*(5), 1197–1209.

Siebenhofer, A., Semlitsch, T., Herborn, T., Siering, U., Kopp, I., & Hartig, J. (2016). Validation and reliability of a guideline appraisal mini-checklist for daily practice use. *BMC Medical Research Methodology, 16*, 39.

Stetler, C. B. (2010). Stetler model. In Rycroft-Malone, & Bucknall (Eds.), *Models and frameworks for implementing evidence-based practice: Linking evidence to action* (pp. 51–77). Wiley-Blackwell.

Stevens, K. R. (2012). *Star model of EBP: Knowledge transformation*. Academic center for evidence-based practice. The University of Texas Health Science Center at San Antonio.

Straus, S. E., Glasziou, P., Richardson, W. S., & Haynes, R. B. (2018). *Evidence-based medicine E-book: How to practice and teach EBM* (5th ed.). Elsevier Health Sciences.

Titler, M. (2014). Overview of evidence-based practice and translation science. *Nursing Clinics of North America, 49*(3), 269–274.

Titler, M. G., Kleiber, C., Steelman, V., Rakel, B., Budreau, G., Everett, L., Buckwalter, K. C., Tripp-Reimer, T., Goode, C. J., & Goode, C. (2001). The Iowa model of evidence-based practice to promote quality care. *Critical Care Nursing Clinics of North America, 13*(4), 497–509.

Tracy, M. & Barnsteiner, J. (2021). Evidence based practice. pp 186–212. In Sherwood, & Barnsteiner, (Eds.). *Quality and safety in nursing: A competency approach to improving outcomes*. John Wiley & Sons.

Tricco, A. C., Straus, S. E., Ghaffar, A., & Langlois, E. V. (2022). Rapid reviews for health policy and systems decision-making: More important than ever before. *Systematic Reviews, 11*(1), 153. https://doi.org/10.1186/s13643-022-01887-7

Wilfling, D., Calo, S., Dichter, M. N., Meyer, G., Möhler, R., & Köpke, S. (2023). Non-pharmacological interventions for sleep disturbances in people with dementia. *The Cochrane Database of Systematic Reviews, 1*(1), CD011881. https://doi.org/10.1002/14651858.CD011881.pub2

World Health Organization (2005). *Bridging the "Know-do" gap: Meeting on knowledge translation in global health*. Retrieved June 20, 2019, from https://www.measureevaluation.org/resources/training/capacity-building-resources/high-impact-research-training-curricula/bridging-the-know-do-gap.pdf

3

Key Concepts and Steps in Qualitative and Quantitative Research

Learning Objectives

1. Provide examples of independent and dependent variables.
2. Discuss the difference between experimental from nonexperimental research.
3. Identify three main disciplinary traditions for qualitative nursing research.
4. Describe the flow and sequence of activities in quantitative and qualitative research and discuss how and why they differ.

INTRODUCTION

This chapter covers a lot of ground—but, for many of you, it is familiar ground. If you have taken an earlier research course, this chapter will be a review of key terms and steps in the research process. If you have no previous exposure to research methods, this chapter offers basic grounding in research terminology.

Research, like any field of study, has its own *jargon*. Some terms are used by both qualitative and quantitative researchers, but others are used mainly by one or the other group. Also, some nursing research jargon has its roots in the social sciences, but sometimes different terms for the same concepts are used in medical research; we cover both.

FUNDAMENTAL RESEARCH TERMS AND CONCEPTS

When researchers address a problem—regardless of the underlying paradigm—they undertake a **study** (or an **investigation**). Studies involve people cooperating with each other in different roles.

The Faces and Places of Research

Studies with humans involve two groups: those doing research and those providing the information. In a quantitative study, the people being studied are called **subjects** or **study participants** (Table 3.1). In a qualitative study, those under study are called study participants or **informants**. Collectively, study participants comprise the **sample**.

The person who conducts a study is the **researcher** or **investigator**. Studies are often done by a team; the person directing the study is the **principal investigator (PI)**. Increasingly nurses are embracing team science in which nurse researchers are either working together in large groups or as part of interdisciplinary research teams. In large-scale projects, dozens of individuals may be involved in planning and conducting the study.

Research can be undertaken in a variety of *settings*—the specific places where information is gathered. Some studies take place in *naturalistic*

TABLE 3.1 • Key Terms in Quantitative and Qualitative Research

CONCEPT	QUANTITATIVE TERM	QUALITATIVE TERM
Person contributing information	Subject Study participant –	– Study participant Informant, key informant
Person undertaking the study	Researcher Investigator	Researcher Investigator
That which is being investigated	– Concepts Constructs Variables	Phenomena Concepts – –
System of organizing concepts	Theory, theoretical framework Conceptual framework, conceptual model	Theory Conceptual framework, sensitizing framework
Information gathered	Data (numerical values)	Data (narrative descriptions)
Connections between concepts	Relationships (cause-and-effect, associative)	Patterns of association
Logical reasoning processes	Deductive reasoning	Inductive reasoning

settings in the field, such as in people's homes, but some studies are done in laboratory or clinical settings. Qualitative researchers are especially likely to engage in **fieldwork** in natural settings because they are interested in the contexts of people's experiences. The *site* is the overall location for the research—it could be an entire community (e.g., a Haitian neighborhood in Miami) or an institution (e.g., a hospital in Toronto). Researchers sometimes undertake **multisite studies** because the use of multiple sites offers a larger or more diverse sample of participants.

The Building Blocks of Research

Phenomena, Concepts, and Constructs

Research involves abstractions. For example, *pain*, *fatigue*, and *obesity* are abstractions of human characteristics. These abstractions are called **concepts** or, in qualitative studies, **phenomena**.

Researchers also use the term **construct**, which refers to an abstraction inferred from situations or behaviors—but often one that is deliberately invented or constructed. For example, *self-care* in Orem's model of health maintenance is a construct. The terms *construct* and *concept* are sometimes used interchangeably, but by convention, a construct typically refers to a more complex abstraction than a concept.

Theories and Conceptual Models

A **theory** is a systematic explanation of some aspect of reality. Theories, which knit concepts together into a coherent system, play a role in both qualitative and quantitative research.

Quantitative researchers may start with a theory or *conceptual model* (distinctions are discussed in Chapter 6). Based on theory, researchers predict how phenomena will behave in the real world *if the theory is true*. Researchers use *deductive reasoning* to go from a theory to specific predictions, which are tested through research; study results are used to support, reject, or modify the theory.

In qualitative research, theories may be used in various ways. Sometimes conceptual or **sensitizing frameworks**, derived from qualitative research traditions we describe later in this chapter, offer an orienting world view. In such studies, the framework helps to guide the inquiry and to interpret the findings. In other qualitative studies, theory is the *product* of the research: the investigators use information from participants *inductively* to develop a theory rooted in the participants' experiences.

Variables

In quantitative studies, concepts often are called **variables**. A variable, as the name implies, is something that varies. Weight, fatigue, and stress are variables—each varies from one person to another. In fact, most aspects of humans are variables. If everyone weighed 150 lb, weight would not be a variable but rather would be a *constant*. It is because people and conditions *do* vary that most research is conducted. Quantitative researchers seek to understand how or why things vary and to learn if differences in one variable are related to differences in another. For example, lung cancer research focuses on the variable of lung cancer, which is a variable because not everyone has this disease. Researchers have studied factors that might be linked to lung cancer, such as cigarette smoking. Smoking is also a variable because not everyone smokes. A variable, then, is any quality of a person, group, or situation that takes on different values.

When an attribute is highly varied in the group under study, the group is **heterogeneous** with respect to that variable. If the amount of variability is limited, the group is **homogeneous**. For example, for the variable height, a sample of 2-year-old children would be more homogeneous than a sample of 21-year-olds.

Characteristics of Variables. Variables may be inherent characteristics of people, such as their age or blood type. Sometimes, however, researchers *create* a variable. For example, if a researcher tests the effectiveness of patient-controlled analgesia as opposed to intramuscular analgesia in relieving pain after surgery, some patients would be given patient-controlled analgesia and others would receive intramuscular analgesia. In the context of the study, method of pain management is a variable because different patients get different analgesic methods.

Some variables take on a wide range of values that can be represented on a continuum. For example, a person's age is a *continuous variable* that can, in theory, assume an infinite number of values between two points. For example, between 1 and 2 lb for the variable *weight*, the number of values is limitless (e.g., 1.05, 1.3333, and so on). Other variables take on only a few values. *Discrete variables* convey quantitative information (e.g., number of children), but *categorical variables* involve placing people into categories (e.g., gender, blood type). Categorical variables with only two categories (e.g., alive/dead) are *dichotomous variables*.

Dependent and Independent Variables. Many studies seek to unravel and understand causes of phenomena. Does a nursing intervention *cause* improvements in patient outcomes? Does smoking *cause* lung cancer? The presumed cause is the **independent variable**, and the presumed effect is the **dependent variable** (or the **outcome variable**). The dependent variable corresponds to the "O" (outcome) of the PICO scheme discussed in Chapter 2. The independent variable corresponds to the "I" (the intervention, influence, or exposure), *plus* the "C" (the comparison). In doing an evidence search, you might want to learn about the effects of an intervention or influence (I), compared with *any* alternative, on an outcome (O). In a study, however, researchers must always specify the comparator (the "C") that they will investigate.

Variation in the dependent variable is presumed to *depend on* variation in the independent variable. For example, researchers study the extent to which lung cancer (the dependent variable) depends on smoking (the independent variable). Or, investigators might study the extent to which patients' pain (the dependent variable) depends on certain nursing actions (the independent variable). The dependent variable is the outcome that researchers want to understand, explain, or predict.

The terms *independent variable* and *dependent variable* are also used to indicate *direction of influence* rather than a causal link. For example, suppose a researcher studied the role of gender in the mental health (O) of spousal caregivers of patients with dementia (P) and found lower depression for wives than for husbands (I and C). We could not conclude that depression was *caused* by gender. Yet the direction of influence clearly runs from gender to depression: patients' level of depression does not influence their gender. Even without a cause-and-effect connection, it is appropriate to consider depression as the outcome variable and gender as an independent variable.

Most outcomes have multiple causes or influences. If we were studying factors that influence obesity, as measured by people's body mass index (the dependent variable), we might consider height, physical activity, and diet as independent variables in this Etiology question. Two or more *dependent* variables also may be of interest. For example, a researcher may compare the effects of alternative nursing interventions for children with cystic fibrosis (a Therapy question). Several dependent variables could be used to assess treatment effectiveness, such as length of hospital stay, number of recurrent respiratory infections, and so on. It is common to design studies with multiple independent and dependent variables.

Variables are not *inherently* dependent or independent. A dependent variable in one study could be an independent variable in another. For example, a study might examine the effect of an exercise intervention versus no intervention (the independent variable) on osteoporosis (the dependent variable) to answer a Therapy question. Another study might investigate the effect of osteoporosis versus no osteoporosis (the independent variable) on bone fracture incidence (the dependent variable) to address a Prognosis question. In short, whether a variable is independent or dependent is a function of the role that it plays in a particular study.

Example of Independent and Dependent Variables

Research question (Etiology/Harm question): Does a nurse-led intervention reduce the incidence and duration of delirium among adults admitted to the intensive care unit? (Lynch et al., 2020)
 Independent variable: Nurse-led intervention versus no intervention.
 Dependent variable: Delirium incidence and duration.

Conceptual and Operational Definitions

Concepts are abstractions of observable phenomena, and researchers' world views shape how those concepts are defined. A **conceptual definition** presents the abstract or theoretical meaning of concepts under study. Even seemingly straightforward terms need to be conceptually defined. The classic example is the concept of *caring*. Morse et al. (1990) examined how researchers and theorists defined *caring* and identified five classes of conceptual definition: as a human trait; a moral imperative; an affect; an interpersonal relationship; and a therapeutic intervention. Smith (2019) identified eight sources in the nursing literature that described caring as core to the discipline of nursing. Further, Smith synthesizes the definition of caring as "the intentions, expressions, behaviors, actions, and experiences, grounded in a moral-ethical-spiritual foundation, that nurture humanization, health, healing, and well-being? (Smith, 2019, p. 11).

In qualitative studies, conceptual definitions of key phenomena may be a major end product, reflecting an intent to have the meaning of concepts defined by those being studied. In quantitative studies, however, researchers must define concepts at the outset because they must decide how the variables will be observed and measured. An **operational definition** specifies what the researchers must do to measure the concept and collect needed information.

Variables differ in the ease with which they can be operationalized. The variable weight, for example, is easy to define and measure. We might operationally define weight as the amount that an object weighs, to the nearest half pound. This definition designates that weight will be measured using one system (pounds) rather than another (grams). We could also specify that weight will be measured using a digital scale with participants fully undressed after 10 hours of fasting. This operational definition clarifies what we mean by the variable *weight*.

Few variables are operationalized as easily as weight. Most variables can be measured in different ways, and researchers must choose the one that best captures the variables as they conceptualize them. Take, for example, *anxiety*, which can be defined in terms of both physiologic and psychological functioning. For researchers choosing to emphasize physiologic aspects, the operational definition might involve a measurement of salivary cortisol. If researchers conceptualize anxiety as a psychological state, the operational definition might be people's scores on a patient-reported test such as the State Anxiety Scale. Readers of research articles may not agree with how variables were conceptualized and measured, but definitional precision is important for communicating exactly what concepts mean within the study.

TIP Operationalizing a concept is often a two-part process that involves deciding (1) how to accurately measure the variable and (2) how to represent it in an analysis. For example, a person's age might be obtained by asking them to report their birthdate but operationalized in an analysis in relation to a threshold (e.g., younger than 65 vs. 65 years or older).

Example of Conceptual and Operational Definitions

Zhai et al. (2023) tested the relationship between organizational culture and thriving at work. In their study, they defined four concepts: thriving at work, culture of care, affective commitment, and work engagement. Each of the concepts was operationalized through existing reliable and valid tools that measured the concepts. Their findings indicated that nurses' work engagement and affective commitment mediated the relationship between the nurses' perceived nursing culture and their thriving at work.

Data

Research **data** (singular, datum) are the pieces of information obtained in a study. In quantitative studies, researchers define their variables and then collect relevant data from study participants. Quantitative researchers collect primarily **quantitative data**—data in numeric form. For example, suppose *depression* was a key variable in a quantitative study. We might ask participants, "Thinking about the past week, how depressed would you say you have been on a scale from 0 to 10, where 0 means 'not at all' and 10 means 'the most possible'?" Box 3.1 presents quantitative data for three fictitious people. Subjects provided a number along a 0 to 10 continuum representing their degree of depression—*9* for subject 1 (a high level of depression), *0* for subject 2 (no depression), and *4* for subject 3 (mild depression). The numeric values for all participants, collectively, would comprise the data on depression in this study.

In qualitative studies, researchers collect **qualitative data**, that is, narrative descriptions.

BOX 3.1 Example of Quantitative Data

Question:	Thinking about the past week, how depressed would you say you have been on a scale from 0 to 10, where 0 means "not at all" and 10 means "the most possible"?
Data:	9 (Subject 1) 0 (Subject 2) 4 (Subject 3)

> **BOX 3.2   Example of Qualitative Data**
>
> **Question:** Tell me about how you've been feeling lately—have you felt sad or depressed at all, or have you generally been in good spirits?
>
> **Data:** "Well, actually, I've been pretty depressed lately, to tell you the truth. I wake up each morning and I can't seem to think of anything to look forward to. I mope around the house all day, kind of in despair. I just can't seem to shake the blues, and I've begun to think I need to go see a shrink." (Participant 1)
>
> "I can't remember ever feeling better in my life. I just got promoted to a new job that makes me feel like I can really get ahead in my company. And I've just gotten engaged to a really great guy who is very special." (Participant 2)
>
> "I've had a few ups and downs the past week, but basically things are on a pretty even keel. I don't have too many complaints." (Participant 3)

Narrative information can be obtained by having conversations with participants, by making detailed notes about how people behave, or by obtaining narrative records, such as diaries. Suppose we were studying depression qualitatively. Box 3.2 presents qualitative data for three people responding conversationally to the question, "Tell me about how you've been feeling lately—have you felt sad or depressed at all, or have you generally been in good spirits?" The data consist of rich narrative descriptions of participant's emotional state.

Relationships

Researchers are rarely interested in isolated concepts, except in descriptive studies. For example, a researcher might describe the percentage of patients receiving intravenous (IV) therapy who experience IV infiltration. In this example, the variable is IV infiltration versus no infiltration. Usually, however, researchers study phenomena in relation to other phenomena—that is, they focus on relationships. A **relationship** is a bond or a connection between phenomena. For example, researchers repeatedly have found a *relationship* between cigarette smoking and lung cancer. Both qualitative and quantitative studies examine relationships, but in different ways.

In quantitative studies, researchers examine the relationship between the independent and dependent variables. Researchers ask whether variation in the dependent variable (the outcome) is systematically related to variation in the independent variable. Relationships are usually expressed in quantitative terms, such as *more than*, *less than*, and so on. For example, let us consider a person's weight as our dependent variable. What variables are related to (associated with) body weight? Some possibilities are height, caloric intake, and exercise. For each independent variable, we can make a prediction about its relationship to the outcome variable:

Height: Taller people will weigh more than shorter people.
Caloric intake: People with higher caloric intake will be heavier than those with lower caloric intake.
Exercise: The lower the amount of exercise, the greater the person's weight.

Each statement expresses a predicted relationship between weight (the dependent variable) and a measurable independent variable. Terms like *more than* and *heavier than* imply that as we observe a change in one variable, we are likely to observe a change in weight. If Alex is taller than Tom, we would predict (in the absence of other information) that Alex is heavier than Tom.

Quantitative studies can address one or more of the following questions about relationships:

- Does a relationship between variables *exist*? (e.g., Is cigarette smoking related to lung cancer?)
- What is the *direction* of the relationship between variables? (e.g., Are people who smoke *more* likely or *less* likely to develop lung cancer than those who do not?)
- How *strong* is the relationship between the variables? (e.g., How great is the risk that smokers will develop lung cancer?)
- What is the *nature* of the relationship between variables? (e.g., Does smoking *cause* lung cancer? Does some other factor *cause* both smoking and lung cancer?)

Variables can be related in different ways. One type of relationship is a **cause-and-effect** (or **causal**) **relationship**. Within the positivist paradigm, natural phenomena have antecedent causes that are presumably discoverable. In our example about a person's weight, we might speculate that there is a causal relationship between caloric intake and weight: we might predict that consuming more calories causes weight gain. Many quantitative studies are *cause-probing*—they seek to illuminate the causes of phenomena.

Example of a Study of Causal Relationships
Lee et al. (2021) evaluated the effect of California's safe patient handling legislation and changes in the experiences of musculoskeletal injury by hospital characteristics.

Not all relationships between variables can be interpreted as causal ones. There is a relationship, for example, between a person's pulmonary artery and tympanic temperatures: people with high readings on one tend to have high readings on the other. We cannot say, however, that pulmonary artery temperature *caused* tympanic temperature, nor vice versa. This type of relationship is a **functional** (or **associative**) **relationship** rather than a causal one.

Example of a Study of Associative Relationships
Khang et al. (2022) examined the symptomatic experiences of patients receiving immunotherapy for lung cancer to determine if symptoms reported during immunotherapy were associated with survival outcomes. They identified 47 symptoms in those receiving immunotherapy. The symptoms of musculoskeletal pain, shortness of breath, lack of appetite, and drowsiness were associated with mortality within 2 years.

Qualitative researchers are not concerned with quantifying relationships nor in testing causal relationships. Qualitative researchers seek patterns of association as a way to illuminate the underlying meaning and dimensionality of phenomena. Patterns of interconnected themes and processes are identified as a means of understanding the whole.

Example of a Qualitative Study of Patterns
You & Yang (2020) explored the patterns and the meaning of health in 21 married Korean immigrant women from various sociocultural circumstances. They identified three patterns: (1) the cultural clash phase: your world; (2) the cultural assimilation phase: our world; and (3) the cultural recreation phase: expanded my world.

MAJOR CLASSES OF QUANTITATIVE AND QUALITATIVE RESEARCH

Researchers usually work within a paradigm that is consistent with their world view and that gives rise to questions that excite their curiosity. The maturity of the focal concept also may lead to one or the other paradigm: when little is known about a phenomenon, a qualitative approach may be more fruitful than a quantitative one. In this section, we briefly describe broad categories of quantitative and qualitative research.

Quantitative Research: Experimental and Nonexperimental Studies

A basic distinction in quantitative studies is between experimental and nonexperimental research. In **experimental research**, researchers actively introduce an intervention or treatment—most often, to address Therapy questions. In **nonexperimental research**, researchers are bystanders—they collect data without intervening (most often, to address Etiology, Prognosis, or Description questions). For example, if a researcher gave bran flakes to one group of people and prune juice to another to evaluate which method facilitated elimination more effectively, the study would be experimental because the researcher intervened in the normal course of things. If, on the other hand, a researcher compared elimination patterns of two groups whose regular eating patterns differed, the study would be nonexperimental because there is no intervention. In medical research, an experimental study usually is called a **clinical trial** and a nonexperimental inquiry is called an **observational study**. A *randomized controlled trial* or RCT is a particular type of clinical trial.

> **TIP** On the evidence hierarchy shown in Figure 2.1, the two levels directly below systematic reviews (RCTs and quasiexperiments) involve interventions.

Experimental studies are explicitly cause-probing—they test whether an intervention *causes* changes in the dependent variable. Sometimes nonexperimental studies also explore causal relationships, but the resulting evidence is usually less conclusive. Experimental studies offer the possibility of greater control over confounding influences than nonexperimental studies, and so causal inferences are more plausible.

Example of Experimental Research
Tz-Han et al. (2022) studied the efficacy of a reminiscence music intervention on cognitive, depressive, and behavioral symptoms in older adults with dementia. They found that the experimental group who received the intervention experienced a significant reduction in depressive symptoms but did not experience a significant change in cognition or behavioral symptoms.

Example of Nonexperimental Research
Riman et al. (2023) found that operational failures were associated with decreased patient satisfaction scores, increased nurse-reported quality and safety issues, and poor nurse job outcomes, and that variation in the hospital work environments explained the relationship.

In this nonexperimental study to address an Etiology/Harm question, the researchers did not intervene in any way—they did not have control over nurse staffing. Their intent was to examine existing relationships rather than to test a potential solution to a problem.

Qualitative Research: Disciplinary Traditions

The majority of qualitative nursing studies can best be described as **qualitative descriptive research**. Many qualitative studies, however, are rooted in research traditions that originated in anthropology, sociology, and psychology. Three such traditions that are prominent in qualitative nursing research are briefly described here. Chapter 22 provides a fuller discussion of these traditions and the methods associated with them.

Grounded theory research, with roots in sociology, seeks to describe and understand the key social psychological processes that occur in social settings. Most grounded theory studies focus on a developing social experience—the social and psychological processes that characterize an event or episode. A major component of grounded theory is the discovery of not only the basic social psychological problem but also a *core variable* that is central in explaining what is going on in that social scene. Grounded theory researchers strive to generate explanations of phenomena that are grounded in reality. Grounded theory was developed in the 1960s by two sociologists, Glaser and Strauss (1967).

Example of a Grounded Theory Study
Vogel et al. (2021) conducted a grounded theory study in Sweden to explore patients' patterns of behavior over the period of becoming critically ill to recovery at home.

Phenomenology is concerned with the lived experiences of humans. Phenomenology is an approach to thinking about what life experiences of people are like and what they mean. The phenomenological researcher asks the questions: What is the *essence* of this phenomenon as experienced by these people? Or, what is the meaning of the phenomenon to those who experience it?

Example of a Phenomenologic Study
Nolan et al. (2022) conducted in-depth interviews with 15 young African American females to explore their experiences in their lives after surviving breast cancer.

Ethnography, the primary research tradition in anthropology, provides a framework for studying the patterns, lifeways, and experiences of a defined cultural group in a holistic manner. Ethnographers typically engage in extensive fieldwork, often participating in the life of the culture under study. Ethnographic research can be concerned with broadly defined cultures (e.g., Syrian refugee communities), but sometimes focuses on more narrowly defined cultures (e.g., the culture of an intensive care unit). Ethnographers strive to learn from members of a cultural group, to understand their world view, and to describe their customs and norms.

Example of an Ethnographic Study
Hirani and Wagner (2022) conducted an ethnographic study with 27 women who were refugees and mothering young children aged 2 years and under in Canada during COVID-19.

MAJOR STEPS IN A QUANTITATIVE STUDY

In quantitative studies, researchers move from the beginning of a study (posing a question) to the end point (obtaining an answer) in a reasonably linear sequence of steps that is broadly similar across studies. In some studies, the steps overlap; in others, some steps are unnecessary. Still, a general flow of activities is typical in a quantitative study (see Figure 3.1). This section describes that flow, and the next section explains how qualitative studies differ.

Phase 1: The Conceptual Phase

Early steps in a quantitative study typically have a strong conceptual element. Activities include reading, conceptualizing, theorizing, and reviewing ideas with colleagues or advisers. During this phase, researchers call on such skills as creativity, deductive reasoning, and a firm grounding in previous research on a topic of interest.

Step 1: Formulating and Delimiting the Problem

Quantitative researchers begin by identifying an interesting, significant research problem and formulating **research questions**. Good research requires starting with good questions. In developing research questions, nurse researchers must attend to substantive issues (What kind of new evidence is needed?); theoretical issues (Is there a conceptual context for understanding this problem?); clinical issues (How could evidence from this study be used in clinical practice?); methodologic issues (How can this question best be studied to yield high-quality evidence?); and ethical issues (Can this question be rigorously addressed in an ethical manner?).

TIP A critical ingredient in developing good research questions is personal interest. Begin with topics that fascinate you or about which you have a passionate interest.

Step 2: Reviewing the Related Literature

Quantitative research is conducted in a context of previous knowledge. Quantitative researchers typically strive to understand what is already known about a topic by undertaking a literature review. A thorough **literature review** provides a foundation on which to base new evidence and usually is conducted before data are collected. For clinical problems, it may also be necessary to learn the "status quo" of current procedures and to review existing practice guidelines.

Step 3: Undertaking Clinical Fieldwork

Unless the research problem originated in a clinical setting, researchers embarking on a clinical nursing study benefit from spending time in relevant clinical settings, discussing the problem with clinicians and administrators, and observing current practices. Clinical fieldwork can provide perspectives on recent clinical trends, diagnostic procedures, and relevant healthcare delivery models; it can also help researchers better understand clients and the settings in which care is provided. Such fieldwork can also be valuable in gaining access to an appropriate site or in developing research strategies. For example, during clinical fieldwork, researchers might discover the need for research staff who are bilingual.

Step 4: Defining the Framework and Developing Conceptual Definitions

Theory transcends the specifics of a particular time, place, and group and characterizes regularities in the relationships among variables. When

Phase 1: The conceptual phase
1. Formulating and delimiting the problem
2. Reviewing the related literature
3. Undertaking clinical fieldwork
4. Defining the framework/developing conceptual definitions
5. Formulating hypotheses

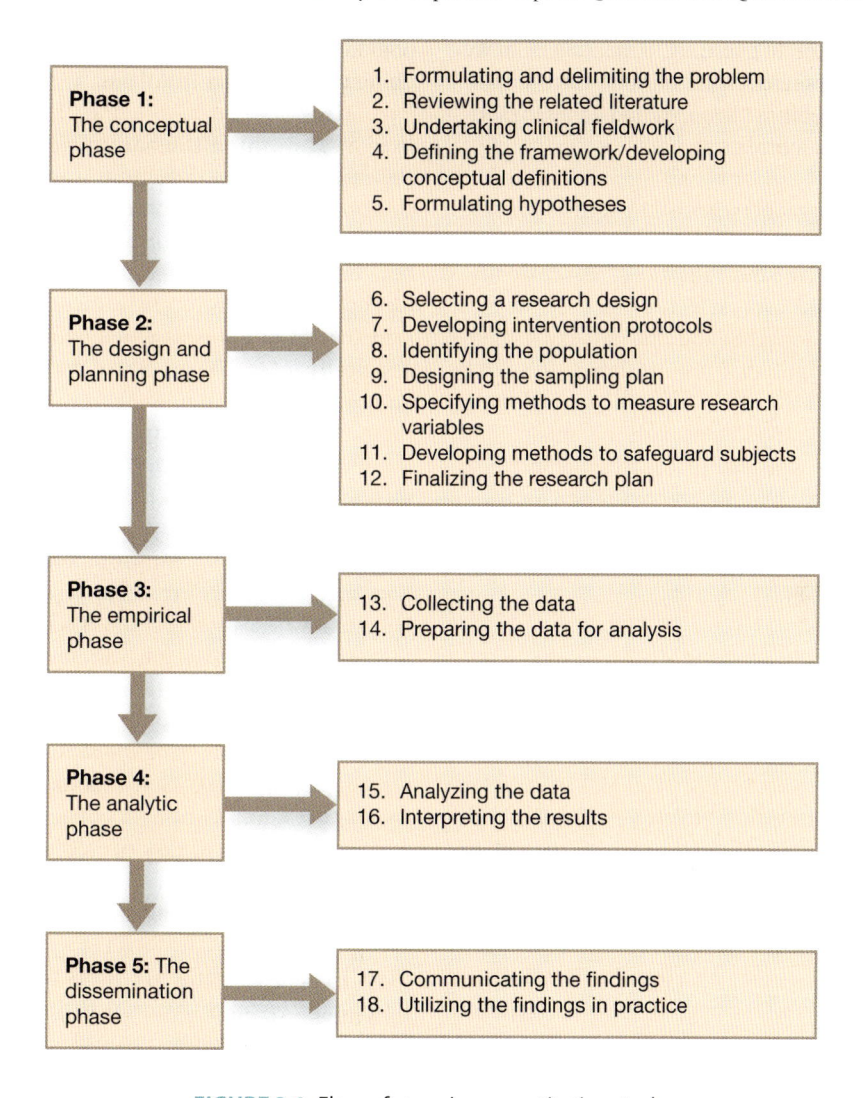

Phase 2: The design and planning phase
6. Selecting a research design
7. Developing intervention protocols
8. Identifying the population
9. Designing the sampling plan
10. Specifying methods to measure research variables
11. Developing methods to safeguard subjects
12. Finalizing the research plan

Phase 3: The empirical phase
13. Collecting the data
14. Preparing the data for analysis

Phase 4: The analytic phase
15. Analyzing the data
16. Interpreting the results

Phase 5: The dissemination phase
17. Communicating the findings
18. Utilizing the findings in practice

FIGURE 3.1 Flow of steps in a quantitative study.

quantitative research is performed within the context of a theoretical framework, the findings often have broader significance and utility. Even when the research question is not embedded in a theory, researchers should have a conceptual rationale and a clear vision of the concepts under study.

Step 5: Formulating Hypotheses

Hypotheses state researcher's predictions about relationships between study variables. The research question identifies the study concepts and asks how the concepts might be related; a hypothesis is the predicted answer. For example, the research question might be: Is preeclamptic toxemia related to stress during pregnancy? This might be translated into the following hypothesis: Females with high levels of stress during pregnancy will be more likely than females with lower stress to experience preeclamptic toxemia. Most quantitative studies involve testing hypotheses through statistical analysis.

Phase 2: The Design and Planning Phase

In the second major phase of a quantitative study, researchers decide on the methods they will use to address the research question. Researchers make many methodologic decisions, which have important implications for the integrity and generalizability of the resulting evidence.

Step 6: Selecting a Research Design
The **research design** is the plan for obtaining answers to the research questions. In designing the study, researchers select a specific design from the many experimental and nonexperimental research designs that are available. Research designs specify how often data will be collected, what types of comparisons will be made, and where the study will take place. Researchers also identify strategies to minimize biases and to maximize the *applicability* of their research to real-life settings. The research design is the architectural backbone of the study.

Step 7: Developing Protocols for the Intervention
In experimental research, researchers create an intervention (the independent variable) and need to articulate its features. For example, if we were interested in testing the effect of biofeedback on hypertension, the independent variable would be exposure to biofeedback compared with either an alternative treatment (e.g., relaxation) or no treatment. An **intervention protocol** for the study must be developed, specifying exactly what the biofeedback treatment would entail (e.g., what type of feedback, who would administer it, how frequently and over how long a period the treatment would last, and so on) *and* what the alternative condition would be. The goal of such protocols is to ensure that all people in each group are treated in the same way. (In nonexperimental research, this step is not necessary.)

Step 8: Identifying the Population
Quantitative researchers need to clarify the group to whom study results can be generalized—that is, they must identify the population to be studied. A **population** is *all* the individuals or objects with common, defining characteristics (the "P" component in PICO questions). For example, the population of interest might be all patients undergoing chemotherapy in Atlanta.

Step 9: Designing the Sampling Plan
Researchers collect data from a sample, which is a subset of the population. Using samples is more feasible than collecting data from an entire population, but the risk is that the sample might not reflect the population's traits. In a quantitative study, a sample's adequacy is assessed by its size and **representativeness**. The quality of the sample depends on how typical, or representative, the sample is of the population. The **sampling plan** specifies how the sample will be selected and recruited and how many subjects there will be.

Step 10: Specifying Methods to Measure Research Variables
Quantitative researchers must identify methods to measure their research variables. The primary methods of data collection are *self-reports* (e.g., interviews), *observations* (e.g., observing the sleep-wake state of infants), and *biophysiologic measurements (biomarkers)*. Self-reports from patients are the largest class of data collection methods in nursing research. The task of selecting measures of research variables and developing a **data collection plan** is complex and challenging.

Step 11: Developing Methods to Safeguard Human/Animal Rights
Most nursing research involves humans, and so procedures need to be developed to ensure that the study adheres to ethical principles. A formal review by an ethics committee is usually required.

Step 12: Reviewing and Finalizing the Research Plan
Before collecting their data, researchers often take steps to ensure that plans will work smoothly. For example, they may evaluate the *readability* of written materials to assess if participants with low reading skills can comprehend them, or they may *pretest* their measuring instruments to see if they work well. Normally, researchers also have their research plan critiqued by peers,

consultants, or other reviewers before implementing it. Researchers seeking financial support submit a **proposal** to a funding source, and reviewers usually suggest improvements.

> **TIP** For major studies, researchers often undertake a small-scale pilot study to test their research plans. Strategies for designing effective pilot studies are described in Chapter 29.

Phase 3: The Empirical Phase

The empirical phase of quantitative studies involves collecting data and preparing the data for analysis. Often, the empirical phase is the most time-consuming part of the investigation. Data collection typically requires months of work.

Step 13: Collecting the Data

The actual collection of data in quantitative studies often proceeds according to a preestablished plan. A *data collection protocol* typically spells out procedures for training data collection staff; for actually collecting data (e.g., the location and timing of gathering the data); and for recording information. Technologic advances have expanded possibilities for automating data collection.

Step 14: Preparing the Data for Analysis

Data collected in a quantitative study must be prepared for analysis. One preliminary step is *coding*, which involves translating verbal data into numeric form (e.g., coding gender as "1" for females, "2" for males, and "3" for other). Another step may involve transferring the data from written documents onto computer files for analysis.

Phase 4: The Analytic Phase

Quantitative data must be subjected to analysis and interpretation, which occur in the fourth major phase of a project.

Step 15: Analyzing the Data

Quantitative researchers analyze their data through **statistical analyses**, which include simple procedures (e.g., computing an average) as well as ones that are complex. Some analytic methods are computationally formidable, but the underlying logic of statistical tests is fairly easy to grasp. Computers have eliminated the need to get bogged down with mathematic operations.

Step 16: Interpreting the Results

Interpretation involves making sense of study results and examining their implications. Researchers attempt to explain the findings in light of prior evidence, theory, and their own clinical experience—and in light of the adequacy of the methods they used in the study. Interpretation also involves drawing conclusions about the *clinical significance* of the results, envisioning how the new evidence can be used in nursing practice, and suggesting what further research is needed.

Phase 5: The Dissemination Phase

In the analytic phase, the researcher comes full circle: questions posed at the outset are answered. Researchers' responsibilities are not completed, however, until study results are disseminated.

Step 17: Communicating the Findings

A study can only contribute evidence to nursing practice if the results are shared. Another—and often final—task of a study is the preparation of a **research report** that summarizes the study. Research reports can take various forms: dissertations, journal articles, conference presentations, and so on. Journal articles—reports appearing in professional journals such as *Nursing Research*—usually are the most useful because they are available to a broad, international audience. We discuss journal articles later in this chapter.

Step 18: Utilizing the Findings in Practice

Ideally, the concluding step of a high-quality study is to plan for the use of the evidence in practice settings. Although nurse researchers may not themselves be able to implement a plan for using research findings, they can contribute to the process by making recommendations for utilizing the evidence, by ensuring that adequate information has been provided for a systematic review, and by pursuing opportunities to disseminate the findings to clinicians.

ACTIVITIES IN A QUALITATIVE STUDY

Quantitative research involves a fairly linear progression of tasks—researchers plan the steps to be taken to maximize study integrity and then follow those steps as faithfully as possible. In qualitative studies, by contrast, the progression is closer to a circle than to a straight line—qualitative researchers continually examine and interpret data and make decisions about how to proceed based on what has already been discovered (Figure 3.2).

Because qualitative researchers have a flexible approach, we cannot show the flow of activities precisely—the flow varies from one study to another, and researchers themselves do not know exactly how the study will unfold. We provide a sense of how qualitative studies are conducted, however, by describing major activities and indicating when they might be performed.

Conceptualizing and Planning a Qualitative Study

Identifying the Research Problem

Qualitative researchers usually begin with a broad topic area, focusing on an aspect of a topic that is poorly understood and about which little is known. Qualitative researchers often proceed with a fairly broad initial question, which may be narrowed and clarified on the basis of self-reflection and discussion with others. The specific focus and questions are usually delineated more clearly once the study is underway.

Doing a Literature Review

Qualitative researchers do not all agree about the value of doing an upfront literature review. Some believe that researchers should not consult the

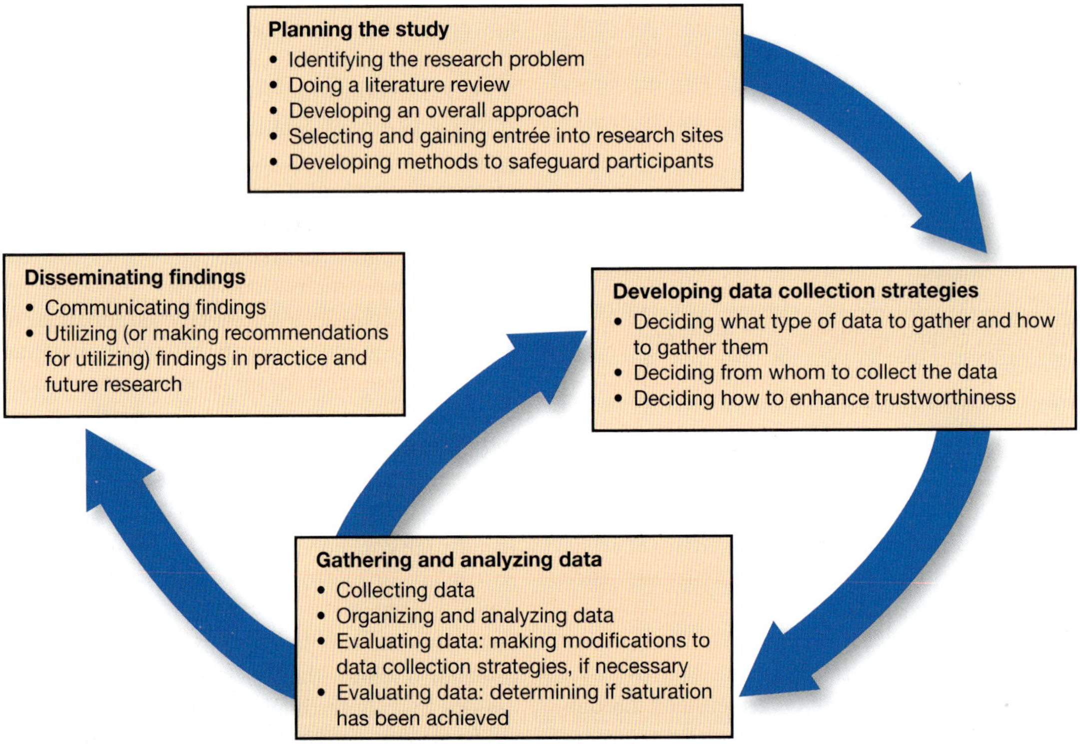

Planning the study
- Identifying the research problem
- Doing a literature review
- Developing an overall approach
- Selecting and gaining entrée into research sites
- Developing methods to safeguard participants

Disseminating findings
- Communicating findings
- Utilizing (or making recommendations for utilizing) findings in practice and future research

Developing data collection strategies
- Deciding what type of data to gather and how to gather them
- Deciding from whom to collect the data
- Deciding how to enhance trustworthiness

Gathering and analyzing data
- Collecting data
- Organizing and analyzing data
- Evaluating data: making modifications to data collection strategies, if necessary
- Evaluating data: determining if saturation has been achieved

FIGURE 3.2 Flow of activities in a qualitative study.

literature before collecting data because prior studies could influence conceptualization of the focal phenomenon. In this view, the phenomena should be explicated based on participants' viewpoints rather than on prior knowledge. Those sharing this opinion often do a literature review at the end of the study. Other researchers conduct a brief preliminary review to get a general grounding. Still others believe that a full early literature review is appropriate. In any case, qualitative researchers typically find a small body of relevant previous work because of the types of question they ask.

Selecting and Gaining Entrée Into Research Sites

Before going into the field, qualitative researchers must identify an appropriate site. For example, if the topic is the health beliefs of the urban population living below the poverty threshold, an inner-city neighborhood with low-income residents must be identified. Researchers may need to engage in anticipatory fieldwork to identify a suitable and information-rich environment for the study. In some cases, researchers have ready access to the study site, but in others, they need to **gain entrée**. A site may be well suited to the needs of the research, but if researchers cannot "get in," the study cannot proceed. Gaining entrée typically involves negotiations with **gatekeepers** who have the authority to permit entry into their world.

> **TIP** The process of gaining entrée is usually associated with doing fieldwork in qualitative studies, but quantitative researchers often need to gain entrée into sites for collecting data as well.

Developing an Overall Approach in Qualitative Studies

Quantitative researchers do not collect data until they have finalized their research design. Qualitative researchers, by contrast, use an **emergent design** that materializes during the course of data collection. Certain design features may be guided by the qualitative research tradition within which the researcher is working, but few qualitative studies follow rigidly structured designs that prohibit changes while in the field. Although qualitative researchers do not always know in advance exactly how the study will progress, they nevertheless must have some sense of how much time is available for fieldwork and must also arrange for and test needed equipment, such as laptop computers or cameras.

Addressing Ethical Issues

Qualitative researchers, like quantitative researchers, must also develop plans for addressing ethical issues—and, indeed, there are special concerns in qualitative studies because of the more intimate nature of the relationship that typically develops between researchers and study participants. Chapter 7 describes these concerns.

Conducting a Qualitative Study

In qualitative studies, the tasks of sampling, data collection, data analysis, and interpretation typically take place iteratively. Qualitative researchers begin by talking with or observing a few people who have first-hand experience with the phenomenon under study. The discussions and observations are loosely structured, allowing for the expression of a full range of beliefs, feelings, and behaviors. Analysis and interpretation are ongoing, concurrent activities that guide choices about the kinds of people to sample next and the types of questions to ask or observations to make.

The process of data analysis involves clustering together related types of narrative information into a coherent scheme. As analysis and interpretation progress, researchers begin to identify **themes** and categories (or stages in a process), which are used to build a rich description or theory of the phenomenon. The kinds of data obtained and the people selected as participants tend to become increasingly purposeful as the conceptualization is developed and refined. Concept development shapes the sampling process—as a conceptualization or theory emerges, the researcher seeks participants who can confirm and enrich the theoretical understandings, as well as participants who can potentially challenge them and lead to further theoretical development.

Quantitative researchers decide upfront how many people to include in a study, but qualitative researchers' sampling decisions are guided by the data. Qualitative researchers use the principle of **data saturation**, which occurs when themes and categories in the data become repetitive and redundant, such that no new information can be gleaned by further data collection.

Quantitative researchers seek to collect high-quality data by measuring their variables with methods that have been found to be reliable and valid. Qualitative researchers, by contrast, are the main data collection instrument and must take steps to demonstrate the *trustworthiness* of the data. The central feature of these efforts is to confirm that the findings accurately reflect the experiences and viewpoints of participants rather than the researcher's perceptions. One confirmatory activity, for example, involves going back to participants and sharing interpretations with them so that they can evaluate whether the researcher's thematic analysis is consistent with their experiences.

Disseminating Qualitative Findings

Qualitative nurse researchers also share their findings with others at conferences and in journal articles. Regardless of researchers' positions about *when* a literature review should be conducted, a summary of prior research is usually offered in qualitative reports as a means of providing context for the study.

Quantitative reports almost never contain **raw data**—that is, data in the form they were collected, which are numeric values. Qualitative reports, by contrast, are usually filled with rich verbatim passages directly from participants. The excerpts are used in an evidentiary fashion to support or illustrate researchers' interpretations and thematic construction.

> **Example of Raw Data in a Qualitative Report**
> Ryan et al. (2022) did an in-depth study of nurses' caring for older patients who are dying from traumatic injuries in the emergency department. Here is an illustrative quote: "Do you go further down the path and expose the patient to unnecessary insult to have the same outcome, or do you give them dignified pain relief and just let them pass?" (pp. 565–566)

Like quantitative researchers, qualitative nurse researchers want their findings used by others. Qualitative findings sometimes are the basis for formulating hypotheses that are tested by quantitative researchers, for developing measuring instruments for both research and clinical purposes, and for designing effective nursing interventions. Qualitative studies help to shape nurses' perceptions of a problem or situation, their conceptualizations of potential solutions, and their understanding of patients' concerns and experiences.

RESEARCH JOURNAL ARTICLES

Research **journal articles**, which summarize the background, design, and results of a study, are the primary method of disseminating research evidence. This section reviews the content and style of research journal articles to ensure that you will be equipped to delve into the research literature. A more detailed discussion of the structure of journal articles is presented in Chapter 32, which provides guidance on writing research reports.

Content of Journal Articles

Many quantitative and qualitative journal articles follow a conventional organization called the **IMRAD format**. This format involves organizing material into four main sections—**I**ntroduction, **M**ethods, **R**esults, **a**nd **D**iscussion. The text of the report is usually preceded by an abstract and followed by cited references.

The Abstract

The **abstract** is a brief description of the study placed at the beginning of the article. The abstract answers, in about 250 words, the following: What were the research questions? What methods did the researcher use to address the questions? What did the researcher find? What are the implications? Readers review abstracts to assess whether the entire report is of interest. Some journals have moved from traditional abstracts—single paragraphs summarizing the study's main features—to longer, structured abstracts with specific headings. For example, in the journal *Nursing Research*, abstracts are organized under the following headings: Background, Objectives, Method, Results, and Discussion.

The Introduction
The introduction communicates the research problem and its context. The introduction, which often is not specifically labeled as "Introduction," follows immediately after the abstract. This section typically describes the following: (1) the central phenomena, concepts, or variables under study; (2) the population of interest; (3) the current state of evidence, based on a brief literature review; (4) the theoretical framework; (5) the study purpose, research questions, or hypotheses to be tested; and (6) the study's significance. Thus, the introduction sets the stage for a description of what the researcher did and what was learned. The introduction corresponds roughly to the conceptual phase of a study.

The Method Section
The method section describes the methods used to answer the research questions. This section lays out methodologic decisions made in the design and planning phase and may offer rationales for those decisions. In a quantitative study, the method section usually describes the following: (1) the research design; (2) the sampling plan for selecting participants from the population of interest; (3) methods of data collection and specific instruments used; (4) study procedures (including ethical safeguards); and (5) analytic procedures and methods.

Qualitative researchers discuss many of the same issues, but with different emphases. For example, a qualitative study often provides more information about the research setting and the study context, and less information on sampling. Also, because formal instruments are not used to collect qualitative data, there is less discussion about data collection methods. Reports of qualitative studies may also include descriptions of the researchers' efforts to enhance the trustworthiness of the study.

The Results Section
The results section presents the **findings** from the data analyses. The text summarizes key findings, and (in quantitative reports) tables provide greater detail. Virtually all results sections contain a description of the participants (e.g., their average age, percentage male/female).

In quantitative studies, the results section provides information about the **statistical tests** used to test hypotheses and to evaluate the believability of the findings. For example, if the percentage of smokers who smoke two packs or more daily is computed to be 40%, how *probable* is it that the percentage is accurate? If the researcher finds that the average number of cigarettes smoked weekly is lower for those in an intervention group than for those not getting the intervention, how *probable* is it that the intervention effect is *real*? Statistical tests help to answer such questions. Researchers typically report the following:

- *The names of statistical tests used.* Different tests are appropriate for different situations but are based on common principles. You do not have to know the names of all statistical tests—there are dozens of them—to comprehend the findings.
- *The value of the calculated statistic.* Computers are used to calculate a numeric value for the statistical test used. The value allows researchers to draw conclusions about the results. The *actual* numeric value of the statistic, however, is not inherently meaningful and need not concern you.
- *The statistical significance.* A critical piece of information is whether the value of the statistic was significant (not to be confused with important or clinically relevant). When researchers say that results are **statistically significant**, it means the findings are probably reliable and replicable with a new sample. Research reports indicate the **level of significance**, which is an index of how probable it is that the findings are reliable. For example, if a report says that a finding was significant at the 0.05 level, this means that only five times out of 100 (5 ÷ 100 = 0.05) would the result be spurious. In other words, 95 times out of 100, similar results would be obtained with a new sample. Readers can have a high degree of confidence—but not total assurance—that the result is reliable.

> **Example From the Results Section of a Quantitative Study**
>
> Jones et al. (2023) examined the pain experience in relation to unique cancer-specific psychosocial factors in 41 cancer survivors after they completed cancer treatment. Using linear regression models and likelihood ratio testing, the team tested the individual and collective contribution of cancer-specific psychosocial factors on the experience of pain. Findings suggest that pain catastrophizing and multisite pain explained a significant degree of variance in pain interference scores ($P < .001$) and pain severity ($P = .005$). However, psychosocial factors specific to cancer did not predict variability in pain interference ($P = .313$) or pain severity ($P = .668$) beyond pain catastrophizing and the number of sites of pain.

Results sections of qualitative reports often have several subsections, the headings of which correspond to the themes, processes, or categories identified in the data. Excerpts from the raw data are presented to support and provide a rich description of the thematic analysis. The results section of qualitative studies may also present the researcher's emerging theory about the phenomenon under study.

The Discussion Section

In the discussion section, researchers draw conclusions about what the results mean, and how the evidence can be used in practice. The discussion in both qualitative and quantitative reports may include the following elements: (1) the degree to which results are consistent with previous research; (2) an interpretation of the results and their clinical significance; (3) implications for clinical practice and for future and research; and (4) study limitations and ramifications for the integrity of the results. Researchers are in the best position to point out sample deficiencies, design problems, weaknesses in data collection, and so forth. A discussion section that presents these limitations demonstrates to readers that the author was aware of these limitations and probably took them into account in interpreting the findings.

The Style of Research Journal Articles

Research reports tell a story. However, the style in which many research journal articles are written—especially reports of quantitative studies—makes it difficult for many readers to figure out the story or become intrigued by it. To unaccustomed audiences, research reports may seem stuffy, pedantic, and overwhelming. Four factors contribute to this impression:

- *Compactness.* Journal space is limited, so authors compress a lot of information into a short space. Interesting, personalized aspects of the study are not reported. Even in qualitative studies, only a handful of supporting quotes can be included.
- *Jargon.* The authors of research reports use terms that may seem esoteric.
- *Objectivity.* Quantitative researchers tell their stories objectively, in a way that may make them sound impersonal. For example, most quantitative reports are written in the passive voice (i.e., personal pronouns are avoided), which tends to make a report less lively than use of the active voice. Qualitative reports, by contrast, are more personal and written in a more conversational style.
- *Statistical information.* Quantitative reports summarize the results of statistical analyses. Numbers and statistical symbols can intimidate readers who do not have statistical training.

In this textbook we try to assist you in dealing with these issues and strive to encourage you to tell *your* research stories in a manner that makes them accessible to practicing nurses.

Tips on Reading Research Reports

As you progress through this book, you will acquire skills for evaluating research reports critically. Some preliminary hints on digesting research reports follow.

- Grow accustomed to the style of research articles by reading them frequently, even though you may not yet understand all the technical points.
- Read from an article that has been downloaded and printed so that you can highlight portions and write marginal notes (or use software that allows you to do this in PDF files).

- Read articles slowly. Skim the article first to get major points and then read it more carefully a second time.
- On the second reading of a journal article, train yourself to be an *active* reader. Reading actively means that you constantly monitor yourself to assess your understanding of what you are reading. If you have problems, go back and reread difficult passages or make notes so that you can ask someone for clarification. In most cases, that "someone" will be your research instructor, but also consider contacting researchers themselves via email.
- Some people find it helpful to use a structured reading method when reading research reports. One such method is called the SQ3R Reading Technique, which involves five steps: *Survey, Question, Read, Recite, and Review.*
- Keep this textbook with you as a reference while you are reading articles so that you can look up unfamiliar terms in the glossary or index.
- Try not to get "turned off" by statistical information. Try to grasp the gist of the story without letting numbers frustrate you.
- Until you become accustomed to research journal articles, you may want to "translate" them by expanding compact paragraphs into looser constructions, by translating jargon into familiar terms, by recasting the report into an active voice, and by summarizing findings with words rather than numbers.

GENERAL QUESTIONS IN REVIEWING A RESEARCH STUDY

Most chapters of this book contain guidelines to help you evaluate different aspects of a research report critically, focusing primarily on the researchers' methodologic decisions. Box 3.3 presents some further suggestions for performing a preliminary overview of a research report, drawing on concepts explained in this chapter. These guidelines supplement those presented in Box 1.1, Chapter 1.

RESEARCH EXAMPLES

In this section, we illustrate the progression of activities and discuss the time schedule of two studies (one quantitative and the other qualitative) conducted by the author of this book.

Project Schedule for a Quantitative Study

Study: One of the authors of this textbook conducted a study: A predictive model of intrinsic factors associated with long-stay nursing home care after hospitalization (Flanagan et al., 2021).

Study purpose: Flanagan and colleagues aimed to build a predictive model with intrinsic factors measured upon admission to skilled nursing facilities (SNFs) postacute care to identify older adults transferred from SNFs to long-term care (LTC) instead of home.

BOX 3.3 Additional Questions for a Preliminary Review of a Research Report

1. What is the study all about? What are the main phenomena, concepts, or constructs under investigation?
2. If the study is quantitative, what are the independent and dependent variables? What are the PICO elements—and for what type of question (Therapy, Prognosis, etc.)?
3. Do the researchers examine relationships or patterns of association among variables or concepts? Does the report imply the possibility of a causal relationship?
4. Are key concepts clearly defined, both conceptually and operationally?
5. What type of study does it appear to be, in terms of types described in this chapter: Quantitative—experimental? nonexperimental? Qualitative—descriptive? grounded theory? phenomenological? ethnographic?
6. Does the report provide any information to suggest how long the study took to complete?
7. Does the format of the report conform to the traditional IMRAD format? If not, in what ways does it differ?

Study methods: This study required a little more than 3 years to complete. Key activities and methodologic decisions included the following:

Phase 1. Conceptual Phase: 6 Months. The team obtained Medicare Provider Analysis and Review data and Resident Assessment Instrument Minimum Data Set 3.0. This was acquired through a Data Use Agreement with the Research Data Assistance Center, which provides Medicare, Medicaid, and Medicare Current Beneficiary Survey data for research. This first phase of obtaining the IRB approval, the data, and safely securing it through HIPPA-protected systems was an involved process that took several months.

Phase 2. Design and Planning Phase: 5 Months. Although the research questions had been formalized during the grant process, the team met several times to discuss the overall aim of the study and to identify which of the hundreds of variables we would focus on to answer our question about developing a predictive model.

Phase 3. Empirical Phase: 0 Months. In this study, the data from 23,662 community-dwelling persons admitted to skilled nursing facilities (SNFs) had already been collected.

Phase 4. Analytic Phase: 12 months. Several statistical analyses were performed. (1) A logistic regression applied to evaluate LTC admission vs. other discharge status, e.g., death considering variables such as dementia, severity of cognitive impairment, gender, race, marital status, diagnoses, vision loss, hearing loss, delirium, depressive symptoms, and pain frequency and severity. (2) The Hosmer-Lemeshow Goodness of Fit test was also performed to assess how well the final model fit the data. (3) To evaluate the predictive accuracy of the final logistic regression model, we generated the receiver operating characteristic (ROC) curve and the AUROC (area under the ROC curve) for the logistic regression model. (4) To assess overfitting, we evaluated the predictive logistic regression using cross-validation ROC Curve and its AUROC. (5) Descriptive statistics were used to describe the sample.

Phase 5. Dissemination Phase: 11 Months. The team submitted a paper to the *Journal of Clinical Nursing*. After peer review and revisions, it was accepted in December of 2020 and published in June 2021.

Project Schedule for a Qualitative Study

Study: Effects of fourth-degree perineal lacerations on women's physical and mental health (Beck, 2021).

Study Purpose: The purpose of this study was to describe the physical and emotional effects of fourth degree perineal lacerations that occurred during childbirth on mothers' daily lives.

Study Methods: This study required a little more than 1 and a half years to complete. Key activities and methodologic decisions included the following:

Phase 1. Conceptual phase: 2 months. This was Beck's first study on fourth degree perineal tears, so she needed time to review relevant studies.

Phase 2. Design and planning phase: 3 months. Beck, one of the authors of this nursing research textbook, chose a phenomenologic design for this study. She had conducted a number of phenomenologic studies so designing this new study did not require a lengthy time period. Once her proposal was finalized, it was submitted to the university's committee on ethics for approval.

Phase 3. Empirical/analytic phrases: 7 months. A recruitment notice was placed on the Facebook support group Mothers with Fourth Degree Tears. Eighteen mothers sent narratives about the impact their fourth-degree perineal tears from a traumatic birth had on their daily lives to Beck's university email address. It took 5 months to recruit the sample. Analysis of the mothers' stories took an additional 2 months. Seven themes emerged from the data analysis: (1) Why wasn't I informed I had this injury? (2) The unthinkable: fecal incontinence and so much more; (3) It has cost me so much; (4) Seeking relief: enduring surgery after surgery; (5) Why didn't anyone ask me about my mental health? (6) To have more children, that is the question; and (7) Are there any positives in all of this?

Phase 4. Dissemination phase: 9 months. It took approximately 2 months to prepare the manuscript reporting this study. It was submitted to the *Journal of Obstetric, Gynecologic, and Neonatal Nursing* (JOGNN) on July 27, 2020. This journal had a rapid response, and 2 months later Beck received a "revise and resubmit" decision from the journal. After Beck submitted her revised manuscript, 1 month later she received notification that her manuscript had been accepted for publication. The article was first published online 2 months later in January 2021 and then it was published in the March 2021 issue of JOGNN.

SUMMARY POINTS

- The people who provide information to the **researchers** (*investigators*) in a study are called **subjects** or **study participants** (in quantitative research) or study participants or **informants** in qualitative research; collectively the participants comprise the **sample.**
- The *site* is the overall location for the research; researchers sometimes engage in **multisite studies.** *Settings* are the types of places where data collection occurs. Settings can range from totally naturalistic environments to formal research locations.
- Researchers investigate **concepts** (or **constructs**) and **phenomena**, which are abstractions or mental representations inferred from behavior or characteristics.
- Concepts are the building blocks of **theories**, which are systematic explanations of some aspect of the real world.
- In quantitative studies, concepts are called variables. A **variable** is an attribute that takes on different values (i.e., that varies from one person to another). Groups that vary with respect to an attribute are **heterogeneous**; groups with limited variability are **homogeneous.**
- The **dependent** (or **outcome**) **variable** is the behavior or characteristic the researcher is interested in explaining, predicting, or affecting (the "O" in the PICO scheme). The **independent variable** is the presumed cause of, antecedent to, or influence on the dependent variable. The independent variable corresponds to the "I" and the "C" components in the PICO scheme.
- A **conceptual definition** describes the abstract or theoretical meaning of a concept being studied. An **operational definition** specifies how the variable will be measured.
- **Data**—information collected during a study—may take the form of narrative information (**qualitative data**) or numeric values (**quantitative data**).
- A **relationship** is a bond or connection between two variables. Quantitative researchers examine the relationship between the independent variable and dependent variable.
- When the independent variable is a cause of the dependent variable, the relationship is a **cause-and-effect** (or **causal**) **relationship.** In an **associative** (*functional*) **relationship**, variables are related, but in a noncausal way.
- A key distinction in quantitative studies is between **experimental research**, in which researchers introduce an intervention, and **nonexperimental** (or **observational**) **research**, in which researchers observe existing phenomena without intervening.
- Qualitative research sometimes is rooted in research traditions that originate in other disciplines. Three such traditions are grounded theory, phenomenology, and ethnography.
- **Grounded theory** seeks to describe and understand key social psychological processes that occur in social settings.
- **Phenomenology** focuses on the lived experiences of humans and is an approach to learning what the life experiences of people are like and what they mean.
- **Ethnography** provides a framework for studying the meanings, patterns, and lifeways of a culture in a holistic fashion.
- Quantitative researchers usually progress in a fairly linear fashion from asking research questions to answering them. The main phases in a quantitative study are the conceptual, planning, empirical, analytic, and dissemination phases.
- The *conceptual phase* involves (1) defining the problem to be studied; (2) doing a **literature review;** (3) engaging in **clinical fieldwork** for clinical studies; (4) developing a framework and conceptual definitions; and (5) formulating **hypotheses** to be tested.
- The *planning phase* entails (6) selecting a **research design**; (7) developing **intervention protocols** if the study is experimental; (8) specifying the **population**; (9) developing

- a **sampling plan**; (10) specifying methods to measure research variables; (11) developing strategies to safeguard the rights of participants; and (12) finalizing the research plan (e.g., *pretesting* instruments).
- The *empirical phase* involves (13) collecting data and (14) preparing data for analysis.
- The *analytic phase* involves (15) analyzing data through **statistical analysis** and (16) interpreting the results.
- The *dissemination phase* entails (17) communicating the findings in a **research report** and (18) promoting the use of the study evidence in nursing practice.
- The flow of activities in a qualitative study is more flexible and less linear. Qualitative studies typically involve an **emergent design** that evolves during data collection.
- Qualitative researchers begin with a broad question regarding a phenomenon, often focusing on a little-studied aspect. In the early phase of a qualitative study, researchers select a site and seek to **gain entrée** into it, which typically involves enlisting the cooperation of **gatekeepers.**
- Once in the field, qualitative researchers select informants, collect data, and then analyze and interpret them in an iterative fashion. Knowledge gained during data collection helps to shape the design of the study and the selection of participants.
- Early analysis in qualitative research leads to refinements in sampling and data collection, until **data saturation** (redundancy of information) is achieved.
- Both qualitative and quantitative researchers disseminate their findings, often in **journal articles** that concisely communicate what the researchers did and what they found.
- Journal articles typically consist of an **abstract** (a brief synopsis) and four major sections in an **IMRAD format**: an **I**ntroduction (explanation of the study problem and its context); **M**ethod section (the strategies used to address the problem); **R**esults section (study findings); **a**nd **D**iscussion (interpretation of the findings).
- Research reports can be difficult to read because they are dense and contain a lot of jargon. Quantitative research reports may be intimidating at first because, compared with qualitative reports, they are more impersonal and include statistical information.
- **Statistical tests** are procedures for testing research hypotheses and evaluating the believability of the findings. Findings that are **statistically significant** are ones that have a high probability of being "real."

REFERENCES CITED IN CHAPTER 3

Beck, C. T. (2021). Effects of fourth-degree perineal lacerations on women's physical and mental health. *Journal of Obstetric, Gynecologic, & Neonatal Nursing, 50*(2), 133–142. https://doi.org/10.1016/j.jogn.2020.10.009

Flanagan, J., Boltz, M., & Ji, M. (2021). A predictive model of intrinsic factors associated with long-stay nursing home care after hospitalization. *Clinical Nursing Research, 30*(5), 654–661. https://doi.org/10.1177/1054773820985276

Glaser, B. G., & Strauss, A. L. (1967). *The discovery of grounded theory: Strategies for qualitative research.* Aldine.

Hirani, S. A. A., & Wagner, J. (2022). Impact of COVID-19 on women who are refugees and mothering: A critical ethnographic study. *Global Qualitative Nursing Research, 9*, 23333936221121335. https://doi.org/10.1177/23333936221121335

Jones, K. F., Wood Magee, L., Fu, M. R., Bernacki, R., Bulls, H., Merlin, J., & McTernan, M. (2023). The contribution of cancer-specific psychosocial factors to the pain experience in cancer survivors. *Journal of Hospice & Palliative Nursing, 25*(5), E85–E93. https://doi.org/10.1097/NJH.0000000000000965

Khang, J., Wang, S., Zhou, Z., Lei, C., Yu, H., Zeng, C., Xia, X., Qiao, G., & Shi, Q. (2022). Unpleasant symptoms of immunotherapy for people with lung cancer: A mixed-method study. *International Journal of Nursing Studies, 139*, 104430.

Lee, S. J., Kang, K. J., & Lee, J. H. (2021). Safe patient handling legislation and changes in programs, practices, perceptions, and experience of musculoskeletal disorders by hospital characteristics: A repeated cross-sectional survey study. *International Journal of Nursing Studies, 113*, 103791. https://doi.org/10.1016/j.ijnurstu.2020.103791

Lynch, J., Rolls, K., Hou, Y. C., Hedges, S., Al Sayfe, M., Shunker, S. A., Brennan, K., Sanchez, D., Bogdanovski, T., Hunt, L., Alexandrou, E., & Frost, S. A. (2020). Delirium in intensive care: A stepped-wedge cluster randomised controlled trial for a nurse-led intervention to reduce the incidence and duration of delirium among adults admitted to the intensive care unit (protocol). *Australian Critical Care, 33*(5), 475–479. https://doi.org/10.1016/j.aucc.2019.12.003

Morse, J. M., Solberg, S. M., Neander, W. L., Bottorff, J. L., & Johnson, J. L. (1990). Concepts of caring and caring as a concept. *Advances in Nursing Science, 13*, 1–14.

Nolan, T. S., Ivankova, N., Carson, T. L., Spaulding, A. M., Dunovan, S., Davies, S., Enah, C., & Meneses, K. (2022). Life after breast cancer: Being a young African American survivor. *Ethnicity & Health, 27*(2), 247–274. https://doi.org/10.1080/13557858.2019.1682524

Riman, K. A., Harrison, J. M., Sloane, D. M., & McHugh, M. D. (2023). Work environment and operational failures associated with nurse outcomes, patient safety, and patient satisfaction. *Nursing Research, 72*(1), 20–29. https://doi.org/10.1097/NNR.0000000000000626

Ryan, K., Windsor, C., & Jack, L. (2022). The phenomenon of caring for older patients who are dying from traumatic injuries in the emergency department: An interpretive phenomenological study. *Journal of Nursing Scholarship, 54*(5), 562–568. https://doi.org/10.1111/jnu.12764

Smith, M. C. (2019). Regenerating nursing's disciplinary perspective. *ANS Advances in Nursing Science, 42*(1), 3–16. https://doi.org/10.1097/ANS.0000000000000241

Tz-Han, L., Wan-Ru, W., I-Hui, C., & Hui-Chuan, H. (2023). Reminiscence music intervention on cognitive, depressive, and behavioral symptoms in older adults with dementia. *Geriatric Nursing, 49*, 127–132. Advance online publication. https://doi.org/10.1016/j.gerinurse.2022.11.014

Vogel, G., Joelsson-Alm, E., Forinder, U., Svensen, C., & Sandgren, A. (2021) Stabilizing life: A grounded theory of surviving critical illness. *Intensive and Critical Care Nursing, 67*: 103096.https://doi.org/10.1016/j.iccn.2021.103096

You, K. S., & Yang, J. (2020). Health as expanding consciousness: Survival trajectory of married immigrant women in Korea. *Applied Nursing Research, 51*, 151230. https://doi.org/10.1016/j.apnr.2019.151230

Zhai, Y., Cai, S., Chen, X., Zhao, W., Yu, J., & Zhang, Y. (2023). The relationships between organizational culture and thriving at work among nurses: The mediating role of affective commitment and work engagement. *Journal of Advanced Nursing, 79*(1), 194–204. https://doi.org/10.1111/jan.15443

Part 2

CONCEPTUALIZING AND PLANNING A STUDY TO GENERATE EVIDENCE FOR NURSING

Chapter 4   Research Problems, Research Questions, and Hypotheses
Chapter 5   Literature Reviews: Finding and Critically Appraising Evidence
Chapter 6   Theoretical Frameworks
Chapter 7   Ethics in Nursing Research
Chapter 8   Planning a Nursing Study

4 Research Problems, Research Questions, and Hypotheses

Learning Objectives

1. Provide examples of the sources of research problems.
2. Describe the steps in the research process.
3. Identify issues related to the feasibility of a study design.
4. Articulate the difference between the purpose statement in a quantitative study as compared to a qualitative study.

OVERVIEW OF RESEARCH PROBLEMS

Studies begin, much like evidence-based practice (EBP) efforts, with a problem that needs to be solved or a question that needs to be answered. This chapter discusses the development of research problems. We begin by clarifying some relevant terms.

Basic Terminology

At a general level, a researcher selects a *topic* or a *phenomenon* on which to focus. Examples of research topics are claustrophobia during MRI tests, pain management for sickle cell disease, and nutrition during pregnancy. Within broad topic areas are many potential research problems. In this section, we illustrate various terms using the topic *side effects of chemotherapy*.

A **research problem** is an enigmatic or troubling condition. Researchers identify a research problem within a broad topic of interest. The purpose of research is to "solve" the problem—or to contribute to its solution—by generating relevant, high-quality evidence. Researchers articulate the problem in a **problem statement** that also presents a rationale for the study.

Many reports include a **statement of purpose** (or purpose statement), which summarizes the goal of the study. **Research questions** are the specific queries researchers want to answer in addressing the problem. Research questions guide the types of data to collect in a study. Researchers who make predictions about answers to research questions pose **hypotheses** that are tested in the study.

These terms are not always consistently defined in research methods textbooks, and differences among them are often subtle. Table 4.1 illustrates the terms as we define them.

Research Problems and Paradigms

Some research problems are better suited to qualitative vs. quantitative methods. Quantitative studies usually focus on concepts that are fairly well developed, about which there is existing evidence, and for which reliable methods of measurement have been (or can be) developed. For example, a quantitative study might be undertaken to explore whether older people with chronic illness who continue working are less (or more) depressed than those who retire. There are relatively good measures of depression

65

TABLE 4.1 • Example of Terms Relating to Research Problems

TERM	EXAMPLE
Topic/focus	Side effects of chemotherapy
Research problem (simple problem statement)	Nausea and vomiting are common side effects among patients on chemotherapy, and interventions to date have been only moderately successful in reducing these effects. One issue concerns the efficacy of alternative means of administering antiemetic therapies.
Statement of purpose	The purpose of the study is to test an intervention to reduce chemotherapy-induced side effects—specifically, to compare the effectiveness of patient-controlled and nurse-administered antiemetic therapy for controlling nausea and vomiting in patients on chemotherapy.
Research questions	What is the relative effectiveness of patient-controlled antiemetic therapy versus nurse-controlled antiemetic therapy with regard to (1) medication consumption and (2) control of nausea and vomiting in patients on chemotherapy?
Hypotheses	Patients receiving antiemetic therapy by a patient-controlled pump will (1) be less nauseous, (2) vomit less, and (3) consume less medication than patients receiving the therapy by nurse administration.

that would yield quantitative information about the level of depression in a sample of employed and retired seniors who are chronically ill.

Qualitative studies are often undertaken because a researcher wants to develop a rich and context-bound understanding of a poorly understood phenomenon. Researchers often initiate a qualitative study to heighten awareness and create a dialogue about a phenomenon. Qualitative methods would not be well suited to comparing levels of depression among employed and retired seniors, but they would be ideal for exploring, for example, the meaning or experience of depression among chronically ill retirees. Thus, the nature of the research question is linked to paradigms and to research traditions within paradigms.

Sources of Research Problems

Where do ideas for research problems come from? At a basic level, research topics originate with researchers' interests. Because research is a time-consuming enterprise, curiosity about and interest in a topic are essential. Research reports rarely indicate the source of researchers' inspiration, but a variety of explicit sources can fuel their interest, including the following:

- *Clinical experience.* Nurses' everyday clinical experience is a rich source of ideas for research inquiries. Immediate problems that need a solution—analogous to problem-focused triggers discussed in Chapter 2—may generate enthusiasm and have high potential for clinical relevance.
- *Patients' involvement.* Increasingly, researchers are turning to patients and other key stakeholders for input in identifying important issues for research. *Patient-centered outcomes research (PCOR)* has become increasingly prominent.
- *Quality improvement efforts.* Important clinical questions sometimes emerge in the context of findings from quality improvement studies. Personal involvement on a quality improvement team can sometimes lead to ideas for a study. In Chapter 12, we discuss a process called *root cause analysis* that can suggest a research focus.
- *Nursing literature.* Ideas for studies sometimes come from reading the nursing literature. Research articles may suggest problems indirectly by stimulating the reader's curiosity and directly by pointing out needed research.
- *Social issues.* Topics are sometimes suggested by global social or political issues of relevance to the healthcare community. For example, the

feminist movement raised questions about such topics as gender equity in healthcare. Public awareness about health disparities has led to research on healthcare access and culturally sensitive interventions.
- *Ideas from external sources.* External sources and direct suggestions can sometimes provide the impetus for a research idea. For example, ideas for studies may emerge from brainstorming with other nurses.

Additionally, researchers who have developed a program of research on a topic area may get inspiration for "next steps" from their own findings or from a discussion of those findings with others.

Example of a Problem Source in a Program of Research
Beck, one of this book's authors, conducted a study with two collaborators (Beck et al., 2015) on secondary traumatic stress among certified nurse midwives (CNMs). Beck has developed a strong research program on postpartum depression and traumatic births. She and Gable had previously conducted a study with labor and delivery nurses and their experiences of secondary traumatic stress caring for females during traumatic births. When Beck presented the findings of this study at conferences, certified CNMs in the audience often said "You should research us too. We are also traumatized."

TIP Personal experiences in clinical settings are a provocative source of research ideas and questions. Here are some hints:
- Watch for a recurring problem and see if you can discern a pattern in situations that lead to the problem. Example: Why do so many patients complain of being tired after being transferred from a coronary care unit to a progressive care unit?
- Think about aspects of your work that are frustrating or do not result in the intended outcome—then try to identify factors contributing to the problem that could be changed. Example: Why is suppertime so frustrating in a nursing home?
- Critically examine your own clinical decisions. Are they based on tradition, or are they based on systematic evidence that supports their efficacy? Example: What would happen if you used the return of flatus to assess the return of GI motility after abdominal surgery, rather than listening to bowel sounds?

DEVELOPING AND REFINING RESEARCH PROBLEMS

Procedures for developing a research problem are difficult to describe. The process is rarely a smooth and orderly one; there are likely to be false starts, inspirations, and setbacks. The few suggestions offered here are not intended to imply that there are techniques for making this first step easy but rather to encourage you to persevere in the absence of instant success.

Selecting a Topic

Developing a research problem is a creative process—and it is a process that is sometimes best done in teams. The teams can include other nurses, mentors, interdisciplinary partners, patients, or other community members.

In the early stages of initiating research ideas, try not to be too self-critical. It is better to relax and jot down topics of interest as they come to mind. It does not matter if the ideas are abstract or concrete, broad or specific, technical or colloquial—the important point is to put ideas on paper.

After this first step, ideas can be sorted in terms of interest, knowledge about the topics, and the perceived feasibility of turning the ideas into a study. When the most fruitful topic area has been selected, the list should not be discarded; it may be necessary to return to it.

TIP The process of selecting and refining a research problem usually takes longer than you might think. The process involves starting with some preliminary ideas; having discussions with colleagues, advisers, or stakeholders; perusing the research literature; looking at what is happening in clinical settings; and a lot of reflection.

Narrowing the Topic

Once you have identified a topic of interest, you can begin to ask some broad questions that can lead you to a researchable problem. Examples of question stems that might help to focus an inquiry include the following:

- What is going on with ...?
- What is the process by which ...?
- What is the meaning of ...?
- What would happen if ...?
- What influences or causes ...?
- What are the consequences of ...?
- What factors contribute to ...?

Early criticism of ideas can be counterproductive. Try not to jump to the conclusion that an idea sounds trivial or uninspired without giving it more careful consideration or exploring it with others. Another potential danger is that new researchers sometimes develop problems that are too broad in scope. The transformation of a general topic into a workable problem often is accomplished in uneven steps. Each step should result in progress toward the goals of narrowing the scope of the problem and sharpening the concepts.

As researchers move from general topics to more specific ideas, several possible research problems may emerge. Consider the following example. Suppose you were working on a medical unit and were puzzled by that fact that some patients always complained about having to wait for pain medication when certain nurses were assigned to them. The general problem is discrepancy in patient complaints regarding pain medications. You might ask: What accounts for the discrepancy? How can I improve the situation? These are not research questions, but they may lead you to ask such questions as the following: How do the two groups of nurses differ? or What characteristics do the complaining patients share? At this point, you may observe that the cultural and ethnic background of the patients and nurses could be relevant. This may lead you to search the literature for studies about culture and ethnicity in relation to nursing care, or it may prompt you to discuss your observations with others. These efforts may result in several research questions, such as the following:

- What is the nature of patient complaints among patients of different cultural backgrounds?
- Is the cultural background of nurses related to the frequency with which they dispense pain medication?
- Does the number of patient complaints increase when patients are of dissimilar cultural backgrounds as opposed to when they are of the same cultural background as nurses?
- Do nurses' dispensing behaviors change as a function of the similarity between their own cultural background and that of patients?

These questions stem from the same problem, yet each would be studied differently. Some suggest a qualitative approach and others suggest a quantitative one. A quantitative researcher might be curious about cultural or ethnic differences in nurses' dispensing behaviors. Both ethnicity and nurses' dispensing behaviors are variables that can be operationalized. A qualitative researcher would likely be more interested in understanding the *essence* of patients' complaints, their *experience* of frustration, or the *process* by which the problem got resolved.

Researchers choose a problem to study based on several factors, including its inherent interest and its compatibility with a paradigm of preference. In addition, tentative problems vary in their feasibility and worth. A critical evaluation of ideas is appropriate at this point.

Evaluating Research Problems

Although there are no rules for selecting a research problem, four important considerations to keep in mind are the problem's significance, researchability, feasibility, and interest to you.

Significance of the Problem

A crucial factor in selecting a problem is its significance to nursing. Evidence from the study should have potential to contribute meaningfully to nursing; the new study should be the right "next step" in building an evidence base. The right next step could be an original study, but it could also be a *replication* to answer previously asked questions with greater rigor or with a different population.

TIP In evaluating the significance of an idea, ask the following kinds of questions: Is the problem important to nursing and its clients? Will patient care benefit from the evidence? Will the findings challenge (or lend support to) existing practices? If the answer to all these questions is "no," then the problem probably should be abandoned.

Researchability of the Problem

Not all problems are amenable to research inquiry. Questions of a moral or ethical nature, although provocative, cannot be researched. For example, should assisted suicide be legalized? There are no *right* or *wrong* answers to this question, only points of view. Of course, related questions could be researched, such as: Do patients living with high levels of pain hold more favorable attitudes toward assisted suicide than those with less pain? What moral dilemmas are perceived by nurses who might be involved in assisted suicide? The findings from studies addressing such questions would have no bearing on whether assisted suicide should be legalized, but they could be useful in developing a better understanding of key issues.

Feasibility of the Problem

A third consideration concerns feasibility, which encompasses several issues. Not all the following factors are universally relevant, but they should be kept in mind in making a decision.

Time. Most studies have deadlines or completion goals, so the problem must be one that can be studied in the allotted time. It is prudent to be conservative in estimating time for the various tasks because research activities typically require more time than anticipated.

Researcher experience. Ideally, the problem should relate to a topic about which you have some prior knowledge or experience. Also, beginning researchers should avoid problems that might require the development of a new measuring instrument or that demand complex analyses.

Availability of study participants. In any study involving humans, researchers need to consider whether people with the desired characteristics will be available and willing to cooperate. Researchers may need to put considerable effort into recruiting participants or may need to offer a monetary incentive.

Cooperation of others. It may be necessary to gain entrée into an appropriate community or setting and to develop the trust of gatekeepers. In institutional settings (e.g., hospitals), access to clients, personnel, or records requires authorization.

Ethical considerations. A research problem may be unfeasible if the study would pose unfair or unethical demands on participants. The ethical issues discussed in Chapter 7 should be reviewed when considering a study's feasibility.

Facilities and equipment. All studies have resource requirements, although needs are sometimes modest. It is prudent to consider what facilities and equipment will be needed and whether they will be available.

Money. Monetary needs for studies vary widely, ranging from $100 or less for small student projects to hundreds of thousands of dollars for large-scale research. If you are on a limited budget, you should think carefully about projected expenses before selecting a problem. Major categories of research-related expenditures include:

- Personnel costs—payments to research assistants (e.g., for interviewing, coding, data entry, transcribing, statistical consulting)
- Participant costs—payments to participants as an incentive for their cooperation or to offset their expenses (e.g., parking, babysitting costs)
- Supplies—paper, memory sticks, postage, and so forth
- Printing and duplication—costs for reproducing forms, questionnaires, and so on
- Equipment—computers and software, audio- or video-recorders, calculators, and the like
- Laboratory fees for the analysis of biophysiologic data
- Transportation costs (e.g., travel to participants' homes)

TIP If your study involves testing a new procedure or intervention, you should also consider the feasibility of ultimately implementing it in real-world settings, should it prove effective. If the innovation requires a lot of resources, there may be little interest in adopting it, even if it results in improvements.

Researcher Interest

Even if a tentative problem is researchable, significant, and feasible, there is one more criterion: your own interest in the problem. Genuine curiosity about a research problem is an important prerequisite to a successful study. A lot of time and energy are expended in a study; there is little sense devoting these resources to a project about which you are not enthusiastic.

> **TIP** New researchers often seek suggestions about a topic area, and such assistance may be helpful in getting started. Nevertheless, it is unwise to be talked into a topic in which you have limited interest. If you do not find a problem appealing at the beginning of a study, you are likely to regret your choice later.

COMMUNICATING RESEARCH PROBLEMS AND QUESTIONS

Every study needs a problem statement—an articulation of what is problematic and is the impetus for the research. Most research reports also present a statement of purpose, research questions, or hypotheses.

Many people do not understand problem statements and may have trouble identifying them in a research article—not to mention developing one. A problem statement often begins with the very first sentence after the abstract. Specific research questions, purposes, or hypotheses appear later in the introduction. Typically, however, researchers *begin* their inquiry by identifying their research question and *then* develop an argument in their problem statement to present the rationale for the new research. This section follows that sequence by describing statements of purpose and research questions, followed by a discussion of problem statements.

Statements of Purpose

Many researchers articulate their research goals in a statement of purpose, worded declaratively. It is usually easy to identify a purpose statement because the word *purpose* is explicitly stated "The purpose of this study was ..."—although sometimes the words *aim*, *goal*, or *objective* are used instead, as in "The goal of this study was ...."

In a quantitative study, a statement of purpose identifies the key study variables and their possible interrelationships, as well as the population of interest (i.e., the PICO elements).

> **Example of a Statement of Purpose from a Quantitative Study**
> "The study objective was to assess the effect of music intervention on level of pain, anxiety and physiological parameters of heart rate, respiratory rate, and oxygen saturation, systolic and diastolic blood pressure among the post-operative sternotomy patients by compare with routine hospital management in control group before and after the music intervention" (Ganesan et al., 2022, p. 140).

In this purpose statement, the population (P) is a patient having a sternotomy. The aim is to assess whether a music intervention (I) compared with no music intervention (C)—which together comprise the independent variable—has an effect on the patient's level of pain, anxiety and physiologic parameters of heart rate, respiratory rate, and oxygen saturation, systolic and diastolic blood pressure, which are the dependent variables (the Os).

In qualitative studies, the statement of purpose indicates the key concept or phenomenon, and the people under study.

> **Example of a Statement of Purpose from a Qualitative Study**
> "In our research, we sought to better understand the interactive challenges faced by breast cancer affected mothers and their daughters from the former's perspective" (Zhu et al., 2022, p. 2).

This statement indicates that the central phenomenon in this study was the experiences of interaction between mothers with breast cancer and their daughters (P).

The statement of purpose communicates more than just the nature of the problem. Researchers' selection of verbs in a purpose statement suggests how they sought to solve the problem, or the state of knowledge on the topic. A study whose purpose is to *explore* or *describe* a phenomenon is likely an investigation of a little-researched topic, sometimes involving a qualitative approach. A purpose statement for a qualitative study may also use verbs such as *understand*, *discover*, or *develop*. Statements of purpose in qualitative studies may "encode" the tradition of inquiry, not only through the researcher's choice of verbs but also through the use of "buzz words" associated with those traditions, as follows:

- *Grounded theory:* Processes; social structures; social interactions
- *Phenomenologic studies:* Experience; lived experience; meaning; essence
- *Ethnographic studies:* Culture; roles; lifeways; cultural behavior

Quantitative researchers also suggest the nature of the inquiry through their selection of verbs. A statement indicating that the study's purpose is to *test* or *evaluate* something (e.g., an intervention) suggests an experimental design. A study whose purpose is to *examine* or *explore* the relationship between two variables likely involves a nonexperimental design. Sometimes the verb is ambiguous: a purpose statement indicating that an intent to *compare* could be referring to a comparison of alternative treatments (using an experimental approach) or a comparison of preexisting groups (using a nonexperimental approach). In any event, verbs such as *test*, *evaluate*, and *compare* suggest an existing knowledge base and quantifiable variables.

The verbs in a purpose statement should connote objectivity. A statement of purpose indicating that the study goal was to *prove*, *demonstrate*, or *show* something suggests a bias. The word *determine* should usually be avoided as well because research methods almost never provide definitive answers to research questions.

TIP Unfortunately, some reports fail to state the study purpose clearly, leaving readers to infer the purpose from such sources as the title of the report. In other reports, the purpose may be difficult to find. Researchers often state their purpose toward the end of the report's introduction.

Research Questions

Research questions are sometimes direct rewordings of purpose statements, phrased interrogatively rather than declaratively, as in the following example:

- *Purpose:* The purpose of this study was to assess the relationship between the functional dependence level of renal transplant recipients and their rate of recovery.
- *Question:* What is the relationship between the functional dependence level (I and C: higher vs. lower levels) of renal transplant recipients (P) and their rate of recovery (O)?

Questions have the advantage of simplicity and directness—they invite an answer and help to focus attention on the kinds of data needed to provide that answer. Some research reports thus omit a statement of purpose and state only research questions. Other researchers use a set of research questions to clarify or lend greater specificity to a global purpose statement.

Research Questions in Quantitative Studies

In Chapter 2, we discussed the framing of clinical foreground questions to guide an EBP inquiry. Many of the EBP question templates in Table 2.2 could yield questions to guide a study as well, but *researchers* tend to conceptualize their questions in terms of their *variables*. Take, for example, the Therapy question in Table 2.2, which states, "In (Population), what is the effect of (Intervention) on (Outcome)?" A researcher would likely think of the question in these terms: "In (population), what is the effect of (independent variable) on (dependent variable)?" Thus, in quantitative studies research questions identify the population (P) under study, the key study variables (I, C, and O components), and possible relationships among the variables. The variables are all quantifiable concepts.

Most research questions concern relationships, so many quantitative research questions could be articulated using a general template: "In (population), what is the relationship between (independent variable or IV) and (dependent variable or DV)?" Variations include the following:

- *Therapy/intervention:* In (population), what is the effect of (IV: intervention vs. an alternative) on (DV)?
- *Prognosis:* In (population), does (IV: presence of disease or illness vs. its absence) affect or increase the risk of (DV: adverse consequences)?

- *Etiology/harm:* In (population), does (IV: exposure vs. nonexposure) cause or increase the risk of (DV: disease, health problem)?

Clinical foreground questions for an EBP-focused search and a question for a study sometimes differ. As shown in Table 2.2, sometimes clinicians ask PICO questions about explicit comparisons (e.g., they want to compare intervention A with intervention B) and sometimes they do not (e.g., they want to learn the effects of intervention A, compared with those of any other intervention or to the absence of an intervention, PIO questions). In a research question, there must *always* be a designated comparison because the independent variable must be operationally defined; this definition would articulate the specific "I" and "C" being studied.

> **TIP** Research questions are sometimes more complex than clinical foreground questions for EBP. They may include, in addition to the independent and dependent variable, elements called moderator variables or mediating variables. A **moderator variable** is a variable that influences the strength or direction of a relationship between two variables (e.g., a person's age might moderate the effect of exercise on physical function). A **mediating variable** is one that acts like a "go-between" in a link between two variables (e.g., a smoking cessation intervention may affect smoking behavior through the intervention's effect on motivation to quit).

Some research questions are primarily descriptive. As examples, here are some descriptive questions that could be addressed in a study on nurses' use of humor:

- What is the frequency with which nurses use humor as a complementary therapy with hospitalized patients with cancer?
- What are the reactions of hospitalized cancer patients to nurses' use of humor?
- What are the characteristics of nurses who use humor as a complementary therapy with hospitalized patients with cancer?
- Is my *Use of Humor Scale* a reliable and valid measure of nurses' use of humor with patients in clinical settings?

Answers to such questions might, if addressed in a methodologically sound study, be useful in developing interventions for reducing stress in patients with cancer.

> **Example of a Research Question from a Quantitative Study**
> Flanagan, one of the authors of this textbook, and colleagues (2022) explored informal caregivers' experiences of participating in a nurse-coached walking program using wireless pedometers. One of the research questions was as follows: What is the effect of the nurse-coached walking program on participants' perceived well-being?

Research Questions in Qualitative Studies

Research questions for qualitative studies state the phenomenon of interest and the group or population of interest. Researchers in the various qualitative traditions vary in their conceptualization of what types of questions are important. Grounded theory researchers are likely to ask *process* questions, phenomenologists tend to ask *meaning* questions, and ethnographers generally ask *descriptive* questions about cultures. Special terms associated with the various traditions, noted previously, are likely to be incorporated into the research questions.

> **Example of a Research Question from a Phenomenological Study**
> What are the experiences of registered nurses working in emergency departments in Jordan who have experienced workplace violence? (Al-Qadi et al., 2022)

Not all qualitative studies are rooted in a specific research tradition. Many researchers use qualitative methods to describe or explore phenomena without focusing on cultures, meaning, or social processes.

> **Example of a Research Question from a Descriptive Qualitative Study**
> In their descriptive qualitative study, Smeltzer et al. (2022) asked, "What are the knowledge, experiences, and perceptions of providing childbirth education to women with physical disability

In qualitative studies, research questions may evolve over the course of the study. Researchers begin with a *focus* that defines the broad boundaries of the study, but the boundaries are not cast in stone. The boundaries "can be altered and, in the typical naturalistic inquiry, will be" (Lincoln and Guba, 1985, p. 228). The naturalist begins with a research question that provides a general starting point but does not prohibit discovery. The emergent nature of qualitative inquiry means that research questions can be modified as new data make it relevant to do so.

Problem Statements

Problem statements express the dilemma or troubling situation that needs investigation and that provide a rationale for a new inquiry. A good problem statement is a well-structured formulation of what is problematic, what "needs fixing," or what is poorly understood. Problem statements, especially for quantitative studies, often have most of the following six components:

1. *Problem identification:* What is wrong with the current situation?
2. *Background:* What is the context of the problem that readers need to understand?
3. *Scope of the problem:* How big a problem is it? How many people are affected?
4. *Consequences of the problem:* What are the costs of *not* fixing the problem?
5. *Knowledge gaps:* What information about the problem is lacking?
6. *Proposed solution:* How would the proposed study contribute to the solution of the problem?

These components, taken together, form the **argument** for the study—researchers try to *persuade* readers that the rationale for undertaking the study is sound.

Suppose our topic was humor as a complementary therapy for reducing stress in hospitalized patients with cancer. Our research question is, "What is the effect of nurses' use of humor on stress and natural killer cell activity in hospitalized patients with cancer?" Box 4.1 presents a rough draft of a problem statement for such a study. This problem statement is a reasonable first draft. The draft has several, but not all, of the six components.

Box 4.2 illustrates how the problem statement could be strengthened by adding information about scope (component 3), long-term consequences (component 4), and possible solutions (component 6). This second draft builds a more compelling argument for new research: millions of people are affected by cancer, and the disease has adverse consequences not only for those diagnosed and their families but also for society. The revised problem statement also suggests a basis for the new study by describing a solution on which the new study might build.

As this example suggests, the problem statement is usually interwoven with supportive evidence from the research literature. In many research articles, it is difficult to disentangle the problem statement from the literature review, unless there is a subsection specifically labeled "Literature Review."

Problem statements for a qualitative study similarly express the nature of the problem, its context, its scope, and information needed to address it, as in the following abridged example:

BOX 4.1   Draft Problem Statement on Humor and Stress

A diagnosis of cancer is associated with high levels of stress. Sizable numbers of patients who receive a cancer diagnosis describe feelings of uncertainty, fear, anger, and loss of control. Interpersonal relationships, psychological functioning, and role performance have all been found to suffer following cancer diagnosis and treatment.

A variety of alternative/complementary therapies have been developed in an effort to decrease the harmful effects of stress on psychological and physiologic functioning, and resources devoted to these therapies (money and staff) have increased in recent years. However, many of these therapies have not been carefully evaluated to determine their efficacy, safety, or cost-effectiveness. For example, the use of humor has been recommended as a therapeutic device to improve quality of life, decrease stress, and perhaps improve immune functioning, but the evidence to support this claim is limited.

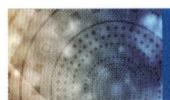

> **BOX 4.2 Some Possible Improvements to Problem Statement on Humor and Stress**
>
> Each year, more than 1 million people are diagnosed with cancer, which remains one of the top causes of death among both males and females (reference citations). Numerous studies have documented that a diagnosis of cancer is associated with high levels of stress. Sizable numbers of patients who receive a cancer diagnosis describe feelings of uncertainty, fear, anger, and loss of control (**citations**). Interpersonal relationships, psychological functioning, and role performance have all been found to suffer following cancer diagnosis and treatment (**citations**). These stressful outcomes can, in turn, adversely affect health, long-term prognosis, and medical costs among cancer survivors (citations).
>
> A variety of alternative/complementary therapies have been developed in an effort to decrease the harmful effects of stress on psychological and physiologic functioning, and resources devoted to these therapies (money and staff) have increased in recent years (**citations**). However, many of these therapies have not been carefully evaluated to determine their efficacy, safety, or cost-effectiveness. For example, the use of humor has been recommended as a therapeutic device to improve quality of life, decrease stress, and perhaps improve immune functioning (**citations**), but the evidence to support this claim is limited. Preliminary findings from a recent small-scale endocrinology study with a healthy sample exposed to a humorous intervention (citation) hold promise for further inquiry with immuno-compromised populations.

Example of a Problem Statement from a Qualitative Study

"Hydrocephalus is a key public health concern which annually affects more than 380,000 individuals worldwide (Dewan et al., 2019). There is a need to understand the unique needs of children with hydrocephalus and their families. There is also a need to assess the availability of resources for supporting these families in dealing with this health condition appropriately. The existing literature showed that mothers of children with hydrocephalus experience many challenges including lack of social support, financial burden, uncertainty, and stigma related to having a child with hydrocephalus (Dorner et al., 2021; Kyarimpa et al., 2020; Ogunleye et al., 2022). However, there is limited literature addressing the mothers' experiences and challenges of having children with hydrocephalus in the Arab world, including Jordan. This study attempts to fill this gap in the literature and hopes to highlight some important aspects of parenting children with hydrocephalus in Jordan" (Shattnawi et al., 2023, p. e127).

Qualitative studies embedded in a particular research tradition usually incorporate terms in their problem statements that foreshadow the tradition. For example, the problem statement in a grounded theory study might refer to the need to generate a theory relating to social processes. A problem statement for a phenomenologic study might note the need to gain insight into people's experiences or the meanings they attribute to those experiences. And an ethnographer might indicate the need to understand how cultural forces affect people's health behaviors.

RESEARCH HYPOTHESES

A hypothesis is a prediction, almost always a prediction about the relationship between variables.[1] In qualitative studies, researchers do not have an a priori hypothesis, in part because there is too little known to justify a prediction and in part because qualitative researchers want the inquiry to be guided by participants' viewpoints rather than by their own hunches. Thus, our discussion here focuses on hypotheses in quantitative research.

Function of Hypotheses in Quantitative Research

Research questions, as we have seen, are usually queries about relationships between variables.

---

[1]Although this does not occur with great frequency, it is possible to make a hypothesis about a specific value. For example, we might hypothesize that the rate of medication compliance in a specific population is 60%. Chapter 18 has an example.

Hypotheses are predicted answers to these queries. For instance, the research question might ask: Does sexual abuse in childhood affect the development of irritable bowel syndrome in females? The researcher might predict the following: Females (P) who were sexually abused in childhood (I) have a higher incidence of irritable bowel syndrome (O) than females who were not (C).

Hypotheses sometimes follow from a theory. Scientists reason from theories to hypotheses and test those hypotheses in the real world. Take, as an example, the theory of reinforcement, which maintains that behavior that is positively reinforced (rewarded) tends to be learned or repeated. Predictions based on this theory could be tested. For example, we could test the following hypothesis: Pediatric patients (P) who are given a reward (e.g., a toy) (I) when they undergo nursing procedures tend to be more cooperative during those procedures (O) than nonrewarded peers (C). This hypothesis can be put to a test, and the theory gains credibility if it is supported with real data.

Even in the absence of a theory, well-conceived hypotheses offer direction and suggest explanations. For example, suppose we hypothesized that cue-based feedings compared with traditional methods of feeding for preterm infants will shorten the time to full oral feedings and discharge from the NICU. We could justify our speculation based on earlier studies or clinical observations, or both. *The development of predictions forces researchers to think logically and to tie together earlier research findings.*

Now let us suppose the preceding hypothesis is not confirmed: We find that time to full oral feedings and discharge is similar for preterm infants on cue-based feedings and traditional methods of feeding. *The failure of data to support a prediction forces researchers to analyze theory or previous research critically, to consider study limitations, and to explore alternative explanations for the findings.* The use of hypotheses tends to induce critical thinking and encourages careful interpretation of the evidence.

To illustrate further the utility of hypotheses, suppose we conducted the study guided only by the research question, Is there a relationship between feeding method in preterm infants and the length of time to full oral feedings and NICU discharge? The investigator without a hypothesis is apparently prepared to accept any results. The problem is that it is almost always possible to explain something superficially after the fact, no matter what the findings are. Hypotheses reduce the risk that spurious results will be misconstrued.

TIP Consider whether it might be appropriate to develop hypotheses that predict different effects of the independent variable on the outcome for different subgroups of people—that is, to consider the effects of *moderator* variables. For example, would you predict the effects of an intervention to be different for males and females? Testing such hypotheses might facilitate greater applicability of the evidence to specific types of patients (Chapter 31).

Characteristics of Testable Hypotheses

Testable hypotheses state the expected relationship between the independent variable (the presumed cause or antecedent) and the dependent variable (the presumed effect or outcome) within a population.

Example of a Research Hypothesis
Coakley and colleagues (2021) hypothesized that a one-time animal-assisted therapy (AAT) visit would reduce the reported anxiety level in patients hospitalized in an acute care setting.

In this example, the population was patients admitted to the acute care setting who received an AAT visit. The independent variable is the animal-assisted therapy visit, and the dependent variable is the anxiety level. The hypothesis predicts that these two variables are related within the population—the animal-assisted therapy visit is predicted to be associated with a decreased anxiety level.

Hypotheses that do not make a relational statement are difficult to test. Take the following example: *Pregnant females who receive prenatal instruction about postpartum experiences are not likely to experience postpartum depression.* This statement expresses no anticipated relationship—there is only one variable (postpartum depression), and a relationship requires at least two variables.

The problem is that without a prediction about an anticipated relationship, the hypothesis is difficult to test using standard statistical procedures. In our example, how would we know whether the hypothesis was supported—what standard could be used to decide whether to accept or reject it? To illustrate this concretely, suppose we asked a group of mothers who had been given instruction on postpartum experiences the following question 1 month after delivery: On the whole, how depressed have you been since you gave birth? Would you say (1) extremely depressed, (2) moderately depressed, (3) a little depressed, or (4) not at all depressed?

Based on responses to this question, how could we compare the actual outcome with the predicted outcome? Would *all* the women have to say they were "not at all depressed?" Would the prediction be supported if 51% of the women said they were "not at all depressed" or "a little depressed?" It is difficult to test the accuracy of the prediction.

A test is simple, however, if we modify the prediction as follows: Pregnant women who receive prenatal instruction are less likely to experience postpartum depression than those with no prenatal instruction. Here, the outcome variable (O) is the women's depression, and the independent variable is receipt (I) vs. nonreceipt (C) of prenatal instruction. The relational aspect of the prediction is embodied in the phrase *less than*. If a hypothesis lacks a phrase such as *more than, less than, greater than, different from, related to, associated with*, or something similar, it is probably not amenable to statistical testing. To test this revised hypothesis, we could ask two groups of women with different prenatal instruction experiences to respond to the question on depression and then compare the average responses of the two groups. The absolute degree of depression of either group would not be at issue.

Hypotheses should be based on justifiable rationales. Hypotheses often follow from previous research findings or are deduced from a theory. When a new area is being investigated, the researcher may have to turn to logical reasoning or clinical experience to justify predictions.

The Derivation of Hypotheses

Many students ask, "How do I go about developing hypotheses?" Two basic processes—induction and deduction—are the intellectual machinery involved in deriving hypotheses.

An **inductive hypothesis** is inferred from observations. Researchers observe certain patterns among phenomena and then make predictions based on the observations. An important source for inductive hypotheses is clinical experiences. For example, a nurse might notice that presurgical patients who ask a lot of questions about pain have a more difficult time than other patients in learning postoperative procedures. The nurse could formulate a hypothesis, such as the following: Patients who are stressed by fear of pain have more difficulty in deep breathing and coughing after surgery than patients who are not stressed. Qualitative studies are an important source of inspiration for inductive hypotheses.

> **Example of Deriving an Inductive Hypothesis**
> LoGiudice and Beck (2016) conducted a phenomenological study of the experience of childbearing from eight survivors of sexual abuse. One of the themes from this study was "Overprotection: Keeping my child safe." A hypothesis that can be derived from this qualitative finding might be as follows: Women who experienced sexual abuse will be more overprotective of their children than mothers who have not experienced sexual abuse.

Inductive hypotheses begin with specific observations and move toward generalizations. **Deductive hypotheses** have theories or prior knowledge as a starting point, as in our earlier example about reinforcement theory. Researchers deduce that if the theory is true, then certain outcomes can be expected. If hypotheses are supported, then the theory is strengthened. The advancement of nursing knowledge depends on both inductive and deductive hypotheses. Researchers need to be organizers of concepts (think inductively), logicians (think deductively), and critics and skeptics of resulting formulations, constantly demanding evidence.

Wording of Hypotheses

A good hypothesis is worded clearly and concisely and in the present tense. Researchers make predictions about relationships that exist in the population and not just about a relationship that will be revealed in a particular sample. There are various types of hypotheses.

Directional Versus Nondirectional Hypotheses

Hypotheses can be stated in a number of ways, as in the following example:

1. Older patients are more likely to fall than younger patients.
2. There is a relationship between the age of a patient and the risk of falling.
3. The older the patient, the greater the risk that they will fall.
4. Older patients differ from younger ones with respect to their risk of falling.
5. Younger patients tend to be less at risk of a fall than older patients.

In each example, the hypothesis indicates the population (patients), the independent variable (patients' age), the dependent variable (a fall), and the anticipated relationship between them.

Hypotheses can be either directional or nondirectional. A **directional hypothesis** is one that specifies not only the existence but the expected direction of the relationship between variables. In our example, hypotheses 1, 3, and 5 are directional because there is an explicit prediction that older patients are more likely to fall than younger ones. A **nondirectional hypothesis** does not state the direction of the relationship, as illustrated by versions 2 and 4. These hypotheses predict that a patient's age and risk of falling are related, but they do not stipulate whether the researcher thinks that *older* patients or *younger* ones are at greater risk.

Hypotheses derived from theory are almost always directional because theories provide a rationale for expecting variables to be related in a certain way. Existing studies also offer a basis for directional hypotheses. When there is no theory or related research, when findings of prior studies are contradictory, or when researchers' own experience leads to ambivalence, nondirectional hypotheses may be appropriate. Some people argue, in fact, that nondirectional hypotheses are preferable because they connote impartiality. Directional hypotheses, it is said, imply that researchers are intellectually committed to certain outcomes, and such a commitment might lead to bias. Yet, researchers typically *do* have hunches about outcomes, whether they state them explicitly or not. We prefer directional hypotheses when there is a reasonable basis for them because they clarify the study's framework and demonstrate that researchers have thought critically about the study variables.

> **TIP** Hypotheses can be either *simple hypotheses* (ones with one independent variable and one dependent variable) or *complex hypotheses* (ones with three or more variables—for example, with multiple independent or dependent variables).

Research Versus Null Hypotheses

Hypotheses can be described as either research hypotheses or null hypotheses. **Research hypotheses** (also called *scientific* hypotheses) are statements of expected relationships between variables. All hypotheses presented thus far are research hypotheses that state actual predictions.

Statistical inference uses a logic that may be confusing. This logic requires that hypotheses be expressed as an expected *absence* of a relationship. **Null hypotheses** (or *statistical hypotheses*) state that there is no relationship between the independent and dependent variables. The null form of the hypothesis used in our example might be as follows: "Patients' age is unrelated to their risk of falling" or "Older patients are just as likely as younger patients to fall." The null hypothesis might be compared with the assumption of innocence of an accused criminal in many justice systems. The variables are assumed to be "innocent" of any relationship until they can be shown "guilty" through appropriate statistical procedures. The null hypothesis represents the formal statement of this assumption of "innocence."

Researchers typically state research rather than null hypotheses. Indeed, you should avoid stating hypotheses in null form in a proposal or a report because this gives an amateurish impression. In statistical testing, underlying null hypotheses are assumed without being stated. If the researcher's *actual* research hypothesis is that no relationship among variables exists, complex procedures are needed to test it.

Hypothesis Testing and Proof

Hypotheses are formally tested through statistical analysis. Researchers use statistics to test whether their hypotheses have a high probability of being correct (i.e., have a $P < .05$). Statistical analysis does not offer proof; it only supports inferences that a hypothesis is *probably* correct (or not. Hypotheses are never *proved* or *disproved*; rather, they are *supported* or *rejected*. Findings are always tentative. Hypotheses come to be increasingly supported with evidence from multiple studies.

Let us look at why this is so. Suppose we hypothesized that height and weight are related. We predict that, on average, tall people weigh more than short people. We then obtain height and weight measurements from a sample and analyze the data. Now suppose we happened by chance to get a sample that consisted of short, heavy people, and tall, thin people. Our results might indicate that there is no relationship between height and weight. But we would not be justified in concluding that this study *proved* or *demonstrated* that height and weight are unrelated.

This example illustrates the difficulty of using observations from a sample to draw definitive conclusions about a population. Issues such as the accuracy of the measures, the effects of uncontrolled variables, and idiosyncrasies of the study sample prevent researchers from concluding that hypotheses are proved.

> **TIP** If a researcher uses any statistical tests (as is true in most quantitative studies), it means that there were underlying hypotheses—regardless of whether the researcher explicitly stated them—because statistical tests are designed to test hypotheses. In planning a quantitative study of your own, do not hesitate to state hypotheses.

CRITICAL APPRAISAL OF RESEARCH PROBLEMS, RESEARCH QUESTIONS, AND HYPOTHESES

In appraising research articles, you need to evaluate whether researchers have adequately communicated their problem. The problem statement, purpose, research questions, and hypotheses set the stage for a description of what the researchers did and what they learned. You should not have to dig deeply to decipher the research problem or the questions.

A critical appraisal of the research problem is multidimensional. Substantively, you need to consider whether the problem has significance for nursing. Studies that build in a meaningful way on existing knowledge are well-poised to contribute to evidence-based nursing practice. Researchers who develop a systematic **program of research**, designing new studies based on their own earlier findings, are especially likely to make important contributions (Conn, 2004). For example, Cheryl Beck's series of studies relating to postpartum depression and traumatic births have influenced women's healthcare worldwide. Also, research problems stemming from established research priorities (Chapter 1) have a high likelihood of yielding important new evidence for nurses because they reflect expert opinion about areas of needed research.

Another dimension in appraising the research problem is methodologic—in particular, whether the research problem is compatible with the chosen research paradigm and its associated methods. You should also evaluate whether the statement of purpose or research questions have been properly worded and lend themselves to empirical inquiry.

In a quantitative study, if the research article does not contain explicit hypotheses, you need to consider whether their absence is justified. If there are hypotheses, you should evaluate whether they are logically connected to the problem and are consistent with existing evidence or relevant theory. The wording of hypotheses should also be assessed. To be testable, the hypothesis should contain a prediction about the relationship between

CHAPTER 4 Research Problems, Research Questions, and Hypotheses • 79

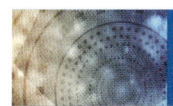

> **BOX 4.3** Guidelines for Critically Appraising Research Problems, Research Questions, and Hypotheses
>
> 1. What is the research problem? Is the problem statement easy to locate and is it clearly stated? Does the problem statement build a cogent and persuasive argument for the new study?
> 2. Does the problem have significance for nursing? How might the research contribute to nursing practice, administration, education, or policy?
> 3. Is there a good fit between the research problem and the paradigm in which the research was conducted? Is there a good fit between the problem and the qualitative research tradition (if applicable)?
> 4. Does the report formally present a statement of purpose, research question, and/or hypotheses? Is this information communicated clearly and concisely, and is it placed in a logical and useful location?
> 5. Are purpose statements or questions worded appropriately? For example, are key concepts/variables identified and is the population of interest specified? Are verbs used appropriately to suggest the nature of the inquiry and/or the research tradition?
> 6. If there are no formal hypotheses, is their absence justified? Are statistical tests used in analyzing the data despite the absence of stated hypotheses?
> 7. Do hypotheses (if any) flow from a theory or previous research? Is there a justifiable basis for the predictions?
> 8. Are hypotheses (if any) properly worded—do they state a predicted relationship between two or more variables? Are they directional or nondirectional, and is there a rationale for how they were stated? Are they presented as research or as null hypotheses?

two or more measurable variables. Specific guidelines for critically appraising research problems, research questions, and hypotheses are presented in Box 4.3.

RESEARCH EXAMPLES

This section describes how the research problem and research questions were communicated in two nursing studies, one quantitative and one qualitative.

Research Example of a Quantitative Study

Study: The effects of a nurse-led integrative medicine-based structured education program on self-management behaviors among individuals with newly diagnosed type 2 diabetes: a randomized controlled trial (Yu, et al., 2022).

Problem statement (Excerpt; citations omitted to streamline presentation): "Culture-tailored interventions have frequently been advocated by healthcare professionals and researchers. However, to date, publications on eligible structured education programs for Chinese individuals with type 2 diabetes are vacant. As China has the largest diabetes population, it is of great significance to develop and evaluate the effectiveness of culturally appropriate structured education programs in Chinese individuals with type 2 diabetes. … Traditional Chinese medicine (TCM), an important branch of alternative medicine that is deeply rooted in the traditional Chinese culture, proposed a variety of lifestyle modifying interventions for individuals with diabetes, such as dietary intervention based on the TCM body constitution theory, exercises including tai chi and ba duan jin (eight-session brocade qigong), and TCM-based psychological care. The effectiveness of such interventions for individuals with type 2 diabetes has been demonstrated in a recent systematic review with meta-analysis. … Integrative medicine, which combines conventional diabetes management with alternative interventions, has gained popularity in type 2 diabetes treatment worldwide (p. 3).

Statement of purpose: "The objectives of this randomized controlled trial were to evaluate the effects of a nurse-led integrative medicine-based structured education program on diabetes self-management behaviors, glycemic control and self-efficacy among individuals with newly diagnosed type 2 diabetes (p. 3)."

Research question: Although not formally stated by the researchers, we can state their Therapy question as follows: Compared to those who do not participate (C), does a nurse-led integrative medicine-based structured education program on diabetes self-management behaviors (I) lead to improvements in glycemic control and self-efficacy (O) among individuals with newly diagnosed type 2 diabetes (P).

Hypotheses: The researchers hypothesized that "compared to the counterparts in the usual care control group, participants who received the structured education program would have significantly higher level of diabetes self-management behaviors, glycemic control (indicated by Glycated Hemoglobin A, HbA1c) and self-efficacy (p. 3).

Study methods: The study was conducted in four tertiary hospitals in China. A total of 128 eligible patients were recruited and allocated, at random, to either receive or not receive the intervention. Those in the intervention group received an 8-session nurse-led integrative medicine-based structured education program. The primary outcome was diabetes self-management behaviors, while the secondary outcomes were HbA1c and self-efficacy.

Key findings: Patients in the intervention group exhibited significant improvements in self-management behaviors, HbA1c, and self-efficacy.

Research Example of a Qualitative Study

Study: Experiences of mothers of NICU preterm infants in milk management out of the hospital: a qualitative study (Yang et al., 2022).

Problem statement (Excerpt; citations omitted to streamline presentation): "In 2018, Chinese researchers found that most (66%) hospitals had no lactation rooms and many (81%) NICUs provided neither hospital-grade milk pumps nor disposable milk storage bags... Mothers could only express milk at home and transport human milk to the hospital via milk storage bags or bottles for the infants. This poses challenges to the human milk feeding and management of hospitalized preterm infants. Paying attention to out-of-hospital human milk management is not only important for ensuring the quality of human milk during the hospitalization of preterm infants, but it is also important for mothers who have to express human milk as well as for their families. Although a health education manual on human milk management is provided to mothers, which covers hand washing, human milk expression (including how to pump human milk, pumping frequency, breast pump cleaning, etc.), human milk storage and transportation, as well as breastfeeding knowledge. However, as the primary implementer of milk management, mothers' experiences remain to be studied. Identifying the experiences of mothers who are conducting human milk management outside the hospital is important for providing support for the continuation of human milk expression" (p. 2).

Statement of purpose: The objective of this study was "to explore the experiences of Chinese mothers providing their newborns in the NICU with human milk expressed outside the hospital (p. 2)."

Research questions: Although not formally stated by the researchers, we can state their question as follows: The mothers' experiences were explored by asking them to describe what it was like for them to provide their newborns in the NICU with human milk expressed outside of the hospital.

Method: This was a qualitative descriptive study that was conducted in a preterm infant care unit in China. Purposive and maximum variation sampling were used to enroll 23 mothers. Study participants were interviewed in-depth, with interviews continuing until data saturation occurred.

Key findings: "Three main themes regarding out-of-hospital human milk management were identified: 1) awareness of human milk management and a willingness to adopt it; 2) lack of standardization regarding expressing, storing, and transporting expressed human milk; and 3) the need for more external support" (p. 3).

SUMMARY POINTS

- A **research problem** is a perplexing or enigmatic situation that a researcher wants to address through disciplined inquiry. Researchers usually

- identify a broad *topic*, narrow the problem scope, and identify questions consistent with a paradigm of choice.
- Common sources of ideas for nursing research problems are clinical experience, patient queries, relevant literature, quality improvement initiatives, social issues, and external suggestions.
- Key criteria in selecting a research problem are that the problem should be clinically important, researchable, feasible, and of personal interest.
- Feasibility involves the issues of time, researcher skills, cooperation of participants and other people, availability of facilities and equipment, adequacy of resources, and ethical considerations.
- Researchers communicate their goals as problem statements, statements of purpose, research questions, or hypotheses.
- **Problem statements,** which articulate the nature, context, and significance of a problem, include several components organized to form an **argument** for a new study: problem identification; the background, scope, and consequences of the problem; knowledge gaps; and possible solutions to the problem.
- A **statement of purpose,** which summarizes the overall study goal, identifies key concepts or variables and the population. Purpose statements often communicate, through the use of verbs and other key terms, the underlying research tradition of qualitative studies, or whether study is experimental or nonexperimental in quantitative ones.
- A **research question** is the specific query researchers want to answer in addressing the research problem. In quantitative studies, research questions usually focus on relationships between variables.
- In quantitative studies, a **hypothesis** is a statement of predicted relationships between two or more variables. Complex hypotheses may involve a **moderator variable** (a variable that alters the strength or direction of a relationship between two variables) or a **mediating variable** that acts as a "go-between" in the link between two variables.
- **Directional hypotheses** predict the direction of a relationship; **nondirectional hypotheses** predict the existence of relationships, not their direction.
- **Research hypotheses** predict the existence of relationships; **null hypotheses**, which express the absence of a relationship, are the hypotheses subjected to statistical testing.
- Hypotheses are never proved or disproved in an ultimate sense—they are accepted or rejected, supported or not supported by the research data.

REFERENCES CITED IN CHAPTER 4

Al-Qadi, M. M., Maruca, A. T., Beck, C. T., & Walsh, S. J. (2022). Exploring Jordanian emergency registered nurses' experiences of workplace violence: A phenomenological study. *International Emergency Nursing*, *65*, 101218. https://doi.org/10.1016/j.ienj.2022.101218

Beck, C. T., LoGiudice, J., & Gable, R. K. (2015). A mixed methods study of secondary traumatic stress in certified nurse-midwives: Shaken belief in the birth process. *Journal of Midwifery & Women's Health*, *60*(1), 16–23.

Coakley, A. B., Annese, C. D., Empoliti, J. H., & Flanagan, J. M. (2021). The experience of animal assisted therapy on patients in an acute care setting. *Clinical Nursing Research*, *30*(4), 401–405. https://doi.org/10.1177/1054773820977198

Conn, V. (2004). Building a research trajectory. *Western Journal of Nursing Research*, *26*(6), 592–594.

Dewan, M. C., Rattani, A., Mekary, R., Glancz, L. J., Yunusa, I., Baticulon, R. E., Fieggen, G., Wellons, J. C., Park, K. B., & Warf, B. C. (2018). Global hydrocephalus epidemiology and incidence: Systematic review and meta-analysis. *Journal of Neurosurgery*, *130*(4), 1065–1079. https://doi.org/10.3171/2017.10.JNS17439

Dorner, R. A., Boss, R. D., Burton, V. J., Raja, K., Robinson, S., & Lemmon, M. E. (2022). Isolated and on guard: Preparing neonatal intensive care unit families for life with hydrocephalus. *American Journal of Perinatology*, *39*(12),1341–1347. https://doi.org/10.1055/S-0040-1722344/ID/JR200894-26

Flanagan, J., Post, K., Hill, R., & DiPalazzo, J. (2022). Feasibility of a nurse coached walking intervention for informal dementia caregivers. *Western Journal of Nursing Research*, *44*(5), 466–476. https://doi.org/10.1177/01939459211001395

Ganesan, P., Manjini, K. J., & Bathala Vedagiri, S. C. (2022). Effect of music on pain, anxiety and physiological parameters among postoperative sternotomy patients: A randomized controlled trial. *Journal of Caring Science*, *11*(3), 139–147. https://doi.org/10.34172/jcs.2022.18

Kyarimpa, R., Muramuzi, D., & Muhwezi, T. (2020). Caregiver's experiences of having a child with hydrocephalus: A phenomenological study at Ruharo mission hospital. *MedRxiv*. https://doi.org/10.1101/2020.06.25.20139683

Lincoln, Y. S., & Guba, E. G. (1985). *Naturalistic inquiry*. Sage.

LoGiudice, J. A., & Beck, C. T. (2016). The lived experience of childbearing from survivors of sexual abuse: "it was the best of times, it was the worst of times." *Journal of Midwifery and Women's Health*, *61*(4), 474–481.

Ogunleye, O., Ismail, N.J., Lasseini, A., & Shehu, B.B. (2022). Management of childhood hydrocephalus in our centre: Parents' knowledge, experiences and expectations. *Global Journal for Research Analysis*, *7*(4), 8–10.

Shattnawi, K. K., Qananbeh, F. S., & Khater, W. (2023). The experiences of mothers of children with hydrocephalus in Jordan: A phenomenological study. *Journal of Pediatric Nursing*, *69*, e127–e135. https://doi.org/10.1016/j.pedn.2022.12.026

Smeltzer, S. C., Tina Maldonado, L., McKeever, A., Amorim, F., Arcamone, A., & Nthenge, S. (2022). Qualitative descriptive study of childbirth educators' perspectives on prenatal education for women with physical disability. *Journal of Obstetric Gynecologic, & Neonatal Nursing*, *51*(3), 302–312. https://doi.org/10.1016/j.jogn.2022.02.002

Yang, R., Chen, D., Wang, H., & Xu, X. (2022). Experiences of mothers of NICU preterm infants in milk management out of the hospital: A qualitative study. *International Breastfeeding Journal*, *17*(1), 95. https://doi.org/10.1186/s13006-022-00540-2

Yu, X., Chau, J. P. C., Huo, L., Li, X., Wang, D., Wu, H., & Zhang, Y. (2022). The effects of a nurse-led integrative medicine-based structured education program on self-management behaviors among individuals with newly diagnosed type 2 diabetes: A randomized controlled trial. *BMC Nursing*, *21*(1), 217. https://doi.org/10.1186/s12912-022-00970-7

Zhu, P., Ji, Q., Liu, X., Xu, T., Wu, Q., Wang, Y., Gao, X., & Zhou, Z. (2022). "I'm walking on eggshells": Challenges faced by mothers with breast cancer in interacting with adolescent daughters. *BMC Women's Health*, *22*(1), 385. https://doi.org/10.1186/s12905-022-01872-1

5 Literature Reviews: Finding and Critically Appraising Evidence

Learning objectives

1. Understand the steps involved in doing a literature review.
2. Identify bibliographic aids for retrieving research reports, and locate references for a research topic.
3. Understand the process of screening, abstracting, appraising, and organizing research evidence.
4. Evaluate the style, content, and organization of a literature review.

INTRODUCTION

A research **literature review** is a written synthesis and appraisal of evidence on a research problem. Researchers typically undertake a literature review as an early step in conducting a study. This chapter describes activities associated with literature reviews, including locating and critically appraising studies.

SOME LITERATURE REVIEW BASICS

Before discussing the steps involved in doing a research-based literature review, we briefly discuss some general issues.

Purposes of Research Literature Reviews

Healthcare professionals are undertaking many different types of research synthesis, several of which are specifically intended to support evidence-based practice. Grant and Booth (2009) identified 14 different types of synthesis. We described one type of synthesis (systematic reviews) in Chapter 2, and several others will be discussed in Chapter 30. In this chapter, we focus primarily on narrative literature reviews that researchers prepare during the conduct of a new study.

TIP A *narrative literature review* is one in which the findings from the studies under review are integrated using the judgments of the reviewers, rather than through statistical integration—as in a meta-analysis. Until meta-analytic techniques were developed, all reviews were narrative reviews.

Once a research problem and research questions have been identified, a thorough literature review is essential. Literature reviews provide researchers with information to guide a high-quality study, such as information about the following:

- The scope and complexity of the identified research problem (for the argument);
- What other researchers have found in relation to the research question;

- The quality and quantity of existing evidence;
- The contexts and locales in which research has been conducted;
- The characteristics of the people who have served as study participants;
- Theoretical underpinnings of completed studies;
- Methodologic strategies that have been used to address the question; and
- Gaps in the existing evidence base—the type of new evidence that is needed.

This list suggests that a good literature review requires thorough familiarity with the available evidence. As Garrard (2020) has advised, you must strive to *own* the literature on a topic to be confident of preparing a high-quality review.

The term "reviewing the literature" is often used to refer to the *process* of identifying, locating, and reading relevant sources of research evidence—that is, conducting a literature review. However, researchers will ultimately need to summarize what they have learned in written form. The length of the product depends on its purpose. Written narrative literature reviews may take the following forms:

- *A review embedded in a research report.* Literature reviews in the introduction to a research report provide readers with an overview of existing evidence and contribute to the argument for new research. These reviews are usually only two to three double-spaced pages, and so only key studies can be cited. The emphasis is on summarizing and critiquing an overall body of evidence and demonstrating the need for a new study.
- *A review in a research proposal.* A literature review in a proposal (often, to request financial support) provides context and illuminates the rationale for new research. The length of such reviews is specified in proposal guidelines; sometimes it is just a few pages. When this is the case, the review must reflect expertise on the topic in a succinct fashion.
- *A review in a thesis or dissertation.* Dissertations in the traditional format (see Chapter 32) often include a thorough, critical literature review. An entire chapter may be devoted to the review, and such chapters are often 20 to 30 pages long.

These reviews typically include an evaluation of the overall body of literature as well as critiques of key individual studies. They may also describe relevant theoretical foundations for the study.

In all three cases, the review is not simply a knowledge synthesis; the review provides a context for readers of the report or proposal and offers a justification for a new inquiry. Such reviews also can demonstrate the researcher's competence and thoroughness.

Additionally, nurses sometimes prepare freestanding narrative reviews that are not necessarily done in connection with a planned new study. A written review may be undertaken as a course requirement in graduate school or for publication in a journal. As an example, King et al. (2022) published a literature review on the impact of early parental loss on children's mental health. Such freestanding reviews are usually 15 to 25 pages long.

Literature Reviews in Qualitative Research

Quantitative researchers usually do an upfront literature review, but qualitative researchers have varying opinions about reviewing the literature before doing a new study. Some of the differences reflect viewpoints associated with qualitative research traditions.

Grounded theory researchers often collect and analyze their data before reviewing the literature. Researchers turn to the literature once the grounded theory is sufficiently developed, seeking to relate the theory to prior findings. Glaser (1978) warned that, "It's hard enough to generate one's own ideas without the 'rich' detailment provided by literature in the same field" (p. 31). Thus, grounded theory researchers may defer doing a literature review, but then later consider how previous research fits with or extends the emerging theory.

Phenomenologists often undertake a search for relevant materials at the outset of a study, looking in particular for experiential descriptions of the phenomenon being studied (Munhall, 2012). The purpose is to expand the researcher's understanding of the phenomenon from multiple perspectives, and this may include an examination of artistic sources in which the phenomenon is described (e.g., in novels or poetry).

Even though "ethnography starts with a conscious attitude of almost complete ignorance" (Spradley, 1979, p. 4), literature relating to the chosen cultural problem is often reviewed before data collection. A second, more thorough literature review is often done during data analysis and interpretation so that findings can be compared with previous findings.

Regardless of tradition, if funding is sought for a qualitative project, an upfront literature review is usually necessary. Proposal reviewers need to understand the context for a proposed study when deciding whether it should be funded.

Sources for a Research Review

Written **source materials** vary in their quality and content. In performing a literature review, you will have to decide what to read and what to include in a written review. You may begin your search with broad reference sources on a topic (e.g., textbooks), but ultimately you will mostly be retrieving information from articles published in professional journals.

Findings from prior completed studies are the most important type of information for a research review. You should rely mostly on **primary source** research reports, which are descriptions of studies written by the researchers who conducted them.

> **TIP** Study *protocols* are an additional type of primary source—they are descriptions of the design and methods for studies that are underway but have not yet been completed. These protocols, which are available in *registries* and sometimes in journals, allow researchers to understand what new evidence will *become* available and hence can help you avoid unwanted duplication.

Secondary sources are descriptions of studies prepared by someone other than the original researcher. Literature reviews, for example, are secondary sources. If reviews are recent, they are very useful because they provide an overview of the topic and a valuable bibliography. Secondary sources are not substitutes for primary sources because they typically fail to provide much detail about studies and may not be completely objective.

In addition to research reports, your search may yield nonresearch references, such as case reports, anecdotes, editorials, or clinical descriptions. Nonresearch materials may broaden understanding of a problem, demonstrate a need for research, or describe aspects of clinical practice. These writings may help in formulating research ideas, but they usually have limited utility in written research reviews because they do not address the central question: What is the current state of *evidence* on this research problem?

Primary and Secondary Questions for a Review

For free-standing literature reviews, reviewers may summarize evidence about a single focused question, such as *Do telehealth visits (I) improve patient satisfaction (O) in receiving follow-up care postoperatively (P)?* For those who are undertaking a literature review as part of a new study, the *primary question* for the literature review is the same as the research question for the new study. The researcher wants to know the following: What is the current state of knowledge on the question that I will be addressing in *my* study?

If you are doing a review for a new study, you inevitably will need to search for current evidence on several *secondary questions* because you need to develop an argument for the new study. An example will clarify this point.

Suppose that we were conducting a study to address the following question: *Among nurses working in hospitals (P), what characteristics of the nurses or their practice settings (I) are associated with their management of children's pain (O)?* Such a question might arise in the context of a perceived problem, such as a concern that nurses' treatment of children's pain is not always optimal. A simplified statement of the problem might be as follows:

Many children are hospitalized annually, and many hospitalized children experience high levels of pain. Although effective analgesic and nonpharmacologic methods of controlling children's pain exist, and although there are reliable methods of assessing children's pain, previous studies have found that nurses do not always manage children's pain effectively.

This rudimentary problem statement suggests several *secondary questions* for which up-to-date evidence needs to be found. Examples of such secondary questions include the following:

- How many children are hospitalized each year?
- What levels of pain do hospitalized children typically experience?
- How can pain in hospitalized children be reliably assessed?
- How knowledgeable are nurses about pain assessment and pain management strategies for children?

Thus, a literature review tends to be a multi-pronged task when it is done in preparation for a new study. It is important to identify all questions for which information from the research literature needs to be retrieved.

Major Steps and Strategies in a Narrative Literature Review

Conducting a literature review is a little like doing a full study, in the sense that reviewers start with a question, formulate and implement a plan for gathering information, and then analyze and interpret the information. The "findings" are then summarized in a written product.

Figure 5.1 outlines key steps in the literature review process. As the figure shows, there are several potential feedback loops, with opportunities to retrace earlier steps in search of more information. This chapter discusses each step, but some steps are elaborated in Chapter 30 in our discussion of systematic reviews.

Conducting a high-quality literature review is more than a mechanical exercise—it is an art and a science. Several qualities characterize a high-quality review. First, the review must be comprehensive, thorough, and up-to-date. To "own" the literature (Garrard, 2020), you must be determined to become an expert on your topic, which means that you need to be diligent in hunting down leads for possible sources of evidence.

TIP Locating all relevant information on a research question is like being a detective. The literature retrieval tools we discuss in this chapter are essential aids, but there inevitably needs to be some digging for the clues to evidence on a topic. Be prepared for sleuthing.

Second, a high-quality review is systematic. Decision rules should be clear, and criteria for including or excluding a study need to be explicit. This is because a third characteristic of a good review is that it is reproducible, which means that another diligent reviewer would be able to apply the same decision rules and criteria and come to similar conclusions about the evidence.

Another desirable attribute of a literature review is the absence of bias. This is more easily achieved when systematic rules for evaluating information

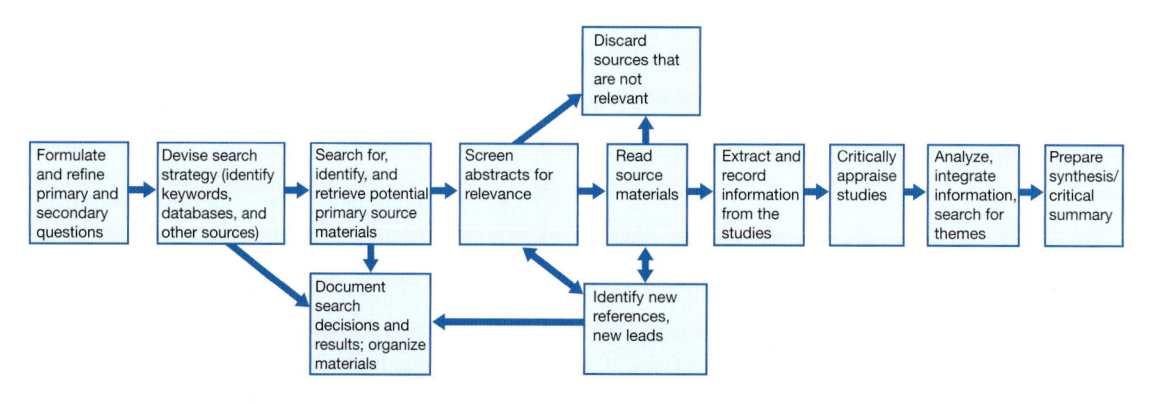

FIGURE 5.1 Flow of tasks in a literature review.

are followed or when a team of researchers participates in the review—as is almost always the case in systematic reviews. Finally, reviewers should strive for a review that is insightful and that is more than "the sum of its parts." Reviewers can contribute to knowledge through an astute synthesis of the evidence.

Doing a literature review is somewhat similar to doing a qualitative study; you will need a flexible and creative approach to "data collection." Leads for relevant studies should be pursued until "saturation" is achieved—that is, until your search strategies yield redundant information about studies to include. Finally, the analysis of your "data" will typically involve the identification of important themes in the literature.

Organization in Literature Reviews

The importance of being well organized in conducting a literature review cannot be overemphasized. As discussed in "Documentation in Literature Retrieval" later in this chapter, we encourage you to document all your decisions and products, and documentation needs to be maintained in an organized framework.

You may prefer to use traditional methods of searching, retrieving, and storing information. For example, you may retrieve a journal article, print or photocopy it, and write notes in the margin. If you do this, you will still need to develop a cataloging system that enables you to find a particular article (e.g., alphabetical filing by last name of the first author).

Increasingly, journal articles are retrieved as portable document files (PDFs) and read online using Adobe software, which permits you to highlight text passages and enter marginal comments. If this is your approach, you should create a folder on your computer or in the cloud to store these articles, naming each file in a manner that will allow you to easily locate it. For example, here is how we named the file storing the previously mentioned King et al. (2022) literature review: King2022NCYPBereavementChildren's MentalHealth.pdf. This file name indicates the last name of the first author, the year of publication, an abbreviation for the journal (NCYP = *Nursing Children and Young People*), and a brief phrase about the topic. This system would result in a document folder with articles listed alphabetically by the first authors' last names.

You may opt to use reference management software that will help you to stay organized—as well as help you retrieve articles, maintain a reference library and notes, insert citations into papers, and create a bibliography when you write up your review. Popular reference management software that that you can use with either Windows for PCs or Macs includes EndNote (free for the Basic version), Mendeley or Zotero (each also free), and RefWorks. Many other reference management software packages are available (for example, see https://en.wikipedia.org/wiki/Comparison_of_reference_management_software).

There is no one way to organize the literature review. However, it is wise to think ahead about the various components of your literature review effort and to have a plan for how to organize them—most likely this will involve the creation of various file folders that will be stored on your computer or in the cloud. For example, if you are not using reference management software, you should create a master folder (e.g., labeled "Mental_Health_Children"), with multiple subfolders. For example, one subfolder could store the source documents (e.g., the PDF journal article files), another could store documentation of your search strategy and results, and another subfolder could save drafts of your actual literature review.

Another effective strategy to organize the literature is by using a spreadsheet. You can import the relevant information into a spreadsheet: title; whether it is a completed manuscript or abstract only; the language in which it is written; authors; sample size; method; and findings. Others rely on software programs to help organize, screen, and create a flowchart. One popular software system is Covidence, but there are several. A listing of these is available here: https://guides.library.illinois.edu/c.php?g=1143681&p=8344820.

Another organizational tool—one that is essential for the reporting of a systematic review—is the

Preferred Reporting Items for Systematic Reviews and Meta-Analyses flow chart that documents your progress in identifying, retrieving, screening, and selecting source materials. Figure 5.2 presents an example of such a flow chart with fictitious numbers (*n=*) shown in each box. This figure shows that the reviewer started with 400 possible source documents, of which only 15 were used in the final literature review.

LOCATING RELEVANT LITERATURE FOR A RESEARCH REVIEW

As shown in Figure 5.1, an early step in a literature review is devising a strategy to locate relevant studies. The ability to locate research documents on a topic is an important skill that requires adaptability. Sophisticated new search strategies and tools are being introduced regularly. We urge you to consult with librarians, colleagues, or faculty for suggestions. Reference librarians in health libraries are especially valuable and often serve on teams conducting systematic reviews.

Formulating a Search Strategy

There are many ways to search for research evidence. Searching is inevitably an iterative process that evolves as you discover new "leads" based on information you have already retrieved.

Search Strategy Options

Cooper (2017) has identified several search strategies, one of which we describe in some detail in this chapter: searching for references in **bibliographic databases**. Database searches, which can be done efficiently from computers and tablets, are likely to yield the largest number of research references—indeed, sometimes the yield can be overwhelming. Databases are searched primarily for key variables (e.g., pain management) but can also be searched for the names of researchers who have played a key role in a field.

Another approach, called the *ancestry approach* (also called *snowballing, footnote chasing,* or *pearl growing*), involves using references cited in recent relevant studies to track down earlier research on the same topic (the "ancestors"). This is an ongoing process that can be used to not only identify earlier

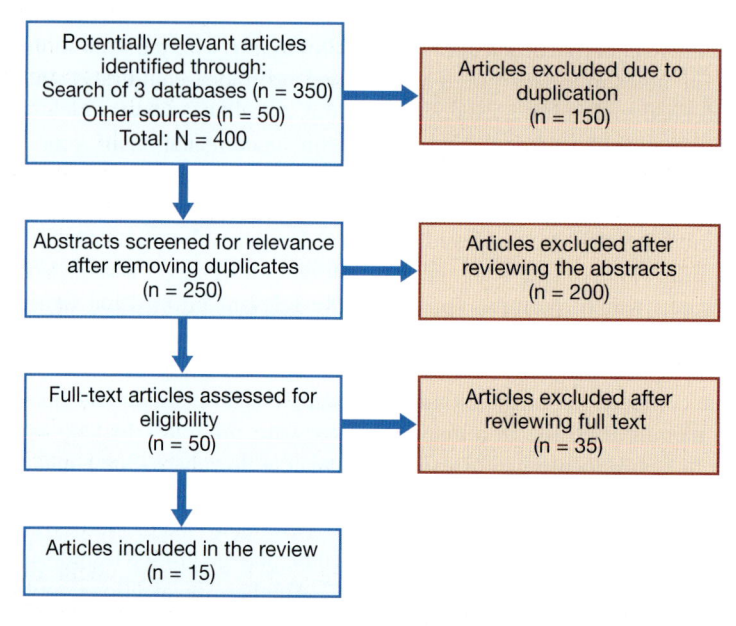

FIGURE 5.2 Example of a flowchart documenting literature search progress.

relevant studies but also to discover new search terms for subsequent electronic searches.

A third method, the *descendancy approach*, is to find a pivotal early study and to search forward in citation indexes to find more recent studies ("descendants") that cited the key study. Other strategies exist for tracking down what is called the *gray literature*, which refers to studies with more limited distribution, such as conference papers, unpublished reports, and so on. We describe these strategies in Chapter 30 on systematic reviews. If your intent is to "own" the literature, then you will likely want to adopt many of these strategies.

TIP You may be tempted to begin a literature search through an Internet search engine, such as Google, Yahoo, or Bing. Such a search is likely to yield several "hits" on your topic but is unlikely to give you full bibliographic information on relevant *research*. However, such searches can provide useful leads for *search terms*. Also, an Internet search may be the appropriate route for finding answers to secondary questions, such as: How many children are hospitalized annually? This information is more likely to be found in government reports, which are available online, than in research articles.

Eligibility Criteria Specifications

Search plans also involve decisions about the criteria that would make a study eligible for your review. These decisions need to be explicit to guide your search of bibliographic databases. Search limits are most often managed in databases through *filters* (or *limiters* in some bibliographic software).

If you are not multilingual, you may need to constrain your search to studies written in your own language. You may want to limit your search to studies conducted within a certain time frame (e.g., within the past 15 years). You may also want to exclude studies with certain types of participants. For instance, in our example of a literature search about nurses' management of children's pain, we might want to exclude studies in which the children were neonates.

Constraining your search might help you to avoid irrelevant material, but be cautious about putting too many restrictions on your search, especially initially. You can always make decisions to exclude studies at a later point.

TIP Be sure not to limit your search to articles exclusively in the nursing literature (e.g., in the nursing subset of records in the database called PubMed). Researchers in many disciplines engage in research relevant to nursing. Also, many nurse researchers publish in nonnursing journals, increasingly as members of interprofessional teams. Moreover, in some databases (e.g., PubMed), some journals with many articles contributed by nurse researchers are not coded as being in the nursing subset (e.g., *Qualitative Health Research*, *Birth*), whereas some journals that are in the nursing subset have articles mostly *not* written by nurse authors (e.g., *Journal of Wound Care*).

Identifying Keywords

Reviewers seeking articles for their reviews begin with a set of search terms, often called **keywords**. Thus, an important early task is to identify and make a written list of the keywords that will be used to search bibliographic databases. The keyword list will be augmented as your search proceeds.

Traditionally, the keywords are your main research variables. Many researchers use the PICO formulation (population, intervention/influence, comparison, outcome) discussed in Chapter 2 as keywords for a literature search, although this may not always be the best strategy for systematic reviews (see Chapter 30).

In developing a list of keywords, it is important to include synonyms and to think broadly about related terms. For example, if we were searching for articles on *teenage smoking*, you should consider other terms for teenage (e.g., *adolescent, children, youth*) and for smoking (e.g., *tobacco, cigarettes*). The use of a thesaurus (available in word processing software) for identifying synonyms is recommended—but take note of keywords specified by researchers themselves in articles you locate.

Searching Bibliographic Databases

Reviewers typically begin by searching bibliographic databases that can be accessed by computer. The databases contain entries for millions of journal articles, and the articles are coded by professional indexers to facilitate retrieval. For example, articles may be coded for language used (e.g., English), subject matter (e.g., pain), journal subset (e.g., nursing), and so on. Some databases can be accessed free of charge (e.g., PubMed, Google Scholar [GS]), whereas others are sold commercially—but they are often available through hospital or university libraries. Most database programs are user-friendly, offering menu-driven systems with on-screen support so that retrieval can proceed with minimal instruction.

Getting Started With a Bibliographic Database

Before searching an electronic database, you should become familiar with the features of the software used to access the database. The software gives you options for limiting your search, combining the results of two searches, saving your search, and sending you notifications of new citations relevant to your search. Most programs have tutorials that can improve the efficiency and effectiveness of your search.

In most databases, there are two major strategies for searching. One method is to search for standardized **subject headings** (subject codes) that are assigned by indexers (usually professionals with master's degrees or higher in relevant disciplines). The subject headings differ from one database to another. It is useful to learn about the relevant subject codes because they offer a path to retrieving articles that use different words to describe the same concept. Another major advantage is that indexers code the articles based on a reading of the entire article (not just the abstract), and they code for *meaning* and not just words. Subject codes for databases can be located in the database's thesaurus or reference tools.

An alternative strategy is to enter your own keywords into a search field. Such a search is an important supplement to searching using the database's controlled vocabulary because indexers are not infallible. However, such keyword searches are limited to searching for words in the article's title or abstract (*not in the full text*), and so if concepts are not mentioned in the title or abstract, the article will not be retrieved.

Most bibliographic software has automatic term mapping capabilities. *Mapping* is a feature that facilitates a search using your own keywords. The software translates ("maps") the keywords you enter into the most plausible subject codes. Nevertheless, it is important to undertake both a keyword search and a subject code search because they yield overlapping but nonidentical results.

General Database Search Features

Some features of an electronic search are similar across databases. One feature is the use of **Boolean operators** to expand or delimit a search. Three widely used Boolean operators are AND, OR, and NOT (in all caps for some databases). The operator AND delimits a search. If we searched for *pain* AND *child,* the software would retrieve only records that have both terms. The operator *OR* expands the search: *pain* OR *child* could be used in a search to retrieve records with either term. Finally, *NOT* narrows a search: *pain NOT child* would retrieve all records with pain that did not include the term child. Note that when using multiple Boolean operators, they are processed from left to right. For example, the search phrase *teenage* AND *smoking* OR *cigarettes* would retrieve (1) records that include both teenage and smoking and (2) *all* records with cigarettes, whether or not the article is about teenage smokers. Parentheses can be used to reorder the terms: *teenage* AND (*smoking* OR *cigarettes*). Boolean operators also can be used to combine searches for keyword terms and the last names of prominent researchers in a field, for example, *teenage* AND (*smoking* OR *cigarettes*) AND Kulbok (a researcher).

> **TIP** Be extremely careful using the "NOT" operator because you run the risk of inadvertently removing relevant articles. For example, if you were searching for studies of female teenage smokers and used "NOT male" in the search field, the software would remove any article that included both male and female participants.

Truncation symbols are another useful tool for searching databases. These symbols vary from one database to another, but their function is to expand the search. A **truncation symbol** (often an asterisk, *) expands a search term to include all forms of a root word. For example, a search for *child** would instruct the computer to search for any word that begins with "child" such as children, childhood, or childrearing. For each database, it is important to learn what these special symbols are and how they work. For example, many databases require at least three letters at the beginning of a search term before a truncation symbol can be used (e.g., *ca** would not be allowed).

Some databases (but not PubMed) allow for a **wildcard symbol**—often a question mark—that can be inserted into the middle of a search term to allow for alternative spellings. For example, in databases that allow wildcards, a search for *behavior* would retrieve records with either *behavior* or *behaviour.*

Although truncation and wildcard symbols can sometimes be useful, they have one major drawback: in most databases, the use of special symbols turns off a software's mapping feature. For example, a search for *child** would retrieve records in which any form of "child" appeared in text fields, but it would not map any of these concepts onto the database's subject heading codes. It may be preferable to use a Boolean operator to list all terms of interest (e.g., *child* OR *children*), which would look for either term in a text word search of the title and abstract *and* would map onto the appropriate subject code.

Another issue concerns phrase searching in which you want words to be kept together (e.g., *blood pressure*). Some bibliometric software would treat this as *blood AND pressure* and would search for records with both terms somewhere in text fields, even if they are not contiguous. Quotation marks sometimes can be used to ensure that the words are searched in combination, as in "blood pressure." PubMed recommends, however, that you do not use quotation marks until you have first tried a search without them. PubMed automatically searches for phrases during its mapping process (i.e., in searching for relevant subject heading codes).

Key Electronic Databases for Nurse Researchers

Two bibliographic databases that are especially useful for nurse researchers are the **C**umulative **I**ndex to **N**ursing and **A**llied **H**ealth **L**iterature (CINAHL) and **Med**ical Literature On-**Line** (MEDLINE, accessed through PubMed), which we discuss in the next sections. We also briefly discuss GS. Other potentially useful bibliographic databases/search engines for nurses include the following:

- **B**ritish **N**ursing **I**ndex (BNI)
- Cochrane Central Register of Controlled Trials (CENTRAL)
- Cochrane Database of Systematic Reviews
- **D**atabase **o**f **P**romoting **H**ealth **E**ffectiveness **R**eviews (DoPHER)
- **E**xcerpta **M**edica data**base** (EMBASE)
- **H**ealth **a**nd **P**sychosocial **I**nstruments database (HaPI)
- **Psyc**hology **Info**rmation (PsycINFO)

In addition, the ISI Web of Knowledge and Scopus are two *citation indexes* for retrieving articles that cite a source article.

Note that a search strategy that works well in one database does not always produce good results in another. Thus, it is important to explore strategies in each database and to understand how each database is structured—for example, what subject codes are used, how they are organized in a hierarchy, and what special features are available.

> **TIP** In the following sections, we provide specific information about using CINAHL and MEDLINE via PubMed. Note, however, that databases and the software through which they are accessed change periodically, and so our instructions may not be up to date.

Cumulative Index to Nursing and Allied Health Literature

CINAHL is an important bibliographic database; it covers references to virtually all English-language nursing and allied health journals, and includes books, dissertations, and selected conference proceedings in nursing and allied health fields. There are several versions of the CINAHL database (e.g., CINAHL Plus, CINAHL Complete), each with somewhat different features relating to full text availability and journal coverage.

The CINAHL database indexes material from more than 3,700 journals dating from 1981 and contains more than 6 million records. In addition to providing bibliographic information for references (i.e., author, title, journal, year of publication, volume, and page numbers), CINAHL provides abstracts of most citations. Links to the actual article are sometimes provided. We illustrate features of CINAHL, but note that some features may be different at your institution.

At the outset, you might begin with a "basic search" by simply entering keywords or phrases relevant to your primary question. As you begin to enter your term into the search box, autocomplete suggestions will display, and you can click on the one that is the best match. In the basic search screen, you can limit your search in a number of ways, for example, limiting the records retrieved to those with certain features (e.g., only ones with abstracts; only research articles); to a specific range of publication dates (e.g., only those from 2010 to the present); or to those in specific languages (e.g., English). The search screen allows you to expand your search by clicking an option labeled "Apply related words."

As an example, suppose we were interested in recent research on the physical and behavioral characteristics of older women who are homeless in the United States, as conducted by a team that included one of the authors of this book (Dickins et al., 2021). If we enter *homeless*, the search yields 10,108 papers, but if we add *AND older women*, the search yields 52 papers. If we then conduct the search using *homeless AND older women AND USA*, the number of papers is further reduced to 11.

An important feature of CINAHL is that it helps you find other relevant references once a good one has been found. Embedded links allow you to click on any of the authors' names to see if they published other related articles. There is also a sidebar link in each record called *Times Cited in This Database* (if there has been a citation), with which you could retrieve records for articles that had cited this paper (for a descendancy search). Another link is labeled *Find Similar Results*, which suggests other relevant references.

In CINAHL, you can also explore the structure of the database's thesaurus to get additional leads for searching. The toolbar at the top of the screen has a tab called *CINAHL Headings*. When you click on this tab, you can enter a term of interest in the *Browse* field and select one of three options: *Term Begins With, Term Contains*, or *Relevancy Ranked* (which is the default). For example, if we entered *homeless women* and then clicked on Browse, we would be shown the major subject headings relating to homeless women; we could then search the database for any of the listed subject codes.

The full records for the 52 references would then be displayed on the monitor in a Search Results list. There is a "sort" option at the top of the list that allows you to sort the references based on several criteria, such as publication date, author's last name, and relevance. From the Results list, we could place promising references into a folder for later scrutiny by clicking on a file icon in the upper right corner of each entry. We could then save the folder, print it, or export it to reference manager software such as EndNote.

An example of an abridged CINAHL record entry for a study identified through the search on the physical and behavioral characteristics of aging homeless women is presented in Figure 5.3. The record begins with the article title, the authors' names and affiliation, and source. The source indicates the following:

- Name of the journal *Archives of Psychiatric Nursing*
- Year and month of publication August 2019
- Volume 33
- Issue 4
- Page numbers 400 to 406

The record also shows the major and minor CINAHL subject headings that were coded by the indexers. Any of these headings could have been used to retrieve this reference. Note that the subject headings include substantive codes (e.g., homeless, women) methodologic codes (e.g., case study, qualitative), person characteristic codes (e.g., middle-aged), and a location code (USA). Next, the abstract for the study is shown. Based on the abstract, we might be able to decide whether this reference was pertinent. Each entry shows an accession number that is the unique identifier for

Title:	A picture of the older homeless female veteran: A qualitative, case study analysis.
Authors:	Kenny, Deborah J.; Yoder, Linda H.
Affiliation:	Helen and Arthur E. Johnson College of Nursing and Health Sciences, University of Colorado, Colorado Springs, 1420 Austin Bluffs Parkway, Colorado Springs, CO 80918, USA; University of Texas at Austin School of Nursing, 1710 Red River, Austin, TX 78712, USA.
Source:	Archives of Psychiatric Nursing (ARCH PSYCHIATR NURS), Aug2019; 33(4): 400-406. (7p)
Publication Type:	Journal Article - research
Language:	English
Major Subjects:	Homeless Persons -- In Middle Age Veterans Women
Minor Subjects:	Human; Female; Middle Age; United States; Qualitative Studies; Case Studies; Interviews; Descriptive Statistics; Sexual Abuse; Substance Abuse; Coping; Mental Health; Funding Source
Abstract:	Homelessness among female veterans is increasing and expected to rise further as more women enter the military. Very few studies qualitatively describe female homeless veterans' needs from their own perspective. Homeless female veterans' perceptions of their homelessness and what they believe is needed for independence and self-sustenance was examined. OA qualitative interpretive interview design was used and findings are reported as a case study. A definitive picture emerged of a homeless female veteran, bounded by several factors they all had in common including age, family upheaval, mental health diagnoses, substance abuse, trauma, and need for information and networking.
Journal Subset:	Core Nursing; Double Blind Peer Reviewed; Editorial Board Reviewed; Expert Peer Reviewed; Nursing; Peer Reviewed; USA
ISSN:	0883-9417
MEDLINE info:	NLM UID: 8708535
Grant Information:	This work was supported through the Carole Schoffstall Endowed Professorship through the University of Colorado, Colorado Springs.
Entry Date:	20190708
Revision Date:	20190708
DOI:	10.1016/j.apnu.2019.05.005
Accession No:	137324343

FIGURE 5.3 Example of a record from a CINAHL (Cumulative Index to Nursing and Allied Health Literature) search. (Excerpt from Kenny, D. J., & Yoder, L. H. (2019). A picture of the older homeless female veteran: A qualitative, case study analysis. *Archives of Psychiatric Nursing*, 33(4), 400–406, with permission of Elsevier.)

each record in the CINAHL database, as well as other identifying numbers.

An important feature of CINAHL helps you to find other relevant references once a good one has been found. In Figure 5.3 you can see that the record offers many embedded links on which you can click. For example, you could click on any of the authors' names to see if they published other related articles. Although not visible in Figure 5.3, there is also a sidebar link in each record called *Times Cited in This Database* (if there has been a citation), with which you could retrieve records for articles that had cited this paper (for a descendancy search). Another link is labeled *Find Similar Results*, which suggests other relevant references.

In CINAHL, you can also explore the structure of the database's thesaurus to get additional leads for searching. The toolbar at the top of the screen has a tab called *CINAHL Headings*. When you click on this tab, you can enter a term of interest in the *Browse* field and select one of three options: *Term Begins With*, *Term Contains*, or *Relevancy Ranked* (which is the default). For example, if we entered *pain management* and then clicked on Browse, we would be shown the major subject headings relating to pain management; we could then search the database for any of the listed subject codes.

> **TIP** Note that the keywords we used to illustrate this simplified search (homeless, women) would not be adequate for a comprehensive retrieval of studies relevant to our review question. For example, we would want to search for several additional terms (e.g., *middle-aged*).

The MEDLINE Database and PubMed

The MEDLINE database was developed by the U.S. National Library of Medicine and is widely recognized as the premier source for bibliographic coverage of the biomedical literature. MEDLINE covers about 5,200 medical, nursing, and health journals published in about 70 countries and contains more than 27 million records dating back to the mid-1940s. In 1999, abstracts of systematic reviews from the Cochrane Collaboration became available through MEDLINE.

The MEDLINE database can be accessed through a commercial vendor, but it can be accessed for free through the PubMed website (http://www.ncbi.nlm.nih.gov/PubMed). This means that anyone, anywhere in the world with Internet access can search for journal articles, and thus PubMed is a lifelong resource. PubMed has excellent tutorials, including a 30-minute tutorial specifically for nurses (PubMed for Nurses). PubMed includes all references in the MEDLINE library plus additional references, such as those that have not yet been indexed.

On the Home page of PubMed, you can launch a basic search that looks for your keywords in text fields of the record. PubMed, like CINAHL, has an autocomplete feature that offers suggestions as you begin to enter your terms.

> **TIP** On the PubMed home page, you can also launch a Clinical Query search, which is a particularly useful tool for searching for evidence in the context of an evidence-based practice (EBP) inquiry.

MEDLINE uses a controlled vocabulary called **MeSH** (Medical Subject Headings) to index articles. Indexers assign as many MeSH headings as appropriate to cover content and features of the article—typically 5 to 15 codes. You can learn about relevant MeSH terms by clicking on the "MeSH database" link on the Home page (under the heading *More Resources*). If, for example, we searched the MeSH database for "pain," we would find that Pain is a MeSH subject heading (a definition is provided) and there are 60 related categories—for example, "Cancer pain," "Back pain," and "Headache." Each category has numerous subheadings, such as "Complications," "Etiology," and "Nursing."

If you begin with a keyword search, you can see how your term mapped onto MeSH terms by looking in the right-hand panel for a section labeled *Search Details*. For example, if we entered "children" as our keyword in the search field of the initial screen, Search Details would show us that PubMed searched for all references that have "child" or "children" in text fields of the database record, *and* it also searched for all references that had been coded "child" as a subject heading because "child" is a MeSH subject heading.

If we did a PubMed search of MEDLINE similar to the one we described earlier for CINAHL on aging homeless women, we would find that a simple search for *homeless* would yield about **2,153** records; a search for *homeless AND women AND middle-aged* would yield nearly 741 records. We can place restrictions on the search using filters that are shown in the left sidebar of the screen. If we limited our search to full text entries, written in English, and published between 2010 and 2023, the search would yield about 415 records. Thus, PubMed search yielded more references than the CINAHL search, in part, because MEDLINE indexes more journals. Another factor is that PubMed does not limit the search to research articles because PubMed does not have a generic category that distinguishes research articles from nonresearch articles.

From the Search Results page, we would then click on links to the citations that suggest a relevant article; this would bring up a new screen that provides the abstract for the article and further details. Figure 5.4 shows the full citation and abstract for the same study we located earlier in CINAHL. Beneath the abstract, the display presents the MeSH terms that were indexed for this study. (Those marked with an asterisk, such as Ill-Housed Persons/psychology, are MeSH subject headings that are a major focus of the article). As you can see, the MeSH terms are different than the subject headings for the same article in CINAHL. As with CINAHL, you can click on highlighted record entries (authors' names and MeSH terms) for possible new leads.

In the right panel of the screen for specific PubMed records, there is a list of *Similar Articles*, which is a useful feature once you have found a study that is a good exemplar of what you are seeking. Further down in the right panel, PubMed provides a list of any articles in the PubMed Central database that have cited this study. PubMed Central is a repository for full-text articles, so you could immediately download any of the articles that appeared in this list. You can also save articles that look pertinent to your review by clicking the button "Add to Favorites" at the top of the right panel.

A useful feature of PubMed is that it provides access to new research by including citations to forthcoming articles in many journals. The records for these not yet published articles have the tag "Epub ahead of print."

TIP Justesen and colleagues (2021) found that the combinations of MEDLINE/PubMed and CINAHL and MEDLINE/PubMed, CINAHL, and Embase resulted in the largest number of references included in systematic reviews of qualitative research regarding diabetes mellitus.

Google Scholar

Launched in 2004, Google Scholar (GS) has become an increasingly popular bibliographic search engine. GS includes articles in journals from scholarly publishers in all disciplines, as well as scholarly books, technical reports, and other documents. GS is accessible free of charge over the Internet. Like other bibliographic search engines, GS allows users to search by topic, by a title, and by author and uses Boolean operators and other search conventions. Like PubMed and CINAHL, GS has a *Cited By* feature for a descendancy search and a *Related Articles* feature to locate other sources with relevant content to an identified article. Because of its expanded coverage of material, GS can provide access to many free full-text publications.

Unlike other scholarly databases, GS does not order the retrieved references by publication date (i.e., most recent ones first). The ordering of records in GS is determined by an algorithm that puts most weight on the number of times a reference has been cited; this in turn means that older references are usually earlier on the list. Another disadvantage of GS is that the search filters are fairly limited.

In the field of medicine, GS has generated considerable controversy, with some arguing that it is of similar utility and quality to popular medical databases and others urging caution in depending primarily on GS (e.g., Bramer et al., 2013; Gusenbauer & Haddaway, 2020). Morshed and Hayden (2020) compared Google Web, GS, PubMed, and PubMed Clinical Queries' search tools for answering clinical questions in the emergency department. PubMed Clinical Queries search had the most relevant hits.

The capabilities and features of GS may improve in the years ahead, but it is not recommended to use GS exclusively. For a full literature review, we think it is best to combine searches using GS with searches of other databases. We note, however, that GS has been of particular interest in efforts to retrieve the so-called *gray literature* (Haddaway et al., 2015).

TIP For most reviews, other resources beyond bibliographic databases should be considered. Other sources include government reports, clinical trial registries (e.g., ClinicalTrials.gov), and records of studies that are in progress such as in NIH RePORTER, which is a searchable database of biomedical projects funded by the U.S. government.

Case Reports > Arch Psychiatr Nurs, 2019 Aug; 33(4):400-406. doi: 10.1016/j.apnu.2019.05.005. Epub 2019 May 22.

A picture of the older homeless female veteran: A qualitative, case study analysis

Deborah J Kenny[1], Linda H Yoder[2]

Affiliations +expand
PMID: 31280786 DOI: 10.1016/j.apnu.2019.05.005
Free article

Abstract:

Background: Homelessness among female veterans is increasing and expected to rise further as more women enter the military. Very few studies qualitatively describe female homeless veterans' needs from their own perspective.

Purpose: Homeless female veterans' perceptions of their homelessness and what they believe is needed for independence and self-sustenance was examined.

Methods: OA qualitative interpretive interview design was used and findings are reported as a case study.

Results: A definitive picture emerged of a homeless female veteran, bounded by several factors they all had in common including age, family upheaval, mental health diagnoses, substance abuse, trauma, and need for information and networking.

Keywords: Homeless persons; Veterans; Vulnerable Populations; Women.

Copyright © 2019 The Authors. Published by Elsevier Inc. All rights reserved.

PubMed Disclaimer

Publication types
- Case Reports
- Research Support, Non-U.S. Gov't

MeSH Terms
- Adult Survivors of Child Abuse / psychology
- Female
- Humans
- Ill-Housed Persons / psychology*
- Middle Aged
- Qualitative Research
- Sex Offenses / psychology
- Southwestern United States
- Substance-Related Disorders / psychology*
- Veterans / psychology*
- Vulnerable Populations

Publication types
MedGen

LinkOut - more resources

Full Text Sources
ClinicalKey Nursing
Elsevier Science
Ovid Technologies, Inc.

Medical
MedlinePlus Consumer Health Information
MedlinePlus Health Information

FIGURE 5.4 Example of a record from a PubMed search. (Excerpt from Kenny, D. J., & Yoder, L. H. (2019). A picture of the older homeless female veteran: A qualitative, case study analysis. *Archives of Psychiatric Nursing, 33*(4), 400–406, with permission of Elsevier.)

Screening and Gathering References

Screening references for relevance is a multiphase process. The first screen is the title of the article itself. For example, suppose our study question was: *Among children in public schools with asthma, what is the impact of disease management knowledge on their asthma-related outcomes?* The PubMed search for *asthma management AND child AND nurse* yielded about 699 references in PubMed. The title of one article identified in this search was "African American parents'/guardians' health literacy and self-efficacy and their child's level of asthma control." Based on this title, we could conclude that this article (which was retrieved because the name of the journal in which it was published included the word "Child," one of our keywords) would provide no evidence about the knowledge needed to influence children's asthma management.

Once this initial screening is completed and the various search lists are also purged of duplicates, we would then examine the abstracts of the remaining references. When there is no abstract, or when the abstract is ambiguous as to its relevance to your review, it is usually necessary to screen the full article. During the screening, keep in mind that some articles judged to be not relevant for your primary question may be useful for a secondary question.

The next step is to retrieve the full text of references you think may have value for your review. If you are affiliated with an institution, you may have online access to most full-text articles, which you should download and file. If you are not so fortunate, more effort will be required to obtain the full-text articles. Consulting with a librarian is a good strategy.

The **open-access journal** movement is gaining momentum in healthcare publishing. Open-access journals provide articles free of charge online, regardless of any institutional subscriptions. Some journals have a hybrid format in which most articles are *not* open-access, but some individual articles *are* designated as open-access. Bibliographic databases indicate which articles are open-access, and for these articles, the full text can be retrieved by clicking on a link. (In PubMed, the link to click on states "Free Article" or "Free PMC article.")

When an article is not available to you online, you may be able to access it by communicating with the lead author. Bibliographic databases usually provide an email address for lead authors. Another alternative is to go to *scholarly collaboration network* websites such as *Research Gate* or *Academia.edu* and do a search for a particular author. Authors sometimes upload articles onto their profile for access by others. If an article has not been uploaded, these network sites provide a mechanism for you to send the author a message so that you can request an article to be sent to you directly.

Documentation in Literature Retrieval

Given your goal is to "own" the literature, you will be using a variety of databases, keywords, subject headings, authors' names, and search strategies in an effort to pursue all leads. As you meander through the complex world of research information, you will likely lose track of your efforts if you do not document your actions from the outset.

It is advisable to use word processing, spreadsheet, or reference manager software to record your search strategies and search results. You should make note of information such as names of the databases searched; limits put on your search; specific keywords, subject headings, or authors used to direct the search; studies used to inaugurate a "Related Articles" or "descendancy" search; websites visited; links pursued; authors contacted to request further information or copies of articles not readily available; and any other information that would help you keep track of what you have done—including information about the dates your searches were undertaken. Part of your strategy usually can be documented by saving your search history from bibliographic databases. Completing a flow chart such as the one shown in Figure 5.2 is recommended if your goal is to publish a freestanding review.

By documenting your actions, you will be able to conduct a more efficient search—that is, you will not inadvertently duplicate a strategy you have already pursued. Documentation will also help you to assess what else needs to be tried—where to go next in your search. Finally, documenting your efforts is a step in ensuring that your literature review is reproducible.

EXTRACTING AND RECORDING INFORMATION

Once you have a set of useful source materials, you need a strategy for making sense of the information. If a literature review is fairly simple, it may be sufficient to jot down notes about key features of the studies under review and to use these notes as the basis for the synthesis.

Many literature reviews are sufficiently complex that a systematic process for extracting and recording information must be developed. In the past, researchers used paper-based data extraction forms to record information about each reference. The use of word processing or spreadsheet software is advantageous, however, because then the forms can be easily searched and sorted. We call them *data extraction forms* because, in a review, the "data" are the information from each study. The data extraction forms are the critical bridge between the information in the original research reports and the synthesis of evidence by reviewers.

An approach that is gaining in popularity is the creation of two-dimensional data collection forms (matrices or *evidence summary tables*) in which rows are used for individual studies and columns are used to insert relevant data about each study, such as sample characteristics, methodologic features, and results. Two-dimensional tables can provide insights into important "themes" in the data across studies.

Information to Extract

It is wise to record key information for each study in a systematic way. Regardless of what approach is used to record data, reviewers should decide in advance what information about each study is important. The key elements will vary from one review to the next, but you should have, as a goal, the creation of a file in which each study in the review is abstracted for a consistent set of features.

Box 5.1 presents a list of some elements that could be considered for your data extraction forms. Not all these elements are needed for each review, and for other reviews, additional elements are likely to be needed. Although many terms in this table may not be familiar to you yet, you will learn about them in later chapters.

Once you have decided on the elements you wish to use in your data extraction form, you should pilot test it with a sample of studies. If you discover later in the extraction process that other elements are needed, you would have to go back to every completed article to retrieve the new information.

We encourage the use of two-dimensional data extraction forms, but you may prefer using a separate form to extract information for each study.

Coding the Studies for Key Variables

In systematic reviews, the review team almost always develops coding systems to support statistical analyses of study findings. Coding may not be necessary in less formal reviews, but coding certain elements can be helpful in organizing the review, and so we offer some suggestions and an example.

We find it useful to code study findings for key variables (quantitative) or themes (qualitative). In our earlier example about the physical and behavioral characteristics of women who were homeless, the independent variables are the demographic characteristics and the dependent variables are the physical and behavioral characteristics. We can assign codes to each type of factor. We find it useful to code study findings for key variables (quantitative) or themes (qualitative). The results of each study can then be coded. You can record these codes in data extraction forms, but it is also useful to note the codes in the margins of the articles themselves, so you can easily find the information. An example of a coding

BOX 5.1 Information to Consider for Data Extraction in a Literature Review

Source
- Citation
- Contact details of lead author

Methods
- Study design
  - Level of evidence

Recruitment and sampling
- Research tradition (qualitative)
- Longitudinal or cross-sectional
- Methods of bias control (e.g., blinding)
- Methods of enhancing trustworthiness (qualitative)
- Statistical analysis
- Type of thematic analysis

Participants
- Number of participants
  - Power analysis information

Setting
- Key characteristics of the sample
  - Age
  - Sex
  - Ethnicity/race
  - Socioeconomic
  - Diagnosis/disease
  - Comorbidities
- Country
- Method of sample selection
- Attrition (percent dropped out)

Intervention/Independent variable(s)
- Independent variable
  - Intervention or influence
  - Comparison
- Number of (intervention) groups
- Specific intervention (e.g., components of a complex intervention)
- Intervention fidelity

Outcomes/Dependent variables
- Outcomes (or phenomena in qualitative studies)
- Time points for outcome data collection

For each key outcome:
- Outcome definition
- Method of data collection (e.g., self-report, observation)
- Specific instrument (if relevant)
  - Reliability, validity information

Results
- Qualitative: Summary of major themes
- Quantitative: for each outcome of interest
- Summary of results
  - Effect size
  - p values
  - Confidence intervals
- Subgroup analyses

Evaluation
- Major strengths
- Major weaknesses
- Overall quality rating

Other
- Theoretical framework
- Funding source
- Key conclusions of the study authors

Broadly adapted with permission from Table 5.3.a Higgins, J. P. T., Thomas, J., Chandler, J. (Eds.). *Cochrane handbook for systematic reviews of interventions version 6.4* (updated August 2023). Cochrane, 2023. Available from www.training.cochrane.org/handbook

scheme is presented in Box 5.2, with the codes of the dependent variables in the study on homeless women by Dickins et al. (2021).

The results of each study can then be coded. You can record these codes in data extraction forms, but it is also useful to note the codes in the margins of the articles themselves, so you can easily find the information. Figure 5.5 provides an example of coding in the margins of the study: A picture of the older homeless female veteran: A qualitative, case study analysis that was referenced in the review by Dickins et al. (2021). In this excerpt, we see the coding scheme related to social and behavioral health as described in Box 5.2.

Coding may not always be necessary or codes that are more fine-tuned could be used in our example. If our research question was focused on the use of sociological interventions for women who are homeless, the outcome categories might be specific sociological approaches, such as the use of social worker interventions used to assist women who are homeless. The point is to use codes to organize information in a way that facilitates retrieval and analysis.

Literature Review Summary Tables

As noted earlier, we recommend using two-dimensional tables (matrices) to extract and record information from the source documents because such tables directly support a thematic analysis of the retrieved evidence. For some literature reviews—for example, in a dissertation—such tables are sometimes included directly in the written product. In other words, these tables can serve not only as a data extraction tool but also as a display of critical information in complex reviews.

As Box 5.1 suggests, the list of potential elements to be extracted from each study can be long. With two-dimensional tables for recording the extracted data, it may be advantageous to create multiple data extraction forms, so that the

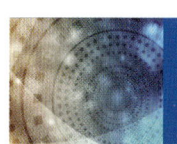

BOX 5.2 Substantive Codes for Physical and Behavioral Health Characteristics of Aging Homeless Women in the United States: An Integrative Review (Dickins et al., 2021)

CODING SCHEME
Code for the independent variables.
Demographics
1. Age
2. Gender
3. Location within the United States
4. Homelessness status—e.g., shelter, streets, unstable housing, e.g., "couch surfing"

Codes for the dependent variable
1. Chronic Physical Conditions with four subdomains:
    a. risk factors for chronic physical conditions
    b. suboptimal nutrition
    c. cancer and cancer screening
    d. geriatric conditions
2. Behavioral Health with two domains
    a. mental health conditions
    b. substance use
    c. trauma experiences (adverse childhood events, adult abuse, sexual coercion).
3. Social Health of aging with two domains
    a. Familial and social dynamics
    b. Socioeconomic disadvantage
4. Spiritual health was a key protective feature among aging homeless women

All the women described coming from very dysfunctional families. However, interestingly, they did not label it as other than their "normal." They matter-of-factly discussed the different dysfunctions experienced within their families. They described the death of a parent or sibling, moving in and out of foster care or being shuffled from relative to relative, then having dysfunctional relationships with spouses and children as if these events were nothing out of the ordinary.	Code 3a Code 2c

FIGURE 5.5 Coded excerpt from the Results section of a research article on homeless women veterans. The codes in the margin correspond to the codes explained in Box 5.2. (Excerpt from Kenny, D. J., & Yoder, L. H. (2019). A picture of the older homeless female veteran: A qualitative, case study analysis. *Archives of Psychiatric Nursing*, *33*(4), 400–406, with permission of Elsevier.)

information can be conveniently displayed on your computer screen without having to scroll right and left. For example, separate forms can be used for source information, methods used, results, and evaluation.

Table 5.1 presents an example of one such matrix for extracting methodologic features of studies in a review. Such tables can be created in word processing or spreadsheet software. This table only shows one illustrative entry: Kenny and Yoder (2019) study, whose CINAHL and PubMed records are shown in Figures 5.3 and 5.4. Complete evidence summary tables would have a row for each study in the review. These tables can be electronically searched, sorted, and resorted (e.g., by authors' names, year of publication, level of evidence, etc.). Although we have only included one entry in this table as an illustration, if this table listed 10 to 15 studies, we would be able to tell at a glance when and where the studies had been done, what sampling methods had been used, and so on. The scrutiny of such tables can tell us not only what *has* been done but also can also point to gaps or problems—for example, overreliance on nurses' self-reported pain management strategies rather than direct observation of nurses' behaviors.

CRITICAL APPRAISAL OF THE EVIDENCE

In drawing conclusions about a body of research, reviewers must record not only factual information about studies—methodologic features and findings—but also must make judgments about the value of the evidence. This section discusses issues relating to the appraisal of studies in the review.

> **TIP** A distinction is sometimes made between a research *critique* and a *critical appraisal*. The latter term is favored by those focusing on the evaluation of evidence for nursing practice. The term *critique* is more often used when individual studies are being evaluated for their scientific merit—for example, when a manuscript is reviewed by two or more **peer reviewers** who make recommendations about publishing the paper, or when a person is preparing a literature review. In both critiques and appraisals, however, the point is to apply knowledge about research methods, theory, and substantive issues to draw conclusions about the validity and relevance of the findings.

Appraisals of Individual Studies

As traditionally defined, a research **critique** is an appraisal of the strengths and weaknesses of a study. A good critique identifies areas of adequacy and inadequacy in an unbiased manner. Literature reviews mainly concern the evaluation of a body of research evidence for a literature review, but we briefly offer some advice about appraisals of individual studies.

We provide support for the critical appraisal of individual studies in several ways. First, suggestions for appraising relevant aspects of a study are included at the end of each chapter.

TABLE 5.1 • Example of an Evidence Summary Table for Methodologic Features of a Study on Homeless Women

AUTHORS	YEAR	COUNTRY	STUDY DESIGN	INDEPENDENT VARIABLES	DEPENDENT VARIABLES	SAMPLE SIZE, CHARACTERISTICS	WOMEN'S AGE	SAMPLING METHOD	DATA COLLECTION METHOD
Kenny and Yoder[a]	2019	USA	Qualitative Study	Women Middle-aged, living in shelter, Southwestern USA	Behavioral (Codes 2 a, b, and Societal); 3 a and b)	Five homeless women veterans	>50 years of age	Convenience	Interpretive interviews, case study analysis

[a]The codes for the independent and dependent variables are shown in Box 5.2.

Second, we offer a set of key critical appraisal questions in this chapter, in Box 5.3 (quantitative studies) and Box 5.4 (qualitative studies). The second column in these two boxes lists appraisal questions. We also suggest you refer to the Critical Assessment Skills Programme (CASP) Checklists found here: https://casp-uk.net/casp-tools-checklists that allow you to appraise the various aspects of each study.

Many questions may be too difficult for you to answer at this point, but your methodologic and appraisal skills will improve as you progress through this book. The questions in these two boxes are relevant for a rapid critical appraisal that would be conducted as part of an EBP effort, as well as for appraisals for a literature review.

A few comments about these guidelines are worth noting. First, the questions in Boxes 5.3 and 5.4 mainly concern the *rigor* with which the researchers conducted their research. For example, there are no questions regarding ethical issues because—while extremely important—the researchers' handling of ethical concerns is unlikely to affect evidence quality.

Second, the questions in these two boxes call for a yes or no answer (although for some, the answer may be "Yes, *but…*"). In all cases, the desirable answer is "yes." A "no" suggests a possible limitation, and a "yes" suggests a likely strength. Therefore, the more "yeses" a study gets, the stronger its evidence is likely to be. These questions can thus cumulatively suggest a global assessment: a report with 10 "yeses" is likely to be superior to one with only 4.

Our simplified guidelines have shortcomings. In particular, they are generic despite the fact that appraisals cannot use a one-size-fits-all list of questions. Some questions that are relevant to, say, clinical trials do not make sense for descriptive studies. Thus, you need to use some judgment about whether the guidelines are appropriate in your situation.

Finally, there are questions in these guidelines for which there are no objective answers. Even experts sometimes disagree about what are the best methodologic strategies for a study.

Students may be asked to critically appraise a study to document their mastery of research concepts. Such appraisals may be expected to be comprehensive, covering substantive, theoretical, ethical, methodologic, and interpretive aspects.

Evaluating a Body of Research

In reviewing the literature, you would not undertake a comprehensive critical appraisal of each study—but you would need to evaluate the evidence quality in each study so that you could aggregate appraisals across studies to draw conclusions about the overall body of evidence.

In preparing a literature review for a new study, the studies under review need to be assessed with an eye to answering some broad questions. First, to what extent do the cumulative findings accurately reflect the *truth* or, conversely, to what extent do methodologic flaws undermine the credibility of the evidence? Another important question to consider follows: For which types of people does the evidence apply—that is, for whom is the evidence applicable?

The use of literature review matrices supports the analysis and evaluation of multiple studies. For example, if there is a column for sample size in the matrix (as in Table 5.1), one could readily see whether, for example, a lot of the evidence is from studies with small, unrepresentative samples.

TIP Formal systems for *grading* a body of evidence have been developed and will be discussed in the chapter on systematic reviews (Chapter 30).

ANALYZING AND SYNTHESIZING INFORMATION

Once all the relevant studies have been retrieved, read, abstracted, and appraised, the information must be analyzed and integrated. A literature review is not simply a summary of each previous study—it is a synthesis that features important patterns. As previously noted, doing a literature review is like

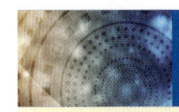

BOX 5.3 Guide to a Focused Critical Appraisal of Evidence Quality in a Quantitative Research Report

SECTION OF THE REPORT	CRITICAL APPRAISAL QUESTIONS	DETAILED GUIDELINES
Method Research design	Was the most rigorous design used, given the purpose of the study? What was the level of evidence for the type of question asked—and is this level the highest possible? Were suitable comparisons made to enhance interpretability? Was the number of data collection points appropriate? Was the period of follow-up (if any) adequate? Did the design minimize threats to the internal validity of the study (e.g., was randomization and blinding used, was attrition minimized)? Did the design enhance the external validity and applicability of the study results? If there was an intervention, did it have a strong theoretical basis?	Box 9.1, page xx; Box 10.1, page xx Box 31.1, page xx
Population and sample	Was the population identified? Was the sample adequately described? Was a good sampling design used to enhance the sample's representativeness of the population? Were sampling biases minimized? Was the sample size adequate? Was a power analysis used?	Box 13.1, page xx
Data collection and measurement	Were key variables operationalized using the best possible methods (e.g., interviews, observations)? Were clinically important and patient-centered outcomes measured? Did the data collection methods yield data that were reliable, valid, and responsive?	Box 14.1, page xx; Box 15.1, page xx
Procedures	If there was an intervention, was it rigorously developed and implemented? Did most participants allocated to the intervention group actually receive it? Were data collected in a manner that minimized bias?	Box 9.1, page xx; Box 10.1, page xx
Results Data analysis	Were appropriate and powerful statistical methods used? Did the analysis help to control for confounding variables? Were Type I and Type II errors avoided or minimized? Were subgroup analyses undertaken to better understand the applicability of the results to different types of people?	Box 17.1, page xx Box 18.1, page xx Box 31.1, page xx
Findings	Were the findings adequately summarized? Was information about effect size and precision of estimates (confidence intervals) presented? Were findings reported in a manner that facilitates a meta-analysis, and with sufficient information needed for EBP?	Box 17.1, page xx

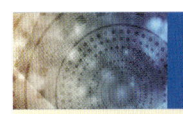

BOX 5.3 Guide to a Focused Critical Appraisal of Evidence Quality in a Quantitative Research Report (*Continued*)

SECTION OF THE REPORT	CRITICAL APPRAISAL QUESTIONS	DETAILED GUIDELINES
Discussion Interpretation of the findings	Were interpretations consistent with the study's limitations? Were causal inferences, if any, justified? Was the clinical significance of the findings discussed? Did the report address the generalizability and applicability of the findings?	Box 21.1, page xx
Summary Assessment	Despite any limitations, do the study findings appear to be valid—do you have confidence in the *truth value* of the results? Does the report inspire confidence about the types of people and settings for whom the evidence is applicable?	

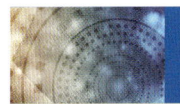

BOX 5.4 Guide to a Focused Critical Appraisal of Evidence Quality in a Qualitative Research Report

SECTION OF THE REPORT	CRITICAL APPRAISAL QUESTIONS	DETAILED GUIDELINES
Method Research design/research tradition	Is the identified research tradition congruent with the methods used to collect and analyze data? Was an adequate amount of time spent with study participants? Was there evidence of reflexivity in the design?	Box 22.1, page xx
Sample and setting	Was the group or population of interest adequately described? Were the setting and sample described in sufficient detail? Was a good method of sampling used to enhance information richness? Was the sample size adequate? Was saturation achieved?	Box 23.1, page xx
Data collection	Were appropriate methods used to gather data? Were data gathered through two or more methods to achieve triangulation? Were the data of sufficient depth and richness?	Box 24.1, page xx
Procedures	Do data collection and recording procedures appear appropriate? Were data collected in a manner that minimized bias?	Box 24.1, page xx
Enhancement of trustworthiness	Did the researchers use effective strategies to enhance the trustworthiness/integrity of the study? Was there "thick description" of the context, participants, and findings, and was it at a sufficient level to support transferability? Do the researchers' methodologic and clinical experience enhance confidence in the study findings and interpretations?	Box 26.1, page xx

(*continued*)

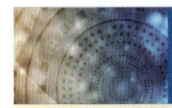

BOX 5.4 Guide to a Focused Critical Appraisal of Evidence Quality in a Qualitative Research Report (Continued)

SECTION OF THE REPORT	CRITICAL APPRAISAL QUESTIONS	DETAILED GUIDELINES
Results Data analysis	Was the data analysis strategy compatible with the research tradition and with the nature and type of data gathered?	Box 25.1, page xx
Findings	Were findings effectively summarized, with good use of excerpts and strong supporting arguments? Did the analysis yield an insightful, provocative, authentic, and meaningful picture of the phenomenon under investigation?	Box 25.1, page xx
Theoretical integration	Were the themes or patterns logically connected to each other to form a convincing and integrated whole?	Box 25.1 page xx
Discussion Interpretation of the findings	Were the findings interpreted within an appropriate social or cultural context, and within the context of prior studies? Were interpretations consistent with the study's limitations? Did the report address the transferability and applicability of the findings?	Box 25.1, page xx
Summary Assessment	Do the study findings appear to be trustworthy—do you have confidence in the *truth* value of the results? Does the report inspire confidence about the types of people and settings for whom the evidence is applicable?	

doing a qualitative study, particularly with respect to the analysis of the data, which in this case is the information from the retrieved studies. In both, the focus is on identifying important *themes*.

A thematic analysis essentially involves detecting regularities, as well as inconsistencies and "holes." Several different types of themes can be identified, as described in Table 5.2. We recommend using literature review summary tables by reading the list of possible themes and questions. It is easier to discern patterns by reading down the columns of the matrices than by flipping through a file of review forms or skimming through articles.

Clearly, it is not possible—even in lengthy free-standing reviews—to address all the questions in Table 5.2. Reviewers must decide which patterns to pursue. In preparing a review as part of a new study, you would need to determine which pattern is of greatest relevance for developing an argument and providing a context for the new research.

PREPARING A WRITTEN LITERATURE REVIEW

Writing literature reviews can be challenging, especially when voluminous information must be condensed into a few pages, as is typical for a journal article or proposal. We offer a few suggestions but acknowledge that skills in writing literature reviews develop over time.

Organizing the Review

Organization is crucial in a written review. Having an outline helps to structure the narrative's flow. If the review is complex, we recommend a written outline. The outline should list the main topics or themes to be discussed and the order of presentation. The important point is to have a plan before starting to write so that the review has a coherent progression of ideas. The goal is to structure the review in such a way that the presentation is

TABLE 5.2 • Thematic Possibilities for a Literature Review

NATURE OF THE THEME	QUESTIONS FOR THEMATIC ANALYSIS
Substantive	What does the pattern of evidence suggest? How much evidence is there? How consistent is the body of evidence across studies? How powerful are observed effects? How persuasive is the evidence? Has the clinical significance of the findings been assessed? What gaps are there in the body of evidence?
Methodologic	What types of research designs or approaches have predominated? What level of evidence is typical? What populations have been studied? Have certain groups been omitted from the research? What data collection methods have been used primarily? Are data typically of high quality? Overall, what are the methodologic strengths and deficiencies?
Theoretical	Which theoretical frameworks have been used—or has most research been atheoretical? How congruent are the frameworks?
Generalizability/ transferability	To what types of people and settings do the findings apply? Do findings vary for different types of people or settings?
Historical	Have there been substantive, methodologic, or theoretical trends over time? Is evidence getting better? When was most research conducted?
Researcher	Who has been doing the research, in terms of discipline, specialty area, and nationality? Do any of the researchers have a systematic program of research devoted to this topic?

logical, demonstrates meaningful thematic integration, and leads to a conclusion about the state of evidence on the topic.

Writing a Literature Review

It is beyond the scope of this book to offer detailed guidance on writing research reviews, but we offer a few comments on their content and style. Additional assistance is provided in books such as the ones by Fink (2020) and Galvan and Galvan (2017).

Content of the Written Literature Review

A written research review should provide readers with an objective, organized synthesis of evidence on a topic. A review should be neither a series of quotes nor a series of abstracts. The central tasks are to digest and critically evaluate the overall evidence to reveal the current state of knowledge—not simply to describe what researchers have done.

Although key studies may be described in some detail, it is seldom necessary to provide particulars for every reference. Studies with comparable findings often are summarized together.

Example of Grouped studies
Kayser et al. (2019) summarized findings from several studies in their introduction to a study of predictors of hospital-acquired pressure injuries: "In a review of 54 studies examining risk factors of pressure injuries … as many as 200 significant risk factors were identified (Coleman et al., 2015). Examples of indirect risk factors studied include incontinence, age, nutrition, diabetes, and vasopressor therapy."

The review should demonstrate that you have considered the cumulative worth of the body of research. The review should be as objective as possible. Studies that are at odds with your hypotheses should not be omitted, and the review should not ignore a study because its findings contradict other studies. Inconsistent results should be analyzed for insights into factors that might have led to discrepancies.

A literature review typically concludes with a concise summary of evidence on the topic and any gaps in the evidence. If the review is undertaken for a new study, this critical summary should demonstrate the need for the research and should clarify the basis for any hypotheses.

> **TIP** As you progress through this book, you will acquire proficiency in critically evaluating studies. We hope you will understand the *mechanics* of doing a review after reading this chapter, but you probably will not be ready to write a state-of-the-art review until you have gained more skills in research methods.

Style of a Research Review

Students preparing their first written research review often struggle with stylistic issues. Students sometimes accept research findings uncritically, perhaps reflecting a common misunderstanding about the conclusiveness of research. You should keep in mind that hypotheses cannot be proved or disproved by empirical testing, and no research question can be answered definitively in a single study. The issue is partly semantic. Hypotheses are not proved; they are *supported* by research findings.

> **TIP** When describing study findings, you should use phrases suggesting that results are tentative, such as the following:
> - Several studies have *found* …
> - Findings thus far *suggest* …
> - The study results *support* the hypothesis that …
> - There *appears* to be good evidence that …

A related stylistic problem is the interjection of opinions into the review. The review should include opinions sparingly and should be explicit about their source. Reviewers' opinions do not belong in a literature review, except for assessments of study quality.

CRITICAL APPRAISAL OF RESEARCH LITERATURE REVIEWS

We conclude this chapter with some advice about appraising a literature review. It is often difficult to critique a research review because the author is almost invariably more knowledgeable about the topic than the readers. It is not usually possible to judge whether the author has included all relevant literature—although you may have suspicions if none of the citations are to recent articles. Several aspects of a review, however, are amenable to evaluation by readers who are not experts on the topic. Some suggestions for appraising written research reviews are presented in Box 5.5. (These questions

---

BOX 5.5   Guidelines for Critically Appraising Literature Reviews

1. Is the review thorough—does it include all major studies on the topic? Does it include *recent* research (studies published within the previous 1-3 years)? Are studies from other related disciplines included, if appropriate?
2. Does the review rely mainly on primary source research articles?
3. Is the review merely a summary of existing work, or does it critically appraise and compare key studies? Does the review identify important trends and gaps in the literature?
4. Is the review well organized? Is the development of ideas clear?
5. Does the review use appropriate language regarding the tentativeness of prior findings? Is the review objective? Does the author paraphrase, or is there an overreliance on quotes from original sources?
6. If the review is part of a research report for a new study, does the review support the need for the study?
7. If it is a review designed to summarize evidence for clinical practice, does the review draw reasonable conclusions about practice implications?

could be used to review your own literature review as well.)

In assessing a literature review, the key question is whether it summarizes the current state of research evidence adequately. If the review is written as part of an original research report, an equally important question is whether the review lays a solid foundation for the new study.

RESEARCH EXAMPLES OF LITERATURE REVIEWS

The best way to learn about the style and organization of a research literature review is to read reviews in nursing journals. We present excerpts from two reviews that were part of the introduction to journal articles about original studies.[1]

Literature Review From a Quantitative Research Report

Study: Disease-related knowledge in people with chronic obstructive pulmonary disease and their informal caregivers: A multilevel modeling analysis (Matarese et al., 2023).

Statement of purpose: The purpose of this study was to assess the level of chronic obstructive pulmonary disease (COPD)-related knowledge within patient and informal caregiver dyads, and to identify factors influencing the knowledge level considering the interdependence within the dyads.

Literature review (excerpt): "Patients with COPD have been shown as having poor knowledge of disease management (Scott et al., 2011), medication use, risk of infections (White et al., 2006) and symptom treatment (Jones et al., 2018). Similarly, informal caregivers presented limited COPD-related knowledge, although greater than that of patients (Ivziku et al., 2018; Wang et al., 2012). Several studies investigated the influence of patient characteristics on their level of COPD-related knowledge, showing that knowledge was higher in patients who attended pulmonary rehabilitation (Jones et al., 2018; Nakken et al., 2017) and lower in those with depressive symptoms (Lee et al., 2013; Zhang et al., 2014). Regarding patient level of COPD knowledge, inconclusive evidence was found on the influence of patient age (Nakken et al., 2017; Scott et al., 2011; White et al., 2006), education level (Ivziku et al., 2018; Nakken et al., 2017; Scott et al., 2011; Wong & Yu, 2016), disease severity and pulmonary function (Ivziku et al., 2018; Lee et al., 2020; Scott et al., 2011; White et al., 2006), years since diagnosis (Nakken et al., 2017; White et al., 2006), patient socioeconomic status (White et al., 2006), self-efficacy (Lee et al., 2014), and gender (Ivziku et al., 2018). A few studies analyzed the influence of caregivers' characteristics on their level of COPD-related knowledge, finding that older caregivers, with lower socioeconomic status (Hsiao et al., 2014) and education level (Hsiao et al., 2014; Ivziku et al., 2018) showed lower COPD-related knowledge.

All of the available studies assessed COPD-related knowledge and its associated characteristics separately in COPD patients and informal caregivers, overlooking the fact that when two individuals interact, they influence each other's cognition, emotions, and motivations, as postulated by the Interdependence Theory (Rusbult & Van Lange, 2003). A model used to assess the interdependence in dyads is the Actor-Partner Interdependence Model (APIM; Cook & Kenny, 2005). APIM describes two different effects occurring when two individuals interact: an actor effect that measures the degree to which an individual's independent variable influences [their] own dependent variable (e.g., [their] level of education influences his/her own level of knowledge); and a partner effect that measures the degree to which an individual's independent variable influences a dependent variable of another individual (e.g., the level of education of one member of the dyad influences the level of knowledge of the other member). Understanding what COPD-related knowledge dyads have in common and what patient and informal caregiver characteristics influence their own knowledge and the knowledge of the other member of the dyad can be useful when designing educational interventions that will benefit both caregivers and patients, promote better adherence by patients to recommended self-care behaviors, and better contributions to patient self-care of informal caregivers. Therefore,

---

[1]Consult the full research reports for references cited within these excerpted literature reviews.

we conducted a study with the following aims: (i) to assess the level of COPD-related knowledge within patient and informal caregiver dyads, and (ii) to identify the patient and informal caregiver characteristics that influence the level of COPD-related knowledge at dyadic level, taking account of the interdependence within the dyads."

(Excerpt reprinted with permission from Matarese, M., Lyons, K. S., Piredda, M., & De Marinis, M. G. (2022). Disease-related knowledge in people with chronic obstructive pulmonary disease and their informal caregivers: A multilevel modeling analysis. *Journal of Clinical Nursing, 32*(13–14), 3543–3556.)

Literature Review From a Qualitative Research Report

Study: Lived experiences of Mongolian immigrant women seeking perinatal care in the United States (McClellan & Madler, 2022).

Statement of purpose: The purpose of this study was to explore the experiences of Mongolian immigrant women seeking perinatal care in the United States in order to inform healthcare providers so they can improve their delivery of culturally informed care.

Literature review (excerpt): "A small, but growing community of Mongolian immigrants has been established in cities across the United States (Pew Research Center, 2017). However, a paucity of information is available on Mongolian culture, placing this growing minority group at high risk of suboptimal healthcare. It is common for information on Asian people to be conglomerated in the literature, but this practice blurs significant differences of economic status, educational levels, and health literacy between first-world Asian countries such as Japan and nomadic and third-world countries such as Mongolia. Lack of distinction prevents cultural understanding, and therefore culturally competent care.

Over the last decade, many articles involving immigrant women seeking perinatal care in the United States have been published. Winn et al. (2017) discuss difficulty in accessing healthcare and differences in cultural expectations as common problems for immigrant women across a wide range of cultures. Trainor et al. (2020) and Lindsay et al. (2016) studied Mexican-born women and Brazilian-born women, respectively, all of whom were seeking perinatal care in the United States. Findings were similar; participants struggled with access to healthcare, language barriers, and financial challenges, Similarly, Chiatti (2018) found Ethiopian women experience linguistic barriers and a perceived lack of caring from healthcare workers. Missal et al. (2015) reported women from Somalia experienced emotional and cultural loss because their mothers were not available to provide support during pregnancy. Researchers also reported that these women experienced difficulty in establishing the desired relationship with healthcare workers. South Korean women have reported struggling to maintain desired cultural perinatal traditions while in the United States (Seo et al., 2014), and Japanese women reported concerns regarding differing standards of care, language and cultural barriers, and lack of support for breastfeeding (Little et al., 2020). Despite the growing body of literature regarding the experiences of immigrant women from a variety of cultures, there remains a paucity of literature regarding Mongolian immigrant women. This knowledge gap leaves Mongolian immigrant women at high risk for disparate healthcare at the critical juncture of childbirth."

(Excerpt reprinted with permission from McClellan, C., & Madler, B. (2022). Lived experiences of Mongolian immigrant women seeking perinatal care in the United States. *Journal of Transcultural Nursing, 33*(5), 594–595.)

SUMMARY POINTS

- A research **literature review** is a written synthesis of evidence on a research problem.
- Major steps in preparing a written research review include formulating a question, devising a search strategy, developing a plan to organize and document review activities, conducting a search, screening and retrieving relevant sources, extracting key data from the sources, appraising studies, analyzing aggregated information for important themes, and writing a synthesis.
- Research articles are the major focus of research reviews. Information in nonresearch references—such as case reports and editorials—may broaden understanding of a research problem but has limited utility in summarizing research evidence.

- A **primary source** is the description of a study prepared by the researcher who conducted it; a **secondary source** is a description of the study written by someone else. Literature reviews should be based on primary source material.
- Strategies for finding studies on a topic include the use of **bibliographic databases**, the *ancestry approach* (tracking down earlier studies cited in a reference list of a report), and the *descendancy approach* (using a pivotal study to search forward to subsequent studies that cited it.)
- Electronic searches of bibliographic databases are a key method of locating references. For nurses, the CINAHL and MEDLINE (via PubMed) databases are especially useful. Google Scholar is also a popular and free resource.
- In searching a database, users can perform a **keyword search** that looks for searcher-specified terms in text fields of a database record (or that *maps* keywords onto the database's subject codes) or they search according to **subject heading** codes themselves.
- Access to many journal articles is becoming easier through online resources, especially for articles available in an **open-access** format.
- References must be screened for relevance, and then pertinent information must be extracted for analysis. Two-dimensional *evidence summary tables* (matrices) facilitate the extraction and organization of data from the studies, as does a good coding scheme.
- A research **critique** (or **critical appraisal**) is a careful evaluation of a study's strengths and weaknesses. Critical appraisals for a research review tend to focus on the methodologic aspects and findings of retrieved studies.
- The analysis of information from a literature search involves the identification of important themes—regularities (and inconsistencies) in the information. Themes can take many forms, including substantive, methodologic, and theoretic themes.
- In preparing a written review, it is important to organize materials logically. The reviewers' role is to describe study findings, the dependability of the evidence, evidence gaps, and (in the context of a new study) contributions that the new study would make.

REFERENCES CITED IN CHAPTER 5

Bramer, W. M., Giustini, D., Kramer, B., & Anderson, P. (2013). The comparative recall of Google scholar versus PubMed in identical searches for biomedical systematic reviews: A review of searches used in systematic reviews. *Systematic Reviews*, 2, 115.

Cooper, H. (2017). *Research synthesis and meta-analysis: A step-by-step approach.* (5th ed.). Sage Publications.

Dickins, K. A., Philpotts, L. L., Flanagan, J., Bartels, S. J., Baggett, T. P., & Looby, S. E. (2021). Physical and behavioral health characteristics of aging homeless women in the United States: An integrative review. *Journal of Women's Health (2002)*, 30(10), 1493–1507. https://doi.org/10.1089/jwh.2020.8557

Fink, A. (2020). *Conducting research literature reviews: From the Internet to paper* (5th ed.). Sage.

Galvan, J. L., & Galvan, M. (2017). *Writing literature reviews: A guide for students of the social and behavioral sciences* (7th ed.). Routledge.

Garrard, J. (2020). *Health sciences literature review made easy: The matrix method* (6th ed.). Jones and Bartlett Publishers.

Glaser, B. (1978). *Theoretical sensitivity.* The Sociology Press.

Grant, M., & Booth, A. (2009). A typology of reviews: An analysis of 14 review types and associated methodologies. *Health Information and Libraries Journal*, 26(2), 91–108.

Gusenbauer, M., & Haddaway, N. R. (2020). Which academic search systems are suitable for systematic reviews or meta-analyses? Evaluating retrieval qualities of Google scholar, PubMed, and 26 other resources. *Research Synthesis Methods*, 11(2), 181–217. https://doi.org/10.1002/jrsm.1378

Haddaway, N., Collins, A., Coughlin, D., & Kirk, S. (2015). The role of Google Scholar in evidence reviews and its applicability to grey literature searching. *PLoS One*, 10(9), e0138237.

He, H. G., Klainin-Yobas, P., Ang, E., Sinnappan, R., Pölkki, T., & Wang, W. (2015). Nurses' provision of parental guidance regarding school-aged children's postoperative pain management: A descriptive correlational study. *Pain Management Nursing*, 16(1), 40–50.

Higgins, J. P. T., Thomas, J., Chandler, J. (Eds.). *Cochrane handbook for systematic reviews of interventions version 6.4* (updated August 2023). Cochrane, 2023. Available from www.training.cochrane.org/handbook

Jones, R., Hollen, P., Wenzel, J., Weiss, G., Song, D., Sims, T., & Petroni, G. (2018). Understanding advanced prostate cancer decision making utilizing an interactive decision aid. *Cancer Nursing*, 41(1), 2–10.

Justesen, T., Freyberg, J., & Schultz, A. N. Ø. (2021). Database selection and data gathering methods in systematic reviews of qualitative research regarding diabetes mellitus - an explorative study. *BMC Medical Research Methodology*, 21(1), 94. https://doi.org/10.1186/s12874-021-01281-2

Kayser, S., VanGilder, C., & Lachenbruch, C. (2019). Predictors of superficial and severe hospital-acquired pressure injuries: A cross-sectional study using the International pressure Ulcer Prevalence™ survey. *International Journal of Nursing Studies*, *89*, 46–52.

Kenny, D. J., & Yoder, L. H. (2019). A picture of the older homeless female veteran: A qualitative, case study analysis. *Archives of Psychiatric Nursing*, *33*(4), 400–406. https://doi.org/10.1016/j.apnu.2019.05.005

King, L. M., Lacey, A., & Hunt, J. (2022). Bereavement and children's mental health: Recognising the effects of early parental loss. *Nursing Children and Young People*, *34*(1), 22–27. https://doi.org/10.7748/ncyp.2021.e1388

Matarese, M., Lyons, K.S., Piredda, M., & De Marinis, M.G.(2023). Disease-related knowledge in people with chronic obstructive pulmonary disease and their informal caregivers: A multilevel modelling analysis. *Journal of Clinical Nursing*, *32*(13–14), 3543–3556, https://doi.org/10.1111/jocn.16433

McClellan, C., & Madler, B. (2022). Lived experiences of Mongolian immigrant women seeking perinatal care in the United States. *Journal of Transcultural Nursing*, *33*(5), 594–602. https://doi.org/10.1177/10436596221091689

Morshed, T., & Hayden, S. (2020). Google versus PubMed: Comparison of Google and PubMed's search tools for answering clinical questions in the emergency department. *Annals of Emergency Medicine*, *75*(3), 408–415.

Munhall, P. L. (2012). *Nursing research: A qualitative perspective* (5th ed.). Jones & Bartlett.

Spradley, J. (1979). *The ethnographic interview*. Holt Rinehart & Winston.

6 Theoretical Frameworks

Learning Objectives

1. Differentiate theories from conceptual models and frameworks.
2. Distinguish the differences between grand, mid-range, and situation-specific theory.
3. Identify several conceptual models or theories frequently used by nurse researchers.
4. Describe how theory and research are linked in quantitative and qualitative studies.
5. Appraise the appropriateness of a conceptual/theoretical framework—or its absence—in a study.

INTRODUCTION

High-quality studies achieve a high level of *conceptual integration*. This means that the methods are appropriate for the research questions, the questions are consistent with existing evidence, and there is a plausible conceptual rationale for hypotheses to be tested or for the design of an intervention.

For example, suppose we hypothesized that a nurse-led smoking cessation intervention would result in reduced rates of smoking among patients with cardiovascular disease. Why would we make this prediction—what is our "theory" (our theoretical rationale) about how the intervention might change people's behavior? Do we predict that the intervention will change patients' knowledge? motivation? sense of control over their decision-making? Our view of how the intervention would "work"—what *mediates* the relationship between intervention receipt and the desired outcome—should guide the design of the intervention and the study.

In designing studies, researchers need to have a conceptualization of people's behaviors or characteristics, and how these aspects affect or are affected by interpersonal, environmental, or biologic forces. In high-quality research, a strong, defensible conceptualization is made explicit. This chapter discusses theoretical and conceptual contexts for nursing research problems.

THEORIES, MODELS, AND FRAMEWORKS

Many terms are used in connection with conceptual contexts for research, such as theories, models, frameworks, schemes, and maps. We offer guidance in distinguishing these terms but note that our definitions are not universal—indeed one confusing aspect of theory-related writings is that there is no consensus about terminology.

Theories

The term *theory* is used in many ways. For example, nursing instructors and students use the term to refer to classroom content, as opposed to the actual

113

practice of performing nursing actions. In both lay and scientific usage, the term *theory* connotes an *abstraction*.

In research, the term theory is used differently by different authors. Classically, **theory** refers to an abstract generalization that explains how phenomena are interrelated. In this definition, a theory embodies at least two concepts that are related in a manner that the theory purports to explain. The purpose of traditional theories is to explain or predict phenomena.

Others, however, use the term *theory* less restrictively to refer to a broad representation that can thoroughly describe a phenomenon. Some authors refer to this type of theory as **descriptive theory**. Broadly speaking, descriptive theories are ones that describe or categorize characteristics of individuals, groups, or situations by abstracting common features observed across multiple manifestations. Descriptive theory plays an important role in qualitative studies. Qualitative researchers often strive to develop conceptualizations of phenomena that are grounded in actual observations. Descriptive theory is sometimes a precursor to predictive and explanatory theories.

Components of a Traditional Theory

Concepts are the basic building blocks of a theory. Classical theories comprise a set of propositions that indicate relationships among the concepts. Relationships are denoted by such terms as "is associated with," "varies directly with," or "is contingent on." The propositions form an interrelated deductive system. Theories provide a mechanism for logically deriving new statements from the original propositions.

Let us illustrate with the **Theory of Planned Behavior** (TPB (Ajzen, 2005)), which is related to another theory called the *Theory of Reasoned Action* (Fishbein & Ajzen, 2015). TPB provides a framework for understanding people's behavior and its psychological determinants. A greatly simplified construction of the TPB consists of the following propositions:

1. Behavior that is volitional is determined by people's intention to perform that behavior.

2. Intention to perform or not perform a behavior is determined by three factors:
   - Attitudes toward the behavior (i.e., the overall evaluation of performing the behavior)
   - Subjective norms (i.e., perceived social pressure to perform or not perform the behavior)
   - Perceived behavioral control (i.e., the anticipated ease or difficulty of engaging in the behavior)

3. The relative importance of the three factors in influencing intention varies across behaviors and situations.

The concepts that form the basis of the TPB include *behaviors, intentions, attitudes, subjective norms*, and *perceived self-control*. The theory, which specifies the nature of the relationship among these concepts, provides a framework for generating hypotheses relating to health behaviors. For example, we might hypothesize that compliance with a medical regimen (the behavior) could be enhanced by changing people's attitudes toward compliance or by increasing their sense of control. The TPB has been used as the underlying theory for studying a wide range of health decision-making behaviors and in developing health-promoting interventions.

> **Example Using the TPB**
> Lareyre et al. (2021) conducted a systematic review using the Theory of Planned Behavior (TPB) to study the characteristics of TPB-based interventions on the impact of smoking behavior.

Levels of Theories

Theories differ in their level of generality and abstraction. The most common labels used in nursing for levels or scope of theory are *grand*, *middle-range*, and *micro* or *practice*.

Grand theories or *macrotheories* purport to describe and explain large segments of human experience. In nursing, several grand theories offer explanations of the whole of nursing and address the nature, goals, and mission of nursing practice, as distinct from the discipline of medicine. An example of a nursing theory that has been described as a grand theory is Parse's Human becoming Paradigm (Parse, 2014).

Theories of relevance to researchers are often more focused than grand theories. **Middle-range theories** attempt to explain such phenomena as decision-making, stress, comfort, and unpleasant symptoms. Middle-range theories are more specific and more amenable to empirical testing than grand theories (Peterson & Bredow, 2020). Dozens of middle-range theories have been developed by or used by nurses, a few of which we briefly describe in this chapter.

The least abstract level of theory is *practice theory* (sometimes called *situation-specific theory* or *micro theory*). Such theories are highly specific, narrow in scope, and have an action orientation. They are not always associated with research, although grounded theory studies can be a source of situation-specific theory (Peterson & Bredow, 2020).

Models

Conceptual models, *conceptual frameworks*, or *conceptual schemes* (we use the terms interchangeably) are a less formal means of organizing phenomena than theories. Like theories, conceptual models deal with abstractions (concepts) that are assembled by virtue of their relevance to a common theme. Conceptual models, however, lack the deductive system of propositions that purport to explain relationships among concepts. Conceptual models provide a perspective regarding interrelated phenomena but are more loosely structured than theories. Conceptual models can serve as springboards for generating hypotheses, but conceptual models in their entirety are not formally "tested." (In actuality, however, the terms *model* and *theory* are sometimes used interchangeably.)

The term *model* is often used in connection with a symbolic representation of a conceptualization. **Schematic models** (or *conceptual maps*), which are visual representations of some aspect of reality, use concepts as building blocks but with a minimal use of words. A visual or symbolic representation of a theory or conceptual framework often helps to express abstract ideas in a concise and accessible format.

Schematic models are common in both qualitative and quantitative research. Concepts and linkages among them are represented through the use of boxes, arrows, or other symbols. Such schematic models can be useful in succinctly communicating linkages among concepts.

Frameworks

A **framework** is the overall conceptual underpinnings of a study. Not every study is based on a formal theory or conceptual model, but every study has a framework—that is, a conceptual rationale. In a study based on a theory, the framework is a **theoretical framework**; in a study with roots in a conceptual model, the framework is a **conceptual framework**.

In most nursing studies, the framework is not an explicit theory or model, and sometimes the underlying conceptual rationale for the inquiry is not explained. Frameworks are often implicit, without being formally described. In studies without an articulated conceptual framework, it may be difficult to figure out what the researchers thought was "going on."

Sometimes researchers fail even to adequately describe key constructs at the conceptual level. The concepts in which researchers are interested are abstractions of observable phenomena, and our world view shapes how those concepts are defined and operationalized. Researchers should make clear the conceptual definition of their key variables, thereby providing information about the study's framework.

In most qualitative studies, the frameworks are part of the research tradition in which the study is embedded. For example, ethnographers usually begin their work within a theory of culture. The questions that most qualitative researchers ask and the methods they use to address those questions inherently reflect certain theoretical formulations.

TIP In recent years, *concept analysis* has become an important enterprise among students and nurse scholars, and several methods have been proposed for undertaking a concept analysis and clarifying conceptual definitions (e.g., Rodgers & Knafl, 2000; Walker & Avant, 2019). Bergdahl and Berterö (2016) have argued that concept analysis is not a suitable approach to theory development while others have indicated the need for concept analyses to move beyond a mere exercise to one with clear linkages to knowledge development and resolution of problems within the discipline (Flanagan, 2021; Rodgers et al., 2018).

Example of Developing a Conceptual Definition
Taghinezhad et al. (2022) used Rodger's six-step concept analysis method to conceptually define humanistic care. Taghinezhad searched and analyzed 75 relevant articles identified through multiple databases and proposed the following: "Clear and practical definition and identification of humanistic care in nursing can be helpful in the further development of existing knowledge, instrumentation, designing guidelines, clinical interventions, knowledge translation, and correction of concept misuse" (p. 83).

THE NATURE OF THEORIES AND CONCEPTUAL MODELS

Theories and conceptual models have much in common, including their origin, general nature, purposes, and role in research. In this section, we examine some characteristics of theories and conceptual models. We use the term *theory* in a broad sense, inclusive of conceptual models.

Origin of Theories and Models

Theories, conceptual frameworks, and models are not *discovered*; they are invented. Theory building depends not only on observable evidence but also on the originator's ingenuity in pulling facts together and organizing them. Theory construction is a creative enterprise that can be undertaken by anyone who is insightful, has a firm grounding in existing evidence, and is able to knit together evidence into an intelligible pattern.

Tentative Nature of Theories and Models

Theories and conceptual models cannot be proved—they represent a theorist's best effort to describe and explain phenomena. Today's flourishing theory may be discredited or revised tomorrow. This may happen if new evidence or observations undermine a previously accepted theory. Or a new theory might integrate new observations into an existing theory to yield a more parsimonious or accurate explanation of a phenomenon.

Theories and models that are not congruent with a culture's values also may fall into disfavor over time. For example, certain psychoanalytic and structural social theories, which had broad support for decades, have come to be challenged as a result of changing views about women's roles. Theories are deliberately invented by humans, and so they are not free from human values, which can change over time.

The Role of Theories and Models

Theories allow researchers to integrate observations and facts into an orderly scheme. The linkage of findings into a coherent structure can make a body of evidence more useful.

In addition to summarizing, theories and models can guide a researcher's understanding of not only the *what* of natural phenomena but also the *why* of their occurrence. Theories often provide a basis for predicting phenomena. Prediction, in turn, has implications for influencing phenomena. A utilitarian theory has potential to bring about desirable changes in people's behavior or health outcomes. Thus, theories are an important resource for developing nursing interventions.

Theories and conceptual models help to stimulate research and the extension of knowledge by providing both direction and impetus. Thus, theories may serve as a springboard for advances in knowledge and the accumulation of evidence for practice.

Relationship Between Theory and Research

Theory and research have a reciprocal relationship. Theories are built inductively from observations, and research evidence is an excellent source for those observations. Concepts and relationships that are validated through research become the foundation for theory development. The theory, in turn, must be tested by subjecting deductions from it (hypotheses) to systematic inquiry. Thus, research plays a dual and continuing role in theory building. Theory guides and generates ideas for research; research assesses the worth of the theory and provides a foundation for new theories.

CONCEPTUAL MODELS AND THEORIES USED IN NURSING RESEARCH

Nurse researchers have used nursing and non-nursing frameworks to provide a conceptual context for their studies. This section briefly discusses several frameworks that have been found useful.

Conceptual Models and Theories of Nursing

Several nurses have formulated theories and models of nursing practice. These models offer formal explanations of what nursing is and what the nursing process entails. As Fawcett and DeSanto-Madeya (2013) have noted, four concepts are central to models of nursing: *human beings*, *environment*, *health*, and *nursing*. The various models, however, define these concepts differently, link them in diverse ways, and emphasize different relationships among them. Moreover, the models view different processes as being central to nursing.

The conceptual models were not developed primarily as a base for nursing research. Most models have had more impact on nursing education and practice than on research. Nevertheless, nurse researchers have been inspired by these conceptual models in formulating research questions and hypotheses. Two nursing models that have generated particular interest as a basis for research are briefly described.

Roy's Adaptation Model
In Roy's **Adaptation Model**, humans are viewed as biopsychosocial adaptive systems who cope with environmental change through the process of adaptation (Roy & Andrews, 2009). Within the human system, there are four subsystems: physiologic/physical, self-concept/group identity, role function, and interdependence. These subsystems constitute adaptive modes that provide mechanisms for coping with environmental stimuli and change. Health is viewed as both a state and a process of becoming integrated and whole that reflects the mutuality of people and environment. The goal of nursing, according to this model, is to promote client adaptation. Nursing also regulates stimuli affecting adaptation. Nursing interventions usually take the form of increasing, decreasing, modifying, removing, or maintaining internal and external stimuli that affect adaptation. Roy's Adaptation Model has been the basis for several middle-range theories and dozens of studies.

> **Example Using Roy's Adaptation Model**
> Zheng and Jin (2022) explored the use of nursing diagnoses informed by Roy's Adaptation Model in regulating the sense of shame in female patients with breast cancer.

Orem's Self-Care Deficit Nursing Theory
Some basic concepts in Orem's **Self-Care Deficit Theory** include self-care, self-care deficit, and self-care agency (Orem et al., 2003). Self-care activities are what people do on their own behalf to maintain their life, health, and well-being. The ability to perform self-care is called self-care agency. Orem's universal self-care requisites to maintain health include air, food, water, elimination, activity and rest, solitude and social interaction, hazard prevention, and promotion of normality. Self-care deficit occurs when self-care agency is not adequate to meet a person's self-care demands. Orem's theory explains that patients need nursing care when their demands for self-care outweigh their abilities.

> **Example Using Orem's Theory**
> Isik and Fredland (2023) examined Orem's self-care deficit theory in relation to children's self-care behaviors. The researchers concluded that self-care programs for children based on Orem's theory were appropriate to improve self-care skills that lead to better self-care practices.

Other Models and Middle-Range Theories Developed by Nurses

In addition to conceptual models that are designed to describe and characterize the nursing process, nurses have developed middle-range theories and models that focus on more specific phenomena of interest to nurses. Examples of middle-range theories that have been used in research include:

- Beck's (2023) Theory of Postpartum Depression;
- Beck's (2015) Traumatic Childbirth Theory;
- Kolcaba's (2003) Comfort Theory;
- Symptom Management Model (Dodd et al., 2001);
- Theory of Transitions (Meleis et al., 2000);
- Peplau's (1997) Theory of Interpersonal Relations;
- Swanson's (1991) Theory of Caring;
- Reed's (1991) Self-Transcendence Theory;
- Pender's Health Promotion Model (Murdaugh et al., 2019); and
- Mishel's Uncertainty in Illness Theory (1990).

The latter two are briefly described here.

The Health Promotion Model

Nola Pender's Health Promotion Model (HPM) focuses on explaining health-promoting behaviors, using a wellness orientation (Murdaugh et al., 2019). According to the model, *health promotion* entails activities directed toward developing resources that maintain or enhance a person's well-being. The model embodies several theoretical propositions that can be used to develop interventions and to gain insight into health behaviors. For example, one HPM proposition is that people commit to behaviors from which they anticipate deriving valued benefits, and another is that perceived competence or self-efficacy relating to a given behavior increases the likelihood of performing it. Greater perceived self-efficacy is viewed as resulting in fewer perceived barriers to a health behavior. The model also incorporates interpersonal and situational influences on a person's commitment to health-promoting actions.

Example Using the HPM
Santi et al. (2022) utilized Pender's Health Promotion Model to guide emancipatory dialogues to understand the perspectives of adolescents' view of health during the COVID-19 pandemic.

Uncertainty in Illness Theory

Mishel's Uncertainty in Illness Theory (Mishel, 1990) focuses on the concept of uncertainty—a person's inability to determine the meaning of illness-related events. According to this theory, people develop subjective appraisals to assist them in interpreting the experience of illness and treatment. Uncertainty occurs when people are unable to recognize and categorize stimuli. Uncertainty results in the inability to obtain a clear conception of the situation, but a situation appraised as uncertain will mobilize individuals to use their resources to adapt to the situation. Mishel's theory as originally conceptualized was most relevant to patients in an acute phase of illness or in a downward illness trajectory, but it has been reconceptualized to include constant uncertainty in chronic or recurrent illness. Mishel's conceptualization of uncertainty, and her Uncertainty in Illness Scale, has been used in many nursing studies.

Example Using Uncertainty in Illness Theory
Reinken and Reed (2022) examined Mishel's uncertainty in illness theory (UIT) to develop an integrated theory-driven practice framework to guide nursing practice aimed at decreasing uncertainty in people with brain cancer.

Other Models and Theories Used by Nurse Researchers

Many concepts of interest to nurse researchers are not unique to nursing, and so their studies are sometimes linked to frameworks that originated in other disciplines. Several of these alternative models have gained special prominence in the development of nursing interventions to promote health-enhancing behaviors. In addition to the previously described TPB, three non-nursing models or theories have often been used in nursing studies: Bandura's Social Cognitive Theory, Prochaska's Transtheoretical (stages of change) Model, and the Health Belief Model (HBM).

Bandura's Social Cognitive Theory

Social Cognitive Theory (Bandura, 1997, 2001), which is sometimes called **self-efficacy theory,** offers an explanation of human behavior using the concepts of self-efficacy and outcome expectations. Self-efficacy concerns people's belief in their own capacity to carry out particular behaviors (e.g., smoking cessation). Self-efficacy expectations influence the behaviors a person chooses to perform, their degree of perseverance, and the quality of the performance. Bandura identified four factors that influence a person's cognitive appraisal of self-efficacy: (1) their own mastery experience; (2) verbal persuasion; (3) vicarious experience; and (4) physiologic and affective cues, such as pain and anxiety. The role of self-efficacy has been studied in relation to numerous health behaviors (e.g., weight control, smoking).

> **TIP** Bandura's self-efficacy construct is a key mediating variable in several theories discussed in this chapter. Self-efficacy has repeatedly been found to explain a significant amount of variation in people's behaviors *and* to be amenable to change. As a result, self-efficacy enhancement is often a goal in interventions designed to change people's health-related behaviors (Conn et al., 2001).

Example Using Social Cognitive Theory
Silveira et al. (2021) examined if social cognitive theory-based change techniques promote physical activity improved symptom clusters in people with multiple sclerosis.

The Transtheoretical (Stages of Change) Model

The **Transtheoretical Model** (Prochaska et al., 2002; Prochaska & Velicer, 1997) has been the basis of numerous interventions designed to change people's problem behavior (e.g., alcohol abuse). The core construct around which other dimensions are organized is *stages of change*, which conceptualizes a continuum of *motivational readiness* to change dysfunctional behavior. The five stages of change are precontemplation, contemplation, preparation, action, and maintenance. Studies have shown that successful self-changers use different processes at each stage, suggesting the desirability of interventions that are individualized to the person's stage of readiness for change. The model incorporates a series of mediating variables, one of which is self-efficacy.

Example Using the Transtheoretical Model
Wang et al. (2022) examined the effect of a mobile health lifestyle modification intervention program for polycystic ovary syndrome.

The Health Belief Model

The **Health Belief Model** (HBM) (Becker, 1978) is a popular framework in nursing studies focused on patient compliance and preventive healthcare practices. The model postulates that health-seeking behavior is influenced by a person's perception of a threat posed by a health problem and the value associated with actions aimed at reducing the threat. The major components of the HBM include perceived susceptibility, perceived severity, perceived benefits and costs, motivation, and enabling or modifying factors. Perceived susceptibility is a person's perception that a health problem is personally relevant or that a diagnosis is accurate. Even when one recognizes personal susceptibility, action will not occur unless the individual perceives the severity to be high enough to have serious implications. Perceived benefits are patients' beliefs that a given treatment will cure the illness or help prevent it, and perceived barriers include the complexity, duration, and accessibility of the treatment. Motivation is the desire to comply with a treatment. Among the modifying factors that have been identified are personality variables, patient satisfaction, and sociodemographic factors.

Example Using the HBM
Firouzbakht and colleagues (2022) used the Health Belief Model as an explanatory model to explain hesitancy about COVID-19 vaccination among pregnant females. Perceived benefits and cues to action helped explain hesitancy among pregnant females but perceived threat did not.

> **TIP** A theoretical framework called the **Theoretical Domains Framework** (TDF) is being used increasingly in implementation science as a way to understand factors influencing the behaviors of healthcare professionals, as well as to facilitate the design of interventions. The TDF, which was

developed by expert consensus, is a framework with 14 domains derived from 33 behavior-change theories (Michie et al., 2005).

Selecting a Theory or Model for Nursing Research

As we discuss in the next section, theory can be used by qualitative and quantitative researchers in various ways. A common challenge, however, is identifying an appropriate model or theory—a task made especially daunting because of the burgeoning number available. There are no rules for how this can be done, but there are two places to start—with the theory or model, or with the phenomenon being studied.

Readings in the theoretical literature often give rise to research ideas, so it is useful to become familiar with a variety of grand and middle-range theories. Several nursing theory textbooks provide good overviews of major nurse theorists (e.g., Alligood, 2021; Butts & Rich, 2018; Morse, 2017). Resources for learning more about middle-range theories include Smith and Liehr (2023) and Peterson and Bredow (2020). Additionally, https://nursology.net/, an online resource, provides a comprehensive listing and synopsis of all nursing theories from grand to middle range to situation-specific ones.

If you begin with a research problem or topic and are looking for a theory, a good strategy is to examine the conceptual contexts of existing studies on a similar topic. You may find that several different theories have been used, and so the next step is to learn as much as possible about the most promising ones so that you can select a theory that is appropriate for your own study.

TIP Although it may be tempting to read about the features of a theory in a secondary source, it is best to consult a primary source and to rely on the most up-to-date reference because models are often revised as research accumulates. However, it is also a good idea to review studies that have used the theory so that you can judge how much empirical support the theory has received and how key variables were measured.

Many writers have offered advice on how to evaluate a theory for use in nursing practice and nursing research (e.g., Chinn & Kramer, 2021; Fawcett & DeSanto-Madeya, 2013; Smith, 2019).

In addition to evaluating the general integrity of the model or theory, it is important to make sure that there is a proper "fit" between the theory and the research question to be studied. A critical issue is whether the theory has done a good job of explaining, predicting, or describing constructs that are key to your research problem. A few additional questions include the following:

- Has the theory been applied to similar research questions, and do the findings from prior research lend credibility to the theory's utility for research?
- Are the theoretical constructs in the model or theory readily operationalized? Do instruments of adequate quality exist?
- Is the theory compatible with your world view and with the world view implicit in the research question?

TESTING, USING, AND DEVELOPING A THEORY OR FRAMEWORK

In this section, we describe how theory is used by qualitative and quantitative researchers. We use the term *theory* broadly to include conceptual models and frameworks.

Theories and Qualitative Research

Theory is almost always present, either peripherally or centrally, in studies that are embedded in a qualitative research tradition such as ethnography, phenomenology, or grounded theory. These research traditions inherently provide an overarching framework that gives qualitative studies a theoretical grounding. However, different traditions involve theory in different ways.

Sandelowski (1993) made a useful distinction between **substantive theory** (conceptualizations of the target phenomenon under study) and theory that reflects a conceptualization of human inquiry.

Some qualitative researchers insist on an atheoretical stance vis-à-vis the phenomenon of interest, with the goal of suspending a priori conceptualizations (substantive theories) that might bias their collection and analysis of data. For example, phenomenologists are in general committed to theoretical naiveté and explicitly try to hold preconceived views of the phenomenon in check. Nevertheless, they are guided in their inquiries by a philosophy of phenomenology that focuses their analysis on certain aspects of a person's lived experiences.

Ethnographers typically bring a strong cultural perspective to their studies, and this perspective shapes their initial fieldwork. Ethnographers often adopt one of two cultural theories: *ideational theories*, which suggest that cultural conditions stem from mental activity and ideas, or *materialistic theories*, which view material circumstances (e.g., resources, money, production) as the source of cultural developments.

The most prominent sociologic theory in grounded theory is **symbolic interaction** (or *interactionism*), which has three underlying premises (Blumer, 1986). First, humans act toward things based on the meanings that the things have for them. Second, the meaning of things arises out of the interaction humans have with other humans. Last, meanings are handled in, and modified through, an interpretive process in dealing with the things that humans encounter. Despite having a theoretical umbrella, grounded theory researchers, like phenomenologists, attempt to hold prior substantive theory (existing knowledge and conceptualizations about the phenomenon) in abeyance until their own substantive theory begins to emerge.

Example of a Grounded Theory Study
Ghafourifard and colleagues (2022) conducted a grounded theory study to develop a model that defined compassionate nursing care. Three main categories were essential to the Compassionate Nursing

BOX 6.1 Some Questions for a Preliminary Assessment of a Model or Theory

Issue	Questions
Theoretical clarity	• Are key concepts defined, and are definitions clear? • Do all concepts "fit" within the theory? Are concepts used in the theory in a manner compatible with conceptual definitions? • Are schematic models helpful, and are they compatible with the text? Are schematic models needed but not presented? • Is the theory adequately explained? Are there ambiguities?
Theoretical complexity	• Is the theory sufficiently rich and detailed? • Is the theory overly complex? • Can the theory be used to explain or predict phenomena, or only to describe them?
Theoretical grounding	• Are the concepts identifiable in reality? • Is there a research basis for the theory? Is the basis a sound one?
Appropriateness of the theory	• Are the tenets of the theory compatible with nursing's philosophy? • Are key concepts within the domain of nursing?
Importance of the theory	• Could research based on this theory answer critical questions for nursing? • Will testing the theory contribute to nursing's evidence base?
General issues	• Are there other theories or models that would do a better job of explaining phenomena of interest? • Is the theory compatible with your world view?

Care Model: (1) contextual factors affecting compassionate care; (2) compassionate care actions; and (3) consequences of compassionate care.

The use of theory in qualitative studies has been the topic of some debate. Morse (2002) called for qualitative researchers to not be "theory ignorant but theory smart" (p. 296) and to "get over" their theory phobia. Morse (2004) elaborated by noting that qualitative research does not necessarily begin with holding in check all prior knowledge of the phenomenon under study. She suggested that if the boundaries of the concept of interest can be identified, a qualitative researcher can use these boundaries as a scaffold to inductively explore the attributes of the concept.

Some qualitative nurse researchers have adopted a perspective known as critical theory as their framework. **Critical theory** is a paradigm that involves a critique of society and societal processes and structures, as we discuss in Chapter 22.

Qualitative researchers sometimes use conceptual models of nursing as an interpretive framework, rather than as a guide for the conduct of a study. For example, some qualitative nurse researchers acknowledge that the philosophic roots of their studies lie in conceptual models of nursing developed by Newman, Parse, or Rogers.

One final note is that a systematic review of qualitative studies on a specific topic is another strategy leading to theory development. In metasyntheses (Chapter 30), qualitative studies on a topic are scrutinized to identify essential elements. The findings from different sources are then used for theory building.

Theories and Models in Quantitative Research

Quantitative researchers, like qualitative researchers, link research to theory or models in several ways. The classic approach is to test hypotheses deduced from an existing theory.

Testing an Existing Theory

Theories sometimes stimulate new studies. For example, a nurse might read about Pender's HPM, and the following type of reasoning might ensue: "If the HPM is valid, then I would expect that patients with osteoporosis who perceived the benefit of a calcium-enriched diet would be more likely to alter their eating patterns than those who perceived no benefits." Such a conjecture can serve as a starting point for testing the model.

In testing a theory or model, quantitative researchers deduce implications (as in the preceding example) and develop hypotheses, which are predictions about the way variables would be interrelated if the theory were sound. The hypotheses are then subjected to testing through systematic data collection and analysis.

The testing process involves a comparison between observed outcomes with those hypothesized. Through this process, a theory is continually subjected to potential disconfirmation. If studies repeatedly fail to disconfirm a theory, it gains support. Testing continues until pieces of evidence cannot be interpreted within the context of the theory but *can* be explained by a new theory that also accounts for previous findings. Theory-testing studies are most useful when researchers devise logically sound deductions from the theory, design a study that reduces the plausibility of alternative explanations for observed relationships, and use methods that assess the theory's validity under maximally heterogeneous situations so that potentially competing theories can be ruled out.

Researchers sometimes base a new study on a theory to explain earlier descriptive findings. For example, suppose several researchers had found that nursing home residents demonstrate greater levels of noncompliance with nursing staff around bedtime than at other times. These findings shed no light on underlying causes of the problem, and so suggest no way to improve it. Explanations rooted in theories of stress might be relevant in explaining the residents' behavior. By directly testing the theory in a study (i.e., deducing hypotheses derived from the theory), a researcher might be able to explain *why* bedtime is a vulnerable period for nursing home residents.

Researchers sometimes combine elements from two theories as a basis for generating hypotheses. In doing this, researchers need to be thoroughly knowledgeable about *both* theories to see if there is an adequate conceptual rationale for conjoining them. If underlying assumptions or conceptual definitions of key concepts are not compatible, the theories should not be combined (although perhaps elements of the two can be used to create a new conceptual framework with its own assumptions and definitions).

Tests of a theory increasingly are taking the form of testing theory-based interventions. If a theory is correct, it has implications for strategies to influence people's health-related attitudes or behavior and hence their health outcomes. The role of theory in the development of interventions is discussed at greater length in Chapter 28.

> **Example of a Theory-Based Intervention**
> Murfield et al. (2022) developed a self-compassion intervention for family caregivers of people with dementia. The intervention was developed using integrated concepts from two theories—The Person-Based Approach (PBA) and the Patient and Public Involvement (PPI) Approach.

Using a Model or Theory as an Organizing Structure

Many researchers who cite a theory or model as their framework are not directly testing it, but rather using the theory as an organizational or interpretive tool. In such studies, researchers begin with a conceptualization of nursing (or stress, health beliefs, and so on) that is consistent with that of a model developer. The researchers *assume* that the model used as a framework is valid and proceed to conceptualize and operationalize constructs with the model in mind. Using models in this fashion can serve a valuable organizing purpose, but such studies do not address the issue of whether the theory itself is sound.

We should note that the framework for a quantitative study need not be a formal theory such as those described in the previous section. Sometimes researchers undertake quantitative studies to further explicate constructs identified in grounded theory or other qualitative research.

Fitting a Problem to a Theory

Researchers sometimes develop a set of research questions or hypotheses and subsequently try to devise a theoretical context in which to frame them. Such an approach may in some case be worthwhile, but we caution that an after-the-fact linkage of theory to a problem does not always enhance a study. An important exception is when the researcher is struggling to make sense of findings and calls on an existing theory to help explain or interpret them.

If it is necessary to find a relevant theory or model after a research problem is selected, the search for such a theory must begin by first conceptualizing the problem on an abstract level. For example, take the following research question: "Do daily telephone conversations between a psychiatric nurse and a patient for 2 weeks after hospital discharge reduce rates of readmission by short-term psychiatric patients?" This is a relatively concrete research problem, but it might profitably be viewed within the context of reinforcement theory, a theory of social support, or a theory of crisis resolution. Part of the difficulty in finding a theory is that a single phenomenon of interest can be conceptualized in ways.

Fitting a problem to a theory after-the-fact should be done with circumspection. Although having a theoretical context can enhance the meaningfulness of a study, artificially linking a problem to a theory is not the route to scientific utility. If a conceptual model is really linked to a problem, then the design of the study, decisions about what to measure and how to measure it, and the interpretation of the findings *flow* from that conceptualization.

> **TIP** If you begin with a research question and then subsequently identify a theory or model, be willing to adapt or augment your original research problem as you gain greater understanding of the theory.

Developing a Framework in a Quantitative Study

Novice researchers may think of themselves as unqualified to develop a conceptual scheme of their own. But theory development depends less on research experience than on powers of observation, grasp of a problem, and knowledge of prior research. Nothing prevents a creative and astute person from formulating an original conceptual framework for a study. The framework may not be a full-fledged theory, but it should place the issues of the study into some broader perspective.

The basic intellectual process underlying theory development is induction—that is, reasoning from particular observations and facts to broader generalizations. The inductive process involves integrating what one has experienced or learned into an organized scheme. For quantitative research, the observations used in the inductive process usually are findings from other studies. When patterns of relationships among variables are derived in this fashion, one has the makings of a theory that can be put to a more rigorous test. The first step in the development of a framework, then, is to formulate a generalized scheme of relevant concepts that is firmly grounded in the research literature.

Let us use as an example a study question identified in Chapter 4, namely, What is the effect of humor on stress in patients with cancer? (See the problem statement in Box 4.2). In undertaking a literature review, we find that researchers and reviewers have suggested a myriad of complex relationships among such concepts as humor, social support, stress, coping, appraisal, immune function, and neuroendocrine function on the one hand and various health outcomes (pain tolerance, mood, depression, health status, and eating and sleeping disturbances) on the other (e.g., Christie & Moore, 2005). While there is a fair amount of research evidence for the existence of these relationships, it is not clear how they all fit together. Without some kind of "map" of what might be going on, it could be challenging to design a strong study—we might, for example, not measure all the key variables or we might not undertake an appropriate analysis. And, if our goal is to design a humor therapy, we might struggle in developing a strong intervention in the absence of a framework.

The conceptual map in Figure 6.1 represents an attempt to put the pieces of the puzzle together for a study involving a test of a humor intervention to improve health outcomes for patients with cancer. According to this map, stress is affected by a cancer diagnosis and treatment both directly and indirectly, through the person's appraisal of the situation. That appraisal, in turn, is affected by the patient's coping skills, personality factors, and available social supports (factors that themselves are interrelated). Stress and physiological function (neuroendocrine and immunologic) have reciprocal relationships.

Note that we have not yet put in a "box" for humor in Figure 6.1. How do we think humor might operate? If we see humor as having primarily a direct effect on physiologic response, we would place humor near the bottom and draw an arrow from the box to immune and neuroendocrine function. But perhaps humor reduces stress because it helps a person cope (i.e., its effects are primarily psychological). Or maybe

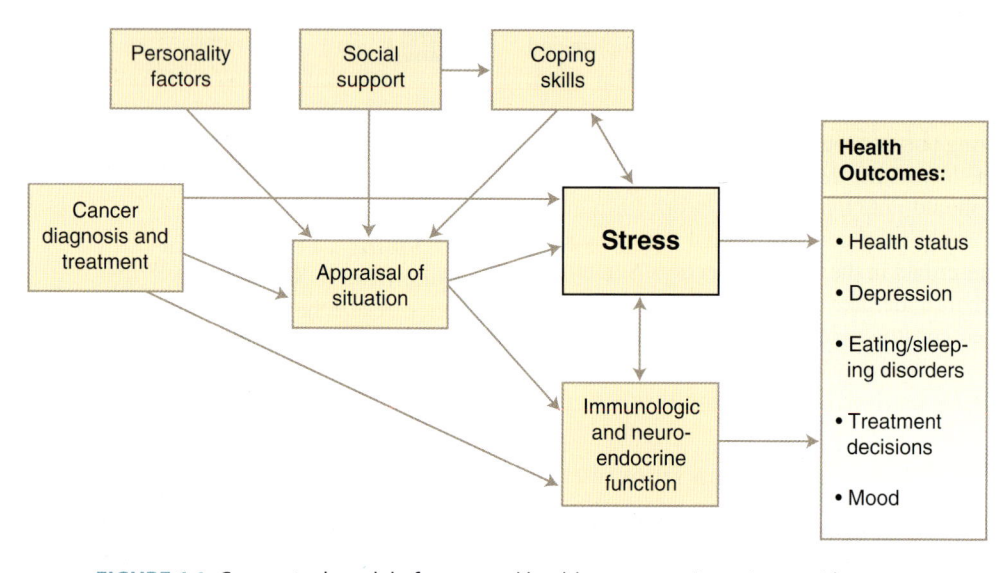

FIGURE 6.1 Conceptual model of stress and health outcomes in patients with cancer.

humor will affect the person's appraisal of the situation. Alternatively, a nurse-initiated humor therapy might have its effect primarily because it is a form of social support. Each conceptualization has a different implication for the design of the intervention and the study. To give but one example, if the humor therapy is viewed primarily as a form of social support, then we might want to compare our intervention with an alternative intervention that involves the presence of a comforting nurse (another form of social support), without any special effort at including humor.

This type of inductive conceptualization based on existing research is a useful means of providing theoretical grounding for a study. Of course, our research question in this example could have been addressed within the context of an existing conceptualization, such as the psychoneuroimmunology framework of McCain et al. (2005), but hopefully our example illustrates how developing an original framework can inform researchers' decisions and strengthen the study. Havenga et al. (2014) offer additional tips on developing a model.

TIP We strongly encourage you to draw a conceptual map before launching an investigation based on either an existing theory or your own inductive conceptualization—even if you do not plan to formally test the entire model or present the model in a report. Such maps are valuable heuristic devices in planning a study.

Example of Developing a New Model
Wand and colleagues (2021) developed and tested the mental health liaison nurse (MHLN) model of care. This new model of care aimed to expedite the care of patients with psychiatric conditions who were presenting to the emergency room.

CRITICAL APPRAISAL OF FRAMEWORKS IN RESEARCH REPORTS

It is often challenging to critically appraise the theoretical context of a published research report—or its absence—but we offer a few suggestions.

In a qualitative study in which a grounded theory is developed and presented, you probably will not be given enough information to refute the proposed theory because only evidence supporting it is presented. You can, however, assess whether the theory seems logical, whether the conceptualization is insightful, and whether the evidence in support of it is persuasive. In a phenomenologic study, you should look to see IF the researcher addressed the philosophical underpinnings of the study. The researcher should briefly discuss the philosophy of phenomenology upon which the study was based.

Critiquing a theoretical framework in a quantitative report is also difficult, especially because you are not likely to be familiar with a range of relevant theories and models. Some suggestions for evaluating the conceptual basis of a quantitative study are offered in the following discussion and in Box 6.2.

The first task is to determine whether the study does, in fact, have a theoretical or conceptual framework. If there is no mention of a theory, model, or framework, you should consider whether the study's contribution is weakened by this absence. In some cases, the research may be so pragmatic that it does not really need a theory to enhance its utility. If, however, the study involves evaluating a complex intervention or testing hypotheses, the absence of a formally stated theoretical framework or rationale suggests conceptual fuzziness.

If the study does have an explicit framework, you must ask whether the particular framework is appropriate. You may not be able to challenge the researcher's use of a particular theory, but you can assess whether the link between the problem and the theory is genuine. Did the researcher present a convincing rationale for the framework used? Do the hypotheses flow from the theory? Will the findings contribute to the validation of the theory? Did the researcher interpret the findings within the context of the framework? If the answer to such questions is no, you may have grounds for criticizing the study's framework, even though you may not be able to articulate how the conceptual basis of the study could be improved.

RESEARCH EXAMPLES

Throughout this chapter, we have mentioned studies that were based on various conceptual and theoretical models. This section presents more detailed examples of the linkages between theory and research from the nursing research literature—one from a quantitative study and the other from a qualitative study.

Research Example From a Quantitative Study: The Health Promotion Model

Study: The effect of exercise training based on the HPM on menopausal symptoms (Polat & Aylaz, 2022).

Statement of purpose: The purpose of this study was to determine the effect of exercise training based on the HPM on menopausal symptoms.

Theoretical framework: The HPM was the guiding framework for the study: "Health promotion is the process of managing people's health in the best and highest quality way. Health promotion according to Pender is the ability of individuals to take up their own health responsibilities, to eat a balanced diet, to do regular physical activity and to manage the stress they experience" (p. 1160).

Method: The sample population included 781 females in menopause who were between the ages of 45 and 60. They were randomly assigned to either the intervention or control group. Study participants completed three measures: a personal information form, the menopause rating scale, and the health-promoting lifestyle profile.

Key findings: The researchers found that "the exercise training based on the health promotion model reduced the severity of menopausal symptoms in women. Twelve-week moderate-intensity walking and aerobic exercise reduced the severity of menopausal symptoms. In the randomized controlled trials using exercise applications, it was determined that exercise reduced menopausal symptoms of women and enhanced their quality of life" (p. 1165).

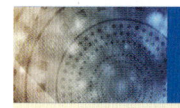

BOX 6.2 Guidelines for Critically Appraising Theoretical and Conceptual Frameworks in a Research Article

1. Did the report describe an explicit theoretical or conceptual framework for the study? If not, does the absence of a framework detract from the usefulness or significance of the research?
2. Did the report adequately describe the major features of the theory or model so that readers could understand the study's conceptual basis?
3. Does the theory or model fit the research problem? Would a different framework have been more appropriate?
4. If there is an intervention, was there a cogent theoretical basis or rationale for how the intervention was expected to "work" to produce desired outcomes?
5. Was the theory or model used as a basis for generating hypotheses, or was it used as an organizational or interpretive framework? Was this appropriate?
6. Did the research problem and hypotheses (if any) naturally flow from the framework, or did the purported link between the problem and the framework seem contrived? Were deductions from the theory logical?
7. Were concepts adequately defined, and in a way that is consistent with the theory? If there was an intervention, were intervention components consistent with the theory?
8. Was the framework based on a conceptual model of nursing or on a model developed by nurses? If it was borrowed from another discipline, is there adequate justification for its use?
9. Did the framework guide the study methods? For example, was the appropriate research tradition used if the study was qualitative? If quantitative, did the operational definitions correspond to the conceptual definitions?
10. Did the researcher tie the study findings back to the framework in the Discussion section? Did the findings support or challenge the framework? Were the findings interpreted within the context of the framework?

Research Example From a Qualitative Study

Study: Family dynamics in dementia care: A phenomenological exploration of the experiences of family caregivers of relatives with dementia (Smith et al., 2022).

Statement of purpose: The purpose of the study was to explore the relationships within families of those caring for a family member experiencing dementia.

Method: A descriptive phenomenological design guided this study.

Key findings: Eight caregivers from South Africa participated in the study. Each of the participants was interviewed four times over a period of 4–6 weeks. Three main themes were identified: "Painting a picture of paradise lost"; "Falling down the rabbit hole"; *and* "A fracture occurred" (Smith et al., 2022, p. 865).

SUMMARY POINTS

- High-quality research requires *conceptual integration*, one aspect of which is having a defensible theoretical rationale for the study. Researchers demonstrate conceptual clarity by delineating a theory, model, or framework on which the study is based.
- A **theory** is a broad characterization of phenomena. As classically defined, a theory is an abstract generalization that systematically explains relationships among phenomena. **Descriptive theory** thoroughly describes a phenomenon.
- Concepts are the basic components of a theory. Classically defined theories consist of a set of propositions about the interrelationships among concepts, arranged in a logical system that permits new statements (hypotheses) to be deduced from them.
- **Grand theories** (*macrotheories*) attempt to describe large segments of the human experience. **Middle-range theories** (e.g., Pender's HPM) are specific to certain phenomena (e.g., stress, uncertainty in illness).
- Concepts are also the basic elements of **conceptual models**, but concepts are not linked in a logically ordered deductive system. Conceptual models, like theories, provide context for nursing studies.
- The goal of theories and models in research is to make findings meaningful, to integrate knowledge into coherent systems, to stimulate new research, and to explain phenomena and relationships among them.
- **Schematic models** (or **conceptual maps**) are graphic, theory-driven representations of phenomena and their interrelationships using symbols or diagrams and a minimal use of words.
- A **framework** is the conceptual underpinning of a study, including an overall rationale and conceptual definitions of key concepts. In qualitative studies, the framework often springs from distinct research traditions.
- Several conceptual models and grand theories of nursing have been developed. The concepts central to models of nursing are *human beings, environment, health*, and *nursing*. Two major conceptual models of nursing used by researchers are Roy's **Adaptation Model** and Orem's **Self-Care Deficit Theory**.
- Non-nursing models used by nurse researchers include Bandura's **Social Cognitive Theory**, Prochaska's **Transtheoretical Model**, and Becker's **HBM.**
- In some qualitative research traditions (e.g., phenomenology), the researcher avoids existing **substantive theories** of the phenomenon under study, but there is a rich theoretical underpinning associated with the tradition itself.
- Some qualitative researchers specifically seek to develop *grounded theories*—data-driven explanations to account for phenomena under study through inductive processes.
- In the classical use of theory, researchers test hypotheses deduced from an existing theory. An emerging trend is the testing of theory-based interventions.
- In both qualitative and quantitative studies, researchers sometimes use a theory or model as an organizing framework or an interpretive tool.
- Researchers sometimes develop a problem, design a study, and *then* look for a conceptual framework; such an after-the-fact selection of a framework usually is less compelling than

- a more systematic application of a particular theory.
- Even in the absence of a formal theory, quantitative researchers can inductively weave together the findings from prior studies into a conceptual scheme that provides methodologic and conceptual direction to the inquiry.

REFERENCES CITED IN CHAPTER 6

Ajzen, I. (2005). *Attitudes, personality and behavior* (2nd ed.). McGraw Hill.

Alligood, M. R. (2021). *Nursing theorists and their work* (10th ed.). Elsevier.

Bandura, A. (1997). *Self-efficacy: The exercise of control*. W. H. Freeman.

Bandura, A. (2001). Social cognitive theory: An agentic perspective. *Annual Review of Psychology*, *52*, 1–26.

Beck, C. T. (2015). Middle range theory of traumatic childbirth: The ever-widening ripple effect. *Global Qualitative Nursing Research*, *2*, 2333393615575313. https://doi.org/10.1177/2333393615575313

Beck, C. T. (2023). Teetering on the edge: A third grounded theory modification of postpartum depression. *Advances in Nursing Science*, *46*(1), 14–27. http://doi.org/10.1097/ANS.0000000000000432

Becker, M. (1978). The health belief model and sick role behavior. *Nursing Digest*, *6*, 35–40.

Bergdahl, E., & Berterö, C. (2016). Concept analysis and the building blocks of theory: Misconceptions regarding theory development. *Journal of Advanced Nursing*, *72*(10), 2558–2566.

Blumer, H. (1986). *Symbolic interactionism: Perspective and method*. University of California Press.

Butts, J., & Rich, K. (2018). *Philosophies and theories for advanced nursing practice* (3rd ed.). Jones & Bartlett.

Chinn, P., & Kramer, M. (2021). *Knowledge development in nursing: Theory and process* (11th ed.). Elsevier.

Christie, W., & Moore, C. (2005). The impact of humor on patients with cancer. *Clinical Journal of Oncology Nursing*, *9*(2), 211–218.

Conn, V. S., Rantz, M. J., Wipke-Tevis, D. D., & Maas, M. L. (2001). Designing effective nursing interventions. *Research in Nursing & Health*, *24*(5), 433–442.

Dodd, M., Janson, S., Facione, N., Faucett, J., Froelicher, E. S., Humphreys, J., Lee, K, Miaskowski, C, Puntillo, K, Rankin, S, Taylor, D, Taylor, D. (2001). Advancing the science of symptom management. *Journal of Advanced Nursing*, *33*(5), 668–676.

Fawcett, J., & DeSanto-Madeya, S. (2013). *Contemporary nursing knowledge: Analysis and evaluation of nursing models and theories* (3rd ed.). Davis Company.

Firouzbakht, M., Sharif Nia, H., Kazeminavaei, F., & Rashidian, P. (2022). Hesitancy about COVID-19 vaccination among pregnant women: A cross-sectional study based on the health belief model. *BMC Pregnancy Childbirth*, *22*(1), 611. https://doi.org/10.1186/s12884-022-04941-3

Fishbein, M., & Ajzen, I. (2015). *Predicting and changing behavior: The reasoned action approach*. Routledge.

Flanagan, J. (2021). From concepts and systematic reviews: A path to enhancing nursing knowledge development. *International Journal of Nursing Knowledge*, *32*(4), 217. https://doi.org/10.1111/2047-3095.12353

Ghafourifard, M., Zamanzadeh, V., Valizadeh, L., & Rahmani, A. (2022). Compassionate nursing care model: Results from a grounded theory study. *Nursing Ethics*, *29*(3), 621–635. https://doi.org/10.1177/09697330211051005

Havenga, Y., Poggenpoel, M., & Myburgh, C. (2014). Developing a model: An illustration. *Nursing Science Quarterly*, *27*(2), 149–156.

Isik, E., & Fredland, N. M. (2023). Orem's self-care deficit nursing theory to improve children's self-care: An integrative review. *The Journal of School Nursing: The Official Publication of the National Association of School Nurses*, *39*(1), 6–17. https://doi.org/10.1177/10598405211050062

Kolcaba, K. (2003). *Comfort theory and practice*. Springer Publishing Co.

Lareyre, O., Gourlan, M., Stoebner-Delbarre, A., & Cousson-Gélie, F. (2021). Characteristics and impact of theory of planned behavior interventions on smoking behavior: A systematic review of the literature. *Preventive Medicine*, *143*, 106327. https://doi.org/10.1016/j.ypmed.2020.106327

McCain, N. L., Gray, D. P., Walter, J. M., & Robins, J. (2005). Implementing a comprehensive approach to the study of health dynamics using the psychoneuroimmunology paradigm. *Advances in Nursing Science*, *28*(4), 320–332.

Meleis, A. I., Sawyer, L. M., Im, E., Hilfinger Messias, D., & Schumacher, K. (2000). Experiencing transitions: An emerging middle-range theory. *Advances in Nursing Science*, *23*(1), 12–28.

Michie, S., Johnston, M., Abraham, C., Lawton, R., Parker, D., & Walker, A., "Psychological Theory" Group. (2005). Making psychological theory useful for implementing evidence-based practice: A consensus approach. *Quality & Safety in Health Care*, *14*(1), 26–33.

Mishel, M. H. (1990). Reconceptualization of the uncertainty in illness theory. *Journal of Nursing Scholarship*, *22*(4), 256–262.

Morse, J. M. (2002). Theory innocent or theory smart? *Qualitative Health Research*, *12*(3), 295–296.

Morse, J. M. (2004). Constructing qualitatively derived theory: Concept construction and concept typologies. *Qualitative Health Research*, *14*(10), 1387–1395.

Morse, J. M. (2017). *Analyzing and conceptualizing the theoretical foundations of nursing*. Springer Publishing Company.

Murdaugh, C., Parsons, M. A., & Pender, N. J. (2019). *Health promotion in nursing practice* (8th ed.). Pearson.

Murfield, J., Moyle, W., & O'Donovan, A. (2022). Planning and designing a self-compassion intervention for family carers of people living with dementia: A person-based and co-design approach. *BMC Geriatrics*, *22*(1), 53. https://doi.org/10.1186/s12877-022-02754-9

Orem, D., Taylor, S., Renpenning, K., & Eisenhandler, S. (2003). *Self-care theory in nursing: Selected papers of Dorothea Orem*. Springer.

Parse, R. R. (2014). *The humanbecoming paradigm: A transformational worldview*. A Discovery International Publication.

Peplau, H. E. (1997). Peplau's theory of interpersonal relations. *Nursing Science Quarterly*, *10*(4), 162–167.

Peterson, S. J., & Bredow, T. S. (2020). *Middle range theories: Applications to nursing research* (5th ed.). Wolters Kluwer.

Polat, F., & Aylaz, R. (2022). The effect of exercise training based on the health promotion model on menopausal symptoms. *Perspectives in Psychiatric Care*, *58*(3), 1160–1169. https://doi.org/10.1111/ppc.12917

Prochaska, J. O., & Velicer, W. F. (1997). The transtheoretical model of health behavior change. *American Journal of Health Promotion*, *12*(1), 38–48.

Prochaska, J. O., Redding, C. A., & Evers, K. E. (2002). The transtheoretical model and stages of changes. In Lewis, F. M. (Ed.), *Health behavior and health education: Theory, research and practice* (pp. 99–120). Jossey Bass.

Reed, P. G. (1991). Toward a nursing theory of self-transcendence: Deductive reformulation using developmental theories. *Advances in Nursing Science*, *13*(4), 64–77.

Reinken, D. N., & Reed, S. M. (2023). Mishel's uncertainty in illness theory: Informing nursing diagnoses and care planning. *International Journal of Nursing Knowledge*, *34*(4), 316, 324, Advance online publication. https://doi.org/10.1111/2047-3095.12406

Rodgers, B., & Knafl, K. (Eds.). (2000). *Concept development in nursing: Foundations, techniques, and applications* (2nd ed.). Saunders.

Rodgers, B. L., Jacelon, C. S., & Knafl, K. A. (2018). Concept analysis and the advance of nursing knowledge: State of the science. *Journal of Nursing Scholarship*, *50*(4), 451–459. https://doi.org/10.1111/jnu.12386

Roy, C. Sr, & Andrews, H. (2009). *The Roy adaptation model* (3rd ed.). Pearson.

Sandelowski, M. (1993). Theory unmasked: The uses and guises of theory in qualitative research. *Research in Nursing & Health*, *16*(3), 213–218.

Santi, D. B., Rossa, R., Bomfim, L. D. S. S., Dias, A. R., Higarashi, I. H., & Baldissera, V. D. A. (2022). Adolescent health in the COVID-19 pandemic: A construction through Nola Pender's model. *Brazilian Nursing Journal*, *75*(6), e20210696. https://doi.org/10.1590/0034-7167-2021-0696

Silveira, S. L., Cederberg, K. L. J., Jeng, B., Sikes, E. M., Sandroff, B. M., Jones, C. D., & Motl, R. W. (2021). Do physical activity and social cognitive theory variable scores differ across symptom cluster severity groups in multiple sclerosis? *Disability and Health Journal*, *14*(4), 101163. https://doi.org/10.1016/j.dhjo.2021.101163

Smith, M. J., & Liehr, P. (2023). *Middle-range theory for nursing* (5th ed.). Springer Publishing Co.

Smith, M. C. (2019). *Nursing theories and nursing practice* (5th ed.). F.A. Davis.

Smith, L., Morton, D., and van Rooyen, D. (2022). Family dynamics in dementia care: A phenomenological exploration of the experiences of family caregivers of relatives with dementia. *Journal of Psychiatric and Mental Health Nursing*, *29*(6), 861–872. https://doi.org/10.1111/jpm.12822

Swanson, K. M. (1991). Empirical development of a middle-range theory of caring. *Nursing Research*, *40*(3), 161–166.

Taghinezhad, F., Mohammadi, E., Khademi, M., & Kazemnejad, A. (2022). Humanistic care in nursing: Concept analysis using Rodgers' Evolutionary approach. *Iranian Journal of Nursing and Midwifery Research*, *27*(2), 83–91. https://doi.org/10.4103/ijnmr.ijnmr_156_

Walker, L. O., & Avant, K. C. (2019). *Strategies for theory construction in nursing* (6th ed.). Prentice Hall.

Wand, T., Collett, G., Cutten, A., Buchanan-Hagen, S., Stack, A., & White, K. (2021). Patient and staff experience with a new model of emergency department based mental health nursing care implemented in two rural settings. *International Emergency Nursing*, *57*, 101013. https://doi.org/10.1016/j.ienj.2021.101013

Wang, L., Liu, Y., Tan, H., & Huang, S. (2022). Transtheoretical model-based mobile health application for PCOS. *Reproductive Health*, *19*(1), 117. https://doi.org/10.1186/s12978-022-01422-w

Zheng, L., & Jin, Q. (2022). Roy adaptation model-based nursing diagnosis and implementation reduces the sense of shame and enhances nursing outcomes in female patients with breast cancer. *American Journal of Translational Research*, *14*(8), 5520–5528.

7 Ethics in Nursing Research

Learning Objectives

1. Discuss the historical background that led to the creation of various codes of ethics.
2. Describe ethical dilemmas that may potentially conflict with research goals.
3. Detail the procedures researchers can adopt to protect study participants in compliance with the three primary ethical principles articulated in the Belmont Report.
4. Provide examples of vulnerable groups who may require extra protections in participating in research.
5. Evaluate the ethical dimensions of a research report.

INTRODUCTION

Researchers who conduct studies with human being or animals must do so ethically. Ethical demands can be challenging because they sometimes conflict with the goal of producing rigorous evidence. This chapter discusses major ethical principles for conducting research.

ETHICS AND RESEARCH

The obligation for ethical conduct with human study participants may strike you as self-evident, but ethics have not always been given adequate attention.

Codes of Ethics

Human rights violations in the name of science have led to the development of various **codes of ethics**. The *Nuremberg Code*, developed after Nazi crimes were made public in the Nuremberg trials, was an international effort to establish ethical standards. The *Declaration of Helsinki*, another international set of ethical principles regarding human experimentation, was adopted in 1964 by the World Medical Association and was most recently revised in 2013.

Most disciplines (e.g., psychology, medicine) have established their own ethical codes. In nursing, the American Nurses Association (ANA) issued *Ethical Guidelines in the Conduct, Dissemination, and Implementation of Nursing Research* (Silva, 1995). The ANA, which declared 2015 the Year of Ethics, published a revised *Code of Ethics for Nurses with Interpretive Statements*, a document that includes principles that apply to nurse researchers. In Canada, the Canadian Nurses Association published a revised version of *Ethical Research Guidelines for Registered Nurses* in 2017. In Australia, three nursing organizations collaborated to develop the *Code of Ethics for Nurses in Australia* (2018). Additionally, the International Council of Nurses (ICN) developed the *ICN Code of Ethics for Nurses*, which was most recently revised in 2021.

Government Regulations for Protecting Study Participants

Governments throughout the world fund research and establish rules for adhering to ethical principles. For example, Health Canada created the *Tri-Council Policy Statement: Ethical Conduct for Research Involving Humans* as the guidelines to protect study participants in all types of research, most recently revised in 2014. In Australia, the National Health and Medical Research Council issued the *National Statement on Ethical Conduct in Human Research,* updated in 2018.

In the United States, the National Commission for the Protection of Human Subjects of Biomedical and Behavioral Research adopted a code of ethics in 1978. The commission issued the *Belmont Report*, which provided a model for many disciplinary guidelines. Regulations affecting research sponsored by the U.S. government, including studies supported by the National Institute of Nursing Research, are based on the Belmont Report. The U.S. Department of Health and Human Services (DHHS) has issued ethical regulations that have been codified as Title 45 Part 46 of the Code of Federal Regulations (45 CFR 46). These regulations were revised most recently in 2018.

Ethical Dilemmas in Conducting Research

Research that violates ethical principles is rarely done to be cruel, but usually reflects a conviction that knowledge is important and beneficial in the long run. There are situations in which participants' rights and study demands are in direct conflict, posing **ethical dilemmas** for researchers. Here are examples of research problems in which the desire for rigor conflicts with ethical considerations:

1. *Research question:* Does a new medication improve mobility in patients with Parkinson disease?
   Ethical dilemma: The best way to test the effectiveness of an intervention is to administer the intervention to some participants but withhold it from others to see if differences between the groups emerge. However, if the intervention is untested (e.g., a new drug), the group receiving the intervention may be exposed to potentially hazardous side effects. On the other hand, the group *not* receiving the drug may be denied a beneficial treatment.

2. *Research question:* Are nurses equally empathic in their care of male and female patients in the intensive care unit (ICU)? *Ethical dilemma:* Ethics require that participants be aware of their role in a study. Yet if the researcher informs nurse participants that their empathy in treating male and female ICU patients will be scrutinized, will their behavior be "normal"? If the nurses' usual behavior is altered because of the known presence of research observers, then the findings will be misleading.

3. *Research question:* How do parents cope if a child has a terminal illness? *Ethical dilemma:* To answer this question, the researcher may need to probe into parents' psychological state at a vulnerable time; such probing could be painful or traumatic. Yet knowledge of the parents' coping mechanisms might help to design effective ways of addressing parents' stress and grief.

4. *Research question:* What is the process by which adult children adapt to the day-to-day stresses of caring for a parent with Alzheimer disease? *Ethical dilemma:* Sometimes, especially in qualitative studies, a researcher may get so close to participants that they become willing to share "secrets" and privileged information. Interviews can become confessions—sometimes of unseemly or illegal behavior. In this example, suppose a woman admitted to physically abusing her mother—how does the researcher respond to that information without undermining a pledge of confidentiality? And, if the researcher divulges the information to authorities, how can a pledge of confidentiality be given in good faith to other participants?

As these examples suggest, researchers are sometimes in a bind. They want to develop good evidence, but they must also protect human rights. Another dilemma can arise if nurse researchers are confronted with conflict-of-interest situations, in which their expected behavior as researchers conflicts with their expected behavior as nurses (e.g., deviating from a research protocol to give assistance to a patient). It is precisely because of such dilemmas that codes of ethics have been developed to guide researchers' efforts.

ETHICAL PRINCIPLES FOR PROTECTING STUDY PARTICIPANTS

The *Belmont Report* articulated three broad principles on which standards of ethical conduct in research in the United States are based: beneficence, respect for human dignity, and justice. We briefly discuss these principles and then describe procedures researchers adopt to comply with them.

Beneficence

Beneficence imposes a duty on researchers to maximize benefits and minimize harm. Human research should be intended to produce benefits for participants or—a more common situation—for others. This principle covers multiple aspects.

> **TIP** The increased involvement of patients and lay people in the development of research questions and protocols has been viewed as an especially ethical approach to research conduct. As noted by Domecq et al. (2014), "there is an overarching ethical mandate for patient participation in research as a manifestation of the 'democratization' of the research process" (p. 1).

The Right to Freedom From Harm and Discomfort

Researchers have an obligation to avoid, prevent, or minimize harm (*nonmaleficence*) in research with humans. Participants should not be subjected to unnecessary risks of harm or discomfort, and their participation must be essential to achieving societally important aims that could not otherwise be realized. In research with humans, *harm* and *discomfort* can be physical (e.g., injury, fatigue), emotional (e.g., stress, fear), social (e.g., diminished social support), or financial (e.g., loss of wages). Ethical researchers must use strategies to minimize all types of harms and discomforts, even ones that are temporary.

Research should be conducted by qualified people, especially if potentially dangerous procedures are used. Ethical researchers must be prepared to terminate a study if they suspect that continuation would result in injury or undue distress to participants. When a new medical procedure or drug is being tested, prior experimentation with animals or tissue cultures is advisable.

Protecting human beings from physical harm may be straightforward, but psychological consequences are often subtle. For example, participants may be asked questions about their personal weaknesses, fears, or concerns. Such queries might lead people to reveal very personal information. The point is not that researchers should refrain from asking questions but that they need to be aware of the intrusion on people's psyches.

The need for sensitivity may be greater in qualitative studies, which often involve in-depth exploration of personal topics. Extensive probing may expose deep-seated anxieties that participants had previously repressed. Qualitative researchers must be vigilant in anticipating potential ethical challenges.

The Right to Protection From Exploitation

Study involvement should not place participants at a disadvantage or expose them to damages. Participants need to be assured that their participation, or information they provide, will not be used against them. For example, people divulging illegal drug use should not fear exposure to criminal authorities.

Study participants enter into a special relationship with researchers, and this relationship should never be exploited. Exploitation may be overt and malicious (e.g., sexual exploitation, commercial use of donated blood) but might be more elusive. For example, suppose people agreed to participate in a study requiring 30 minutes of their time, but the time commitment was actually 2 hours. In such a situation, the researcher might be accused of exploiting the researcher–participant relationship.

Because nurse researchers may have a nurse–patient (in addition to a researcher–participant) relationship, special care may be required to avoid exploiting that bond. Patients' consent to participate in a study may result from their understanding of the researcher's role as *nurse*, not as *researcher*.

In qualitative research, psychological distance between researchers and participants often declines as the study progresses. The emergence of a pseudotherapeutic relationship is not uncommon, which can heighten the risk that exploitation could occur inadvertently (Eide & Kahn, 2008). On the other hand, qualitative researchers often are in a better position than quantitative researchers to *do good*, rather than just to avoid doing harm.

> **Example of Therapeutic Research Experiences**
> Some of the participants in Beck et al.'s (2015) study on secondary traumatic stress among certified nurse-midwives told the researchers that writing about the traumatic births they had attended was therapeutic for them. One participant wrote, "I think it's fascinating how little respect our patients and coworkers give to the traumatic experiences we suffer. It is healing to be able to write out my experiences in this study and actually have researchers interested in studying this topic."

Respect for Human Dignity

Respect for human dignity is the second ethical principle in the *Belmont Report*. This principle includes the right to self-determination and the right to full disclosure.

The Right to Self-Determination

Humans should be treated as autonomous agents. **Self-determination** means that prospective participants can voluntarily decide whether to take part in a study, without risk of prejudicial treatment. It also means that people have the right to ask questions, to refuse to give information, and to withdraw from the study.

A person's right to self-determination includes freedom from **coercion**, which involves threats of penalty for failing to participate in a study or excessive rewards for agreeing to participate. Protecting people from coercion requires careful thought when the researcher is in a position of authority or influence over potential participants, as is often the case in a nurse–patient relationship. The issue of coercion may require scrutiny even when there is not a pre-established relationship. For example, a generous monetary incentive (or **stipend**) offered to encourage participation among an economically disadvantaged group (e.g., the homeless) might be considered mildly coercive because such incentives might pressure prospective participants into cooperation.

The Right to Full Disclosure

People's right to make informed, voluntary decisions about study participation requires full disclosure. **Full disclosure** means that the researcher has fully described the study, the right to refuse participation, the researcher's responsibilities, and likely risks and benefits. The right to self-determination and the right to full disclosure are the two major elements of *informed consent*, discussed later in this chapter.

Full disclosure can, however, create biases and sample recruitment problems. Suppose we were testing the hypothesis that high school students with a high rate of absenteeism are more likely to have substance abuse disorder than students with good attendance. If we approached potential participants and fully explained the study purpose, some students likely would refuse to participate, and nonparticipation would be selective; those least likely to volunteer might well be students with substance abuse disorder—the group of primary interest. Moreover, by knowing the research question, those who *do* participate might not give candid responses. In such a situation, full disclosure could undermine the study.

A technique that is sometimes used in such situations is **covert data collection** (*concealment*), which is the collection of data without participants' knowledge and consent. This might happen, for example, if a researcher wanted to observe people's behavior in real-world settings and worried that doing so openly would affect the behavior of interest. Researchers might choose to obtain the information through concealed methods, such as by videotaping with hidden equipment or observing while pretending to be engaged in other activities. Covert data collection may in some cases be acceptable if risks are negligible and participants' right to privacy has not been violated. Covert data collection is least likely to be ethically tolerable if the study is focused on sensitive aspects of people's behavior, such as drug use or sexual conduct.

A more controversial technique is the use of **deception**, which involves deliberately withholding information about the study or providing participants with false information. For example, in studying high school students' use of drugs, we might describe the research as a study of students' health practices, which is a mild form of misinformation.

Deception and concealment are problematic ethically because they interfere with people's right to make informed decisions about personal costs and benefits of participation. Some people argue that deception is never justified. Others, however, believe that if the study involves minimal risk to participants and if there are anticipated benefits to society, then deception may be justified as a means of enhancing the validity of the findings.

Another issue that has emerged in this era of electronic communication concerns data collection over the Internet. For example, some researchers analyze the content of messages posted to social media sites. The issue is whether such messages can be treated as research data without permission and informed consent. Some researchers believe that messages posted electronically are in the public domain and can be used without consent for research purposes. Others, however, feel that standard ethical rules should apply in cyberspace research and that researchers must carefully protect the rights of those who participate in "virtual" communities. Guidance for the ethical conduct of health research on the internet is offered by Mahon (2014) and Martin et al. (2020).

Justice

The third broad principle articulated in the *Belmont Report* concerns justice, which includes participants' right to fair treatment and their right to privacy.

The Right to Fair Treatment

One aspect of justice concerns the equitable distribution of benefits and burdens of research. Participant selection should be based on study requirements and not on a group's vulnerability. Participant selection has been a key ethical issue historically, with researchers sometimes selecting groups with lower social standing (e.g., prisoners) as participants. The principle of justice imposes special obligations toward individuals who are unable to protect their own interests (e.g., dying patients) to ensure that they are not exploited.

Distributive justice also imposes duties to not discriminate against individuals or groups who may benefit from research. During the 1980s and 1990s, it became evident that females and underrepresented groups were being unfairly excluded from many clinical studies in the United States. This led to the promulgation of regulations requiring that researchers who seek funding from the National Institutes of Health (NIH) include females and underrepresented groups as participants. The regulations also require researchers to examine whether clinical interventions have differential effects (e.g., whether benefits are different for males than for females), although this provision has had limited adherence (Polit & Beck, 2009, 2013).

The fair treatment principle covers issues other than participant selection. The right to fair treatment means that researchers must treat people who decline to participate (or who withdraw from the study) in a nonprejudicial manner; that they must honor all agreements with participants; that they demonstrate respect for the beliefs and lifestyles of people from different backgrounds or cultures; that they give participants access to research staff for desired clarification; and that they treat participants courteously and tactfully at all times.

The Right to Privacy

Research with humans involves intrusions into personal lives. Researchers should ensure that their research is not more intrusive than it needs to be and that participants' privacy is maintained. Participants have the right to expect that their data will be kept in strict confidence.

Privacy issues have become especially salient in the U.S. healthcare community since the passage of the Health Insurance Portability and Accountability Act of 1996 (HIPAA), which articulates federal standards to protect patients' health information. In response to the HIPAA legislation, the U.S. DHHS issued the regulations *Standards for Privacy of Individually Identifiable Health Information*.

TIP Some information relevant to HIPAA compliance is presented in this chapter, but you should confer with organizations that are involved in your research (if they are covered entities) regarding their practices and policies relating to HIPAA provisions. Here is a website that provides information about the implications of HIPAA for health research: https://privacyruleandresearch.nih.gov.

PROCEDURES FOR PROTECTING STUDY PARTICIPANTS

Now that you are familiar with fundamental ethical principles in research, you need to understand procedures that researchers use to adhere to them.

Risk/Benefit Assessments

One strategy that researchers use to protect participants is to conduct a **risk/benefit assessment.** Such an assessment is designed to evaluate whether the benefits of participating in a study are in line with the costs, be they financial, physical, emotional, or social—that is, whether the *risk/benefit ratio* is acceptable. A summary of risks and benefits should be communicated to recruited individuals so that they can evaluate whether it is in their best interest to participate. Box 7.1 summarizes some potential costs and benefits of research participation.

The risk/benefit ratio should take into account whether risks to participants are commensurate with benefits to society. A broad guideline is that the degree of risk by participants should never exceed the potential humanitarian benefits of the evidence to be gained. Thus, the selection of a significant topic that has the potential to improve patient care is the first step in ensuring that research is ethical. Geller and colleagues (2021) provide guidance on this topic.

All research involves some risks, but risk is sometimes small. **Minimal risk** is defined as risks no greater than those ordinarily encountered in daily life or during routine procedures. When the risks are not minimal, researchers must proceed with caution, taking every step possible to diminish risks and maximize benefits.

BOX 7.1 Potential Benefits and Risks of Research to Participants

Major Potential Benefits to Participants
- Access to a potentially beneficial intervention that might otherwise be unavailable
- Comfort in being able to discuss their situation or problem with a friendly, objective person
- Increased knowledge about themselves or their conditions, either through opportunity for introspection and self-reflection or through direct interaction with researchers
- Escape from normal routine
- Satisfaction that information they provide may help others with similar conditions
- Direct monetary or material gains through stipends or other incentives

Major Potential Risks to Participants
- Physical harm, including unanticipated side effects
- Discomfort, fatigue, or boredom
- Emotional distress as a result of self-disclosure, introspection, discomfort with strangers, fear of repercussions, anger, or embarrassment at the questions being asked
- Social risks, such as the risk of stigma, adverse effects on personal relationships, loss of status
- Loss of privacy
- Loss of time
- Monetary costs (e.g., for transportation, childcare, time lost from work)

In quantitative studies, most details of the study usually are spelled out in advance, and so a reasonably accurate risk/benefit assessment can be developed. Qualitative studies, however, usually evolve as data are gathered, and so it may be difficult to assess all risks at the outset. Qualitative researchers must remain sensitive to potential risks throughout the study.

Example of Ongoing Vigilance and Assessment
Sperlich and Gabriel (2022) sought to understand the reasons for choosing and out of hospital birth or unattended birth in two different groups of females: Black females and those who had experienced adverse childhood events associated with physical and/or sexual abuse. Recognizing that interviewing these people could trigger painful emotional reactions, the interviewers were vigilant for signs of emotional distress and allowed participants to opt out of a recorded interview. Although all 18 participants endorsed a history of trauma, all participants recruited completed the interviews and opted to be recorded.

One potential benefit to participants is monetary. Stipends offered to prospective participants are rarely viewed as an opportunity for financial gain, but there is ample evidence that stipends are useful incentives to participant recruitment and retention (Edwards et al., 2009). Financial incentives are especially effective when the group under study is difficult to recruit, when the study is time-consuming or tedious, or when participants incur study-related costs (e.g., for childcare or transportation). Stipends can range from $1 to hundreds of dollars, but many are in the $25 to $75 range.

TIP In evaluating the anticipated risk/benefit ratio of a study design, you might want to consider how comfortable *you* would feel about being a study participant.

Informed Consent and Participant Authorization

A particularly important procedure for safeguarding participants is to obtain their informed consent. **Informed consent** means that participants have adequate information about the research, comprehend that information, and can consent to or decline participation voluntarily. This section discusses procedures for obtaining informed consent and for complying with HIPAA rules regarding accessing patients' health information.

The Content of Informed Consent

Fully informed consent typically involves communicating the following pieces of information to participants:

1. *Participant status.* Prospective participants need to understand the distinction between *research* and *treatment*. They should be told which healthcare activities are routine and which are implemented specifically for the study. They also should be informed that data they provide will be used for research purposes.
2. *Study goals.* The overall goals of the research should be stated, in lay rather than technical terms. The use to which the data will be put should be described.
3. *Type of data.* Prospective participants should be told what type of data (e.g., self-reports, laboratory tests) will be collected.
4. *Procedures.* Prospective participants should be given a description of the data collection procedures and procedures to be used regarding any innovative treatment.
5. *Nature of the commitment.* Participants should be told the expected time commitment at each point of contact and the number of contacts within a given time frame.
6. *Sponsorship.* Information on who is sponsoring or funding the study should be noted; if the research is part of an academic requirement, this information should be shared.
7. *Participant selection.* Prospective participants should be told how they were selected for recruitment and how many people will be participating.
8. *Potential risks.* Foreseeable risks (physical, psychological, social, or economic) or discomforts should be communicated, as well as efforts that will be made to minimize risks. The possibility of unforeseeable risks should be discussed, if appropriate. If injury is possible, treatments that will be made available to participants should be described. When risks are

more than minimal, prospective participants should be encouraged to seek advice before consenting.
9. *Potential benefits.* Specific benefits to participants, if any, should be described, as well as possible benefits to others.
10. *Alternatives.* If appropriate, participants should be told about alternative procedures or treatments that might be advantageous to them.
11. *Compensation.* If stipends or reimbursements are to be paid (or if treatments are offered without any fee), these arrangements should be discussed.
12. *Confidentiality pledge.* Prospective participants should be assured that their privacy will be protected. If anonymity can be guaranteed, this should be stated.
13. *Voluntary consent.* Researchers should indicate that participation is strictly voluntary and that failure to volunteer will not result in any penalty or loss of benefits.
14. *Right to withdraw and withhold information.* Prospective participants should be told that, after consenting, they have the right to withdraw from the study or to withhold any specific piece of information. Researchers may need to describe circumstances under which researchers would terminate the study.
15. *Contact information.* The researcher should tell participants whom they could contact in the event of questions, comments, or complaints.

In qualitative studies, especially those requiring repeated contact with participants, it may be difficult to obtain meaningful informed consent at the outset. Qualitative researchers do not always know in advance how the study will evolve. Because the research design emerges during data collection, researchers may not know the exact nature of the data to be collected, the risks and benefits to participants, or how much of a time commitment they will be expected to make. Thus, in a qualitative study, consent is often viewed as an ongoing, transactional process, which is sometimes called **process consent**. With this type of consent, the researcher continually renegotiates the consent, allowing participants to play a collaborative role in making decisions about ongoing participation.

Example of Process Consent
Klykken (2022) used an ethnographic approach to study the everyday educational activities in a Norwegian upper secondary classroom. Before initiation of the study, informed consent from the students was obtained. As the study progressed, Klykken noted students were discussing various understandings of the study to which they had consented. As a result, Klykken implemented a process consent that allowed the students to continue with participation or not. Although all students continued with the study, during the reconsent process, one student declined to be videotaped.

Comprehension of Informed Consent

Consent information is typically presented to prospective participants while they are being recruited, either orally or in writing. Written notices should not, however, take the place of spoken explanations, which provide opportunities for elaboration and for participants to question and "screen" the researchers.

Because informed consent is based on a person's evaluation of the potential risks and benefits of participation, the information must not only be communicated but understood. Researchers may have to play a "teacher" role in conveying consent information. They should use simple language and avoid technical terms whenever possible. Written statements should be consistent with the participants' reading levels. For participants from a general population (e.g., patients in a hospital), statements should be at about the seventh or eighth grade reading level.

TIP Innovations to improve understanding of consent are being developed. Nishimura et al. (2013) did a systematic review of 54 of them.

For some studies, especially those involving more than minimal risk, researchers need to ensure that prospective participants understand what participation will entail. This might involve testing participants' comprehension of informed consent material before deeming them eligible. Such efforts are especially warranted with participants whose native tongue is not the same as the researchers or who have cognitive impairments (Fields & Calvert, 2015; Simpson, 2010).

Example of Ensuring Comprehension in Informed Consent

Tyrrell and colleagues (2021) studied older people's experience of undergoing a cognitive assessment and the possible experience of neuropsychiatric symptoms related to neurocognitive diagnosis. To assure their comprehension for consent participants were asked to repeat what the study was about. They were also required to score >15 on the Mini Mental State Examination. The authors suggest that research indicates that 15 is the cutoff for informed consent and the ability to converse and communicate.

Documentation of Informed Consent

Researchers usually document informed consent by having participants sign a **consent form**. In the United States, federal regulations for studies funded by the government require written consent of participants, except under certain circumstances. When the study does not involve an intervention and data are collected anonymously—or when existing data from records or specimens are used without linking identifying information to the data—regulations requiring written informed consent usually do not apply. HIPAA legislation is explicit about the type of information that must be eliminated from patient records for the data to be considered **deidentified**. The consent form should contain all the information essential to informed consent. Prospective participants (or their *legally authorized representatives*) should have ample time to review the document before signing it. The consent form should also be signed by the researcher, and a copy should be retained by both parties.

TIP In developing a consent form, the following suggestions might prove helpful:
1. Organize the form coherently so that prospective participants can follow the logic of what is being communicated. If the form is complex, use headings as an organizational aid.
2. Use a large enough font so that the form can be easily read, and use spacing that avoids making the document appear too dense. Make the form attractive and inviting.
3. In general, simplify. Avoid technical terms if possible, and if they are needed, include definitions.
4. Assess the form's reading level by using a **readability formula** to ensure an appropriate level for the group under study. There are several such formulas, including the Flesch Reading Ease score and Flesch–Kincaid grade level score (Flesch, 1948). Microsoft Word provides Flesch readability statistics.
5. Test the form with people similar to those who will be recruited, and ask for feedback.

In certain circumstances (for example, with non–English-speaking participants), researchers have the option of presenting the full information orally and then summarizing essential information in a **short form**. If a short form is used, however, the oral presentation must be witnessed by a third party and the witness's signature must appear on the short consent form. The signature of a third-party witness is also advisable in studies involving more than minimal risk, even when a comprehensive consent form is used.

When the primary means of data collection is through self-administered questionnaires, some researchers do not obtain written informed consent because they assume **implied consent** (i.e., that the return of the completed questionnaire reflects voluntary consent to participate). In such situations, researchers often provide an *information sheet* that contains all the elements of an informed consent form but does not require a signature. An example of such an information sheet used in a study of Cheryl Beck (an author of this book) is presented in Figure 7.1. The numbers in the margins of this figure correspond to the types of information for informed consent outlined earlier.

TIP Most universities offer templates of informed consent forms and provide guidance on documenting the research process.

Authorization to Access Private Health Information

Under HIPAA regulations in the United States, a covered entity such as a hospital can disclose *individually identifiable health information* from its records if the patient signs an authorization. The

Principal Investigator: Cheryl Tatano Beck, DNSc, CNM, FAAN
Study Title: Impact of Traumatic Childbirth on Mothers' Experiences Caring for Their Children

1. **Introduction** You are invited to participate in a research study so that we can better understand the impact of traumatic childbirth on mothers' experiences interacting with and caring for their infants and older children.

2. **Why is this study being done?** For decades now researchers have studied the long-term effects that postpartum depression can have on mother-infant interactions and child development. Much less attention has focused on the possible effects of posttraumatic stress on mother-infant interaction and attachment and children's emotional and cognitive development. The purpose of this study is to help understand the experiences of mothers who have had a traumatic birth and how this may impact their interactions with their infants and older children.

3. **What are the study procedures? What will I be asked to do?** If you agree to take part in this survey you will be asked to complete (1) a participant Profile Form which includes questions about yourself such as your age, education, and type of delivery, and (2) to describe in as much detail as you wish your
4. experiences of caring for and interacting with your infant and any older children you may have. Depending on how in depth you write about your experiences, participation in the study could take between 30- 60
5. minutes. Your participation will be anonymous and you will not be contacted again in the future. You will not be paid for being in this study.

8. **What are the risks or inconveniences of the study?** We believe there are no known risks associated with this research study; however, if you become anxious remembering your traumatic childbirth please know you can stop participating in the study. You do not have to complete the study. One possible inconvenience to you may be the time it takes to complete this survey.

9. **What are the benefits of the study?** You may not directly benefit from this research; however, we hope your participation in this survey will help healthcare professionals provide better care to mothers who have experienced a traumatic childbirth.

11. **Will I receive payment for participation? Are there costs to participate?** There are no costs and you will not be paid to be in this study.

12. **How will my personal information be protected?** The following procedures will be used to protect the confidentiality of your data. The researchers will keep all study records indefinitely in a locked file in a secure location. Research records will be labeled with a code. The code will be derived from a sequential 3 digit number that reflects how many people have enrolled in the study. All electronic files (e.g., database, spreadsheet, etc.) will be password protected. Any computer hosting such files will also have password protection to prevent access by unauthorized users. Only the members of the research staff will have access to the passwords. At the conclusion of this study, the researchers may publish their findings. Information will be presented in summary format and you will not be identified in any publications or presentations.

   "We will do our best to protect the confidentiality of the information we gather from you but we cannot guarantee 100% confidentiality. Your confidentiality will be maintained to the degree permitted by the technology used. Specifically, no guarantees can be made regarding the interception of data sent via the Internet by any third parties."

   You should also know that the UConn Institutional Review Board (IRB) and Research Compliance Services may inspect study records as part of its auditing program, but these reviews will only focus on the researchers and not on your responses or involvement. The IRB is a group of people who review research studies to protect the rights and welfare of research participants.

13. **Can I stop being in the study and what are my rights?** You do not have to be in this study if you do not want to. If you agree to be in the study, but later change your mind, you may drop out at any time.
14. There are no penalties or consequences of any kind if you decide that you do not want to participate.

15. **Whom do I contact if I have questions about the study?** Take as long as you like before you make a decision. We will be happy to answer any question you have about this study. If you have further questions about this project or if you have a research-related problem, you may contact the principal investigator, (Dr. Cheryl Beck, 860-xxx-xxx). If you have any questions concerning your rights as a research subject, you may contact the University of Connecticut Institutional Review Board (IRB) at 860-xxx-xxxx

FIGURE 7.1 Example of an information sheet for study participants.

authorization can be incorporated into the consent form, or it can be a separate document. Using a separate authorization form may be advantageous to protect the patients' confidentiality because the form does not need to provide detailed information about the study purpose. If the research purpose is not sensitive, or if the entity is already cognizant of the study purpose, an integrated form may suffice. The authorization, whether obtained separately or as part of the consent form, must include the following: (1) who will receive the information; (2) what type of information will be disclosed; and (3) what further disclosures the researcher anticipates.

Confidentiality Procedures

Study participants have the right to expect that data they provide will be kept in strict confidence. Participants' right to privacy is protected through various confidentiality procedures.

Anonymity

Anonymity, the most secure means of protecting confidentiality, occurs when the researcher cannot link participants to their data. For example, if questionnaires were distributed to a group of nursing home residents and were returned without any identifying information, responses would be anonymous. As another example, if a researcher reviewed hospital records from which all identifying information had been expunged, anonymity would protect participants' right to privacy. Whenever it is possible to achieve anonymity, researchers should strive to do so.

> **Example of Anonymity**
> Post et al. (2021) conducted a study to explore the relationship between sociodemographic factors, survivorship variables, and patient engagement in breast cancer survivors. A sample of 303 people who recovered from breast cancer responded to an anonymous online survey.

Confidentiality in the Absence of Anonymity

When anonymity is not possible, other confidentiality procedures are needed. A promise of **confidentiality** is a pledge that any information participants provide will not be reported in a manner that identifies them and will not be accessible to others. This means that research information should not be shared with strangers nor with people known to participants (e.g., relatives, doctors, other nurses), unless participants give explicit permission to do so.

Researchers can take a number of steps to ensure that a **breach of confidentiality** does not occur, including the following:

- Obtain identifying information (e.g., name, address) from participants only when essential.
- Assign an **identification** (ID) **number** to each participant and attach the ID number rather than other identifiers to actual data forms.
- Maintain identifying information in a locked file.
- Restrict access to identifying information to only a few people on a need-to-know basis.
- Enter identifying information onto computer files that are encrypted.
- Destroy identifying information as quickly as practical.
- Make research personnel sign confidentiality pledges if they have access to identifying information.
- Report research information in the aggregate; if information for a person is reported, disguise the person's identity, such as through the use of a fictitious name.

> **TIP** Researchers who plan to collect data from participants multiple times (or who use multiple forms that need to be linked) do not have to forgo anonymity. A technique that has been successful is to have participants themselves generate an ID number. They might be instructed, for example, to use the first three letters of their mother's middle names and their birth year as their ID code (e.g., FRA1983). This code would be put on every form so that forms could be linked, but researchers would not know participants' identities.

Qualitative researchers may need to take extra steps to safeguard participants' privacy. Anonymity is rarely possible in qualitative studies because researchers typically become closely involved with participants. Moreover, because of the in-depth nature of qualitative studies, there may be a greater invasion of privacy than is true in quantitative research. Researchers who spend time in the home of a participant may, for example, have difficulty segregating the public behaviors that the participant is willing to share from private behaviors that unfold during data collection. A final issue concerns disguising participants in reports. Because the number of participants is small, qualitative researchers need to take special precautions to safeguard identities. This may mean more than simply using a fictitious name. Qualitative researchers may have to slightly distort identifying information or provide broad descriptions. For example, a 49-year-old antique dealer with ovarian cancer might be described as "a middle-aged cancer patient who was a shop owner" to avoid identification that could occur with the more detailed description.

Example of Confidentiality Procedures in a Qualitative Study
Walsh et al. (2020) conducted a narrative inquiry exploring caregivers' experiences of the last days of a family member dying from cancer. Oral informed consent was obtained from the caregivers. To assure confidentiality, Walsh assured participants that pseudonyms would be used in the transcribing and reporting of the data and that all data would be kept on an encrypted secured computer.

Certificates of Confidentiality

In some situations, confidentiality can create tensions between researchers and legal or other authorities, especially if participants engage in criminal activity (e.g., substance abuse). To avoid the possibility of forced, involuntary disclosure of sensitive research information (e.g., through a court order or subpoena), researchers in the United States can apply for a **Certificate of Confidentiality** from the NIH (Lutz et al., 2000; Wolf et al., 2015). Any research that involves the collection of personally identifiable, sensitive information is potentially eligible for a Certificate. Information is considered sensitive if its release might damage participants' financial standing, employability, or reputation. Information about a person's mental health, as well as genetic information, is also considered sensitive. A Certificate allows researchers to refuse to disclose identifying information on study participants in any civil, criminal, administrative, or legislative proceeding at the federal, state, or local level.

A Certificate of Confidentiality helps researchers to achieve their research objectives without threat of involuntary disclosure and can be helpful in recruiting participants. Researchers who obtain a Certificate should inform prospective participants about this valuable protection in the consent form and should state any planned exceptions to those protections. For example, a researcher might decide to voluntarily comply with state child abuse reporting laws even though the Certificate would prevent authorities from punishing researchers who chose not to comply.

Example of Obtaining a Certificate of Confidentiality
Marraccini and colleagues (2022) conducted a study exploring the school-related risk and protective factors of suicidal thoughts and behaviors among youth with suicide-related crises. They interviewed adolescents with a history of suicide-related crises, their parents, school professionals, and hospital professionals. The National Institute of Mental Health provided a certificate of confidentiality.

Debriefings, Communications, and Referrals

Researchers can show their respect—and proactively minimize emotional risks—by carefully attending to the nature of their interactions with participants. For example, researchers should always be gracious and polite, should phrase questions tactfully, and should be considerate with regard to cultural and linguistic diversity.

Researchers can also use formal strategies to communicate respect for participants' well-being. For example, it is sometimes useful to offer **debriefing** sessions after data collection is completed to permit participants to ask questions or air complaints. Debriefing is especially important when the data collection has been stressful or when ethical guidelines had to be "bent" (e.g., if any deception was used in explaining the study).

> **Example of Debriefing**
> The previously mentioned study by Marraccini and colleagues (2022) also provides an example of debriefing during which the researchers debriefed by providing a summary of the interview while paying attention to respondents' reactions.

It is also thoughtful to communicate with participants after the study is completed, to let them know that their participation was appreciated. Researchers sometimes offer to share study findings with participants once the data have been analyzed (e.g., by emailing them a summary). The National Academies of Science, Engineering and Medicine in the United States (2018) has published guidance on returning individual results to participants.

Finally, in some situations, researchers may need to assist study participants by referring them to appropriate health, social, or psychological services.

> **Example of Referrals**
> Johnson and colleagues (2022) researched the associations between trauma, mental health symptomatology, and infectious disease outcomes (HIV/STI/HCV) among females who were enrolled in a program to support their transition to the community postincarceration. If requested or deemed necessary by the research team, participants received referrals to substance use and mental health counseling services.

Treatment of Vulnerable Groups

Adherence to ethical standards is often straightforward, but additional procedures may be required to protect special **vulnerable groups**. Vulnerable populations may be incapable of giving fully informed consent (e.g., cognitively impaired people) or may be at risk of unintended side effects because of their circumstances (e.g., pregnant females). Researchers interested in studying high-risk groups should understand guidelines governing informed consent, risk/benefit assessments, and acceptable research procedures for such groups. Research with vulnerable groups should be undertaken only when the risk/benefit ratio is low or when there is no alternative (e.g., studies of prisoners' health behaviors require inmates as participants).

Among the groups that nurse researchers should consider vulnerable are the following:

- *Children.* Legally and ethically, children do not have competence to give informed consent, so the informed consent of their parents or legal guardians must be obtained. It is appropriate, however—especially if the child is at least 7 years old—to obtain the child's assent as well. **Assent** refers to the child's agreement to participate. If the child is mature enough to understand basic informed consent information, it is advisable to obtain written consent from the child and the parent, as evidence of respect for the child's right to self-determination. Research suggests that children at the age of 12 years are competent to give consent (Hein et al., 2015). The U.S. government has issued special regulations (Code of Federal Regulations, 2009; Subpart D) for additional protections of children as study participants.

> **TIP** Crane and Broome (2017) have prepared a systematic review on the ethical aspects of research participation from the perspective of participating children and adolescents.

- *Mentally or emotionally disabled people.* Individuals whose disability makes it impossible for them to weigh the risks and benefits of participation (e.g., people who are in a coma) also cannot legally or ethically provide informed consent. In such cases, researchers should obtain the written consent of a legal guardian. If possible, informed consent or assent from participants themselves should be sought as a supplement to a guardian's consent. NIH guidelines stipulate that studies involving people whose autonomy is compromised by disability should focus directly on their condition.
- *Severely ill or physically disabled people.* For patients who are very ill, it might be prudent to assess their ability to make reasoned decisions about study participation. For certain disabilities, special procedures for obtaining consent may be required. For example, with deaf participants, the entire consent process may need to be in writing.

For people who have a physical impairment preventing them from writing or for participants who cannot read, alternative procedures for documenting informed consent (e.g., video recording consent proceedings) should be used.

- *The terminally ill.* Terminally ill people seldom expect to benefit personally from participating in research, and so the risk/benefit ratio needs to be carefully assessed. Researchers must take steps to ensure that the care and comfort of terminally ill participants are not compromised.
- *Institutionalized people.* Prudence is required in recruiting institutionalized people because their dependence on healthcare personnel may make them feel pressured into participating; they may believe that their treatment would be jeopardized by failure to cooperate. Prison inmates, who have lost autonomy in many spheres of activity, may also feel constrained in their ability to withhold consent. The U.S. government has issued specific regulations for the protection of prisoners as study participants (see Code of Federal Regulations, 2009; Subpart C). Researchers studying institutionalized groups need to emphasize the voluntary nature of participation.
- *Pregnant females.* The U.S. government has issued additional requirements governing research with pregnant females and fetuses (Code of Federal Regulations, 2009; Subpart B). These requirements reflect a desire to safeguard both the pregnant female, who may be at heightened physical and psychological risk, and the fetus, who cannot give informed consent. The regulations stipulate that a pregnant female cannot be involved in a study unless its purpose is to meet the health needs of the pregnant female and risks to the mother and the fetus are minimized or there is only a minimal risk to the fetus.

Example of Research With a Vulnerable Group
Mburu et al. (2020) qualitatively explored the factors influencing Kenyan females' decision to inject illicit drugs during pregnancy. Researchers conducted in-depth interviews with 45 females who injected drugs during pregnancy along with five key stakeholders who provide care to drug users in Kenya. Participation was voluntary.

Researchers need to proceed with extreme caution in conducting research with people who fall into two or more vulnerable categories (e.g., incarcerated youth).

External Reviews and the Protection of Human Rights

Researchers, who have a commitment to their research, may not be objective in their risk/benefit assessments or in their plans to protect participants' rights. Because a biased self-evaluation is possible, the ethical dimensions of a study normally should be subjected to external review.

Most institutions where research is conducted have formal committees for reviewing proposed research plans. These committees are sometimes called *human subjects committees*, *ethical advisory boards*, or *research ethics committees*. In the United States, the committee usually is called an **Institutional Review Board (IRB)**; in Canada, it is called a **Research Ethics Board**.

TIP You should find out early what an institution's requirements are regarding ethics, in terms of its forms, procedures, and review schedules. It is wise to allow a generous amount of time for negotiating with IRBs, which may require modifications and rereview.

Institutional Review Boards

In the United States, federally sponsored studies are subject to strict guidelines for evaluating the treatment of human participants. Before undertaking such a study, researchers must submit research plans to the IRB and must also go through formal training on ethical conduct and a certification process.

The duty of the IRB is to ensure that the proposed plans meet federal requirements for ethical research. An IRB can approve, require modifications to, or disapprove the proposed plans. The main requirements governing IRB decisions may be summarized as follows (Code of Federal Regulations, 2009; §46.111):

- Risks to participants are minimized.
- Risks to participants are reasonable in relation to anticipated benefits, if any, and the importance

of the knowledge that may reasonably be expected to result.
- Selection of participants is equitable.
- Informed consent will be sought, as required, and appropriately documented.
- Adequate provision is made for monitoring the research to ensure participants' safety.
- Appropriate provisions are made to protect participants' privacy and confidentiality of the data.
- When a vulnerable group is involved, appropriate additional safeguards are included to protect the rights and welfare of participants.

Example of Institutional Review Board Approval
Tabloski et al. (2021) examined the association of patient factors such as health and well-being, patient/caregiver relationships, and living arrangements with caregiver burden due to delirium. The study was approved by the IRBs of the Beth Israel Deaconess Medical Center and Hebrew SeniorLife in Boston, the study coordinating center.

Many studies require a full IRB review at a meeting with a majority of IRB members present. An IRB must have five or more members, at least one of whom is not a researcher (e.g., a lawyer or someone from the patient population). One IRB member must be a person who is not affiliated with the institution and is not a family member of an affiliated person. To protect against potential biases, the IRB cannot comprise entirely males, females, or members from a single profession.

For certain research involving no more than minimal risk, the IRB can use expedited review procedures, which do not require a meeting. In an **expedited review**, a single IRB member (usually the IRB chairperson) carries out the review. An example of research that qualifies for an expedited IRB review is minimal-risk research "… employing survey, interview, oral history, focus group, program evaluation, human factors evaluation, or quality assurance methodologies" (Code of Federal Regulations, 2009; §46.110).

Federal regulations also allow certain types of research in which there are no apparent risks to participants to be exempt from IRB review. The website of the Office for Human Research Protections, in its policy guidance section, includes decision charts designed to clarify whether a study is exempt.

TIP Researchers seeking a Certificate of Confidentiality must first obtain IRB approval, which is a prerequisite for the Certificate. Applications for the Certificate should be submitted at least 3 months before participants are expected to enroll in the study.

Data and Safety Monitoring Boards

In addition to IRBs, researchers in the United States may have to communicate information about ethical aspects of their studies to other groups. For example, some institutions have established separate **Privacy Boards** to review researchers' compliance with provisions in HIPAA, including review of authorization forms and requests for waivers.

For researchers evaluating interventions in clinical trials, NIH also requires review by a **data and safety monitoring board** (DSMB). The purpose of a DSMB is to oversee the safety of participants, to promote data integrity, and to review accumulated outcome data on a regular basis to evaluate whether study protocols should be altered or if the study should be stopped altogether. Members of a DSMB are selected based on their clinical, statistical, and methodologic expertise. The degree of monitoring by the DSMB should be proportionate to the degree of risk involved. Slimmer and Andersen (2004) offer suggestions on developing a DSM plan. Artinian et al. (2004) provided good descriptions of their data and safety monitoring plan for a study of a nurse-managed telemonitoring intervention and discussed how IRBs and DSMBs differ.

Building Ethics Into the Design of the Study

Researchers need to give thought to ethical requirements while planning a study and should ask themselves whether intended safeguards are sufficient. They must continue their vigilance throughout the course of the study as well, because unforeseen ethical dilemmas may arise. Of course, first steps in doing ethical research include asking clinically important questions and using rigorous methods—it can be construed as unethical to do poorly designed research because it would be a poor use of participants' time.

Another issue concerns dissemination: it can be considered unethical and wasteful of people's time to not communicate research findings to others.

The remaining chapters of the book offer advice on how to design studies that yield high-quality evidence for practice. Methodologic decisions about rigor, however, must be made within the context of ethical requirements. Box 7.2 presents examples of questions that might be posed in thinking about ethical aspects of study design.

TIP After study procedures have been developed, researchers should evaluate those procedures to determine if they meet ethical requirements. Box 7.3 later in this chapter provides guidelines that can be used for such a self-evaluation.

OTHER ETHICAL ISSUES

In discussing ethical issues relating to the conduct of nursing research, we have given primary consideration to the protection of human participants. Two other ethical issues also deserve mention: the treatment of animals in research and research misconduct.

Ethical Issues in Using Animals in Research

Some nurse researchers work with animal subjects. Despite opposition to such research by animal rights activists, researchers in health fields likely will continue to use animals to explore physiologic mechanisms and interventions that could pose risks to humans.

Ethical considerations are clearly different for animals and humans: the concept of *informed consent* is not relevant for animal subjects. Guidelines have been developed governing treatment of animals in research. In the United States, the Public Health Service has issued a policy statement on the humane care and use of laboratory animals. The guidelines articulate nine principles for the proper treatment of animals used in biomedical and behavioral research. These principles cover such issues as alternatives to using animals, pain and distress

---

BOX 7.2 Examples of Questions for Building Ethics Into the Design of a Study

RESEARCH DESIGN
- Will participants be assigned fairly to different treatment groups?
- Will the study setting minimize participants' discomfort or anxiety?

INTERVENTION
- Is the intervention designed to maximize benefits and minimize harms?
- Under what conditions could the intervention be withdrawn or altered?

SAMPLE
- Is the population under study defined so as to minimize the risk that certain types of people (e.g., females, underrepresented groups) will be excluded or underrepresented?
- Will potential participants be recruited into the study equitably and without the use of coercion?

DATA COLLECTION
- Will respondent burden be minimized? Will participants' time be used efficiently?
- Will procedures for ensuring confidentiality of data be adequate?
- Will data collection staff be trained to be courteous, respectful, and caring?

REPORTING
- Will participants' identities be adequately protected?

> **BOX 7.3** Guidelines for Critically Appraising the Ethical Aspects of a Study
>
> 1. Was the study approved and monitored by an Institutional Review Board, REB, or other similar ethics review committee?
> 2. Were participants subjected to any physical harm, discomfort, or psychological distress? Did the researchers take appropriate steps to remove, prevent, or minimize harm?
> 3. Did the benefits to participants outweigh any potential risks or actual discomfort they experienced? Did the benefits to society outweigh the costs to participants?
> 4. Was any type of coercion or undue influence used to recruit participants? Did they have the right to refuse to participate or to withdraw without penalty?
> 5. Were participants deceived in any way? Were they fully aware of participating in a study and did they understand the purpose and nature of the research?
> 6. Were appropriate informed consent procedures used? If not, were there valid and justifiable reasons?
> 7. Were adequate steps taken to safeguard participants' privacy? How was confidentiality maintained? Were Privacy Rule procedures followed (if applicable)? Was a Certificate of Confidentiality obtained? If not, *should* one have been obtained?
> 8. Were vulnerable groups involved in the research? If yes, were special precautions used because of their vulnerable status?
> 9. Were groups omitted from the inquiry without a justifiable rationale, such as females (or males), underrepresented groups, or older people?

in animal subjects, researcher qualifications, use of appropriate anesthesia, and conditions for euthanizing animals. In Canada, researchers who use animals in their studies must adhere to the policies and guidelines of the Canadian Council on Animal Care as articulated in their *Guide to the Care and Use of Experimental Animals* (2020). Holtzclaw and Hanneman (2002) noted several important considerations in the use of animals in nursing research, and Osier et al. (2016) discussed the use of animal models in genomic nursing research.

Example of Research With Animals
Mitchell and Colleagues (2019) investigated the impact of intermittent fasting on the health and survival of male mice. All animal protocols were approved by the Animal Care and Use Committee (352-TGB-2018) of the National Institute on Aging at the National Institutes of Health. Specifications around the mice, husbandry, and diets were provided (e.g., the dimensions of the cages and bedding).

Research Misconduct

Ethics in research involves not only the protection of human and animal subjects but also protection of the public trust. The issue of **research misconduct** has received greater attention in recent years as incidents of researcher fraud and misrepresentation have come to light. Currently, the agency in the United States responsible for overseeing efforts to improve research integrity and for handling allegations of research misconduct is the Office of Research Integrity. Researchers seeking funding from NIH must demonstrate that they have received training on research integrity and the responsible conduct of research.

Research misconduct is defined by U.S. Public Health Service regulation (42 CFR Part 93.103) as "fabrication, falsification, or plagiarism in proposing, performing, or reviewing research, or in reporting research results." To be construed as misconduct, there must be a significant departure from accepted practices in the research community, and the misconduct must have been committed intentionally and knowingly. *Fabrication* involves making up data or study results. *Falsification* involves manipulating research materials, equipment, or processes; it also involves changing or omitting data or distorting results. *Plagiarism* involves the appropriation of someone's ideas, results, or words without giving due credit, including information obtained as a reviewer of research proposals or manuscripts.

> **Example of Research Misconduct**
> In 2020, the U.S. Office of Research Integrity ruled that a researcher engaged in scientific misconduct in a study supported by the NINR. The researcher falsified and/or fabricated data that were reported in six grant applications submitted to the NINR.

Although the official definition focuses on only three types of misconduct, there is widespread agreement that research misconduct covers many other issues including improprieties of authorship, poor data management, conflicts of interest, inappropriate financial arrangements, failure to comply with governmental regulations, and unauthorized use of confidential information.

Research integrity is an important concern. Research misconduct includes protocol violations, consent violations, fabrication, falsification, conflicts of interest, and issues around unethical publication (Abd ElHafeez et al., 2022). Some of these violations can be attributed to a lack of training related to the responsible conduct of research. It is critical that nurses conducting research activities keep up to date with training about the ethical conduct of research.

CRITICAL APPRAISAL OF ETHICS IN RESEARCH

Guidelines for critically appraising the ethical aspects of a study are presented in Box 7.3. Members of an ethics committee should be provided with sufficient information to answer all these questions. Research journal articles, however, do not always include detailed information about ethics because of space constraints. Thus, it is not always possible to evaluate researchers' adherence to ethical guidelines, but we offer a few suggestions for considering a study's ethical aspects.

Many research reports acknowledge that study procedures were reviewed by an IRB or ethics committee, and some journals require such statements. When a report specifically mentions a formal review, it is usually safe to assume that a group of concerned people did a conscientious review of the study's ethical issues.

You can also come to some conclusions based on a description of the study methods. There may be sufficient information to judge, for example, whether participants were subjected to harm or discomfort. Reports do not always state whether informed consent was secured, but you should be alert to situations in which the data could not have been gathered as described if participation were purely voluntary (e.g., if data were gathered unobtrusively).

In thinking about ethical issues, you should also consider who the study participants were. For example, if a study involved vulnerable groups, there should be more information about protective procedures. You might also need to consider who the study participants were *not*. For example, there has been considerable concern about the omission of certain groups (e.g., minorities) from clinical research. It is often difficult to determine whether the participants' privacy was safeguarded unless the researcher mentions pledges of confidentiality or anonymity.

RESEARCH EXAMPLES

Two research examples that highlight ethical issues are presented in the following sections. Increasingly researchers are publishing study protocols. These are helpful to review as they allow you to see all the anticipated steps necessary in the research process. The quantitative example reports a study protocol.

Research Example From a Quantitative Study Protocol

Study: The perinatal bereavement project: development and evaluation of supportive guidelines for families experiencing stillbirth and neonatal death in Southeast Brazil—a quasi-experimental before-and-after study (Salgado et al., 2021).

Study purpose: The purpose of this study is to assess the effects that supportive guidelines have on the mental health of grieving parents and their families who have undergone perinatal loss in public maternities in Brazil.

Research methods: The study is planned as a quasi-experimental study. The intervention is the implementation of bereavement supportive guidelines for females who experienced a stillbirth or a neonatal death. The goal is to enroll 40 participants, 20 of whom will be enrolled before the guidelines are in place and 20 will be enrolled once they are in place. A semistructured questionnaire capturing demographics and three scales, the *Perinatal Grief Scale*, *Edinburgh Postnatal Depression Scale*, *and Depression Anxiety Stress Scales*, will be used to assess the effects of the guidelines.

Ethics-related procedures: The investigators report that this study is in accordance with the Helsinki Declaration and follows the guidelines and norms of the National Health Council. They emphasize that the data collected will be exclusively used for academic research. They state that the identity and privacy of the participants will be assured through the coding of the data.

Anticipated findings: It is anticipated that findings will support the use of specific guidelines for females and families who lost their babies during gestation, labor, or the postpartum period. The investigators also anticipate that the guidelines must be adapted for Brazilian maternity wards.

Research Example From a Qualitative Study

Study: Factors associated with the decision to prescribe and administer antipsychotics for older people with delirium: a qualitative descriptive study (Tomlinson et al., 2021).

Study purpose: "To explore factors associated with decision-making of nurses and doctors in prescribing and administering as required antipsychotic medications to older people with delirium."

Study methods: The researchers used a qualitative descriptive approach. Data for the study were gathered through in-depth interviews with 25 nurses and 17 doctors from 4 hospitals. The interviews were conducted at each of the hospitals and lasted between 25 and 40 minutes. All interviews were audio-recorded, digitally stored, and transcribed verbatim.

Ethics-related procedures: The study was approved by human research ethics committees in the relevant facilities. Participants signed written informed consent forms, and verbal consent was reaffirmed throughout the interview process. The interviews were either individually or through focus groups. Confidentiality was assured through the process of the researcher deidentifying all data in the reporting of the results. Confidentiality was assured through the secure storing of signed consent forms in a locked cabinet and office at the researchers' university. Before the commencement of the interviews, the investigators reminded participants that these discussions were not aimed at critiquing their clinical practice but rather to understand their decision-making process.

Key findings: The researchers identified five themes associated with the participants' decision to provide antipsychotic medications: "(1) *safety*, (2) *a last resort*, (3) *nursing workload (can't do my job)*, (4) *dilemma to medicate*, and (5) *anticipating worsening behaviors (p. 4)*."

SUMMARY POINTS

- Researchers sometimes face **ethical dilemmas** in designing studies that are rigorous *and* ethical. **Codes of ethics** have been developed to guide researchers.
- Three major ethical principles from the *Belmont Report* are incorporated into most guidelines: beneficence, respect for human dignity, and justice.
- **Beneficence** involves the performance of some good and the protection of participants from physical and psychological harm and exploitation.
- **Respect for human dignity** involves participants' **right to self-determination**, which means they are free to control their own actions, including voluntary participation.
- **Full disclosure** means that researchers have fully divulged participants' rights and the risks and benefits of the study. When full disclosure could bias the results, researchers sometimes use **covert data collection** (the collection of information without the participants' knowledge or consent) or **deception** (providing false information).

- **Justice** includes the **right to fair treatment** and the **right to privacy.** In the United States, privacy has become a major issue because of the Privacy Rule regulations that resulted from the HIPAA.
- Various procedures have been developed to safeguard study participants' rights. For example, researchers can conduct a **risk/benefit assessment** in which the potential benefits of the study to participants and society are weighed against the risks.
- **Informed consent** procedures, which provide prospective participants with information needed to make a reasoned decision about participation, normally involve signing a **consent form** to document voluntary and informed participation.
- In qualitative studies, consent may need to be continually renegotiated with participants as the study evolves, through **process consent** procedures.
- Privacy can be maintained through **anonymity** (wherein not even researchers know participants' identities) or through formal **confidentiality procedures** that safeguard the information participants provide. Researchers must guard against a **breach of confidentiality.**
- U.S. researchers can seek a **Certificate of Confidentiality** that protects them against the forced disclosure of confidential information (e.g., by a court order).
- Researchers sometimes offer **debriefing** sessions after data collection to provide participants with more information or an opportunity to air complaints.
- **Vulnerable groups** require additional protection. These people may be vulnerable because they are unable to make a truly informed decision about study participation (e.g., children); because of diminished autonomy (e.g., prisoners); or because circumstances heighten the risk of physical or psychological harm (e.g., pregnant females).
- External review of the ethical aspects of a study by an ethics committee or **Institutional Review Board (IRB)** is often required by the agency funding the research and the organization from which participants are recruited.
- In studies in which risks to participants are minimal, an **expedited review** by a single member of the IRB may be substituted for a full board review; in cases in which there are no anticipated risks, the research may be exempted from review.
- Researchers need to give careful thought to ethical requirements throughout the study's planning and implementation and to ask themselves continually whether safeguards for protecting humans are sufficient.
- Ethical conduct in research involves not only protection of the rights of human and animal subjects, but also efforts to maintain high standards of integrity and avoid such forms of **research misconduct** as *plagiarism*, *fabrication* of results, or *falsification* of data.

REFERENCES CITED IN CHAPTER 7

Abd ElHafeez, S., Salem, M., & Silverman, H. J. (2022). Reliability and validation of an attitude scale regarding responsible conduct in research. *PloS One*, *17*(3), e0265392. https://doi.org/10.1371/journal.pone.0265392

Artinian, N., Froelicher, E., & Vander Wal, J. S. (2004). Data and safety monitoring during randomized controlled trials of nursing interventions. *Nursing Research*, *53*(6), 414–418.

Beck, C. T., LoGiudice, J., & Gable, R. K. (2015). A mixed methods study of secondary traumatic stress in certified nurse-midwives: Shaken belief in the birth process. *Journal of Midwifery & Womens Health*, *60*(1), 16–23.

Crane, S., & Broome, M. (2017). Understanding ethical issues of research participation from the perspective of participating children and adolescents: A systematic review. *Worldviews on Evidence-Based Nursing*, *14*(3), 200–209.

Domecq, J., Prutsky, G., Elraiyah, T., Wang, Z., Nabhan, M., Shippee, N., Brito, J. P., Boehmer, K., Hasan, R., Firwana, B., Erwin, P., Eton, D., Sloan, J., Montori, V., Asi, N., Dabrh, A. M. A., Murad, M. H., & Murad, M. H. (2014). Patient engagement in research: A systematic review. *BMC Health Services Research*, *14*, 89.

Edwards, P., Roberts, I., Clarke, M., Diguiseppi, C., Woolf, B., Perkins, C., & Pratap, S. (2023). Methods to increase response to postal and electronic questionnaires. *Cochrane Database of Systematic Reviews*, *11*(11), MR000008.

Eide, P., & Kahn, D. (2008). Ethical issues in the qualitative researcher-participant relationship. *Nursing Ethics*, *15*(2), 199–207.

Fields, L., & Calvert, J. (2015). Informed consent procedures with cognitively impaired patients: A review of ethics and best practices. *Psychiatry and Clinical Neurosciences*, 69(8), 462–471.

Flesch, R. (1948). New readability yardstick. *Journal of Applied Psychology*, 32, 221–223.

Gelling, L., Ersser, S., Heaslip, V., Tait, D., & Trenoweth, S. (2021). Ethical conduct of nursing research. *Journal of Clinical Nursing*, 30(23–24), e69–e71. https://doi.org/10.1111/jocn.16038

Hein, I., DeVries, M., Troost, P., Meynen, G., Van Goudoever, J., & Lindauer, R. (2015). Informed consent instead of assent is appropriate in children from the age of twelve: Policy implications of new findings on children's competence to consent to clinical research. *BMC Medical Ethics*, 16(1), 76.

Holtzclaw, B. J., & Hanneman, S. (2002). Use of non-human biobehavioral models in critical care nursing research. *Critical Care Nursing Quaterly*, 24(4), 30–40.

Johnson, K. A., Hunt, T., Puglisi, L. B., Maeng, D., Epa-Llop, A., Elumn, J. E., Nguyen, A., Leung, A., Chen, R., Shah, Z., Wang, J., Johnson, R., Chapman, B. P., Gilbert, L., El-Bassel, N., & Morse, D. S. (2022). Trauma, mental health distress, and infectious disease prevention among women recently released from incarceration. *Frontiers in Psychiatry*, 13, 867445. https://doi.org/10.3389/fpsyt.2022.867445

Klykken, F. H. (2022). Implementing continuous consent in qualitative research. *Qualitative Research*, 22(5), 795–810.

Lutz, K. F., Shelton, K., Robrecht, L., Hatton, D., & Beckett, A. (2000). Use of certificates of confidentiality in nursing research. *Journal of Nursing Scholarship*, 32(2), 185–188.

Mahon, P. Y. (2014). Internet research and ethics: Transformative issues in nursing education research. *Journal of Professional Nursing*, 30(2), 124–129. https://doi.org/10.1016/j.profnurs.2013.06.007

Marraccini, M. E., Pittleman, C., Griffard, M., Tow, A. C., Vanderburg, J. L., & Cruz, C. M. (2022). Adolescent, parent, and provider perspectives on school-related influences of mental health in adolescents with suicide-related thoughts and behaviors. *Journal of School Psychology*, 93, 98–118. https://doi.org/10.1016/j.jsp.2022.07.001

Martin, C. L., Kramer-Kostecka, E. N., Linde, J. A., Friend, S., Zuroski, V. R., & Fulkerson, J. A. (2020). Leveraging interdisciplinary teams to develop and implement secure websites for behavioral research: Applied tutorial. *Journal of Medical Internet Research*, 22(9), e19217. https://doi.org/10.2196/19217

Mburu, G., Ayon, S., Mahinda, S., & Kaveh, K. (2020). Determinants of women's drug use during pregnancy: Perspectives from a qualitative study. *Maternal and Child Health Journal*, 24(9), 1170–1178. https://doi.org/10.1007/s10995-020-02910-w

Mitchell, S. J., Bernier, M., Mattison, J. A., Aon, M. A., Kaiser, T. A., Anson, R. M., Ikeno, Y., Anderson, R. M., Ingram, D. K., & de Cabo, R. (2019). Daily fasting improves health and survival in male mice independent of diet composition and calories. *Cell Metabolism*, 29(1), 221–228.e3. https://doi.org/10.1016/j.cmet.2018.08.011

Mwalabu, G., Evans, C., & Redsell, S. (2017). Factors influencing the experience of sexual and reproductive healthcare for female adolescents with perinatally-acquired HIV: A qualitative case study. *BMC Women's Health*, 17(1), 125.

National Academies of Sciences, Engineering, and Medicine. (2018). *Returning individual research results to participants: Guidance for a new research paradigm*. National Academies.

Nishimura, A., Carey, J., Erwin, P., Tilburt, J., Murad, M., & McCormick, J. (2013). Improving understanding in the research informed consent process: A systematic review of 54 interventions tested in randomized control trials. *BMC Medical Ethics*, 14, 28.

Osier, N., Pham, L., Savarese, A., Sayles, K., & Alexander, S. (2016). Animal models in genomic research: Techniques, applications, and roles for nurses. *Applied Nursing Research*, 32, 247–256.

Polit, D. F., & Beck, C. T. (2009). International gender bias in nursing research, 2005–2006: A quantitative content analysis. *Internationa Journal of Nursing Studies*, 46(8), 1102–1110.

Polit, D. F., & Beck, C. T. (2013). Is there still gender bias in nursing research? An update. *Research in Nursing Health*, 36(1), 75–83.

Post, K. E., Berry, D. L., Shindul-Rothschild, J., & Flanagan, J. (2021). Patient engagement in breast cancer survivorship care. *Cancer Nursing*, 44(5), E296–E302. https://doi.org/10.1097/NCC.0000000000000853

Salgado, H. d. O., Andreucci, C. B., Gomes, A. C. R., & Souza, J. P. (2021). The perinatal bereavement project: Development and evaluation of supportive guidelines for families experiencing stillbirth and neonatal death in Southeast Brazil-a quasi-experimental before-and-after study. *Reproductive Health*, 18(1), 5. https://doi.org/10.1186/s12978-020-01040-4

Silva, M. C. (1995). *Ethical guidelines in the conduct, dissemination, and implementation of nursing research*. American Nurses Association.

Simpson, C. (2010). Decision-making capacity and informed consent to participate in research by cognitively impaired individuals. *Applied Nursing Research*, 23(4), 221–226.

Slimmer, L., & Andersen, B. (2004). Designing a data and safety monitoring plan. *Western Journal of Nursing Research*, 26(7), 797–803.

Sperlich, M., & Gabriel, C. (2022). "I got to catch my own baby": A qualitative study of out of hospital birth. *Reproductive Health*, 19(1), 43. https://doi.org/10.1186/s12978-022-01355-4

Tabloski, P. A., Arias, F., Flanagan, N., Webb, M., Gregas, M., Schmitt, E. M., Travison, T. G., Jones, R. N., Inouye, S. K., & Fong, T. G. (2021). Predictors of caregiver burden in delirium: Patient and caregiver factors. *Journal of Gerontological Nursing*, 47(9), 32–38. https://doi.org/10.3928/00989134-20210803-03

Tomlinson, E. J., Rawson, H., Manias, E., Phillips, N. N. M., Darzins, P., & Hutchinson, A. M. (2021). Factors associated with the decision to prescribe and administer antipsychotics for older people with delirium: A qualitative descriptive study. *BMJ Open*, 11(7), e047247. https://doi.org/10.1136/bmjopen-2020-047247

Tyrrell, M., Hedman, R., Fossum, B., Skovdahl, K., Religa, D., & Hillerås, P. (2021). Feeling valued versus abandoned: Voices of persons who have completed a cognitive assessment. *International Journal of Older People Nursing*, *16*(6), e12403. https://doi.org/10.1111/opn.12403

Walsh, E. P., Flanagan, J. M., & Mathew, P. (2020). The last day narratives: An exploration of the end of life for patients with cancer from a caregivers' perspective. *Journal of Palliative Medicine*, *23*(9), 1172–1176. https://doi.org/10.1089/jpm.2019.0648

Wolf, L. E., Patel, M., Williams-Tarver, B., Austin, J., Dame, L., & Beskow, L. (2015). Certificates of confidentiality: Protecting human subject research data in law and practice. *Journal of Law, Medicine & Ethics*, *43*(3), 594–609.

8 Planning a Nursing Study

Learning Objectives

1. Describe the criteria for assessing the quality of the findings for quantitative and qualitative research.
2. Identify strategies researchers use to manage bias and enhance validity in quantitative studies.
3. Summarize the strategies used to promote the trustworthiness of qualitative research
4. Explain the importance of reflexivity in research.
5. Provide examples of research designs that researchers use to develop evidence that is accurate and interpretable.

INTRODUCTION

Advance planning is required for all research. This chapter provides advice for planning qualitative and quantitative studies.

TOOLS AND CONCEPTS FOR PLANNING RIGOROUS RESEARCH

This section discusses key methodologic concepts and tools in meeting the challenges of doing rigorous research.

Inference

Inference is an integral part of doing and evaluating research. An **inference** is a conclusion drawn from the study evidence, considering the methods used to generate that evidence. Inference is the attempt to come to conclusions based on limited information, using logical reasoning processes.

Inference is necessary because researchers use proxies that "stand in" for the things that are fundamentally of interest. A sample of participants is a proxy for an entire population. A study site is a proxy for all relevant sites in which the phenomena of interest could unfold. A control group that does not receive an intervention is a proxy for what would happen to those receiving the intervention if they did not receive it.

Researchers face the challenge of using methods that yield persuasive evidence in support of inferences they wish to make.

Reliability, Validity, and Trustworthiness

Researchers want their inferences to correspond with the *truth*. Research cannot contribute evidence to guide clinical practice if the findings are biased or fail to represent the experiences of the target group. Consumers of research need to assess the quality of a study's evidence by evaluating the conceptual and methodologic decisions the researchers made, and those who do research must strive to make decisions that result in high-quality evidence.

Quantitative researchers use several criteria to assess the rigor of a study, sometimes referred to as its **scientific merit**. Two especially important criteria are reliability and validity. **Reliability** refers to the accuracy and consistency of information obtained in a study. The term is most often associated with the methods used to measure variables. For example, if a thermometer measured Alan temperature as 98.1°F 1 minute and as 102.5°F the next minute, the reliability of the thermometer would be suspect.

Validity is a more complex concept that broadly concerns the *soundness* of the study's evidence—whether the findings are unbiased and well grounded. Like reliability, validity is a key criterion for evaluating methods to measure variables. In this context, the validity question is whether the methods are really measuring the concepts that they purport to measure. Is a self-reported measure of depression *really* measuring depression? Or is it measuring something else, such as loneliness? Researchers strive for solid conceptualizations of research variables and valid methods to operationalize them.

Validity is also relevant with regard to inferences about the effect of the independent variable on the dependent variable. Did a nursing intervention *really* bring about improvements in patients' outcomes—or were other factors responsible for patients' progress? Researchers make numerous methodologic decisions that influence this type of study validity. Yet another validity question concerns whether the evidence can validly be extrapolated to people who did not participate in the study.

Qualitative researchers use different criteria (and different terminology) in evaluating a study's quality. Qualitative researchers pursue methods of enhancing the **trustworthiness** of the study evidence (Lincoln & Guba, 1985). Trustworthiness encompasses several dimensions—credibility, transferability, confirmability, dependability, and authenticity—which are described in Chapter 26.

Credibility, an especially important aspect of trustworthiness, is achieved to the extent that the research methods inspire confidence that the results and interpretations are truthful. Credibility can be enhanced in various ways, but one strategy merits early discussion because it has implications for the design of all studies, including quantitative ones. **Triangulation** is the use of multiple sources or referents to draw conclusions about what constitutes the truth. In a quantitative study, this might mean using multiple measures of an outcome variable to see if predicted effects are consistent. In a qualitative study, triangulation might involve trying to reveal the complexity of a phenomenon by using multiple means of data collection to converge on the truth (e.g., having in-depth discussions with participants, as well as watching their behavior in natural settings). Or it might involve triangulating the interpretations of multiple researchers working together as a team. Nurse researchers are increasingly triangulating across paradigms—that is, integrating both qualitative and quantitative data in a **mixed methods study** to enhance the validity of the conclusions (Chapter 27).

Example of Triangulation
Torkar et al. (2022) assessed the needs of patients with severe mental illness who were attending follow-up day hospitals. Interviews were conducted with three key stakeholders whose views helped to triangulate the findings. Sources of data were the patient, relatives, and clinical experts.

Nurse researchers need to design their studies so that the reliability, validity, and trustworthiness of their studies are maximized. This book offers advice on how to do this.

Bias

A **bias** is an influence that produces a distortion or error. Bias can threaten a study's validity and trustworthiness and is a major concern in designing a study. Bias can result from factors that need to be considered in planning a study. These include the following:

- *Participants' lack of candor.* Sometimes people distort their behavior or statements—consciously or subconsciously—to present themselves in the best light.
- *Researcher subjectivity.* Investigators may distort inferences in the direction of their expectations or in line with their own experiences—or they may unintentionally communicate their expectations to participants and thereby induce biased responses.

- *Sample imbalances.* The sample itself may be biased; for example, if a researcher studying abortion attitudes included only members of right-to-life (or pro-choice) groups in the sample, the results would be distorted.
- *Faulty methods of data collection.* Inadequate methods of capturing concepts can lead to biases; for example, a flawed measure of patient satisfaction with nursing care may exaggerate or underestimate patients' concerns.
- *Inadequate study design.* A researcher may structure the study in such a way that an unbiased answer to the research question cannot be achieved.
- *Flawed implementation.* Even a well-designed study can sustain biases if the study protocols are not carefully implemented.

A researcher's job is to reduce or eliminate bias to the extent possible, to establish mechanisms to detect or measure it when it exists, and to take known biases into account in interpreting study findings. The job of consumers is to scrutinize methodologic decisions to reach conclusions about whether biases undermined the study evidence.

Unfortunately, bias can seldom be avoided totally because the potential for its occurrence is pervasive. Some bias is haphazard. **Random bias** (or *random error*) is essentially "noise" in the data. When error is random, distortions are as likely to bias results in one direction as the other. **Systematic bias**, on the other hand, is consistent and distorts results in a single direction. For example, if a scale consistently measured people's weights as being 2 lb heavier than their true weight, there would be systematic bias in the data on weight.

Researchers adopt a variety of strategies to eliminate or minimize bias and strengthen study rigor. Triangulation is one such approach, the idea being that multiple sources of information or points of view can help counterbalance biases and offer avenues to identify them. Methods that quantitative researchers use to combat bias often involve research control.

Research Control

Quantitative researchers usually make efforts to control aspects of the study. **Research control** typically involves holding constant other influences on the dependent variable so that the true relationship between the independent and dependent variables can be understood. In other words, research control attempts to eliminate contaminating factors that might obscure the relationship between the variables of central interest.

Contaminating factors—called **confounding** (or **extraneous**) **variables**—can best be illustrated with an example. Suppose we were studying whether urinary incontinence (UI) affects depression. Prior evidence suggests a link, but the question is whether UI itself (the independent variable) contributes to higher levels of depression, or whether other factors account for the relationship between UI and depression. We need to design a study to control other determinants of depression that are also related to the independent variable, UI.

One confounding variable in this situation is age. Levels of depression tend to be higher in older people; people with UI tend to be older than those without this problem. In other words, perhaps age is the *real* cause of higher depression in people with UI. If age is not controlled, then any observed relationship between UI and depression could be caused by UI or by age.

Three possible explanations might be portrayed schematically as follows:

1. UI → depression
2. Age → UI → depression
3.
   Age ↘
   ↓   depression
   UI ↗

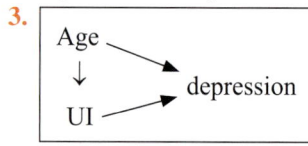

The arrows here symbolize a causal mechanism or an influence. In Model 1, UI directly affects depression, independent of any other factors. In Model 2, UI is a **mediating variable**—the effect of age on depression is *mediated* by UI. According to this representation, age affects depression *through* the effect that age has on UI. In Model 3, both age and UI have separate effects on depression and age also increases the risk of UI. Some research is specifically designed to test paths of mediation and multiple causation, but in the present example, age is extraneous to the research question. We want to design a study so that the first explanation can be tested. Age must be controlled if our goal is to explore the validity of Model 1, which posits that, no matter what a person's age, having UI makes a person more vulnerable to depression.

How can we impose such control? There are several ways (Chapter 10), but the general principle is that confounding variables must be *held constant*. The confounding variable must somehow be handled so that, in the context of the study, it is not related to the independent variable or the outcome. As an example, let us say we wanted to compare the average scores on a depression scale for those with and without UI. We would want to design a study in such a way that the ages of those in the UI and non-UI groups are comparable, even though, in general, the groups are not comparable in terms of age.

By exercising control over age, we would have more confidence in explaining the relationship between UI and depression. The world is complex; many variables are interrelated in complicated ways. When studying a problem in a quantitative study, it is difficult to examine this complexity directly; researchers analyze only a few relationships at a time. The value of the evidence in quantitative studies is often related to how well researchers controlled confounding influences. In the present example, we identified one variable (age) that could affect depression, but dozens of others might be relevant (e.g., social support, self-efficacy). Researchers need to isolate the independent and dependent variables in which they are interested and then identify confounding variables that need to be controlled.

> Confounding variables need to be controlled only if they are simultaneously related to both the dependent and independent variables.

Research control is a critical tool for managing bias and enhancing validity in quantitative studies. Sometimes, however, too much control can introduce bias. If researchers tightly control the ways in which key study variables are manifested, the true nature of those variables may be obscured. In studying phenomena that are poorly understood or whose dimensions have not been clarified, a qualitative approach that allows flexibility and exploration is more appropriate.

Randomness

For quantitative researchers, bias reduction often involves **randomness**—having features of the study established by chance rather than by researcher preference. When people are selected at random to participate in the study, for example, each person in the initial pool has an equal probability of being selected—which means that there are no systematic biases in the sample's makeup. Similarly, if participants are assigned randomly to groups that will be compared (for example, intervention and "usual care" groups), then there would be no systematic biases in the groups' composition. Randomness is a compelling method of controlling confounding variables and reducing bias.

> **Example of Randomness**
> Flanagan, one of the authors of this textbook, and colleagues (2022) tested the feasibility of a nurse-coached walking intervention for informal caregivers of people with dementia. Thirty-two participants were randomly assigned to either a nurse-coached group or a control group. The two groups were compared in terms of steps, walked well-being, and perceived stress.

Qualitative researchers almost never consider randomness a desirable tool. Qualitative researchers tend to use information obtained early in the study in a purposeful (nonrandom) fashion to guide their inquiry and to pursue information-rich sources that can help them expand or refine their conceptualizations. Researchers' judgments are viewed as indispensable vehicles for uncovering the complexities of phenomena of interest.

Reflexivity

Qualitative researchers do not use research control or randomness, but they are as interested as quantitative researchers in discovering the truth about human experience. Qualitative researchers often rely on reflexivity to guard against personal bias in making judgments. **Reflexivity** is the process of reflecting critically on the self and of analyzing and recording personal values that could affect data collection and interpretation.

Schwandt (2007) has described reflexivity as having two aspects. The first concerns an acknowledgment that the researcher is part of the setting or context under study. The second involves self-reflection about one's own biases, preferences, and fears about the research. Qualitative researchers are encouraged to explore these issues, to be reflexive about decisions made during the inquiry, and to note their reflexive thoughts in personal journals. As Patton (2015) noted, "To excel in qualitative inquiry requires keen and astute self-awareness" (p. 71).

Reflexivity can be a useful tool in quantitative as well as qualitative research. Self-awareness and introspection can enhance the quality of any study. It is important to note that reflexivity is now a required part of any publication of qualitative research as indicated in the CASP checklist found here: https://casp-uk.net/images/checklist/documents/CASP-Qualitative-Studies-Checklist/CASP-Qualitative-Checklist-2018_fillable_form.pdf.

Example of Reflexivity
Cousin et al. (2022) explored the experience of living with chronic pain from the perspective of Black females living in the Deep South. The authors provide the following statement on reflexivity. "The methodological design and results of any study, particularly qualitative, are enhanced when the epistemological underpinning and authors' identity and positionality (e.g., social location and educational status, assumptions, and power/privilege) are clearly noted; these reflexive strategies along with bracketing and field notes helped bring attention to the authors' assumptions and biases that could influence analysis. As demonstrated by the introductory story, the PI's experiences are intricately woven into the conceptualization and approach to nursing research with an older racial minority population. The research described herein uses critical constructivist and pragmatic perspectives to construct and present the realities of older Black women with chronic pain living in the South" (p. 132).

Generalizability and Transferability

Nurses increasingly rely on evidence from research in their clinical practice. Evidence-based practice is based on the assumption that study findings are not unique to the people, places, or circumstances of the original research (Polit & Beck, 2010).

Generalizability is a criterion used in quantitative studies to assess the extent to which findings can be applied to people and settings beyond those used in a study. How do researchers enhance the generalizability of a study? First and foremost, they must design studies strong in reliability and validity. There is no point in wondering whether results are generalizable if they are not accurate or valid. In selecting participants, researchers must also give thought to the types of people to whom the results might be generalized—and then select participants in such a way that the sample reflects the population of interest. If a study is intended to have implications for male and female patients, then males and females should be included as participants. Several chapters in this book describe strategies for enhancing generalizability.

Qualitative researchers do not specifically aim for generalizability, but they do want to generate knowledge that could be useful in other situations. Lincoln and Guba (1985), in their influential book on naturalistic inquiry, discussed the concept of **transferability**, the extent to which qualitative findings can be transferred to other settings, as an aspect of a study's trustworthiness. An important mechanism for promoting transferability is the amount of rich descriptive information qualitative researchers provide about study contexts. Transferability in qualitative research is discussed in Chapter 26.

TIP Researchers are increasingly paying attention to the *applicability* of their findings—that is, the extent to which findings can be applied to individuals or small subgroups. We discuss this issue at length in Chapter 31.

Stakeholder Engagement

There is growing agreement within the healthcare community that greater **stakeholder** engagement is needed in all phases of research, beginning in the planning phase—or even earlier, during the identification of a research problem. Proponents of stakeholder involvement during the planning and implementation of health research argue that it enhances the relevance and transparency of the research and accelerates the adoption of research evidence in practice.

TIP In Europe, advocates often use the term **patient and public involvement** (**PPI**). In the United States, the Patient-Centered Outcomes Research Institute (PCORI) was established in 2010 to fund research that can help patients make better healthcare choices, and patients play a role in guiding the research agenda.

Although patients have been identified as key stakeholders, researchers can consider involving others in planning a study. Concannon et al. (2012) developed a taxonomy to guide researchers in this new era of stakeholder-engaged research and proposed this definition of "engagement" of stakeholders: "A bi-directional relationship between the stakeholder and the researcher that results in informed decision-making about the selection, conduct, and use of research" (p. 986). They created a framework called the 7Ps to aid in the identification of stakeholders: Patients and the public; providers (e.g., nurses, physicians); purchasers; payers; policy makers; product makers; and principal investigators. Researchers need to identify key stakeholders and determine how best to involve them in the planning process.

OVERVIEW OF RESEARCH DESIGN FEATURES

A study's research design spells out the basic strategies that researchers adopt to develop evidence that is accurate and interpretable. The research design incorporates some of the most important methodologic decisions that researchers make, particularly in quantitative studies.

Table 8.1 describes seven design features that need to be considered in planning a quantitative

TABLE 8.1 • Key Research Design Features in Quantitative Studies

FEATURE	KEY QUESTIONS	DESIGN OPTIONS
Intervention	Will there be an intervention? What will the intervention entail? What specific design will be used?	Experimental (randomized controlled trial), quasiexperimental, nonexperimental (observational) design
Control over confounding variables	How will confounding variables be controlled? Which confounding variables will be controlled?	Matching, homogeneity, blocking, crossover, randomization, statistical control
Blinding (masking)	From whom will critical information be withheld to avoid bias?	Open vs. closed study; single-blind, double-blind (with blinded groups specified)
Relative timing	When will information on independent and dependent variables be collected—looking backward or forward?	Retrospective, prospective design
Comparisons	What type of comparisons will be made to illuminate key processes or relationships? What is the nature of the comparison?	Within-subject design, between-subject design, mixed design, external comparisons
Location	Where will the study take place?	Single site vs. multisite; in the field vs. controlled setting
Timeframes	How often will data be collected? When, relative to other events, will data be collected?	Cross-sectional, longitudinal design; repeated measures design

Note: Many terms in this table are explained in subsequent chapters.

study; several are also pertinent in qualitative studies. These features include:

- whether or not there will be an *intervention*;
- how confounding variables will be *controlled*;
- whether *blinding* will be used to avoid biases;
- what the *relative timing* for collecting data on dependent and independent variables will be;
- what types of *comparisons* will be made to enhance interpretability;
- what the *location* of the study will be; and
- what *timeframes* will be adopted.

This section discusses the last three features because they are relevant in planning both qualitative and quantitative studies. Chapters 9 and 10 elaborate on the first four.

TIP Design decisions affect the integrity of your findings. These decisions may influence whether you receive funding (if you seek financial support) or whether your findings will be published (if you submit to a journal). Therefore, a great deal of care and thought should go into these decisions during the planning phase.

Comparisons

In most quantitative (and some qualitative) studies, researchers incorporate comparisons into their design to provide a context for interpreting results. Most quantitative research questions involve either an explicit or an implicit comparison. For example, if our research question asks about the effect of massage on anxiety in hospitalized patients, the implied comparison is massage versus no massage, which is the independent variable.

Researchers can structure their studies to make various types of comparison, the most common of which are as follows:

1. *Comparison between two or more groups.* For example, if we were studying the emotional consequences of having a mastectomy, we might compare the emotional status of females who had a mastectomy with that of females with breast cancer who did not have a mastectomy. Or we might compare those receiving a special intervention with those receiving "usual care." In a qualitative study, we might compare mothers and fathers with respect to their experience of having a child diagnosed with leukemia.

2. *Comparison of one group's status at two or more points in time.* For example, we might want to compare patients' levels of stress before and after introducing a procedure to reduce preoperative stress. Or we might want to compare coping processes among caregivers of patients with AIDS early and later in the caregiving experience.

3. *Comparison of one group's status under different circumstances.* For example, we might compare people's heart rates during two different types of exercise.

4. *Comparison based on relative rankings.* If, for example, we hypothesized a relationship between the pain level and degree of hopefulness in patients with cancer, we would be asking whether those with high levels of pain felt less hopeful than those with low levels of pain. This research question involves a comparison of those with different rankings—higher versus lower—on both variables.

5. *Comparison with external data.* Researchers may compare their results with those from other studies or with **norms** (standards from a large and representative sample). This type of comparison often supplements rather than replaces other comparisons. In quantitative studies, this approach is useful primarily when the dependent variable is measured with a reliable, well-accepted method (e.g., blood pressure readings, scores on a respected measure of depression).

Example of Using Comparative Data From External Sources
Logan and colleagues (2020) examined the rates of (1) mental health diagnoses, (2) outpatient mental health visits, and (3) prescriptions for antidepressants and anxiolytics among parents, 6 months before and 6 months after their child's pediatric intensive care admission. Each parent served as their own control. The researchers compared their findings to national U.S. Centers for Disease Control and Prevention estimates.

Research designs for quantitative studies can be categorized based on the type of comparisons that are made. Studies that compare different people (as in examples 1 and 4) are **between-subjects designs**. Sometimes, however, it is preferable to make comparisons for the *same* participants at different times or under difference circumstances, as in examples 2 and 3. Such designs are **within-subjects designs**. When two or more groups of people are followed over time, the design is sometimes called a **mixed design** because comparisons can be both within groups over time and between different groups at a given point in time.

Comparisons provide a context for interpreting the findings. In example 1 regarding the emotional status of females who had a mastectomy, it would be difficult to know whether the females' emotional state was worrisome without comparing it with that of others—or comparing it to their state at an earlier time (for example, prior to diagnosis). In designing a study, quantitative researchers choose comparisons that will best illuminate answers to the research question.

Qualitative researchers sometimes plan to make comparisons when they undertake an in-depth study, but comparisons are rarely their primary focus. Nevertheless, patterns emerging in the data often suggest that certain comparisons have rich descriptive value.

TIP Try not to make design decisions single-handedly. Seek the advice of faculty or colleagues; patient input may also be desirable. Once you have made design decisions, consider writing out a rationale for your choices and sharing it with others to see if they can suggest improvements.

Research Location

An important planning task is to identify sites for the study. In some situations, the study site is a "given," as might be the case for a clinical study conducted in a hospital or institution with which researchers are affiliated, but in other studies, the identification of an appropriate site involves considerable effort. The closer the setting is to the "real world," the more relevant the evidence is likely to be to clinical practice (Chapter 31).

Planning the study location involves two types of activities—selecting the site or sites and gaining access to them. Although some of the issues we discuss here are of particular relevance to qualitative researchers working in the field, many quantitative studies also need to attend to these matters in planning a project, especially in intervention studies.

Site Selection

The primary consideration in site selection is whether the site has people with the behaviors, experiences, or characteristics of interest. The site must also have a sufficient *number* of these kinds of people and adequate *diversity* or mix of people to achieve research goals. In addition, the site must be one in which access to participants will be granted. Both methodologic goals (e.g., ability to impose needed controls) and ethical requirements (e.g., ability to ensure privacy and confidentiality) need to be achieved in the chosen site.

Researchers sometimes must decide *how many* sites to include. Having multiple sites is advantageous for enhancing the generalizability of the study findings, but multisite studies are complex and challenging. Multiple sites are a good strategy when several coinvestigators from different institutions are working together on a project.

Site visits to potential sites and clinical fieldwork are useful to assess the "fit" between what the researcher needs and what the site has to offer. During site visits, the researcher makes observations and converses with key gatekeepers or stakeholders at the site to better understand its characteristics and constraints. Gustavson et al. (2019) describe issues that make research in nursing homes challenging. They detail lessons learned and outline how to form mutually beneficial partnerships between researchers and nursing homes to advance research within these settings.

Gaining Entrée

Researchers must gain entrée into the sites deemed suitable for the study. If the site is an entire community, a multitiered effort of gaining acceptance from gatekeepers may be needed. For example, it may be necessary to enlist the cooperation first of community leaders and subsequently of administrators and staff in specific institutions (e.g., domestic violence organizations) or leaders of specific groups (e.g., support groups).

Because establishing *trust* is a central issue, gaining entrée requires strong interpersonal skills, as well as familiarity with the site's customs and language. Researchers' ability to gain the gatekeepers' trust can best occur if researchers are candid about research requirements and express genuine interest in and concern for people in the site. Gatekeepers are most likely to be cooperative if they believe that there will be direct benefits to them or their constituents.

Information to help gatekeepers make a decision about granting access usually should be put in writing, even if the negotiation takes place in person. An information sheet should cover the following points: (1) the purpose and significance of the research; (2) why the site was chosen; (3) what the research would entail (e.g., study timeframes, how much disruption there might be, what resources are required); (4) how ethical guidelines would be maintained, including how results would be reported; and (5) what the gatekeeper or others at the site have to gain from cooperating in the study. Figure 8.1 presents an example of a letter of inquiry for gaining entrée into a facility.

Ms. Wendy Smith, R.N.
Family Birth Place
General Hospital
Hartford, CT

Dear Ms. Smith:

I am the Principal Investigator of a study whose primary goal is to improve the detection of postpartum depression in Hispanic mothers. The study will involve testing a standard Spanish version of the Postpartum Depression Screening Scale (PDSS). Postpartum depression is a cross-cultural mental illness that can have devastating effects for 10%–15% of new mothers and their families. It has been estimated that up to 50% of all cases go undetected. Non–English-speaking women in this country may be even more disadvantaged and isolated in their environments and may thus be at even higher risk for depression than English-speaking women, and thus effective screening with a valid instrument may be especially important.

Your hospital would be a desirable site for this research because of the high percentage of Hispanic women who deliver at your Family Birth Place. The research would require a sample of 75 Hispanic mothers 18 years of age or older who have given birth within the past 3 months. Each mother would complete the PDSS-Spanish Version and would participate in a diagnostic interview for *DSM-IV* depressive disorders, conducted by a female Hispanic psychologist. If a woman is diagnosed with postpartum depression, she would be referred for psychiatric follow-up. Each mother would be given a gift certificate for $25.00 for participating in the study.

If feasible, I would like to approach the 75 Hispanic women to invite them to participate in the study soon after delivery, while they are on the postpartum unit. The mothers would be recruited by a Hispanic research assistant who is an RN. Prospective participants will be asked to sign an informed consent form, which will be available in both English and Spanish (whichever language version participants prefer). Confidentiality will be strictly maintained. No name or identifying information will be written on any of the data collection forms. All data will be kept in a locked file cabinet in my office at the University of Connecticut.

Results of the study will be presented at research conferences and in a nursing research journal. The study findings will provide you with a more complete picture of your own Hispanic population and the percentage suffering from postpartum depression. A Spanish version of the PDSS will be made available for your use for screening Hispanic mothers at your hospital.

If it is possible, I would like to schedule an appointment with you so that we can discuss the possibility of my conducting this research on your unit.

Sincerely,
Cheryl Tatano Beck, DNSc, CNM, FAAN
Distinguished Professor

FIGURE 8.1 Sample letter of inquiry for gaining entrée into a research site (fictitious).

Gaining entrée may be an ongoing process of establishing relationships and rapport with people at the site, including prospective informants. The process might involve *progressive entry*, in which certain privileges are negotiated at first and then are subsequently expanded. Ongoing communication with gatekeepers between the time that access is granted and the start-up of the study is recommended—this may be a lengthy period if funding requests are involved. It is not only courteous to keep people informed, but it may also prove critical to the project's success because circumstances (and leadership) at the site can change.

Timeframes

Research designs designate when, and how often, data will be collected. In many studies, data are collected at one point in time. For example, patients might be asked on a single occasion to describe their health-promoting behaviors. Some designs, however, call for multiple contacts with participants, often to assess changes over time. Thus, in planning a study, researchers must decide on the number of data collection points needed to address the research question properly. The research design also designates *when*, relative to other events, data will be collected. For example, the design might call for weight measurements 4 and 8 weeks after an exercise intervention.

Designs can be categorized in terms of study time frames. The major distinction, for both qualitative and quantitative researchers, is between cross-sectional and longitudinal designs.

Cross-Sectional Designs

Cross-sectional designs involve the collection of data once: the phenomena under study are captured at a single time point. Cross-sectional studies are appropriate for describing the status of phenomena or for describing relationships at a fixed point in time. For example, we might be interested in examining whether psychological symptoms in females going through menopause correlate contemporaneously with physiologic symptoms.

Example of a Cross-Sectional Study
Using a cross-sectional design, Gode et al. (2022) studied the self-care practices among adults who had type 2 diabetes with and without peripheral neuropathy in Ethiopia. A total 216 patients, half with and half without diabetic neuropathy, completed measures related to diabetes self-care practices, self-evaluated peripheral neuropathy, self-efficacy, diabetes knowledge, and social support.

Inferences about causal relationships are tricky when cross-sectional designs are used. For example, we might test the hypothesis, using cross-sectional data, that a determinant of excessive alcohol consumption is low impulse control, as measured by a psychological test. When both alcohol consumption and impulse control are measured concurrently, however, it is difficult to know which variable influenced the other, if either.

Cross-sectional data can best be used to infer time sequence under two circumstances: (1) when a cogent theoretical rationale guides the analysis or (2) when evidence or logic indicates that one variable preceded the other. For example, in a study of the effects of low birth weight on morbidity in school-aged children, it is clear that birth weight came first.

Cross-sectional studies can be designed to permit inferences about processes evolving over time, but such designs are weaker than longitudinal ones. Suppose, for example, we were studying changes in children's health promotion activities between the ages of 10 and 13 years. One way to study this would be to interview children at the age of 10 years and then 3 years later at the age of 13 years—a longitudinal design. On the other hand, we could use a cross-sectional design by interviewing *different* children of ages 10 and 13 years and then comparing their responses. If 13-year-olds engaged in more health-promoting activities than 10-year-olds, we might infer that children improve in making healthy choices as they age. To make this kind of inference, we would have to assume that the older children would have responded like the younger ones had they been questioned 3 years earlier, or, conversely, that 10-year-olds would report more health-promoting activities if they were questioned again 3 years later. Such a design, which involves a comparison of multiple age cohorts, is sometimes called a *cohort comparison design*.

Cross-sectional studies are economical but inferring changes over time with such designs is problematic. In our example, 10- and 13-year-old children may have different attitudes toward health promotion, independent of maturation. Rapid social and technologic changes make it risky to assume that differences in the behaviors or traits of different age groups are the result of time passing rather than of cohort differences. In cross-sectional studies designed to explore change, there are often alternative explanations for the findings—and that is precisely what good research design tries to avoid.

> **Example of a Cross-Sectional Study With Inference of Change Over Time**
> Gianella et al. (2022) studied the differential effects of age and duration of HIV infection on depression and anxiety among in people with HIV. Findings indicate that younger person with HIV had the highest levels of depression and anxiety. The researchers suggest that older people with HIV may have adaptive skills that help them deal with the stressors of the illness.

Longitudinal Designs

A study in which researchers collect data at more than one point in time *over an extended period* is a **longitudinal design**. There are four situations in which a longitudinal design is appropriate:

1. *Studying time-related processes.* Some research questions specifically concern phenomena that evolve over time (e.g., wound healing).
2. *Determining time sequences.* It is sometimes important to establish how phenomena are sequenced. For example, if it is hypothesized that infertility affects depression, then it would be important to ascertain that the depression did not precede the fertility problem.
3. *Assessing changes over time.* Some studies examine whether changes have occurred over time. For example, an intervention study might examine both short-term and long-term changes in health outcomes. A qualitative study might explore the evolution of grieving in the spouses of palliative care patients.
4. *Enhancing research control.* Quantitative researchers sometimes collect data at multiple points to enhance the interpretability of the results. For example, when two groups are being compared with regard to the effects of alternative interventions, the collection of preintervention data allows the researcher to assess group comparability initially.

There are several types of longitudinal designs. Most involve collecting data from one group of participants multiple times, but others involve different samples. **Trend studies**, for example, are investigations of a specific phenomenon using different samples from the same population over time (e.g., every 2 years). Trend studies permit researchers to examine patterns and rates of change and to predict future developments. Many trend studies document trends in public health issues, such as smoking, obesity, and so on.

> **Example of a Trend Study**
> In conducting a secondary analysis of longitudinal data from a clinical trial assessing the efficacy of a 6-month parental stress management intervention, Margolis et al. (2022) studied the relationship among stressful life events, caregiver depression, and asthma symptom-free days in publicly insured Black children aged 4 to 12 years with persistent asthma. Findings indicated that caregiver depression, but not stressful life events, was negatively associated with children's symptom-free days.

In a more typical longitudinal study, the *same* people provide data at two or more points in time. Longitudinal studies of general (nonclinical) populations are sometimes called **panel studies**. The term *panel* refers to the sample of people providing data. Because the same people are studied over time, researchers can examine diverse patterns of change (e.g., those whose health improved or deteriorated). Panel studies are intuitively appealing as an approach to studying change, but they are expensive.

> **Example of a Panel Study**
> From a sample of 123,330 postmenopausal females initially free of cardiovascular disease (CVD) who were enrolled in the Women's Health Initiative from 1993 through 2017, Glen and colleagues (2021) examined the association of the Portfolio Diet with cardiovascular outcomes.

Follow-up studies are undertaken to examine the subsequent development of individuals who have a specified condition or who have received a specific treatment. For example, patients who have received a special nursing intervention may be followed to ascertain long-term effects. Or, in a qualitative study, patients interviewed shortly after a diagnosis of prostate cancer may be followed to assess their experiences after treatment decisions have been made.

> **Example of a Qualitative Follow-Up Study**
> Hearn and colleague (2020) conducted a follow-up qualitative study with 19 fathers 4 to 5 years after their infants' initial NICU stay. Interviews were conducted using the telephone.

In some longitudinal studies, called **cohort studies**, a group of people (the cohort) is tracked over time to see if subsets with exposure to different factors diverge in terms of subsequent outcomes. For example, in a cohort of females, those with or without a history of childbearing could be tracked to examine differences in rates of ovarian cancer. This type of study, sometimes called a *prospective study,* is discussed in Chapter 9.

Longitudinal studies are appropriate for studying the trajectory of a phenomenon over time, but a major problem is **attrition**—the loss of participants after initial data collection. Attrition is problematic because those who drop out of the study often differ in systematic ways from those who continue to participate, resulting in potential biases and difficulty in generalizing to the original population. The longer the interval between data collection points, the greater the risk of attrition and resulting biases.

In longitudinal studies, researchers make decisions about the number of data collection points and the intervals between them. When change or development is rapid, numerous time points at short intervals may be needed to document it. Researchers interested in outcomes that may occur years after the original data collection must use longer-term follow-up—*or* use **surrogate outcomes**. For example, in evaluating the effectiveness of a smoking cessation intervention, the main outcome of interest might by lung cancer incidence or age at death, but the researcher would likely use subsequent smoking (e.g., 3 months after the intervention) as the surrogate outcome.

Repeated Measures Designs

Studies with multiple points of data collection are sometimes described as having a **repeated measures design**, which usually signifies a study in which data are collected three or more times. Longitudinal studies, such as follow-up and cohort studies, sometimes use a repeated measures design.

Repeated measures designs, however, can also be used in studies that are essentially cross-sectional. For example, a study involving the collection of postoperative patient data on vital signs hourly over a 6-hour period would not be described as longitudinal because the study does not involve an extended time perspective. Yet, the design could be characterized as repeated measures. Researchers are especially likely to use the term *repeated measures design* when they use a repeated measures approach to statistical analysis (see Chapter 18).

> **Example of a Repeated Measures Design**
> In a randomized control design study using repeated measures, Anderson and Brown (2021) studied the effect of animal-assisted therapy on nursing student anxiety prior to the medication calculation exam. They found that animal-assisted therapy reduced students' anxiety.

> **TIP** In making design decisions, you will need to balance various considerations, such as time, cost, ethics, and study rigor. Try to understand your "upper limits" before finalizing your design. That is, what is the *most* money that can be spent on the project? What is the *maximum amount* of time available for conducting the study? What is the limit of acceptability with regard to attrition? These limits often eliminate some design options. With these constraints in mind, the central focus should be on designing a study that maximizes the rigor or trustworthiness of the study.

PLANNING DATA COLLECTION

In planning a study, researchers must select methods to gather their research data. This section provides an overview of various methods of data collection for qualitative and quantitative studies.

Overview of Data Collection and Data Sources

A broad array of data collection methods can be used in research. In some cases, researchers may be able to use data from existing sources, such as records. Most often, however, researchers collect new data, and one key planning decision concerns the types of data to gather. Three approaches have been used most frequently by nurse researchers: self-reports, observation, and biophysiologic measures.

Self-Reports (Patient-Reported Outcomes)

A good deal of information can be gathered by questioning people directly, a method known as **self-report**. In the medical literature, self-reports are often called **patient-reported outcomes** or **PROs**, but some self-reports are not about patients (e.g., self-reports about nurses' burnout) and some are not *outcomes* (self-reports about prior hospitalizations). Most nursing studies involve self-report data. The unique ability of humans to communicate verbally makes direct questioning a particularly important part of nurse researchers' data collection repertoire.

Self-reports are versatile. If we want to know what people think, believe, or plan to do, the most efficient approach is to ask them. Self-reports can yield information that would be impossible to gather by other means. Behaviors can be observed but only if participants engage in them publicly. Furthermore, observers can observe only those behaviors occurring at the time of the study. Through self-reports, researchers can gather *retrospective data* about events occurring in the past or information about behaviors in which people plan to engage in the future. Self-reports can also capture psychological attributes such as motivation or resilience.

Nevertheless, verbal report methods have some weaknesses. The most serious issue concerns their validity and accuracy: Can we be sure that people feel or act the way they say they do? We all have a tendency to present ourselves positively, and this may conflict with the truth. Researchers who gather self-report data should recognize this limitation and take it into consideration when interpreting the results.

> **Example of a Study Using Self-Reports**
> Abozaid et al. (2022) implemented and evaluated the effectiveness of training on workplace violence delivered to nurses in Cairo. The training aimed to empower them with skills needed to effectively identify and manage workplace violence. The self-reported measures of Confidence in Coping with Patient Aggression and Nurses' Attitudes Toward Violence/Aggressive Behavior Questionnaire were delivered pre and post the training session.

Self-report methods depend on respondents' willingness to share personal information. **Projective techniques** are sometimes used to obtain data about people's psychological states indirectly. Projective techniques present participants with a stimulus of low structure, permitting them to "read in" and describe their interpretations. The Rorschach (inkblot) test is an example of a projective technique. Other projective methods encourage self-expression through the construction of a product (e.g., drawings). The assumption is that people express their needs, motives, and emotions by working with or manipulating materials. Projective methods are used by nurse researchers mainly in studies exploring sensitive topics with children.

> **Example of a Study Using Projective Methods**
> West et al. (2022) conducted a grounded theory study on family experiences of pediatric hematopoietic stem cell transplant in which the researchers simultaneously adapted and studied a "dialoguing with images," an art-based method.

Observation

An alternative to self-reports is **observation** of study participants. Observation can be done directly through the human senses or with technical apparatus, such as video equipment, X-rays, and so on. Observational methods can be used to gather information about a wide range of phenomena, such as (1) people's characteristics and conditions (e.g., patients' sleep–wake state); (2) verbal communication (e.g., nurse–patient dialogue); (3) nonverbal communication (e.g., facial expressions); (4) activities and behavior (e.g., geriatric patients' self-grooming); (5) skill attainment (e.g., skill of patients with diabetes in testing their urine); and (6) environmental conditions (e.g., architectural barriers in nursing homes).

Observation in healthcare settings is an important data-gathering strategy. Nurses are in an advantageous position to observe, relatively unobtrusively, the behaviors of patients, their families, and hospital staff. Moreover, nurses may, by training, be especially sensitive observers.

Observational methods are especially useful when people are unaware of their own behavior (e.g., manifesting preoperative symptoms of anxiety), when people are embarrassed to report activities (e.g., aggressive actions), when behaviors are emotionally laden (e.g., grieving), or when people cannot describe their actions (e.g., young children). A shortcoming of observation is potential behavior distortions when participants are aware of being observed—a problem called **reactivity**. Reactivity can be eliminated if observations are made without people's knowledge, through concealment—but this may pose ethical concerns. Another problem is **observer biases**. Several factors (e.g., prejudices, emotions, fatigue) can undermine objectivity. Observational biases can be minimized through careful training.

> **Example of a Study Using Observation**
> Kuamoto et al. (2021) studied the skin-to-skin contact practice of mothers with their full-term newborns in the first hour after birth. The time mothers spent providing skin-to-skin contact was observed by a member of the research team.

Biophysiologic Measures/Biomarkers

Many clinical studies rely on the use of **biophysiologic measures** or biomarkers. **Biomarkers** are objective, quantifiable characteristics of biologic processes (Strimbu & Tavel, 2010). Biophysiologic and physical variables typically are measured using specialized technical instruments and equipment. Because such equipment is available in healthcare settings, the costs of these measures to nurse researchers may be small or nonexistent.

A major strength of biophysiologic measures is their objectivity. Nurse A and nurse B, reading from the same spirometer output, are likely to record the same forced expiratory volume (FEV) measurements. Furthermore, two different spirometers are likely to produce the same FEV readouts. Another advantage of physiologic measurements is the relative precision they normally offer. By *relative*, we are implicitly comparing physiologic instruments with measures of psychological phenomena, such as self-report measures of anxiety or pain. Biophysiologic measures usually yield data of exceptionally high quality.

> **Example of a Study Using Biomarkers**
> Coakley et al. (2021) studied the effects of an animal-assisted visitation program on patients. A single group pre-post quasiexperimental design evaluated the effect of pet therapy on hospitalized patients. Biomarkers measures included salivary cortisol, respiratory, and heart rate.

Records

Most researchers create original data for their studies, but sometimes they take advantage of information available in **records**. Electronic health records and other records constitute rich data sources to which nurse researchers may have access. Research data obtained from records are advantageous because they are economical: the collection of original data can be time-consuming and costly. Also, records avoid problems stemming from people's reaction to study participation.

On the other hand, when researchers are not responsible for collecting data, they may be unaware of the records' limitations and biases, such as the biases of *selective deposit* and *selective survival*. If the available records are not the entire set of all possible such records, researchers must question how representative existing records are. Many record keepers *intend* to maintain an entire universe of records but may not succeed. Careful researchers should attempt to learn what biases might exist. Alzu'bi and colleagues (2021) discuss various abstraction methods and the advantages and disadvantages of each. Ehsani-Moghaddam and Queenan (2021) discuss the iterative strategies to assure accuracy, precision, completeness, comprehensiveness, consistency, timeliness, uniqueness, data cleaning, and coherence of data quality.

Other difficulties also may be relevant. Sometimes records have to be verified for their authenticity or accuracy, which may be difficult if the records are old. In using records to study trends, researchers should be alert to possible changes in record-keeping procedures. Another problem is the increasing difficulty of gaining access to institutional records. Thus, although records may be plentiful and inexpensive, they should not be used without paying attention to potential problems.

> **TIP** Nurse researchers are increasingly using information from "Big Data" sources, such as large administrative databases or *registries*. Registries are collections of large amounts of data about a particular disease or patient population, such as trauma or cancer registries. Gephart et al. (2018) and Perazzo and colleagues (2019) have written about doing research with large databases.

Example of a Study Using Records
Banister and colleagues (2022) audited the electronic health records of patients hospitalized with COVID-19 to identify types and frequency of nurse-sensitive indicators, including social determinants of health.

Dimensions of Data Collection Approaches

Data collection methods vary along three key dimensions: structure, researcher obtrusiveness, and objectivity. In planning a study, researchers make decisions about where on these dimensions the data collection methods should fall.

Structure

In structured data collection, information is gathered from participants in a comparable, prespecified way. Most self-administered questionnaires are structured: They include a fixed set of questions, usually with predesignated response options (e.g., agree/disagree). Structured methods give participants limited opportunities to qualify their answers or to explain the meaning of their responses. By contrast, qualitative studies rely mainly on unstructured methods of data collection.

Structured methods often take considerable effort to develop, but they yield data that are relatively easy to analyze because the data can be readily quantified. Structured methods are not appropriate for an in-depth examination of a phenomenon, however. Consider the following two methods of asking people about their levels of stress:

Structured. During the past week, would you say you felt stressed:

1. rarely or none of the time,
2. some or a little of the time,
3. occasionally or a moderate amount of the time, or
4. most or all of the time?

Unstructured. How stressed or anxious have you been this past week? Please tell me about any tensions and stresses you experienced.

The structured question allows us to compute what percentage of respondents felt stressed most of the time but provides no information about the circumstances of the stress. The unstructured question allows for deeper and more thoughtful responses but may not be useful for people who are not good at expressing themselves; moreover, the resulting data are more difficult to analyze.

Researcher Obtrusiveness

Data collection methods differ in the degree to which people are aware of the data-gathering process. If people know they are under scrutiny, their behavior and responses may not be "normal," and distortions can undermine the value of the research. When data are collected unobtrusively, however, ethical problems may emerge.

Study participants are most likely to distort their behavior and their responses to questions under certain circumstances. Researcher obtrusiveness is likely to be most problematic when (1) a program is being evaluated and participants have a vested interest in the evaluation outcome; (2) participants engage in socially unacceptable or unusual behavior; (3) participants have not complied with medical and nursing instructions; and (4) participants are the type of people who have a strong need to "look good." When researcher obtrusiveness is unavoidable under these circumstances, researchers should make an effort to put participants at ease, to emphasize the importance of candor, and to adopt a nonjudgmental demeanor.

Objectivity

Objectivity refers to the degree to which two independent researchers can arrive at similar "scores" or make similar observations regarding concepts of interest. Objectivity is a mechanism for avoiding biases. Some data collection approaches require more subjective judgment than others. Researchers with a positivist orientation usually strive for a reasonable amount of objectivity. In research based on the constructivist paradigm, however, the subjective judgment of investigators is considered essential for understanding human experiences.

Developing a Data Collection Plan

In planning a study, researchers make decisions about the type and amount of data to collect. Several factors, including costs, must be weighed, but a key goal is to identify the kinds of data that will yield accurate, valid, and trustworthy information for addressing the research question.

Most researchers face the issue of balancing information needs against the risk of overburdening participants. In many studies, more data are collected than are needed or analyzed. Although it is better to have adequate data than to have unwanted omissions, minimizing *participant burden* should be an important goal. Specific guidance on data collection plans is offered in Chapter 14 for quantitative studies and Chapter 24 for qualitative studies.

ORGANIZATION OF A RESEARCH PROJECT

Studies typically take many months to complete and longitudinal studies require years of work. During the planning phase, it is a good idea to make preliminary estimates of how long various tasks will require. Having deadlines helps to restrict tasks that might otherwise continue indefinitely, such as a literature review.

Chapter 3 presented a sequence of steps that quantitative researchers follow in a study. The steps represented an idealized conception: the research process rarely follows a neatly prescribed sequence of procedures, even in quantitative studies. Decisions made in one step, for example, may require alterations in a previous activity. For example, sample size decisions may require rethinking how many sites are needed. Nevertheless, preliminary time estimates are valuable. In particular, it is important to have a sense of how much total time the study will require and when it will begin.

> **TIP** We could not suggest even approximations for the percentage of time that should be spent on each task. Some projects need many months to recruit participants, whereas other studies can rely on an existing group. Clearly, not all steps are equally time-consuming.

Researchers sometimes develop visual timelines to help them organize a study. These devices are especially useful if funding is sought because the schedule helps researchers to understand when and for how long staff support is needed (e.g., for transcribing interviews). This can best be illustrated with an example, in this case of a hypothetical quantitative study.

Suppose a researcher was studying the following problem: Is a female's decision to have an annual mammogram related to her perceived susceptibility to breast cancer? Using the organization of steps outlined in Chapter 3, here are some of the tasks that might be undertaken:[1]

1. The researcher is concerned that many older females do not get mammograms regularly. The specific *research question* is whether mammogram practices are different for females with different perceptions about their susceptibility to breast cancer.
2. The researcher *reviews the research literature* on breast cancer, mammography use, and factors affecting mammography decisions.
3. The researcher does *clinical fieldwork* by discussing the problem with nurses and other healthcare professionals in various clinical

---
[1]This is only a partial list of tasks and is designed to illustrate the flow of activities; the flow in this example is more orderly than would ordinarily be true.

settings and by having informal discussions with females in a support group for breast cancer patients.
4. The researcher *seeks theories* and models for the problem. The researcher finds that the Health Belief Model is relevant, which helps her to develop a conceptual definition of susceptibility to breast cancer.
5. Based on the framework, the following *hypothesis is developed*: Females (P) who perceive themselves as susceptible to breast cancer (I) are more likely than other females (C) to get an annual mammogram (O).
6. The researcher adopts a nonexperimental, cross-sectional, between-subjects *research design*. The comparison strategy will be to compare females with different rankings on a measure of susceptibility to breast cancer. The researcher designs the study to control the confounding variables of age, marital status, and health insurance status. The research site will be Pittsburgh.
7. There is no *intervention* in this study and so this step is unnecessary.
8. The researcher designates that the *population* of interest is females between the ages of 50 and 65 years living in Pittsburgh who have not been previously diagnosed as having any form of cancer.
9. The researcher will recruit 250 females living in Pittsburgh as the *research sample*; they are identified at random using a procedure known as *random-digit dialing,* and so the researcher does not need to gain entrée into any institution.
10. *Research variables will be measured* by self-report; the independent variable (perceived susceptibility), dependent variable (mammogram history), and confounding variables will be measured by asking participants a series of questions.
11. The Institutional Review Board (IRB) at the researcher's institution is asked to review the plans to ensure that the study *adheres to ethical standards.*
12. *Plans for the study are finalized*: the methods are reviewed by colleagues with clinical and methodologic expertise and by the IRB; the data collection instruments are pretested; and interviewers who will collect the data are trained.
13. *Data are collected* by means of telephone interviews with females in the research sample.
14. *Data are prepared for analysis* by coding them and entering them onto a computer file.
15. *Data are analyzed* using statistical software.
16. The results indicate that the hypothesis is supported; however, the researcher's *interpretation* must take into consideration that many females who were asked to participate declined to do so.
17. The researcher presents an early report on their findings and interpretations at a conference of Sigma Theta Tau International. The researcher subsequently publishes the report in the *International Journal of Nursing Studies.*
18. The researcher seeks out clinicians to discuss how the study findings can be *used in practice.*

The researcher plans to conduct this study over a 2-year period. Figure 8.2 presents a hypothetical schedule. Many steps overlap or are undertaken concurrently; some steps are projected to involve little time, whereas others require months of work.

In developing a schedule, several considerations should be kept in mind, including methodologic expertise and the availability of funding. In the present example, if the researcher needed financial support to pay for the cost of interviewers, the timeline would need to be expanded to accommodate the time required to prepare a proposal and await the funding decision. It is also important to consider the practical aspects of performing the study, which were not noted in the preceding section. Securing permissions, hiring staff, and holding meetings are all time-consuming, but necessary, activities.

In large-scale studies—especially studies in which there is an intervention—it is wise to undertake a **pilot study**. A pilot study is a trial run designed to test planned methods and procedures. Results and experiences from pilot studies help to inform many of decisions for larger projects.

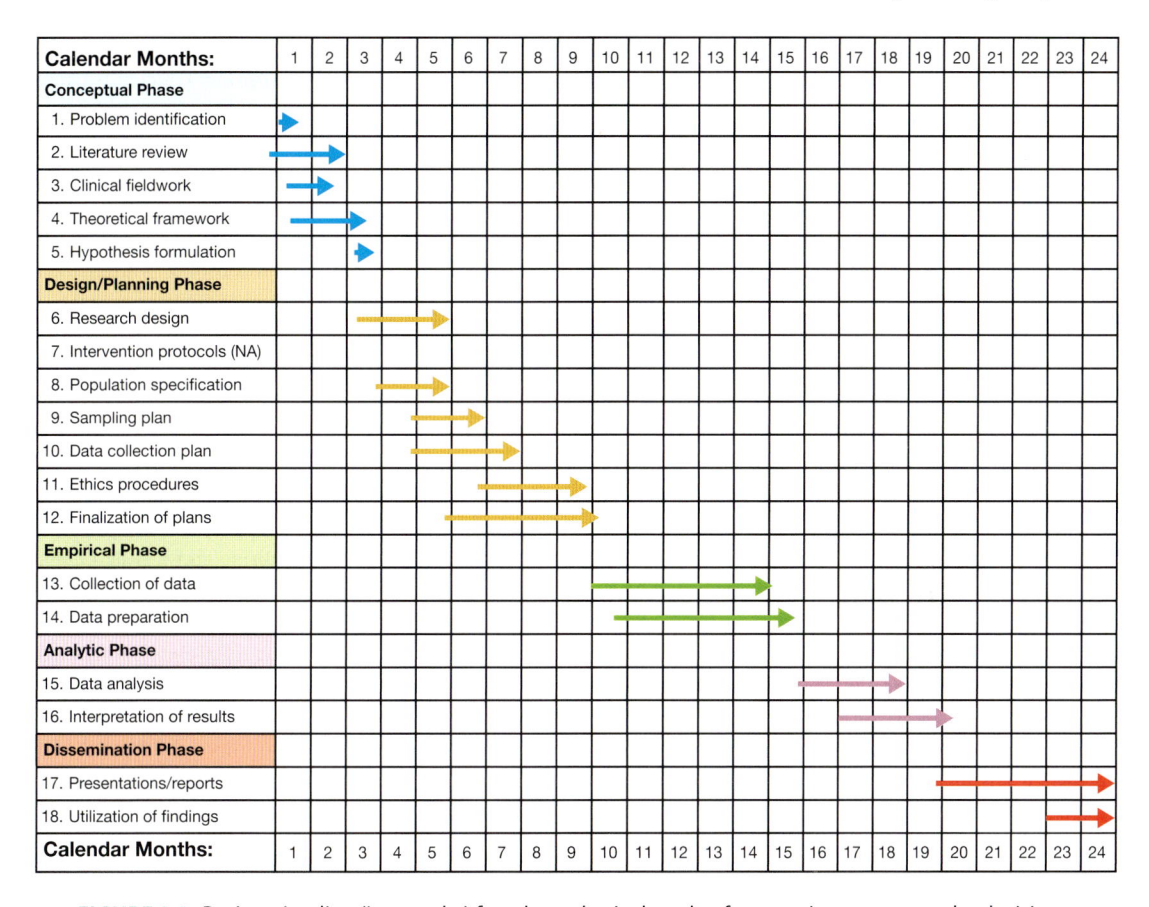

Calendar Months:	1	2	3	4	5	6	7	8	9	10	11	12	13	14	15	16	17	18	19	20	21	22	23	24
Conceptual Phase																								
1. Problem identification																								
2. Literature review																								
3. Clinical fieldwork																								
4. Theoretical framework																								
5. Hypothesis formulation																								
Design/Planning Phase																								
6. Research design																								
7. Intervention protocols (NA)																								
8. Population specification																								
9. Sampling plan																								
10. Data collection plan																								
11. Ethics procedures																								
12. Finalization of plans																								
Empirical Phase																								
13. Collection of data																								
14. Data preparation																								
Analytic Phase																								
15. Data analysis																								
16. Interpretation of results																								
Dissemination Phase																								
17. Presentations/reports																								
18. Utilization of findings																								

FIGURE 8.2 Project timeline (in months) for a hypothetical study of women's mammography decisions.

We discuss the important role of pilot studies in Chapter 29.

Individuals differ in the kinds of tasks that appeal to them. Some people enjoy the preliminary phase, which has an intellectual component; others are more eager to collect the data, which is more interpersonal. Researchers should, however, allocate a sensible amount of time to do justice to each activity.

TIP Getting organized for a study has many dimensions beyond having a timeline. Two important issues concern having the right team and mix of skills for a research project, and developing plans for hiring and monitoring research staff (Nelson & Morrison-Beedy, 2008).

CRITICAL APPRAISAL OF THE PLANNING ASPECTS OF A STUDY

Researchers typically do not describe the planning process or problems that arose during the study in journal articles. Thus, there is typically little that readers can do to critically appraise the researcher's planning efforts. What *can* be appraised, of course, are the outcomes of the planning—that is, the methodologic decisions themselves. Guidelines for critically appraising those decisions are provided throughout this book.

Readers can, however, be alert to a few things relating to research planning. First, evidence of careful conceptualization provides a clue that the project was well planned. If a conceptual map is presented (or implied) in the report, it means that the researcher had a "road map" that facilitated planning.

Second, readers can consider whether the researcher's plans reflect adequate attention to concerns about evidence-based practice. For example, was the comparison group strategy designed to reflect a realistic practice concern? Was the setting one that maximizes potential for the generalizability of the findings? Did the timing of data collection correspond to clinically important milestones? Was the intervention sensitive to the constraints of a typical practice environment?

Finally, a report might provide clues about whether the researcher devoted sufficient time and resources in preparing for the study. For example, if the report indicates that the study grew out of earlier research on a similar topic, or that the researcher had previously used the same instruments, or had completed other studies in the same setting, this suggests that the researcher was not plunging into unfamiliar waters. Unrealistic planning can sometimes be inferred from a discussion of sample recruitment. If the report indicates that the researcher was unable to recruit the originally hoped-for number of participants, or if recruitment took months longer than anticipated, this suggests that the researcher may not have done adequate homework during the planning phase.

RESEARCH EXAMPLE

In this section, we describe a pilot study and the "lessons learned" by the researchers. This is a good example of the importance of strong advance planning for a study.

Study: Stigma as a Barrier to Participant Recruitment of Minority Populations in Diabetes Research: Development of a Community-Centered Recruitment Approach (Mitchell et al., 2021).

Purpose: The purpose of the article was the researchers' discovery of diabetes-related stigma as an underrecognized impediment to recruitment for the Women in Control 2.0 virtual diabetes self-management education study.

Methods: The researchers' initial recruitment plan was to use traditional strategies to recruit underrepresented females with uncontrolled type 2 diabetes. This included letters and phone calls to targeted patients, referrals from clinicians, and posted flyers.

Findings: Despite some initial success in the recruitment of 46 participants, the team was unable to reach their enrollment target. They found that clinician referral was challenging as was community-based recruitment. The research team then consulted with a patient advisory group and experts in community advocacy; they found that diabetes-related stigma emerged as a prominent barrier to recruitment. As a result, the team revised recruitment materials and outreach scripts. With these changes, the team was able to not only reach their target goal of 212 participants but to exceed it, recruiting a total of 309 participants,

Conclusions: The researchers concluded that diabetes has a stigma associated with it. Those with T2 diabetes struggle with the perception of being labeled as "lazy" or having "a lack of self-control" and feeling "responsible" for causing their diabetes. Being sensitive to these concerns while employing strategies for recruitment such as empowering messaging and fostering community helped to improve the number of people interested in study participation.

SUMMARY POINTS

- Researchers face numerous challenges in planning a study, including the challenge of designing a study that is strong with respect to reliability and validity (quantitative studies) or trustworthiness (qualitative studies).
- **Reliability** refers to the accuracy and consistency of information obtained in a study. **Validity** is a more complex concept that broadly concerns the *soundness* of the study's evidence—that is, whether the findings are cogent and well grounded.
- **Trustworthiness** in qualitative research encompasses several different dimensions, including dependability, confirmability, authenticity, transferability, and credibility.
- **Credibility** is achieved to the extent that the research methods engender confidence in the truth of the data and in the researchers' interpretations. **Triangulation**, the use of multiple

- sources or referents to draw conclusions about what constitutes the truth, is one approach to enhancing credibility.
- A **bias** is an influence that distorts study results. **Systematic bias** results when a bias operates in a consistent direction.
- In quantitative studies, **research control** is used to *hold constant* outside influences on the outcome variable so that its relationship to the independent variable can be better understood. Researchers use various strategies to control **confounding variables,** which are extraneous to the study aims and can obscure understanding.
- In quantitative studies, a powerful tool to eliminate bias is **randomness**—having certain features of the study established by chance rather than by researchers' intentions.
- **Reflexivity,** the process of reflecting critically on the self and of scrutinizing personal values that could affect interpretation, is an important tool in qualitative research.
- **Generalizability** in a quantitative study concerns the extent to which findings can be applied to people or settings other than the ones used in the research. **Transferability** is the extent to which qualitative findings can be transferred to other settings.
- During the planning phase, researchers need to consider the extent to which key **stakeholders** will be involved in the research and who the key stakeholders are.
- In planning a study, researchers make many design decisions, including whether to have an intervention, how to control confounding variables, what type of comparisons will be made, where the study will take place, and what the study time frames will be.
- Quantitative researchers often incorporate comparisons into their designs to enhance interpretability. In **between-subjects designs**, different groups of people are compared. **Within-subjects designs** involve comparisons of the same people at different times or under different circumstances, and **mixed designs** involve both types of comparison.
- Site selection for a study often requires **site visits** to evaluate suitability and feasibility. Gaining entrée into a site involves developing and maintaining trust with gatekeepers.
- **Cross-sectional designs** involve collecting data at one point in time, whereas **longitudinal designs** involve data collection two or more times over an extended period.
- **Trend studies** have multiple points of data collection with different samples from the same population. **Panel studies** gather data from the same people, usually from a general population, more than once. In a **follow-up study,** data are gathered two or more times from a well-defined group (e.g., those with a particular health problem). In a **cohort study**, a cohort of people is tracked over time to see if subsets with different exposures to risk factors differ in terms of subsequent outcomes.
- A **repeated measures design** typically involves collecting data three or more times, either in a longitudinal fashion or in rapid succession over a shorter timeframe.
- Longitudinal studies are typically expensive and time-consuming, and have risk of **attrition** (loss of participants over time) but are essential for illuminating time-related phenomena.
- Researchers also develop a **data collection plan.** In nursing, the most widely used methods are self-report, observation, biophysiologic measures, and existing records.
- **Self-report** data (sometimes called **patient-reported outcomes** or **PROs**) are obtained by directly questioning people. Self-reports are versatile and powerful, but a drawback is the potential for respondents' deliberate or inadvertent misrepresentations.
- A wide variety of human activity and traits are amenable to direct **observation.** Observation is subject to **observer biases** and distorted participant behavior (**reactivity**).
- **Biophysiologic measures** (**biomarkers**) tend to yield high-quality data that are objective and valid.
- Existing **records** and documents are an economical source of research data, but two potential biases in records are *selective deposit* and *selective survival.*
- Data collection methods vary in terms of structure, researcher obtrusiveness, and objectivity,

- and researchers must decide on these dimensions in their plan.
- Planning efforts should include the development of a timeline that provides estimates of when important tasks will be completed.

REFERENCES CITED IN CHAPTER 8

Abozaid, D. A., Momen, M., Ezz, N. F. A. E., Ahmed, H. A., Al-Tehewy, M. M., El-Setouhy, M., El-Shinawi, M., Hirshon, J. M., & Houssinie, M. E. (2022). Patient and visitor aggression de-escalation training for nurses in a teaching hospital in Cairo, Egypt. *BMC Nursing*, *21*(1), 63. https://doi.org/10.1186/s12912-022-00828-y

Alzu'bi, A. A., Watzlaf, V. J. M., & Sheridan, P. (2021). Electronic Health Record (EHR) abstraction. *Perspectives in Health Information Management*, *18*(Spring), 1g.

Anderson, D., & Brown, S. (2021). The effect of animal-assisted therapy on nursing student anxiety: A randomized control study. *Nurse Education in Practice*, *52*, 103042. https://doi.org/10.1016/j.nepr.2021.103042

Banister, G., Carroll, D. L., Dickins, K., Flanagan, J., Jones, D., Looby, S. E., & Cahill, J. E. (2022). Nurse-sensitive indicators during COVID-19. *International Journal of Nursing Knowledge*, *33*(3), 234–244. https://doi.org/10.1111/2047-3095.12372

Coakley, A. B., Annese, C. D., Empoliti, J. H., & Flanagan, J. M. (2021). The experience of animal assisted therapy on patients in an acute care setting. *Clinical Nursing Research*, *30*(4), 401–405. https://doi.org/10.1177/1054773820977198

Concannon, T., Meissner, P., Grunbaum, J., McElwee, N., Guise, J. M., Santa, J., Conway, P. H., Daudelin, D, Morrato, E. H., Leslie, L. K., & Leslie, L. (2012). A new taxonomy for stakeholder engagement in patient-centered outcomes research. *Journal of General Internal Medicine*, *27*(8), 985–991.

Cousin, L., Johnson-Mallard, V., & Booker, S. Q. (2022). "Be strong My Sista'": Sentiments of strength from Black women with chronic pain living in the deep South. *Advances in Nursing Science*, *45*(2), 127–142. https://doi.org/10.1097/ANS.0000000000000416

Ehsani-Moghaddam, B., Martin, K., & Queenan, J. A. (2021). Data quality in healthcare: A report of practical experience with the Canadian primary care sentinel surveillance network data. *Health Information Management Journal*, *50*(1–2), 88–92. https://doi.org/10.1177/1833358319887743

Flanagan, J., Post, K., Hill, R., & DiPalazzo, J. (2022). Feasibility of a nurse coached walking intervention for informal dementia caregivers. *Western Journal of Nursing Research*, *44*(5), 466–476. https://doi.org/10.1177/01939459211001395

Gephart, S., Davis, M., & Shea, K. (2018). Perspectives on policy and the value of nursing science in a Big Data era. *Nursing Science Quaterly*, *31*(1), 78–81.

Gianella, S., Saloner, R., Curtin, G., Little, S. J., Heaton, A., Montoya, J. L., Letendre, S. L., Marquine, M. J., Jeste, D. V., & Moore, D. J. (2022). A cross-sectional study to evaluate the effects of age and duration of HIV infection on anxiety and depression in cisgender men. *AIDS and Behaviour*, *26*(1), 196–203. https://doi.org/10.1007/s10461-021-03373-y

Gode, M., Aga, F., & Hailu, A. (2022). Self-care practices among adult type 2 diabetes patients with and without peripheral neuropathy: A cross-sectional study at tertiary healthcare settings in Ethiopia. *The Canadian Journal of Nursing Research*, *54*(3), 345–356. https://doi.org/10.1177/08445621211020653

Gustavson, A. M., Drake, C., Lakin, A., Daddato, A. E., Falvey, J. R., Capell, W., Lum, H. D., Jones, C. D., Unroe, K. T., Towsley, G. L., Stevens-Lapsley, J. E., Levy, C. R., Boxer, R. S., & PACRATS Investigators. (2019). Conducting clinical research in post-acute and long-term nursing home care settings: Regulatory challenges. *Journal of the American Medical Directors Association*, *20*(7), 798–803. https://doi.org/10.1016/j.jamda.2019.04.022

Hearn, G., Clarkson, G., & Day, M. (2020). The role of the NICU in father involvement, beliefs, and confidence: A follow-up qualitative study. *Advances in Neonatal Care*, *20*(1), 80–89. https://doi.org/10.1097/ANC.0000000000000665

Kuamoto, R. S., Bueno, M., & Riesco, M. L. G. (2021). Skin-to-skin contact between mothers and full-term newborns after birth: A cross-sectional study. *Revista Brasileira de Enfermagem*, *74*(Suppl. 4), e20200026. https://doi.org/10.1590/0034-7167-2020-0026

Lincoln, Y. S., & Guba, E. G. (1985). *Naturalistic inquiry*. Sage.

Logan, G. E., Sahrmann, J. M., Gu, H., & Hartman, M. E. (2020). Parental mental health care after their child's pediatric intensive care hospitalization. *Pediatric Critical Care Medicine*, *21*(11), 941–948. https://doi.org/10.1097/PCC.0000000000002559

Margolis, R. H. F., Shelef, D. Q., Gordish-Dressman, H., Masur, J. E., & Teach, S. J. (2023). Stressful life events, caregiver depressive symptoms, and child asthma symptom-free days: A longitudinal analysis. *Journal of Asthma*, *60*(3), 508–515. https://doi.org/10.1080/02770903.2022.2062674

Mitchell, S., Bragg, A., Moldovan, I., Woods, S., Melo, K., Martin-Howard, J., & Gardiner, P. (2021). Stigma as a barrier to participant recruitment of minority populations in diabetes research: Development of a community-centered recruitment approach. *JMIR Diabetes*, *6*(2), e26965. https://doi.org/10.2196/26965

Nelson, L. E., & Morrison-Beedy, D. (2008). Research team training: Moving beyond job descriptions. *Applied Nursing Research*, *21*(3), 159–164.

Patton, M. Q. (2015). *Qualitative research & evaluation methods* (4th ed.). Sage.

Perazzo, J., Rodriguez, M., Currie, J., Salata, R., & Webel, A. R. (2019). Creation of data repositories to advance nursing science. *Western Journal of Nursing Research*, *41*(1), 78–95. https://doi.org/10.1177/0193945917749481

Polit, D. F., & Beck, C. T. (2010). Generalization in quantitative and qualitative research: Myths and strategies. *International Journal of Nursing Studies*, *47*(11), 1451–1458.

Schwandt, T. (2007). *The Sage dictionary of qualitative inquiry* (3rd ed.). Sage.

Strimbu, K., & Tavel, J. (2010). What are biomarkers? *Current Opinion in HIV and AIDS*, *5*(6), 463–466.

Torkar, T., Homar, V., & Švab, V. (2023). Triangulation study of needs assessment of people with severe mental illness in "follow-up" day hospital settings. *Nursing Open*, *10*(5), 2859–2868. Advance online publication. https://doi.org/10.1002/nop2.1527

West, C. H., Dusome, D. L., Winsor, J., Winther Klippenstein, A., & Rallison, L. B. (2022). Dialoguing with images: An expressive arts method for health research. *Qualitative Health Research*, *32*(7), 1055–1070. https://doi.org/10.1177/10497323221084924

Part 3

DESIGNING AND CONDUCTING QUANTITATIVE STUDIES TO GENERATE EVIDENCE FOR NURSING

Chapter 9 Quantitative Research Design
Chapter 10 Rigor and Validity in Quantitative Research
Chapter 11 Specific Types of Quantitative Research
Chapter 12 Quality Improvement and Improvement Science
Chapter 13 Sampling in Quantitative Research
Chapter 14 Data Collection in Quantitative Research
Chapter 15 Measurement and Data Quality
Chapter 16 Developing and Testing Self-Report Scales
Chapter 17 Descriptive Statistics
Chapter 18 Inferential Statistics
Chapter 19 Multivariate Statistics
Chapter 20 Processes of Quantitative Data Analysis
Chapter 21 Clinical Significance and Interpretation of Quantitative Results

9 Quantitative Research Design

Learning Objectives

1. Discuss the concept of causality and identify criteria for causal relationships.
2. Identify different choices researchers have for a control group.
3. Articulate various types of randomization.
4. Describe experimental, quasi-experimental, and nonexperimental designs.
5. Understand the strengths and limitations of various quantitative designs.

GENERAL DESIGN ISSUES

This chapter describes options for designing quantitative studies. We begin by discussing several broad issues.

Causality

Several types of research questions are relevant to evidence-based nursing practice—questions about interventions (Therapy); Diagnosis and assessment; Prognosis; Etiology (causation) and prevention of harm; Description; and Meaning or process. Questions about meaning or process call for qualitative approaches (Chapter 22). Questions about diagnosis or assessment, as well as questions about the status quo of health-related situations, are typically descriptive. Many research questions, however, are about *causes* and *effects*:

- Does a telephone therapy intervention (I) for patients diagnosed with prostate cancer (P) *cause* improvements in their decision-making skills (O)? (Therapy question)
- Do birthweights less than 1,500 g (I) *cause* developmental delays (O) in children (P)? (Prognosis question)
- Does a high-carbohydrate diet (I) *cause* cognitive impairment (O) in older adults (P)? (Etiology [causation]/prevention of harm question)

Causality is a hotly debated issue, and yet we all understand the general concept of a **cause**. For example, we understand that lack of sleep *causes* fatigue and that high caloric intake *causes* weight gain.

Most phenomena have multiple causes. Weight gain, for example, can be the effect of high caloric consumption, but many other factors can cause weight gain. Causes of health-related phenomena usually are not *deterministic*, but rather are *probabilistic*—that is, the causes increase the probability that an effect will occur. For example, there is ample evidence that smoking is a cause of lung cancer, but not everyone who smokes develops lung cancer, and not everyone with lung cancer has a history of smoking.

The Counterfactual Model

While it might be easy to grasp what researchers mean when they talk about a *cause*, what exactly is an **effect**? Shadish et al. (2002), who wrote a seminal book on research design and causal inference, explained that a good way to grasp the meaning of an effect is to conceptualize a counterfactual. In a research context, a **counterfactual** is what would have happened *to the same people* exposed to a causal factor if they *simultaneously* were *not* exposed to the causal factor. An effect is the difference between what actually did happen with the exposure and what would have happened without it. A counterfactual clearly can never be realized, but it is a good model to keep in mind in designing a study to answer cause-probing questions.

Criteria for Causality

Several writers have proposed criteria for establishing a *cause-and-effect relationship*. Three criteria are attributed to 19th-century philosopher John Stuart Mill:

1. *Temporal:* A cause must precede an effect in time. If we test the hypothesis that smoking causes lung cancer, we need to show that cancer occurred *after* smoking commenced.
2. *Relationship:* An *empirical relationship* between the presumed cause and the presumed effect must exist. In our example, an association between smoking and cancer must be found—that is, a higher percentage of smokers than nonsmokers get lung cancer.
3. *No confounders:* The relationship cannot be explained as being *caused by a third variable*. Suppose that most smokers lived in urban environments. The relationship between smoking and lung cancer might then reflect an underlying causal link between the environment and lung cancer.

Additional criteria were proposed by Bradford-Hill (1965)—precisely as part of the discussion about the causal link between smoking and lung cancer. Two of Bradford-Hill's criteria foreshadow the importance of meta-analyses, techniques for which had not been developed to conduct a meta-analyses when the criteria were proposed. The criterion of *coherence* involves having similar evidence from multiple sources, and the criterion of *consistency* involves having similar levels of statistical relationship in several studies. Another important criterion is *biologic plausibility*, that is, evidence from laboratory or basic physiologic studies that a causal pathway is credible.

Causality and Research Design

Researchers testing hypotheses about casual relationships seek to provide persuasive evidence that these various criteria have been met. Some research designs are better at revealing cause-and-effect relationships than others. True experimental designs are the best possible designs for illuminating causal relationships, but it is not always possible to use such designs.

Design Terminology

Research design terms can be confusing because there is inconsistency among writers. Also, design terms used by medical researchers are often different from those used by social scientists. Early nurse researchers got research training in social science fields such as psychology before doctoral training became available in nursing schools, and so social scientific terms have prevailed in the nursing literature.

Nurses interested in establishing an evidence-based practice must comprehend studies from many disciplines. We use both medical and social science terms in this book. The first column of Table 9.1 shows design terms used by social scientists and the second shows corresponding terms used by medical researchers.

EXPERIMENTAL DESIGN

A basic distinction in quantitative research design is between experimental and nonexperimental research. In an **experiment** (typically called a **randomized controlled trial, RCT**), researchers are active agents, not simply observers. Early physical scientists learned that although observation is valuable, complexities in nature often made it difficult to disentangle relationships. This problem was addressed by isolating phenomena and controlling the conditions under which they occurred. The 20th century witnessed the acceptance of experimental methods by researchers interested in human physiology and behavior.

TABLE 9.1 • Research Design Terminology in the Social Scientific and Medical Literature

SOCIAL SCIENTIFIC TERM	MEDICAL RESEARCH TERM
Experiment, true experiment, experimental study	Randomized controlled trial, randomized clinical trial, RCT
Quasi-experiment, quasi-experimental study	Controlled clinical trial; clinical trial without randomization
Nonexperimental study; correlational study	Observational study
Retrospective study	Case–control study
Prospective nonexperimental study	Cohort study
Group or condition (e.g., experimental or control group/condition)	Group or arm (e.g., intervention or control arm)
Experimental group	Treatment or intervention group
Dependent variable	Outcome or endpoint

Controlled experiments are considered the *gold standard* for yielding reliable evidence about causes and effects. Experimenters can be relatively confident in the veracity of causal relationships because they are observed under controlled conditions and meet the criteria for causality. Hypotheses are never *proved* by scientific methods, but RCTs offer the most convincing evidence about whether one variable has a casual effect on another.

A true experimental or RCT design is characterized by the following properties:

- *Manipulation:* the researcher *does* something to at least some participants—there is some type of intervention
- *Control:* the researcher introduces controls, including devising a counterfactual approximation—usually, a control group that does not receive the intervention
- *Randomization:* the researcher assigns participants to a control or experimental condition on a random basis

Design Features of True Experiments

Researchers have many options in designing an experiment. We begin by discussing several features of experimental designs.

Manipulation: The Experimental Intervention

Manipulation involves *doing* something to study participants. Experimenters manipulate the independent variable by administering a **treatment** (or **intervention** [I]) to some people and withholding it from others (C), or by administering alternative treatments to two or more groups. Experimenters deliberately *vary* the independent variable (the presumed cause) and observe the effect on the outcome (O)—which is sometimes referred to as an **endpoint** in the medical literature.

For example, suppose we hypothesized that gentle massage is an effective pain relief strategy for nursing home residents (P). The independent variable, receipt of gentle massage, can be manipulated by giving some patients the massage intervention (I) and withholding it from others (C). We would then compare pain levels (O) in the two groups to see if receipt of the intervention resulted in group differences in average pain levels.

In designing RCTs, researchers make many decisions about what the experimental condition entails. To get a fair test, the intervention should be appropriate to the problem, consistent with a theoretical rationale, and of sufficient intensity and duration that effects might reasonably be expected.

The full nature of the intervention must be delineated in formal **intervention protocols** that spell out exactly what the treatment is. Here are some questions intervention researchers need to address:

- What *is* the intervention, and how does it differ from usual methods of care?
- What is the dosage or intensity of the intervention?
- Over how long a period will the intervention be administered, how frequently will it be administered, and when will the treatment begin (e.g., 2 hours after surgery)?
- Who will administer the intervention? What are their credentials? What type of special training will they need?
- Under what conditions will the intervention be withdrawn or altered?

The goal in most RCTs is to have an identical intervention for all people in the treatment group. For example, in most drug studies, those in the experimental group are given the exact same ingredient, in the same dose, and administered in exactly the same manner. There has, however, been a growing interest in precision health, **tailored interventions** or **patient-centered interventions** (PCIs), whose purpose is to enhance personalized health and well-being by taking people's characteristics such as the microbiome, genetics, genomics into account considering (Fu et al., 2019). With tailored interventions, each person receives an intervention customized to certain characteristics, such as genetics (family history), demographic traits (e.g., gender), or cognitive factors (e.g., reading level). Behavioral interventions based on the Transtheoretical (Stages of change) Model (Chapter 6) usually are PCIs because the intervention is tailored to fit people's readiness to change their behavior. While evidence suggests that tailored interventions can be effective, special challenges face those conducting PCI research (Beck et al., 2010).

TIP Although PCIs are not universally standardized, they are administered according to well-defined procedures; intervention agents are trained in making systematic decisions about who should get which type of treatment.

Manipulation: The Control Condition

Evidence about relationships requires a comparison. If we were to supplement the diet of premature infants (P) with a special nutrient (I) for 2 weeks, their weight (O) at the end of 2 weeks would tell us nothing about treatment effectiveness. At a bare minimum, we would need to compare posttreatment weight with pretreatment weight to determine if, at least, their weight had increased. But let us assume that we find an average weight gain of 1 lb. Does this gain support the conclusion that the nutrition supplement (the independent variable) caused weight gain (the outcome)? No, it does not. Babies normally gain weight as they mature. Without a control group—a group that does *not* receive the supplement (C)—it is hard to separate the effects of maturation from those of the treatment.

The term **control group** refers to a group of participants whose performance on an outcome is used to evaluate the performance of the treatment group on the same outcome. Researchers with training in the social sciences use the term "group" or "condition" (e.g., the control group or control condition), but medical researchers often use the term "arm," as in the "intervention arm" or the "control arm" of the study.

The control condition is a proxy for an ideal counterfactual. Researchers have choices about what to use as the counterfactual. Possibilities for the counterfactual include the following:

1. An alternative intervention—for example, participants could receive alternative therapies for pain, such as music vs. massage.
2. Standard methods of care—that is, the usual procedures used to care for patients. This is the most typical control condition in nursing studies.
3. A **placebo** or pseudointervention is presumed to have no therapeutic value—for example, in drug studies, some patients get the experimental drug and others get an innocuous substance. Placebos are used to control for the nonpharmaceutical effects of drugs, such as extra attention. There can, however, be **placebo effects**—changes in the outcome attributable to the placebo condition—because of participants' expectations of benefits or harms.

Example of a Placebo Control Group
Zhang et al. (2022) tested the effect of an intervention bundle to relieve thirst and dry mouth in critically ill patients in China. The intervention bundle included vitamin C sprays, peppermint water mouthwash, and a lip moisturizer, while the control group received a placebo intervention that included saline sprays, water mouth wash, and wetting the lips with water.

4. Sometimes researchers use an **attention control group** when they want to rule out the possibility that intervention effects are caused by the special attention given to those receiving the intervention, rather than by the actual treatment itself. The idea is to separate the "active ingredients" of the treatment from the "inactive ingredient" of special attention.

Example of an Attention Control Group
Doering and Dogan (2018) did a pilot test of an intervention for postpartum sleep and fatigue. Participants were randomized to the theory-guided intervention that focused on self-management or to an attention control group that received general information about healthy eating and sleep.

5. Different doses or intensities of treatment wherein all participants get some type of intervention, but the experimental group gets an intervention that is richer, more intense, or longer. This approach is attractive when there is a desire to analyze **dose–response effects**, that is, to test whether larger doses are associated with larger benefits, or whether a smaller (and less costly or burdensome) dose would suffice.

Example of an Alternative Dose Design
Cai et al. (2022) studied the effects of vitamin D supplementation on frailty in older adults at risk for fall. In a randomized controlled trial, 688 community dwelling adults aged 70 and older were initially randomized to 200 IU/d (control dose; n = 339) or a higher dose (1,000 IU/d, 2,000 IU/d, or 4,000 IU/d; n = 349). Once the 1,000 IU/d was selected as the best higher dose, other higher dose groups were reassigned to the 1,000 IU/d group. New enrollees were randomized to either 1,000 IU/d group or to the control group.

6. **Wait-list control group**, with delayed treatment; the control group eventually receives the full intervention after all outcomes are assessed.

In terms of inferential conclusiveness, the best test is between two conditions that are as different as possible, as when the experimental group gets a strong treatment and the control group gets no treatment. Ethically, the wait-list approach (number 6) is appealing, but may be hard to do pragmatically. Testing two competing interventions (number 1) also has ethical appeal but runs the risk of ambiguous results if both interventions are moderately effective. This option is, however, the preferred approach in **comparative effectiveness research (CER)**, which strives to produce evidence that is especially useful for clinical decision-making. CER is described in Chapters 11 and 31.

Some researchers combine several comparison strategies. For example, they might test two alternative treatments (option 1) against a placebo (option 3). The use of three or more comparison groups is often attractive but adds to the cost and complexity of the study.

Example of a Three-Group Randomized Design
Rodrìguez-Blanco and an interdisciplinary team (2022) compared the effectiveness of two different exercise-based programs through telerehabilitation in patients with coronavirus disease. Subjects were randomized into three groups: breathing exercises group, strength exercises group, and no treatment/control group.

The control group decision should be based on an underlying conceptualization of how the intervention might "cause" the intended effect and should also reflect what needs to be controlled. For example, if attention control groups are being considered, there should be an underlying conceptualization of the construct of "attention" (Gross, 2005).

Researchers need to carefully spell out their control group strategy. In research reports, researchers sometimes say that the control group got "usual care" without explaining what usual care entailed. In drawing on evidence for practice, nurses need to understand exactly what happened to study participants in different conditions. Barkauskas et al. (2005) and Shadish et al. (2002) offer useful advice about developing a control group strategy.

Randomization

Randomization (also called **random assignment** or **random allocation**) involves assigning participants to treatment conditions at random. *Random* means that participants have an equal chance of being assigned to any group. If people are placed in groups randomly, there is no systematic bias in the groups with respect to preintervention attributes that are potential confounders that could affect outcomes.

Randomization Principles. The purpose of random assignment is to approximate the ideal—but impossible—counterfactual of having the same people exposed to two or more conditions simultaneously. For example, suppose we wanted to study the effectiveness of a contraceptive counseling program for multiparous females (P) who wish to avoid another pregnancy (O). Two groups of females are included—one will be counseled (I) and the other will not (C). Females in the sample are likely to be diverse in terms of age, marital status, income, and so on. Any of these characteristics could affect a female's contraceptive use, independent of whether she receives counseling. We need to have the "counsel" and "no counsel" groups equal with respect to confounding traits to assess the impact of counseling on subsequent pregnancies. Random assignment of people to one group or the other is designed to perform this equalization function.

Although randomization is the preferred method for equalizing groups, there is no *guarantee* that the groups will be equal. The risk of unequal groups is high when sample size is small. For example, with a sample of only 10—five males and five females—it is possible that all five males would be assigned to one group and all five females to the other. The likelihood of getting markedly unequal groups is reduced as the sample size increases.

You may wonder why we do not consciously control characteristics that are likely to affect the outcome through **matching**. For example, if matching were used in the contraceptive counseling study, we could ensure that if there were a married, 38-year-old female with three children in the experimental group, there would be a married, 38-year-old female with three children in the control group. To match effectively, however, we must know the characteristics that are likely to affect the outcome, but this knowledge is often imperfect. Even if we knew the relevant traits, the complications of matching on more than two or three confounders simultaneously are prohibitive. With random assignment, *all* personal characteristics—age, income, health status, and so on—are likely to be equally distributed in all groups. Over the long run, randomized groups tend to be counterbalanced with respect to an infinite number of biologic, psychological, economic, and social traits.

Basic Randomization. The most straightforward randomization procedure for a two-group design is to simply allocate each person as they enroll into a study on a random basis—for example, by flipping a coin. If the coin comes up "heads," a participant would be assigned to one group; if it comes up "tails," the participant would be assigned to the other group. This type of randomization, with no restrictions, is sometimes called *complete randomization*. Each successive person has a 50-50 chance of being assigned to the intervention group. The problem with this approach is that large imbalances in group size can occur, especially when the sample size is small. For example, with a sample of 10 subjects, there is only a 25% probability that perfect balance (5 per group) would result. In other words, three times out of four, the intervention and control groups would be of unequal size, by chance alone. This method is not recommended with sample sizes less than 200 (Lachin et al., 1988).

Researchers often want treatment groups of equal size or with predesignated proportions. *Simple randomization* involves starting with a known sample size, and then prespecifying the proportion of subjects who will be randomly allocated to different treatment conditions. To illustrate simple randomization, suppose we were testing two interventions to reduce the anxiety of children who are about to undergo tonsillectomy. One intervention involves giving structured information about the surgical team's activities (procedural information); the other involves structured information about what the child will feel (sensation information). A third control group receives no special intervention. We have a sample of 15 children, and five will be randomly assigned to each group.

Before widespread availability of computers, researchers used a **table of random numbers** to randomize. A small portion of such a table is shown in Table 9.2. In a table of random numbers, any digit from 0 to 9 is equally likely to follow any other digit. Going in any direction from any point in the table produces a random sequence.

In our example, we would number the 15 children from 1 to 15, as shown in column 2 of Table 9.3, and then draw numbers between 01 and 15 from the random number table. To find a random starting point, you can close your eyes and let your finger fall at some point on the table. For this example, assume that our starting point is at number 52, bolded in Table 9.2. We can move in any direction from that point, selecting numbers that fall between 01 and 15. Let us move to the right, looking at two-digit combinations. The number to the right of 52 is 06. The person whose number is 06, Alexander, is assigned to group I. Moving along, the next number within our range is 11. (To find numbers in the desired range, we bypass numbers between 16 and 99.) Violet, whose number is 11, is also assigned to group I. The next three numbers are 01, 15, and 14. Thus, Alaine, Christopher, and Paul are assigned to group I. The next five numbers between 01 and 15 in the table are used to assign five children to group II, and the remaining five are

TABLE 9.2 • Small Table of Random Digits

46	85	05	23	26	34	67	75	83	00	74	91	06	43	45
69	24	89	34	60	45	30	50	75	21	61	31	83	18	55
14	01	33	17	92	59	74	76	72	77	76	50	33	45	13
56	30	38	73	15	16	**52**	06	96	76	11	65	49	98	93
81	30	44	85	85	68	65	22	73	76	92	85	25	58	66
70	28	42	43	26	79	37	59	52	20	01	15	96	32	67
90	41	59	36	14	33	52	12	66	65	55	82	34	76	41
39	90	40	21	15	59	58	94	90	67	66	82	14	15	75
88	15	20	00	80	20	55	49	14	09	96	27	74	82	57
45	13	46	35	45	59	40	47	20	59	43	94	75	16	80
70	01	41	50	21	41	29	06	73	12	71	85	71	59	57
37	23	93	32	95	05	87	00	11	19	92	78	42	63	40
18	63	73	75	09	82	44	49	90	05	04	92	17	37	01
05	32	78	21	62	20	24	78	17	59	45	19	72	53	32
95	09	66	79	46	48	46	08	55	58	15	19	02	87	82
43	25	38	41	45	60	83	32	59	83	01	29	14	13	49
80	85	40	92	79	43	52	90	63	18	38	38	47	47	61
81	08	87	70	74	88	72	25	67	36	66	16	44	94	31
84	89	07	80	02	94	81	03	19	00	54	10	58	34	36

TABLE 9.3 • Example for Random Assignment Procedure

CHILD'S NAME	NUMBER	GROUP ASSIGNMENT
Alaine	01	I
Kristina	02	III
Julia	03	III
Lauren	04	II
Grace	05	II
Alexander	06	I
Norah	07	III
Cormac	08	III
Ronan	09	II
Cullen	10	III
Violet	11	I
Maren	12	II
Leo	13	II
Paul	14	I
Christopher	15	I

put into group III. Note that numbers often reappear in the table before the task is completed. For example, the number 15 appeared four times during this randomization. This is normal because the numbers are random.

We can look at the three groups to see if they are similar for one discernible trait, gender. We started out with eight girls and seven boys. Randomization did a fairly good job of allocating boys and girls similarly across the three groups: there are 2, 3, and 3 girls and 3, 2, and 2 boys in groups I through III, respectively. We must hope that other characteristics (e.g., age, initial anxiety) are also well distributed in the randomized groups. The larger the sample, the stronger the likelihood that the groups will be balanced on all factors that could affect the outcome.

Researchers usually assign participants proportionately to groups being compared. For example, a sample of 300 participants in a two-group design would generally be allocated 150 to the treatment group and 150 to the control group. If there were three groups, there would be 100 per group. It is also possible (and sometimes desirable ethically) to have a different allocation. For example, if an especially promising treatment were developed, we could assign 200 to the treatment group and 100 to the control group. Such an allocation does, however, make it more difficult to detect treatment effects at statistically significant levels—or, to put it another way, the overall sample size must be larger to attain the same level of statistical reliability.

Computerized resources are available for free on the Internet to help with randomization (e.g., www.randomizer.org, which has a useful tutorial). Standard statistical software packages (e.g., SPSS or SAS) can also be used.

TIP There is considerable confusion—even in research methods textbooks—about random assignment vs. random sampling. Randomization is a *signature* of an experimental design. If participants are not randomly allocated to conditions, then the design is not a true experiment. Random *sampling*, by contrast, is a method of selecting people for a study (see Chapter 13). Random sampling is *not* a signature of an experiment. In fact, most RCTs do *not* involve random sampling.

Randomization Procedures. The success of randomization depends on two factors. First, the allocation process should be truly random. Second, there must be strict adherence to the randomization schedule. The latter can be achieved if the allocation is *unpredictable* (for both participants and those enrolling them) and *tamperproof*. Random assignment should involve **allocation concealment** that prevents those who enroll participants from knowing upcoming assignments, to avoid potential biases. As an example, if the person doing the enrollment knew that the next person would be assigned to a promising intervention, they might defer enrollment until a needier patient enrolled.

Several methods of allocation concealment have been devised, several of which involve developing a randomization schedule before the study begins. This is advantageous when people do not enter a study simultaneously, but rather on a *rolling enrollment* basis. One method is to have *sequentially numbered, opaque sealed envelopes* (*SNOSE*) containing assignment information. Participants entering the study receive the next envelope in the sequence (for procedural suggestions, see (Doig & Simpson, 2005). The gold standard approach is to have treatment allocation performed by an agent unconnected with enrollment and communicated to researchers by telephone or e-mail. Herbison et al. (2011) found, however, that trials with a SNOSE system had a comparable risk of bias as trials with centralized randomization.

Timing of randomization is important. Study eligibility—whether a person meets the criteria for inclusion—should be ascertained before randomization. If **baseline data** (preintervention data on outcomes) are collected, this should occur before randomization to rule out any possibility that knowledge of the group assignment might distort baseline measurements. Randomization should occur as closely as possible to the intervention start-up, to increase the likelihood that participants will actually receive the condition to which they have been assigned. Figure 9.1 illustrates the sequence of steps that occurs in most RCTs, including the timing for obtaining informed consent.

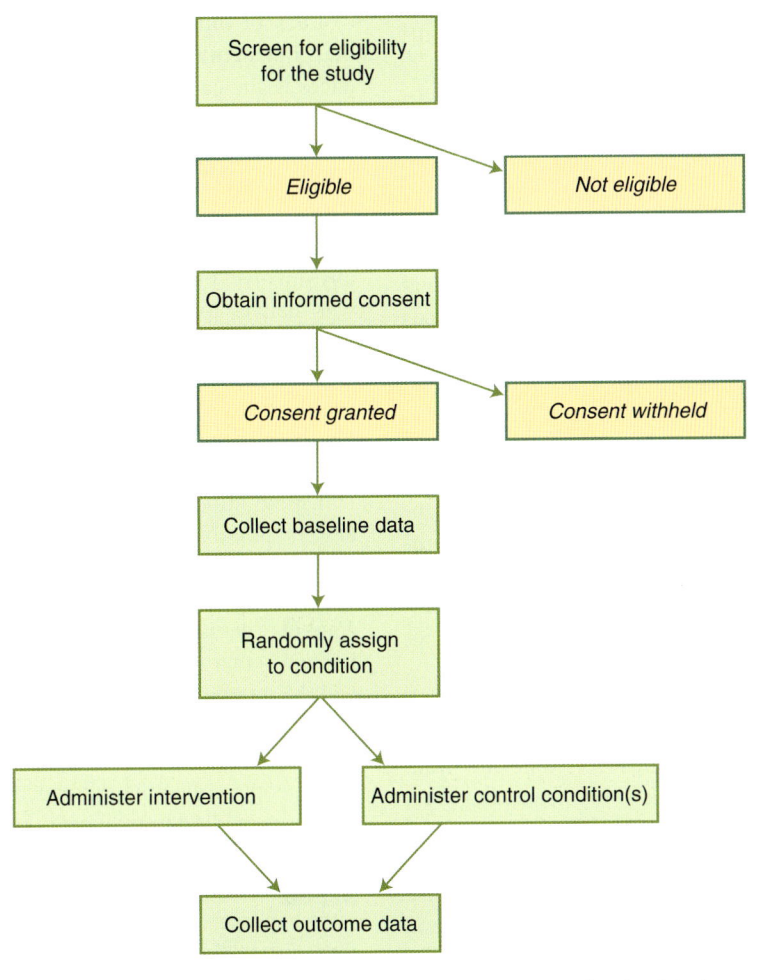

FIGURE 9.1 Sequence of steps in a standard two-arm randomized design.

> **TIP** Some studies use **quasi-randomization**, which is a method of allocating participants in a manner that is not strictly random. For example, participants may be assigned to groups on an alternating basis (every other person to a group) or based on whether their birthdate is an odd or even number. These are not true methods of randomization.

Randomization Variants. Simple or complete randomization is used in many nursing studies, but variants of randomization offer advantages in terms of ensuring group comparability or minimizing certain biases. These variants include the following:

- **Stratified randomization**, in which randomization occurs separately for distinct subgroups (e.g., males and females);
- **Permuted block randomization**, in which people are allocated to groups in small, randomly sized blocks to ensure a balanced distribution in each block;
- **Urn randomization**, in which group balance is continuously monitored and the allocation probability is adjusted when an imbalance occurs (i.e., the probability of assignment becomes higher for the condition with fewer participants);
- **Randomized consent**, in which randomization occurs prior to obtaining informed consent (also called a **Zelen design**);
- **Partial randomization**, in which only people without a strong treatment preference are randomized—sometimes called **partially randomized patient preference (PRPP)**; and
- **Cluster randomization**, which involves randomly assigning clusters (e.g., hospitals) rather than people to different treatment groups.

Blinding or Masking

People usually want things to turn out well. Researchers want their ideas to work, and they want their hypotheses supported. Participants want to be helpful and want to present themselves in a positive light. These tendencies can lead to biases because they can affect what participants do and say (and what researchers ask and perceive) in ways that distort the truth.

A procedure called **blinding** (or **masking**) is often used in RCTs to prevent biases stemming from *awareness*. Blinding involves concealing information from participants, data collectors, care providers, intervention agents, or data analysts to enhance objectivity and minimize **expectation bias**. For example, if participants are not aware of whether they are getting an experimental drug or a placebo, then their outcomes cannot be influenced by their expectations of its efficacy. Blinding typically involves disguising or withholding information about participants' status in the study (e.g., whether they are in the experimental or control group) but can also involve withholding information about study hypotheses or baseline performance on outcomes.

Lack of blinding can result in several types of bias. **Performance bias** refers to systematic differences in the care provided to members of different groups of participants, apart from any intervention. For example, those delivering an intervention might treat participants in groups differently (e.g., with greater attentiveness), apart from the intervention itself. Efforts to avoid performance bias usually involve blinding participants and the agents who deliver treatments. **Detection** (or **ascertainment**) bias, which concerns systematic differences between groups in how outcome variables are measured, verified, or recorded, is addressed by blinding those who collect the outcome data or, in some cases, those who analyze the data.

Unlike allocation concealment, blinding is not always possible. Drug studies often lend themselves to blinding but many nursing interventions do not. For example, if the intervention were a smoking cessation program, participants would know whether they were receiving the intervention, and the interventionist would be aware of who was in the program. However, it is usually possible, and desirable, to mask participants' treatment status from people collecting outcome data and from clinicians providing normal care.

> **TIP** Blinding may not be necessary if subjectivity in measuring the outcome is low. For example, participants' ratings of pain are susceptible to biases stemming from their own or data collectors'

awareness of treatment group status. Hospital readmission and length of hospital stay, on the other hand, are less likely to be affected by people's awareness.

When blinding is not used, the study is an *open study*, in contrast to a *closed study*. When blinding is used with only one group of people (e.g., study participants), it is sometimes called a **single-blind study**. When it is possible to mask with two groups (e.g., those delivering an intervention and those receiving it), it is sometimes called **double blind**. However, recent guidelines recommend that researchers not use these terms without explicitly stating which groups were blinded because the term "double blind" has been used to refer to many different combinations of blinded groups (Moher et al., 2010).

The term *blinding*, though widely used, has been criticized because of possible pejorative connotations. The American Psychological Association, for example, has recommended using masking instead. Medical researchers appear to prefer *blinding* unless the people in the study have vision impairments (Schulz et al., 2002). Most nurse researchers use the term *blinding* rather than *masking* (Polit et al., 2011).

Example of an Experiment With Blinding
Kim and Park (2023) conducted a single, blind, randomized, placebo-controlled trial to study the effects of auricular acupressure on blood pressure, stress, and sleep in older adults with essential hypertension. Participants were blinded to whether they were in the experimental or control group. The experimental group (*n* = 23) received 8 weeks of auricular acupressure intervention on specific acupoints related to blood pressure, pulse rate, stress, and sleep, whereas the control group (*n* = 23) received auricular acupressure on nonspecific acupoints.

Specific Experimental Designs

Some popular experimental designs are described in this section. We illustrate some of them using design notation from a classic monograph (Campbell & Stanley, 1963). In this system, R means random assignment; O represents outcome measurements; and X stands for exposure to the intervention. Each row designates a different group.

Basic Experimental Designs

Earlier in this chapter, we described a study that tested the effect of gentle massage on pain in nursing home residents. This example illustrates a simple design that is sometimes called a **posttest-only design** (or *after-only design*) because data on the outcome are collected only once—after randomization and completion of the intervention. Here is the notation for this design, which shows that both groups are randomized (R), but only the first group gets the intervention (X):

| R | X | O |
| R | | O |

A second basic design involves collecting baseline data, like the design in Figure 9.1. Suppose we hypothesized that convective airflow blankets are more effective than conductive water-flow blankets in cooling critically ill febrile patients. Our design involves assigning patients to the two blanket types (the independent variable) and measuring the outcome (body temperature) twice, before and after the intervention. Here is a diagram for this design:

| R | O_1 | X | O_2 |
| R | O_1 | | O_2 |

This design allows us to examine whether one blanket type is more effective than the other in *reducing* fever; with this design researchers can examine *change*. This design is a **pretest–posttest design** (*before–after design*), which are mixed designs: analyses can examine both differences *between* groups and changes *within* groups over time. Some pretest–posttest designs include data collection at multiple postintervention points (i.e., *repeated measures designs*). These basic designs can be "tweaked" in various ways—for example, the design could involve comparison of three or more groups.

> **Example of a Pretest–Posttest Experimental Design**
> Tanriverdi and Kilic (2022) examined the effect of progressive muscle relaxation on abdominal pain and distension in colonoscopy patients using a pretest–posttest experimental design. After the colonoscopy, pretests included assessing abdominal pain (Visual Analogue Scale (VAS) pain) and distension (VAS distension). Next, progressive muscle relaxation was applied for 30 minutes to the experimental group but not the control group. Posttests for pain and distension were repeated after the intervention was completed.

Factorial Design

Most experimental designs involve manipulating only one independent variable, but it is possible to manipulate two or more variables simultaneously. Suppose we wanted to compare two therapies for premature infants: tactile vs. auditory stimulation. We also want to learn if the daily *amount* of stimulation (15, 30, or 45 minutes) affects infants' progress. The outcomes are measures of infant development (e.g., weight gain). Figure 9.2 illustrates the structure of this RCT.

This **factorial design** allows us to address three research questions:

1. Does auditory stimulation have a more beneficial effect on premature infants' weight gain than tactile stimulation, or vice versa?
2. Is amount of stimulation (independent of type) related to infants' weight gain?
3. Is auditory stimulation most effective when linked to a certain dose and tactile stimulation most effective when coupled with a different dose?

The third question shows the strength of factorial designs: they permit us to test not only **main effects** (effects from the manipulated variables, as in questions 1 and 2) but also **interaction effects** (effects from combining treatments). Our results may indicate that 30 minutes of auditory stimulation is the most beneficial treatment. We could not have learned this by conducting two separate studies that manipulated one independent variable and held the second one constant.

In factorial experiments, participants are randomly assigned to a specific combination of conditions. In our example (Figure 9.2), infants would be assigned randomly to one of six **cells** (i.e., six treatment conditions). The two independent variables in a factorial design are the **factors**. Type of stimulation is factor A, and amount of daily exposure is factor B. Level 1 of factor A is auditory and level 2 is tactile. When describing the dimensions of the design, researchers refer to the number of **levels**. The design in Figure 9.2 is a 2 × 3 design: two levels in factor A times three levels in factor B. Factorial experiments with more than two factors are rare.

> **Example of a Factorial Design**
> Mojtehedi et al. (2022) conducted a randomized controlled trial with a factorial design to study the effect of two factors, aromatherapy with essential oil of lavender-bergamot and mindfulness, on sexual function, anxiety, and depression in 132 postmenopausal females with sexual dysfunction.

Crossover Design

Thus far, we have described RCTs in which different people are randomly assigned to different conditions. For instance, in the previous example, infants who received auditory stimulation were not the same infants as those who received tactile stimulation. A **crossover design** involves exposing the same people to more than one condition. This within-subjects design has the advantage of ensuring the highest possible equivalence among participants exposed to different conditions—the groups being compared are equal with respect to age, weight, and so on because they are composed of the same people.

Type of stimulation

		Auditory A1	Tactile A2
Daily dose	15 min. B1	A1 B1	A2 B1
	30 min. B2	A1 B2	A2 B2
	45 min. B3	A1 B3	A2 B3

FIGURE 9.2 Example of a 2 × 3 factorial design.

Because randomization is a signature of an experiment, participants in a crossover design must be randomly assigned to different *orderings* of treatments. For example, if a crossover design were used to compare the effects of auditory and tactile stimulation on infant development, some infants would be randomly assigned to receive auditory stimulation first, and others would be assigned to receive tactile stimulation first. When there are three or more conditions to which participants will be exposed, the procedure of **counterbalancing** can be used to rule out ordering effects. For example, if there were three conditions (A, B, C), participants would be randomly assigned to one of six counterbalanced orderings:

A, B, C	A, C, B
B, C, A	B, A, C
C, A, B	C, B, A

Although crossover designs are powerful, they are inappropriate for certain research questions because of possible **carry-over effects**. When people are exposed to two different conditions, they may be influenced in the second condition by their experience in the first one. Drug studies, for example, rarely use a crossover design because drug B administered *after* drug A is not necessarily the same treatment as drug B administered *before* drug A. When carry-over effects are a potential concern, researchers often have a **washout period** in between the treatments (i.e., a period of no treatment exposure).

Example of a Crossover Design
Fernández-Gutiérrez et al. (2022) used a randomized three period crossover design to test the effect of a multimodal simulation intervention to improve empathy and attitudes toward older adults in 70 nursing students in Spain.

TIP New experimental designs are emerging in response to growing interest in personalized health care. Several of these designs, such as **N-of-1 trials** and **adaptive trials**, are discussed in Chapter 31, which focuses on the applicability and relevance of research evidence.

Strengths and Limitations of Experiments

In this section, we explore why experimental designs are held in high esteem and examine some limitations.

Experimental Strengths

Experimental designs are the gold standard for testing interventions because they yield strong evidence about intervention effectiveness. Experiments offer greater corroboration than other approaches that, *if* the independent variable (e.g., diet, drug, teaching approach) is varied, *then* certain consequences to the outcomes (e.g., weight loss, recovery, learning) will ensue. The great strength of RCTs, then, lies in the confidence with which causal relationships can be inferred. Through the controls imposed by manipulation, comparison, and randomization, alternative explanations can be discredited. It is because of this strength that meta-analyses of RCTs, which integrate evidence from multiple experiments, are at the pinnacle of evidence hierarchies for Therapy questions (Figure 2.2 of Chapter 2).

Experimental Limitations

Despite the benefits of experiments, they also have limitations. First, constraints—which we discuss later in this chapter—often make an experimental approach impractical or impossible.

Experiments are sometimes criticized for their artificiality, which partly stems from the requirements for comparable treatment within randomized groups, with strict adherence to protocols. In ordinary life, by contrast, we interact with people in nonformulaic ways. A related concern is that the rigidity of the research process can undermine translation into real-world settings, an issue we address in Chapter 31.

Problems also emerge when participants "opt out" of the intervention. Suppose, for example, that we randomly assigned patients with HIV to a support group intervention or to a control group. Intervention subjects who elect not to participate in the support groups, or who participate infrequently, are in a "condition" that looks more like the control condition than the experimental one. The treatment is diluted through nonparticipation, and it may be difficult to detect treatment effects, no matter how effective it might otherwise have been.

Another potential problem is the **Hawthorne effect**, which is caused by people's expectations. The term is derived from a series of experiments conducted at the Hawthorne plant of the Western Electric Corporation in which various environmental conditions, such as light and working hours, were varied to test their effects on worker productivity. Regardless of what change was introduced, that is, whether the light was made better or worse, productivity increased. Knowledge of being in the study (not just knowledge of being in a particular group) appears to have affected people's behavior, obscuring the effect of the intervention.

In sum, despite the superiority of RCTs for testing causal hypotheses, they have several limitations, some of which may make them difficult to apply to real clinical problems. Nevertheless, with the growing demand for strong evidence for practice, experimental designs are increasingly being used to test the effects of nursing interventions.

QUASI-EXPERIMENTS

Quasi-experiments, sometimes called *controlled trials without randomization* in the medical literature, involve an intervention, but they lack randomization, the signature of a true experiment. Some quasi-experiments even lack a control group. The signature of a quasi-experimental design, then, is an intervention in the absence of randomization.

Quasi-Experimental Designs

We describe a few widely used quasi-experimental designs in this section, and for some we use the schematic notation introduced earlier.

Nonequivalent Control Group Designs

The **nonequivalent control group pretest–posttest design** (sometimes called a *controlled before–after design* in the medical literature) involves two groups of participants, for whom outcomes are measured before and after the intervention. For example, suppose we wished to study the effect of a new chair yoga intervention for older people. The intervention is being offered to everyone at a community senior center, and randomization is not workable. For comparative purposes, we collect outcome data at a different senior center that is not instituting the intervention. Data on health-related quality of life are collected from both groups at baseline and again 10 weeks after implementing the intervention. Here is a schematic representation of this design:

O_1	X	O_2
O_1		O_2

The top line represents those receiving the intervention (X) at the experimental site and the second row represents the group at the comparison site. This diagram is identical to the experimental pretest–posttest design depicted earlier *except* there is no "R"—participants have not been randomized to groups. The quasi-experimental design is weaker because *it cannot be assumed that the experimental and comparison groups are initially equivalent*. Because there is no randomization, quasi-experimental comparisons provide a weaker counterfactual than experimental comparisons. The design is nevertheless strong because baseline data allow us to assess whether patients in the two centers had similar quality-of-life scores at the outset. If the two groups are similar, on average, at baseline, we could be relatively confident inferring that posttest differences in outcomes were the result of the yoga intervention. If quality-of-life scores are different initially, however, it will be difficult to interpret posttest differences. Note that in quasi-experiments, the term **comparison group** is used in lieu of *control group* to refer to the group with whom the treatment group is compared.

Now suppose we had been unable to collect baseline data:

X	O
	O

This design has a major flaw. We no longer have information about initial equivalence of people in the two senior centers. If quality of life in the experimental center is higher than that in the control site at posttest, can we conclude that the intervention *caused* improved quality of life? An alternative explanation for posttest differences is that the people in the two centers differed at the outset. This *nonequivalent control group posttest-only design* is a much weaker quasi-experimental design.

> **Example of a Nonequivalent Control Group Pretest–Posttest Design**
> Kim and Kim (2022) used a quasi-experimental design to test the effects of a nonviolent communication-based anger management program on self-esteem, anger, and aggression on psychiatric inpatients in Korea. The sample of 44 psychiatric inpatients consisted of 21 participants in the experimental group and 24 participants in the control group.

In lieu of using a contemporaneous comparison group, researchers sometimes use a **historical comparison group**. That is, comparison data are gathered from other people *before* implementing the intervention. Even when the people are from the same institutional setting, however, it is risky to assume that the two groups are comparable, or that the environments are comparable except for the new intervention. The possibility remains that something other than the intervention could account for observed differences in outcomes.

> **Example of a Historical Comparison Group**
> Zhong et al. (2022) conducted a historical comparative study in China to analyze the application value of multidisciplinary diagnosis and treatment nursing mode based on doctor–nurse integration for stroke patients undergoing emergency intervention surgery.

Time Series Designs

In the designs just described, a control group was used but randomization was not, but some quasi-experiments have neither. Suppose that a hospital implemented rapid response teams (RRTs) in its acute care units. Administrators want to examine the effects on patient outcomes (e.g., unplanned ICU admissions, mortality rate). For the purposes of this example, assume no other hospital could serve as a good comparison. One comparison that can be made is a before–after contrast. If RRTs were to be implemented in January, the mortality rate (for example) during the 3 months before RRTs could be compared with the mortality rate during the subsequent 3-month period. The schematic representation of such a study is:

O_1	X	O_2

This one-group pretest–posttest design seems straightforward, but it has several weaknesses. What if either of the 3-month periods is atypical, apart from the innovation? What about the effects of other policy changes inaugurated during the same period? What about the effects of external factors that influence mortality, such as a flu outbreak? This design cannot control these factors.

In our RRT example, the design could be modified so that some alternative explanations for changes in mortality could be ruled out. One such design is the **time series design** (or *interrupted time series design*). In a time series, data are collected over an extended period during which an intervention is introduced, as in this diagram:

O_1	O_2	O_3	O_4	X	O_5	O_6	O_7	O_8

Here, O_1 through O_4 represent four separate instances of preintervention outcome measurement, X is the introduction of the intervention, and O_5 through O_8 represent four posttreatment measurements. In our example, O_1 might be the number of deaths in January through March in the year before the new RRT system, O_2 the number of deaths in April through June, and so forth. After RRTs are introduced, data on mortality are collected for four consecutive 3-month periods, giving us observations O_5 through O_8.

Even though the time series design does not eliminate all interpretive challenges, the extended time period strengthens our ability to attribute change to the intervention. Figure 9.3 demonstrates why this is so. The line graphs (*A* and *B*) in the figure show two possible outcome patterns for eight mortality observations. The vertical dotted line in the center represents the introduction of the RRT system. Patterns *A* and *B* both reflect a feature common to time series studies—fluctuation from one data point to another. These fluctuations are normal. One would not expect that, if 480 patients died in a hospital in 1 year, the deaths would be spaced

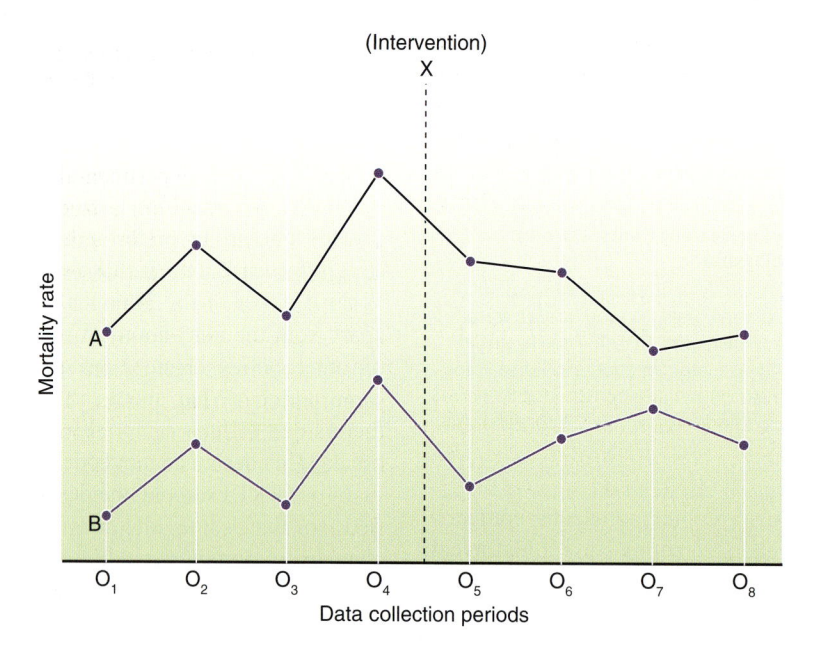

FIGURE 9.3 Two possible time series outcome patterns for quarterly mortality data.

evenly with 40 per month. It is precisely because of these fluctuations that the one-group pretest–posttest design, with only one observation before and after the intervention, is so weak.

Let us compare the interpretations for the outcomes shown in Figure 9.3. In both patterns *A* and *B*, mortality decreased between O_4 and O_5, immediately after RRTs were implemented. In *B*, however, the number of deaths rose at O_6 and continued to rise at O_7. The decrease at O_5 looks similar to other apparently haphazard fluctuations in mortality. In *A*, on the other hand, the number of deaths decreased at O_5 and remained relatively low for subsequent observations. There may well be other explanations for a change in the mortality rate, but the time series design permits us to rule out the possibility that the data reflect unstable measurements of deaths at only two points in time. If we had used a simple pretest–posttest design, it would have been analogous to obtaining the measurements at O_4 and O_5 of Figure 9.3 only. The outcomes in both *A* and *B* are the same at these two time points. The broader time perspective leads us to draw different conclusions about the effects of RRTs. Nevertheless, the absence of a comparison group means that the design does not yield an ideal counterfactual.

Example of a Time Series Design
Warjri et al. (2022) conducted a quasi-experimental time series pretest–posttest group design. These researchers studied the impact of a white noise app on sleep quality among critically ill patients in India. Sleep quality was measured daily for 3 days while the patients were in the intensive care unit.

One drawback of a time series design is that many data points—100 or more—are recommended for a traditional analysis (Shadish et al., 2002), and the analysis tends to be complex. Nurse researchers have, however, begun to use a versatile approach called **statistical process control (SPC)** to assess effects when they have collected data sequentially over a period of time before and after implementing a practice change (Polit & Chaboyer, 2012). Time series designs with SPC analyses are important in *quality improvement (QI)* projects because randomization is rarely possible in QI (see Chapter 12).

A particularly powerful quasi-experimental design results when the time series and nonequivalent control group designs are combined. In the example just described, a time series nonequivalent control group design would involve collecting data over an extended period from both the hospital introducing the RRTs and another similar hospital not implementing the system. Information from another comparable hospital would make any inferences regarding the effects of RRTs more convincing because other external factors influencing the trends (e.g., a flu outbreak) would likely be similar in both cases.

Numerous variations on the simple time series design are possible. For example, additional evidence regarding the effects of a treatment can be achieved by instituting the treatment at several different points in time, strengthening the treatment over time, or instituting the treatment at one point in time and then withdrawing it at a later point, sometimes with reinstitution.

Other Quasi-Experimental Designs

Earlier in this chapter, we mentioned the PRPP design. Those without a strong treatment preference are randomized, but those *with* a preference are given the condition they prefer and are followed up as part of the study. The two randomized groups are part of the true experiment, but the two groups who get their preference are part of a quasi-experiment. This type of design can yield valuable information about the kind of people who prefer one condition over another and may help persuade people to participate in a study. However, evidence of treatment effectiveness is weak in the quasi-experimental segment because the people who elected a certain treatment likely differ from those who opted for the alternative—and these preintervention differences, rather than the alternative treatments, could account for observed differences in outcomes. Yet, evidence from the quasi-experiment could usefully support or qualify evidence from the experimental portion of the study.

Example of a PRPP Design
Parsons et al. (2022) assessed the feasibility of a prenatal and postnatal lifestyle intervention for females with gestational diabetes to decrease type 2 diabetes risk. Participants were initially randomized to either the intervention group or control group. Females who declined randomization were allowed to choose a preference for either condition.

Another quasi-experimental approach—sometimes embedded within a true experiment—is a **dose–response** design in which the outcomes of those receiving different doses of an intervention (not as a result of randomization) are compared. For example, in lengthy interventions, some people attend more sessions or get more intensive treatment than others. The rationale for a quasi-experimental dose–response analysis is that if a larger dose corresponds to better outcomes, the results provide supporting evidence that the treatment caused the outcome. The difficulty, however, is that people tend to get different treatment doses because of differences in motivation, physical function, or other characteristics that could be the true cause of outcome differences. Nevertheless, dose–response evidence may yield useful information.

Example of a Dose–Response Analysis
One of the aims in a study by Sanders et al. (2020) was to determine the dose–response effects of low- and high-intensity combined aerobic and strength exercise on physical and cognitive functions.

Quasi-Experimental and Comparison Conditions

Researchers using a quasi-experimental approach should develop intervention protocols that document what the interventions entail. Researchers need to be especially careful in understanding and documenting the counterfactual. In the case of nonequivalent control group designs, this means understanding the conditions to which the comparison group is exposed (e.g., activities at the senior center without the yoga intervention in our example). In time series designs, the counterfactual is the conditions existing before implementing the intervention, and these should be understood. Blinding should be used, to the extent possible—indeed, this may be more feasible in a quasi-experiment than in an RCT.

Strengths and Limitations of Quasi-Experiments

A major strength of quasi-experiments is that they are practical. In clinical settings, it may be impossible to conduct true experimental tests of nursing interventions. Strong quasi-experimental designs introduce some research control when full experimental rigor is not possible.

Another advantage of quasi-experiments is that patients are not always willing to relinquish control over their treatment condition. Indeed, people are increasingly unwilling to volunteer to be randomized in clinical trials (Vedelø & Lomborg, 2011). Quasi-experimental designs, because they do not involve random assignment, are likely to be acceptable to a broader group of people. This, in turn, has positive implications for the generalizability of the results—but the problem is that the evidence may be less conclusive.

Researchers using quasi-experimental designs should realize their weaknesses and take them into account in interpreting results. When a quasi-experimental design is used, there usually are **rival hypotheses** competing with the intervention as explanations for the results. (This issue relates to *internal validity*, discussed in Chapter 10.) Take as an example the case in which we administer a special diet to frail nursing home residents to assess its effects on weight gain. If we use no comparison group or a nonequivalent control group and then observe a weight gain, we must ask: Is it *plausible* that some other factor caused the gain? Is it *plausible* that pretreatment differences between the intervention and comparison groups resulted in differential gain? Is it *plausible* that the older adults on average gained weight because the frailest patients died? If the answer is "yes" to such questions, then inferences about the causal effect of the intervention are weakened. The plausibility of any particular rival explanation typically cannot be known unequivocally, but nevertheless a careful *plausibility analysis* should be undertaken.

TIP The *Journal of Clinical Epidemiology* has published an excellent 13-paper series on quasi-experimental designs. Examples include papers by Geldsetzer and Fawzi (2017) and Bärnighausen et al. (2017).

NONEXPERIMENTAL/OBSERVATIONAL RESEARCH

Many research questions—including ones seeking to establish causal relationships—cannot be addressed with an experimental or quasi-experimental design. For example, at the beginning of this chapter we posed this Prognosis question: Do birthweights less than 1,500 g *cause* developmental delays in children? Clearly, we cannot manipulate birthweight, the independent variable. One way to answer this question is to compare developmental outcomes for two groups of infants—babies with birthweights above and below 1,500 g. When researchers do not intervene by manipulating the independent variable, the study is **nonexperimental**, or, in the medical literature, **observational**.

Most nursing studies are nonexperimental because most human characteristics (e.g., weight, lactose intolerance) cannot be manipulated. Also, many variables that could *technically* be manipulated cannot be manipulated ethically. For example, if we were studying the effect of prenatal care on infant mortality, it would be unethical to provide such care to one group of pregnant females while deliberately depriving females in a randomized control group. We would need to locate naturally occurring groups of pregnant females who had or had not received prenatal care, and then compare their birth outcomes. The problem, however, is that the two groups of females are likely to differ in terms of other characteristics, such as age, education, and income, any of which individually or in combination could affect infant mortality, independent of prenatal care. Nevertheless, many nonexperimental studies explore cause-and-effect relationships when an experimental design is not possible.

Correlational Cause-Probing Research

When researchers study the effect of a potential *cause* that they cannot manipulate, they use **correlational designs** to examine relationships between variables. A **correlation** is a relationship or association between two variables, that is, a tendency for variation in one variable to be related to variation in another. For example, in human adults, height and weight are correlated because there is a tendency for taller people to weigh more than shorter people.

As mentioned earlier, one criterion for causality is that an empirical relationship (correlation) between variables must be demonstrated. It is risky, however, to infer causal relationships in correlational research. A famous research dictum is relevant: *correlation does not prove causation*. The mere existence of a relationship between variables is not enough to conclude that one variable caused the other, even if the relationship is strong. In experiments, researchers directly control the independent variable; the experimental treatment can be administered to some and withheld from others, and the two groups can be equalized through randomization with respect to everything except the independent variable. In correlational research, investigators do not control the independent variable, which often has already occurred. Groups being compared often differ in ways that affect outcomes of interest—that is, there are usually confounding variables. Although correlational studies are inherently weaker than experimental studies in confirming causal relationships, different designs offer differing degrees of supportive evidence.

Retrospective Designs

Studies with a **retrospective design** are ones in which a phenomenon existing in the present is linked to phenomena that occurred in the past. The signature of a retrospective study is that the researcher begins with the dependent variable (the effect) and then examines whether it is correlated with one or more previously occurring independent variables (potential causes).

Most early studies of the smoking–lung cancer link used a retrospective **case–control design**, in which researchers began with a group of people who had lung cancer (*cases*) and another group who did not (*controls*). The researchers then looked for differences between the two groups in antecedent circumstances or behaviors, such as smoking.

In designing a case–control study, researchers try to identify controls without the disease or condition who are as similar as possible to the cases on key confounding variables (e.g., age, gender). Researchers sometimes use matching or other techniques to control for confounding variables. To the degree that researchers can demonstrate comparability between cases and controls regarding confounding traits, inferences regarding the presumed cause of the disease are enhanced. The difficulty, however, is that the two groups are almost never totally comparable on factors influencing the outcome. Grimes and Schulz (2005) offer guidance on identifying controls for case–control studies.

Example of a Case–Control Design
Tom et al. (2022) conducted a matched case–control study of adults aged ≥18 years to determine the association between probiotic use and invasive infections caused by probiotic organisms. The sample consisted of a total of 112 cases (28 who used probiotics and 84 controls) who were admitted to Oregon Health & Science University. The researchers conducted a regression analysis. Findings indicated that those who used probiotics had a 127 times greater chance of invasive infections than the control group patients.

Not all retrospective studies can be described as using a case–control design. Sometimes researchers use a retrospective approach to identify risk factors for different *amounts* of an outcome rather than "caseness." For example, a retrospective design might be used to identify factors predictive of the length of time new mothers breastfed their infants. Such a design often is intended to understand factors that *cause* females to make different breastfeeding decisions (i.e., an Etiology question).

Many retrospective studies are cross-sectional, with data on both the dependent and independent variables collected at a single point in time. In such studies, data for the independent variables often are based on recollection (retrospection)—or the researchers "assume" that the independent variables occurred before the outcome. One problem, however, is that recollection can be biased by subsequent events or memory lapses.

Example of a Retrospective Design
Flanagan, one of the authors of this textbook, and colleagues (2020) used a retrospective design to analyze publicly available data to determine the association between various hospital-related factors and rates of sepsis after surgery in Massachusetts hospitals. They explored the relationship between independent variables of nurse and physician staffing levels and the dependent variable of sepsis rates.

Prospective Nonexperimental Designs

In correlational studies with a **prospective design** (called a **cohort design** in medical circles), researchers start with a presumed cause and then go forward in time to the presumed effect. For example, in prospective lung cancer studies, researchers start with a cohort of adults (P) that includes smokers (I) and nonsmokers (C), and then compare the two groups in terms of subsequent lung cancer incidence (O). The best design for Prognosis questions, and for Etiology questions when randomization is impossible, is a cohort design. A particularly strong design for Prognosis questions is an **inception cohort design**, which involves the study of a group assembled at a common time early in a health disorder or exposure to a putative "cause" of an outcome (e.g., immediately after a traumatic brain injury), and then followed thereafter to assess the outcomes.

Prospective studies are more costly than retrospective studies, in part because prospective studies require at least two rounds of data collection. A lengthy follow-up period may be needed before the outcome of interest occurs, as is the case in prospective studies of cigarette smoking and lung cancer. Also, prospective designs require large samples if the outcome of interest is rare. Another issue is that in a good prospective study, researchers take steps to confirm that all participants are free from the effect (e.g., the disease) at the time the independent variable is measured, and this may be difficult or expensive to do. For example, in prospective smoking/lung cancer studies, lung cancer may be present initially but not yet diagnosed.

Despite these issues, prospective studies are considerably stronger than retrospective studies. Any ambiguity about whether the presumed cause occurred before the effect is resolved in prospective research if the researcher has confirmed the initial absence of the effect. In addition, samples are more likely to be representative, and investigators may be able to impose controls to rule out competing explanations for the results.

TIP The term "prospective" is not synonymous with "longitudinal." Although most nonexperimental prospective studies *are* longitudinal, prospective studies are not *necessarily* longitudinal. Prospective means that information about a possible cause is obtained prior to information about an effect. RCTs are inherently prospective because researchers introduce the intervention and then determine its effect. An RCT that collected outcome data 1 hour after an intervention would be prospective, but not longitudinal.

Some prospective studies are exploratory. Researchers sometimes measure a wide range of possible "causes" at one point in time (e.g., foods consumed), and then examine an outcome of interest at a later point (e.g., a cancer diagnosis). Such studies are usually more convincing than retrospective studies if it can be determined that the outcome was not present initially because time sequences are clear. They are not, however, as powerful as prospective studies that involve specific *a priori* hypotheses and the comparison of cohorts known to differ on a presumed cause. Researchers doing exploratory retrospective or prospective studies are sometimes accused of going on "fishing expeditions" that can lead to erroneous conclusions because of spurious or idiosyncratic relationships in a particular sample of participants.

Example of a Prospective Nonexperimental Study
Senecal and Jurgens (2022) sought to (1) describe heart-failure symptom burden at hospital discharge and (2) examine the relationship of that symptom burden at discharge to 30-day clinical events. They found that heart-failure symptoms such as fatigue, a need to rest, nocturia, and shortness of breath at discharge predicted 30-day clinical events such as emergency department visits, hospital admission, and death.

Natural Experiments

Researchers are sometimes able to study the outcomes of a **natural experiment** in which a group exposed to a phenomenon with potential health consequences is compared with a nonexposed group. Natural experiments are nonexperimental because the researcher does not intervene, but they are called "natural *experiments*" if people are affected essentially at random. For example, the psychological well-being of people living in a community struck with a natural disaster (e.g., a volcanic eruption) could be compared with the well-being of people living in a similar but unaffected community to assess the toll exacted by the disaster (the independent variable).

Example of a Natural Experiment
Baird et al. (2022) aimed to understand the causal impact of the adoption and discontinuation of telehealth on hospital performance over 2 years compared to hospitals in the control group who had similar characteristics but made no changes to telehealth adoption/discontinuation. Outcomes such as emergency department visits, total ambulatory visits, outpatient services revenue, total facility expenses, and total hospital revenue were studied in this natural experiment.

Path Analytic Studies

Researchers interested in testing theories of causation using nonexperimental data often use a technique called **path analysis** (or similar *causal modeling* techniques). Using sophisticated statistical procedures, researchers test a hypothesized causal chain among a set of independent variables, mediating variables, and a dependent variable. Path analytic procedures allow researchers to test whether nonexperimental data conform sufficiently to the underlying model to justify causal inferences. Path analytic studies can be done within the context of both cross-sectional and longitudinal designs, the latter providing a stronger basis for causal inferences because of the ability to verify time sequences.

Example of a Path Analytic Study
Li et al. (2022) conducted a path analysis to determine if the relationship between job strain and organizational commitment could be moderated by social support. The data were obtained from a convenience sample of 509 operating room nurses from across 30 hospitals in Beijing, China. The findings support that social support moderated job strain and organizational commitment among the operating room nurses in this study.

Descriptive Research

Descriptive research is a second broad class of nonexperimental research. The purpose of descriptive studies is to observe, describe, and document a situation as it naturally occurs. Sometimes descriptive studies are a starting point for hypothesis generation or theory development.

Descriptive Correlational Studies

Some research problems are cast in noncausal terms. We may ask, for example, whether males are less likely than females to seek assistance for depression, not whether configurations of sex chromosomes *caused* differences in health behavior. Unlike other types of correlational research—such as the cigarette smoking and lung cancer investigations—the aim of **descriptive correlational research** is to describe relationships among variables rather than to support inferences of causality.

Example of a Descriptive Correlational Study
Wan et al. (2021) conducted a descriptive correlational study to examine the relationship between financial toxicity (out-of-pocket treatment expenses) and patient preference for shared decision-making in females with metastatic breast cancer who received care at two academic hospitals in the state of Alabama, United States.

Studies designed to address Diagnosis/assessment questions—that is, whether a tool or procedure yields accurate assessment or diagnostic information about a condition or outcome—often involve descriptive correlational designs—although sometimes two procedures or tools are tested against each other for accuracy in RCTs.

Univariate Descriptive Studies

The aim of some descriptive studies is to describe the frequency of occurrence of a behavior or condition, rather than to study relationships. **Univariate descriptive studies** are not necessarily focused on a single variable. For example, a researcher interested in female's experiences during menopause might gather data about the frequency of various symptoms and the use of medications to alleviate symptoms. The study involves multiple variables, but the primary purpose is to describe the status of each, not to study correlations among them.

Two types of descriptive study come from the field of epidemiology. **Prevalence studies** are done to estimate the prevalence rate of some condition (e.g., a disease or a behavior, such as smoking) at a particular point in time. Prevalence studies rely on cross-sectional designs in which data are obtained from the population at risk of the condition. The researcher takes a "snapshot" of the population at risk to determine the extent to which the condition is present. The formula for a **prevalence rate** (PR) follows:

$$\frac{\text{Number of cases with the condition or disease at a given point in time}}{\text{Number in the population at risk of being a case}} \times K$$

K is the number of people for whom we want to have the rate established (e.g., per 100 or per 1,000 population). When data are obtained from a sample, the denominator is the size of the sample, and the numerator is the number of cases identified with the condition. If we sampled 500 adults living in a community, administered a measure of depression, and found that 80 people met the criteria for clinical depression, then the estimated prevalence rate of clinical depression would be 16 per 100 adults in that community.

Incidence studies estimate the frequency of *new* cases. Longitudinal designs are needed to estimate incidence because the researcher must first establish who is at risk of becoming a new case—that is, who is free of the condition at the outset. The formula for an **incidence rate** (IR) follows:

$$\frac{\text{Number of new cases with the condition or disease over a given time period}}{\text{Number in the population at risk of being a case (free of the condition at the outset)}} \times K$$

Continuing with our previous example, suppose in July 2022 we found that 80 in a sample of 500 people were clinically depressed (PR = 16 per 100). To determine the 1-year incidence rate, we would reassess the sample in July 2020. Suppose that, of the 420 previously deemed *not* to be clinically depressed in 2020, 21 were now found to meet the criteria for depression. In this case, the estimated 1-year incidence rate would be 5 per 100 ([21 ÷ 420] × 100 = 5).

Prevalence and incidence rates can be calculated for subgroups of the population (e.g., for males vs. females). When this is done, it is possible to calculate another important descriptive index. **Relative risk** is an estimated risk of "caseness" in one group compared with another. Relative risk is computed by dividing the rate for one group by the rate for another. Suppose we found that the 1-year incidence rate for depression was 6 per 100 females and 4 per 100 males. Females' relative risk for developing depression over the 1-year period would be 1.5; that is, females would be estimated to be 1.5 times more likely to develop depression than males. Relative risk (discussed in Chapter 17) is an important index in assessing the contribution of risk factors to a disease or condition.

Example of a Prevalence Study
Kovacic et al. (2021) used data from Medicaid Databases from Arizona, Wisconsin, and a nationwide private insurance database to assess the prevalence of pediatric feeding disorders in children in the United States.

TIP The quality of studies that test hypothesized causal relationship is heavily dependent on design decisions—that is, how researchers design their studies to rule out competing explanations for the outcomes. Methods of enhancing the rigor of such studies are described in the next chapter. The quality of descriptive studies, by contrast, depends more on having a good sample (Chapter 13) and strong measures (Chapter 15).

Strengths and Limitations of Correlational Research

The quality of a study is not necessarily related to its approach; there are many excellent nonexperimental studies as well as flawed RCTs. Nevertheless, nonexperimental correlational studies have several drawbacks if causal explanations are sought.

Limitations of Correlational Research

Relative to experimental and quasi-experimental research, nonexperimental studies are weak in their ability to support causal inferences. In correlational studies, researchers work with preexisting groups that were not formed at random, but rather through **self-selection**. A researcher doing a correlational study cannot assume that groups being compared were similar before the occurrence of the hypothesized cause (i.e., the independent variable). Preexisting differences may be a plausible alternative explanation for any group differences on the outcome variable.

The difficulty of interpreting correlational findings stems from the fact that, in the real world, behaviors and characteristics are interrelated (correlated) in complex ways. An example may help to clarify the problem. Suppose we conducted a cross-sectional study that examined the relationship between level of depression in cancer patients and their level of social support (i.e., assistance and emotional support from others). We hypothesize that social support (the independent variable) affects levels of depression (the outcome). Suppose we find that the patients with weak social support are significantly more depressed than patients with strong support. We could interpret this finding to mean that patients' emotional state is influenced by the adequacy of their social supports. This relationship is diagrammed in Figure 9.4, row A. Yet, there are alternative explanations. Perhaps a third variable influences *both* social support and depression, such as the patients' marital status. It may be that having a spouse is a powerful influence on how depressed cancer patients feel *and* on the quality of their social support. This set of relationships is diagrammed in Figure 9.4, row B. In this scenario, social support and depression are correlated simply because marital status affects both. A third possibility is reversed causality (Figure 9.4, row C). Depressed patients with cancer may find it more difficult to elicit needed support from others than patients who are more cheerful or amiable. In this interpretation, the person's depression causes the amount of received social support, and not the other way around. Thus, interpretations of most correlational results should be considered tentative, particularly if the research has no theoretical basis and if the design is cross-sectional.

Strengths of Correlational Research

Earlier, we discussed constraints that limit the application of experimental designs. Correlational research will continue to play a crucial role in nursing research because many interesting problems cannot be addressed any other way.

Correlational research is often efficient in that it may involve collecting a large amount of data about a problem. For example, it would be possible to collect extensive information about the health histories and eating habits of a large number of individuals. Researchers could then examine which health problems were associated with which diets and could discover a large number of interrelationships in a relatively short amount of time. By contrast, an experimenter looks at only a few variables at a time. One experiment might manipulate foods high in cholesterol, whereas another might manipulate salt, for example.

Finally, correlational research is often strong in realism. Unlike many experimental studies, correlational research is seldom criticized for its artificiality.

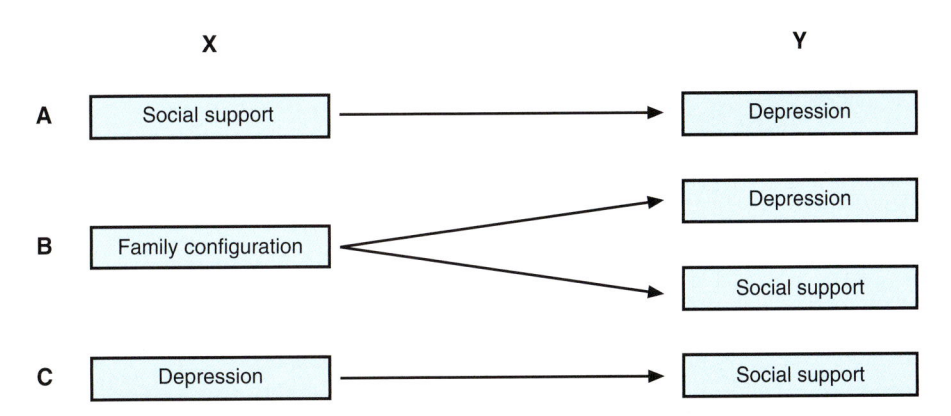

FIGURE 9.4 Alternative explanations for relationship between depression and social support in patients with cancer.

> **TIP** It can be useful to design a study with several relevant comparisons. In nonexperimental studies, multiple comparison groups can be effective in dealing with self-selection, especially if groups are chosen to address competing biases. For example, in case–control studies of potential causes of lung cancer, cases would be people with lung cancer, one comparison group could be people with a different lung disease, and a second could be those with no pulmonary disorder.

DESIGNS AND RESEARCH EVIDENCE

Evidence for nursing practice depends on descriptive, correlational, and experimental research. There is often a progression to evidence expansion that begins with rich description, including description from qualitative research. In-depth qualitative research may suggest causal links that could be the focus of controlled quantitative research. For example, Dwyer et al. (2020) explored communication patterns around family cancer history and genetic risk. Their findings based on interviews with 97 females with a positive BRCA genetic history suggest that gender role influenced family communication about genetic risk and the need for screening. Based on the findings from this work and the Theory of Planned Behavior, the team suggested the need for interventions. Subsequently, several members of the team advanced this work by conducting another study that integrated quantitative and qualitative findings to develop tailored interventions to enhance the health of females of reproductive age who have a positive BRCA genetic risk (Hesse-Biber et al., 2022). Thus, although qualitative studies are low on the standard evidence hierarchy for *confirming* causal connections, they serve an important function in stimulating ideas.

Correlational studies also play a role in developing evidence for causal inferences. Retrospective case–control studies may pave the way for more rigorous (but more expensive) prospective studies. As the evidence base builds, conceptual models may be developed and tested using path analytic designs and other theory-testing strategies. These studies can provide hints about how to structure an intervention, who can most profit from it, and when it can best be instituted.

Different questions relating to causality (Therapy, Prognosis, Etiology) have different evidence hierarchies for ranking designs according to the risk of bias, as we show in Table 9.4, which augments the evidence hierarchy presented in Figure 2.2 (Chapter 2). For Therapy questions (and some Etiology questions), experimental designs are the gold standard (Level II), superseded only by systematic reviews of RCTs on level-of-evidence scales (Level I). On the next rung of the hierarchy for Therapy questions are quasi-experimental designs (and even at this rung, some designs have a lower risk of bias than others). Further down the hierarchy are observational and qualitative studies, which tend not to be strong in corroborating causal hypotheses.

For Prognosis questions, by contrast, randomization to groups is not possible (e.g., for the question of whether low birthweight causes developmental delays). In the hierarchy for Prognosis questions, the best design for an individual study is a prospective cohort design. Path analytic studies with longitudinal data and a strong theoretical basis can also be powerful. Retrospective case–control studies are relatively weak in addressing questions about causality. Systematic reviews of multiple prospective studies, together with support from theories or biophysiologic research, represent the strongest evidence for these types of question.

In terms of Etiology questions, RCTs are sometimes feasible (e.g., Does low salt intake cause reductions in blood pressure levels?). For such questions, the hierarchy is the same as that for Therapy questions. Many important Etiology questions will never be answered using evidence from RCTs, however. A good example is the Etiology question of whether smoking causes lung cancer. Despite the inability to randomize people to smoking and nonsmoking groups, few people doubt that this causal connection exists. Thinking about the criteria for causality discussed early in this chapter, there is abundant evidence that smoking cigarettes

TABLE 9.4 • Level of Evidence Rankings for Different Cause-Probing Research Questions

LEVEL	TYPE OF QUESTION	
	THERAPY/INTERVENTION AND ETIOLOGY (CAUSATION)/PREVENTION OF HARM[a]	PROGNOSIS
I	Systematic review of RCTs[b]	Systematic review of nonexperimental studies
II	Randomized controlled trial	Prospective cohort study
III	Quasi-experimental study	Path analytic/theory-based study
IV	Systematic review of nonexperimental studies	Retrospective/case–control study
V	Nonexperimental/observational study a. Prospective cohort study b. Path analytic/theory-based study c. Retrospective case/control study d. Descriptive correlational study	Descriptive correlational study
VI	Metasynthesis of qualitative studies	Metasynthesis of qualitative studies
VII	Qualitative study	Qualitative study
VIII	Nonresearch source	Nonresearch source

[a]RCTs and quasi-experimental designs can sometimes be used for Etiology (causation)/prevention of harm questions (e.g., the effect of salt intake on blood pressure levels). If intervening is not possible (e.g., testing smoking as a cause of lung cancer), the level of evidence rankings would be the same as for Prognosis questions.

[b]Systematic reviews (Level I) sometimes include RCTs and quasi-experimental studies.

is correlated with lung cancer and, through prospective studies, that smoking precedes lung cancer. Researchers have been able to control for, and thus rule out, other possible "causes" of lung cancer. There has been a great deal of consistency and coherence in the findings, and the criterion of biologic plausibility has been met through basic physiologic research.

TIP Some early studies found that evidence from experimental and observational studies often do not yield the same results. The relationship between "causes" and "effects" was found to be stronger in nonexperimental studies than in randomized studies. However, other studies have found that well-designed observational studies do not overestimate the magnitude of effects in comparison with RCTs, especially when the criteria for participating in the study are similar (e.g., Concato et al., 2000).

CRITICAL APPRAISAL OF QUANTITATIVE RESEARCH DESIGNS

The research design used in a quantitative study strongly influences the quality of its evidence, and so should be carefully scrutinized. Researchers' design decisions have more of an impact on study quality than any other methodologic decision when the research question is about causal relationships.

Actual designs and some control techniques (randomization, blinding, allocation concealment) were described in this chapter, and the next chapter explains in greater detail specific strategies for enhancing research control. The guidelines in Box 9.1 are questions that will help you in critically appraising quantitative research designs.

BOX 9.1 Guidelines for Critically Appraising Quantitative Research Designs

1. What type of question (Therapy, Prognosis, etc.) was being addressed in this study? Is the research question cause-probing, that is, does it concern a hypothesized causal relationship between the independent and dependent variables?
2. What would be the strongest design for the research question? How does this compare to the design actually used?
3. Was there an intervention or treatment? Was the intervention adequately described? Was the control or comparison condition adequately described? Was an experimental or quasi-experimental design used?
4. If the study was an RCT (a true experiment), what specific design was used? Was this design appropriate?
5. In RCTs, what type of randomization was used? Were randomization procedures adequately explained and justified? Was allocation concealment confirmed?
6. If the design was quasi-experimental, what specific quasi-experimental design was used? Was there adequate justification for deciding not to randomize participants to treatment conditions? Did the report provide evidence that any groups being compared were equivalent prior to the intervention?
7. If the design was nonexperimental, was the study inherently nonexperimental? If not, is there adequate justification for not manipulating the independent variable? What specific nonexperimental design was used? If a retrospective design was used, is there good justification for not using a prospective design? What evidence did the report provide that any groups being compared were similar with regard to important confounding characteristics?
8. What types of comparisons were specified in the design (e.g., before–after? between groups?) Did these comparisons adequately illuminate the relationship between the independent and dependent variables? If there were no comparisons, or faulty comparisons, how did this affect the study's integrity and the interpretability of the results?
9. Was the study longitudinal? Was the timing of the collection of data appropriate? Was the number of data collection points reasonable?
10. Was blinding/masking used? If yes, who was blinded—and was this adequate? If not, was there a justifiable rationale for failure to mask? Was the intervention a type that could raise participants' expectations that, in and of themselves, could affect the outcomes?

RESEARCH EXAMPLES

In this section we present descriptions of an experimental, quasi-experimental, and nonexperimental study.

Research Example of an RCT

Study: A Randomized Trial of a Multifactorial Strategy to Prevent Serious Fall Injuries (Bhasin et al., 2020).

Statement of Purpose: The purpose of this study was to determine the clinical effectiveness of a patient-centered intervention implemented by specially trained nurses that was aimed at preventing the risk of falls at 86 different primary care settings across the United States.

Treatment Group: In this trial, there were one intervention group and one control group.

Method: Nurses delivered a fall intervention strategy in partnership with the participants and their primary care providers. The intervention had five components: (1) an assessment of modifiable fall risk factors; (2) a standardized protocol delivered to the participants or their caregiver using motivational interviewing with the goal of managing the risk factors; (3) the development of an individualized care plan that was approved by the primary care providers and focused on one to three fall risk factors; (4) included the implementation of the care plan; and (5) follow-up care that was conducted by telephone or in person. The control group and intervention groups each had access to a webinar about fall prevention. In addition, participants in the control group received an informational pamphlet about fall prevention developed by the Centers for Disease Control Prevention and were encouraged to discuss fall prevention with their primary care provider.

Key Findings: The rate of all serious fall injuries, and serious adverse events did not differ significantly between the two groups.

Research Example of a Quasi-Experimental Study

Study: The Mindful Path to Nursing Accuracy: A Quasi-Experimental Study on Minimizing Medication Administration Errors (Ekkens & Gordon, 2021).

Statement of Purpose: The purpose of the study was to determine if training nurses in mindfulness thinking reduced the frequency and severity of medication administration errors.

Treatment Groups: This study included one intervention group and one control group. The intervention group received a manual on mindfulness thinking and a 2-hour recorded training in mindfulness by a psychologist with this expertise. The control group received an article on the impact of emerging technologies in nursing care. The participants in each group self-reported frequency and severity of medication errors over 3 months.

Method: This study had one intervention and one control group. Participants in each group had similar educational backgrounds, certifications, and work experience and were alternately assigned to the groups. In total, 119 participated in the study (51 treatment, 60 control).

Key Findings: The intervention group had a 73.3% decrease in the number of medical errors, whereas the control group did not significantly decrease medication errors or severity of errors.

Research Example of a Correlational Study

Study: Psychological Distress in Parents of Children with Cancer: A Descriptive Correlational Study (Isabel Tan et al., 2020).

Statement of Purpose: The purpose of the study was to determine the levels of distress and the contributing factors among parent caregivers of pediatric cancer patients in Singapore.

Method: The study participants in this descriptive correlational study were recruited through convenience sampling from a children's cancer center within a large, academic tertiary hospital in Singapore. In total, 81 parent caregivers participated. Study participation involved completing a self-administered demographic survey and the Distress Thermometer for Parents tool.

Key Findings: More than half of the parent caregivers (67.9%) were distressed. The mean distress score was 5.07 out of a maximum of 10 and with 4 being the cutoff score for not being distressed. The researchers concluded that there is a need to support parent caregivers' adjustment to their child's cancer as an important aspect of providing quality care for pediatric cancer patients.

SUMMARY POINTS

- Many quantitative nursing studies aim to facilitate inferences about *cause-and-effect relationships*.
- One criterion for causality is that the cause must precede the effect. Two other criteria are that a relationship between a presumed cause (independent variable) and an effect (dependent variable) exists and cannot be explained as being caused by other (confounding) variables.
- In an idealized model, a **counterfactual** is what would have happened to the same people simultaneously exposed *and* not exposed to a causal factor. The *effect* is the difference between the two. The goal of research design is to find a good approximation to the idealized (but impossible) counterfactual.
- **Experiments** (or **randomized controlled trials, RCTs**) involve **manipulation** (the researcher manipulates the independent variable by introducing a **treatment** or **intervention**); control (including use of a **control group** that does not receive the intervention and represents the comparative counterfactual); and **randomization/random assignment** (with people allocated to experimental and control groups at random so that they are equivalent at the outset).
- Participants in the experimental group usually all get the same intervention as delineated in formal protocols, but some studies involve **patient-centered interventions (PCIs)** that are *tailored* to meet individual needs or characteristics.

- Researchers can expose the control group to various conditions, including no treatment; an alternative treatment; standard treatment ("usual care"); a **placebo** or pseudointervention; different doses of the treatment; or a *delayed treatment* (for a **wait-list** group).
- Random assignment is done by methods that give every participant an equal chance of being in any group, such as by flipping a coin or using a **table of random numbers**. Randomization is the most reliable method for equalizing groups on all characteristics that could affect study outcomes. Randomization should involve **allocation concealment** that prevents foreknowledge of upcoming assignments.
- Several variants to simple randomization exist, such as **permuted block randomization**, in which randomization is done for blocks of people—for example, 6 or 8 at a time, in randomly selected block sizes.
- **Blinding** (or **masking**) is often used to avoid biases stemming from participants' or research agents' awareness of group status or study hypotheses. In **double-blind studies**, two groups (e.g., participants and investigators) are blinded.
- Many specific experimental designs exist. A **posttest-only** (*after-only*) **design** involves collecting data after an intervention only. In a **pretest–posttest** (*before–after*) **design**, data are collected both before and after the intervention, permitting an analysis of change.
- **Factorial designs**, in which two or more independent variables are manipulated simultaneously, allow researchers to test both **main effects** (effects from manipulated independent variables) and **interaction effects** (effects from combining treatments).
- In a **crossover design**, subjects are exposed to more than one condition, administered in a randomized order, and thus they serve as their own controls.
- Experimental designs are the *gold standard* because they come closer than any other design in meeting criteria for inferring causal relationships.
- **Quasi-experimental designs** (*trials without randomization*) involve an intervention but lack randomization. Strong quasi-experimental designs incorporate features to support causal inferences.
- The **nonequivalent control group pretest–posttest design** involves using a nonrandomized **comparison group** and the collection of pretreatment data so that initial group equivalence can be assessed.
- In a **time series design**, information on the dependent variable is collected multiple times before and after the intervention in a single group. The extended time period for data collection enhances the ability to attribute change to the intervention.
- Other quasi-experimental designs include nonrandomized **dose–response analyses** and the nonrandomized **arms** of a **partially randomized patient preference** (**PRPP**) design (i.e., groups with strong preferences).
- In evaluating the results of quasi-experiments, it is important to ask whether it is plausible that factors other than the intervention caused or affected the outcomes (i.e., whether there are credible **rival hypotheses** for explaining the results).
- **Nonexperimental** (or **observational**) **research** includes **descriptive research**—studies that summarize the status of phenomena—and **correlational** studies that examine relationships among variables but involve no manipulation of independent variables (often because they *cannot* be manipulated).
- Designs for cause-probing correlational studies include **retrospective (case–control) designs** (which look back in time for antecedent causes of "caseness" by comparing **cases** that have a disease or condition with controls who do not); **prospective (cohort) designs** (studies that begin with a presumed cause and look forward in time for its effect); **natural experiments** (in which a group is affected by a random event, such as a disaster); and **path analytic studies** (which test causal models developed on the basis of theory).
- **Descriptive correlational studies** describe how phenomena are interrelated without invoking a causal explanation. **Univariate descriptive studies** examine the frequency or average value of variables.

- Descriptive studies include **prevalence studies** that document the **prevalence rate** of a condition at one point in time and **incidence studies** that document the frequency of *new* cases, over a given time period. When the **incidence rates** for two subgroups are estimated, researchers can compute the **relative risk** of "caseness" for the two.
- The primary weakness of correlational studies for cause-probing questions is that they can harbor biases, such as **self-selection** into groups being compared.

REFERENCES CITED IN CHAPTER 9

Baird, A., Cheng, Y., & Xia, Y. (2022). Telehealth adoption and discontinuation by US hospitals: Results from 2 quasi-natural experiments. *JMIR Formative Research*, 6(2), e28979. https://doi.org/10.2196/28979

Barkauskas, V. H., Lusk, S. L., & Eakin, B. L. (2005). Selecting control interventions for clinical outcome studies. *Western Journal Nursing Research*, 27(3), 346–363.

Bärnighausen, T., Røttingen, J. A., Rockers, P., Shemilt, I., Tugwell, P., Geldsetzer, P., & Atun, R. (2017). Quasi-experimental study designs series-paper 1: Introduction—two historical lineages. *Journal of Clinical Epidemiology*, 89, 4–11.

Beck, C., McSweeney, J., Richards, K., Roberson, P. K., Tsai, P., & Souder, E. (2010). Challenges in tailored intervention research. *Nursing Outlook*, 58(2), 104–110.

Bhasin, S., Gill, T. M., Reuben, D. B., Latham, N. K., Ganz, D. A., Greene, E. J., Dziura, J., Basaria, S., Gurwitz, J. H., Dykes, P. C., McMahon, S., Storer, T. W., Gazarian, P., Miller, M. E., Travison, T. G., Esserman, D., Carnie, M. B., Goehring, L., Fagan, M., … STRIDE Trial Investigators, (2020). A randomized trial of a multifactorial strategy to prevent serious fall injuries. *New England Journal of Medicine*, 383(2), 129–140. https://doi.org/10.1056/NEJMoa2002183

Bradford-Hill, A. (1965). The environment and disease: Association or causation. *Proceedings of the Royal Society of Medicine*, 58, 295–300.

Cai, Y., Wanigatunga, A. A., Mitchell, C. M., Urbanek, J. K., Miller, E. R., Juraschek, S. P., Michos, E. D., Kalyani, R. R., Roth, D. L., Appel, L. J., & Schrack, J. A. (2022). The effects of vitamin D supplementation on frailty in older adults at risk for falls. *BMC Geriatrics*, 22 (1), 312. https://doi.org/10.1186/s12877-022-02888-w

Campbell, D. T., & Stanley, J. C. (1963). *Experimental and quasi-experimental designs for research*. Rand McNally.

Concato, J., Shah, N., & Horwitz, R. (2000). Randomized, controlled trials, observational studies, and the hierarchy of research designs. *New England Journal of Medicine*, 342(25), 1887–1892.

Doering, J., & Dogan, S. (2018). A postpartum sleep and fatigue intervention feasibility pilot study. *Behavioral Sleep Medicine*, 16(2), 185–201.

Doig, G., & Simpson, F. (2005). Randomization and allocation concealment: A practical guide for researchers. *Journal of Critical Care*, 20(2), 187–193.

Dwyer, A. A., Hesse-Biber, S., Flynn, B., & Remick, S. (2020). Parent of origin effects on family communication of risk in *BRCA+* women: A qualitative investigation of human factors in cascade screening. *Cancers*, 12(8), 2316. https://doi.org/10.3390/cancers12082316

Ekkens, C. L., & Gordon, P. A. (2021). The mindful path to nursing accuracy: A quasi-experimental study on minimizing medication administration errors. *Holistic Nursing Practice*, 35(3), 115–122. https://doi.org/10.1097/HNP.0000000000000440

Fernández-Gutiérrez, M., Bas-Sarmiento, P., Pino-Chinchilla, H. D., Poza-Méndez, M., & Marìn-Paz, A. J. (2022). Effectiveness of a multimodal intervention and the simulation flow to improve empathy and attitudes towards older adults in nursing students: A crossover randomized controlled trial. *Nurse Education in Practice*, 64, 1033430. https://doi.org/10.1016/j.nepr.2022.103430

Flanagan, J. M., Read, C., & Shindul-Rothschild, J. (2020). Factors associated with the rate of sepsis after surgery. *Critical Care Nursing*, 40(5), e1–e9. https://doi.org/10.4037/ccn2020171

Fu, M. R., Kurnat-Thoma, E., Starkweather, A., Henderson, W. A., Cashion, A. K., Williams, J. K., Katapodi, M. C., Reuter-Rice, K., Hickey, K. T., Barcelona de Mendoza, V., Calzone, K., Conley, Y. P., Anderson, C. M., Lyon, D. E., Weaver, M. T., Shiao, P. K., Constantino, R. E., Wung, S. F., Hammer, M. J., … Coleman, B. (2020). Precision health: A nursing perspective. *International Journal of Nursing Science*, 7(1), 5–12. https://doi.org/10.1016/j.ijnss.2019.12.008

Geldsetzer, P., & Fawzi, W. (2017). Quasi-experimental study designs series-paper 2: Complementary approaches to advancing global health knowledge. *Journal of Clinical Epidemiology*, 89, 12–16.

Grimes, D., & Schulz, K. (2005). Compared to what? Finding controls for case-control studies. *The Lancet*, 365(9468), 1429–1433.

Gross, D. (2005). On the merits of attention control groups. *Research in Nursing Health*, 28(2), 93–94.

Herbison, P., Hay-Smith, J., & Gillespie, W. (2011). Different methods of allocation to groups in randomized trials are associated with different levels of bias. A meta-epidemiological study. *Journal of Clinical Epidemiology*, 64(10), 1070–1075.

Hesse-Biber, S., Seven, M., Jiang, J., Schaik, S. V., & Dwyer, A. A. (2022). Impact of *BRCA* status on reproductive decision-making and self-concept: A mixed-methods study informing the development of tailored interventions. *Cancers*, 14(6), 1494. https://doi.org/10.3390/cancers14061494

Isabel Tan, X. W., Mordiffi, S. Z., Lopez, V., & Leong, K. (2021). Psychological distress in parents of children with cancer: A descriptive correlational study. *Asia-Pacific Journal of Oncology Nursing*, 8(1), 94–102. https://doi.org/10.4103/apjon.apjon_46_20

Kim, J., & Kim, S. (2022). Effects of a nonviolent communication-based anger management program on psychiatric inpatients. *Archives of Psychiatric Nursing*, *41*, 87–95. https://doi.org/10.1016/j.apnu.2022.07.004

Kim, B., & Park, H. (2023). The effects of auricular acupressure on blood pressure, stress, and sleep in elders with essential hypertension: A randomized single-blind sham-controlled trial. *European Journal of Cardiovascular Nursing*, *22*(6), 610–619. https://doi.org/10.1093/eurjcn/zvad005

Kovacic, K., Rein, L. E., Szabo, A., Kommareddy, S., Bhagavatula, P., & Goday, P. S. (2021). Pediatric feeding disorder: A nationwide prevalence study. *The Journal of Pediatrics*, *228*, 126–131.e3. https://doi.org/10.1016/j.jpeds.2020.07.047

Lachin, J. M., Matts, J., & Wei, L. (1988). Randomization in clinical trials: Conclusions and recommendations. *Controlled Clinical Trials*, *9*(4), 365–374.

Li, N., Zhang, L., Li, X., & Lu, Q. (2022). Moderated role of social support in the relationship between job strain, burnout, and organizational commitment among operating room nurses: A cross-sectional study. *International Journal of Environmental Research and Public Health*, *19*(17), 10813. https://doi.org/10.3390/ijerph191710813

Moher, D., Hopewell, S., Schulz, K. F., Montori, V., Gøtzsche, P. C., Devereaux, P., Elbourne, D., Egger, M., Altman, D. G., Altman, D. G. (2010). CONSORT 2010 explanation and elaboration: Updated guidelines for reporting parallel-group randomised trials. *BMJ*, *340*, c869.

Mojtehedi, M., Salehi-Pourmehr, H., Ostadrahimi, A., Asnaashari, S., Esmaeilpour, K., & Farshbaf-Khalili, A. (2022). Effect of aromatherapy with essential oil of Lavandula angustifolia mill-citrus bergamia and mindfulness-based intervention on sexual function, anxiety, and depression in postmenopausal women: A randomized controlled trial with factorial design. *Iranian Journal of Nursing and Midwifery Research*, *27*(5), 392–405. https://doi.org/10.4103/ijnmr.ijnmr_129_21

Parsons, J., Forde, R., Brackenridge, A., Hunt, K. F., Ismail, K., Murrells, T., Reid, A., Rogers, H., Rogers, R., & Forbes, A. (2022). The gestational diabetes future diabetes prevention study (GODDESS): A partially randomised feasibility controlled trial. *PLoS ONE*, *17*(12), e0273992. https://doi.org/10.1371/journal.pone.0273992

Polit, D. F., & Chaboyer, W. (2012). Statistical process control in nursing research. *Reseach in Nursing & Health*, *35*(1), 82–93.

Polit, D., Gillespie, B., & Griffin, R. (2011). Deliberate ignorance: A systematic review of the use of blinding in nursing clinical trials. *Nursing Research*, *61*, 9–16.

Rodrìguez-Blanco, C., Bernal-Utrera, C., Anarte-Lazo, E., Saavedra-Hernandez, M., De-La-Barrera-Aranda, E., Serrera-Figallo, M. A., Gonzalez-Martin, M., & Gonzalez-Gerez, J. J. (2022). Breathing exercises versus strength exercises through telerehabilitation in coronavirus disease 2019 patients in the acute phase: A randomized controlled trial. *Clinical Rehabilitation*, *36*(4), 486–497. https://doi.org/10.1177/02692155211061221

Sanders, L. M. J., Hortobágyi, T., Karssemeijer, E. G. A., Van der Zee, E. A., Scherder, E. J. A., & van Heuvelen, M. J. G. (2020). Effects of low- and high-intensity physical exercise on physical and cognitive function in older persons with dementia: A randomized controlled trial. *Alzheimer's Research & Therapy*, *12*(1), 28. https://doi.org/10.1186/s13195-020-00597-3

Schulz, K. F., Chalmers, I., & Altman, D. G. (2002). The landscape and lexicon of blinding in randomized trials. *Annals of Internal Medicine*, *136*(3), 254–259.

Senecal, L., & Jurgens, C. (2022). Persistent heart failure symptoms at hospital discharge predicts 30-day clinical events. *Journal of Cardiovascular Nursing*, *37*(2), 158–166. https://doi.org10.1097/JCN.0000000000000767

Shadish, W. R., Cook, T. D., & Campbell, D. T. (2002). *Experimental and quasi-experimental designs for generalized causal inference*. Houghton Mifflin.

Tanriverdi, S., & Parlar Kılıç, S. (2023). The effect of progressive muscle relaxation on abdominal pain and distension in colonoscopy patients. *Journal of PeriAnesthesia Nursing*, *38*(2), 224–231. https://doi.org/10.1016/j.jopan.2022.04.013

Tom, F. S., Tucker, K. J., McCracken, C. M., McGregor, J. C., & Gore, S. J. (2022). Infectious complications of probiotic use: A matched case-control study. *Infection Control & Hospital Epidemiology*, *43*(10), 1498–1500. https://doi.org/10.1017/ice.2021.261

Vedelø, T. W., & Lomborg, K. (2011). Reported challenges in nurse-led randomised controlled trials: An integrative review of the literature. *Scandinavian Journal of Caring Sciences*, *25*(1), 194–200.

Wan, C., Williams, C. P., Nipp, R. D., Pisu, M., Azuero, A., Aswani, M. S., Ingram, S. A., Pierce, J. Y., & Rocque, G. B. (2021). Treatment decision making and financial toxicity in women with metastatic breast cancer. *Clinical Breast Cancer*, *21*(1), 37–46. https://doi.org/10.1016/j.clbc.2020.07.002

Warjri, E., Dsilva, F., Sanal, T. S., & Kumar, A. (2022). Impact of a white noise app on sleep quality among critically ill patients. *Nursing in Critical Care*, *27*(6), 815–823. https://doi.org/10.1111/nicc.12742

Zhang, W., Gu, Q., Gu, Y., Zhao, Y., & Zhu, L. (2022). Symptom management to alleviate thirst and dry mouth in critically ill patients: A randomised controlled trial. *Australian Critical Care*, *35*(2), 123–129. https://doi.org/10.1016/j.aucc.2021.04.002

Zhong, H., Liang, A., Luo, H., Hu, X., Xu, S., Zheng, Z., & Zhu, X. (2022). Application analysis of multidisciplinary diagnosis and treatment nursing mode based on doctor-nurse-integration for stroke patients undergoing emergency intervention surgery. *Emergency Medical International*, *2022*, 6299676. https://doi.org/10.1155/2022/6299676

10 Rigor and Validity in Quantitative Research

Learning Objectives

1. Recognize the threats to validity in quantitative research.
2. Identify and evaluate the various methods of controlling confounding variables.
3. Describe strategies to assure treatment fidelity.
4. Evaluate a quantitative study in terms of its research design and methods of controlling confounding variables.

VALIDITY AND INFERENCE

This chapter describes strategies for controlling sources of bias in quantitative studies. Many of these strategies strengthen inferences that can be made about cause-and-effect relationships.

Validity and Validity Threats

In designing a study, it is useful to anticipate factors that could undermine the **validity** of inferences. Shadish et al. (2002) define validity in the context of research design as "the approximate truth of an inference" (p. 34). For example, inferences that a *cause* results in a hypothesized *effect* are valid to the extent that researchers can marshal strong supporting evidence. Validity is always a matter of degree, not an absolute.

Validity is a property of an inference, not of a research design, but design elements profoundly affect the inferences that can be made. **Threats to validity** are reasons that an inference could be wrong. When researchers introduce design features to minimize potential threats, the validity of the inference about relationships under study is strengthened.

Types of Validity

Shadish and colleagues (2002) proposed a taxonomy that identified four types of validity and cataloged dozens of validity threats. This chapter describes the taxonomy and summarizes major threats, but we urge researchers to consult this seminal work for further guidance.

The first type of validity, **statistical conclusion validity**, concerns the validity of inferences that there truly is an empirical relationship, or correlation, between the presumed cause and the effect. The researcher's job is to provide strong evidence that an observed relationship is *real*.

Internal validity concerns the validity of inferences that, given that an empirical relationship exists, it is the independent variable, rather than something else, that caused the outcome. Researchers must develop strategies to rule out the plausibility that some factor other than the independent variable accounts for the observed relationship.

Construct validity involves the validity of inferences "from the observed persons, settings, and cause-and-effect operations included in the study to the constructs that these instances might represent" (p. 38). One aspect of construct validity concerns the degree to which an intervention is a good representation of the underlying construct that was theorized as having the potential to cause beneficial outcomes. Another issue concerns whether the measures of the outcomes are good operationalizations of the constructs for which they are intended.

External validity concerns whether inferences about observed relationships will hold over variations in people, setting, or time. External validity, then, relates to the generalizability of inferences—a critical concern for evidence-based nursing practice.

These four types of validity and their associated threats are discussed in this chapter. Many validity threats result from inadequate control over confounding variables, and so we briefly review methods of controlling confounders associated with participants' characteristics.

Controlling Confounding Participant Characteristics

This section describes six methods of controlling participant characteristics—characteristics that could compete with the independent variable as the cause of an outcome.

Randomization

As noted in Chapter 9, randomization is the most effective method of controlling individual characteristics. The function of randomization is to secure comparable groups—i.e., to equalize groups with respect to confounding variables. A distinct advantage of random assignment, compared with other strategies, is that it can control *all* possible sources of confounding variation, *without any conscious decision about which variables need to be controlled*.

Crossover

Randomization within a crossover design is an especially powerful method of ensuring equivalence between groups being compared—participants serve as their own controls. Moreover, fewer participants usually are needed in such a design. Fifty people exposed to two treatments in random order yield 100 data points (50 × 2); 50 people randomly assigned to two different groups yield only 50 data points (25 × 2). Crossover designs are not appropriate for all studies, however, because of possible carry-over effects: people exposed to two different conditions may be influenced in the second condition by their experience in the first.

Homogeneity

When randomization and crossover are not feasible, alternative methods of controlling confounding characteristics are needed. One method is to use only people who are homogeneous with respect to confounding variables. Suppose we were testing the effectiveness of a physical fitness program on the cardiovascular functioning of older people. In our quasiexperimental design, older adults from two different nursing homes are recruited, with adults in one of them receiving the intervention. If gender were a key confounding variable—and if the two nursing homes had different proportions of males and females—we could control gender by using only males (or only females) as participants.

The price of homogeneity is that research findings cannot be generalized to types of people who did not participate in the study. If the physical fitness intervention was found to have beneficial effects on the cardiovascular status of a sample of females 65 to 75 years of age, its usefulness for improving the cardiovascular status of males in their 80s would require a separate study. Indeed, one criticism of this approach is that researchers sometimes exclude people who are extremely ill, which means that the findings cannot be generalized to those who may be most in need of interventions.

> **Example of Control Through Homogeneity**
> Choi and colleagues (2022) used a nonequivalent control group to develop a posttraumatic growth program for breast cancer survivors. Several variables were controlled through homogeneity including being a breast cancer survivor from one of two outpatient departments at two university hospitals in South Korea, having stage 1 to 3 breast cancer, and being age greater than 20 years.

> **TIP** The principle of homogeneity is often used to control (hold constant) *external* factors known to influence outcomes. For example, it may be important to collect outcome data at the same time of the day for all participants if time could affect the outcome (e.g., fatigue). As another example, it may be desirable to maintain **constancy of conditions** in terms of data collection locale—e.g., interviewing all respondents in their homes, rather than some in their places of work, because context can influence responses to questions.

Stratification/Blocking

Another approach to controlling confounders is to include them in the research design through stratification. To pursue our example of the physical fitness intervention with gender as the confounding variable, we could use a *randomized block design* in which males and females are assigned separately to treatment groups. This approach can enhance the likelihood of detecting differences between our experimental and control groups because the effect of the blocking variable (gender) on the outcome is eliminated. In addition, if the blocking variable is of interest substantively, researchers have the opportunity to study differences in the subgroups created by the stratifying variable (e.g., males vs. females).

Matching

Matching (also called **pair matching**) involves using information about people's characteristics to create comparable groups. If matching were used in our physical fitness example and age and gender were the confounding variables, we would match a person in the intervention group with one in the comparison group with respect to age and gender.

Matching is often problematic: to use matching, researchers must know the relevant confounders in advance. Also, it is difficult to match on more than two or three variables. This problem is sometimes addressed with a sophisticated matching technique, called **propensity matching.** This method, which requires some statistical sophistication, involves the creation of a **propensity score** that captures the conditional probability of exposure to a treatment given various preintervention characteristics. Members of the groups being compared (either in an observational or quasiexperimental study) can then be matched on the propensity score (Qin et al., 2008). Both conventional and propensity matching are most easily implemented when there is a large pool of potential comparison group participants from which good matches to treatment group members can be selected. Nevertheless, matching as the primary control technique should be used only when other, more powerful procedures are not feasible.

Sometimes, as an alternative to matching, researchers use a **balanced design** with regard to key confounders. In such situations, researchers attempt only to ensure that the groups being compared have similar proportional representation on confounding variables, rather than matching on a one-to-one basis. For example, if gender and age were the two variables of concern, we would strive to ensure that the same percentage of males and females were in the two groups and that the average age was comparable. Such an approach is less cumbersome than matching but has similar limitations. Nevertheless, both matching and balancing are preferable to failing to control participant characteristics at all.

> **Example of Control Through Matching**
> Aranda-Gallardo and colleagues (2022) used a case–control design to study associations between hyponatremia and the risk of falls in hospitalized patients. The sample included adult patients hospitalized at a Spanish hospital who had a fall recorded in their hospital health record during a 2-year period. Each case included was matched by the following controls: age, gender, hospital unit, and date of stay (within a week of the person who had a recorded fall). Findings indicate that hyponatremia is a predictor of falls in hospitalized patients.

Statistical Control

Another method of controlling confounding variables is through statistical analysis rather than research design. A detailed description of powerful **statistical control** mechanisms will be postponed until Chapter 19, but we will explain underlying

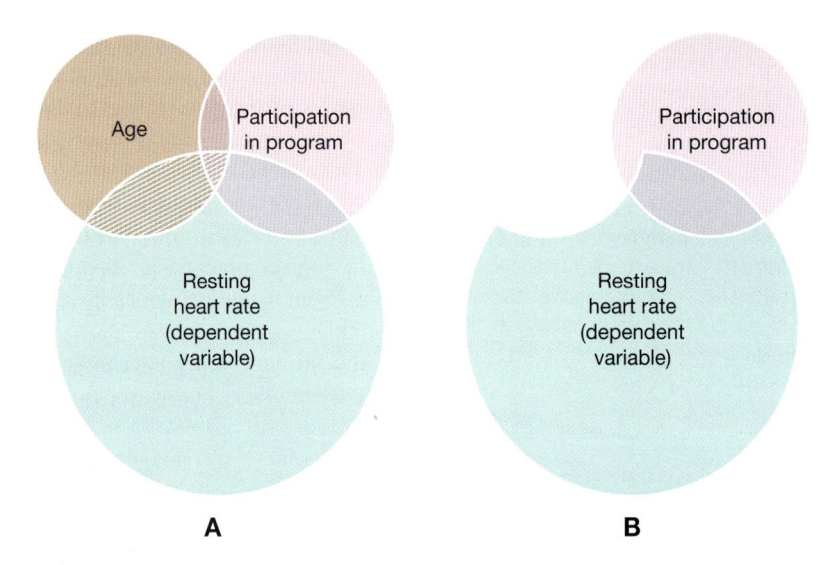

FIGURE 10.1 Schematic diagram illustrating principles of analysis of covariance conceptually.

principles with a simple illustration of a procedure called **analysis of covariance (ANCOVA)**.

In our physical fitness example, suppose we used a nonequivalent control group design with older adults from two nursing homes, and resting heart rate was an outcome. Individual differences in heart rate in the sample would be expected—that is, heart rate would vary from one person to the next. The research question is, "Can some of the differences in heart rate be attributed to program participation?" We know that differences in heart rate are also related to other traits, such as age. In Figure 10.1, the large circles represent the total amount of variation for resting heart rate. A certain amount of variation can be explained by a person's age, depicted as the small circle on the left in Figure 10.1A. Other variation may be explained by participation or nonparticipation in the program, represented as the small circle on the right. The two small circles (age and program participation) overlap, indicating a relationship between the two. In other words, people in the physical fitness group are, on average, either older or younger than those in the comparison group. Age should be controlled; otherwise, we could not determine whether postintervention differences in resting heart rate are due to differences in age or program participation.

ANCOVA statistically removes the effect of confounding variables on the outcome. In the illustration, the portion of heart rate variability attributable to age (the hatched area of the large circle in A) is removed through ANCOVA. Figure 10.1B shows that the final analysis tests the effect of program participation on heart rate *after removing the effect of age*. By controlling heart rate variability resulting from age, we get a more accurate estimate of the effect of the program on heart rate. Note that even after removing variability due to age, there is still individual variation not associated with the program treatment—the bottom half of the large circle in B. This means that the study can probably be improved by controlling additional confounders, such as gender, smoking history, and so on. ANCOVA and other sophisticated procedures can control multiple confounding variables.

Example of Statistical Control
Yu et al. (2022) conducted a secondary analysis examining the longitudinal associations of mental health and behavior change skills with eating behaviors in a cohort of women who were over 18 months postpartum. In their analysis, the researchers controlled for the following covariates: the intervention arm, race, ethnicity, number of children, gestational weight gain, and 6-month age, marital status, employment, income, education, breastfeeding, drinking, smoking, and BMI.

TIP Confounding participant characteristics that need to be controlled vary from one study to another, but we can offer some guidance. The best variable is the outcome variable itself, measured before the independent variable occurs. In our physical fitness example, controlling preprogram measures of cardiovascular functioning would be a good choice. Major demographic variables (e.g., age, race/ethnicity, education) and health indicators are usually good candidates for statistical control. Confounding variables that correlate with the outcomes should be identified through a literature review.

Evaluation of Control Methods

Table 10.1 summarizes benefits and drawbacks of the six control mechanisms. Randomization is the most effective method of managing confounding variables—that is, of approximating the ideal but unattainable counterfactual discussed in Chapter 9—because it tends to cancel out individual differences on all possible confounders. Crossover designs are a useful supplement to randomization but are not always appropriate. The remaining alternatives have common disadvantages: Researchers must know in advance the relevant confounding

TABLE 10.1 • Methods of Control Over Participant Characteristics

METHOD	BENEFITS	LIMITATIONS
Randomization	• Controls all preintervention confounding variables • Does not require advance knowledge of which variables need to be controlled	• Constraints (ethical, practical) on which variables can be manipulated • Possible artificiality of conditions • Resistance to being randomized by many people
Crossover	• If done with randomization, very strong approach: subjects serve as their own controls and thus are perfectly "matched"	• Cannot be used if there are possible carry-over effects from one condition to the next • History threat may be relevant if external factors change over time
Homogeneity	• Easy to achieve in all types of research • Could enhance interpretability of relationships	• Limits generalizability • Requires knowledge of which variables to control • Range restriction could lower statistical conclusion validity
Stratification/blocking	• Enhances the ability to detect and interpret relationships • Offers opportunity to examine stratifying variable as an independent variable	• Usually restricted to a few stratifying variables • Requires knowledge of which variables to control
Matching	• Enhances ability to detect and interpret relationships • May be easy if there is a large "pool" of potential available comparison subjects	• Usually restricted to a few matching variables (except with propensity matching) • Requires knowledge of which variables to match • May be difficult to find comparison group matches, especially if there are more than two matching variables
Statistical control	• Enhances ability to detect and interpret relationships • Relatively economical means of controlling several confounding variables	• Requires knowledge of which variables to control, as well as measurement of those variables • Requires some statistical sophistication

variables and can rarely control all of them. To use homogeneity, stratify, match, or perform ANCOVA, researchers must know which variables need to be measured and controlled. Yet, when randomization is impossible, the use of any of these strategies is better than no control strategy.

STATISTICAL CONCLUSION VALIDITY

One criterion for establishing causality is demonstrating that there is a relationship between the independent and dependent variable. Statistical methods are used to support inferences about whether relationships exist. Researchers can make design decisions that protect against reaching false statistical conclusions. Shadish and colleagues (2002) discussed nine threats to statistical conclusion validity. We focus here on three especially important threats.

Low Statistical Power

Detecting existing relationships among variables requires **statistical power**. Adequate statistical power can be achieved in various ways, the most straightforward of which is to use a sufficiently large sample. When small samples are used, statistical power tends to be low, and the analyses may fail to show that the independent and dependent variables are related—*even when they are*. Power and sample size are discussed in Chapters 13 and 18.

Another aspect of a powerful design concerns how the independent variable is defined. Both statistically and substantively, results are clearer when differences between groups being compared are large. Group differences on the outcomes can be enhanced by maximizing differences on the independent variable. Conn and colleagues (2001) offered good suggestions for enhancing the power and effectiveness of nursing interventions. Note that strengthening group differences is easier in randomized controlled trials (RCTs) than in nonexperimental research. In experiments, investigators can devise treatment conditions that are as distinct as money, ethics, and practicality permit.

Maximizing **precision**, another facet of statistical power, is achieved through accurate measuring tools, controls over confounding variables, and powerful statistical methods. Precision can best be explained with an example. Suppose we were studying the effect of admission into a nursing home on depression by comparing people who were or were not admitted. Depression varies from one older person to another for various reasons. We want to isolate—as precisely as possible—variation in depression attributable to a person's entry into a nursing home. The following ratio expresses what we wish to assess in this example:

$$\frac{\text{Variability in depression due to nursing home admission}}{\text{Variability in depression due to other factors (e.g., age, pain, medical condition)}}$$

This ratio, greatly simplified here, captures the essence of many statistical tests. We want to make variability in the numerator (the upper half) as large as possible relative to variability in the denominator (the lower half), to evaluate precisely the relationship between nursing home admission and depression. The smaller the variability in depression due to confounding variables (e.g., age, pain), the easier it will be to detect differences in depression between older people who were or were not admitted to a nursing home. Thus, reducing variability caused by confounders can increase statistical conclusion validity. As a purely hypothetical illustration, we will attach some numeric values[1] to the ratio as follows:

$$\frac{\text{Variability due to nursing home admission}}{\text{Variability due to all confounding variables}} = \frac{10}{4}$$

If we can make the bottom number smaller, say by changing it from 4 to 2, we will have a more precise estimate of the effect of nursing home admission on depression, relative to other influences. Control mechanisms such as those described earlier help reduce variability caused by extraneous variables. We illustrate this by continuing our example, singling out age as a key confounding variable.

---

[1]You should not be concerned with how these numbers can be obtained. Analytic procedures are explained in Chapter 18.

Total variability in levels of depression can be conceptualized as having the following components:

Total variability in depression = Variability due to nursing home admission + Variability due to age + Variability due to other confounding variables

This equation can be taken to mean that part of the reason why older adults differ in depression is that some were admitted to a nursing home and others were not; some were older, and some were younger; and other factors (e.g., pain) also affect depression.

One way to increase precision in this study would be to control age, thereby removing the variability in depression that results from age differences. We could do this, for example, by restricting age to older people younger than 80 years, thereby reducing the variability in depression due to age. As a result, the effect of nursing home admission on depression becomes greater, relative to the remaining variability. Thus, this design decision (homogeneity) enabled us to get a more precise estimate of the effect of nursing home admission on level of depression (although, of course, this limits generalizability). Research designs differ in the sensitivity with which effects under study can be detected statistically. Lipsey (1990) has prepared a good guide to enhancing the sensitivity of research designs.

Restriction of Range

The control of extraneous variation through homogeneity is easy to use and can help to clarify the relationship between key research variables, but it can be risky. Not only does this approach limit generalizability, but it can also sometimes undermine statistical conclusion validity. When the use of homogeneity restricts the range of values on the outcome variable, relationships between the outcome and the independent variable will be *attenuated* and may therefore lead to the erroneous conclusion that the variables are unrelated. For example, if *everyone* in the sample had a depression score of 50, scores would be unrelated to age, nursing home admission, and so on.

In our example, we suggested limiting the sample of nursing home residents to people younger than 80 years to reduce variability in the denominator. Our aim was to enhance the variability in depression scores attributable to nursing home admission, relative to depression variability due to other factors. But what if few people younger than 80 years were depressed? With limited variability, relationships cannot be detected. Therefore, in designing a study, you should consider whether there will be sufficient variability to support the statistical analyses envisioned. The issue of *floor effects* and *ceiling effects*, which involve range restrictions at the lower and upper end of a measure, respectively, is discussed later in this book.

Unreliable Implementation of a Treatment

The strength of an intervention—and statistical conclusion validity—can be undermined if an intervention is not as powerful in reality as it is "on paper." **Intervention fidelity** (or **treatment fidelity**) concerns the extent to which the implementation of an intervention is faithful to its plan. Intervention fidelity and considerable advice on how to achieve it are discussed by Bova et al. (2017), Rixon et al. (2016), and Siedlecki (2018).

Interventions can be weakened by various factors, which researchers can often influence. One issue concerns whether the intervention is similar from one person to the next. Usually, researchers strive for constancy of conditions in implementing a treatment because lack of standardization adds extraneous variation. Even in tailored, patient-centered interventions, there are protocols, though different protocols are used with different people. Using the notions just described, when standard protocols are not followed, variability due to the intervention (i.e., in the numerator) can be suppressed, and variability due to other factors (i.e., in the denominator) can be inflated, possibly leading to the erroneous conclusion that the intervention was ineffective. This suggests the need for some standardization, the use of procedures manuals, thorough training of personnel, and vigilant monitoring (e.g., observing delivery of the intervention) to ensure that the intervention is being implemented as planned—and that control group members have not gained access to the intervention.

Assessing whether the intervention was delivered as intended may need to be supplemented with efforts to ensure that the intervention was *received* as intended. This may involve a **manipulation check** to assess whether the treatment was perceived in an expected manner. For example, if we were testing the effect of soothing versus jarring music on anxiety, we might want to learn whether participants themselves perceived the music as soothing and jarring. Another aspect of treatment fidelity for behavior change interventions concerns the concept of enactment (Bellg et al., 2004). *Enactment* refers to participants' performance of the treatment-related skills, behaviors, and cognitive strategies in relevant real-life settings.

Example of Attention to Intervention Fidelity
Palese et al. (2022) described fidelity challenges while implementing an intervention aimed at increasing eating among nursing home residents with cognitive decline. Assessments were made after every session of the intervention delivery on the following five dimensions of fidelity: adherence, dose or exposure, intervention quality, participant responsiveness, and program differentiation.

Treatment adherence can be another problem. It is not unusual for those in the intervention group to elect not to participate fully in the treatment—for example, they may stop going to treatment sessions. Researchers should take steps to encourage participation among those in the treatment group. This might mean making the intervention as enjoyable as possible, offering incentives, and reducing burden in terms of data collection (Polit & Gillespie, 2010). Nonparticipation in an intervention is rarely random. Researchers should document which people got what amount of treatment so that individual differences in "dose" can be examined in the analysis or interpretation of results.

TIP Except for small-scale studies, every study should have a **procedures manual** that delineates the protocols and procedures for implementation.

INTERNAL VALIDITY

Internal validity refers to the extent to which it is possible to make an inference that the independent variable, rather than another factor, truly had a causal effect on the outcome. We infer from an effect to a cause by eliminating other potential causes. The control mechanisms reviewed earlier are strategies for improving internal validity. If researchers do not manage confounding variation, the conclusion that the outcome was caused by the independent variable is open to challenge.

Threats to Internal Validity

Experiments possess a high degree of internal validity because manipulation and random assignment allows researchers to rule out most alternative explanations for the results. Researchers who use quasiexperimental or correlational designs must contend with competing explanations of what caused the outcomes. Major threats to internal validity are examined in this section.

Temporal Ambiguity

One criterion for inferring a causal relationship is that the cause must precede the effect. In RCTs, researchers create the independent variable and then observe subsequent performance on an outcome, so establishing temporal sequencing is never a problem. In correlational studies, however, it may be unclear whether the independent variable preceded the dependent variable, or vice versa—and this is especially true in cross-sectional studies.

Selection

Selection (self-selection) encompasses biases resulting from preexisting differences between groups. When individuals are not assigned to groups randomly, the groups being compared are seldom completely equivalent. Differences on the outcomes could then reflect initial group differences rather than the effect of the independent variable. For example, if we found that men who were overweight were more likely to be depressed than men who were not overweight, it would be impossible to conclude that the two groups differed in depression *because* of their weight. The problem of selection is reduced if researchers can collect data on participants' characteristics before the occurrence of the independent variable. In our example, if we could measure men's level of depression *before* they became overweight, then the study could be designed to control earlier levels of depression. Selection bias is the most problematic and frequent threat to internal validity in studies not using an experimental design.

History

The **history threat** concerns the occurrence of external events that take place concurrently with the independent variable and that can affect the outcomes. For example, suppose we were studying the effectiveness of an outreach program to encourage pregnant females in rural areas to improve health practices (e.g., smoking cessation, prenatal care). The program might be evaluated by comparing the average birth weight of infants born in the 12 months before the outreach program with the average birth weight of those born in the 12 months after the program was introduced, using a time series design. However, suppose that 1 month after the new program was launched, a well-publicized TV program about the importance of healthy lifestyles during pregnancy was aired. Infants' birth weight might now be affected by both the intervention and the messages in the TV program, and it would be difficult to disentangle the two effects.

In a true experiment, history is not as likely to be a threat to a study's internal validity because we can often assume that external events are as likely to affect the intervention group as the control group. When this is the case, group differences on the dependent variables represent effects over and above those created by outside factors. There are, however, exceptions. For example, when a crossover design is used, an event external to the study may occur during the first half (or second half) of the experiment, and so treatments would be contaminated by the effect of that event. That is, some people would receive treatment A with the event and others would receive treatment A without it, and the same would be true for treatment B.

Selection biases sometimes interact with history to compound the threat to internal validity. For example, if the comparison group is different from the treatment group, then the characteristics of the members of the comparison group could lead them to have different intervening experiences, thereby introducing both history and selection biases into the design.

Maturation

In a research context, **maturation** refers to processes occurring during the study as a result of the passage of time rather than as a result of the independent variable. Examples of such processes include physical growth, emotional maturity, and fatigue. For instance, if we wanted to evaluate the effects of a sensorimotor program for developmentally delayed children, we would have to consider that progress occurs in these children even without special assistance. A one-group pretest–posttest design is highly susceptible to this threat.

Maturation is often a relevant consideration in health research. Maturation does not refer just to aging but rather to any change that occurs as a function of time. Thus, maturation in the form of wound healing, postoperative recovery, and other bodily changes could be a rival explanation for the independent variable's effect on outcomes.

Mortality/Attrition

Mortality is the validity threat that arises from attrition in groups being compared. If different kinds of people remain in the study in one group versus another, then these differences, rather than the independent variable, could account for observed differences on the outcomes. Severely ill patients might drop out of an experimental condition because it is too demanding, or they might drop out of the control group because they see no advantage to participating. In a prospective cohort study, there may be differential attrition between groups being compared because of death, illness, or geographic relocation. Attrition bias can also occur in single-group quasiexperiments if those dropping out of the study are a biased subset that makes it look like a change in average values resulted from a treatment.

The risk of attrition is especially great when the length of time between points of data collection is long. A 12-month follow-up of participants, for example, tends to produce higher rates of attrition than a 1-month follow-up (Polit & Gillespie, 2009). In clinical studies, the problem of attrition may be especially acute because of patient death or disability.

If attrition is random (i.e., those dropping out of a study are comparable to those remaining in it), then there would not be bias. However, attrition is rarely random. In general, the higher the rate of attrition, the greater the likelihood of bias.

> **TIP** In longitudinal studies, attrition may occur because researchers cannot locate participants, not because they dropped out of the study. An effective strategy for **tracing** people is to obtain **contact information** from participants at each point of data collection. Contact information should include the names, addresses, telephone numbers, and email addresses of two to three people with whom the participant is close (e.g., siblings)—people who could provide information if participants moved.

Testing and Instrumentation

Testing refers to the effects of taking a pretest on people's performance on a posttest. It has been found, particularly in studies of attitudes, that the mere act of collecting data from people changes them. Suppose a sample of nursing students completed a questionnaire about attitudes toward assisted suicide. We then teach them about various arguments for and against assisted suicide, outcomes of court cases, and the like. Then we give them the same attitude measure and observe whether their attitudes have changed. The problem is that the first questionnaire might sensitize students, resulting in attitude changes regardless of whether instruction follows. If a comparison group is not used, it may be impossible to segregate the effects of the instruction from the pretest effects. Sensitization, or testing, problems are more likely to occur when people are exposed to controversial or novel material in the pretest.

A related threat is **instrumentation**. This bias reflects changes in measuring instruments or methods of measurement between two points of data collection. For example, if we used one measure of stress at baseline and a revised measure at follow-up, any differences might reflect changes in the measuring tool rather than the effect of an independent variable. Instrumentation effects can occur even if the same measure is used. For example, if the measuring tool yields more accurate measures on a second administration (e.g., if data collectors are more experienced) or less accurate measures the second time (e.g., if participants become bored and answer haphazardly), then these differences could bias the results.

Internal Validity and Research Design

Quasiexperimental and correlational studies are especially susceptible to threats to internal validity. Table 10.2 lists specific designs that are *most* vulnerable to the threats just described—but it should not be assumed that threats are irrelevant in designs not listed. Each threat represents an alternative explanation that competes with the independent variable as a cause of the outcome. The aim of

TABLE 10.2 • Research Designs and Threats to Internal Validity

THREAT	DESIGNS MOST SUSCEPTIBLE
Temporal ambiguity	Case–control
	Other retrospective/cross-sectional studies
Selection	Nonequivalent control group (especially, posttest-only)
	Case–control
	"Natural" experiments with two groups
	Time series, if the population undergoes a change
History	One-group pretest–posttest
	Time series
	Prospective cohort
	Crossover
Maturation	One-group pretest–posttest
Mortality/ attrition	Prospective cohort
	Longitudinal studies (experimental and observational)
	One-group pretest–posttest
Testing	All pretest–posttest designs
Instrumentation	All pretest–posttest designs

a strong research design is to rule out competing explanations.

An experimental design normally rules out most rival hypotheses, but even in RCTs, researchers must exercise caution. For example, if there is treatment infidelity or contamination between treatments, then history might be a rival explanation for any group differences (or lack of differences). Mortality can be a salient threat in true experiments. Because the experimenter does things differently with the experimental and control groups, people in the groups may drop out of the study differentially. This is particularly apt to happen if the experimental treatment is painful or inconvenient or if the control condition is boring or bothersome. When this happens, participants remaining in the study may differ from those who left, thereby nullifying the initial equivalence of the groups. In short, researchers should consider how best to guard against and detect all possible threats to internal validity, no matter what design is used.

TIP Traditional evidence hierarchies or level of evidence scales (e.g., Figure 2.2) rank evidence sources almost exclusively based on the risk of internal validity threats.

Internal Validity and Data Analysis

The best strategy for enhancing internal validity is to use a strong research design that includes control mechanisms and design features discussed in this chapter. Even when this is possible (and, certainly, when this is *not* possible), it is advisable to conduct analyses to assess the nature and extent of biases. When biases are detected, the information can be used to interpret the substantive results. Moreover, in some cases, biases can be statistically controlled.

Researchers need to be self-critics. They need to consider fully and objectively the types of biases that could have arisen—and then systematically search for evidence of their existence (while hoping, of course, that no evidence can be found). To the extent that biases can be ruled out or controlled, the quality of causal evidence will be strengthened.

Selection biases should always be examined. Typically, this involves comparing groups on pretest measures when pretest data have been collected. For example, if we were studying depression in females who gave birth to a baby by cesarean delivery versus those who gave birth vaginally, selection bias could be assessed by comparing depression scores in these two groups during or before the pregnancy. If there are significant predelivery differences, then any postdelivery differences would have to be interpreted with initial differences in mind (or with differences controlled). In designs with no pretest measure of the outcome, researchers should assess selection biases by comparing groups with respect to key background variables, such as age, health status, and so on.

Whenever the research design involves multiple points of data collection, researchers should analyze attrition biases. This is typically achieved by comparing those who did and did not complete the study on baseline measures of the outcome or on other baseline characteristics.

Example of Assessing Internal Validity Threats
Feeley and colleagues (2020) used a quasiexperimental design to compare stress symptoms and readiness for discharge in mothers of infants cared for in an open-ward neonatal intensive care unit to those cared for in a unit that includes both six-bed pods and single-family rooms. There were no significant differences between groups in stress symptoms. The two groups were comparable when considering infant and mother characteristics except for the mother's education level. Using ANCOVA, they controlled for education level and noted significant differences on readiness for discharge based on maternal education in that mothers in the six-bed pods or single-family rooms perceived their infant's readiness for discharge to be greater than those who were in the open wards.

When people withdraw from an intervention study, researchers are in a dilemma about whom to "count" as being "in" a condition. One approach is a **per-protocol analysis**, which includes members in a treatment group only if they actually received the treatment. Such an analysis is problematic, however, because not receiving the treatment involves self-selection that can undo initial group comparability. This type of analysis will almost always be biased toward finding positive treatment effects. The "gold standard" approach is to use an

intention-to-treat analysis, which involves keeping participants who were randomized in the groups to which they were assigned even if they drop out (Polit & Gillespie, 2009, 2010). An intention-to-treat analysis may yield an underestimate of the effects of a treatment if many participants did not actually get the assigned treatment—but may better reflect what would happen in the real world. One difficulty with an intention-to-treat analysis is that it is often difficult to obtain outcome data for people who have dropped out of a treatment, but there are strategies for estimating outcomes for those with missing data, as we discuss in Chapter 20.

> **Example of an Intention-to-treat Analysis**
> Conradie and colleagues (2020) investigated the treatment of three oral agents in 109 people with treatment-intolerant or nonresponsive multidrug-resistant tuberculosis. In the intent-to-treat analysis, the team found that 98 patients had a favorable outcome to one of the oral agents at the primary endpoint of 6 months after the end of treatment.

In a crossover design, history is a potential threat both because an external event could differentially affect people in different treatment orderings and because the different orderings are in themselves a kind of differential history. *Substantive* analyses of the data involve comparing outcomes under treatment A versus treatment B. The analysis of bias, by contrast, involves comparing participants in the different orderings (e.g., A then B vs. B then A). Significant differences between the two orderings are evidence of an **ordering bias**.

In summary, efforts to enhance the internal validity of a study should not end once the design strategy has been put in place. Researchers should seek additional opportunities to understand (and possibly to correct) the various threats to internal validity that can arise.

CONSTRUCT VALIDITY

Researchers conduct a study with specific exemplars of treatments, outcomes, settings, and people, which are stand-ins for broad constructs. Construct validity involves inferences from study particulars to the higher-order constructs that they are intended to represent. Constructs are the means for linking the operations used in a study to mechanisms for translating the resulting evidence into practice. If studies contain construct errors, the evidence may be misleading.

Enhancing Construct Validity

The first step in fostering construct validity is a careful explication of the treatment, outcomes, setting, and population constructs of interest; the next step is to select instances that match those constructs as closely as possible. Construct validity is further cultivated when researchers assess the match between the exemplars and the constructs and the degree to which any "slippage" occurred.

Construct validity has most often been a concern to researchers in connection with the measurement of outcomes, an issue we discuss in Chapter 15. There is a growing interest, however, in the careful conceptualization and development of theory-based interventions in which the treatment itself has strong construct validity (see Chapter 28). It is just as important for the independent variable (whether it be an intervention or something not amenable to manipulation) to be a strong instance of the construct of interest as it is for the measured outcome to have strong correspondence to the outcome construct. In nonexperimental research, researchers do not create and manipulate the hypothesized cause, so ensuring construct validity of the independent variable is often difficult.

Shadish and colleagues (2002) broadened the concept of construct validity to cover people and settings as well as outcomes and treatments. For example, some nursing interventions specifically target groups that are characterized as "disadvantaged," but there is not always agreement on how this term is defined and operationalized. Researchers select specific people to represent the construct of a disadvantaged group about which inferences will be made, and so it is important that the specific people are good exemplars of the underlying construct. The construct "disadvantaged" must be carefully delineated before a sample is selected. Similarly, if a researcher is interested in such settings as "immigrant neighborhoods" or "school-based clinics," these are constructs that require careful description and the selection of good exemplars that match those constructs.

Threats to Construct Validity

Threats to construct validity are reasons that inferences from a particular study exemplar to an abstract construct could be erroneous. Such a threat could occur if the operationalization of the construct fails to incorporate all the relevant characteristics of the underlying construct or if it includes extraneous content—both of which are instances of a mismatch. Shadish and colleagues (2002) identified 14 threats to construct validity (their Table 3.1) and several additional threats specific to case–control designs (their Table 4.3). Among the most noteworthy threats are the following:

1. *Reactivity to the study situation.* Participants may behave in a particular manner because they are aware of their role in a study (the Hawthorne effect). When people's responses reflect, in part, their perceptions of study participation, those perceptions become an unwanted part of the treatment construct under study. Strategies to reduce this problem include blinding, the use of outcome measures not susceptible to reactivity (e.g., from hospital records), and the use of preintervention strategies to satisfy participants' desire to look competent or please the researcher.

   Example of a Possible Hawthorne Effect
   Lobo et al. (2022) examined the adherence of hand hygiene practices and central line hub disinfection through direct and indirect (video) observation before and after an educational intervention in an adult intensive care unit in Brazil. While both hand hygiene and central line disinfection improved after the education intervention, the indirect observation improvement was less than the direct observation. These findings suggest the Hawthorne effect impacted the results.

2. *Researcher expectancies.* A similar threat stems from the researcher's influence on participant responses through subtle (or not-so-subtle) communication about desired outcomes. When this happens, the researcher's expectations become part of the treatment construct that is being tested. Blinding can reduce this threat, but another strategy is to make observations to detect verbal or behavioral signals of research staff's expectations and correct them.

3. *Novelty effects.* When a treatment is new, participants and research agents alike might alter their behavior. People may be either enthusiastic or skeptical about new methods of doing things. Results may reflect reactions to the novelty rather than to the intrinsic nature of an intervention, and so the intervention construct is clouded by novelty content.

4. *Compensatory effects.* In intervention studies, *compensatory equalization* can occur if healthcare staff or family members try to compensate for the control group members' failure to receive a perceived beneficial treatment. The compensatory goods or services are then part of the construct description of study conditions. *Compensatory rivalry* is a related threat arising from the control group members' desire to demonstrate that they can do as well as those receiving a special treatment.

5. *Treatment diffusion or contamination.* Alternative treatment conditions can become blurred, which can impede good construct descriptions of the independent variable. This may occur when participants in a control group condition receive services similar to those in the treatment condition. More often, blurring occurs when those in a treatment condition essentially put themselves into the control group by dropping out of the intervention. This threat can also occur in nonexperimental studies. For example, in case–control comparisons of smokers and nonsmokers, care must be taken during screening to ensure that participants are appropriately categorized (e.g., some people may consider themselves nonsmokers even though they smoke regularly, but only on weekends).

Construct validity requires careful attention to what we *call* things (i.e., construct labels) so that appropriate construct inferences can be made. Enhancing construct validity in a study requires careful thought before a study is undertaken, in terms of a well-considered explication of constructs, and requires poststudy scrutiny to assess the degree to which a match between operations and constructs was achieved.

EXTERNAL VALIDITY

External validity concerns the extent to which it can be inferred that relationships observed in a study hold true over variations in people, conditions, and settings. External validity has emerged as a major concern in an evidence-based practice (EBP) world in which there is an interest in generalizing evidence from tightly controlled research settings to real-world clinical practice settings.

External validity questions may take several different forms. We may ask whether relationships observed in a study sample can be generalized to a larger population—for example, whether results from a smoking cessation program found effective with pregnant teenagers in Boston can be generalized to pregnant teenagers throughout the United States. Other external validity questions are about generalizing to types of people, settings, or treatments unlike those in the research (Polit & Beck, 2010). For example, can findings about a pain reduction treatment in a study of Australian women be generalized to men in Canada? Sometimes new studies are needed to answer questions about external validity, but external validity often can be enhanced by researchers' design decisions.

Enhancements to External Validity

One aspect of external validity concerns the *representativeness* of the participants used in the study. For example, if the sample is selected to be representative of a population to which the researcher wishes to generalize the results, then the findings can more readily be applied to that population (Chapter 13). Similarly, if the settings in which the study occurs are representative of the clinical settings in which the findings might be applied, then inferences about relevance in those other settings can be strengthened.

An important concept for external validity is *replication*. Multisite studies are powerful because more confidence in the generalizability of the results can be attained if findings are replicated in several sites—particularly if the sites are different on important dimensions (e.g., size, nursing skill mix, and so on). Studies with a diverse sample of participants can test whether study results are replicated for subgroups of the sample—for example, whether benefits from an intervention apply to males *and* females. Systematic reviews are a crucial aid to external validity precisely because they illuminate the consistency of results in studies replicated with different groups and settings.

Threats to External Validity

In the previous chapter, we discussed *interaction effects* that can occur in a factorial design when two treatments are simultaneously manipulated. The interaction question is whether the effects of treatment A hold (are comparable) for all levels of treatment B. Conceptually, questions regarding external validity are similar to this interaction question. Threats to external validity concern ways in which relationships between variables might interact with or be moderated by variations in people, settings, time, and conditions. Shadish and colleagues (2002) described several threats to external validity, such as the following two:

1. *Interaction between relationship and people.* An effect observed with certain types of people might not be observed with other types of people. A common complaint about RCTs is that many people are excluded—not because they would not benefit from the treatment, but because they cannot provide needed research data (e.g., cognitively impaired patients, non-English speakers) or because they would not allow the "best test" of the intervention (e.g., they have complex comorbidities).
2. *Interaction between causal effects and treatment variation.* An innovative treatment might be effective because it is paired with other elements, and sometimes those elements are intangible—e.g., an enthusiastic project director. The same "treatment" could never be fully replicated, and thus different results might be obtained in subsequent tests.

Shadish and colleagues (2002) noted that moderators of relationships are the norm, not the exception. With interventions, it is normal for a treatment to "work better" for some people than for others. We address this issue in Chapter 31.

TRADEOFFS AND PRIORITIES IN STUDY VALIDITY

Quantitative researchers strive to design studies that are strong with respect to all four types of study validity. Sometimes, efforts to increase one type of validity also benefit another type. In many instances, however, addressing one type of validity increases threats to others.

For example, suppose we were scrupulous in maximizing intervention fidelity in an RCT. Our efforts might include strong training of staff, careful monitoring of intervention delivery, and steps to maximize participants' adherence to treatment. Such efforts would have positive effects on statistical conclusion validity because the treatment was made powerful. Internal validity would be enhanced if attrition biases were minimized. Intervention fidelity would also improve the construct validity of the treatment because the content delivered and received would better match the underlying construct. But what about external validity? All of the actions undertaken to ensure that the intervention is strong, construct-valid, and administered according to plan are not consistent with the realities of clinical settings. People are not normally paid to adhere to treatments; nurses are not monitored and corrected to ensure that they are following a script; training in the use of new protocols is usually brief; and so on.

This example illustrates that researchers need to give careful thought to how design decisions may affect various types of study validity. Of particular concern are tradeoffs between internal and external validity.

Internal Validity and External Validity

Tension between the goals of achieving internal validity and external validity is pervasive. Many control mechanisms that are designed to rule out competing explanations for hypothesized cause-and-effect relationships make it difficult to infer that the relationships hold true in uncontrolled real-life settings.

Internal validity was long considered the "sine qua non" of experimental research (Campbell & Stanley, 1963). The rationale was this: If there is insufficient evidence that an intervention really caused an effect, why worry about generalizing the results? This high priority given to internal validity, however, is somewhat at odds with the current emphasis on evidence-based practice. A reasonable question might be: If study results cannot be generalized to real-world clinical settings, who *cares* if an intervention is effective? Clearly, both internal and external validity are important to building an evidence base for nursing practice.

There are several "solutions" to the conflict between internal and external validity. The first (and most prevalent) approach is to emphasize one and sacrifice the other. Most often, it is external validity that is sacrificed. For example, external validity is not even considered in ranking evidence in level of evidence scales (Chapter 2).

A second approach is to use a phased series of studies. In the earlier phase, there are tight controls, strict intervention protocols, and stringent criteria for including people in the RCT. Such studies are **efficacy studies**. Once the intervention has been deemed to be effective under tightly controlled conditions in which internal validity was the priority, it is tested with larger samples in multiple sites under less restrictive conditions, in **effectiveness studies** that emphasize external validity.

A third approach is to compromise. There has been recent interest in promoting designs that aim to achieve a balance between internal and external validity in a single intervention study. We describe such *pragmatic clinical trials* in Chapter 31, a new chapter that discusses the *applicability* of research findings.

Prioritization and Design Decisions

It is impossible to avoid all possible threats to study validity. By understanding the various threats, however, you can pinpoint the tradeoffs you are willing to make to achieve study goals. Some threats are more worrisome than others in terms of likelihood of occurrence and dangers to inferences you would like to make. Moreover, some threats are costlier to avoid than others. Resources available for a study must be allocated to address the most important validity issues. For example, with a fixed budget, you need to decide whether it is better to increase the size of the sample and hence power (statistical conclusion validity) or to use the money on efforts to reduce attrition (internal validity).

The point is that you should make conscious decisions about how to structure a study to address validity concerns. Every design decision has both a "payoff" and a cost in terms of study integrity.

> **TIP** A useful strategy is to create a matrix that lists various design decisions in the first column (e.g., randomization, crossover design), and then use the next four columns to identify the potential impact of those options on the four types of study validity.

CRITICAL APPRAISAL OF STUDY VALIDITY

In critically appraising a research report to evaluate its potential contribution to nursing practice, it is crucial to make judgments about the extent to which threats to validity were minimized—or, at least, assessed and taken into consideration in interpreting the results. From an EBP perspective, it is important to remember that drawing inferences about causal relationships relies not only on how high up on the evidence hierarchy a study is (Figure 2.2), but also, for any given level of the hierarchy, how successful the researcher was in managing study validity and balancing competing validity demands.

RESEARCH EXAMPLE

We conclude this chapter with an example of a study in which careful attention was paid to many aspects of study validity. The design being used in this research is explained more fully in Chapter 31.

Study: Reflexology and meditative practices for symptom management among people with cancer (Wyatt et al., 2021).

BOX 10.1 Guidelines for Critically Appraising Design Elements and Study Validity in Quantitative Studies

1. Was there adequate statistical power? Did the manner in which the independent variable was operationalized create strong contrasts that enhanced statistical power? Was precision enhanced by controlling confounding variables? If hypotheses were not supported (e.g., a hypothesized relationship was not found), is it possible that statistical conclusion validity was compromised and the results are wrong?
2. In intervention studies, did the researchers attend to intervention fidelity? For example, were staff adequately trained? Was the implementation of the intervention monitored? Was attention paid to both the delivery and receipt of the intervention?
3. What evidence does the report provide that selection biases were eliminated or minimized? What steps were taken to control confounding participant characteristics that could affect the equivalence of groups being compared? Were these steps adequate?
4. To what extent did the research design rule out the plausibility of other threats to internal validity, such as history, attrition, maturation, and so on? What are your overall conclusions about the internal validity of the study?
5. Were there any major threats to the construct validity of the study? In intervention studies, was there a good match between the underlying conceptualization of the intervention and its operationalization? Was the intervention confounded with extraneous content, such as researcher expectations? Was the setting or site a good exemplar of the type of setting envisioned in the conceptualization?
6. Was the context of the study sufficiently described to enhance its capacity for external validity? Were the settings or participants representative of the types to which results were designed to be generalized?
7. Overall, did the researcher appropriately balance validity concerns? Was attention paid to certain types of threats (e.g., internal validity) at the expense of others (e.g., external validity)?

Statement of purpose: The purpose of the study was to evaluate the efficacy of a Sequential Multiple Assignment Randomized Trial (SMART) of interventions to improve symptom management among patients with cancer.

Treatment groups: The study was testing two evidence-based practices: reflexology and meditative (mindfulness) practices. Dyads of solid tumor cancer patients and their caregivers were initially assigned to one of these interventions, which are offered in the patients' homes, or to a control group of usual care. After 4 weeks, intervention group dyads that showed little improvement in fatigue were rerandomized to either continuing in the original intervention or adding the alternative intervention.

Method: The researchers were using a design that addresses many validity concerns. Randomization (both initially and at rerandomization) was achieved by using a computer minimization algorithm that is designed to balance the arms for the patient's site of a solid tumor cancer (e.g., breast, lung, colon), stage of cancer, and type of treatment. The researchers estimated how large a sample was needed to achieve adequate power for statistical conclusion validity, using a procedure called power analysis (Chapter 13).

Additional study validity efforts: For dyads in the reflexology group, caregivers were trained by a study reflexologist. For dyads in the meditative group, both the patient and the caregiver were trained by a study meditation provider. All intervention agents were carefully trained and monitored throughout the study. Patients and caregivers in all groups were interviewed twice by telephone, at baseline and then at study week 12. The interviewers were blinded to the dyad's group assignments. The interviewers gathered information about patients' fatigue, pain, depression, and anxiety using instruments known to be of high quality. A study coordinator called patients weekly to ask about their symptoms and also asked caregivers in the intervention groups about the number of sessions conducted with the patients.

The researchers implemented extensive procedures to ensure intervention fidelity. For example, both the intervention agents and the caregivers had to show proficiency in their therapies. The analysis included statistically controlling for demographic and baseline clinical characteristics. The researchers also undertook an attrition analysis to compare the characteristics of those who did or did not drop out of the study.

Findings: There were 347 dyads with 150 dyads in the meditation arm, 150 dyads in the reflexology arm, and 47 in the control. Findings indicated that there were no statistical differences in symptom experience in either the mediation or reflexology group except in the summed symptom score at 8-week point for the group assigned to reflexology.

Conclusions: The researchers concluded that nurses may recommend either meditation or reflexology alone since no differences were found among the therapies, and these study findings indicated that adding an additional therapy at 4 weeks was not warranted.

SUMMARY POINTS

- Study validity concerns the extent to which appropriate inferences can be made. **Threats to validity** are reasons that an inference could be wrong. A key function of quantitative research design is to rule out validity threats.

- Control over confounding participant characteristics is key to managing many validity threats. The best control method is randomization to treatment conditions, which effectively controls all confounding variables—especially in the context of a crossover design.

- When randomization is not possible, other control methods include **homogeneity** (the use of a homogeneous sample to eliminate variability on confounding characteristics); blocking or stratifying, as in the case of a *randomized block design*; **pair matching** participants on key variables to make groups more comparable (or by using **propensity matching**, which involves matching on a **propensity score** for each participant); **balancing** groups to achieve comparability; and **statistical control** to remove the effect of a confounding variable statistically (e.g., through **analysis of covariance**).

- Homogeneity, stratifying, matching, and statistical control share two disadvantages: Researchers must know in advance which confounding

- variables to control, and they can rarely control all of them.
- Four types of validity affect the rigor of a quantitative study: statistical conclusion validity, internal validity, construct validity, and external validity.
- **Statistical conclusion validity** concerns the validity of the inference that a relationship between variables really exists.
- Threats to statistical conclusion validity include low **statistical power** (the ability to detect true relationships among variables); low **precision** (the exactness of the relationships revealed after controlling confounding variables); and factors that weaken the operationalization of the independent variable.
- **Intervention** (or **treatment**) **fidelity** concerns the extent to which the implementation of a treatment is faithful to its plan. Intervention fidelity is enhanced through standardized treatment protocols, careful training of intervention agents, monitoring of the delivery and receipt of the intervention, **manipulation checks,** and steps to promote **treatment adherence** and avoid **contamination of treatments.**
- **Internal validity** concerns the inference that outcomes were caused by the independent variable, rather than by confounding factors. Threats to internal validity include temporal ambiguity (lack of clarity about whether the presumed cause preceded the outcome); **selection** (preexisting group differences); **history** (the occurrence of external events that could affect outcomes); **maturation** (changes resulting from the passage of time); **mortality** (effects attributable to attrition); **testing** (effects of a pretest); and **instrumentation** (changes in the way data are gathered).
- Internal validity can be enhanced through judicious design decisions but can also be addressed analytically (e.g., through an analysis of selection or attrition biases). When people withdraw from a study, an **intention-to-treat analysis** (analyzing outcomes for all people in their original treatment conditions) is preferred to a **per-protocol analysis** (analyzing outcomes only for those who received the full treatment) for maintaining the integrity of randomization.
- **Construct validity** concerns inferences from the particular exemplars of a study (e.g., the specific treatments, outcomes, and settings) to the higher-order constructs that they are intended to represent. The first step in fostering construct validity is a careful explication of those constructs.
- Threats to construct validity can occur if the operationalization of a construct fails to incorporate all relevant characteristics of the construct, or if it includes extraneous content. Examples of such threats include *subject reactivity, researcher expectancies, novelty effects, compensatory effects*, and *treatment diffusion.*
- **External validity** concerns inferences about the extent to which study results can be generalized—i.e., whether relationships observed in a study hold true over variations in people, settings, time, and treatments. External validity can be enhanced by selecting *representative* people and settings and through replication.
- Researchers need to prioritize and recognize tradeoffs among the various types of validity, which sometimes compete with each other. Tensions between internal and external validity are especially prominent. One solution has been to begin with a study that emphasizes internal validity (**efficacy studies**) and then if a causal relationship can be inferred, to undertake **effectiveness studies** that emphasize external validity.

REFERENCES CITED IN CHAPTER 10

Aranda-Gallardo, M., Gonzalez-Lozano, A., Oña-Gil, J. I., Morales-Asencio, J. M., Mora-Banderas, A., & Canca-Sanchez, J. C. (2022). Relation between hyponatraemia and falls by acute hospitalised patients: A case-control study. *Journal of Clinical Nursing, 31*(7–8), 958–966. https://doi.org/10.1111/jocn.15952

Bellg, A., Borrelli, B., Resnick, B., Hecht, J., Minicucci, D., Ory, M, Ogedegbe, G., Orwig, D., Ernst, D., Czajkowski, S., & Treatment Fidelity Workgroup of the NIH Behavior Change Consortium. (2004). Enhancing treatment fidelity in health behavior change studies: Best practices and recommendations from the NIH Behavior Change Consortium. *Health Psychology, 23*(5), 443–451.

Bova, C., Jaffarian, C., Crawford, S., Quintos, J., Lee, M., & Sullivan-Bolyai, S. (2017). Intervention fidelity: Monitoring drift, providing feedback, and assessing the control condition. *Nursing Research*, 66(1), 54–59.

Campbell, D. T., & Stanley, J. C. (1963). *Experimental and quasi-experimental designs for research*. Rand McNally.

Choi, S. H., Lee, Y. W., Kim, H. S., Kim, S. H., Lee, E. H., Park, E. Y., & Cho, Y. U. (2022). Development and effects of a post-traumatic growth program for patients with breast cancer. *European Journal of Oncology Nursing*, 57, 102100. https://doi.org/10.1016/j.ejon.2022.102100

Conn, V. S., Rantz, M. J., Wipke-Tevis, D. D., & Maas, M. L. (2001). Designing effective nursing interventions. *Research in Nursing & Health*, 24(5), 433–442.

Conradie, F., Diacon, A. H., Ngubane, N., Howell, P., Everitt, D., Crook, A. M., Mendel, C. M., Egizi, E., Moreira, J., Timm, J., McHugh, T. D., Wills, G. H., Bateson, A., Hunt, R., Van Niekerk, C., Li, M., Olugbosi, M., Spigelman, M., & Nix-TB Trial Team. (2020). Treatment of highly drug-resistant pulmonary tuberculosis. *New England Journal of Medicine*, 382(10), 893–902. https://doi.org/10.1056/NEJMoa1901814

Feeley, N., Robins, S., Genest, C., Stremler, R., Zelkowitz, P., & Charbonneau, L. (2020). A comparative study of mothers of infants hospitalized in an open ward neonatal intensive care unit and a combined pod and single-family room design. *BMC Pediatrics*, 20(1), 38. https://doi.org/10.1186/s12887-020-1929-1

Lipsey, M. W. (1990). *Design sensitivity: Statistical power for experimental research*. Sage.

Lobo, R. D., Oliveira, M. S., Colella, J. J., Silva, N. D. D., Pastore Junior, L., & Souza, R. C. D. S. (2022). Assessment of the Hawthorne effect during central venous catheter manipulation. *Revista da Escola de Enfermagem da USP*, 56, e20220125. https://doi.org/10.1590/1980-220X-REEUSP-2022-0125en

Morrison, J., Becker, H., & Stuifbergen, A. (2017). Evaluation of intervention fidelity in a multisite clinical trial in persons with multiple sclerosis. *Journal of Neuroscience Nursing*, 49(6), 344–348.

Palese, A., Achbani, B., Hayter, M., & Watson, R. (2022). Fidelity challenges while implementing an intervention aimed at increasing eating performance among nursing home residents with cognitive decline: A multicentre, qualitative descriptive study design. *Journal of Clinical Nursing*, 31(13–14), 1835–1849. https://doi.org/10.1111/jocn.15507

Polit, D. F., & Beck, C. T. (2010). Generalization in quantitative and qualitative research: Myths and strategies. *International Journal of Nursing Studies*, 47(11), 1451–1458.

Polit, D. F., & Gillespie, B. (2009). The use of the intention-to-treat principle in nursing clinical trials. *Nursing Research*, 58(6), 391–399.

Polit, D. F., & Gillespie, B. (2010). Intention-to-treat in randomized controlled trials: Recommendations for a total trial strategy. *Research in Nursing & Health*, 33(4), 355–368.

Qin, R., Titler, M., Shever, L., & Kim, T. (2008). Estimating effects of nursing intervention via propensity score analysis. *Nursing Research*, 57(6), 444–452.

Rixon, L., Baron, J., McGale, N., Lorencatto, F., Francis, J., & Davies, A. (2016). Methods used to address fidelity of receipt in health intervention research: A citation analysis and systematic review. *BMC Health Services Research*, 16(1), 663.

Shadish, W. R., Cook, T. D., & Campbell, D. T. (2002). *Experimental and quasi-experimental designs for generalized causal inference*. Houghton Mifflin Co.

Siedlecki, S. L. (2018). Research intervention fidelity: Tips to improve internal validity of your intervention studies. *Clinical Nurse Specialist*, 32(1), 12–14. https://doi.org/10.1097/nur.0000000000000342

Wyatt, G., Lehto, R., Guha-Niyogi, P., Brewer, S., Victorson, D., Pace, T., Badger, T., & Sikorskii, A. (2021). Reflexology and meditative practices for symptom management among people with cancer: Results from a sequential multiple assignment randomized trial. *Research in Nursing & Health*, 44(5), 796–810. https://doi.org/10.1002/nur.22169

Yu, Y., Ma, Q., Fernandez, I. D., & Groth, S. W. (2022). Mental health, behavior change skills, and eating behaviors in postpartum women. *Western Journal of Nursing Research*, 44(10), 932–945. https://doi.org/10.1177/01939459211021625

11 Specific Types of Quantitative Research

Learning Objectives

1. Describe the various types of quantitative studies.
2. Articulate several ways to evaluate research.
3. Distinguish the various ways to demonstrate the impact of research.
4. Understand the importance of health services outcome research.
5. Identify types of research other than clinical trials, evaluation, and health services outcomes research.

INTRODUCTION

All quantitative studies can be categorized as experimental, quasiexperimental, or nonexperimental in design. This chapter describes the types of research that vary in study purpose rather than research design. The first two types (clinical trials and evaluations) involve interventions, but methods for each have evolved separately because of their disciplinary roots. Clinical trials are associated with healthcare and medicine, and evaluation research is associated with the fields of education, social work, and public policy. There is overlap in approaches, but to acquaint you with relevant terms, we discuss each separately. Later sections of this chapter describe comparative effectiveness research (CER), outcomes research, survey research, and several other types relevant to nursing.

CLINICAL TRIALS

Clinical trials are studies designed to assess clinical interventions. Many nurse researchers are involved in clinical trials, often as members of interprofessional teams.

Phases of a Clinical Trial

In medical and pharmaceutical research, clinical trials often adhere to a planned sequence of studies—often a series of four phases, as follows:

Phase I occurs after initial development of the drug or therapy and is designed primarily to establish safety and tolerance and to determine optimal dose. This phase typically involves small-scale studies using simple designs, such as a one group pretest–posttest design. The focus is on developing the best possible (and safest) treatment.

Phase II involves gathering preliminary evidence about the intervention's practicability. During this phase, researchers assess the feasibility of launching a rigorous test, seek evidence that the treatment holds promise, and identify refinements to improve the intervention. This phase, a pilot test of the treatment, may be designed either as a small-scale experiment or as a quasiexperiment. Pilot tests of interventions are described in Chapter 29.

Example of an Early Phase Clinical Trial
Heyland and colleagues (2018) described a protocol for a Phase II trial of two alternative approaches to partnering with family members in the care of critically ill long-stay ICU patients. A total of 150 families were randomly assigned to a control group or to one of the two approaches of supporting families in shared decision-making (50 per group).

Phase III is a full test of the intervention—a randomized controlled trial (RCT) with randomization to treatment groups under controlled conditions. The goal of this phase is to develop evidence about treatment *efficacy*—i.e., whether the treatment is more efficacious than usual care (or an alternative counterfactual). Adverse effects are also monitored. Phase III RCTs often involve a fairly large sample of participants, sometimes selected from multiple sites to ensure that findings are not unique to a single setting. Phase III (and Phase IV) efforts may also examine the cost-effectiveness of the intervention.

Example of a Multisite RCT
Dionne-Odom and colleagues (2020) undertook a single-blind randomized clinical trial. They examined the impact of a nurse-led palliative care telehealth intervention on family caregiver's quality of life, mood, and burden. The team recruited 158 family caregivers from several outpatient heart failure clinics affiliated with a large academic center and one Veterans Affairs medical center.

Phase IV trials are studies of the *effectiveness* of an intervention in a general population. The emphasis is on the external validity of an intervention that has shown promise of efficacy under controlled (but often artificial) conditions.

TIP Researchers should record their trials in a **clinical trials registry**. These registries provide transparency about research and offer information for accessing the trial. Most registries are searchable online (e.g., by disease, location of the trial). The largest registry is ClinicalTrials.gov; another important registry is the International Clinical Trials Registry of the World Health Organization. Some journals refuse to publish reports of trials unless they have been registered. Protocols for clinical trials are often registered before the study gets underway.

Superiority, Noninferiority, and Equivalence Trials

The vast majority of RCTs are **superiority trials,** in which researchers hypothesize that the intervention is "superior" to (more effective than) the control condition. Standard statistical analysis does not permit a straightforward testing of the null hypothesis (i.e., the hypothesis that the effects of two treatments are comparable). Yet, there are circumstances in which it is desirable to test whether a new (and perhaps less costly or less painful) intervention results in similar outcomes to a standard intervention. In a **noninferiority trial**, the goal is to assess whether a new intervention is no worse than a reference treatment (typically, the standard of care). Other trials are called **equivalence trials,** in which the goal is to test the hypothesis that the outcomes from two interventions are equal. In a noninferiority trial, it is necessary to specify in advance the smallest margin of inferiority on a primary outcome (e.g., 1%) that would be tolerated to accept the hypothesis of noninferiority. In equivalence trials, a *tolerance* must be established for the nonsuperiority of one treatment over the other, and the statistical test is two-sided—meaning that equivalence is accepted if the two are not different (in either direction) by no more than the specified tolerance. Both noninferiority and equivalence trials require statistical sophistication and very large samples to ensure statistical conclusion validity. Further information is provided by Christensen (2007) and Piaggio et al. (2012).

Example of an Equivalence Trial
Verdes-Montenegro-Atalaya et al. (2021) conducted an equivalence trial to compare the effectiveness of two different types of mindfulness-based stress reduction (MBSR) programs. They enrolled a total of 122 primary care providers in Spain and enrolled them into one of three groups: control, abbreviated 4-week MBSR or standard 8-week MBSR. The primary outcome was perceived stress. The results indicated that the standard 8-week program resulted in significant improvements of perceived stress as compared to the 4-week intervention or the control group.

> **TIP** In a traditional Phase III trial, it may take months to recruit and randomize a sufficiently large sample and years to draw conclusions about efficacy (i.e., after all data have been collected and analyzed). In a **sequential clinical trial,** experimental data are continuously analyzed as they become available, and the trial can be stopped when the evidence is strong enough to support a conclusion about the intervention's efficacy. More information about sequential trials is provided by Bartroff et al. (2013).

Pragmatic Clinical Trials

One problem with traditional Phase III RCTs is that, in efforts to enhance internal validity in support of a causal inference, the designs are so tightly controlled that their relevance to real-life applications can be questioned. Concern about this situation has led to a call for **pragmatic** (or *practical*) **clinical trials,** in which researchers strive to maximize external validity with minimal negative effect on internal validity. Pragmatic clinical trials address practical questions about the benefits and risks of an intervention as they would unfold in routine clinical practice. We elaborate on pragmatic clinical trials in Chapter 31.

EVALUATION RESEARCH

Evaluation research focuses on developing information needed by decision-makers about whether to adopt, modify, or abandon a program, practice, procedure, or policy. Patton (2015) distinguishes *research* and *evaluation,* stating that "research has as its primary purpose contributing to knowledge, and evaluation has as its primary purpose informing action" (p. 86). However, evaluations often generate knowledge that can be used in other settings. Concepts from evaluation research are embedded in many efforts to test healthcare interventions.

Evaluations often try to answer broader questions than whether a program is effective—for example, they may involve efforts to improve the program or to learn how the program actually "works" in practice. Evaluations sometimes address *black box questions*—that is, what specifically is it about a multifaceted program that is driving observed effects? Good resources for learning more about evaluation research include the books by Patton (2012) and Rossi and colleagues (2019).

> **TIP** Evaluations can be threatening. Even though the focus of most evaluations is on a nontangible entity (e.g., a program), it is *people* who implement it. People may think that they, or their work, are being evaluated and may feel that their jobs or reputation are at stake. Thus, evaluation researchers need to have more than methodologic skills—they need to be adept in interpersonal relations.

Evaluation Components

Evaluations may involve several components to answer a range of questions, as we describe in this section.

Process/Implementation Analyses

A **process** or **implementation analysis** provides descriptive information about the manner in which a program gets implemented and how it actually functions. A process analysis typically addresses questions such as the following: Does the program operate the way its designers intended? How does the program differ from traditional practices? What were the barriers to its implementation? What do staff and clients like most/least about the program?

A process analysis may be undertaken with the aim of improving a program (a *formative evaluation*). In other situations, the purpose of the process analysis is primarily to describe a program carefully so that it can be replicated—or so that people can understand why the program was or was not effective in meeting its objectives. In either case, a process analysis involves an in-depth examination of the operation of a program, often requiring the collection of both qualitative and quantitative data. Process evaluations sometimes overlap with efforts to monitor intervention fidelity.

> **Example of a Process Analysis**
> Teupen et al. (2021) undertook a process analysis to explore the unsatisfactory results of an intervention aimed at reducing the problem behaviors of dementia in nursing home residents with dementia. They were able to explain the factors and circumstances that impacted the implementation of a complex intervention trial including organizational readiness, resources, and a need for more tailored interventions.

Outcome and Impact Analyses

Evaluations may focus on whether a program or policy is meeting its objectives. The intent of such evaluations is to help people decide whether the program should be continued or replicated. Some evaluation researchers distinguish between an outcome analysis and an impact analysis. An **outcome analysis** (or *outcome evaluation*) simply documents the extent to which the goals of the program are attained, that is, the extent to which positive outcomes occur. For example, a program may be designed to encourage females in a poor rural community to obtain prenatal care. In an outcome analysis, the researchers might document the percentage of pregnant females who had obtained prenatal care, the average month in which prenatal care was begun, and so on, and perhaps compare this information to preintervention community data.

An **impact analysis** assesses a program's **net impacts**—impacts that can be attributed to the program, over and above effects of a counterfactual (e.g., standard care). Impact analyses use an experimental or strong quasiexperimental design because their aim is to facilitate causal inferences about program effects. In our example, suppose that the program to encourage prenatal care involved having nurses make home visits to females in rural areas to explain the benefits of early care. If the visits could be made to pregnant females randomly assigned to the program, the outcomes of the group of females receiving the home visits could be compared with those not receiving them to assess the intervention's net impacts—for example, the percentage *increase* in receipt of prenatal care among the experimental group relative to the control group.

Example of an Impact Analysis
Barreveld and colleagues (2021) tested the impact of an interprofessional case-based learning module that aimed to improve interprofessional students' (pharmacy, dental, medical, nursing, physician assistants) assessment and treatment of pain in a simulated case. Findings indicated that there was no difference in assessment and pain management for the students who were exposed to the case-based learning module as compared to a control group. The authors conclude that more structured education may be required to impact outcomes.

Cost/Economic Analyses

New programs are often expensive to implement, and existing programs also may be costly. In our current situation of spiraling healthcare costs, evaluations (and clinical trials) may include a **cost analysis** (**economic analysis**) to examine whether program benefits outweigh the monetary costs. Administrators make decisions about resource allocations for health services based not only on whether something "works," but also on whether it is economically viable. Cost analyses are typically done in connection with impact analyses and Phase III clinical trials, that is, alongside rigorous tests of a program's or an intervention's efficacy.

Two types of economic analysis are cost–benefit and cost-effectiveness analyses:

- **Cost–benefit analysis,** in which monetary estimates are established for both costs and benefits. One difficulty, however, is that it is sometimes difficult to quantify benefits of health services in monetary terms. There is also controversy about methods of assigning dollar amounts to the value of human life.
- **Cost-effectiveness analysis,** which is used to compare health outcomes and resource costs of alternative interventions. Costs are measured in monetary terms, but outcome effectiveness is not. Such analyses estimate what it costs to produce impacts on outcomes that cannot easily be valued in dollars, such as quality of life. Without information on monetary benefits, however, such research may face challenges in persuading decision-makers to make changes.

Example of a Cost-Effectiveness Analysis
Muir et al. (2022) undertook a cost-effectiveness analysis using three different hypothetical examples: (1) a hospital with static numbers of nurse burnout; (2) a hospital with a nurse burnout reduction program; and (3) a hospital experiencing a decrease in nurse burnout.

Cost–utility analyses are a third type of economic analysis. This approach is preferred when morbidity and mortality are outcomes of interest or when quality of life is a major concern. An index called the **quality-adjusted life year (QALY)** is an important outcome indicator in cost–utility analyses. As a measure of disease burden, QALY includes both the quality and quantity of life lived. One QALY equates to 1 year in perfect health; zero QALY is associated with death.

> **Example of a Cost–Utility Analysis**
> Javanbakht and colleagues (2022) conducted a cost–utility analysis in two groups of patients admitted to a hospital for pneumonia in the United Kingdom. In one group, the respiratory rate was monitored through the use of noninvasive wearable sensors as well as intermittent nurse-led respiratory rate monitoring. They were compared to a group that was only monitored by intermittent nurse-led respiratory rate monitoring. The team found that the approach using both noninvasive sensors and intermittent nurse monitoring was a cost-saving and cost-effective intervention.

In doing economic analyses, researchers must think about possible short-term costs (e.g., clients' days of work missed within 6 months) and long-term costs (e.g., lost years of productive work life). Often the cost analyst examines economic gains and losses from different accounting perspectives—for example, for the target group; the hospitals implementing the program; taxpayers; and society as a whole. Distinguishing these different perspectives is crucial if a program effect is a loss for one group (e.g., taxpayers) but a gain for another (e.g., the target group).

Nurse researchers are increasingly becoming involved in cost analyses—although Cook and colleagues (2017) recently found many deficiencies in the quality of economic evaluations in nursing research in the United States. A useful resource for further guidance is the internationally acclaimed textbook by Drummond and colleagues (2015).

> **TIP** Among those planning an evidence-based practice improvement, the costs of an innovation may be a concern. A key question might be whether there is the potential for **return on investment (ROI)**, that is, whether the innovation might save money (or at least be cost neutral) in the long run, relative to the time and resources that will be expended to implement it in routine practice.

Realist Evaluations

Some nurse researchers have begun to undertake **realist evaluations,** which constitute a theory-driven approach to evaluating programs—especially complex programs or interventions. The realist approach acknowledges that interventions are not always effective for everyone, because people are diverse and embedded in complicated social and cultural contexts. In a realist evaluation, consideration is given to the theoretical mechanisms underlying the effects of an intervention. The focus is on understanding why certain groups benefitted from an intervention while others did not benefit.

Pawson and Tilley (1997), who are key proponents of realist evaluations, argued that to be useful to decision-makers, evaluators need to identify "What works for whom and under what circumstances?" rather than simply, "Does this work?" Realist evaluations are not undertaken with a prescribed set of methods; decisions about design, data collection, and analysis are guided by the types of data needed to answer the evaluation questions and test the initial program theory. Most often, realist evaluations involve the collection of both quantitative and qualitative data, and qualitative approaches play an especially important role.

> **Example of a Realist Evaluation**
> Malcolm and Knighting (2022) used a realist evaluation framework in their study of a home-based, end-of-life pediatric care program in Scotland to understand what worked for whom, why, how it worked, and in what circumstances.

> **TIP** Health technology assessments (HTAs) are systematic evaluations of the effects of health technologies and interventions. HTA is a form of health policy research that examines the health and social consequences of the application of technology. A central goal of such evaluations is to provide policy-makers with evidence on policy alternatives. Ramacciati (2013) has written a useful review about HTAs in nursing.

COMPARATIVE EFFECTIVENESS RESEARCH

Comparative effectiveness research (CER) involves direct comparisons of two or more health interventions. Like realist approaches, CER seeks insights into which intervention works best, for which patients. CER has emerged as a major force in health research; disappointment with some of the methods favored for evidence-based practice—especially the strong reliance on tightly controlled RCTs with placebo comparators—has led to the development of new ideas, new models, and new methods of research that fall within the umbrella of CER.

In the United States, CER gained ground in the early 2000s and the impetus crystallized with the publication of a report by the Institute of Medicine (IOM) in (2009). The IOM, which proposed initial priorities for comparative effectiveness research, defined CER as: "the generation and synthesis of evidence that compares the benefits and harms of alternative methods to prevent, diagnose, treat, and monitor a clinical condition or to improve the delivery of care. The purpose of CER is to assist consumers clinicians, purchasers, and policy makers to make informed decisions that will improve healthcare at both the individual and population level" (Chapter 2, p. 41).

Another major stimulus for CER in the United States was the creation of the independent nonprofit organization called the **Patient-Centered Outcomes Research Institute (PCORI)**, which was authorized by the U.S. Congress in 2010. PCORI specifically sponsors CER—in fact, CER is sometimes referred to as **patient-centered outcomes research**. PCORI funds research that is designed to help patients select the healthcare options that best meet their needs. CER studies often incorporate outcomes that are especially important to patients and their caregivers. The standard outcomes used in medical research (e.g., blood pressure, mortality) are increasingly being supplemented by outcomes in which patients have a strong interest, such as functional limitations, quality of life, and experiences with care. Barksdale and colleagues (2014) have described the relevance of PCORI to nursing, including funding opportunities.

Designs for CER vary widely. Some studies are RCTs involving a comparison of two or more active (nonplacebo) treatments. Some CER projects, however, are observational studies using data from large databases, such as patient registries. CER is described at greater length in Chapter 31, which focuses on methods to enhance the applicability of research to individual patients in real-world clinical settings.

> **Example of Comparative Effectiveness Research**
> Chen et al. (2022) conducted a comparative effectiveness analysis to compare the effects of nonpharmacological interventions aimed at reducing the incidence and duration of delirium in intensive care units. They found that multicomponent strategies, such as early ambulation and family involvement, were most effective in reducing delirium incidence and duration.

HEALTH SERVICES AND OUTCOMES RESEARCH

Health services research is the broad interdisciplinary field that studies how organizational structures and processes, social factors, and personal behaviors affect access to healthcare, the cost and quality of healthcare, and, ultimately, people's health and well-being.

Outcomes research, a subset of health services research, comprises efforts to understand the end results of the structures and processes of healthcare and to assess the effectiveness of healthcare services. While evaluation research focuses on a specific program or policy, outcomes research is a more global assessment of the value of healthcare services. In nursing, outcomes research addresses the question, "What effect does nursing have on patient outcomes?" Outcomes research seeks evidence about the nursing profession's contribution to care.

Outcomes research represents a response to the increasing demand from policy-makers, insurers, and the public to justify care practices and systems in terms of costs and improved patient outcomes. Outcomes research reflects a shift in emphasizing outcome-based healthcare (what do healthcare staff *accomplish*?) rather than task-based healthcare (what do healthcare staff *do* for patients?). The focus of outcomes research in the 1980s and 1990s was predominantly on patient health status and costs associated with medical care, but there is a growing interest in studying broader patient outcomes and an awareness that nursing practice can play a role in quality improvement and healthcare safety, despite the many challenges.

> **TIP** Interest in improving care quality and documenting key health outcomes has led to several initiatives in nursing. For example, the Quality and Safety Education for Nurses project is part of the effort to transform the quality of nursing care by strengthening the competencies of nurses (Sherwood & Barnsteiner, 2017).

Although many nursing studies examine patient outcomes, specific efforts to appraise and document the impact of nursing care—as distinct from the care provided by the overall healthcare system—are less common. A major obstacle is *attribution*—that is, linking patient outcomes to specific nursing actions, distinct from the actions of other members of the healthcare team. Outcomes research has used a variety of traditional nonexperimental designs and methodologic strategies (primarily quantitative ones) but is also developing new methods.

Models of Healthcare Quality

In appraising quality in nursing services, various factors need to be considered. Donabedian (1987) whose pioneering efforts created a framework for outcomes research, emphasized three factors: structure, process, and outcomes. The underpinning of this framework is that good structures will support good processes, which in turn will result in desirable patient outcomes. The *structure* of care refers to broad organizational features. For example, structure can be appraised in terms of such attributes as size and range of services. *Processes* involve aspects of clinical management, decision-making, and clinical interventions (e.g., discharge planning). *Outcomes* refer to the specific clinical end results of patient care, such as quality of life and functional status. Mitchell and coauthors (1998) noted that "the emphasis on evaluating quality of care has shifted from structures (having the right things) to processes (doing the right things) to outcomes (having the right things happen)" (p. 43).

Several modifications to Donabedian framework for appraising healthcare quality have been proposed. One noteworthy framework is the Quality Health Outcomes Model developed by the American Academy of Nursing (Mitchell et al., 1998). This model is less linear and more dynamic than Donabedian original framework and takes client and system characteristics into account. This model does not link actions and processes directly to outcomes. Rather, the effects of actions are seen as mediated by client and system characteristics. This model and others like it are increasingly used as the conceptual framework for studies that evaluate quality of care (Baernholdt et al., 2018). Another quality framework has been developed with specific reference to nursing performance: the Nursing Care Performance Framework or NCPF (Dubois et al., 2013). Outcomes research usually focuses on various linkages within such models, rather than on testing the overall model.

Structure of Care

Several studies have examined the effect of nursing structures on various patient outcomes. Numerous indicators of structure of relevance to nursing care have been identified. For example, nurse staffing levels, nursing skill mix, nursing staff experience, nursing care hours per patient, and continuity of nurse staffing are structural variables that have been found to correlate with patient outcomes. These structural variables can be reliably measured, and data for these variables are generally routinely available.

Efforts have been made to measure a more complex structural variable, nurses' practice environments. The most well-known measure, which has been translated into several languages, is the Nursing Work Index-Revised (Anunciada et al., 2022), particularly its Practice Environment Scale (Harolds & Miller, 2022).

Example of Research on Structure of Care
Hong and Cho (2021) studied the relationship between patient experience scores and hospital characteristics and nurse staffing levels in South Korea. They found that tertiary hospitals in the capital region that had the best scores on nurse staffing were associated with the better patient experience scores.

Nursing Processes and Actions

To demonstrate nurses' effects on health outcomes, nurses' clinical actions and behaviors must be described and documented. Examples of nursing process variables include nurses' problem-solving; clinical decision-making; clinical competence; and specific activities or interventions (e.g., communication, touch, ambulation assistance).

The work that nurses do has been documented in classification systems and taxonomies. Several research-based classification systems of nursing interventions have been developed, refined, and tested. Among the most prominent are the Nursing Diagnoses Taxonomy of NANDA-International as described by Herdman and Kamitsuru (2021) and the Nursing Intervention Classification or NIC developed at the University of Iowa (Wagner et al., 2023). NIC consists of more than 400 interventions, and each is associated with a definition and a detailed set of activities that a nurse undertakes to implement the intervention.

Patient Risk Adjustment

Patient outcomes vary not only because of the care they receive, but also because of differences in patient conditions and comorbidities. Adverse outcomes can occur no matter what nursing intervention is used. Thus, in evaluating the effects of nursing actions on outcomes, there needs to be some way of taking into account patients' risks for poor outcomes or the mix of risks in a caseload.

Risk adjustments have been used in many nursing outcomes studies. These studies typically adopt global measures of patient risks or patient acuity, such as the Acute Physiology and Chronic Health Evaluation (APACHE I, II, III, or IV) system for critical care environments.

Example of Outcomes Research With Risk Adjustment
Using a database that captured all trauma patients who were admitted to an acute care facility in Western Australia between 2009 and 2019, Ravindranath and colleagues (2021) aimed to validate the Geriatric Trauma Outcome Score (GTOS) I and II. They examined age, severity of injury, and blood transfusion in the first 24 hours to unfavorable discharge including death, long-term care placement, or hospice. In those admitted to intensive care units, they examined the GTOS with the APACHE III and the Australian and New Zealand Risk of Death (ANZROD). They found that while the GTOS measures were able to predict survival, they overestimated negative outcomes; were inferior to APACHE and ANZROD; and were no better than age alone in predicting discharge outcome.

Nursing-Sensitive Outcomes

Understanding the link between patient outcomes and nursing actions is critical in making improvements to nursing quality. Outcomes of relevance to nursing can be defined in terms of physical or physiologic function (e.g., heart rate, blood pressure), psychological function (e.g., comfort, satisfaction with care), or health behaviors (e.g., self-care, exercise). Outcomes may be either temporary (e.g., postoperative body temperature) or longer-term (e.g., return to employment). Furthermore, outcomes may be the end results to individual patients receiving care or to broader units such as a family or a community.

Nursing-sensitive outcomes are patient outcomes that improve if there is greater quantity or quality of nurses' care, and this is an area that Aiken and colleagues have researched extensively (Aiken & Sloane, 2020). Examples include pressure ulcers, sepsis, and cardiac arrest. Several nursing-sensitive outcome classification systems have been developed. The American Nurses Association has developed a database of such outcomes, the National Database of Nursing Quality Indicators or NDNQI (Harolds & Miller, 2022; Montalvo, 2007). Also, the Nursing-Sensitive Outcomes Classification has been developed by nurses at the University of Iowa College of Nursing to complement the Nursing Intervention Classification (Moorhead et al., 2023).

> **Example of Research With Nursing-Sensitive Outcomes**
>
> Shin et al. (2023) conducted a retrospective descriptive study to investigate in residents of long-term care facilities in Korea, the linkage between the nursing diagnosis as described by the nurse to the nursing interventions and nursing outcomes using smartphone technology. They found that the top five nursing diagnoses were linked to nursing interventions and outcomes.

Challenges in Outcomes Research

The nursing profession faces several challenges in efforts to document the effects of nursing practice on patient outcomes. As noted by Jones (2016), "empirical evidence to support the unique contribution to quality outcomes is currently lacking" (p. 1). One challenge is that nursing care is more difficult to conceptualize and measure than medical actions. Nursing interventions are often more diffuse than medical interventions—for example, nursing surveillance does not involve a single discrete act, or even a single nurse.

Perhaps for this reason, nursing-sensitive indicators have tended not to be endorsed by bodies that legislate and make policy relating to healthcare quality. For example, in the United States, consensus standards for measures of quality need the endorsement of the National Quality Forum (NQF). As of this writing, the NQF has endorsed only 15 new nursing-sensitive indicators out of the 150 potential measures that were submitted to the NQF for review, and it has not endorsed any such indicators since 2004. Examples of NQF-approved nursing outcome indicators include falls prevalence, pressure ulcer prevalence, and restraint prevalence (Namburi & Lee, 2023). Further research documenting the link between nursing actions and patient outcomes may eventually lead to a greater appreciation of nursing's important role in improving health outcomes.

Another challenge is developing and validating nursing-sensitive *process* variables (Heslop & Lu, 2014; Jones, 2016). Efforts are needed to identify and measure the active ingredients of nursing care. The NQF endorsed only three nursing-sensitive process indicators—all of them relating to smoking cessation counseling for three different disease populations. Clearly, the full scope of nursing practice is not captured in these three NQF indicators.

Dubois and others (2017) have identified a set of indicators that "have sufficient breadth and depth to capture the whole spectrum of nursing care" (p. 3154), and they envision their effort as setting the stage for new initiatives in operationalizing nursing care performance.

One other challenge deserves mention, and that is the difficulty of ensuring full documentation of nursing actions. Reliable nurse process measures that can be assessed for their impact on patient outcomes require comprehensive documentation. The documentation burden for nurses is traditionally high, and the introduction of electronic health records does not necessarily decrease that burden or produce more comprehensive documentation.

SURVEY RESEARCH

A **survey** is designed to obtain information about the prevalence, distribution, and interrelations of phenomena within a population. Political opinion polls are examples of surveys. When a survey involves a sample, as is usually the case, it may be called a **sample survey** (as opposed to a **census**, which covers an entire population). Survey research relies on participants' **self-reports**—participants respond to a series of questions posed by investigators. Surveys, which yield quantitative data primarily, may be cross-sectional or longitudinal (e.g., panel studies). Surveys are especially appropriate for answering Description questions, but longitudinal surveys are also used to address Etiology and Prognosis questions. The quality of evidence from surveys for descriptive and correlational purposes is highly dependent on the quality of the sample used (Chapter 13) and the quality of the data collected (Chapter 15).

Survey research is flexible: it can be applied to many populations; it can focus on a wide range of topics; and its information can be used for many purposes. Information obtained in most surveys, however, tends to be relatively superficial: surveys rarely probe deeply into human complexities.

Any information that can reliably be obtained by direct questioning can be gathered in a survey, although surveys include mostly questions that require brief responses (e.g., yes/no, always/sometimes/never). Surveys often focus on what people do: what they eat, how they care for their health, and so forth. In some instances, the emphasis is on what people plan to do—for example, health screenings they plan to have done—or what they have done in the past.

Survey data can be collected in various ways. The most respected method is through **personal interviews** (or *face-to-face interviews*), in which interviewers meet in person with respondents. Personal interviews tend to be costly because they involve a lot of personnel time. Nevertheless, personal interviews are regarded as the best method of collecting survey data because of the quality of information they yield and because refusal rates tend to be low.

Example of a Survey With Personal Interviews
Schuster and colleagues (2020) conducted a cross-sectional survey involving patients, caregivers, and psychiatrists. They used open-ended questions to understand caregivers' descriptions of when and how they report being involved in care treatment and to identify which topics are mainly discussed.

Telephone interviews are less costly than in-person interviews, but respondents may be difficult to reach on the telephone. Telephoning can be an acceptable method of collecting data if researchers have had prior personal contact with respondents. For example, some researchers conduct in-person interviews in clinical settings at baseline and then conduct follow-up interviews on the telephone. Telephone interviews may be difficult for certain groups of respondents, including those who may have hearing problems.

Questionnaires, unlike interviews, are self-administered. Respondents read the questions and then give their answers in writing. Respondents differ in their reading levels and in their ability to communicate in writing, so care must be taken in a questionnaire to word questions clearly and simply. Questionnaires are economical but are not appropriate for surveying certain populations (e.g., children). In survey research, questionnaires can be distributed in person in clinical settings or through the mail (sometimes called a *postal survey*), but are increasingly being distributed over the Internet. Further guidance on surveys, including mailed and web-based ones is provided in Chapter 14.

Example of an E-Mailed Survey
O'Reilly-Jacob and colleagues (2021) emailed surveys to a sample of nurse practitioners (NP) working in Massachusetts, to examine the impact of temporarily waived state-practice restrictions on NP care delivery during the initial phase of the COVID-19 pandemic. The survey included open and closed questions, including one related to the NPs' perception of the waived restrictions on their clinical work.

Survey researchers are using new technologies to assist in data collection. Most major telephone surveys now use **computer-assisted telephone interviewing (CATI)**, and some in-person surveys use **computer-assisted personal interviewing (CAPI)** with laptop computers. Both procedures involve developing computer programs that present interviewers with the questions to be asked on the monitor; interviewers then enter coded responses directly onto a computer file. CATI and CAPI surveys, although costly, greatly facilitate data collection and improve data quality because there is less opportunity for interviewer error.

Audio-CASI or **ACASI** (*computer-assisted self-interview*) technology is an approach for giving respondents more privacy than is possible in an interview (e.g., when asking about drug abuse) and is useful for populations with literacy problems (Brown et al., 2013). With audio-CASI, respondents sit at a computer and listen to questions over headphones. Respondents enter their responses directly onto the keyboard, without the interviewer seeing the responses. This approach is also being extended to surveys with tablets and smartphones.

Example of Audio-CASI
Lor (2020) conducted a survey with interviews with 30 older Hmong adults from the Midwest using an Audio-CASI tool with both color encoded and text-based responses as well as help from a helper. Findings indicated that some colors had strong cultural connotations while others had none.

There are many excellent resources for learning more about survey research, including the classic books by Fowler (2014) and Dillman et al. (2014).

OTHER TYPES OF RESEARCH

The majority of quantitative studies that nurse researchers have conducted are the types described thus far in this chapter or in Chapter 9, but nurse researchers have pursued other specific types of research. In this section, we provide a brief description of some of them.

- **Translational research.** Translational research (sometimes called *translation science*) is an interdisciplinary field that involves systematic efforts to convert basic research knowledge into practical applications to enhance human well-being.
- **Implementation research.** The goal of implementation research is to solve problems in the implementation of healthcare improvements, such as new programs, policies, or practices.
- **Secondary analysis.** Secondary analyses involve the use of data from a previous study (or from large databases) to test hypotheses or answer questions that were not initially envisioned. Secondary analyses often are based on quantitative data from a large data set (e.g., from national surveys), but secondary analyses of data from qualitative studies have also been undertaken (Beck, 2019).
- **Needs assessments.** Researchers conduct needs assessments to understand the needs of a group, community, or organization. The aim of such studies is to assess the need for special services or to see if standard services are meeting the needs of intended beneficiaries.
- **Delphi surveys.** Delphi surveys were developed as a tool for short-term forecasting. The technique involves a panel of experts who are asked to complete several rounds of questionnaires focusing on their judgments about a topic of interest. Multiple iterations are used to achieve consensus.
- **Replication studies.** Researchers sometimes undertake a replication study, which is an explicit attempt to see if findings obtained in one study can be duplicated in another setting.
- **Methodologic studies.** Nurse researchers have undertaken many methodologic studies, which are aimed at gathering evidence about strategies of conducting high-quality, rigorous research.

CRITICAL APPRAISAL OF STUDIES DESCRIBED IN THIS CHAPTER

It is difficult to provide guidance on critically appraising the types of studies described in this chapter because they are so varied and because many of the fundamental methodologic issues that require an appraisal concern the overall design. Guidelines for appraising design-related issues were presented in the previous two chapters.

Box 11.1 offers a few specific questions for appraising the kinds of research included in this chapter.

BOX 11.1 Some Guidelines for Critically Appraising Studies Described in Chapter 11

1. Does the study purpose match the study design? Was the best possible design used to address the study purpose?
2. If the study was a clinical trial, was adequate attention paid to developing a strong, carefully conceived intervention? Was the intervention adequately pilot tested?
3. If the study was a clinical trial or evaluation, was there an effort to understand how the intervention was implemented (i.e., a process-type analysis)? Were the financial costs and benefits assessed? If not, should they have been?
4. If the study was an evaluation, to what extent do the study results serve the practical information needs of key decision-makers or intended users?
5. If the study was outcomes research, were nursing-sensitive indicators used? Were the hypothesized linkages (e.g., between nursing structures and outcomes or nursing processes and outcomes) cogent in terms of the potential to illuminate nursing's unique contribution to care?
6. If the study was a survey, was the most appropriate method used to collect the data (i.e., in-person interviews, telephone interviews, or mail or Internet questionnaires)?

RESEARCH EXAMPLE

This section describes a clinical trial and several studies that informed the development of this research study.

Study: Results from Project GOLD: A pilot randomized controlled trial of a psychoeducational HIV/STI prevention intervention for black youth, Brawner et al. (2021).

Synopsis: Although HIV prevention interventions exist, there have been barriers to implementation, and this is a particular concern for Black youth for whom the incidence and prevalence of HIV/STI is high. Also concerning is the lack of studies examining the role of mental illness and emotion regulation in sexual risk behaviors and HIV/STI prevention. Studies that do exist are not geared toward Black youth or the sociostructural factors that may contribute mental health concerns and sexual risk behaviors among Black youth. Brawner and colleagues (2021) conducted a pilot randomized control trial of a psychoeducational HIV/STI prevention intervention designed to address the role of mental illness and emotion regulation to reduce the sexually transmitted disease risk among heterosexually active Black youth aged 14 to 17. Findings suggest that program participants reported an increase in condom use, fewer sexual partners, and less depressive symptomatology.

Earlier work by Brawner et al. (2012) was focused on the link between HIV risk behaviors and depression in Black females ages 13 to 19. This study used both a survey and personal interviews to explore these issues. Respondents who reported depression also reported a higher frequency of having sex, more sexual partners, and sexual encounters under the influence of drugs and/or alcohol.

Other work by Brawner (Baker et al., 2012) included being part of a team that conducted focus group interviews with 48 males ages 18 to 24 to understand the sexual risks (e.g., condom use, number of sexual partners) in this population. In further work, Brawner et al. (2013) used focus groups to explore barbers' attitudes and beliefs about delivering HIV prevention strategies to their clients, particularly young Black males.

To develop the intervention that would later be integrated into the clinical trial described above, Brawner conducted seven focus group interviews with a total of 33 Black adolescents who also reported having mental illness. The team explored the influences of HIV/STI risk in this population including social, cultural, and psychological factors.

SUMMARY POINTS

- **Clinical trials** to assess the effectiveness of clinical interventions can unfold in a series of phases. Features of the intervention are finalized in *Phase I*. *Phase II* involves seeking opportunities for refinements and preliminary evidence of feasibility and efficacy. *Phase III* is a full experimental test of treatment *efficacy*. In *Phase IV*, researchers focus primarily on generalized *effectiveness*.

- Most trials are **superiority trials**, in which researchers hypothesize that an intervention will result in better outcomes than the counterfactual. In a **noninferiority trial**, the goal is to test whether a new intervention is no worse than a reference treatment. In **equivalence trials**, the goal is to test the hypotheses that the outcomes from two treatments are equal, within a specified level of tolerance.

- **Evaluation research** assesses the effectiveness of a program, policy, or procedure and often involves several components. **Process** or **implementation analyses** describe the process by which a program gets implemented and how it functions in practice. **Outcome analyses** describe the status of outcomes after the introduction of a program. **Impact analyses** test whether a program caused **net impacts** on key outcomes, relative to a counterfactual. **Cost (economic) analyses** assess whether the monetary costs of a program are outweighed by benefits and include **cost–benefit analyses, cost-effectiveness analyses**, and **cost–utility analyses**. **Realist evaluations** constitute a theory-driven approach to evaluating programs; the theoretical

mechanisms underlying the effects of an intervention are a key concern.
- **Comparative effectiveness research (CER)** involves direct comparisons of clinical and public health interventions to gain insights into which work best for which patients—as well as which have greater risks of harm. The **Patient-Centered Outcomes Research Institute (PCORI)** is a major funder of CER.
- **Outcomes research** (a subset of **health services research**) examines the quality and effectiveness of healthcare and nursing services. Models of healthcare and nursing quality typically encompass several broad concepts, including *structure* (factors such as nursing skill mix); *process* (e.g., nursing actions); client risk factors (e.g., illness severity, comorbidities); and *outcomes*. In nursing, researchers often focus on the effects of nursing structure and processes on **nursing-sensitive outcomes**—patient outcomes that benefit from greater quantity or quality of nurse care (e.g., patient falls, pressure ulcers).
- **Survey research** involves gathering data about people's characteristics, behaviors, and intentions by asking them questions. One survey method is through **personal interviews**, in which interviewers meet respondents face-to-face and question them. **Telephone interviews** are less costly but are inadvisable if the interview is long or if questions are sensitive. **Questionnaires** are self-administered (i.e., questions are read by respondents, who then give written responses) and are usually distributed by mail or over the Internet.
- Other specific types of research include the following: **translational research** (which involves systematic efforts to convert basic research knowledge into practical applications); **implementation research** (in which researchers seek methods to improve the implementation of innovative program, policies, or interventions); **secondary analysis** (in which researchers analyze previously collected data); **needs assessments** (which are designed to understand and document the needs of a group or community); **Delphi surveys** (which involve several rounds of questioning with an expert panel to achieve consensus); **replication studies** (which duplicate prior studies to test whether results can be repeated); and **methodologic studies** (in which the focus is to develop and test methodologic tools or strategies).

REFERENCES CITED IN CHAPTER 11

Aiken, L. H., & Sloane, D. M. (2020). Nurses matter: More evidence. *BMJ Quality & Safety*, *29*(1), 1–3. https://doi.org/10.1136/bmjqs-2019-009732

Anunciada, S., Benito, P., Gaspar, F., & Lucas, P. (2022). Validation of psychometric properties of the Nursing Work Index Revise Scale in Portugal. *International Journal of Environmental Research and Public Health*, *19*(9), 4933. https://doi.org/10.3390/ijerph19094933

Baernholdt, M., Dunton, N., Hughes, R., Stone, P., & White, K. (2018). Quality measures: A stakeholder analysis. *Journal of Nursing Care Quality*, *33*(2), 149–156.

Baker, J. L., Brawner, B., Cederbaum, J. A., White, S., Davis, Z. M., Brawner, W., & Jemmott, L. S. (2012). Barbershops as venues to assess and intervene in HIV/STI risk among young, heterosexual African American men. *American Journal of Mens Health*, *6*(5), 368–382. https://doi.org/10.1177/1557988312437239

Barksdale, D., Newhouse, R., & Miller, J. (2014). The Patient-Centered Outcomes Research Institute (PCORI): Information for academic nursing. *Nursing Outlook*, *62*(3), 192–200.

Barreveld, A. M., Flanagan, J. M., Arnstein, P., Handa, S., Hernández-Nuño de la Rosa, M. F., Matthews, M. L., & Shaefer, J. R. (2021). Results of a team Objective Structured Clinical Examination (OSCE) in a patient with pain. *Pain Medicine*, *22*(12), 2918–2924. https://doi.org/10.1093/pm/pnab199

Bartroff, J., Lai, T. L., & Shih, M. (2013). *Sequential experimentation in clinical trials*. Springer.

Beck, C. T. (2019). *Secondary qualitative data analysis in the health and social sciences*. Routledge.

Brawner, B. M., Baker, J. L., Stewart, J., Davis, Z. M., Cederbaum, J., & Jemmott, L. S. (2013). "The black man's country club": Assessing the feasibility of an HIV risk-reduction program for young heterosexual African American men in barbershops. *Family & Community Health*, *36*(2), 109–118. https://doi.org/10.1097/FCH.0b013e318282b2b5

Brawner, B. M., Gomes, M. M., Jemmott, L. S., Deatrick, J. A., & Coleman, C. L. (2012). Clinical depression and HIV risk-related sexual behaviors among African-American adolescent females: Unmasking the numbers. *AIDS Care*, *24*(5), 618–625. https://doi.org/10.1080/09540121.2011.630344

Brawner, B. M., Jemmott, L. S., Hanlon, A. L., Lozano, A. J., Abboud, S., Ahmed, C., & Wingood, G. (2021). Results from project GOLD: A pilot randomized controlled trial of a psychoeducational HIV/STI prevention intervention for black youth. *AIDS Care, 33*(6), 767–785. https://doi.org/10.1080/09540121.2021.1874273

Brown, J., Swartzendruber, A., & DiClemente, R. J. (2013). Application of audio computer-assisted self-interviews to collect self-reported health data: An overview. *Caries Research, 47*(suppl 1)(0 1), S40–S45.

Wagner, C., Butcher, H., & Clarke, M. (2023). *Nursing interventions classification (NIC)* (8th ed.). Elsevier.

Chen, T. J., Traynor, V., Wang, A. Y., Shih, C. Y., Tu, M. C., Chuang, C. H., Chiu, H. Y., & Chang, H. C. R. (2022). Comparative effectiveness of non-pharmacological interventions for preventing delirium in critically ill adults: A systematic review and network meta-analysis. *International Journal of Nursing Studies, 131*, 104239. https://doi.org/10.1016/j.ijnurstu.2022.104239

Christensen, E. (2007). Methodology of superiority vs. equivalence trials and non-inferiority trials. *Journal of Hepatology, 46*(5), 947–954.

Cook, W., Morrison, M., Eaton, L., Theodore, B., & Doorenbos, A. (2017). Quantity and quality of economic evaluations in U.S. Nursing research, 1997–2015: A systematic review. *Nursing Research, 66*(1), 28–39.

Dillman, D. A., Smyth, J., & Christian, L. (2014). *Internet, phone, mail, and mixed-mode surveys: The tailored design method* (4th ed.). John Wiley.

Dionne-Odom, J. N., Ejem, D. B., Wells, R., Azuero, A., Stockdill, M. L., Keebler, K., Sockwell, E., Tims, S., Engler, S., Kvale, E., Durant, R. W., Tucker, R. O., Burgio, K. L., Tallaj, J., Pamboukian, S. V., Swetz, K. M., & Bakitas, M. A. (2020). Effects of a telehealth early palliative care intervention for family caregivers of persons with advanced heart failure: The ENABLE CHF-PC randomized clinical trial. *JAMA Network Open, 3*(4), e202583. https://doi.org/10.1001/jamanetworkopen.2020.2583

Donabedian, A. (1987). Some basic issues in evaluating the quality of health care. In Rinke, L. T., (Ed.), *Outcome measures in home care* (Vol. 1, pp. 3–28). National League for Nursing.

Drummond, M., Sculpher, M., Claxton, G., Stoddart, G., & Torrance, G. (2015). *Methods for the economic evaluation of health care programs* (4th ed.). Oxford Medical Publications.

Dubois, C., D'Amour, D., Brault, I., Dallaire, C., Dery, J., Duhoux, A., Lavoie-Tremblay, M., Mathieu, L., Karemere, H., Zufferey, A., & Zufferey, A. (2017). Which priority indicators to use to evaluate nursing care performance? A discussion paper. *Journal of Advanced Nursing, 73*(12), 3154–3167.

Dubois, C., D'Amour, D., Pomey, M., Girard, F., & Brault, I. (2013). Conceptualizing performance of nursing care as a prerequisite for better measurement: A systematic and interpretive review. *BMC Nurs, 12*, 7.

Fowler, F. J. (2014). *Survey research methods* (5th ed.). Sage.

Harolds, J. A., & Miller, L. B. (2022). Quality and safety in health care, part LXXX: The national database for nursing quality indicators and the practice environment scale of the nursing work index. *Clinical Nuclear Medicine, 47*(6), e472–e474.

Herdman, T. H., & Kamitsuru, S. (2021). *NANDA International nursing diagnoses: Definitions & classification, 2021–2023,* 12th ed.). Thieme Publishers.

Heslop, L., & Lu, S., Xu, X (2014). Nursing-sensitive indicators: A concept analysis. *Journal of Advanced Nursing, 70*(11), 2469–2482.

Heyland, D., Davidson, J., Skrobik, Y., des Ordons, A., Van Scoy, L., Day, A., Vandall-Walker, V., Marshall, A. P., & Marshall, A. (2018). Improving partnerships with family members of ICU patients: Study protocol for a randomized controlled trial. *Trials, 19*(1), 3.

Hong, K. J., & Cho, S. H. (2021). Associations between nurse staffing levels, patient experience, and hospital rating. *Healthcare, 9*(4), 387. https://doi.org/10.3390/healthcare9040387

Institute of Medicine of the National Academies. (2009). *Initial priorities for comparative effectiveness research.* IOM.

Javanbakht, M., Moradi-Lakeh, M., Mashayekhi, A., & Atkinson, J. (2022). Continuous monitoring of respiratory rate with wearable sensor in patients admitted to hospital with pneumonia compared with intermittent nurse-led monitoring in the United Kingdom: A cost-utility analysis. *Pharmacoeconomics Open, 6*(1), 73–83. https://doi.org/10.1007/s41669-021-00290-7

Jones, T. (2016). Outcome measurement in nursing: Imperatives, ideals, history, and challenges. *The Online Journal of Issues in Nursing, 21*, 1.

Lor, M. (2020). Color-encoding visualizations as a tool to assist a nonliterate population in completing health survey responses. *Informatics for Health and Social Care, 45*(1), 31–42. https://doi.org/10.1080/17538157.2018.1540422

Malcolm, C., & Knighting, K. (2022). A realist evaluation of a home-based end of life care service for children and families: What works, for whom, how, in what circumstances and why? *BMC Palliative Care, 21*(1), 31. https://doi.org/10.1186/s12904-022-00921-8

Mitchell, P., Ferketich, S., & Jennings, B. (1998). Quality health outcomes model. American Academy of Nursing Expert Panel on Quality Health Care. *Image—The Journal of Nursing Scholarship, 30*(1), 43–46.

Montalvo, I. (2007). The National Database of Nursing Quality Indicators® (NDNQI®). *The Online Journal of Issues in Nursing, 12*(3). https://doi.org/10.3912/OJIN.Vol12No03Man02

Moorhead, S., Swanson, E., & Johnson, M. (2023). *Nursing outcomes classification(NOC): Measurement of health outcomes* (7th ed.). Elsevier.

Muir, K. J., Wanchek, T. N., Lobo, J. M., & Keim-Malpass, J. (2022). Evaluating the costs of nurse burnout-attributed turnover: A Markov modeling approach. *Journal of Patient Safety, 18*(4), 351–357. https://doi.org/10.1097/PTS.0000000000000920

Namburi, N., & Lee, L. S. (2023). *National quality forum.* StatPearls Publishing.

O'Reilly-Jacob, M., Perloff, J., Sherafat-Kazemzadeh, R., & Flanagan, J. (2022). Nurse practitioners' perception of temporary full practice authority during a COVID-19 surge: A qualitative study. *International Journal of Nursing Studies*, *126*, 104141. https://doi.org/10.1016/j.ijnurstu.2021.104141

Patton, M. Q. (2012). *Essentials of utilization-focused evaluation*. Sage.

Patton, M. Q. (2015). *Qualitative research and evaluation methods* (4th ed.). Sage.

Pawson, R., & Tilley, N. (1997). *Realistic evaluation*. Sage.

Piaggio, G., Elbourne, D., Pocock, S., Evans, S., Altman, D., CONSORT Group. (2012). Reporting of noninferiority and equivalence randomized trials: Extension of the CONSORT 2010 statement. *Journal of the American Medical Association*, *308*(24), 2594–2604.

Ramacciati, N. (2013). Health technology assessment in nursing: A literature review. *International Nursing Review*, *60*(1), 23–30.

Ravindranath, S., Ho, K. M., Rao, S., Nasim, S., & Burrell, M. (2021). Validation of the geriatric trauma outcome scores in predicting outcomes of elderly trauma patients. *Injury*, *52*(2), 154–159. https://doi.org/10.1016/j.injury.2020.09.056

Rossi, P., Lipsey, M., & Henry, G. (2019). *Evaluation: A systematic approach* (8th ed.). Sage.

Schuster, F., Holzhüter, F., Heres, S., & Hamann, J. (2020). Caregiver involvement in psychiatric inpatient treatment—a representative survey among triads of patients, caregivers and hospital psychiatrists. *Epidemiology and Psychiatric Sciences*, *29*, e129. https://doi.org/10.1017/S2045796020000426

Sherwood, G., & Barnsteiner, J. (2017). *Quality and safety in nursing: A competence approach to improving outcomes*, 2nd ed. Wiley-Blackwell.

Shin, J. H., Jung, S. O., & Lee, J. S. (2024). *35*(1), 46–68, Identification of North American Nursing Diagnosis Association—Nursing Interventions Classification—Nursing Outcomes Classification of nursing home residents using on-time data by android smartphone application by registered nurses. *International Journal of Nursing Knowledge*, *2*, 90. https://doi.org/10.1111/2047-3095.12419

Teupen, S., Holle, D., & Roes, M. (2021). Types of implementation of the dementia-specific case conference concept WELCOME-IdA in nursing homes: A qualitative process evaluation of the FallDem effectiveness trial. *Implementation Science Communication*, *2*(1), 90. https://doi.org/10.1186/s43058-021-00191-0

Verdes-Montenegro-Atalaya, J. C., Pérula-de Torres, L. Á., Lietor-Villajos, N., Bartolomé-Moreno, C., Moreno-Martos, H., Rodríguez, L. A., Grande-Grande, T., Pardo-Hernández, R., León-Del-Barco, B., Santamaría-Peláez, M., Mínguez, L. A., González-Santos, J., Soto-Cámara, R., González-Bernal, J. J., & On Behalf of the Minduudd Collaborative Study Group. (2021). Effectiveness of a mindfulness and self-compassion standard training program versus an abbreviated training program on stress in tutors and resident intern specialists of family and community medicine and nursing in Spain. *International Journal of Environmental Research and Public Health*, *18*(19), 10230. https://doi.org/10.3390/ijerph181910230

12 | Quality Improvement and Improvement Science

Learning Objectives

1. Understand the role of quality improvement (QI) to make changes in practice.
2. Distinguish the difference between QI and original research.
3. Articulate how QI may improve patient outcomes and result in better system performance.
4. Describe the various approaches to QI.
5. Identify the advantages and disadvantages of each approach to QI.

INTRODUCTION

The improvement of healthcare services and patient outcomes is a goal shared by all health disciplines. Several forces converged around the turn of the century that led to the emergence of new endeavors and lines of inquiry relating specifically to healthcare improvement. Quality improvement (QI) and improvement science are rapidly evolving and are still in their early stages of development, leaving abundant opportunity for nurses to participate as leaders in this field. This chapter highlights a few key features of quality improvement initiatives; we urge you to consult other references (e.g., Finkelman, 2018) for more comprehensive presentations.

QUALITY IMPROVEMENT BASICS

In this section, we describe how quality improvement (QI) differs from research, discuss the QI movement, and review basic features of QI.

Quality Improvement vs. Research

A decade ago, there was a lot of discussion in nursing journals about the differences and similarities between quality improvement, research, and evidence-based practice (EBP) projects. All three have a lot in common, notably the use of systematic methods of solving health problems with an overall aim of fostering improvements in health care. Often, the methods used overlap: patient data and statistical analysis—sometimes combined with analysis of qualitative data—are also used in all three.

Although the definitions proposed for QI, research, and EBP are distinct, it is not always easy to distinguish them in real-world projects; as a result, there is sometimes confusion. According to the U.S. Centers for Medicare and Medicaid Services (CMS, 2021) "**quality improvement** is the framework used to systematically improve care. Quality improvement seeks to standardize processes and structure to reduce variation, achieve predictable results, and improve outcomes for patients, healthcare systems, and organizations. Structure includes things like technology, culture, leadership, and physical capital; process includes knowledge capital (e.g., standard operating procedures) or human capital (e.g., education and training)." Under the code of U.S. Federal Regulations, *research* is defined as a "systematic investigation, including research development, testing and evaluation, designed to develop or contribute to generalizable knowledge" (U.S. Code of Federal Regulations). EBP projects are efforts to translate "best evidence" into protocols to guide the actions of healthcare staff to maximize good outcomes for clients.

A key difference between research and QI concerns how patients are exposed to risk—in QI projects, risks are usually minimal. As a result, most QI efforts (as well as EBP projects) are not subject to the regulations protecting human subjects in research, and patient informed consent is typically not obtained.

In the past, the expectation for QI was that results would be internally disseminated; publication in professional journals was not considered necessary. However, not only are many QI projects now described in professional journals, but several journals are now devoted specifically to improvement activities.

An important consideration of QI, EBP, and research is the generalizability of the knowledge gained from the respective project. The growing interest in healthcare improvement has led to efforts to inspire more systematic, rigorous, theoretical, and replicable improvement activity—in short, to develop and advance **improvement science** (Marshall et al., 2015). Increasingly, improvement researchers are developing their own base of QI evidence. Systematic reviews of QI evidence are being published and will facilitate **evidence-based quality improvement** (**EBQI**).

The Impetus for Improvement in Health Care

In 1999, the U.S. Institute of Medicine (IOM) published an influential report, *To Err Is Human*, which highlighted the large number of deaths in the United States attributable to medical errors—nearly 100,000 deaths annually. Two years later, IOM (2001) published another report, *Crossing the Quality Chasm*, which outlined six goals to address quality problems, sometimes referred to by the acronym **STEEEP** (Finkelman, 2020):

1. *Safe.* Avoiding injuries to patients from the care intended to help them
2. *Timely.* Reducing waits and harmful delays
3. *Effective.* Providing services based on knowledge (i.e., evidence-based) and avoiding the provision of services not likely to benefit patients
4. *Efficient.* Avoiding waste of resources and energy
5. *Equitable.* Providing care that does not vary in quality because of patients' personal characteristics
6. *Patient-centered.* Providing care that is respectful of individual patient preferences and ensuring that patient values guide clinical decisions

Yet another IOM report, *Health Professions Education: A Bridge to Quality*, was published in 2003. The expert panel that prepared this report identified five core competencies for healthcare professionals to reach a desired level of quality of care: (1) providing patient-centered care, (2) working in interprofessional teams, (3) employing EBP, (4) applying quality improvement, and (5) using information technology.

These and other IOM "Quality Chasm" reports have galvanized diverse sectors of the healthcare system (e.g., providers, policy-makers, the public) and various healthcare disciplines with a sense of urgency to address quality problems. Perspectives on responsibility for quality health care began to shift from healthcare administrators to *all* healthcare providers. Batalden and Davidoff (2007) proposed defining quality improvement as "the combined and unceasing efforts of everyone—healthcare professionals, patients and their families, researchers, payers, planners and educators—to make changes that will lead to better patient outcomes (health), better system performance (care), and better professional development (learning)" (p. 2).

Features of Quality Improvement and Improvement Science

Quality improvement projects typically have as their primary goal the swift attainment of positive change in a healthcare service. QI projects are practical and are often focused on a specific problem identified in a local context. Quality improvement can also involve an ongoing process in which interprofessional teams collaborate to improve systems and processes, with the goals of reducing waste, increasing efficiency, and increasing satisfaction. The ongoing nature of such efforts is integral to a quality management philosophy called **continuous quality improvement** (**CQI**). CQI encourages members of healthcare teams to continuously ask such questions as, "How are we doing?" and "Can we do this better?" (National Learning Consortium, 2013).

Several features characterize many QI projects. For example, the intervention or protocol for an improvement project can change as it is being evaluated to incorporate new ideas and insights—unlike what occurs in quantitative studies. Another feature is that QI projects are designed to achieve an improvement that is sustainable. Typically, QI projects are interprofessional, involving a team with diverse perspectives on a problem.

> **TIP** The Agency for Healthcare Research and Quality (AHRQ) in the United States offers training in a teamwork system (TeamSTEPPS) designed to improve communication and teamwork skills and eliminate barriers to quality and safety.

The field of healthcare improvement is an emergent one characterized by debate and differences of opinion. In particular, there have been discussions about whether improvement efforts can be simultaneously practical (aimed at producing change in local contexts) and scientific (aimed at producing knowledge that is more generalizable) (Portela et al., 2015). The dividing line is increasingly blurry, and our view is that QI will inevitably serve both purposes.

Marshall and colleagues (2015) are among a growing group of advocates promoting improvement science as a distinct discipline. They have argued that improvement science "aims to generate local wisdom and generalizable or transferable knowledge with robust, well established research methods applied in highly pragmatic ways" (p. 419). They have noted—as have many other commentators—that QI projects are often methodologically weak, relying on poor strategies and unverified data to reach conclusions. They called for the adoption of a more scientific approach to healthcare improvement and for increased efforts to draw on and contribute to theories of how change happens in complex adaptive systems. Others have noted the importance of carefully studying the role of contextual factors on quality improvement initiatives (Coles et al., 2017).

> **TIP** A Delphi survey was conducted (by a team that included nurses) with experts in seven European countries to arrive at a consensus definition of *improvement science*. The definition is closely aligned with the aims articulated in IOM's Quality Chasm reports (i.e., STEEEP): "The generation of knowledge to cultivate change and deliver person-centered care that is safe, effective, efficient, equitable and timely. It improves patient outcomes, health system performance and population health" (Skela-Savič, 2017).

Despite great enthusiasm for improvement initiatives, QI teams are often confronted with numerous challenges. For example, Tappen and colleagues (2017) described several critical barriers to implementing a widely publicized change initiative in long-term care settings (INTERACT). Major barriers included the magnitude and complexity of the change, leadership instability, competing demands, stakeholder resistance, scarce resources, and technical problems.

Nursing and Improvement Science

Seidl and Newhouse (2012) have argued that "quality improvement skills and engagement are central to nurses' responsibility in healthcare settings" (p. 299). Indeed, quality improvement is one of the six core competencies identified by the Quality and Safety Education for Nurses (QSEN) project. (The six QSEN core competencies directly map to the five competencies identified in the 2003 IOM report on healthcare education, with the exception of the additional QSEN competency category for *safety*.)

Nurses are being encouraged to not only participate in QI efforts but also to play a lead role. As Johnson (2012) observed, "Who better to lead the effort to improve healthcare delivery and outcomes than the professionals delivering the majority of health care…?" (p. 113). To play such a role, nurses must learn new skills and become familiar with new tools—which we hope to facilitate in this chapter.

Indeed, nurses have been prominent in several organizations devoted to QI. For example, the Improvement Science Research Network (ISRN) is a group whose mission is to accelerate interprofessional improvement science in a systems context. ISRN was funded by the National Institutes of Nursing Research, beginning in 2009 with a grant to researchers at the University of Texas. As another example, a leading and cutting-edge organization in improvement science, the Institute for Healthcare Improvement (IHI), had several nurses on its staff.

Nurses have worked on QI teams within local healthcare organizations and have also been involved in several large-scale improvement projects. The Robert Wood Johnson Foundation (RWJF) has been an especially strong supporter of nurses' efforts in this area. For example, the QSEN project was funded by the foundation, and the Nursing Alliance for Quality Care was started in 2010 with support from RWJF. An important quality initiative, called Transforming Care at the Bedside (TCAB), was implemented by the foundation in collaboration with the IHI. The TCAB initiative developed, tested, and disseminated a process for empowering nurses to take the lead in improving the quality of patient care on medical-surgical units. TCAB-related projects have been undertaken in several countries.

Example of a TCAB Project
Adams and colleagues (2022) implemented a TCAB program to minimize nurse distractions during the chemotherapy verification process. They found that using a clear and concise checklist, both nurses' distractions during the chemotherapy verification process and medication administration errors decreased.

Types of Quality Improvement Interventions

Efforts to improve quality and safety in healthcare organizations have involved a wide variety of approaches to achieving positive change. Ting and colleagues (2009) have identified eight types of QI intervention:

1. *Provider education.* Many QI projects involve teaching members of healthcare teams about how best to manage particular situations or conditions. Educational interventions might involve workshops, the distribution of educational material, or other forms of educational outreach.

Example of a Provider Education Quality Improvement Project
Aqtash and colleagues (2022) undertook a QI project in the United Arab Emirates (UAE). The structured nursing leadership program was implemented with the aim of improving nurse managers' professional abilities and perception of their management and leadership competencies. They found that the structured program did improve nurses' leadership scores based on the Management Competency Self-Assessment.

2. *Provider reminders.* QI projects sometimes involve the development of reminders or decision support materials designed to prompt healthcare professionals to undertake some action. The reminders can be paper-based or electronic.

Example of Reminders to Nurses in a Quality Improvement Project
In a quality improvement project aimed at reducing hospital acquired pressure injuries, Gupta et al. (2020) implemented a bundle and used reminders such as signs, turning clocks, calendars reporting pressure injury. The incidence of pressure injuries was reduced by >80% and further, this was sustained over a 4-year period.

3. *Audit and feedback.* This approach to QI involves providing a summary of clinical performance delivered by individual healthcare providers or units back to those providers. The feedback is often accompanied by recommended targets or benchmarks.

Example of the Use of Audits in Quality Improvement

In describing the implementation of the Focus of Care Initiatives to improve patient care in New Zealand, Aspinall et al. (2023) described the importance of audits/peer review by peers and leaders throughout the implementation process. The program is multifaceted and includes strategies to improve communication, clinical monitoring and management, the clinical environment, comfort and pain management, respect, privacy and dignity, nutrition and hydration, safety prevention, personal care, and self-care.

4. *Patient education.* Quality improvement efforts sometimes involve interventions designed to increase patients' understanding of specific prevention or treatment strategies.
5. *Promotion of patient self-management.* Other QI initiatives develop resources to promote patient self-management and compliance with recommended treatment plans. This approach sometimes involves providing patients with access to resources that support their day-to-day decisions.
6. *Patient reminders.* QI initiatives sometimes involve developing methods (e.g., phone calls, text messages) to encourage patients to keep appointments or to adhere to self-care regimens.

Example of a Patient-Focused Quality Improvement Initiative

Ziyar et al. (2022) implemented a QI project to improve patients' understanding of epinephrine autoinjectors, their usage, and the frequency of patients carrying them with them at all times. After the implementation of the project that included both education and reminders, they noted an 80% improvement in the knowledge of the use of and carrying of the epinephrine injector.

7. *Structural changes and case management programs.* QI efforts may involve structural changes, such as the creation of case management systems or disease management teams. Systems can be implemented to coordinate diagnosis, treatment, and follow-up.

Example of a Care Coordination Quality Improvement Initiative

Matiz and colleagues (2021) conducted a quality improvement initiative. Over a 4-month period, they implemented and evaluated the impact of nurse care managers' longitudinal care in the home on children with special health care needs. The results indicated that there was a statistically significant reduction in the number of emergency department visits and inpatient admissions postintervention ($p < .05$).

8. *Financial incentives, regulation, and policy.* QI projects sometimes involve financial incentives offered to clinicians for performing certain care processes or achieving specific outcomes.

Example of a Financial Incentive Quality Improvement Program

Berry and colleagues (2022) describe an incentive program implemented in nursing homes during COVID-19 with nursing home staff. They compared those who were offered rewards such as T-shirts to those who were not. Those units who were offered incentives had vaccination champions and set vaccination goals as well as other low-cost incentives were more likely to have staff with higher rates of vaccination.

Ting and colleagues (2009) have pointed out that, based on systematic reviews, these QI strategies have typically yielded small to modest effects. Like other commentators, they advocated for a more thoughtful approach to QI: "One important reason for the generally poor performance of these established quality improvement interventions is that they are often lifted off the shelf with little thought to the degree that the selected solution matches the target quality problem" (p. 1968). Similarly, Shojania and Grimshaw (2005) have noted that "the choices of particular interventions lack compelling theories predicting their success or informing specific features of their development" (p. 148). Ting et al. have also observed that the limited impact of QI interventions could reflect inattention to mediating factors and to contextual factors related to the implementation setting.

TIP For many years, the concept known as The Triple Aim was a popular way to conceptualize the optimization of health system performance. The Triple Aim guided health system improvement in three dimensions of performance simultaneously: improving the health of populations, enhancing patients' experience of care, and reducing costs. In 2014, Bodenheimer and Sinsky urged the inclusion of a fourth dimension, resulting in The Quadruple Aim: the improvement of the work life of healthcare providers. Thus, some QI projects now involve efforts to improve the wellbeing and satisfaction of clinicians and other health staff as a path to improving patient care.

QUALITY IMPROVEMENT MODELS

Quality improvement projects typically are based on one of several general models to guide processes and activities. We briefly review four prominent models and provide examples of QI projects linked to these models in which nurses have played a role.

The Lean Approach

Many quality improvement initiatives in healthcare use process improvement methods adapted from industry. The **Lean approach,** also called the *Toyota Production System*, is an important example. Lean thinking has been used in industry and health care in efforts to achieve improved quality and efficiency at lower costs (Institute for Healthcare Improvement, 2005). A major feature of Lean is that it strives to eliminate three types of waste: (1) unnecessary actions, waiting, overproduction; (2) unevenness and variability in product or in flow of information; and (3) unreasonableness of a process for a person's (or equipment's) capability. The goal of a Lean process is to eliminate non–value-added steps, to identify what "value" means to customers (patients) and to serve customers' needs.

Lean approaches generally focus on an entire system or process—for example, from the time a patient enters a healthcare setting to the time the patient leaves. Lean thinking involves systematically analyzing steps in the process of providing a care service and rethinking the process to make it more efficient. Flow diagrams are used to critically analyze processes to look for inefficiencies, redundancies, and opportunities to improve workflow. The goal is continuous improvement and standardization of work practices. In nursing and health care, the Lean approach has been used to improve patient flow in clinical areas (e.g., in the emergency department, in the operating room) and to reduce waiting times (Johnson et al., 2012).

Six Sigma

The **Six Sigma** approach was developed by the Motorola Corporation in the 1980s (Pyzdek & Keller, 2014). "Sigma" refers to the Greek letter (σ), which is used as the representation of a statistical index of variation—the standard deviation (Chapter 17). When a product or process is almost perfect, there is minimum variation; the boundaries for performance are three standard deviations above and below an average—that is, six sigma. The Six Sigma standard is 3.4 problems (e.g., medication errors) per million "opportunities."

The Six Sigma model uses a systematic framework to understand and improve performance. The model involves five steps (DMAIC): define, measure, analyze, improve, and control. The goal is to improve outputs by minimizing variation, which is assessed using *control charts* with data collected multiple times before and after QI changes are made. Six Sigma methods have been widely adopted in quality improvement efforts, often used jointly with other methods such as Lean (sometimes called Lean Six Sigma) or Plan-Do-Study-Act (PDSA)/Plan-Do-Check-Act (PDCA), which we discuss next.

> **Example of a Lean Six Sigma Quality Improvement Project**
> Martin and colleagues (2022) used Lean and Six Sigma tools and methodology to identify why patients were not being screened for delirium in the emergency room and then to provide an education program aimed at improving screening. The multidisciplinary team found that the program resulted in a change from 16% of patients being screened at baseline to 92% being screened at 17 weeks post the intervention.

Plan-Do-Study-Act. The most widely used QI model in health care is **Plan-Do-Study-Act (PDSA),**

which is sometimes referred to as **Plan-Do-Check-Act (PDCA)**. The PDSA cycle, part of the IHI's Model for Improvement, was originally introduced by Deming and Shewhart as a framework for CQI in business and manufacturing (Hughes, 2008). Typically, PDSA relies on multiple **rapid cycles** of investigating and acting on a problem. The idea underpinning rapid cycle improvement is to first try an improvement strategy on a small scale to see how well it works and then modify it and try it again until there is confidence in the effectiveness of the change.

Deming (1988) used the acronym FOCUS along with PDSA to guide process improvements:

- **F:** Find a process with opportunity for improvement
  - Finding a process typically involves brainstorming, reviewing information about trends and events, and preparing an *opportunity statement* that identifies the key issue and its importance.
- **O:** Organize a team that understands the process
  - Key stakeholders in the process from all relevant disciplines need to be identified, and representatives need to be recruited.
- **C:** Clarify current knowledge about the process
  - Current best practices should be examined by doing a literature review. Also, current workflow in the institution is often analyzed by creating flowchart diagrams, which can help identify why the current process might be problematic.
- **U:** Understand causes of variation or poor quality
  - In this step, the team examines why variations exist or why current practices deviate from best practices.
- **S:** Select a part of the process to improve
  - The last step is to consider what specific aspects of a problem will be addressed.

As shown in Figure 12.1, these five steps lead to PDSA cycles. PDSA allows the QI team to test improvement strategies in a controlled manner, to measure results of these strategies, and to drive further improvements. The PDSA/PDCA process involves the following:

1. **Plan:** The QI team initially works on developing explicit strategies or interventions to address the problem identified during the FOCUS work. During this phase, the team also develops a

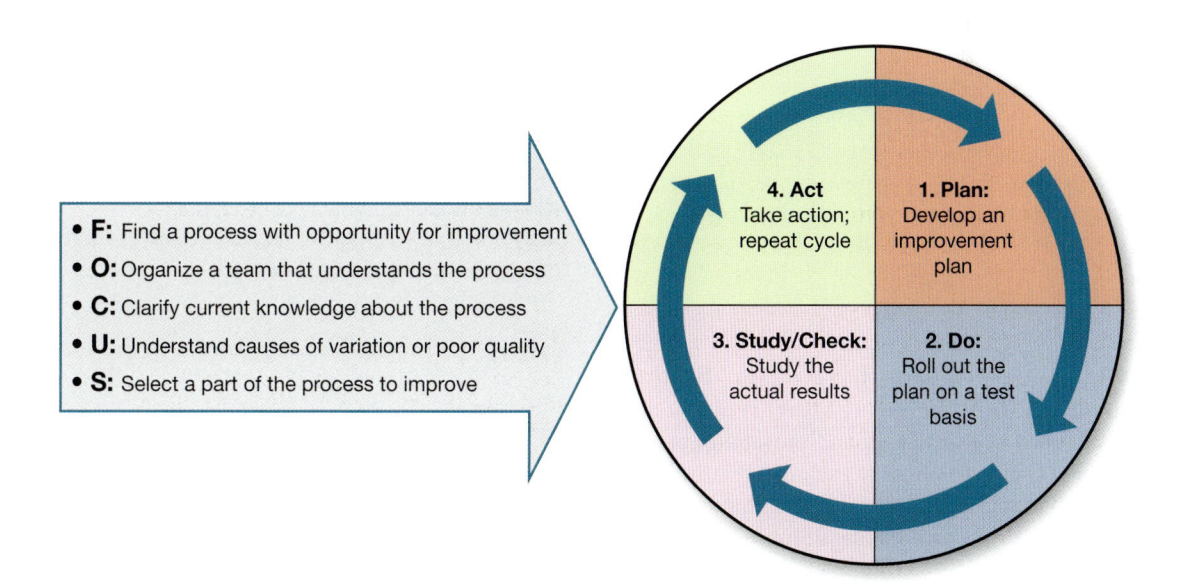

FIGURE 12.1 The FOCUS-PDSA (Plan-Do-Study-Act) Model.

plan for data collection and identifies key measures that will be used to assess improvement. Baseline (pre-QI intervention) data typically are collected during this phase.
2. **Do:** The team then implements the process improvement and collects data on key outcomes to assess whether improvement occurred. In a PDSA cycle, each improvement is tested on a fairly small scale.
3. **Study/Check:** Data from the trial run are analyzed to see if a positive change occurred.
4. **Act:** If the QI project resulted in improved outcomes, the team considers how best to sustain (and perhaps disseminate) the practice change. If no improvements were observed, or were modest, the team would work through the PDSA/PDCA model again, starting with decisions on what changes to make next.

Ideally, multiple PDSA cycles are used in fairly quick succession (rapid cycle), with the easiest changes made early in the initiative, and more difficult ones tested later.

TIP The U.S. Agency for Healthcare Research and Quality (AHRQ) offers PDSA worksheets and other tools and resources for QI projects (http://www.innovations.ahrq.gov/content.aspx?id=2398).

Example of a PDSA Project
Yuzeng and Hui (2020) used a series of plan, do, study, act cycles with the goal of improving the wait time to triage in an emergency department in Singapore within 1 year. They implemented several interventions and found a sustained reduction in triage wait time from 18 minutes preimplementation to 13 minutes postintervention.

Failure Mode and Effect Analysis. The **Failure Mode and Effect Analysis (FMEA)** is a systematic approach to identifying and preventing problems and failures *before* they occur. FMEA is used to assess complex processes using a standardized approach, with the aim of identifying factors that carry a risk of causing harm. Like Lean, the FMEA process has its origins in industry. In the United States, The Joint Commission (which accredits and certifies hospitals and other healthcare organizations) introduced the FMEA model in 2001. Accredited facilities are required to conduct at least one FMEA-type project each year.

TIP Worksheets and templates for an FMEA analysis (and for other QI analyses) are widely available online. A particularly useful resource is the Institute for Healthcare Improvement's (2017) "QI Essential Toolkit."

An FMEA project involves a review of the following: Failure modes (What could go wrong?), failure causes (Why would the failure happen?), and failure effects (What would be the consequences of a failure?). The analysis of processes for possible failure allows healthcare teams to prevent them by making proactive corrections, rather than waiting for adverse events to occur. DeRosier and coauthors (2002) described the use of FMEA in the U.S. Department of Veterans Affairs Center for Patient Safety as a five-step process:

1. Define the FMEA topic in a high-risk or high-vulnerability area
2. Assemble an interdisciplinary team
3. Graphically describe the process under consideration using process flow diagrams
4. Conduct a hazard analysis, listing all possible failure modes for each part of the process under examination
5. Develop a description of action for each failure mode cause and identify outcome measures

Example of a Failure Mode and Effect Analysis
Lu et al. (2021) did a retrospective observational study to explore the effects of the failure mode and effect analysis (FMEA) on the limb posture positioning on patients with severe burns. Two groups of patients were observed over 5 months, those who received usual limb positioning and those who received limb positioning using FMEA limb positioning.

SPECIFIC QUALITY IMPROVEMENT TOOLS AND METHODS

Quality improvement projects often involve the use of many of the same designs, methods, measures, and procedures that are used in research studies. Yet, tools and methods that are distinctive to QI have been developed. Some of these tools are especially useful in the planning stage. Most of these tools can be used in any of the QI models just described.

Quality Improvement Planning Tools: Root Cause Analysis

During the planning of QI initiatives, a major issue is the identification of a problem on which to focus. This is likely to involve informal discussions with key stakeholders, brainstorming, a review of institutional trends, a search for relevant evidence, and the creation of flowcharts and process maps.

Once a problem or process has been selected for improvement, the QI team usually tries to investigate the *causes* of the problem. It is difficult to develop solutions to institutional problems without understanding the underlying factors contributing to it. QI teams often undertake what is called a **root cause analysis (RCA)** that involves efforts to identify underlying process deficiencies (Haxby & Shuldham, 2018). RCA can involve the use of various tools and processes; only a few of which will be described here.

TIP Root cause analyses are often undertaken by looking globally at factors that contribute to a quality problem. In some QI initiatives, however, separate root cause analyses are undertaken for *each* occurrence of a problem. For example, Sharma and colleagues (2022) conducted a study that involved a root cause analysis to understand why patients across five California safety net hospitals delayed having a colonoscopy after having a positive fecal occult blood test.

The 5 Whys

One tool for identifying the root cause of a problem is a process called the "**5 Whys**." Figure 12.2 shows a template for a 5-whys analysis. The process begins by identifying the specific problem, then asking why the problem happens. If the answer fails to get to the underlying cause, "Why" is asked again. The process may be completed in fewer than five rounds of "Whys" or may require additional probing. Here is an example (Chambers et al., 2014):

Problem: Patient falls while toileting.

1. Why do patients fall while toileting? → *Because nurses do not stay in the bathroom with their patients.*
2. Why don't nurses stay in the bathroom with patients? → *Because patients don't understand that a nurse should stay with them.*
3. Why don't patients understand why a nurse should stay? → *Because they don't know that*

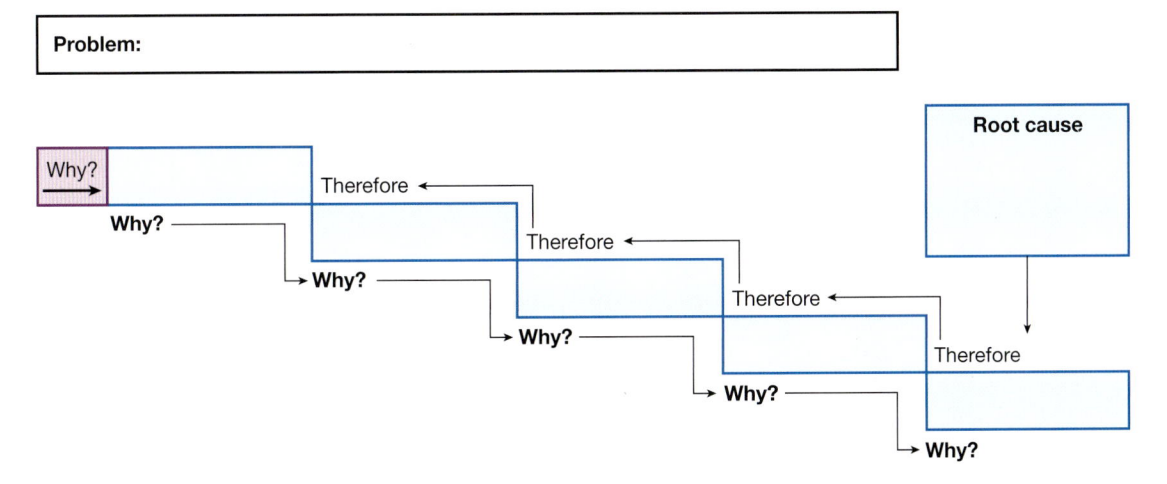

FIGURE 12.2 Template for a 5-whys analysis.

they might be unstable and that nurses can prevent them from falling if they stay in the room.
4. Why don't patients know this? → *Because nurses have not explained this safety precaution to them.*
5. Why don't nurses explain this safety precaution to them? → *Because current training and practice do not address this strategy.*

Some advice for carrying out the 5 Whys properly includes the following: (1) Focus on the process, not on people—do not be tempted to arrive at a root cause that is "human error" or "Mary's fault," (2) distinguish causes from symptoms, (3) identify successive causes step-by-step without jumping to conclusions, and (4) continue asking "Why" until you identify the root cause, the elimination of which will minimize the risk that the problem will recur.

Fishbone Analysis

Another tool for root cause analyses is called a **fishbone analysis**, which may be undertaken alongside the 5-Whys process. A fishbone analysis uses a *fishbone diagram* (also called a *cause-and-effect diagram* or an *Ishikawa diagram*) to visualize causal processes and identify opportunities for improvement (Phillips & Simmonds, 2013).

As shown in Figure 12.3, the "head" of the fishbone, at the tip of the diagram, specifies the "effect," which is the problem under consideration. Each "bone" represents a broad category that can be used to identify potential causes of the problem. Commonly used categories are (1) people (which could be healthcare staff, patients, family members, and so on); (2) equipment; (3) environmental factors; (4) processes/methods; (5) materials; and (6) management (Johnson, 2012). However, additional categories (e.g., regulations) might be relevant or

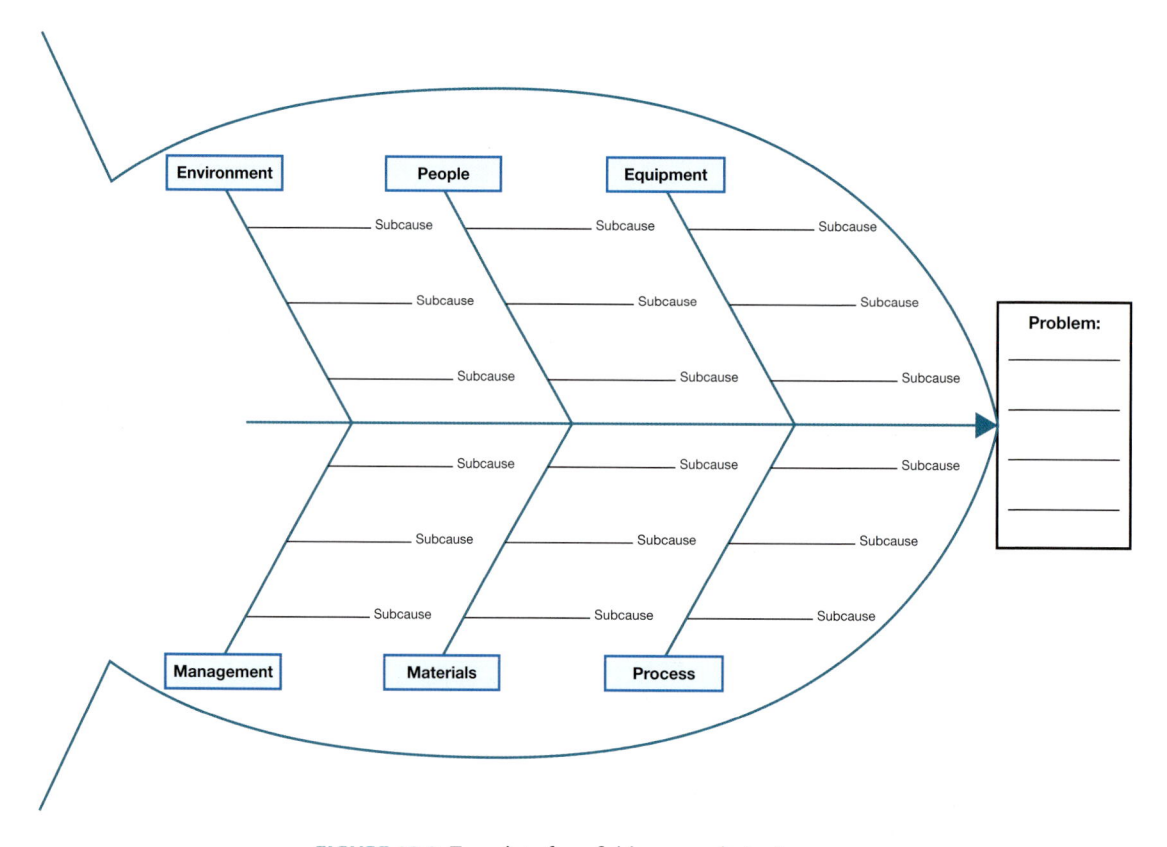

FIGURE 12.3 Template for a fishbone analysis diagram.

fewer categories might be needed, depending on the problem.

The diagram facilitates discussion—usually in interdisciplinary brainstorming sessions that encourage collaboration—and provides a tool for detecting a wide range of possible causes of a problem. The group collaboratively should identify the category headings, and each main category should be explored in detail. The goal is to illuminate causal factors for which the healthcare staff might find solutions that they had not previously considered.

Example of Using a Fishbone Diagram
Lipprandt and colleagues (2022) undertook a QI initiative to identify the causes of adverse events in patients on mechanical ventilation in the home setting. They interviewed key stakeholders including staff nurses and professional clinical educators. After analyzing the data, they created a root cause fishbone diagram outlining the causes of adverse events. Lastly, based on the findings, they developed efforts to reduce the risk of adverse events of risk mitigation measures to help avoid adverse events.

Pareto Charts

Sometimes QI teams graph the "root causes" of a problem on a **Pareto chart** that shows graphically the distribution of factors contributing to the targeted problem. Vilfredo Pareto, an Italian economist, observed that about 80% of the "effects" (occurrences of a problem) come from 20% of the causes—this is the so-called *80-20 rule*. Pareto charts are designed to visually portray the "vital few" causes against the "trivial many" causes. Pareto diagrams are useful when there are many possible courses of action, and the QI team wants to select ones that will yield the best improvement benefit. These charts, in other words, can be a good priority-setting tool (Chambers et al., 2014).

Pareto charts have a series of bars on the horizontal axis, each of which represents an identified cause of (or factor in) a problem (Figure 12.4). Frequencies (number of times a given cause resulted in the problem) are on the left vertical axis; the right vertical axis portrays cumulative percentages. The "causes" (bars) are arranged from left to right in decreasing order of frequency. A dot associated with each bar is added, and then the dots are connected to show cumulative percentages with successive causal factors. In the fictitious example in Figure 12.4, nearly 80% of patient falls occurred while patients were engaged in four activities.

Example of a Quality Improvement Project Using Pareto Charts
Boyar and Galiczewski (2021) conducted a QI project to reduce the incidence of peripheral intravenous catheter extravasation in neonates. They obtained baseline data on extravasations over a 6-month period. In addition, they surveyed the nurses on knowledge of intravenous care and randomly assessed intravenous stabilization techniques. They created a Pareto chart to identify the most common causes of extravasation prior to implementing four plan-do-study-act cycles. They found that post implementation extravasation decreased by 54%.

TIP Pareto charts can be created within Microsoft Excel and other spreadsheet programs.

Designs for Quality Improvement Projects

Most QI projects use simple designs that tend to be at risk of bias and misinterpretation. Conducting projects within real-world healthcare settings makes it challenging to use strong designs, but those who are promoting a more rigorous approach (i.e., those advocating for *improvement science*) are urging QI teams to consider stronger designs.

Randomized controlled trials (RCTs) are rare in the field of QI, but they do exist and are important for widespread implementation.

Example of a Quality Improvement Randomized Controlled Trial
An example of a QI project that used a randomized control design was conducted by Adisso et al. (2022). They explored the effect of a web-based tutorial and a workshop on housing decision-making provided for one group of healthcare workers that were randomized to the intervention group as opposed to the control group of healthcare workers who were recipients of passively distributed information. They examined the impact the interventions had on the older adult patients and/or caregivers housing decision-making. They found little difference in the two groups in terms of patients' and caregivers' housing decision-making.

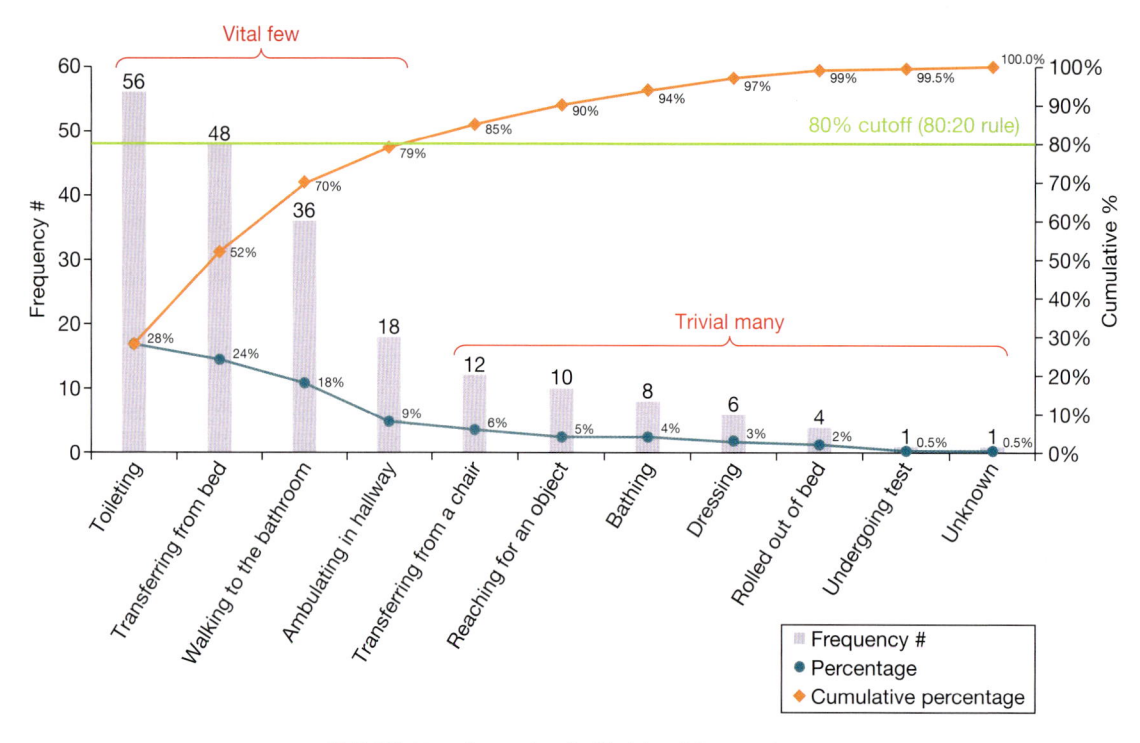

FIGURE 12.4 Example of a (fictitious) Pareto chart.

Most QI teams, however, rely on quasi-experimental designs to test the effectiveness of changes to systems or processes of care. Before–after designs, which measure changes to key outcomes after implementing a QI intervention, are especially common, but they are notably weak designs. They do not, for example, take into account secular trends in the population or the outcomes.

The nonequivalent control group design, which would involve comparisons with an institution not implementing the QI intervention, is a much stronger design option. Portela and colleagues (2015) have noted that it may be challenging to find a suitable comparison but also warned not to select a comparison site solely on superficial structural characteristics such as size or location: "The choice of relevant characteristics should be made based on anticipated hypotheses concerning the mechanisms of changes involved in the intervention and the contextual influences on how they work (e.g., … organizational culture)" (p. 348).

Time series type designs are especially useful for sorting out the effects of seasonal or cyclical trends from QI intervention effects. Time series designs involve the collection of outcome data over an extended time period, with multiple measurements before and after introducing an intervention. Traditional time series studies require enormous sample sizes, but an option pursued by many QI projects is the use of **statistical process control (SPC)**. SPC is often associated with the Six Sigma approach to QI but is also used in other improvement models. SPC uses **control charts** to map variation in the outcome of interest over time, typically using data from existing health records (Polit & Chaboyer, 2012).

Figure 12.5 presents an example of an SPC control chart used in a nurse-led quality improvement project. Gillespie and colleagues (2019) implemented a training intervention designed to improve nontechnical skills (communication, teamwork, decision-making) in surgical teams. Surgical teams were observed and assigned a score on a measure of proficiency in nontechnical skills (NOTECS) for about 25 weeks before the intervention and 20 to 25 weeks after the intervention. Figure 12.5 plots the mean scores for one of the four surgical teams who received the QI intervention—the cardiac team. Even without training in SPC methods, it is easy to see in this graph that noteworthy improvements in nontechnical skills were observed after the intervention was introduced. These improvements, according to SPC rules, were statistically significant.

Example of a Quality Improvement Project Using Statistical Process Control

Reynolds et al. (2022) tested a nurse-driven protocol to reduce indwelling urinary catheter utilization and catheter-associated urinary tract infection (CAUTI) rates at a large academic health system. The researchers used statistical process control to monitor the impact of their nurse-driven protocol on the number of CAUTIs and indwelling urinary catheter utilization. No reduction in urinary catheter utilization was found.

Quality Improvement and Measurement

Quality improvement relies on the ability of the team to assess whether the QI effort yielded a positive change. Measurement of healthcare performance variables is integral to quality improvement—indeed, it is sometimes said that measures *drive* improvement.

In the United States, the National Quality Forum (NQF) plays a critical role in endorsing performance measures for quality improvement efforts. Each measure in the NQF portfolio is carefully assessed, using four criteria: the importance of the measure to healthcare quality; its scientific soundness, based on evidence of the measure's reliability and validity (see Chapter 15); the usability and relevance of the measure to intended users; and the feasibility of collecting data on the measure without undue burden.

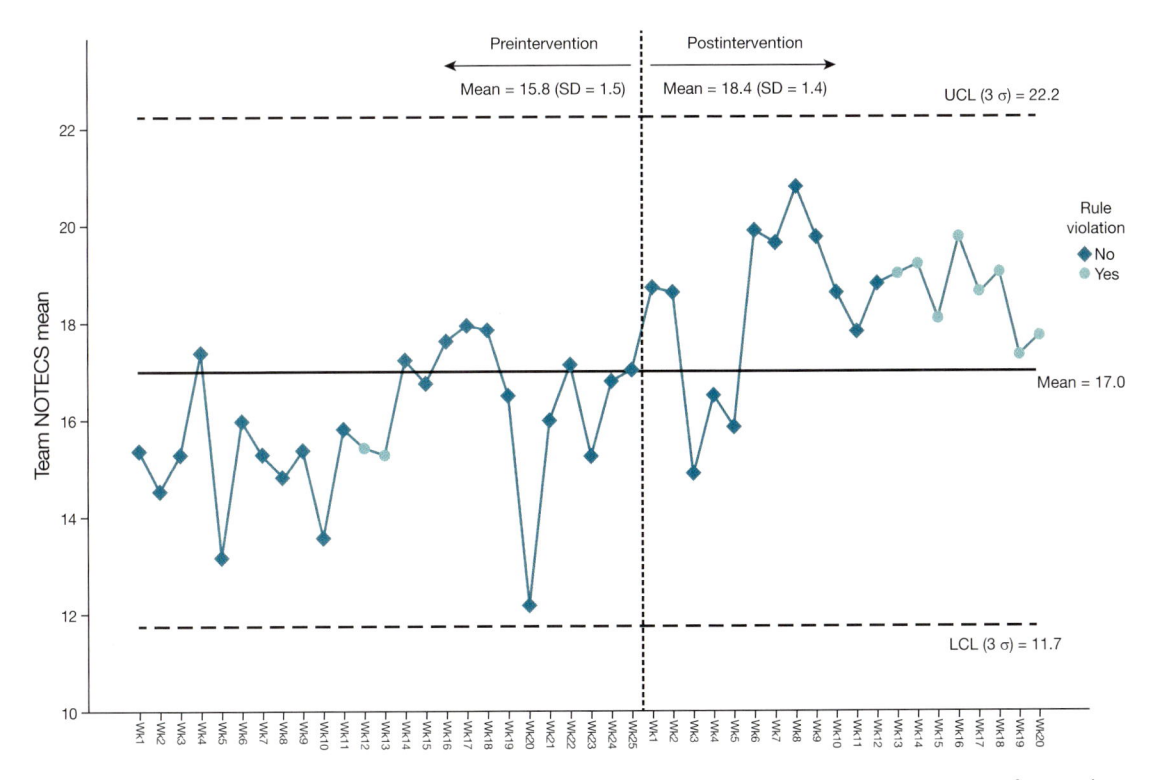

FIGURE 12.5 Example of a statistical process control (SPC) chart plotting mean scores on a measure of nontechnical skills (NOTECS) over a 25-week preintervention period and a 20-week postintervention period for cardiac teams. (Adapted with permission from Gillespie, B., Harbeck, E., Kang, E., Steel, C., Fairweather, N., Pamwatwanich, K., & Chaboyer, W. Effects of a brief team training program on surgical teams' nontechnical skills: An interrupted time-series design. *Journal of Patient Safety, 17*(5), e448–e454. https://doi.org/10.1097/PTS.0000000000000361.)

The NQF has endorsed measures in five categories, building on the Donabedian (1987) framework discussed in Chapter 11 in connection with outcomes research. The five categories are:

- *Process measures* that capture whether an action was completed or appropriate steps were taken and followed correctly;
- *Structural measures* that reflect the conditions in which providers care for their patients (e.g., staffing);
- *Outcome measures* that capture the actual results of care (these are usually the measures that providers are most interested in improving);
- *Patient experience measures* that capture patients' perspectives on their care; and
- *Composite measures* that combine multiple performance measures.

TIP As noted in Chapter 11, NQF has been slow to endorse nursing-sensitive measures, but that situation is likely to change as more nurses play leadership roles in QI initiatives.

Increasingly, data for QI projects are being retrieved from electronic health records (EHRs). However, several commentators have expressed concerns about the challenges of using EHR data, including the extensive time needed to document actions and outcomes, the failure of EHRs to include some relevant quality measures, the structure of the EHR, presentational challenges, problems of missing data, and problems in the availability of resources to guide data extraction (Baernholdt et al., 2018; Samuels et al., 2015). It can be expected that considerable progress in making EHRs more responsive to QI needs will occur in the future. One promising trend is the growing interest in data visualization to convey complex information (Caban & Gotz, 2015; Monsen et al., 2015).

TIP Many QI projects use mixed-methods designs that involve collecting both qualitative and quantitative data. Qualitative methods are especially well-suited during the planning phase and during the "Act" phase when the QI team must consider what to do next.

CRITICAL APPRAISAL OF QUALITY IMPROVEMENT STUDIES

Box 12.1 offers several questions for critically appraising quality improvement reports. Due to page constraints in journals, the reports may not

---

BOX 12.1 Guidelines for Critically Appraising Quality Improvement Studies

1. Was the nature and significance of the problem adequately described? Was the purpose of the QI initiative clear?
2. Did the project draw on existing evidence about solutions to similar problems? Was the initiative linked to a theory of change?
3. Who was on the QI team? Was interprofessional collaboration an important aspect of the project?
4. What methods were used to identify the root causes of the problem? Were those methods adequate?
5. What model of QI was used (e.g., Lean, PDSA)? Was it used appropriately?
6. What specific QI interventions were implemented? Were the interventions sufficiently described so that others could reproduce them?
7. What research design was used to assess the effects of the QI changes? Did the design rule out alternative explanations for the findings (i.e., was there good internal validity)? If statistical process control was used, were there enough data points before and after the intervention?
8. What outcome measures were used to assess the effects of the QI effort? Were these measures appropriate, and was there evidence that the measures were of good quality?
9. Were the results clearly explained? Was the interpretation of the results consistent with the rigor of the methods used?
10. Did the report discuss any limitations to the generalizability of the QI study?

provide rich description of all aspects of a QI project. In particular, many QI reports do not provide a lot of detail about the tools they used to identify root causes of the problem being targeted, focusing instead on the interventions they introduced and what they learned in efforts to evaluate the intervention. However, the authors should ideally offer a rationale (a theoretical explanation) for why they believed the intervention would lead to improved outcomes, and this rationale should guide the interpretation of the results.

As with research studies, the design of QI projects should be scrutinized to assess internal validity, as well as construct and statistical conclusion validity. Ideally, the report would provide fairly detailed information about the context so that readers could assess whether a similar quality improvement strategy could work in their setting.

RESEARCH EXAMPLE

This section describes a quality improvement project.

Study: Implementing a Standardized Workflow Process to Increase the Palliative Care to Hospice Admission Rate (Boyd et al., 2023)

Background: The authors, Boyd and colleagues (2023) noted that hospice referrals and subsequently the care provided are underutilized. This is despite the benefits of hospice care in improving quality of life, pain and symptom management, and decreasing the cost of care at the end of life. While patients enrolled in palliative care potentially have a smoother transition to hospice care, they noted in their institution there were increased wait times for people transitioning from palliative care to hospice care.

The QI Initiative: The QI initiative was to implement and evaluate a standardized workflow process with chart completion mandates to determine if this reduced wait times and increased the admission rate of patients transferring to hospice services from palliative care within their organization.

The PDSA model was used to continuously improve the process of timely transfers to hospice.

The new standardized workflow process included the following steps. The palliative care provider (1) assigned an urgency level to the hospice referral and (2) deactivated the patient's electronic health record to signal that the hospice referral was appropriate and complete. This process alerted the hospice referral specialist to know that the patient was ready for admission.

Results: The new standardized workflow process increased the palliative care to hospice admission rate by 11.5%. These findings suggest the standardized process was effective in providing improved access to hospice care services for patients in their palliative care program.

SUMMARY POINTS

- **Quality improvement (QI)** in health care is the collaborative effort of healthcare professionals to make changes that will improve patient outcomes and result in better system performance.
- **Improvement science** is the discipline devoted to the systematic and rigorous generation and evaluation of evidence to cultivate positive change in healthcare processes and outcomes.
- Research is considered distinct from QI projects, but distinctions are becoming blurred because QI is no longer considered exclusively a "local" enterprise. QI projects are increasingly being reported in journals, and the evidence from QI studies is the focus of systematic reviews—with an eye to facilitating the use of **evidence-based quality improvement (EBQI)** in other settings.
- In the United States, the IOM's *Quality Chasm* reports galvanized interest in making systematic healthcare improvements and in adopting a quality management philosophy called **continuous quality improvement (CQI)** that encourages ongoing scrutiny of quality. Nurses are playing an increasingly important role in improvement science.
- Various types of QI interventions have been implemented, including provider education, provider reminders, provider feedback, patient education, patient reminders, patient supports for self-management, case management and care coordination, and financial incentives.

- Several quality improvement models, many originating in industry, have been used in healthcare initiatives. The **Lean approach** (also known as the *Toyota Production System*) strives to eliminate waste, inefficiencies, and redundancies. The goal is continuous improvement and the standardization of work practices.
- The **Failure Mode and Effect Analysis (FMEA)** model is a systematic approach to identifying and preventing problems before they occur. An FMEA project seeks answers to such questions as: What could go wrong? Why would a failure occur? and What could be the consequences of a failure?
- **Six Sigma** is an approach designed to standardize processes and reduce variation. The model involves five steps (DMAIC): Define, measure, analyze, improve, and control.
- The most widely used QI model in health care is called **Plan-Do-Study-Act (PDSA)** (or **Plan-Do-Check-Act [PDCA]**), which involves multiple **rapid cycles** of improvements and testing. The PDSA cycles are guided by **FOCUS** steps: Find a process for improvement, Organize a team, Clarify current knowledge about the process, Understand causes of variation or poor quality, and Select a part of the process to improve.
- During the planning phase of a QI study, the team can use a variety of tools, such as flowcharts, process maps, and methods for doing a **root cause analysis (RCA)**. RCA involves efforts to review and understand underlying process deficiencies.
- One tool for an RCA is called the **5 Whys**, which probes for fundamental reasons for a problem by asking "Why" multiple times in response to the answers to previous "Whys."
- Another RCA tool is a **fishbone analysis** that seeks to portray diagrammatically all potential causes of a problem on a chart that resembles a fish skeleton.
- Causes of a problem can be graphed on a **Pareto chart** that visually portrays the causes of a problem in descending order of occurrence. Pareto charts can facilitate prioritizing QI efforts; the so-called *80-20 rule* articulates the expectation that about 80% of a problem is attributable to about 20% of the causes.
- Many QI studies use weak before–after designs that are at risk to various biases and confounders. One of the strongest designs for QI is the time series design, which is often used with an analytic strategy called **statistical process control (SPC).**
- SPC involves the use of **control charts** that map variation in the outcome of interest over time, with many points of data collection before and after introducing the QI intervention.
- Although QI projects can involve the collection of both qualitative and quantitative data, performance measures play a key role in QI projects, and increasingly those performance measures are being extracted from electronic health records (EHRs).

REFERENCES CITED IN CHAPTER 12

Adisso, É. L., Taljaard, M., Stacey, D., Brière, N., Zomahoun, H. T. V., Durand, P. J., Rivest, L. P., & Légaré, F. (2022). Shared decision-making training for home care teams to engage frail older adults and caregivers in housing decisions: Stepped-wedge cluster randomized trial. *JMIR Aging, 5*(3), e39386. https://doi.org/10.2196/39386

Aqtash, S., Alnusair, H., Brownie, S., Alnjadat, R., Fonbuena, M., & Perinchery, S. (2022). Evaluation of the impact of an education program on self-reported leadership and management competence among nurse managers. *SAGE Open Nursing, 8*, 23779608221106450. https://doi.org/10.1177/23779608221106450

Aspinall, C., Johnstone, P., & Parr, J. M. (2023). Reflections on the implementation and evaluation of a system-wide improvement programme based on the fundamentals of care: Lessons learned. *Journal of Advanced Nursing, 79*(3), 980–990. https://doi.org/10.1111/jan.15389

Baernholdt, M., Dunton, N., Hughes, R., Stone, P., & White, K. (2018). Quality measures: A stakeholder analysis. *Journal of Nursing Care Quality, 33*(2), 149–156.

Batalden, P., & Davidoff, F. (2007). What is "quality improvement" and how can it transform healthcare? *Quality and Safety in Health Care, 16*(1), 2–3.

Berry, S. D., Baier, R. R., Syme, M., Gouskova, N., Bishnoi, C., Patel, U., Leitson, M, Gharpure, R, Stone, N. D., Link-Gelles, R., Gifford, D. R., & Gifford, D. R. (2022). Strategies associated with COVID-19 vaccine coverage among nursing home staff. *Journal of the American Geriatric Society, 70*(1), 19–28.

Bodenheimer, T., & Sinsky, C. (2014). From triple to quadruple aim: Care of the patient requires care of the provider. *Annals of Family Medicine*, 12(6), 573–576.

Boyar, V., & Galiczewski, C. (2021). Reducing peripheral intravenous catheter extravasation in neonates: A quality improvement project. *Journal of Wound Ostomy and Continence Nursing*, 48(1), 31–38. https://doi.org/10.1097/WON.0000000000000728

Boyd, C., DiBartolo, M. C., Helne, D., & Everett, K. (2023). Implementing a standardized workflow process to increase the palliative care to hospice admission rate. *Journal of Nursing Care Quality*, 38(2), 185–189. https://doi.org/10.1097/NCQ.0000000000000682

Caban, J., & Gotz, D. (2015). Visual analytics in healthcare—opportunities and research challenges. *Journal of the American Medical Informatics Association*, 22(2), 260–262.

Centers for Medicare & Medicaid Services. (2021). *Quality measurement and quality improvement what is quality improvement?* Retrieved from https://www.cms.gov/Medicare/Quality-Initiatives-Patient-Assessment-Instruments/MMS/Quality-Measure-and-Quality-Improvement

Chambers, C., Petrie, J., Lindsie, S., & Makic, M. B. (2014). How to use quality improvement processes to implement evidence-based practice. In Fink, R., Oman, K., & Makic, B. B. (Eds.). *Research & evidence-based practice manual* (3rd ed., pp. 37–48). University of Colorado Hospital Authority.

Coles, E., Wells, M., Maxwell, M., Harris, F., Anderson, J., Gray, N., Milner, G., MacGillivray, S., & McGillivray, S. (2017). The influence of contextual factors on healthcare quality improvement initiatives: What works, for whom and in what setting? *Systematic Review*, 6(1), 168.

Deming, W. E. (1988). *Out of the crisis*. Massachusetts Institute of Technology Center for Advanced Engineering Study xiii, 1991;507.

DeRosier, J., Stalhandske, E., Bagian, J., & Nudell, T. (2002). Using health care failure mode and effect analysis: The VA National center for patient safety's prospective risk analysis system. *Joint Communication Journal on Quality Improvement*, 28(5), 248–209.

Donabedian, A. (1987). Some basic issues in evaluating the quality of health care. In Rinke, L. T. (Ed.), *Outcome measures in home care* (Vol. I, pp. 3–28). National League for Nursing.

Finkelman, A. (2020). *Quality improvement: A guide for integration in nursing* (2nd ed.). Jones & Bartlett.

Gillespie, B., Harbeck, E., Kang, E., Steel, C., Fairweather, N., Panuwatwanich, K., & Chaboyer, W. (2021). Effects of a brief team training program on surgical teams' nontechnical skills: An interrupted time-series study. *Journal of Patient Safety*, 17(5), e448–e454. https://doi.org/10.1097/PTS.0000000000000361

Gupta, P., Shiju, S., Chacko, G., Thomas, M., Abas, A., Savarimuthu, I., Omari, E., Al-Balushi, S., Jessymol, P., Mathew, J., Quinto, M., McDonald, I., & Andrews, W. (2020). A quality improvement programme to reduce hospital-acquired pressure injuries. *BMJ Open Quality*, 9(3), e000905. https://doi.org/10.1136/bmjoq-2019-000905

Haxby, E., & Shuldham, C. (2018). How to undertake a root cause analysis investigation to improve patient safety. *Nursing Standard*, 32(20), 41–46.

Hughes, R. G. (2008). Tools and strategies for quality improvement and patient safety. In Hughes, R. G. (Ed.). *Patient safety and quality: An evidence-based handbook for nurses*. Agency for Healthcare Research and Quality.

Institute for Healthcare Improvement. (2005). *Going Lean in health care*. IHI.

Institute for Healthcare Improvement. (2017). *Quality essentials Toolkit*. IHI.

Institute of Medicine. (1999). *To err is human: Building a safer health system*. National Academies Press.

Institute of Medicine. (2001). *Crossing the quality chasm: A new health system for the 21st century*. National Academies Press.

Institute of Medicine. (2003). *Health professions education: A bridge to quality*. National Academies Press.

Johnson, J. (2012). Quality improvement. In Sherwood, G., & Barnsteiner, J., (Eds.), *Quality and safety in nursing: A competency approach to improving outcomes* (pp. 113–132). John Wiley & Sons.

Johnson, J. E., Smith, A., & Mastro, K. (2012). From Toyota to the bedside: Nurses can lead the lean way in health care reform. *Nursing Administration in Quarterly*, 36(3), 234–242.

Kuwaiti, A. A., & Subbarayalu, A. V. (2017). Reducing patients' falls rate in an academic medical center (AMC) using Six Sigma "DMAIC" approach. *International Journal of Health Care Quality Assurance*, 30(4), 373–384.

Lipprandt, M., Liedtke, W., Langanke, M., Klausen, A., Baumgarten, N., & Röhrig, R. (2022). Causes for adverse events in home ventilation: A nursing perspective. *BMC Nursing*, 21(1), 264.

Lu, Y., Zhou, Q., Wang, L. N., He, T., Zhao, H. Y., & Cao, X. Q. (2021). Application effects of failure mode and effect analysis on the limb posture positioning nursing of extremely severe burn patients. *Journal of Burns*, 37(11), 1078–1084. https://doi.org/10.3760/cma.j.cn501120-20210412-00126

Marshall, M., Pronovost, P., & Dixon-Woods, M. (2015). Promotion of improvement as science. *The Lancet*, 381, 419–421.

Martin, L., Lyons, M., Patton, A., O Driscoll, M., McLoughlin, K., Hannon, E., & Deasy, C. (2022). Implementing delirium screening in the emergency department: A quality improvement project. *BMJ Open Quality*, 11(2), e001676. https://doi.org/10.1136/bmjoq-2021-001676

Matiz, L. A., Kostacos, C., Robbins-Milne, L., Chang, S. J., Rausch, J. C., & Tariq, A. (2021). Integrating nurse care managers in the medical home of children with special health care needs to improve their care coordination and impact health care utilization. *Journal of Pediatric Nursing*, 59, 32–36. https://doi.org/10.1016/j.pedn.2020.12.018

Monsen, K., Peterson, J., Mathiason, M., Kim, E., Lee, S., Chi, C., & Pieczkiewicz, D. (2015). Data visualization techniques to showcase nursing care quality. *Computers, Informatics, Nursing*, 33(10), 417–426.

National Learning Consortium. (2013). *Continuous quality improvement (CQI) strategies to optimize your practice*. NLC.

Phillips, J., & Simmonds, L. (2013). Using fishbone analysis to investigate problems. *Nursing Times*, *109*(15), 18–20.

Polit, D., & Chaboyer, W. (2012). Statistical process control in nursing research. *Research in Nursing Health*, *35*(1), 82–93.

Portela, M., Pronovost, P., Woodcock, T., Carter, P., & Dixon-Woods, M. (2015). How to study improvement interventions: A brief overview of possible study types. *BMJ Quality & Safety*, *24*(5), 325–336.

Pyzdek, T., & Keller, P. (2014). *The six Sigma handbook* (4th ed.). McGraw Hill.

Reynolds, S. S., Lozano, H., Fleurant, M., & Bhandari, K. (2022). Using statistical process control charts to measure changes from a nurse-driven protocol to remove urinary catheters. *American Journal of Infection Control*, *50*(12), 1355–1359. https://doi.org/10.1016/j.ajic.2022.03.005

Samuels, J., McGrath, R., Fetzer, S., Mittal, P., & Bourgoine, D. (2015). Using the electronic health record in nursing research: Challenges and opportunities. *Western Journal of Nursing Research*, *37*(10), 1284–1294.

Seidl, K., & Newhouse, R. (2012). The intersection of evidence-based practice with 5 quality improvement methodologies. *The Journal of Nursing Administration*, *42*(6), 299–304.

Sharma, A. E., Lyson, H. C., Cherian, R., Somsouk, M., Schillinger, D., & Sarkar, U. (2022). A root cause analysis of barriers to timely colonoscopy in California safety-net health systems. *Journal of Patient Safety*, *18*(1), e163–e171. https://doi.org/10.1097/PTS.0000000000000718

Shojania, K., & Grimshaw, J. (2005). Evidence-based quality improvement: The state of the science. *Health Affairs Journal*, *24*(1), 138–150.

Skela-Savič, B., MacRae, R., Lillo-Crespo, M., & Rooney, K. (2017). The development of a consensus definition for healthcare improvement science (HIS) in seven European countries: A consensus methods approach. *Zdravstveno Varstvo*, *56*(2), 82–90.

Tappen, R., Wolf, D., Rahemi, Z., Engstrom, G., Rojido, C., Shutes, J., & Ouslander, J. (2017). Barriers and facilitators to implementing a change initiative in long-term care using the INTERACT® quality improvement program. *Health Care Manag*, *36*(3), 219–230.

Ting, H., Shojania, K., Montori, V., & Bradley, E. (2009). Quality improvement: Science and action. *Circulation*, *119*(14), 1962–1974.

United States Code of Federal Regulations, 45CFR 46.102 (d). Accessed July 23, 2019. http://www.hhs.gov/ohrp/humansubjects/guidance/45cfr46

Yuzeng, S., & Hui, L. L. (2020). Improving the wait time to triage at the emergency department. *BMJ Open Quality*, *9*(1), e000708. https://doi.org/10.1136/bmjoq-2019-000708

Ziyar, A., Kwon, J., Li, A., Naderi, A., & Jean, T. (2022). Improving epinephrine autoinjector usability and carriage frequency among patients at risk of anaphylaxis: A quality improvement initiative. *BMJ Open Quality*, *11*(3), e001742. https://doi.org/10.1136/bmjoq-2021-001742

13 Sampling in Quantitative Research

Learning Objectives

1. Recognize the importance and limitations of eligibility criteria for studies.
2. Understand the differences between nonprobability and probability sampling.
3. Distinguish the different types of sampling designs in quantitative studies.
4. Describe the advantages and disadvantages of the various types of random sampling.

INTRODUCTION

Researchers almost always obtain data from samples. In testing the efficacy of a new fall prevention program for hospital patients, for example, researchers reach conclusions without testing it with *every* hospitalized patient worldwide, or even with every patient in a specific hospital. But researchers must be careful not to draw conclusions based on a flawed sample.

Quantitative researchers seek to select samples that will allow them to achieve statistical conclusion validity and to generalize their results beyond the sample used. They develop a **sampling plan** that specifies in advance how participants are to be selected and how many to include. Qualitative researchers, by contrast, make sampling decisions during the course of data collection and use different criteria to evaluate sampling adequacy. This chapter discusses sampling for quantitative studies.

BASIC SAMPLING CONCEPTS

We begin by reviewing some terms associated with sampling—terms that are used primarily (but not exclusively) in quantitative research.

Populations

A **population** (the "P" of PICO questions) is the entire aggregation of cases in which a researcher is interested. For instance, if we were studying American nurses with doctoral degrees, the population could be defined as all U.S. citizens who are registered nurses (RNs) and who have a PhD, DNSc, DNP, or other doctoral-level degree. Other possible populations might be all patients who had cardiac surgery at Memorial Hospital in 2021, all females with irritable bowel syndrome in Sweden, or all children in Canada with cystic fibrosis. Populations are not restricted to humans. A population might consist of all blood samples at a particular laboratory. Whatever the basic unit, the population comprises the aggregate of the elements of interest.

It is sometimes useful to distinguish between target and accessible populations. The **accessible population** is the aggregate of cases that conform to designated criteria *and* that are accessible for a study. The **target population** is the aggregate of cases about which the researcher would like to generalize. A target population might consist of all diabetic people in California, but the accessible population might consist of all patients with diabetes being treated at clinics in Los Angeles. Researchers usually sample from an accessible population and hope to generalize to a target population.

> **TIP** Many quantitative researchers fail to identify their target population or to discuss the generalizability of the results. Evidence for nursing practice must come from research that is relevant to particular clinical populations. Thus, the population of interest needs to be carefully considered in planning and reporting a study.

Eligibility Criteria

Researchers must specify criteria that define who is in the population. Consider the population, American nursing students. Does this population include students in all types of nursing programs? Do foreign students enrolled in American nursing programs qualify? Researchers must indicate the exact criteria by which it could be decided whether a person would or would not be classified as a member of the population. The criteria that specify population characteristics are the **eligibility criteria** or **inclusion criteria**. Sometimes, a population is also defined in terms of characteristics that people must *not* possess (i.e., **exclusion criteria**). For example, the population may be defined to exclude people who do not speak English.

In thinking about ways to define the population, it is important to consider whether the resulting sample is likely to be a good exemplar of the population construct in which you are interested. A study's construct validity is enhanced when there is a good match between the eligibility criteria and the population construct.

Of course, eligibility criteria for a study often reflect considerations other than substantive concerns. Eligibility criteria may reflect one or more of the following:

- *Costs.* Some criteria reflect cost constraints. For example, when non–English-speaking people are excluded, this likely does not mean that researchers are uninterested in non-English speakers, but rather that they cannot afford to hire translators or multilingual staff.
- *Practical constraints.* Sometimes, there are other practical constraints, such as difficulty including people from rural areas, people who are hearing impaired, and so on.
- *People's ability to participate in a study.* The health condition of some people may preclude their participation. For example, people with cognitive impairments, who are in coma, or who are in an unstable medical condition may need to be excluded.
- *Design considerations.* As noted in Chapter 10, it is sometimes advantageous to define a homogeneous population, as a means of controlling confounding variables.

The criteria used to define a population for a study have implications for the interpretation and generalizability of the findings. In fact, a growing concern about the sampling plans for randomized controlled trials is that researchers often use exclusion criteria that make it impossible to apply the results to the people who are most in need of the intervention (e.g., excluding people with a comorbidity). Exclusion criteria may reflect a desire to strengthen internal validity, at the expense of external validity, as we discuss in Chapter 31.

> **Example of Inclusion and Exclusion Criteria**
> Faulkner and colleagues (2022) conducted a secondary analysis to explore if there were distinct patterns of dyspnea reported by patients from preimplantation of a left ventricular assistive device (LVAD) to 6 months postimplantation and if so, to determine what factors predicted patterns of dyspnea over time. Inclusion criteria included all females and males with advanced heart failure who were greater than age 21, and who enrolled in a prior study at a clinic in the northwest USA and were awaiting a LVAD implant. There were several exclusion criteria such as those who did not understand English or Spanish at the fifth-grade level, or had significant uncorrected hearing or vision impairments.

Samples and Sampling

Sampling is the process of selecting cases to represent an entire population, to permit inferences about the population. A **sample** is a subset of population

elements, which are the most basic units about which data are collected. In nursing research, elements most often are humans.

Samples and sampling plans vary in quality. *Two key considerations in assessing a sample in a quantitative study are its representativeness and size.* A **representative sample** is one whose key characteristics closely approximate those of the population. If the population in a study of patients is 50% male and 50% female, then a representative sample would have a similar gender distribution. If the sample is not representative of the population, the study's external validity and construct validity are at risk.

Certain sampling methods are less likely to result in biased samples than others, but a representative sample can never be guaranteed. Researchers operate under conditions in which error is possible. Quantitative researchers strive to minimize errors and, when possible, to estimate their magnitude.

Sampling designs are classified as either probability sampling or nonprobability sampling. **Probability sampling** involves random selection of elements. In probability sampling, researchers can specify the probability that an element of the population will be included in the sample. Greater confidence can be placed in the representativeness of probability samples. In **nonprobability samples**, elements are selected by nonrandom methods. There is no way to estimate the probability that each element has of being included in a nonprobability sample, and every element usually does *not* have a chance for inclusion.

Strata

Sometimes, it is useful to think of populations as consisting of subpopulations or **strata**. A stratum is a mutually exclusive segment of a population, defined by one or more characteristics. For instance, suppose our population was all RNs in the United Kingdom. This population could be divided into three strata based on gender (male, female, other). Or we could specify two age strata: nurses younger than 40 years or nurses 40 years or older. Strata are often used in sample selection to enhance the sample's representativeness. Using strata in the sampling design can also facilitate the analysis of data for subgroups, to see if results differ for people with different characteristics.

Staged Sampling

Samples are sometimes selected in multiple phases, in what is called **multistage sampling**. In the first stage, large units (such as hospitals or nursing homes) are selected. Then, in the next stage, smaller units (e.g., individuals) are sampled. In staged sampling, it is possible to combine probability and nonprobability sampling. For example, the first stage could involve the deliberate (nonrandom) selection of study sites. Then, people within the selected sites could be selected through random procedures.

Sampling Bias

Researchers seldom have the resources to study all members of a population. It is possible to obtain fairly accurate information from a sample, but data from samples *can* be erroneous. Finding 100 people willing to participate in a study may be easy, but it is often hard to select 100 people who are an unbiased subset of the population. **Sampling bias** refers to the systematic overrepresentation or underrepresentation of a population subgroup on a characteristic relevant to the research question.

As an example of consciously biased selection, suppose we were investigating patients' responsiveness to nurses' touch and decide to recruit the first 50 patients meeting eligibility criteria. We decide, however, to omit Mr. Z from the sample because he has been hostile to nursing staff. Mrs. X, who has just lost her spouse, is also bypassed. These decisions to exclude certain people do not reflect bona fide eligibility criteria. Such decisions can lead to bias because responsiveness to nurses' touch (the outcome variable) may be affected by patients' feelings about nurses or their emotional state.

Sampling bias often occurs unconsciously, however. If we were studying nursing students and systematically interviewed every 10th student who entered the nursing school library, the sample would be biased in favor of library-goers, even if we are conscientious about including every 10th student regardless of age, gender, or other traits.

> **TIP** Internet surveys are attractive because they can be distributed to geographically dispersed people. However, there is an inherent bias in such surveys, unless the population is defined as people who have easy access to, and comfort with, computers and the Internet.

Sampling bias is partly a function of population homogeneity. If population elements were all identical on key attributes, then any sample would be as good as any other. Indeed, if the population were completely homogeneous—exhibited no variability at all—then a *single* element would be sufficient. For many physiologic attributes, it may be safe to assume reasonably high homogeneity. For example, the blood in a person's veins is relatively homogeneous and so a single blood sample is adequate. For most human attributes, however, homogeneity is the exception rather than the rule. Age, stress, resilience—all these attributes reflect human heterogeneity. When variation occurs in the population, then similar variation should be reflected, to the extent possible, in a sample.

NONPROBABILITY SAMPLING

Nonprobability sampling is less likely than probability sampling to produce representative samples. Despite this fact, the vast majority of studies in nursing and other health disciplines rely on nonprobability samples.

Convenience Sampling

Convenience sampling entails using the most conveniently available people as participants. For example, a nurse who conducts a study of teenage risk-taking by recruiting students from a local youth organization is relying on a convenience sample. The problem with convenience sampling is that those who participate might be atypical of the population with regard to critical variables.

Sometimes, researchers seeking people with certain characteristics place an ad in a newspaper, put up signs in clinics, or post messages on online social media. These "convenient" approaches are subject to bias because people who respond to posted notices likely differ from those who do not volunteer or do not see the notices.

Snowball sampling (also called *network sampling* or *chain sampling*) is a variant of convenience sampling. With this approach, early sample members (called **seeds**) are asked to refer other people who meet the eligibility criteria. This approach is often used when the population involves people who might otherwise be difficult to identify (e.g., people who have recurrent nightmares).

Convenience sampling is the weakest form of sampling. In heterogeneous populations, no other sampling approach faces a greater risk of sampling bias. Yet, convenience sampling is the most commonly used method in many disciplines.

> **Example of a Convenience Sample**
> Rahmani et al. (2022) sought to investigate the factors associated with family caregiver burden of patients with schizophrenia. They used convenience sampling techniques to recruit 215 family caregivers from outpatient psychiatric clinics.

> **TIP** Rigorous methods of sampling *hidden populations*, such as people who are homeless or who use injection drug, are emerging. Because standard probability sampling is inappropriate for such hidden populations, a method called **respondent-driven sampling (RDS),** a variant of snowball sampling, has been developed. RDS, unlike traditional snowballing, allows the assessment of relative inclusion probabilities based on mathematical models. Abdella et al. (2022) used RDS in their cross-sectional study of HIV prevalence and associated factors among female sex workers in Ethiopia.

Quota Sampling

A **quota sample** is one in which the researcher identifies population strata and determines how many participants are needed from each stratum. By using information about population characteristics, researchers can ensure that diverse segments are represented in the sample, in the proportion in which they occur in the population.

Suppose we were interested in studying nursing students' attitudes toward working with AIDS patients. The accessible population is a nursing school with 500 undergraduate students; a sample of 100 students is desired. The easiest procedure would be to distribute questionnaires in classrooms through convenience sampling. Suppose, however, that we suspect that male and female students have different attitudes. A convenience sample might result in too many males or too many females. Table 13.1 presents fictitious data showing the gender distribution for the population (column 2) and for a convenience sample (column 3). In this example, the convenience sample underrepresents males. We can, however, establish "quotas" so that the sample includes the appropriate number of cases from both strata. The far-right column of Table 13.1 shows the number of males and females required for a quota sample.

You may better appreciate the dangers of sampling bias with a concrete example. Suppose a key question for study participants was, "Would you be willing to work on a unit that cared exclusively for AIDS patients?" The number and percentage of students in the population who would respond "yes" are shown in the first column of Table 13.2. We would not know these values—they are shown to illustrate a point. Within the population, males are more likely than females to say they would work on a unit with AIDS patients, yet males were underrepresented in the convenience sample. As a result, population and sample values on this key question are discrepant: Nearly twice as many students in the population (20%) are favorable toward working with AIDS patients than we would conclude based on results from the convenience sample (11%). The quota sample does a better job of reflecting the views of the population (19%). In actual research situations, the distortions from a convenience sample may be smaller than in this example but could be larger as well.

Stratification should be based on variables that would reflect important differences in the outcome, such as gender in our fictitious example. Variables such as age, ethnicity, gender, education, and medical diagnosis may be good stratifying variables.

Procedurally, quota sampling is like convenience sampling. The people in any subgroup are a convenience sample from that population stratum. For example, the initial sample of 100 students in Table 13.1 constituted a convenience sample from the population of 500. In the quota sample, the 20 males are a convenience sample of the 100 males in the population. Quota sampling can share similar weaknesses as convenience sampling. For instance, if a researcher is required by a quota sampling plan to interview 10 males between the ages of 65 and 80 years, a trip to a nursing home might be the most convenient method of obtaining participants. Yet this approach would fail to represent older males living independently in the community.

Despite its limitations, quota sampling is a major improvement over convenience sampling. Quota sampling does not require sophisticated skills or a lot of effort. Many researchers who use a convenience sample could profitably use quota sampling.

Example of a Quota Sample
To understand nurses' perception about structural empowerment in their work setting, Saleh and colleagues (2022) used quota sampling to recruit 200 registered nurses from two hospitals in Jordan.

TABLE 13.1 • **Numbers and Percentages of Students in Strata of a Population, Convenience Sample, and Quota Sample**

STRATA	POPULATION	CONVENIENCE SAMPLE	QUOTA SAMPLE
Male	100 (20%)	5 (5%)	20 (20%)
Female	400 (80%)	95 (95%)	80 (80%)
Total	500 (100%)	100 (100%)	100 (100%)

TABLE 13.2 • Students Willing to Work on an AIDS Unit, in the Population, Convenience Sample, and Quota Sample

	POPULATION	CONVENIENCE SAMPLE	QUOTA SAMPLE
Willing males (number)	28	2	6
Willing females (number)	72	9	13
Total number of willing students	100	11	19
Total number of all students	500	100	100
Percentage willing	20%	11%	19%

Consecutive Sampling

Consecutive sampling involves recruiting *all* the people from an accessible population who meet the eligibility criteria over a specific time interval or for a specified sample size. For example, in a study of ventilated-associated pneumonia in intensive care unit (ICU) patients, if the accessible population were patients in an ICU of a specific hospital, a consecutive sample might consist of all eligible patients admitted to that ICU over a 6-month period. Or it might be the first 250 eligible patients admitted to the ICU, if 250 were the targeted sample size.

Consecutive sampling is a far better approach than sampling by convenience, especially if the sampling period is sufficiently long to deal with potential biases that reflect seasonal or other time-related fluctuations. When all members of an accessible population are invited to participate in a study over a fixed time period, the risk of bias is greatly reduced. Consecutive sampling is often a good choice for a sampling design when there is "rolling enrollment" into a contained accessible population.

Example of a Consecutive Sample
Using consecutive sampling, Zúñiga and colleagues (2022) did a retrospective chart review of 1,276 visits by nursing home residents to Swiss emergency rooms. The researchers aimed to explore the factors associated with use of services and possibly avoidable emergency room visits.

Purposive Sampling

Purposive sampling uses researchers' knowledge about the population to make selections. Researchers might decide purposely to select people who are judged to be particularly knowledgeable about the issues under study, for example, as in the case of a Delphi survey. A drawback is that this approach may not result in a typical or representative sample. Purposive sampling is sometimes used to good advantage in two-staged sampling. For example, sites can first be sampled purposively, with efforts made to select sites that reflect divergent population characteristics; then people can be sampled from the sites in some other fashion, such as by using consecutive sampling.

Example of Purposive Sampling
Janatolmakan and Khatony (2022) used purposive sampling to recruit 14 nurses working in a hospital to qualitatively explore these nurses experience of missed nursing care.

Evaluation of Nonprobability Sampling

Except for some consecutive samples, nonprobability samples are rarely representative of the population. When every element in the population does not have a chance of being included in the sample, it is likely that some segment of it will be systematically underrepresented. When there is sampling bias, the results could be misleading, and efforts to generalize to a broader population could be misguided.

Nonprobability samples will continue to predominate, however, because of their practicality. Probability sampling requires time, skill, and resources, so using a probability approach might not be an option. Convenience sampling without explicit efforts to enhance representativeness, however, should be avoided. We would argue that quantitative researchers would do better at achieving representative samples for generalizing to a population if they had an approach that was more purposeful (Polit & Beck, 2010).

Quota sampling is a semipurposive sampling strategy that is far superior to convenience sampling because it seeks to ensure sufficient representation within key strata of the population. Another purposive strategy for enhancing generalizability is deliberate multisite sampling. For instance, a convenience sample could be obtained from two communities known to differ socioeconomically, so that the sample would reflect the experiences of both lower- and middle-class participants. In other words, if the population is known to be heterogeneous, you should take steps to capture important variation in the sample.

Even in one-site studies in which convenience sampling is used, researchers can make an effort to explicitly add cases to correspond more closely to population traits. For example, if half the population is known to be male, then the researcher can check to see if approximately half the sample is male and then use outreach to recruit more males if they are underrepresented.

Quantitative researchers using nonprobability samples must be cautious about the inferences they make, especially if they do not make efforts to deliberately (purposively) enhance representativeness. Purposive approaches, although not usually held in high esteem in quantitative research, can be used to great advantage to improve the relevance of research evidence to real-world clinical settings.

PROBABILITY SAMPLING

Probability sampling involves the random selection of elements from a population. **Random sampling** involves a selection process in which each element in the population has an equal, independent chance of being selected. Probability sampling is a complex, technical topic; books such as those by Thompson (2012) offer further guidance for advanced students.

> **TIP** Random sampling should not be (but often is) confused with random assignment, which was described in connection with experimental designs (Chapter 9). Random assignment is the process of allocating people to different treatment conditions at random. Random *assignment* is unrelated to how people in an RCT were selected in the first place. Indeed, random sampling is rarely used in RCTs.

Simple Random Sampling

The most basic probability sampling is **simple random sampling**. Researchers using simple random sampling establish a **sampling frame,** the technical name for the list of elements from which the sample will be randomly chosen. If nursing students at the University of Connecticut were the accessible population, then a roster of those students would be the sampling frame. If the sampling unit were 300-bed or larger hospitals in Taiwan, then a list of all such hospitals would be the sampling frame. Sometimes a population is defined in terms of an existing sampling frame. For example, if we wanted to use a voter registration list as a sampling frame, we would have to define the community population as residents who had registered to vote.

Once a sampling frame has been developed, elements are numbered consecutively. A table of random numbers or computer software would then be used to draw a random sample of the desired size. An example of a sampling frame for a population of 50 people is shown in Table 13.3. Assume we wish to randomly sample 20 people. We could find a starting place in a random numbers table by blindly placing our finger at some point on the page to find a two-digit combination between 01 and 50. For this example, suppose that we began with the first two-digit number in the random number table of Table 9.2 (p. xx), which is 46, the person corresponding to that number, D. Abraham, is the first person selected to participate in the study. Number 05, H. Edelman, is the second selection, and number 23, J. Yepsen, is the third. This process would continue until 20 participants were chosen. The selected elements are circled in Table 13.3.

A sample selected randomly in this fashion is unbiased. Although there is no guarantee that a random sample will be representative, random selection ensures that differences in the attributes of the sample and the population are purely a function of chance. The probability of selecting an unrepresentative sample decreases as the size of the sample increases.

Simple random sampling tends to be laborious. Developing a sampling frame, numbering all elements, and selecting elements are time-consuming chores, particularly if the population is large. In actual practice, simple random sampling is used infrequently because it is relatively inefficient. Furthermore, it is not always possible to get a listing of every element in the population, so other methods are often required.

Example of a Simple Random Sample
Feng et al. (2022) explored near-miss organizational learning in a Chinese nursing organization. To do so, they used both quantitative and qualitative approaches. For the quantitative arm, they used simple random sampling to survey 600 nurses.

Stratified Random Sampling

In **stratified random sampling**, the population is first divided into two or more homogeneous strata (e.g., based on gender), from which elements are selected at random. Unlike quota sampling, stratified random sampling requires that a person's status in a stratum be known before making selections, which can be problematic. Patient listings or organizational directories may contain information for meaningful stratification, but many lists do not.

The most common procedure for drawing a stratified random sample is to group together elements belonging to a stratum and to select the desired number of elements randomly. To illustrate, suppose that the list in Table 13.3 consisted of 25 males (numbers 1 through 25) and 25 females (numbers 26 through 50). Using gender as the stratifying variable, we could guarantee a sample of 10 males and 10 females by randomly sampling 10 numbers from the first half of the list and 10 from the second half. As it turns out, simple random sampling did result in 10 people being chosen from each half-list, but this was purely by chance. It would not have been unusual to draw, say, 8 names

TABLE 13.3 • Sampling Frame for Simple Random Sampling Example

①.	N. Alexander	㊉.	C. Ball
2.	D. Brady	27.	L. Chodos
3.	D. Carroll	28.	K. DiSanto
4.	M. Dakes	29.	B. Eddy
⑤.	H. Edelman	㉚.	J. Fishon
⑥.	L. Forester	㉛.	R. Griffin
7.	J. Galt	32.	B. Hebert
8.	L. Hall	㉝.	C. Joyce
9.	R. Ivry	㉞.	S. Kane
10.	A. Janosy	35.	C. Lace
11.	J. Kettlewell	36.	M. Montanari
12.	L. Lack	37.	B. Nicolet
⑬.	B. Mastrianni	㊳.	T. Opitz
⑭.	K. Nolte	39.	J. Portnoy
15.	N. O'Hara	40.	G. Queto
16.	T. Piekarz	41.	A. Ryan
⑰.	J. Quint	42.	S. Singleton
⑱.	M. Riggi	㊸.	L. Tower
19.	M. Solomons	44.	V. Vaccaro
20.	S. Thompson	45.	B. Wilmot
㉑.	C. VanWagner	㊻.	D. Abraham
22.	R. Walsh	47.	V. Brusser
㉓.	J. Yepsen	48.	O. Crampton
㉔.	M. Zimmerman	49.	R. Davis
25.	A. Arnold	㊿.	C. Eldred

from one half and 12 from the other. Stratified sampling can guarantee the appropriate representation of different population segments.

Stratification usually divides the population into unequal subpopulations. For example, if the person's race were used to stratify the population of U.S. citizens, the subpopulation of White people would be larger than that of other populations. In **proportionate stratified sampling,** participants are selected in proportion to the size of the population stratum. If the population was students in a nursing school that had 20% African American, 20% Hispanic, 10% Asian, and 50% White students, then a proportionate stratified sample of 100 students, with race/ethnicity as the stratifier, would draw 20, 20, 10, and 50 students from the respective strata.

Proportionate sampling may result in insufficient numbers for making comparisons between strata. In our example, it would be risky to draw conclusions about Asian nursing students based on only 10 cases. For this reason, researchers may use **disproportionate sampling** when comparisons are sought between strata of greatly unequal size. In our example, the sampling proportions might be altered to select 20 African American, 20 Hispanic, 20 Asian, and 40 White students. This design would ensure more adequate coverage of Asian nurses. When disproportionate sampling is used, however, it is necessary to make an adjustment to arrive at the best estimate of *overall* population values. This adjustment, called **weighting**, is a simple mathematic computation described in textbooks on sampling.

Stratified random sampling enables researchers to sharpen a sample's representativeness. Stratified sampling, however, may be impossible if information on the critical variables is unavailable. Furthermore, a stratified sample requires even more labor and effort than simple random sampling because the sample must be drawn from multiple enumerated listings.

Example of Stratified Random Sampling
Jadoon et al. (2022) used a stratified random sampling technique to recruit 195 nursing students. The researchers aimed to explore these students' knowledge, attitudes, and readiness to assess people's sexuality.

Multistage Cluster Sampling

For many populations, it is impossible to obtain a listing of all elements. For example, the population of full-time nursing students in Canada would be difficult to list and enumerate for the purpose of drawing a random sample. Large-scale surveys almost never use simple or stratified random sampling; they usually rely on multistage sampling, beginning with clusters.

Cluster sampling involves selecting broad groups (clusters), rather than selecting individuals, as the first stage of a multistage approach. For a sample of nursing students, we might first draw a random sample of nursing schools and then draw a sample of students from the selected schools. The usual procedure for selecting samples from a general population in the United States is to sample successively such administrative units as census tracts, then households, and then household members. The resulting design can be described in terms of the number of stages (e.g., three-stage sampling). Clusters can be selected by simple or stratified methods. For instance, in selecting nursing schools, we could stratify on geographic region.

For a specified number of cases, multistage sampling tends to be less accurate than simple or stratified random sampling. Yet, multistage sampling is more practical than other types of probability sampling, particularly when the population is large and widely dispersed.

Example of Multistage Sampling
Using focus groups and qualitative interviews Abel and colleagues (2023) engaged females who were enrolled in the original Migrant Women's Health Care Needs for Chronic Illness Services in Switzerland. The parent study explored females' access to and quality of healthcare, whereas the sub study utilized a multistage sampling process to explore females' suggestions for improving care services and policy recommendations.

Systematic Sampling

Systematic sampling involves selecting every *k*th case from a list, such as every 10th person on a patient listing or every 25th person on a student roster. When this sampling method is applied to a sampling frame, an essentially random sample can be drawn, using the following procedure.

The desired sample size is established at some number (n). The size of the population must be known or estimated (N). By dividing N by n, a sampling interval (k) is established. The **sampling interval** is the standard distance between sampled elements.

In other words, every 200th element on the list would be sampled. The first element should be selected randomly. Suppose that we randomly selected number 73 from a random number table. People corresponding to numbers 73, 273, 473, and so on would be sampled.

Systematic sampling yields essentially the same results as simple random sampling but involves less work. Problems can arise if a list is arranged in such a way that a certain type of element is listed at intervals coinciding with the sampling interval. For instance, if every 10th nurse listed in a nursing staff roster was a head nurse and the sampling interval was 10, then head nurses would either always or never be included in the sample. Problems of this type are rare, fortunately. Systematic sampling can also be applied to lists that have been stratified.

TIP Systematic sampling is sometimes used to sample every *k*th person entering a store or leaving a hospital. In such situations, unless the population is narrowly defined as all those people entering or leaving, the sample is essentially a sample of convenience.

Example of a Systematic Sample
Jara and colleagues (2022) in investigated the factors associated with consistent condom use in sexually active military personnel in Eastern Ethiopia. To obtain a sample of 314 study subjects, the team used systematic sampling techniques. Using a list of all 3,650 military personnel, they enrolled every 12th person into the study.

Evaluation of Probability Sampling

Probability sampling is the best method of obtaining representative samples. If all the elements in a population have an equal probability of being selected, then the resulting sample is likely to do a good job of representing the population. Another advantage is that probability sampling allows researchers to estimate the magnitude of sampling error. **Sampling error** refers to differences between sample values (e.g., the average age of the sample) and population values (the average age of the population).

The drawback of probability sampling is its impracticality. It is typically not possible to select a probability sample, unless the population is narrowly defined—and if it *is* narrowly defined, probability sampling might be "overkill." Probability sampling is the preferred and most respected method of obtaining sample elements but is often unfeasible.

TIP The quality of the sampling plan is of particular importance in survey research, because the purpose of surveys is to obtain information about the prevalence or average values for a population. All national surveys, such as the National Health Interview Survey in the United States, use probability samples. Probability samples are almost never used in intervention studies.

SAMPLE SIZE IN QUANTITATIVE STUDIES

Quantitative researchers typically identify how large a sample they need at the outset of a study. A procedure called **power analysis** (Cohen, 1988) can be used to estimate sample size needs, but some statistical knowledge is needed before this procedure can be explained. In this section, we offer guidelines to beginning researchers; advanced students can read about power analysis in Chapter 18.

Sample Size Basics

There are no simple formulas that can tell you how large a sample you will need in study, but as a general recommendation, you should use as large a sample as possible. The larger the sample, the more representative of the population it is likely to be. Every time researchers calculate a percentage or an average based on sample data, they are estimating a population value. Larger samples yield smaller sampling errors.

Let us illustrate this with an example of monthly aspirin consumption in a nursing home (Table 13.4). The population consists of 15 residents whose aspirin consumption averages 16.0 aspirins per month, as shown in the top row of the table. We drew 8 simple random samples—two each with sample sizes of 2, 3, 5, and 10. Each sample average represents an estimate of the population average (here, 16.0). With a sample size of two, our estimate might have been wrong by as many as eight aspirins (sample 1B, average of 24.0), which is 50% greater than the population value. As the sample size increases, the averages get closer to the true population value, *and the differences in the estimates between samples A and B get smaller as well.* As sample size increases, the probability of getting a deviant sample diminishes. Large samples provide an opportunity to counterbalance atypical values. In the absence of a power analysis, the safest procedure is to obtain data from as large a sample as is feasible.

Large samples are no assurance of accuracy, however. When nonprobability sampling is used, even large samples can harbor bias. A famous example is the 1936 American presidential poll conducted by the magazine *Literary Digest*, which predicted that Alfred Landon would defeat Franklin D. Roosevelt by a landslide. About 2.5 million people participated in this poll. Biases resulted from the fact that this large sample was drawn from telephone directories and automobile registrations during a depression year when only the affluent (who preferred Landon) had a car or telephone. Thus, a large sample cannot correct for a faulty sampling design, but a large nonprobability sample is preferable to a small one.

Most nursing studies use samples of convenience, and many are based on samples that are too small to provide an adequate test of research hypotheses. Research reports often offer no justification for sample size. When samples are too small, quantitative researchers run the risk of gathering data that will not support their hypotheses, *even when their hypotheses are correct*, thereby undermining statistical conclusion validity.

Factors Affecting Sample Size Requirements in Quantitative Research

The number of participants needed in a study is affected by various factors, including effect size, homogeneity of the population, cooperation and attrition, and subgroup analysis.

TABLE 13.4 • Comparison of Population and Sample Values and Averages: Nursing Home Aspirin Consumption Example

NUMBER OF PEOPLE IN GROUP	GROUP	INDIVIDUAL DATA VALUES (NUMBER OF ASPIRINS CONSUMED, PRIOR MONTH)	AVERAGE
15	Population	2, 4, 6, 8, 10, 12, 14, 16, 18, 20, 22, 24, 26, 28, 30	16.0
2	Sample 1A	6, 14	10.0
2	Sample 1B	20, 28	24.0
3	Sample 2A	16, 18, 8	14.0
3	Sample 2B	20, 14, 26	20.0
5	Sample 3A	26, 14, 18, 2, 28	17.6
5	Sample 3B	30, 2, 26, 10, 4	14.4
10	Sample 4A	22, 16, 24, 20, 2, 8, 14, 28, 20, 4	15.8
10	Sample 4B	12, 18, 8, 10, 16, 6, 28, 14, 30, 22	16.4

Effect Size

Power analysis builds on the concept of an **effect size**, which expresses the strength of relationships among research variables. If there is reason to expect that the independent and dependent variables are strongly correlated, then a relatively small sample may be adequate to reveal the relationship statistically. Typically, however, nursing interventions have moderate effects. When there is no a priori reason for believing that relationships are strong, then small samples are risky.

Homogeneity of the Population

If the population is relatively homogeneous, a small sample may be adequate. The greater the variability, the greater is the risk that a small sample will not adequately capture the full range of variation. For most nursing studies, it is probably best to assume a fair degree of heterogeneity.

Cooperation and Attrition

In most studies, not everyone invited to participate in a study agrees to do so. Therefore, in developing a sampling plan, it is good to begin with a realistic, evidence-based estimate of the percentage of people likely to cooperate. Thus, if your targeted sample size is 200 but you expect a 50% refusal rate, you would have to recruit about 400 eligible people.

In longitudinal studies, the number of participants usually declines over time. Attrition is most likely to occur if the time lag between data collection points is great, if the population is mobile, or if the population is at risk of death or disability. Participants might be less likely to drop out if they have an ongoing relationship with the researchers, but it is rarely 0%. Thus, in estimating sample size needs, attrition needs to be considered.

Attrition problems are not restricted to longitudinal studies. People who initially agree to cooperate in a study may be subsequently unable or unwilling to participate for various reasons, such as death, deteriorating health, early discharge, or simply a change of heart. Researchers should expect participant loss and recruit accordingly.

Subgroup Analyses

Researchers sometimes wish to test hypotheses not only for an entire population but for subgroups. For example, suppose we were interested in assessing whether a structured exercise program is effective in improving infants' motor skills. We might also want to test whether the intervention is more effective for certain infants (e.g., low-birthweight vs. normal-birthweight infants). When a sample is divided to test for **subgroup effects**, the sample must be large enough to support analyses with subsets of the sample.

IMPLEMENTING A QUANTITATIVE SAMPLING PLAN

This section provides some practical guidance about implementing a sampling plan.

Steps in Sampling in Quantitative Studies

The steps to be undertaken in drawing a sample vary somewhat from one sampling design to the next, but a general outline of procedures can be described.

1. *Identify the population.* You should begin with a clear idea about the population to which you would like to generalize your results. Unless you have extensive resources, you are unlikely to have access to the full target population, so you will also need to identify the population that is accessible to you. Researchers sometimes *begin* by identifying an accessible population and then decide how best to characterize the target population.

2. *Specify the eligibility criteria.* The criteria for eligibility should then be spelled out. The criteria should be as specific as possible with regard to characteristics that might exclude potential participants (e.g., extremes of poor health, inability to read English). The criteria might lead you to redefine the target population.

3. *Specify the sampling plan.* Next, you must decide the method of drawing the sample and how large it will be. If you can perform a power analysis to estimate the needed number of participants,

we highly recommend that you do so. Similarly, if probability sampling is a viable option, that option should be exercised. If you are not in a position to do either, we recommend using as large a sample as possible and taking steps to build representativeness into the design (e.g., by using quota or consecutive sampling).
4. *Recruit the sample.* The next step is to recruit prospective participants (after any needed institutional permissions have been obtained) and ask for their cooperation. Issues relating to participant recruitment are discussed next.

Sample Recruitment

Recruiting people to participate in a study typically involves two major tasks: identifying eligible candidates and persuading them to participate. Researchers must consider the best sources for recruiting potential participants. Researchers must ask such questions as, Where do large numbers of people matching my population construct live or obtain care? Will I have direct access, or will I need to work through gatekeepers? Will there be sufficiently large numbers in one location, or will multiple sites be necessary? During the recruitment phase, it may be necessary to create a **screening instrument**, which is a brief form that allows researchers to determine whether a prospective participant meets the study's eligibility criteria.

The next task involves gaining the cooperation of people who have been deemed eligible. There is considerable evidence that the percentage of people willing to cooperate in clinical trials and surveys is declining, and so it is critical to have an effective recruitment strategy.

TIP Technologic innovations have made it possible to access research samples for certain kinds of studies. Participants can be recruited through social media outlets and specialized crowdsourcing platforms, such as Amazon's Mechanical Turk. Studies comparing these approaches to typical approaches to community sampling indicate that this sort of crowdsourcing is cost effective and comparable (Mortensen & Hughes, 2018). Further, others indicate that this sort of approach may contribute to an ability to recruit more diverse and some hard-to-reach samples (Lee et al., 2022). Others support the use of these platforms but also caution that they may not be generalizable and in the case of older adults may overrepresent a healthy, technologically savvy, and better educated population (Turner et al., 2021).

Studies involving biobanking have proliferated in the past few years. The National Institute of Health has a biobank, *All of Us*. Some of the data available include the following: survey responses, physical measurements, electronic health records, genotyping arrays, genome sequences, and Fitbit records (NIH, 2023). *All of Us* is just one example of a biobank; there are numerous others, many of which are private entities. Access to biobanks is variable in terms of cost. While all require permissions and data use agreements, some are available publicly, others at a cost per specimen and if your organization has a biobank, you are typically able to apply for access without cost. For further reading, Annaratone and colleagues (2021) provide more information about biobanking, including its history and potential.

A lot of recent methodologic research in health fields has focused on strategies for effective recruitment. Researchers have found that rates of cooperation can often be enhanced by means of the following: face-to-face recruitment; multiple contacts and requests; monetary and nonmonetary incentives; brief data collection; inclusion of questions perceived as having high relevance to participants; assurances of anonymity; and endorsement of the study by a respected person or institution. Researchers have also anticipated recruitment benefits from the involvement of patients in the research process, but the evidence about the success of such efforts is mixed (Brett et al., 2014; Dawson et al., 2018).

Participant recruitment often proceeds at a slower pace than researchers anticipate. This makes it useful to develop contingency plans for recruiting more people, should the initial plan prove overly optimistic. For example, a contingency plan might involve relaxing the eligibility criteria, identifying another institution through which participants could be recruited, offering incentives to make participation more attractive, or lengthening the recruitment period. When such plans are developed at the outset, it reduces the likelihood that you will have to settle for a less-than-desirable sample size.

Generalizing From Samples

Ideally, the sample is representative of the accessible population, and the accessible population is representative of the target population. By using a strong sampling plan, researchers can be reasonably confident that the first part of this ideal has been realized. The second part of the ideal entails greater risk. Are diabetic patients in Boston representative of diabetic patients in the United States? Researchers must exercise judgment in assessing the degree of similarity.

The best advice is to be realistic and conservative and to ask challenging questions: Is it reasonable to assume that the accessible population is representative of the target population? In what ways might they differ? How would such differences affect the conclusions? If differences are great, it would be prudent to specify a more restricted target population to which the findings could be meaningfully generalized.

Interpretations about the generalizability of findings can be strengthened by comparing sample characteristics with population characteristics, when this is possible. Published information about the characteristics of many populations may be available to help in evaluating sampling bias. For example, if you were studying low-income children in Chicago, you could obtain information on the Internet about salient characteristics (e.g., race/ethnicity, age distribution) of low-income American children from the U.S. Bureau of the Census. Population characteristics could then be compared with sample characteristics and differences taken into account in interpreting the findings.

> **Example of Comparing Sample and Population Characteristics**
> Yu and colleagues (2022) aimed to study potential predictors of attrition in a longitudinal study examining health-related quality of life. Wave one included 2,734 respondents, whereas wave two had 1,467 and wave three had 964. In comparing factors such as health-related quality of life, COVID-19 experience, and demographics over time, they were able to determine the predictors of attrition such as younger age.

We encourage further reading on the important topic of sampling. For example, Sousa et al. (2004) have provided suggestions for drawing conclusions about whether a convenience sample is representative of the population. Greenhouse et al. (2008) described an approach for making what they call "generalizability judgments" from clinical trial data. Sen et al. (2016) proposed a multitrait metric to explore how a study's eligibility criteria affect its generalizability.

CRITICAL APPRAISAL OF SAMPLING PLANS

In coming to conclusions about the quality of evidence that a study yields, you should carefully scrutinize the sampling plan. If the sample is too small or likely to be biased, the findings may be misleading or just plain wrong.

You should consider two issues in your appraisal of a study's sampling plan. The first is whether the researcher adequately described the sampling strategy. Reports of nursing studies have been found to be deficient in their descriptions of sampling plans (e.g., Suhonen et al., 2015). Ideally, research reports should include a description of the following:

- The type of sampling approach used (e.g., convenience, simple random)
- The study population and eligibility criteria for sample selection
- The number of participants and a rationale for the sample size, including whether a power analysis was performed
- A description of the main characteristics of sample members (e.g., age, gender, medical condition, and so forth) and, ideally, of the population
- The number and characteristics of potential participants who declined to participate in the study and/or who did not participate in later rounds of data collection

If the description of the sample is insufficient, you may not be able to come to conclusions about whether the researcher made good sampling decisions. And, if the description is incomplete, it will be difficult to know whether the evidence is of use in your clinical practice.

Sampling plans should be scrutinized with respect to their effects on the construct, internal, external, and statistical conclusion validity of the study. If a sample is small, statistical conclusion validity may be undermined. If the eligibility criteria are restrictive, this could benefit internal validity—but possibly to the detriment of construct and external validity.

You will never know for sure if a study sample adequately represents the population, but if the sampling design is weak or if the sample size is small, there is reason to suspect some bias. When researchers adopt a sampling plan in which the risk for bias is high, they should take steps to estimate the direction and degree of this bias so that readers can draw informed conclusions.

Even with a rigorous sampling plan, the sample may be biased if not all people invited to participate in a study agree to do so—which is almost always the case. If certain segments of the population refuse to participate, then a biased sample can result, even when probability sampling is used. Research reports should provide information about **response rates** (i.e., the number of people participating in a study relative to the number of people sampled) and about possible **nonresponse bias** (sometimes called *response bias*), which reflects differences between participants and those who declined to participate. In longitudinal studies, attrition bias should be reported.

One of your jobs in appraising studies is to come to conclusions about the reasonableness of generalizing the findings from the researcher's sample to the accessible population and from the accessible population to a target population. If the sampling plan is flawed, it may be risky to generalize the findings without replicating the study with another sample.

Box 13.1 presents some guiding questions for critically appraising the sampling plan of a quantitative research report.

BOX 13.1 Guidelines for Critically Appraising Quantitative Sampling Plans

1. Was the study population identified and described? Were eligibility criteria specified? Were the sample selection procedures clearly delineated?
2. Do the sample and population specifications (eligibility criteria) support an inference of construct validity with regard to the population construct?
3. What type of sampling plan was used? Was the sampling plan one that could be expected to yield a representative sample? Would an alternative sampling plan have yielded a better sample?
4. If sampling was stratified, was a useful stratification variable selected? If a consecutive sample was used, was the time period long enough to address seasonal or temporal variation? In a multisite study, were sites selected in a manner that improved representativeness?
5. How were people recruited into the sample? Does the method suggest potential biases? Were strategies used to strengthen recruitment?
6. Is it likely that some factor other than the sampling plan (e.g., a low response rate, recruitment difficulties) affected the representativeness of the sample?
7. Are possible sample biases or other sampling deficiencies identified by the researchers?
8. Are key characteristics of the sample described (e.g., average age, percent female)?
9. Is the sample size sufficiently large to enhance statistical conclusion validity? Was the sample size justified on the basis of a power analysis or other rationale?
10. Does the sample support inferences of external validity? To whom can the study results reasonably be generalized?

RESEARCH EXAMPLE

In this section, we describe the sampling plan of a quantitative nursing project.

Study: Active Engagement, Protective Buffering, and Depressive Symptoms in Young-Midlife Couples Surviving Cancer: The Roles of Age and Sex (Lyons et al., 2022.)

Purpose: To explore in couples, where one partner is surviving cancer, the roles that survivor age and sex have on active engagement, protective buffering, and depressive symptoms.

Method: This study used an exploratory descriptive design to engage cancer survivors and their partners 1 to 3 years post the diagnosis.

Sampling plan: The study team used the Oregon State Cancer Registry to recruit potential participants. Targeted mailings describing the study were sent by registry staff to survivors meeting initial eligibility criteria. Zip codes were used so as to recruit from both urban and rural areas of Oregon. Letters (N = 700) were sent within equal numbers sent to survivors age (aged 21–39 at the time of diagnosis) and survivors (aged 40–56 at the time of diagnosis). Other sampling techniques include posting flyers in an oncology clinic at Oregon Health and Science University.

Research staff used eligibility criteria to screen potential participants. They were eligible if the survivor had a primary diagnosis of invasive cancer in the past 1 to 3 years, the couple was cohabiting in Oregon and age 21 to 56 at the time of the cancer diagnosis, could read and speak English, had access to a telephone, and not considering retirement at time of diagnosis. There was no requirement for the couples to be married and the study was open to couples of any sexual orientation.

Two survivors responded from the oncology office postings and 158 from registry mailings. While 21% of those who responded could not be reached despite several attempts, a total of 77 couples were eligible and consented to be in the study.

Key findings:

- There were no significant differences in the level of depressive symptoms between survivors and their partners.
- At 1 to 3 years post the cancer diagnosis, 33% of survivors had depressive symptoms warranting further assessment.
- Between the survivors and partners, there was not a significant difference in depressive symptoms based on age or sex.
- There were group differences by survivor sex in active engagement and protective buffering behaviors with male survivors reporting significantly higher levels of active engagement by their partners and female survivors reporting significantly more protective buffering by their partners.
- Lastly, the findings indicate that older partners and female survivors seemed to experience more positive effects than younger partners and male survivors indicating age and sex were moderators.

SUMMARY POINTS

- **Sampling** is the process of selecting a portion of the **population,** which is an entire aggregate of cases, for a study. An **element** is the most basic population unit about which information is collected—usually humans in nursing research.
- **Eligibility criteria** are used to establish population characteristics and to determine who can participate in a study—either who can be included (**inclusion criteria**) or who should be excluded (**exclusion criteria**).
- Researchers usually sample from an **accessible population** but should identify the **target population** to which they would like to generalize their results.
- In quantitative studies, a key quality criterion for a sample is its **representativeness**—the extent to which the sample is similar to the population and free from bias. **Sampling bias** refers to the systematic overrepresentation or underrepresentation of some segment of the population.
- Methods of **nonprobability sampling** (wherein elements are selected by nonrandom methods) include convenience, quota, consecutive, and purposive sampling. Nonprobability sampling designs are practical but usually have strong potential for bias.

- **Convenience sampling** uses the most readily available or convenient group of people for the sample. **Snowball sampling** is a type of convenience sampling in which referrals for potential participants are made by those already in the sample.
- **Quota sampling** divides the population into homogeneous **strata** (subpopulations) to ensure representation of subgroups; within each stratum, people are sampled by convenience.
- **Consecutive sampling** involves taking *all* of the people from an accessible population who meet the eligibility criteria over a specific time interval or for a specified sample size.
- In **purposive sampling**, elements are hand-picked to be included in the sample based on the researcher's knowledge about the population.
- **Probability sampling** designs, which involve the random selection of elements from the population, yield more representative samples than nonprobability designs and permit estimates of the magnitude of **sampling error.**
- **Simple random sampling** involves the random selection of elements from a **sampling frame** that enumerates all population elements. **Stratified random sampling** divides the population into homogeneous strata from which elements are selected at random, either *proportionately* relative to the size of the subgroup in the population or *disproportionately* to ensure an adequate sample size for small subgroups.
- **Cluster sampling** involves sampling of large units. In **multistage random sampling,** there is a successive, multistaged selection of random samples from larger units (clusters) to smaller units (individuals) by either simple random or stratified random methods.
- **Systematic sampling** is the selection of every *k*th case from a list. By dividing the population size by the desired sample size, the researcher establishes the **sampling interval,** which is the standard distance between the selected elements.
- In quantitative studies, researchers ideally should use a **power analysis** to estimate **sample size** needs. Large samples are preferable to small ones because larger samples enhance statistical conclusion validity and tend to be more representative, but even large sample do not *guarantee* representativeness.
- The recruitment of study participants is increasingly challenging. **Response rates** are often low, which can lead to a biased sample and to problems reaching the desired sample size.

REFERENCES CITED IN CHAPTER 13

Abdella, S., Demissie, M., Worku, A., Dheresa, M., & Berhane, Y. (2022). HIV prevalence and associated factors among female sex workers in Ethiopia, east Africa: A cross-sectional study using a respondent-driven sampling technique. *EClinicalMedicine*, *51*, 101540. https://doi.org/10.1016/j.eclinm.2022.101540

Abel, T., Tadesse, L., Frahsa, A., & Sakarya, S. (2023). Integrating Patient-Reported Experience (PRE) in a multistage approach to study access to health services for women with chronic illness and migration experience. *Health Expectations*, *26*(1), 237–244. https://doi.org/10.1111/hex.13649

Annaratone, L., De Palma, G., Bonizzi, G., Sapino, A., Botti, G., Berrino, E., Mannelli, C., Arcella, P., Di Martino, S., Steffan, A., Daidone, M. G., Canzonieri, V., Parodi, B., Paradiso, A. V., Barberis, M., Marchiò, C., & Alleanza Contro il Cancro ACC Pathology and Biobanking Working Group. (2021). Basic principles of biobanking: From biological samples to precision medicine for patients. *Virchows Archiv*, *479*(2), 233–246. https://doi.org/10.1007/s00428-021-03151-0

Brett, J., Staniszewska, S., Mockford, C., Herron-Marx, S., Hughes, J., Tysall, C., & Suleman, R. (2014). Mapping the impact of patient and public involvement on health and social care research: A systematic review. *Health Expectations*, *17*(5), 637–650.

Cohen, J. (1988). *Statistical power analysis for the behavioral sciences* (2nd ed.). Lawrence Erlbaum Associates.

Dawson, S., Campbell, S. M., Giles, S. J., Morris, R. L., & Cheraghi-Sohi, S. (2018). Black and minority ethnic group involvement in health and social care research: A systematic review. *Health Expectations*, *21*(1), 3–22. https://doi.org/10.1111/hex.12597

Faulkner, K. M., Jurgens, C. Y., Denfeld, Q. E., Chien, C. V., Thompson, J. H., Gelow, J. M., Grady, K. L., & Lee, C. S. (2022). Patterns and predictors of dyspnoea following left ventricular assist device implantation. *European Journal of Cardiovascular Nursing*, *21*(7), 724–731. https://doi.org/10.1093/eurjcn/zvac007

Feng, T., Zhang, X., Tan, L., Su, Y., & Liu, H. (2022). Near-miss organizational learning in nursing within a tertiary hospital: A mixed methods study. *BMC Nursing*, *21*(1), 315. https://doi.org/10.1186/s12912-022-01071-1

Greenhouse, J., Kaizar, E., Kelleher, K., Seltman, H., & Gardner, W. (2008). Generalizing from clinical trial data: A case study. The risk of suicidality among pediatric antidepressant users. *Statistics in Medicine*, *27*(11), 1801–1813.

Jadoon, S. B., Nasir, S., Victor, G., & Pienaar, A. J. (2022). Knowledge attitudes and readiness of nursing students in assessing peoples' sexual health problems. *Nurse Education Today*, *113*, 105371. https://doi.org/10.1016/j.nedt.2022.105371

Janatolmakan, M., & Khatony, A. (2022). Explaining the experience of nurses on missed nursing care: A qualitative descriptive study in Iran. *Applied Nursing Research*, *63*, 151542. https://doi.org/10.1016/j.apnr.2021.151542

Jara, H., Damena, M., Urgessa, K., Deressa, A., Debella, A., Mussa, I., Mohammed, A., & Weldegebreal, F. (2022). Consistent condom use and associated factors among sexually active military personnel in Eastern Ethiopia: Cross-sectional study Design. *Risk Management and Healthcare Policy*, *15*, 2057–2070. https://doi.org/10.2147/RMHP.S375340

Lee, J. J., Aguirre Herrera, J., Cardona, J., Cruz, L. Y., Munguía, L., Leyva Vera, C. A., & Robles, G. (2022). Culturally tailored social media content to reach Latinx immigrant sexual minority men for HIV prevention: Web-based feasibility study. *JMIR Formative Research*, *6*(3), e36446. https://doi.org/10.2196/36446

Lyons, K. S., Gorman, J. R., Larkin, B. S., Duncan, G., & Hayes-Lattin, B. (2022). Active engagement, protective buffering, and depressive symptoms in young-midlife couples surviving cancer: The roles of age and sex. *Frontiers in Psychology*, *13*, 816626. https://doi.org/10.3389/fpsyg.2022.816626

Mortensen, K., & Hughes, T. L. (2018). Comparing Amazon's Mechanical Turk Platform to conventional data collection methods in the health and medical research literature. *Journal of General Internal Medicine*, *33*(4), 533–538. https://doi.org/10.1007/s11606-017-4246-0

National institute of Health. (2023). *Opportunities for researchers*. Retrieved from https://allofus.nih.gov/get-involved/opportunities-researchers

Polit, D. F., & Beck, C. T. (2010). Generalization in quantitative and qualitative research: Myths and strategies. *International Journal of Nursing Studies*, *47*(11), 1451–1458.

Rahmani, F., Roshangar, F., Gholizadeh, L., & Asghari, E. (2022). Caregiver burden and the associated factors in the family caregivers of patients with schizophrenia. *Nursing Open*, *9*(4), 1995–2002. https://doi.org/10.1002/nop2.1205

Saleh, M. O., Eshah, N. F., & Rayan, A. H. (2022). Empowerment predicting nurses' work motivation and occupational mental health. *SAGE Open Nursing*, *8*. https://doi.org/10.1177/23779608221076811

Sen, A., Chakrabarti, S., Goldstein, A., Wang, S., Ryan, P., & Weng, C. (2016). GIST 2.0: A scalable multi-trait metric for quantifying population representativeness of individual clinical studies. *Journal of Biomedical Informatics*, *63*, 325–336.

Sousa, V., Zauszniewski, J. A., & Musil, C. (2004). How to determine whether a convenience sample represents the population. *Applied Nursing Research*, *17*(2), 130–133.

Suhonen, R., Stolt, M., Katajisto, J., & Leino-Kilpi, H. (2015). Review of sampling, sample and data collection procedures in nursing research-An example of research on ethical climate as perceived by nurses. *Scandinavian Journal of Caring Science*, *29*(4), 843–858.

Thompson, S. K. (2012). *Sampling* (3rd ed.). John Wiley.

Turner, A. M., Engelsma, T., Taylor, J. O., Sharma, R. K., & Demiris, G. (2020). Recruiting older adult participants through crowdsourcing platforms: Mechanical Turk versus Prolific Academic. *AMIA Annual Symposium Proceedings*, *2020*, 1230–1238.

Yu, T., Chen, J., Gu, N. Y., Hay, J. W., & Gong, C. L. (2022). Predicting panel attrition in longitudinal HRQoL surveys during the COVID-19 pandemic in the US. *Health and Quality of Life Outcomes*, *20*(1), 104. https://doi.org/10.1186/s12955-022-02015-8

Zúñiga, F., Gaertner, K., Weber-Schuh, S. K., Löw, B., Simon, M., & Müller, M. (2022). Inappropriate and potentially avoidable emergency department visits of Swiss nursing home residents and their resource use: A retrospective chart-review. *BMC Geriatrics*, *22*(1), 659. https://doi.org/10.1186/s12877-022-03308-9

14 Data Collection in Quantitative Research

Learning Objectives

1. Understand the process of developing a data collection plan.
2. Recognize the various types of structured self-report instruments.
3. Describe the differences between open and closed-ended questionnaires.
4. Explain the advantages and disadvantages of various mechanisms to distribute surveys.
5. Appreciate the skills required of interviewers to put respondents at ease and build rapport and skillfully probe for additional information when respondents give incomplete responses.

INTRODUCTION

Quantitative researchers typically collect data that are highly structured. The goal is to achieve consistency for each variable, in an effort to reduce biases and facilitate analysis. Major methods of collecting structured data are discussed in this chapter.

DEVELOPING A DATA COLLECTION PLAN

Data collection plans for quantitative studies ideally yield accurate, valid, and meaningful data. This is a challenging goal, requiring considerable effort to achieve. Steps in developing a data collection plan are described in this section.

TIP Researchers sometimes cannot measure the "real" outcomes in which they are interested. For example, mortality is an important clinical outcome, but it is rarely used in nursing research because it is too distal. When there are impediments to using a desired ultimate outcome, researchers use **surrogate outcomes**. Surrogate outcomes are not important clinical events (e.g., malnutrition), but they *predict* such events (e.g., nonuse of nutritional supplements). Although the use of surrogate outcomes is inevitable in clinical research, potential problems have been noted (e.g., Fleming & Powers, 2012; Weintraub et al., 2015).

Identifying Data Needs

Researchers usually begin by identifying the types of data needed for their study. In quantitative studies, researchers need data for several of the following purposes:

1. Testing hypotheses, addressing research questions. Researchers must include one or more measures of all key variables.
2. *Describing the sample.* Information is usually gathered about demographic and health characteristics of sample members. We advise gathering data about participants' age, gender, race or ethnicity, and education or income. This information is critical in understanding the population to whom findings can be generalized. If the

275

sample includes participants with a health problem, data on the nature of that problem should be gathered (e.g., severity, time since diagnosis).
3. *Controlling confounding variables.* Some approaches to controlling confounding variables require measuring them. For example, researchers must gather data for variables that will be statistically controlled.
4. *Analyzing potential biases.* Data for testing potential biases should be collected. For example, researchers should gather information that can shed light on selection or attrition biases.
5. *Understanding subgroup effects.* It is often desirable to answer research questions for key subgroups of participants. For example, we may wish to know if an intervention for pregnant women is equally effective for primiparas and multiparas. In such a situation, we would need to collect data about participants' childbearing history.
6. *Assessing treatment fidelity.* In intervention studies, it is useful to gather data on whether the intended treatment was actually received.
7. *Assessing costs.* In intervention studies (and in some quality improvement projects), information about costs and monetary benefits of alternative interventions is useful.
8. *Documenting administrative features.* Administrative data often need to be gathered (e.g., dates of data collection, participants' contact information).

The list of possible data needs may seem daunting, but many categories overlap. For example, participant characteristics for sample description are often used for analyzing bias, controlling confounders, or creating subgroups. If resource constraints make it impossible to collect data for the full range of variables, then researchers must prioritize data needs.

Selecting Types of Measures

After data needs have been identified, a data collection method (e.g., self-report) must be selected for each variable. It is common to combine methods (self-reports, observations, biomarkers, records) in a single study.

Data collection decisions must be guided by ethical considerations (e.g., whether covert data collection is warranted), cost constraints, availability of assistants to help with data collection, and other issues discussed in the next section. Data collection is often the costliest and lengthiest part of a study, and so compromises about the type or amount of data collected must sometimes be made.

Selecting and Developing Instruments

After making preliminary data collection decisions, researchers search for **instruments** to measure study variables (or determine whether data are available in existing records). Potentially useful data collection instruments then need to be assessed. The primary consideration is conceptual relevance: Does the instrument correspond to your conceptual definition of the variable? Another important criterion is whether the instrument will yield high-quality data. Approaches to evaluating data quality are discussed in Chapter 15. Additional factors that may affect decisions in selecting an instrument are as follows:

1. *Resources.* Resource constraints sometimes prevent the use of the highest-quality instruments. There may be direct costs (e.g., some instruments must be purchased), but the biggest expense is likely to be compensation for data collectors if you cannot collect data single-handedly. In such a situation, the instrument's length may affect its practicability. The use of costly methods may mean that you will be forced to cut costs elsewhere (e.g., using a smaller sample), so data collection expenses must be estimated.
2. *Population appropriateness.* Instruments must be chosen with the characteristics of the target population in mind. Participants' age and literacy levels are especially important. If there is concern about participants' reading skills, the *readability* of a prospective instrument should be assessed. If participants include members of minority groups, you should strive to find instruments that are culturally appropriate. If non–English-speaking participants are included in the sample, then the selection of an instrument may be based on the availability of a translated version.

3. *Norms and comparisons.* It may be desirable to select an instrument that has relevant norms. **Norms** indicate the "normal" values on the measure for a specified population, and thus offer a useful comparison. Also, it may be advantageous to select an instrument because it was used in other similar studies, which could facilitate interpretation of study findings.
4. *Clinical significance.* As we discuss in Chapter 21, efforts are increasingly being made to identify thresholds for clinically significant change on outcome measures. It might be beneficial to select an instrument for which such thresholds have been established (i.e., measures for which a *minimal important change* benchmark is available).
5. *Administration issues.* Some instruments have special requirements. For example, measuring the developmental status of children may require the skills of a professional psychologist. Some instruments require stringent conditions with regard to administration time limits, privacy, and so on. In such a case, requirements for obtaining valid measures must match attributes of the research setting.
6. *Reputation.* Two measures of the same construct may differ in the reputation they enjoy among specialists in a field, even if they are comparable with regard to data quality. Thus, it may be useful to seek the advice of people with experience using the instruments. Also, some instruments have been evaluated by special expert panels. For example, the U.S. Agency for Healthcare Research and Quality maintains a National Quality Measures Clearinghouse with recommended measures that are especially useful for outcomes research and quality improvement projects (https://www.qualitymeasures.ahrq.gov/). As another example, the COMET Initiative is an effort to standardize outcome measures used in randomized controlled trials (Williamson et al., 2017).

If existing instruments are not suitable for some variables, you may be faced with either adapting an instrument or developing a new one. Creating a new instrument should be a last resort, especially for novice researchers, because it is challenging to develop accurate and valid measuring tools (see Chapter 15).

If you locate a suitable instrument, your next step likely will be to obtain the authors' permission to use it. Instruments that have been developed under a government grant are often in the public domain, but when in doubt, it is best to obtain permission. By contacting the instrument's author, you can also request more information about the instrument and its quality.

TIP In finalizing decisions about instruments, you may need to consider tradeoffs between data quality and data quantity (i.e., how much data are collected). If compromises have to be made, it is preferable to forgo quantity: long data collection instruments tend to depress participant cooperation.

Pretesting the Data Collection Package

Researchers who develop a new instrument usually subject it to rigorous **pretesting** so that it can be evaluated and refined. Even when the data collection plan involves existing instruments, however, it is wise to conduct a pretest with a small sample of people (usually 10 to 15) who are similar to actual participants.

One purpose of a pretest is to see how much time it takes to administer the entire instrument package. Time estimates are often required for informed consent purposes, for developing a budget, and for assessing participant burden. Pretests (especially pretests of self-report instruments) can serve many other purposes, including the following:

- Identifying parts of the instrument that are hard for participants to read or understand
- Identifying questions that participants find objectionable or offensive
- Assessing whether the sequencing of questions or instruments is sensible
- Evaluating the training needs of data collectors
- Evaluating whether the measures yield data with sufficient variability

With regard to the last purpose, researchers need to ensure that there is adequate variation on key variables. For example, in a study of the link between depression and a miscarriage, depression would be compared for women who had or had not experienced a miscarriage. If the entire pretest sample looked very depressed (or not at all depressed), however, it would be advisable to pretest a different measure of depression because the original measure might not be sufficiently sensitive to detect varying levels of depression.

> **Example of Pretesting**
> Kumari et al. (2021) conducted a study to understand COVID-19 vaccine hesitancy. Based on a literature review, they developed an instrument to assess knowledge, attitude, practices, and concerns regarding the COVID-19 vaccine. They also used techniques such as focus group discussions, expert evaluation, and pretesting of the survey before administering it to 201 participants.

Developing Data Collection Forms and Procedures

After finalizing the instruments, researchers face several administrative tasks, such as developing various forms (e.g., screening forms to assess eligibility, informed consent forms, records of attempted contacts with participants). It is prudent to design forms that are attractively formatted, legible, and inviting to use; they should also be designed to ensure confidentiality. For example, identifying information (e.g., name, address) should be recorded on a page that can be detached and kept separate from other data.

> **TIP** Whenever possible, try to avoid reinventing the wheel. It is seldom necessary to start from scratch—not only in developing instruments but also in creating forms, training materials, and protocols. Ask seasoned researchers if they have materials that you could borrow or adapt.

In most quantitative studies, researchers develop **data collection protocols** that spell out procedures to be used in data collection. These protocols describe such things as the following:

- Conditions for collecting the data (e.g., Can others be present during data collection? Where must data collection occur?)
- Specific requirements for collecting the data (e.g., sequencing instruments, recording information)
- Answers to questions participants might ask (i.e., answers to FAQs). Examples of such questions include the following: How will information from this study be used? How did you get my name? How long will this take? Who will have access to this information? Can I see the study results? Whom can I contact if I have a complaint? Will I be paid or reimbursed for expenses?
- Procedures to follow if a participant becomes distraught, or for any other reason cannot complete the data collection process.

Researchers also need to decide how to actually gather, record, and manage their data. Technological advances continue to offer new options, some of which we discuss later in the chapter. Suggestions about new technology for data collection are offered by Coons et al. (2015), Schick-Makaroff and Molzahn (2015), and Udtha et al. (2015).

> **TIP** Document all major actions and decisions as you develop and implement your data collection plan. You may need the information later when you write your research report, request funding for a follow-up study, or help other researchers with a similar study.

STRUCTURED SELF-REPORT INSTRUMENTS

The most widely used data collection method by nurse researchers is structured self-reports, which involve formal instruments. The instrument is an **interview schedule** when questions are asked orally in face-to-face or telephone interviews. It is called a **questionnaire** or an SAQ (self-administered questionnaire) when respondents complete the instrument themselves, either in a paper-and-pencil format or on a computer. This section discusses the development and administration of structured self-report instruments.

Types of Structured Questions

Structured self-report instruments consist of a set of questions (often called **items**) in which the wording of both the questions and, in most cases, **response options** are predetermined. Participants are asked to respond to the same questions, in the same order, and with a fixed set of response alternatives. Researchers developing structured instruments must carefully attend to the content, form, and wording of questions.

Open- and Closed-Ended Questions

Instruments vary in degree of structure through different combinations of open-ended and closed-ended questions. **Open-ended questions** allow people to respond in their own words, in narrative fashion. The question "What was your biggest challenge after your surgery?" is an example of an open-ended question. In questionnaires, respondents are asked to give a written reply to open-ended items, and so adequate space must be provided to permit a full response. Interviewers are expected to quote oral responses verbatim.

Closed-ended (or *fixed-alternative*) **questions** offer response options, from which respondents choose the one that most closely matches their answer. The alternatives may range from a simple *yes* or *no* ("Have you smoked a cigarette today?") to complex expressions of opinion or behavior.

Both open- and closed-ended questions have certain strengths and weaknesses. Good closed-ended items are often difficult to construct but easy to administer and, especially, to analyze. With closed-ended questions, researchers need only to tabulate the number of responses to each alternative to gain descriptive insights. The analysis of open-ended items is more difficult and time-consuming. The usual procedure is to develop categories and code open-ended responses into the categories. That is, researchers essentially transform open-ended responses to fixed categories in a post hoc fashion so that tabulations can be made.

Closed-ended items are more efficient than open-ended questions: respondents can answer more closed- than open-ended questions in a given amount of time. In questionnaires, participants may be less willing to compose written responses than to check off a response alternative. Closed-ended items are also preferred if respondents cannot express themselves well verbally. Furthermore, some questions are less intrusive in closed form than in open form. Take the following example:

1. What was your family's total annual income last year?
2. In what range was your family's total annual income last year?
   ☐ 1. Under $50,000,
   ☐ 2. $50,000 to $99,999, or
   ☐ 3. $100,000 or more.

The second question gives respondents greater privacy than the open-ended question and is less likely to go unanswered.

A drawback of closed-ended questions is the risk of failing to include important response options. Such omissions can lead to inadequate understanding of the issues or to outright error if respondents choose an alternative that misrepresents their position. Another issue is that closed-ended items tend to be superficial. Open-ended questions allow for a richer and fuller perspective on a topic, if respondents are verbally expressive and cooperative. Some of this richness may be lost when researchers tabulate answers they have categorized, but direct excerpts from open-ended responses can be valuable in imparting the flavor of the replies. Finally, some people object to being forced to choose from response options that do not exactly reflect their opinions.

Decisions about the mix of open- and closed-ended questions are based on such considerations as the sensitivity of the questions, respondents' verbal ability, and the amount of time available. Combinations of both types can be used to offset the strengths and weaknesses of each. Questionnaires typically use closed-ended questions primarily, to minimize respondents' writing burden. Interview schedules, on the other hand, tend to be more variable in their mixture of these two question types.

Specific Types of Closed-Ended Questions

The analytic advantages of closed-ended questions are often compelling. Various types of closed-ended questions, illustrated in Table 14.1, are described here.

- **Dichotomous questions** require respondents to make a choice between two response alternatives, such as yes/no. Dichotomous questions are most useful for gathering factual information.
- **Multiple-choice questions** offer three or more response alternatives. Graded alternatives are preferable to dichotomous items for attitude questions because researchers get more information (intensity as well as direction of opinion).
- **Rank-order questions** ask respondents to rank concepts on a continuum, such as most to least important. Respondents are asked to assign a 1 to the concept that is most important, a 2 to the concept that is second in importance, and so on. Rank-order questions can be useful, but some respondents misunderstand them so good instructions are needed. Rank-order questions should involve 10 or fewer rankings.

TABLE 14.1 • Examples of Closed-Ended Questions

QUESTION TYPE	EXAMPLE
1. Dichotomous question	Have you ever been pregnant? 1. Yes 2. No
2. Multiple-choice question	How important is it to you to avoid a pregnancy at this time? 1. Extremely important 2. Very important 3. Somewhat important 4. Not important
3. Rank-order question	People value different things in life. Below is a list of things that many people value. Please indicate their order of importance to you by placing a "1" beside the most important, "2" beside the second-most important, and so on. _____ Career achievement/work _____ Family relationships _____ Friendships, social interactions _____ Health _____ Money _____ Religion
4. Forced-choice question	Which statement most closely represents your point of view? 1. What happens to me is my own doing. 2. Sometimes I feel I don't have enough control over my life.
5. Rating question	On a scale from 0 to 10, where 0 means "extremely dissatisfied" and 10 means "extremely satisfied," how satisfied were you with the nursing care you received during your hospitalization? 0　1　2　3　4　5　6　7　8　9　10 Extremely dissatisfied　　　　　　　　　　Extremely satisfied

The next question is about things that may have happened to you personally. Please indicate how recently, if ever, these things happened to you:

	Yes, within past 12 mo	Yes, 2–3 years ago	Yes, more than 3 years ago	No, never
a. Has someone ever yelled at you all the time or put you down on purpose?	1	2	3	4
b. Has someone ever tried to control your every move?	1	2	3	4
c. Has someone ever threatened you with physical harm?	1	2	3	4
d. Has someone ever hit, slapped, kicked, or physically harmed you?	1	2	3	4

FIGURE 14.1 Example of a checklist (matrix question).

- **Forced-choice questions** require respondents to choose between two statements that represent polar positions.
- **Rating scale questions** ask respondents to evaluate something on an ordered dimension. Rating questions are typically on a **bipolar scale**, with end points specifying opposite extremes on a continuum. The end points and sometimes intermediary points along the scale are verbally labeled. The number of gradations or points along the scale can vary but is preferably an odd number, such as 5, 7, 9, or 11, to allow for a neutral midpoint. (In the example in Table 14.1, the rating question has 11 points, numbered 0-10.)
- **Checklists** include multiple questions with the same response options. A checklist is a two-dimensional matrix in which questions are listed on one dimension (usually vertically) and response options are listed on the other. Checklists are relatively efficient and easy to understand but are difficult to communicate orally, so they are used more often in SAQs than in interviews. Figure 14.1 presents an example of a checklist.
- **Visual analog scales** (**VASs**) are used to measure subjective experiences, such as pain, dyspnea, or fatigue. The VAS is a straight line, the end anchors end points of which are labeled as the extreme limits of the sensation or feeling being measured. People are asked to mark a point on the line corresponding to the amount of sensation experienced. Traditionally, the VAS line is 100 mm in length, which facilitates the derivation of a score from 0 to 100 through simple measurement by simply measuring the distance from one end of the scale to the person's mark on the line. An example of a VAS is shown in Figure 14.2.

Researchers sometimes collect information about activities and dates using an **event history calendar** (Vanhoutte & Nazroo, 2016). Such calendars are matrices that plot time on one dimension (usually horizontally) and events or activities on the other. The person recording the data (either the participant or an interviewer) draws lines to indicate the stop and start dates of the specified events or behaviors. Event history calendars are especially useful in collecting information about the occurrence and sequencing of events retrospectively. Data quality about past occurrences is enhanced

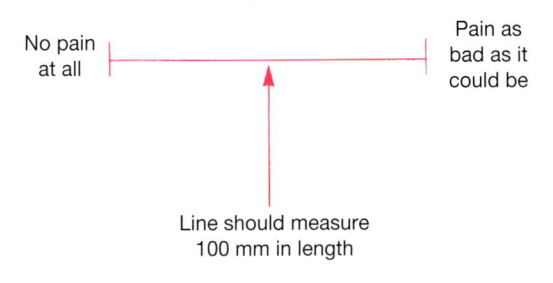

FIGURE 14.2 Example of a visual analog scale.

because the calendar helps participants relate the timing of some events to the timing of others.

An alternative to collecting event history data retrospectively is to ask participants to maintain information in an ongoing structured **diary** over a specified time period. This approach is often used to collect quantitative information about sleeping, eating, exercise behavior, or symptom experiences.

> **Example of a Structured Diary**
> Gonella and colleagues (2020) studied the challenges encountered by researchers conducting studies on end-of-life discussions. They conducted in-depth interviews and had the participants keep diaries to record their reflections. Collectively, the data were analyzed to describe the challenges.

Composite Scales and Other Structured Self-Reports

Multi-item composite scales are an important type of structured self-report. A **scale** yields a numeric score that places respondents on a continuum with respect to an attribute, much like a scale for measuring people's weight. Scales are used to discriminate quantitatively among people with different attitudes, symptoms, conditions, and needs. In the medical literature, a self-report scale completed by patients is typically called a **patient-reported outcome (PRO)**.

Likert-Type Summated Rating Scales

A widely used scaling technique is the **Likert scale**, named after the psychologist Rensis Likert. A traditional Likert scale consists of several declarative items that express a viewpoint on a topic. Respondents are asked to indicate the degree to which they agree or disagree with the opinion expressed in the item.

Table 14.2 illustrates a six-item Likert-type scale for measuring attitudes toward condom use. Likert-type scales often have more than six items; our example simply illustrates key features. After respondents complete a Likert scale, their responses are scored. Typically, agreement with positively worded statements and disagreement with negatively worded ones are assigned higher scores (see Chapter 16, however, regarding problems in including both positive and negative items on a scale).

The first statement in Table 14.2 is positively worded; agreement indicates a favorable attitude toward condom use. Thus, a higher score would be assigned to those agreeing with this statement than to those disagreeing. With five response options, we would give a score of 5 to those strongly agreeing, 4 to those agreeing, and so forth. The responses of two hypothetical respondents are shown by a check or an X; item scores are shown in far-right columns. Person 1, who agreed with the first statement, has an item score of 4, whereas person 2, who strongly disagreed, has a score of 1. The second statement is negatively worded, and so scoring is reversed—a 1 is assigned to those who strongly agree, and so on. This reversal is needed so that a high score consistently reflects positive attitudes toward condom use. A person's total score is computed by adding together individual item scores. Such scales are often called **summated rating scales** because of this feature. The total scores of both respondents are shown at the bottom of Table 14.2. The scores reflect a much more positive attitude toward condom use for person 1 (score = 26) than person 2 (score = 11).

The summation feature of such scales makes it possible to finely discriminate among people with different viewpoints. A single question from our scale would allow people to be put in only five categories. A six-item scale, such as the one in Table 14.2, permits finer gradation—from a minimum possible score of 6 (6 × 1) to a maximum possible score of 30 (6 × 5).

Summated rating scales can be used to measure a wide array of attributes. The bipolar scale is not always on an agree/disagree continuum—it might be always/never, likely/unlikely, and so on. Constructing a good summated rating scale requires considerable skill and work. Chapter 16 describes the steps involved in developing and testing such scales.

> **Example of a Likert Scale**
> Flanagan and colleagues (2022) used a visual analogue Likert scale to measure caregivers' of people with dementia perceived number of steps walked daily by. The responses were on a scale of 1–8: 1 reflected 0–499 steps/0.25 miles and a rating of 8 reflected 8,000–10,000 steps/4–5 miles per day.

TABLE 14.2 • Example of a Likert Scale

SCORING DIRECTION[a]	ITEM	RESPONSES[b]					SCORE	
		SA	A	?	D	SD	PERSON 1 (✓)	PERSON 2 (✗)
+	1. Using a condom shows you care about your partner.		✓			✗	4	1
−	2. My partner would be angry if I talked about using condoms.				✗	✓	5	3
−	3. I wouldn't enjoy sex as much if my partner and I used condoms.		✗		✓		4	2
+	4. Condoms are a good protection against AIDS and other sexually transmitted diseases.				✓	✗	3	2
+	5. My partner would respect me if I insisted on using condoms.	✓				✗	5	1
−	6. I would be too embarrassed to ask my partner about using a condom.		✗			✓	5	2
	Total score						26	11

[a]Researchers would not indicate the direction of scoring on a Likert scale administered to study participants. The scoring direction is indicated in this table for illustrative purposes only.
[b]SA, strongly agree; A, agree; ?, uncertain; D, disagree; SD, strongly disagree.

Most nurse researchers use existing scales rather than developing their own. A place to look for existing instruments is in the Health and Psychosocial Instruments database. Systematic reviews of instruments for specific constructs also appear in the healthcare literature. For example, Jiang and colleagues (2023) reviewed instruments that measure self-reported compassion.

Cognitive and Neuropsychological Tests

Nurse researchers sometimes assess or study cognitive functioning. Several different types of **cognitive tests** are available. For example, *intelligence tests* evaluate a person's global ability to solve problems and *aptitude tests* measure potential for achievement. Nurse researchers are most likely to use ability tests in studies of high-risk groups, such as low-birthweight children.

Some cognitive tests are specially designed to assess neuropsychological functioning among people with potential cognitive impairments, such as the Mini-Mental Status Examination. These tests capture varying types of competence, such as the ability to concentrate and the ability to remember. A good source for learning more about ability tests is the book by the Buros Institute (Carlson et al., 2021), which is updated every 3 years.

Example of a Study Assessing Neuropsychological Function
In a study examining the feasibility of a physical training intervention with music in older adults with mid cognitive impairment, Domínguez-Chávez et al. (2022) used several cognitive measures. To screen the participants for eligibility, the team used the Montreal Cognitive Assessment (MoCA). To measure the impact of the intervention, two of the pre-post measures assessed neuropsychological function: the Wechsler Memory Scale, which tested immediate memory and the Frontal Assessment Battery which was used to test executive function.

Other Types of Structured Self-Reports

Nurse researchers sometimes use other types of structured self-report methods. A brief description of these data collection methods is offered here:

- **Semantic differential (SD) scales** are a technique for measuring attitudes—an alternative to Likert scales. With the SD, respondents are asked to rate concepts (e.g., dieting, exercise) on a series of *bipolar adjectives*, such as good/bad, effective/ineffective, important/unimportant.
- **Q sorts** present participants with a set of cards on which statements are written. Participants are asked to sort the cards along a specified dimension, such as most helpful/least helpful, never true/always true.
- **Vignettes** are brief descriptions of events or situations (fictitious or actual) to which respondents are asked to react and provide information about how they would handle the situation described.
- **Ecological momentary assessments** involve repeated assessments of people's current behaviors, feelings, and experiences in real time, within their natural environment, using contemporary technologies such as text messaging.

Questionnaires Versus Interviews

In developing data collection plans, researchers must decide whether to collect self-report data through interviews or questionnaires. Each method has advantages and disadvantages.

Advantages of Questionnaires

Self-administered questionnaires, which can be distributed in person, by mail, or over the internet, offer some advantages, such as the following:

- *Cost.* Questionnaires, relative to interviews, are much less costly. Distributing questionnaires to groups (e.g., nursing home residents) is inexpensive and expedient. And, with a fixed amount of funds or time, a larger and more geographically diverse sample can be obtained with mailed or internet questionnaires than with interviews.
- *Anonymity.* Unlike interviews, questionnaires offer the possibility of complete anonymity. A guarantee of anonymity can be crucial in obtaining candid responses to sensitive questions. Anonymous questionnaires often result in a higher proportion of responses revealing socially undesirable viewpoints or traits than interviews.
- *Interviewer bias.* The absence of an interviewer ensures that there will be no interviewer bias. Interviewers ideally are neutral agents through whom questions and answers are passed. Studies have shown, however, that this ideal is difficult to achieve. Respondents and interviewers interact as humans, and this interaction can affect responses.

Internet data collection is especially economical and can yield a dataset directly amenable to analysis, without requiring someone to enter data onto a file; the same is also true for computer-assisted personal and telephone interviews—CAPI and CATI. Internet surveys also provide opportunities for providing participants with customized feedback and prompts that can minimize missing responses.

Advantages of Interviews

It is true that interviews are costly, prevent anonymity, and bear the risk of interviewer bias. Nevertheless, interviews are considered superior to questionnaires for most research purposes because of the following advantages:

- *Response rates.* Response rates tend to be high in face-to-face interviews. People are less likely to refuse to talk to an interviewer who seeks their cooperation than to ignore a mailed questionnaire or an email. A well-designed interview study normally achieves response rates in the vicinity of 80% to 90%, whereas mailed and internet questionnaires typically achieve response rates of less than 50%. Because nonresponse is not random, low response rates can introduce bias. However, if questionnaires are personally distributed—for example, to patients in a clinic—reasonably good response rates often can be achieved.
- *Audience.* Many people cannot fill out a questionnaire. Examples include young children and blind or illiterate individuals. Interviews, on the other hand, are feasible with most people. An important drawback for internet questionnaires is that not everyone has access to computers or uses them regularly—but this problem is declining.
- *Clarity.* Interviews offer some protection against ambiguous or confusing questions. Interviewers can provide needed clarifications. With questionnaires, misinterpreted questions can go undetected.
- *Depth of questioning.* Information obtained from questionnaires tends to be more superficial than from interviews, largely because questionnaires usually contain mostly closed-ended items. Furthermore, interviewers can enhance the quality of self-report data through *probing*, a topic we discuss later in this chapter.
- *Missing information.* Respondents are less likely to give "don't know" responses or to leave a question unanswered in an interview than on a questionnaire.
- *Supplementary data.* Face-to-face interviews can yield additional data through observation. Interviewers can observe and assess respondents' level of understanding, degree of cooperativeness, living conditions, and so forth. Such information can be useful in interpreting responses.

Some advantages of face-to-face interviews also apply to telephone interviews. Long or detailed interviews or ones with sensitive questions are not well suited to telephone administration, but for relatively brief instruments, telephone interviews are economical and tend to yield higher response rates than mailed or internet questionnaires.

Designing Structured Self-Report Instruments

We discussed major steps for developing structured self-report instruments earlier in this chapter, but a few additional considerations should be mentioned. For example, related constructs should be clustered into *modules* or areas of questioning. For example, an interview schedule may consist of a module on demographic information, another on health symptoms, and a third on health-promoting activities.

Thought needs to be given to sequencing modules, and questions within modules, to arrive at an order that is psychologically meaningful and encourages candor. The schedule should begin with questions that are interesting and not too sensitive. Whenever both general and specific questions about a topic are included, general questions should be placed first to avoid "coaching."

Instruments should be prefaced by introductory comments about the nature and purpose of the study. In interviews, introductory information is communicated by the interviewer, who typically follows a script. In questionnaires, the introduction takes the form of a **cover letter** (or cover email). The introduction should be carefully constructed because it is the earliest point of contact with potential respondents. An example of a cover letter for a mailed questionnaire is presented in Figure 14.3.

When a first draft of the instrument is in reasonably good order, it should be reviewed by experts in questionnaire construction, by substantive content area specialists, and by someone capable of detecting spelling mistakes or grammatical errors. When feedback is incorporated into the instrument, it can then be pretested.

In the remainder of this section, we offer some specific suggestions for designing high-quality self-report instruments. Additional guidance is offered

> Dear Mr. O'Hara,
>
> We are doing a study to understand how men who are nearing retirement age (55-65 years old) manage their health. This study, sponsored by the National Institutes of Health, will enable health care providers to better meet the needs of men in your age group.
>
> Would you please assist us by completing the enclosed questionnaire? Your input is needed
> to give an accurate picture of men's health.
>
> Your name was selected at random from a list of residents in your area. The questionnaire is completely anonymous, so we hope you will feel comfortable giving your honest opinions. If you have concerns about any questions, feel free to contact me by e-mail (dfp1@grifuni.edu) or by phone (518-587-3994).
>
> The questionnaire should only take about 10 minutes of your time. A postage-paid return envelope is enclosed for your convenience. Please return your questionnaire by May 12. In appreciation for your help, I am enclosing $2.
>
> Your participation in the study is completely voluntary. By returning your booklet, you will be consenting to participate in the study. Thank you in advance for your assistance.
>
> Sincerely,
> Denise F. Polit, Ph.D.
> Professor

FIGURE 14.3 Example of a cover letter for a mailed questionnaire. This cover letter could be readily adapted for an email message inviting people to participate in a web-based survey.

in the book by DeVillis and Thorpe (2022), entitled *Scale Development: Theory and Applications*.

Tips for Wording Questions

We all are accustomed to asking questions, but the proper phrasing of questions for a study is not easy. In wording questions, researchers should keep four important considerations in mind.

1. *Clarity*. Questions should be worded clearly and unambiguously. This is usually easier said than done. Respondents do not always have the same mind-set as the researchers.
2. *Ability of respondents to give information*. Researchers need to consider whether respondents can be expected to understand the question or are qualified to provide meaningful answers.
3. *Bias*. Questions should be worded in a manner that minimizes the risk of response bias.
4. *Sensitivity*. Researchers should strive to be courteous, considerate, and sensitive to respondents' circumstances, especially when asking questions of a private nature.

Here are some specific suggestions with regard to these four considerations:

- Clarify in your own mind the information you are seeking. The question, "When do you usually eat your evening meal?" might elicit such responses as "around 6 p.m.," or "when my son gets home from soccer practice," or "when I feel like cooking." The question itself contains no words that are difficult, but the question is unclear because the researcher's intent is not apparent.
- Avoid jargon or technical terms (e.g., edema) if lay terms (e.g., swelling) are equally appropriate. Use words that are simple enough for the *least* educated sample members.
- Do not assume that respondents will be aware of, or informed about, issues in which you are interested—and avoid giving the impression that they *ought* to be informed. Questions on complex issues can be worded in such a way that respondents will be comfortable admitting ignorance (e.g., "Many people have not read about factors that increase the risk of diabetes. Do you

happen to know of any risk factors?"). Another approach is to preface a question by a short explanation about terminology or issues.
- Avoid leading questions that suggest a particular answer. A question such as, "Do you agree that nurse-midwives play an indispensable role in the health team?" is not neutral.
- State a range of alternatives within the question itself when possible. For instance, the question, "Do you like to get up early on weekends?" is more suggestive of the "right" answer than "Do you prefer to get up early or to sleep late on weekends?"
- For questions that ask about socially undesirable behavior (e.g., excessive drinking), closed-ended questions may be preferred. It is easier to check off having engaged in socially disapproved actions than to verbalize those actions in response to open-ended questions. When controversial behaviors are presented as options, respondents are more likely to believe that their behavior is commonplace, and admissions of such behavior become less awkward.
- Impersonal wording of questions is sometimes useful in encouraging honesty. For example, compare these two statements with which respondents might be asked to agree or disagree: (1) "I am dissatisfied with the nursing care I received during my hospitalization," (2) "The quality of nursing care in this hospital is unsatisfactory." A respondent might feel more comfortable admitting dissatisfaction with nursing care in the less personally worded second question.

Tips for Preparing Response Options

If closed-ended questions are used, researchers also need to develop response alternatives. Below are some suggestions for preparing them.

- Response options should cover all significant alternatives. If respondents are forced to choose from options provided by researchers, the available options should be reasonably inclusive. As a precaution, researchers often have a final response option with a phrase such as "Other—please specify."
- Alternatives should be mutually exclusive. The following categories for a question on a person's age are *not* mutually exclusive: 30 years or younger, 30 to 50 years, or 50 years or older. People who are exactly 30 or 50 would qualify for two categories.
- Response options should be ordered rationally. Options often can be placed in order of decreasing or increasing favorability, agreement, or intensity (e.g., strongly agree, agree, etc.). When options have no "natural" order, alphabetic ordering can avoid leading respondents to a particular response (e.g., see the rank-order question, Table 14.1).
- Response options should be brief. One sentence or phrase for each option is usually sufficient to express a concept. Response alternatives should be about equal in length.

Tips for Formatting an Instrument

The appearance and layout of an instrument may seem a matter of minor administrative importance. Yet, a poorly designed format can have substantive consequences if respondents (or interviewers) become confused, miss questions, or answer questions they should have omitted. The format is especially important in questionnaires because respondents cannot ask for help. The following suggestions may be helpful in laying out an instrument:

- Do not compress questions into too small a space. An extra page of questions is better than a form that appears dense and confusing and that provides inadequate space for responses to open-ended questions.
- Set off the response options from the question or stem. Response alternatives are often aligned vertically (see Table 14.1).
- Give care to formatting **filter questions**, which route respondents through different sets of questions depending on their responses. In interview schedules, **skip patterns** instruct interviewers to skip to a specific question for a given response (e.g., SKIP TO Q10). In SAQs, skip instructions can be confusing. It is often better to put questions appropriate to a subset of respondents apart from the main series of questions, as illustrated in Box 14.1, part B. An important advantage of CAPI, CATI, audio-CASI, and internet surveys is that skip patterns are built into the computer program, leaving no room for human error.

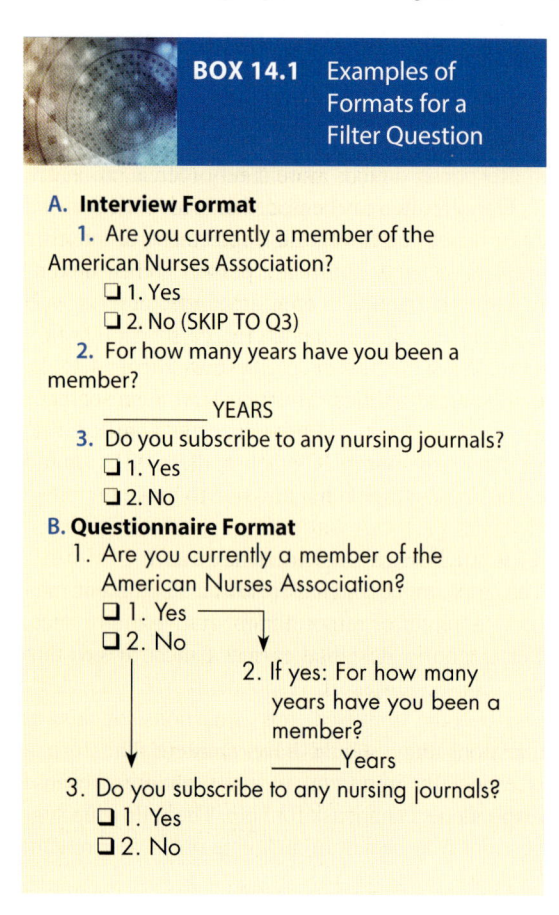

> **BOX 14.1 Examples of Formats for a Filter Question**
>
> **A. Interview Format**
>   1. Are you currently a member of the American Nurses Association?
>   ❏ 1. Yes
>   ❏ 2. No (SKIP TO Q3)
>   2. For how many years have you been a member?
>   _____ YEARS
>   3. Do you subscribe to any nursing journals?
>   ❏ 1. Yes
>   ❏ 2. No
>
> **B. Questionnaire Format**
>   1. Are you currently a member of the American Nurses Association?
>   ❏ 1. Yes
>   ❏ 2. No
>   2. If yes: For how many years have you been a member?
>   _____ Years
>   3. Do you subscribe to any nursing journals?
>   ❏ 1. Yes
>   ❏ 2. No

- Avoid forcing all respondents to go through inapplicable questions in an SAQ. Suppose question 2 in Box 14.1, part B had been worded as follows: "If you are a member of the American Nurses Association, for how long have you been a member?" Nonmembers may not be sure how to handle this question and may be annoyed at having to read irrelevant material.

Administering Structured Self-Report Instruments

Administering interview schedules and questionnaires involves different issues and skills.

Collecting Interview Data

The quality of interview data relies on interviewer proficiency. Interviewers for large survey organizations receive extensive training. Although we cannot cover all the principles of good interviewing, we can identify some major issues.

A primary task of interviewers is to put respondents at ease so that they feel comfortable in expressing their views honestly. Interviewers should always be punctual (if an appointment has been made), courteous, and friendly. Interviewers should strive to appear unbiased and to create an atmosphere that encourages candor. All opinions of respondents should be accepted as natural; interviewers should not express surprise, disapproval, or even approval.

> **Example of Well-Trained Interviewers**
> Hubbard et al. (2022) conducted a study to explore the barriers to initiating antiviral therapy in males who were HIV positive and their female partners. The interviews guides were piloted with four respondents (two males and two females) and refined based on interviewee feedback. The interviewers, one male and one female research assistant who were fluent in the local language, were trained in research techniques. They conducted the interviews in quiet, private locations in the community or near the facilities where care was provided. The participants were paired by gender (e.g., male interviewer with male participant).

Interviewers should follow question wording in the interview schedule precisely. Interviewers should not offer spontaneous explanations of what questions mean. Repetition of a question is usually adequate to dispel misunderstandings, especially if the instrument has been pretested. Interviewers should not read questions mechanically. A natural, conversational tone is essential in building rapport, and this tone is impossible to achieve if interviewers are not thoroughly familiar with the questions.

When closed-ended questions have lengthy response alternatives or when a series of questions has the same response options, interviewers should hand respondents a **show card** that lists the options. People cannot be expected to remember detailed unfamiliar material and may choose the last response option if they cannot recall earlier ones.

Interviewers record answers to closed-ended items by checking or circling the appropriate alternative, but responses to open-ended questions must either be written out in full or recorded for later transcription. Interviewers should not paraphrase or summarize respondents' replies.

Obtaining complete, relevant responses to questions is not always easy. Respondents may reply to seemingly straightforward questions with partial answers. Some may say, "I don't know" to avoid giving their opinions on sensitive topics, or to stall while they think. In such cases, the interviewers' job is to **probe**. The purpose of a probe is to elicit more useful information than respondents volunteered initially. A probe can take many forms. Sometimes it involves repeating the question and sometimes it is a long pause intended to communicate to respondents that they should continue. It may be necessary to encourage a more complete response to open-ended questions by using a nondirective supplementary question, such as, "How is that?" Interviewers must be careful to use only *neutral* probes that do not influence the content of a response. Box 14.2 gives examples of neutral, nondirective probes used by professional interviewers to stimulate more complete responses to questions. The ability to probe well is perhaps the greatest test of an interviewer's skill. To know when to probe and which probe to use, interviewers must understand the purpose of each question.

Guidelines for telephone or video interviews are essentially the same as those for face-to-face interviews. While there can sometimes be technology-related issues, these approaches are more commonly used since the COVID-19 pandemic. Some have reported that the anonymity of an interview conducted by telephone allowed the person to speak more freely (Flanagan et al., 2022). Others have noted that video interviews allow the interviewer the opportunity to observe more closely times when a person seems uncomfortable or is at ease about the interview as well as other important characteristics such as family presence (Cahill et al., 2021; Land et al., 2022). Lastly, these approaches often allow the researcher to sample more widely promoting greater diversity in the sample (Cahill, et al., 2021). In all cases, interviewers should strive to make the interview a pleasant and satisfying experience in which respondents come to understand that the information they are providing is valued. Saarijärvi and Bratt (2021) offer tips on various types of interviews and the advantages and disadvantages that should be considered.

Example of a Telephone Survey Interview
Flanagan and colleagues (2022) conducted a telephone survey of caregivers of people with dementia. The purpose of the study was to understand these caregivers' perspective of participating in a walking program to address their health and well-being.

Collecting Questionnaire Data Through In-Person Distribution

Questionnaires can be distributed by personal delivery, through the mail, and over the internet on various devices. The most convenient procedure is to distribute questionnaires to a group of people who complete the instrument at the same time. This approach has the obvious advantages of maximizing the number of completed questionnaires and allowing respondents to ask questions. Group administrations may be possible in some clinical and educational settings.

Researchers can also hand out questionnaires to individual respondents. Personal contact has a positive effect on response rates, and researchers can answer questions. Individual distribution of questionnaires in clinical settings is often inexpensive and efficient.

BOX 14.2　Examples of Neutral, Nondirective Probes

- Is there anything else?
- Go on.
- Are there any other reasons?
- How do you mean?
- Could you please tell me more about that?
- Would you tell me what you have in mind?
- There are no right or wrong answers; I'd just like to get your thinking.
- Could you please explain that?
- Could you please give me an example?

Collecting Questionnaire Data Through the Mail

For surveys of a broad population, questionnaires can be mailed. A *mail* (or *postal*) *survey* approach was once considered a cost-effective for reaching geographically dispersed respondents, but it has been increasingly replaced with surveys that are emailed. Mailed surveys have the advantage of not requiring a person to have an email account, but overall mailed surveys tend to yield low response rates, often lower than 50%. The risk of bias in such cases is great. Response rates can be affected by how the questionnaires are designed and mailed. The recommended procedure is to include a stamped, addressed return envelope.

People are more likely to complete a mailed questionnaire if they are encouraged to do so by someone whose name they recognize. If possible, obtain an endorsement of a well-known person or write the cover letter on the stationery of a respected organization, such as a university.

Collecting Questionnaire Data via the Internet

The internet provides an economical means of distributing questionnaires. It allows researchers to access large groups of people who are interested in specific topics.

Researchers can administer internet surveys in several ways. One method is to design a questionnaire in a word processing program, similar to mailed questionnaires. The researcher attaches the file with the questionnaire to an email message for distribution. Respondents can complete the questionnaire, and return it as an email attachment or print it and return it by mail or fax. This method may be problematic if respondents have trouble opening attachments or if they use a different word processing program. Surveys sent via email also run the risk of not getting delivered to the intended party, either because email addresses have changed or because the email messages are blocked by security filters.

Increasingly, researchers collect data through **web-based surveys**. This approach requires researchers to have a website on which the survey is placed or to use survey platforms such as Survey Monkey (http://www.surveymonkey.com/) or Qualtrics (www.qualtrics.com/). Respondents typically access the website by clicking on a hypertext link. For example, respondents may be invited to participate in the survey through an email message that includes the link to the survey, or they may be invited to participate when they enter a website related in content to the survey (e.g., the website of a cancer support organization).

Web-based forms often can be programmed to include interactive features. By having dynamic features, respondents can receive as well as give information—a feature that can increase motivation to participate. For example, respondents can be given information about their own responses (e.g., how they scored on a scale) or aggregated information about responses from previous participants.

A major advantage of web-based surveys is that they are able to reach wide geographic areas, increase the diversity of the sample, and the data are directly amenable to analysis. However, a disadvantage of web-based surveys includes the potential for what is known as bots. That is the falsifying of information to receive the compensation that is sometimes provided as an incentive to increase the response rate. While the easiest way to avoid this is to not compensate respondents, incentives such as gift cards do help increase response rates. Hallberg (2022) provides several strategies that can be easily added to surveys to avoid bots such as time-stamps, branching logic, and attention questions—all of which are described in more detail here: https://lifespan.ku.edu/online-surveys-and-data-collection-tools.

Follow-up reminders are critical in improving response rates for mailed and internet questionnaires. This involves additional mailings urging nonrespondents to complete and return their forms. Follow-up reminders should be sent about 5 to 10 days after the initial mailing. Sometimes reminders simply involve sending an email or a postcard of encouragement to nonrespondents, but it may be necessary to send another questionnaire because many nonrespondents will have misplaced or discarded the original. With anonymous questionnaires, researchers may not be able to distinguish respondents and nonrespondents for the purpose of sending follow-up letters. In such a situation, the best procedure is to send out a follow-up notice to everyone, thanking those who have already answered and asking others to cooperate.

Example Distributing Questionnaires in Various Ways
Gavurova and colleagues (2021) used surveys to examine patient satisfaction with inpatient care in the Czech Republic. They distributed both paper versions at the hospital, but they also allowed patients to opt into an electronic version through a request to fill in the questionnaire. The total sample of participants was 1,425.

TIP When sending out an email invitation, avoid using the word "survey" or "questionnaire" in the subject line—these words tend to discourage people from opening the email. There is some evidence that the best time to send out email invitations is Monday mornings.

Internet surveys have proliferated. They are inexpensive and can reach a broad audience. However, samples are almost never representative, and response rates tend to be low—even lower than mailed questionnaires. Several references are available to help researchers who wish to launch an internet survey. For example, the book by Bethlehem and Biffignandi (2021), entitled *Handbook of Web Surveys*, provides useful information.

A project funded by the National Institutes of Health offers another option for gathering PROs over the internet. The Patient-Reported Outcomes Measurement Information System (**PROMIS®**) initiative (Cella et al., 2010) makes it possible to measure a broad range of PROs online, using measures that have been rigorously developed and tested. Examples of patient outcomes in PROMIS® include those in the physical health domain (e.g., fatigue, physical functioning, sleep disturbance), in the mental health domain (e.g., anxiety, depression, anger), and in the social health domain (e.g., social support). Measures are available for both adult and pediatric populations and can be administered online and scored, with normed information provided instantly.

Example of a Study Using PROMIS®
Huang and colleagues (2021) examined whether anxiety was a mediator between coping and healthcare transition readiness. They used the PROMIS Anxiety scale to measure the level of anxiety in the children and their parents.

Evaluation of Structured Self-Reports

Structured self-reports are a powerful data collection method. They are versatile and yield information that can be readily analyzed statistically. Structured questions can be carefully worded and rigorously pretested. On the other hand, structured questions tend to be more superficial than questions in unstructured interviews.

Structured self-reports are susceptible to the risk of various **response biases**—some of which can also occur with unstructured self-reports. Respondents may give biased answers in reaction to the interviewers' behavior or appearance, for example. Perhaps the most pervasive problem is people's tendency to present a favorable image of themselves. **Social desirability response bias** refers to the tendency of some individuals to misrepresent themselves by giving answers that are congruent with prevailing social values. This problem is often difficult to combat. Subtle, indirect, and delicately worded questioning sometimes can help to minimize this response bias. Creating a nonjudgmental atmosphere and providing anonymity also encourage frankness. In an interview situation, interviewer training is essential.

Some response biases, called **response sets**, are most commonly observed in composite scales. **Extreme responses** are a bias reflecting consistent selection of extreme alternatives (e.g., "strongly agree"). These extreme responses distort the findings because they do not necessarily reflect the most intense feelings about the phenomenon under study, but rather capture a trait of the respondent.

Some people have been found to agree with statements regardless of content. Such people are called **yea-sayers**, and the bias is known as the **acquiescence response set**. A less common problem is the opposite tendency for other individuals, called **nay-sayers**, to disagree with statements independently of question content.

Researchers who construct scales should try to eliminate or minimize response set biases. If an instrument or scale is being developed for use by others, evidence should be gathered to demonstrate that the scale is sufficiently free from response biases to measure the critical variable.

STRUCTURED OBSERVATION

Structured observation is used to record behaviors, interactions, and events in a systematic way. Structured observation involves using formal instruments and protocols that specify what to observe, how long to observe it, and how to record information. Although observations often focus on patients or their caretakers, observations are also used to record the behaviors of nurses and other healthcare professionals, especially in quality improvement studies.

Methods of Recording Structured Observations

Researchers recording structured observations often use either a checklist or a rating scale. Both types of record-keeping instruments are designed to produce numeric information.

Category Systems and Checklists

Structured observation often involves constructing a category system to classify observed phenomena. A **category system** represents a method of capturing consistently the qualitative behaviors and events transpiring in the observational setting.

Some category systems are constructed so that *all* observed behaviors within a specified domain (e.g., speech) can be classified into one and only one category. In such an exhaustive system, the categories are mutually exclusive.

Example of Exhaustive Categories
Liu et al. (2023) conducted a secondary analysis on mealtime behaviors between residents with dementia and staff in nine nursing homes. They examined previously recorded videotapes to observe 25 residents with dementia and 29 staff and coded the behaviors using the refined Cue Utilization and Engagement in Dementia mealtime video-coding scheme. They captured resident mealtime behaviors into mutually exclusive categories such as positive verbal behaviors or resistiveness to care for residents and in staff, task-oriented care, or verbal person-centered care.

When all behaviors of a certain type (e.g., verbal exchanges) are observed and recorded, researchers usually need to carefully define categories so that observers know when one behavior ends and a new one begins. The assumption in using such a category system is that behaviors, events, or actions that are allocated to a particular category are equivalent to every other behavior, event, or action in that same category.

Another approach is to develop a system in which only certain behaviors (which may or may not occur) are recorded. For example, if we were studying aggressive behavior in children with autism, we might specify categories such as "strikes another child" or "kicks/hits walls or floor." In such a category system, many behaviors—all the ones that are nonaggressive—would not be classified. Such nonexhaustive systems may be adequate, but one risk is that resulting data might be difficult to interpret. Problems may arise if a large number of behaviors are not categorized or if segments of the observation sessions do not involve the target behaviors. In such situations, investigators should record the amount of time in which the target behaviors occurred, relative to the total time under observation.

Example of Nonexhaustive Categories
Libster and colleagues (2023) explored the meaning of friendship and feelings of loneliness in 58 children with autism and 42 children who did not have autism. Findings were coded for the perceived experience of loneliness and four categories that children used to define friendships including personality, companionship, dependability, and intimacy. Behaviors unrelated to friendship or the experience of loneliness were not explored.

A good category system requires the careful definition of behaviors or characteristics to be observed. Each category must be explained carefully so that observers have unambiguous criteria for identifying the occurrence of a specified phenomenon. Even with detailed definitions of categories, virtually all category systems require observer inference, to a greater or lesser degree. For instance, coding children's experience of friendship or loneliness in the study mentioned in the previous example (Libster et al., 2023) would require considerable inference, even with good training materials.

Category systems are the basis for a **checklist**, which is the instrument observers use to record observed phenomena. The checklist is usually formatted with behaviors or events from the category system listed vertically on the left and space for recording the frequency, duration, or intensity of behavior occurrences on the right. With nonexhaustive category systems, the behaviors of interest, which may or may not be manifested, are listed on the checklist. The observer's tasks are to watch for instances of these behaviors and to record their occurrence.

With exhaustive checklists, the observers' task is to place all behaviors in only one category for each element. By **element**, we refer to either a unit of behavior, such as a sentence in a conversation, or a specified time interval. To illustrate, suppose we were studying the problem-solving behavior of a group of public health staff discussing an intervention for the homeless. Our category system involves eight categories: (1) seeks information, (2) gives information, (3) describes problem, (4) offers suggestion, (5) opposes suggestion, (6) supports suggestion, (7) summarizes, and (8) miscellaneous. Observers would be required to classify every group member's contribution—using, for example, each sentence as the element—into one of these eight categories.

Another approach with exhaustive systems is to categorize relevant behaviors at regular time intervals. For example, in a category system for infants' motor activities, the researcher might use 10-second time intervals as the element; observers would categorize infant movements within 10-second periods.

Rating Scales

An alternative to a checklist for recording structured observations is a **rating scale** that requires observers to rate a phenomenon along a descriptive continuum that is typically bipolar. Observers may be required to rate behaviors or events at specified intervals throughout the observational period (e.g., every 5 minutes). Alternatively, observers may rate entire events or transactions after observations are completed. Post observation ratings require observers to integrate a number of activities and to judge which point on a scale most closely fits their interpretation of the situation. For example, suppose we were observing children's behavior during a scratch test for allergies. After each session, observers might be asked to rate the children's overall anxiety during the procedure on a graphic rating scale such as the following:

Rate how calm or nervous the child appeared to be during the procedure:

1	2	3	4	5	6	7
Extremely calm		Neither calm nor nervous			Extremely nervous	

TIP Observational rating scales are sometimes incorporated into structured interviews.

Rating scales can also be used as an extension of checklists, wherein observers record not only the occurrence of a behavior but also rate some qualitative aspect of it, such as its intensity. When rating scales are coupled with a category scheme, considerable information about a phenomenon can be obtained, but it places a large burden on observers, particularly if there is extensive activity.

Example of Observational Ratings

Döra and Büyük (2021) conducted a study to examine the effect of white noise and lullabies on the perception of pain during blood sampling procedures in premature babies. Infant pain was measured using the Premature Infant Pain Profile, a widely used measure that incorporates both observers' ratings of infant behaviors and physiological indicators (e.g., vital signs).

In the Premature Infant Pain Profile (PIPP) system, observers watch an infant for 30 seconds and score certain behaviors, such as *eye squeeze* and *behavioral state*. Table 14.3 shows the PIPP rating system for the four observer-rated behaviors.

TIP It is often advisable to spend some time with participants before observations and data recording begin. Having a warm-up period helps to relax people, especially if audio or video equipment is being used and can be helpful to observers (for example, if participants have a strong accent or speech patterns to which they must adjust).

Constructing Versus Borrowing Structured Observational Instruments

Compared to the abundance of books that provide guidance in developing self-report instruments, there are relatively few resources for healthcare researchers who want to design their own observational instruments. Yoder and colleagues (2018) provide one resource for observational measurements of behavior.

As with self-report instruments, however, we encourage you to search for an available observational instrument, rather than creating one yourself. The use of an existing instrument saves considerable work and time and facilitates cross-study comparisons. The best source for existing instruments is recent research literature on the study topic. For

TABLE 14.3 • Observer-Rated Categories for the Premature Infant Pain Profile (PIPP)

INDICATOR	OBSERVATION[a]	POINTS
Behavioral state	Active/awake, eyes open, facial movements	0
	Quiet/awake, eyes open, no facial movements	1
	Active/sleep, eyes closed, facial movements	2
	Quiet/sleep, eyes closed, no facial movements	3
Brow bulge	None (<9% of time)	0
	Minimum (10%–39% of time)	1
	Moderate (40%–69% of time)	2
	Maximum (>70% of time)	3
Eye squeeze	None (<9% of time)	0
	Minimum (10%–39% of time)	1
	Moderate (40%–69% of time)	2
	Maximum (>70% of time)	3
Nasolabial furrow	None (<9% of time)	0
	Minimum (10%–39% of time)	1
	Moderate (40%–69% of time)	2
	Maximum (>70% of time)	3

Adapted with permission from Stevens, B., Johnston, C., Petryshen, P., & Taddio, A. (1996). Premature infant pain profile: Development and initial validation. *Clinical Journal of Pain, 12,* 13–22.

[a]Observations are made in a 15-second baseline period and in a 30-second period immediately after a painful event.

example, if you were conducting an observational study of infant pain, a good place to begin would be to read recent research on this topic to learn how infant pain was operationalized.

Sampling for Structured Observations

Researchers must decide when, and for how long, structured observations will be undertaken. Observations are typically done for a specific amount of time, and the amount of time is standardized across participants. Sampling may be needed to obtain representative examples of behaviors. *Observational sampling* concerns the selection of behaviors or activities to be observed, not the selection of participants.

With **time sampling**, researchers select time periods during which observations occur. The time frames may be selected systematically (e.g., 60 seconds at 5-minute intervals) or at random. For example, suppose we were studying mothers' interactions with their children in a clinic. During a 30-minute observation period, we sample moments to observe, rather than observing continuously. Let us say that observations are made in 2-minute segments. If we used systematic sampling, we would observe for 2 minutes, then cease observing for a prespecified period, say 3 minutes. With this scheme, a total of six 2-minute observations would be made for each dyad. A second approach is to sample 2-minute periods at random from the total of 15 such periods in a half hour; a third is to use all 15 periods. Decisions about the length and number of periods for creating a good sample must be consistent with research aims. In establishing time units, a key consideration is determining a psychologically meaningful time frame. Pretesting with different sampling plans is advisable.

> **Example of Time Sampling**
> Page and colleagues (2021) explored the impact of visitor restrictions and staff wearing protective equipment during COVID on the well-being of patients with mental health issues and moderate to severe dementia. To determine patient well-being, the researchers used the Dementia Care Mapping tool to observe and record behaviors. The analysis included 500 time frames representing 41.6 observed patient hours. Findings indicated that patients' well-being was better than expected given the restrictions.

Event sampling uses integral behavior sets or events for observation. Event sampling requires that the investigator either have knowledge about the occurrence of events or be in a position to wait for (or arrange) their occurrence. Examples of integral events suitable for event sampling include nurses' shift changes and cast removals of pediatric patients. This approach is preferable to time sampling when events of interest are widely spaced in time. When phenomena of interest are frequent, time sampling can enhance the representativeness of observed behaviors.

> **Example of Event Sampling**
> Bertolazzi and Perroca (2020) examined interruptions during nursing interventions on a nursing care unit focused on providing chemotherapy to oncology patients. The observer recorded the number of interruptions and used a stopwatch to record the duration of the interruptions and the total time elapsed to complete the interventions.

Technical Aids in Observations

A wide array of technical devices is available for recording behaviors and events, making analysis or categorization at a later time possible. When the target behavior is auditory (e.g., verbal interactions), recordings can be used to obtain a permanent record. Technologic advances have vastly improved the quality, sensitivity, and unobtrusiveness of recording equipment. Auditory recordings can also be analyzed using speech software to obtain objective quantitative measures of certain features (e.g., volume, pitch).

Video recording can be used when permanent visual records are desired. Video records can capture complex behaviors that might elude on-the-spot observers. Videos make it possible to check coders' accuracy and are useful in observer training. Finally, cameras are often less obtrusive than a human observer. Video records have a few drawbacks, some of which are technical, such as lighting requirements, lens limitations, and so on. Sometimes the camera angle can present a lop-sided view of an event. Also, some participants may be self-conscious in front of a video camera. Still, for many applications, visual records offer unparalleled opportunities to expand the scope of observational studies. Haidet and colleagues (2009) offer valuable advice on improving data quality of video-recorded observations.

There is a growing technology for assisting with the encoding and recording of observations known as m-health. For example, mobile apps and wearable devices equipment can record physiologic data into a computer system as the activity occurs.

Example of Using Equipment
In the aforementioned study by Flanagan and colleagues (2022), the study participants were provided wearable devices that measured steps walked, time being active per day, heart rate, and sleep. These were inputted directly into an online platform so participants could observe their progress over time.

Structured Observations by Nonresearch Observers

The observations discussed thus far are undertaken by research team members. Sometimes, however, researchers ask people not connected with the research to provide structured data, based on their observations of others. This method has much in common (in terms of format and scoring) with self-report instruments; the primary difference is that the person answering questions is asked to describe the behaviors of *another* person. For example, mothers might be asked to describe their children's behavior problems.

Obtaining observational data from nonresearchers is economical compared with using trained observers. For example, observers might have to watch children for hours or days to capture the nature and intensity of behavior problems, whereas parents or teachers could do this readily. Some behaviors might never lend themselves to outsider observation because they occur in private situations.

On the other hand, such methods may have the same problems as self-reports (e.g., response set biases) in addition to observer bias. Observer bias may in some cases be extreme, such as may happen when parents provide information about their children. Nonresearch observers are typically not trained, and interobserver agreement usually cannot be assessed. Thus, this approach has some problems but will continue to be used because, in many cases, there are no alternatives.

Example of Observations by Nonresearch Personnel
Arias and colleagues (2022) examined the effectiveness a parent-mediated, social skills intervention. They had the parent's/caregivers record behaviors after the 14-week intervention using the Child Behavior Checklist as a measure of the children's externalizing and internalizing behaviors.

Evaluation of Structured Observation

Structured observation is an important data collection method, particularly for recording aspects of people's behaviors when they are incapable of reliable self-report. Observational methods are particularly valuable for gathering data about infants and children, older people who are confused or agitated, or people whose communication skills are impaired.

Observations, like self-reports, are vulnerable to biases. One source of bias comes from those being observed. Participants may distort their behaviors in the direction of "looking good." They may also behave atypically because of their awareness of being observed (*reactivity*), or their shyness in front of strangers or a camera.

Biases can also reflect observers' perceptual errors. To make and record observation in a completely objective fashion is challenging. The risk of bias is especially great when a high degree of observer inference is required.

Several types of observational bias may occur. With **assimilatory biases**, observers distort observations in the direction of identity with previous inputs. This bias would have the effect of miscategorizing information in the direction of regularity and orderliness. Assimilation to the observer's expectations and attitudes also occurs.

With regard to rating scales, the **halo effect** is the tendency of observers to be influenced by one characteristic in judging other, unrelated characteristics. For example, if we had a positive general impression of a person, we might rate that person as intelligent and dependable simply because these traits are positively valued. Ratings may reflect observers' personality. The **error of leniency** is the tendency for observers to rate everything positively, and the **error of severity** is the contrasting tendency to rate too harshly.

The careful pretesting of checklists and rating scales and the thorough training of observers are essential in minimizing biases. Training should include practice sessions in which the comparability of observers' classifications and ratings is assessed. That is, two or more independent observers should watch a trial situation and observational coding should then be compared. *Interrater reliability* of structured observations is described in the next chapter.

> **TIP** People being observed are less likely to behave typically if they think they are being appraised. Even positive cues (such as nodding approval) should be avoided because approval may induce repetition of a behavior that might not otherwise have occurred.

BIOMARKERS

As defined by the Biomarker Working Group at the National Institutes of Health (2001), a **biomarker** is "a characteristic that is objectively measured and evaluated as an indicator of normal biological processes, pathogenic processes, or pharmacologic response to a therapeutic intervention" (p. 90). Examples of biomarkers include routine clinical measurements (e.g., blood pressure) and complex laboratory tests of blood, other body fluids, and tissue.

Settings in which nurses work are typically filled with a wide variety of technical instruments for measuring physiologic functions. Nurse researchers have used biomarkers for a wide variety of purposes. Examples include studies of basic biophysiologic processes, explorations of the ways in which nursing actions and interventions affect physiologic outcomes, and studies of the correlates of physiologic functioning in patients with health problems. Corwin and Ferranti (2016) have urged nurse researchers to integrate biomarkers into their studies to be "better able to precisely tailor and test nursing interventions" (p. 293).

It is beyond the scope of this book to describe the many kinds of biomarkers available to nurse researchers. Our goals are to present an overview of biophysiologic measures, to illustrate their use in research and to note considerations in decisions to use them.

Types of Biomarkers

Physiologic measurements are either in vivo or in vitro. **In vivo measurements** are performed directly in or on living organisms. Examples include measures of oxygen saturation, blood pressure, and body temperature. An **in vitro measurement**, by contrast, is performed outside the organism's body, for example, measuring serum potassium concentration in the blood.

In vivo instruments have been developed to measure all bodily functions, and technologic improvements continue to advance our ability to measure biophysiologic phenomena more accurately, conveniently, and rapidly than ever before.

> **Example of a Study With In Vivo Measures**
> In a systematic review of five randomized clinical control trials examining the impact of singing in people with stable chronic obstructive lung disease, Fang and colleagues (2022) found that singing improved respiratory muscles and quality of life.

With in vitro measures, data are gathered by extracting physiologic material from people and submitting it for laboratory analysis. Usually, labs establish a *reference range* of normal values for each measurement, which helps in interpreting the results. Several classes of laboratory analysis have been used by nurse researchers, including chemical measurements (e.g., measures of potassium levels), microbiologic measures (e.g., bacterial counts), cytologic *or* histologic measures (e.g., tissue biopsies), and genetic testing. Laboratory analyses of blood and urine samples are the most frequently used in vitro measures in nursing investigations.

> **Example of a Study With In Vitro Measures**
> Roberts et al. (2020) tested the impact of a mindfulness-based stress reduction program delivered over 8 weeks on parents of children with developmental delays. Measures of psychological stress by self-report and cortisol levels were taken pre-post and at 6 months post the intervention.

Selecting a Biomarker

The most basic issue in selecting a biomarker is whether it will yield good information about key research variables. In some cases, researchers need to consider whether the variable should be measured by observation or self-report instead of (or in addition to) using biophysiologic equipment. For example, stress could be measured by asking people questions (e.g., using the State-Trait Anxiety Inventory), by observing their behavior during exposure to stressful stimuli, or by measuring heart rate, blood pressure, or levels of adrenocorticotropic hormone in urine samples.

TIP There has been considerable debate in the medical community about the use of biomarkers as surrogates for clinical end points in clinical trials. A critical issue is whether treatment effects on a biomarker reliably predict treatment effects on end points that are more clinically meaningful (Fleming & Powers, 2012).

Several other considerations should be kept in mind in selecting a biophysiologic measure. Some key questions include the following:

- Is the necessary equipment or laboratory analysis readily available to you?
- Will you have difficulty obtaining permission from an Institutional Review Board or other institutional authority?
- Is a single measure of the outcome sufficient, or are multiple measures needed for a reliable estimate? If the latter, what burden does this place on participants?
- Are your measures likely to be influenced by reactivity (participants' awareness of their status)?
- Are you thoroughly familiar with safety precautions, such as grounding procedures?

Evaluation of Biomarkers

Biophysiologic measures offer the following advantages to nurse researchers:

- Biomarkers are accurate and precise compared with psychological measures (e.g., self-report measures of anxiety).
- Biomarkers are objective. Two nurses reading from the same sphygmomanometer are likely to obtain the same blood pressure measurements, and two different sphygmomanometers are likely to produce the same readouts. Patients cannot easily distort measurements of biophysiologic functioning.
- Biophysiologic instruments provide valid measures of targeted variables: thermometers can be depended on to measure temperature and not blood volume, and so forth. For self-report and observational measures, it is more difficult to be certain that the instrument is really measuring the target concept.

Biomarkers also have a few disadvantages:

- The cost of collecting some types of biophysiologic data may be low or nonexistent, but when laboratory tests are involved, they may be more expensive than other methods (e.g., assessing smoking status by means of cotinine assays vs. self-report).
- The measuring tool may affect the variables it is attempting to measure. The presence of a sensing device, such as a transducer, located in a blood vessel partially blocks that vessel and, hence, alters the pressure–flow characteristics being measured.
- Energy must often be applied to the organism when taking the biophysiologic measurements; caution must be exercised to avoid the risk of damaging cells by high-energy concentrations.
- Laboratory protocols can vary between independent research labs and clinical or commercial labs, and these differences can lead to variations in results.
- Normed values of biological markers are often based on information from Caucasian males, and normal values may vary by sex, age, race, and ethnicity.

The difficulty in choosing biomarkers for nursing studies lies not in their shortage nor in their inferiority to other methods. Indeed, they are plentiful, often highly reliable and valid, and extremely useful in clinical nursing studies. Care must be exercised, however, in selecting instruments or laboratory analyses with regard to practical, ethical, medical, and technical considerations.

> **Example of a biophysiological measure**
> Chen and colleagues (2022) investigated the effect of sex on the weekly development of preterm neonatal gut microbiome profiles in the first 4 weeks of NICU hospitalization.

PHYSICAL PERFORMANCE TESTS

Patients' abilities and skills are sometimes measured with **performance tests**. For example, the 6-Minute Walk Test (6MWT) is a widely used measure of physical functioning for patients with various cardiovascular, respiratory, or neurologic diseases or those in need of surgical or rehabilitative intervention. The measure is the distance walked in a 6-minute period, sometimes involving the use of a treadmill. Many other physical performance tests have been devised to measure such attributes as balance, mobility, endurance, and flexibility.

> **Example of Performance Testing**
> Fernández-Sevillano and colleagues (2021) examined the association of altered cognition that may contribute to suicidal behavior. They conducted neurocognitive testing in four groups: those who were depressed with a recent attempt, those who were depressed with a history of suicide attempt, those who were depressed but had no history of suicide attempt, and healthy controls.

DATA EXTRACTED FROM RECORDS

In many nursing studies, especially quality improvement and outcome-based studies, data are more commonly retrieved from electronic health records (EHRs). Even though data from EHRs are available, researchers should consider a team that includes an expert in natural language processing (NLP). Together, the team can develop a strategy for data retrieval with nurses clarifying the language used within the EHR and the NLP team member creating the algorithm for data extraction. For example, the nurse may need to clarify that a patient who "seems anxious" and "appears distressed" are describing the same psychological reaction.

Whereas physicians and mental health providers do have standardized languages (ICD-11 and DSM-5 respectively), nursing has yet to adopt the widespread use of a single standardized language. As a result, there is less work by nursing extracting data from the EHR using NLP. Despite the availability of the EHR as a source of data, nurses still often rely on creating a paper-based tool or a spreadsheet abstraction tool to assure that there is accuracy and consistency in the data retrieved.

Alzu'bi and colleagues (2021) have suggested some useful strategies to enhance data quality when extracting data from medical records:

- The tool developed should be validated through a consensus of the clinicians with expert knowledge of the phenomenon being studied;
- Data abstractors should be carefully trained;
- If the study is beyond the scope of a descriptive study, the abstractors should be blinded to study hypotheses;
- Inclusion and exclusion criteria for the records to be abstracted should be explicit;
- The variables of interest should be carefully defined, and, if relevant, the possible range of values should be communicated (e.g., on a measure that should be coded 1 or 0, a 2 would be out of range);
- Clear guidelines about how to deal with missing data should be established at the outset;
- Clear-cut rules should be established about how to deal with conflicting data (i.e., when there are two or more versions of the same variable in the database);
- Data abstractors should be trained, the training should be reinforced throughout the process;
- Data abstractors findings need to be checked for accuracy during the process; and
- The accuracy of the abstraction should, indeed, be verified in random samples of records.

IMPLEMENTING A DATA COLLECTION PLAN

Data quality in a quantitative study is affected by both the data collection plan and how the plan is implemented.

Selecting Research Personnel

An important decision concerns who will actually collect the research data. In small studies, the lead researcher usually collects the data personally, but in large studies this is not feasible. When data are collected by others, it is important to select appropriate people. In general, they should be neutral agents—their characteristics or behavior should not affect the data. Here are some considerations to keep in mind when selecting research personnel:

- *Experience.* Research staff ideally have had relevant prior experience (e.g., prior interviewing experience). If this is not feasible, look for people who can readily acquire needed skills (e.g., interviewers should have good verbal and social skills).
- *Congruence with sample characteristics.* If possible, data collectors should match participants with respect to racial or cultural background and gender. The greater the sensitivity of the questions, the greater the desirability of congruence.
- *Unremarkable appearance.* Extremes of appearance should be avoided. For example, data collectors should not dress very casually (e.g., in tee shirts) nor formally (e.g., in designer clothes). Data collectors should not wear anything that conveys their political, social, or religious views.
- *Personality.* Data collectors should be pleasant (but not effusive), sociable (but not overly chatty), and nonjudgmental (but not unfeeling). The goal is to have nonthreatening data collectors who can put participants at ease.

In some situations, researchers cannot select research personnel. For example, the data collectors may be staff nurses employed at a hospital. Training of the data collection staff is particularly important in such situations. When researchers collect their own data, they should self-monitor their demeanor and prepare for their role with care.

Training Data Collectors

Depending on prior experience, training needs to cover both general procedures (e.g., how to probe in an interview) and ones specific to the study (e.g., how to ask a particular question or how to categorize a behavior). Complex projects may require several days of training. The lead researcher is usually the best person to develop training materials and to conduct the training.

Data collection protocols usually are a good foundation for a **training manual**. The manual normally includes background materials (e.g., the study aims), general instructions, specific instructions, and copies of all data forms.

Training often includes demonstrations of high-quality fictitious data collection sessions, performed live or on video. Training may involve having trainees do trial runs of data collection (*mock interviews*) in front of the trainers to demonstrate their understanding of the instructions. Thompson and colleagues (2005) provide additional tips about the training of research personnel.

Another issue concerns blinding. Ideally, the data collectors would be blinded to study hypotheses and to participants' membership in groups being compared. Data collectors should understand the study *variables* and the *population* but not researchers' expectations.

> **Example of Data Collector Training and Potential Issues**
> Rajamani et al. (2021) did a study on the influence of data training on the predictive risk of death models. They provided trained and untrained providers in 19 Australian intensive care units with three patient scenarios and asked study participants to rate the severity of illness and risk of death. They found large variations within the groups, but in addition, the nontrained providers overestimated both the severity of illness and risk of death. The authors cited the importance providing training for all staff, reinforcing training during the data collection and auditing data as they are submitted.

CRITICAL APPRAISAL OF STRUCTURED METHODS OF DATA COLLECTION

Researchers make many decisions about data collection methods and procedures that can affect data quality and hence overall study quality. These decisions should be critically appraised in evaluating the study's evidence, to the extent possible. The guidelines in Box 14.3 focus on broad issues relating to the design and implementation of a data collection plan in quantitative studies. Note, however, that data collection procedures are often not thoroughly described in research reports, owing to space constraints in journals. A full appraisal of data collection plans is seldom feasible.

A second set of critical appraisal guidelines is presented in Box 14.4. These questions focus on structural methods of collecting data in quantitative studies. Further guidance on drawing conclusions about data quality is provided in the next chapter.

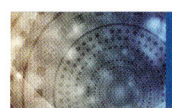

BOX 14.3 Guidelines for Critically Appraising Data Collection Plans in Quantitative Studies

1. Was the collection of structured data (vs. unstructured data) consistent with study aims?
2. Were appropriate methods used to collect the data (self-report, observation, etc.)? Was triangulation of different methods used appropriately? Should additional data collection methods have been used?
3. Was the right amount of data collected? Were data collected to address the varied needs of the study? Were *too much* data collected, resulting in high participant burden; if so, how might this have affected data quality?
4. Did the researcher select good instruments, in terms of congruence with underlying constructs, data quality, reputation, efficiency, and so on? Were new instruments developed without a justifiable rationale?
5. Were data collection instruments adequately pretested?
6. Did the report provide sufficient information about data collection procedures?
7. Who collected the data? Were data collectors judiciously chosen, with traits that were likely to enhance data quality?
8. Was the training of data collectors described? Was the training adequate? Were steps taken to improve data collectors' ability to produce high-quality data, or to monitor their performance?
9. Where and under what circumstances were data gathered? Was the setting for data collection appropriate?
10. Were other people present during data collection? Could the presence of others have resulted in biases?
11. Were data collectors blinded to study hypotheses or to participants' group status?

BOX 14.4 Guidelines for Critically Appraising Structured Data Collection Methods

1. If self-report data were collected, did the researcher make good decisions about the specific method used to solicit self-report information (e.g., a mix of open- and closed-ended questions, use of composite scales, and so on)?
2. Was the instrument package adequately described in terms of conceptual appropriateness, reading level of the questions, length of time to complete it, and so on?
3. Was the mode of obtaining the self-report data appropriate (e.g., in-person interviews, mailed questionnaires, web-based questionnaires)?
4. Were self-report data gathered in a manner that promoted high-quality and unbiased responses (e.g., in terms of privacy, efforts to put respondents at ease, etc.)?
5. If observational methods were used, did the report adequately describe the specific constructs that were observed?
6. Was a category system or rating system used to record observations? Was the category system exhaustive? How much inference was required of the observers? Were decisions about exhaustiveness and degree of observer inference appropriate?
7. What methods were used to sample observational units? Was the sampling approach a good one—that is, did it likely yield a representative sample of behavior?
8. To what degree were observer biases controlled or minimized?
9. Were biomarkers used in the study, and was this appropriate? Did the researcher appear to have the skills necessary for proper interpretation of biomarkers?
10. Were performance measures used in the study, and was this appropriate?
11. Were data extracted from records? If so, were appropriate steps taken to ensure high-quality data?

RESEARCH EXAMPLE

In the study described next, a variety of data collection approaches were used to measure study variables.

Study: Factors associated with resident-to-resident mistreatment of older people in nursing homes (Pillemer et al., 2022).

Study Purpose: The aim of this study was to explore the individual and environmental factors that contribute to resident-to-resident mistreatment of older people.

Design: In this multisite observational study resident-to-resident mistreatment included any aggressive physical, sexual, or verbal interactions between two or more long-term care residents that would likely be construed as unwelcome and potentially distressful. Ten nursing homes in New York were randomly selected based on their size and location and included five urban and five suburban facilities. The researchers used several strategies to collect a wide variety of data based on potential risk categories including resident factors and environmental level factors that may contribute to resident-to resident mistreatment. Data were collected using the following techniques.

Observational Data: The research team captured direct observations of residents and staff members' shift reports.

Qualitative Interviews: The research team conducted semistructured interviews with both with residents and staff. Each was asked about 22 forms of physical, verbal, or sexually aggressive events in a 1-month period and during the past year.

Retrospective Data: The research team collected data via chart reviews and reviews of incident reports.

Resident factors included measures of the following:

1. Cognition, which a member of the study team administered to residents using the Comprehensive Assessment and Referral Evaluation Diagnostic Cognitive Disorder Scale.
2. Behavioral symptoms captured using the Barrett Behavior Index, which staff used to rate resident's behavior on such items as wandering and aggression.
3. Communication was determined by research assistants' observations and ratings of expression, reception, and speech.
4. Functional status was captured using the Performance Activities of Daily Living Scale, which measures a person's inability to perform activities of daily living independently and was recorded by staff in the health record.
5. Depression, which was measured by the research team who administered the Feeling Tone Questionnaire to residents.
6. Hearing and vision which were assessed by the research assistants based on their observation of the respondent during the interview.
7. Gender, age, and race

Measures for environmental factors included two items:

1. Living in special care unit, which is a unit dedicated to residents with severe cognitive impairment.
2. Staffing, which was determined by the ratio of certified nursing assistants to the number of residents on the day shift.

Key Findings: Residents with less severe cognitive impairment and less severe functional issues exhibited more behavioral symptoms. Those with more severe dementia and who are placed in special units intended to protect them, may be at higher risk for resident-to-resident mistreatment of older people.

SUMMARY POINTS

- Quantitative researchers develop a **data collection plan** before they begin to collect their data. For structured data, researchers use formal data collection **instruments** that place constraints on those collecting data and those providing them.
- An early step in developing a data collection plan is the identification and prioritization of data needs. Then, measures of the variables must be located. The selection of existing instruments should be based on such factors as conceptual suitability, data quality, population appropriateness, cost, and reputation.
- Even when existing instruments are used, the instruments should be **pretested** to assess length, clarity, and overall adequacy.

- Structured self-report instruments, which are sometimes referred to as **patient-reported outcomes** or PROs, can include open- and closed-ended questions. **Open-ended questions** permit respondents to reply in narrative fashion, whereas **closed-ended** (*fixed-alternative*) **questions** offer **response options** from which respondents must choose.
- Types of closed-ended questions include (1) **dichotomous questions**, which require a choice between two options (e.g., yes/no), (2) **multiple-choice questions**, which offer a range of alternatives, (3) **rank-order questions**, in which respondents are asked to rank concepts on a continuum, (4) **forced-choice questions**, which require respondents to choose between two competing options, (5) **rating questions**, which ask respondents to make graded ratings along a bipolar dimension, (6) **checklists** that include several questions with the same response format, and (7) **visual analog scales (VASs)**, which are continua used to measure subjective experiences such as fatigue. **Event history calendars** and *diaries* are used to capture data about the occurrence of events.
- Composite psychosocial **scales** are multiquestion self-report tools for measuring the degree to which individuals possess or are characterized by target attributes. Traditional **Likert scales** (**summated rating scales**) comprise a series of statements (**items**) about a phenomenon (e.g., abortions). Respondents rate their reaction to the item along a *bipolar continuum* (e.g., strongly agree/disagree). A total score is computed by summing item scores, each of which is scored for the intensity and direction of favorability expressed.
- Other self-report methods include **SDs**, which consist of a set of bipolar rating scales on which respondents indicate reactions toward a phenomenon; **Q sorts**, in which people sort a set of card statements into piles according to specified criteria; **vignettes**, which are descriptions of an event or situation to which respondents are asked to react; and **ecological momentary assessments**, which involve repeated assessments of people's current behaviors or experiences in real time.

- Structured self-report instruments are administered either orally (via **interview schedules**) or in written form (**questionnaires**). Questionnaires are less costly and time-consuming than interviews and offer the possibility of anonymity. Interviews have higher response rates, are suitable for a wider variety of people, and tend to yield richer data than questionnaires.
- Data quality in interviews depends on interviewers' interpersonal skills. Interviewers must put respondents at ease and build rapport and need to **probe** skillfully for additional information when respondents give incomplete responses.
- Group administration is the most economical way to distribute questionnaires. Another approach is to mail them. Self-administered questionnaires (SAQs) can be distributed via the internet, most often as a **web-based survey** that is accessed through a hypertext link. Questionnaires, especially those distributed over the internet, tend to have low **response rates**, which can result in bias. Techniques such as **follow-up reminders** and good **cover letters** increase response rates to questionnaires.
- Structured self-reports are vulnerable to the risk of biases. **Response set biases** reflect the tendency of some people to respond to questions in characteristic ways, independently of content. Common response sets include **social desirability**, **extreme response**, and **acquiescence** (**yea-saying**).
- Methods of **structured observation** impose limits on what observers watch for and record, to enhance the accuracy and consistency of observations and to obtain an adequate representation of phenomena of interest.
- **Checklists** are used in observations to record the occurrence, frequency, duration, or intensity of designated behaviors, events, or actions. Checklists are based on **category systems** for encoding observed phenomena into discrete categories. When using **rating scales**, observers rate phenomena along a dimension that is typically bipolar (e.g., passive/aggressive).
- In collecting observational data, observers use different sampling approaches. **Time sampling** involves specifications of the duration and

frequency of observational periods and inter-session intervals. **Event sampling** selects integral behaviors or events of a special type for observation.
- Observational methods are an excellent way to operationalize some constructs but are subject to various biases. The greater the degree of observer inference, the more likely that distortions will occur.
- **Biomarkers** comprise **in vivo measurements** (those performed within or on living organisms, such as blood pressure measurement) and **in vitro measurements** (those performed outside the organism's body, such as blood tests).
- Biomarkers are objective, accurate, and precise, but care must be taken in using such measures with regard to practical, technical, and ethical considerations.
- Physical **performance tests** are sometimes used to gather outcome data relating to patients' physical functioning.
- Data for research or quality improvement projects are increasingly drawn from medical records, especially EHRs. The extraction of records data requires the development of explicit rules and procedures.
- When researchers cannot collect the data without assistance, they should select data collection staff with care and devote resources to formally train them.

REFERENCES CITED IN CHAPTER 14

Alzu'bi, A. A., Watzlaf, V. J. M., Sheridan, P. (2021). Electronic health record (EHR) abstraction. *Perspectives in Health Information Management*, 18(Spring), 1g.

Arias, A. A., Rea, M. M., Adler, E. J., Haendel, A. D., & Van Hecke, A. V. (2022). Utilizing the child behavior checklist (CBCL) as an autism spectrum disorder preliminary screener and outcome measure for the PEERS® intervention for autistic adolescents. *Journal of Autism and Developmental Disorders*, 52(5), 2061–2074. https://doi.org/10.1007/s10803-021-05103-8

Bertolazzi, L. G., & Perroca, M. G. (2020). Impact of interruptions on the duration of nursing interventions: A study in a chemotherapy unit. *Revista da Escola de Enfermagem da USP*, 54, e03551. https://doi.org/10.1590/S1980-220X2018047503551

Bethlehem, J., & Biffignandi, S. (2021). *Handbook of web surveys* (2nd ed.). John Wiley & Sons, INC.

Biomarkers Definitions Working Group. (2001). Biomarkers and surrogate endpoints: Preferred definitions and conceptual framework. *Clinical Pharmacological & Therapeutics*, 69(3), 89–95.

Cahill, S. R., Wang, T. M., Fontenot, H. B., Geffen, S. R., Conron, K. J., Mayer, K. H., Johns, M. M., Avripas, S. A., Michaels, S., & Dunville, R. (2021). Perspectives on sexual health, sexual health education, and HIV prevention from adolescent (13-18 Years) sexual minority males. *Journal of Pediatric Health Care*, 35(5), 500–508. https://doi.org/10.1016/j.pedhc.2021.04.008

Carlson, J. F., Geisinger, K. F., & Jonson, J. L. (Eds.). (2021). *The twenty-first mental measurements yearbook*. Buros Center for Testing, The University of Nebraska-Lincoln.

Cella, D., Riley, W., Stone, A., Rothrock, N., Reeve, B., Yount, S., Amtmann, D., Bode, R., Buysse, D., Choi, S., Cook, K., Devellis, R., DeWalt, D., Fries, J. F., Gershon, R., Hahn, E. A., Lai, J. S., Pilkonis, P., Revicki, D., ... PROMIS Cooperative Group. (2010). The Patient-Reported Outcomes Measurement Information System (PROMIS) developed and tested its first wave of adult self-reported health outcome item banks. *Journal of Clinical Epidemiology*, 63(11), 1179–1194.

Chen, J., Li, H., Maas, K., Starkweather, A., Chen, M., & Cong, X. (2022). Sex-specific gut microbiome profiles among preterm infants during the neonatal intensive care hospitalization. *Interdisciplinary Nursing Research*, 1(1), 6-13. https://doi.org/10.1097/nr9.0000000000000004

Coons, S., Eremenco, S., Lundy, J., O'Donohoe, P., O'Gorman, H., & Malizia, W. (2015). Capturing patient-reported outcome (PRO) data electronically: The past, present, and promise of ePRO measurement in clinical trials. *Patient*, 8(4), 301–309.

Corwin, E., & Ferranti, E. (2016). Integration of biomarkers to advance precision nursing interventions for family research across the lifespan. *Nursing Outlook*, 64(4), 292–298.

DeVillis, R. F., & Thorpe, C. T. (2022). *Scale development: Theory and application* (5th ed.). Sage.

Domínguez-Chávez, C. J., Benavides-Torres, R. A., Gallegos-Cabriales, E. C., & Salazar-González, B. C. (2022). Feasibility of a physical training intervention with music in community-dwelling older women: A quasi-experimental study. *Journal of Gerontological Nursing*, 48(11), 37–43. https://doi.org/10.3928/00989134-20221003-05

Döra, Ö., & Büyük, E. T. (2021). Retracted: Effect of white noise and lullabies on pain and vital signs in invasive interventions applied to premature babies. *Pain Management Nursing*, 22(6), 724–729. https://doi.org/10.1016/j.pmn.2021.05.005

Fang, X., Qiao, Z., Yu, X., Tian, R., Liu, K., & Han, W. (2022). Effect of singing on symptoms in stable COPD: A systematic review and meta-analysis. *International Journal of Chronic Obstructive Pulmononary Disease*, 17, 2893–2904. https://doi.org/10.2147/COPD.S382037

Fernández-Sevillano, J., Alberich, S., Zorrilla, I., González-Ortega, I., López, M. P., Pérez, V., Vieta, E., González-Pinto,

A., & Saíz, P. (2021). Cognition in recent suicideattempts: Altered executive function. *Frontiers in Psychiatry*, *12*, 701140. https://doi.org/10.3389/fpsyt.2021.701140

Flanagan, J., Post, K., Hill, R., & DiPalazzo, J. (2022). Feasibility of a nurse coached walking intervention for informal dementia caregivers. *Western Journal of Nursing Research*, *44*(5), 466–476. https://doi.org/10.1177/01939459211001395

Fleming, T., & Powers, J. (2012). Biomarkers and surrogate endpoints in clinical trials. *Statistics in Medicine*, *31*(25), 2973–2984.

Gavurova, B., Dvorsky, J., & Popesko, B. (2021). Patient satisfaction determinants of inpatient healthcare. *International Journal of Environmental Research and Public Health*, *18*(21), 11337. https://doi.org/10.3390/ijerph182111337

Gonella, S., Di Giulio, P., Palese, A., Dimonte, V., & Campagna, S. (2021). Qualitative research on end-of-life communication with family carers in nursing homes: A discussion of methodological issues and challenges. *Nursing Open*, *8*(1), 180–190. https://doi.org/10.1002/nop2.617

Haidet, K. K., Tate, J., Divirgilio-Thomas, D., Kolanowski, A., & Happ, M. (2009). Methods to improve reliability of video-recorded behavioral data. *Research in Nursing Health*, *32*(4), 465–474.

Hallberg, L. (2022). *Understanding survey bots and tools for data validation: Strategies for identifying possibly fraudulent responses*. Retrieved from https://lifespan.ku.edu/online-surveys-and-data-collection-tools

Huang, Y., Faldowski, R., Burker, E., Morrison, B., & Rak, E. (2021). Coping, anxiety, and health care transition readiness in youth with chronic conditions. *Journal of Pediatric Nursing*, *60*, 281–287. https://doi.org/10.1016/j.pedn.2021.07.027

Hubbard, J. A., Mphande, M., Phiri, K., Balakasi, K., Hoffman, R. M., Daniels, J., Choko, A., Coates, T. J., & Dovel, K. (2022). Improving ART initiation among men who use HIV self-testing in Malawi: A qualitative study. *Journal of the International AIDS Society*, *25*(6), e25950. https://doi.org/10.1002/jia2.25950

Jiang, H., Wang, W., Mei, Y., Zhao, Z., Lin, B., & Zhang, Z. (2023). A scoping review of the self-reported compassion measurement tools. *BMC Public Health*, *23*, 2323. https://doi.org/10.1186/s12889-023-17178-2

Kumari, A., Ranjan, P., Chopra, S., Kaur, D., Upadhyay, A. D., Kaur, T., Bhattacharyya, A., Arora, M., Gupta, H., Thrinath, A., Prakash, B., & Vikram, N. K. (2021). Development and validation of a questionnaire to assess knowledge, attitude, practices, and concerns regarding COVID-19 vaccination among the general population. *Diabetes & Metabolic Syndrome*, *15*(3), 919–925. https://doi.org/10.1016/j.dsx.2021.04.004

Land, LPW, Chenoweth, L, Zhang, YG. Exploring adoption and satisfaction with self-service health technology in older age: Perspectives of healthcare professionals and older people. *Healthcare*. 2022;*10*(4):738. https://doi.org/10.3390/healthcare10040738

Lee, R. Y., Kross, E. K., Torrence, J., Li, K. S., Sibley, J., Cohen, T., Lober, W. B., Engelberg, R. A., & Curtis, J. R. (2023). Assessment of natural language processing of electronic health records to measure goals-of-care discussions as a clinical trial outcome. *JAMA Network Open*, *6*(3), e231204. https://doi.org/10.1001/jamanetworkopen.2023.1204

Libster, N., Knox, A., Engin, S., Geschwind, D., Parish-Morris, J., & Kasari, C. (2023). Sex differences in friendships and loneliness in autistic and non-autistic children across development. *Molecular Autism*, *14*(1), 9. https://doi.org/10.1186/s13229-023-00542-9

Liu, W., Jao, Y. L., Paudel, A., & Yoon, S. O. (2023). Mealtime interactions between nursing home staff and residents with dementia: a behavioral analysis of Language characteristics. *BMC Geriatrics*, *23*(1), 588. https://doi.org/10.1186/s12877-023-04320-3

Page, S., Davies-Abbott, I., & Jones, A. (2021). Dementia care from behind the mask? Maintaining well-being during COVID-19 pandemic restrictions: Observations from dementia care mapping on NHS mental health hospital wards in Wales. *Journal of Psychiatric and Mental Health Nursing*, *28*(6), 961–969. https://doi.org/10.1111/jpm.12763

Pillemer, K., Silver, S., Ramirez, M., Kong, J., Eimicke, J. P., Boratgis, G. D., Meador, R., Schultz, L., Lachs, M. S., Nolte, J., Chen, E. K., & Teresi, J. A. (2022). Factors associated with resident-to-resident elder mistreatment in nursing homes. *Journal of American Geriatric Society*, *70*(4), 1208–1217. https://doi.org/10.1111/jgs.17622

Rajamani, A., Huang, S., Subramaniam, A., Thomson, M., Luo, J., Simpson, A., McLean, A., Aneman, A., Madapusi, T. V., Lakshmanan, R., Flynn, G., Poojara, L., Gatward, J., Pusapati, R., Howard, A., & Odlum, D. (2021). Evaluating the influence of data collector training for predictive risk of death models: An observational study. *BMJ Quality & Safety*, *30*(3), 202–207. https://doi.org/10.1136/bmjqs-2020-010965

Roberts, L. R., Boostrom, G. G., Dehom, S. O., & Neece, C. L. (2020). Self-reported parenting stress and cortisol awakening response following mindfulness-based stress reduction intervention for parents of children with developmental delays: A pilot study. *Biological Research for Nursing*, *22*(2), 217–225. https://doi.org/10.1177/1099800419890125

Saarijärvi, M., & Bratt, E. L. (2021). When face-to-face interviews are not possible: Tips and tricks for video, telephone, online chat, and email interviews in qualitative research. *European Journal of Cardiovascular Nursing*, *20*(4), 392–396. https://doi.org/10.1093/eurjcn/zvab038

Schick-Makaroff, K., & Molzahn, A. (2015). Strategies to use tablet computers for collection of electronic patient-reported outcomes. *Health and Quality of Life Outcomes*, *13*, 2.

Stevens, B., Johnston, C., Petryshen, P., & Taddio, A. (1996). Premature infant pain profile: Development and initial validation. *The Clinical Journal of Pain*, *12*(1), 13–22.

Thompson, A., Pickler, R., & Reyna, B. (2005). Clinical coordination of research. *Applied Nursing Research*, *18*(2), 102–105.

Udtha, M., Nomie, K., Yu, E., & Sanner, J. (2015). Novel and emerging strategies for longitudinal data collection. *Journal of Nursing Scholarship*, *47*(2), 152–160.

Vanhoutte, B., & Nazroo, J. (2016). Life-history data. *Public Health Research & Practice*, 26, e2631630.

Weintraub, W., Lüscher, T., & Pocock, S. (2015). The perils of surrogate endpoints. *European Heart Journal*, 36(33), 2212–2218.

Williamson, P., Altman, D., Bagley, H., Barnes, K., Blazeby, J., Brookes, S., Clarke, M., Gargon, E., Gorst, S., Harman, N., Kirkham, J. J., McNair, A., Prinsen, C. A. C., Schmitt, J., Terwee, C. B., Young, B., & Young, B. (2017). The COMET Handbook: Version 1.0. *Trials*, 18(Suppl. 3), 280.

Yoder, P., Lloyd, B., & Symons, F. (2018). *Observational measurement of behavior* (2nd ed.). Paul H. Brooks Publishing Co.

15 | Measurement and Data Quality

Learning Objectives

1. Understand the criteria for evaluating the quality of data used in measurement.
2. Recognize several types of error of measurement.
3. Articulate the importance of the property domains and interpretability aspects of measurement.
4. Distinguish the four different approaches to reliability assessment.
5. Realize the various statistical tests for determining reliability.
6. Differentiate the various types of validity.

INTRODUCTION

In quantitative studies, an ideal data collection procedure is one that measures a construct accurately, soundly, and with precision. Biomarkers are better at attaining these goals than self-report or observational methods, but no method is flawless. In this chapter, we discuss criteria for evaluating the quality of data obtained through formal measurements. A more detailed presentation of statistical issues in measurement is provided in Polit and Yang (2016). We begin by discussing principles of measurement.

MEASUREMENT

Quantitative researchers obtain data through the measurement of constructs. **Measurement** involves assigning numbers to represent the amount of an attribute present in a person or object. Attributes are not constant: They vary from day to day or from one person to another. Variability is capable of a numeric expression signifying *how much* of an attribute is present. The purpose of assigning numbers is to distinguish people with different amounts of the attribute.

Rules and Measurement

Measurement involves assigning numbers according to rules. *Rules* promote consistency and interpretability. The rules for measuring temperature, weight, and other physical attributes are familiar to us. Rules for measuring constructs such as nausea or quality of life, however, must be invented. Whether the data are collected by observation, self-report, or some other method, researchers must specify criteria for assigning numeric values to the characteristic of interest. Researchers create a **measure** of a construct when they invent rules to quantify it. Measures yield **scores**—numeric values that communicate *how much* of an attribute is present or whether it is present at all.

Rules for measuring constructs should be evaluated to see if they are *good* rules. The rules must yield quantitative information that accurately corresponds to different amounts of the targeted trait. New measurement rules reflect hypotheses about how attributes vary. The adequacy of the hypotheses—the worth of the measures—needs to be assessed empirically.

Advantages of Measurement

What exactly does measurement accomplish? Consider how disadvantaged clinicians would be without measurements. For example, what if there were no measures of body temperature or blood pressure? A major strength of measurement is that it removes subjectivity. Because measurement is based on explicit rules, resulting information tends to be objective—it can be independently verified. Two people measuring a person's weight using the same scale would likely get identical results. Most measures incorporate mechanisms for minimizing subjectivity.

Measurement also makes it possible to obtain reasonably precise information. Instead of describing Alex as "rather tall," we can depict him as being 6 feet 3 inches tall.

Finally, measurement is a language of communication. Numbers are less vague than words. If a researcher reported that the average temperature of a sample of patients was "high," different readers might interpret the sample's physiologic state differently. However, if the researcher reported an average temperature of 99.8°F, there would be no ambiguity.

Theories of Measurement

Psychometrics is a field of inquiry concerned with the theory and methods of psychological measurement. Health measurement has been strongly influenced by psychometrics, although differences in aims and conceptualizations are emerging. When new measures are developed and tested, researchers often say that they are undertaking a *psychometric assessment*.

Within psychometrics (and health measurement), two theories of measurement have been influential. **Classical test theory (CTT)** is a theory of measurement that has been dominant until fairly recently. CTT has been used as a basis for developing multi-item measures of health constructs and is also appropriate for conceptualizing all types of measurements (e.g., biomarkers). An alternative measurement theory (**item response theory** or **IRT**) is gaining in popularity, as discussed in Chapter 16. Unlike CTT, IRT is an appropriate measurement framework only for multi-item scales and tests.

Errors of Measurement

Procedures for obtaining measurements, as well as the objects being measured, are susceptible to influences that can alter the resulting data. Some biasing influences can be controlled or minimized, but such efforts are rarely completely successful.

Instruments that are not perfectly accurate yield measurements containing some error. Within CTT, an **observed** (or **obtained**) **score** can be conceptualized as having two parts—an error component and a true component. This can be written as follows:

$$\text{Obtained score} = \text{True score} \pm \text{Error}$$

or

$$X_O = X_T \pm X_E$$

The first term in the equation is an observed score—for example, a score on an anxiety scale. X_T is the value that would be obtained with an infallible measure. The **true score** is hypothetical—it can never be known because measures are *not* infallible. The final term is the **error of measurement**. The difference between true and obtained scores results from factors that distort the measurement.

When researchers measure an attribute, they are also "measuring" attributes that are not of interest. The true score component is what they wish to isolate; the error component is a composite of other factors that are also being measured, contrary to their wishes. We illustrate with an exaggerated example. Suppose a researcher measured the weight of 10 people on a spring scale. As participants step on the scale, the researcher places a hand on their shoulders and applies pressure. The resulting measures (the X_Os) will be biased upward because scores reflect both actual weight (X_T) and pressure (X_E). Errors of measurement are problematic because their value is unknown and because they often are variable. In this example, the amount of pressure applied likely would vary from one person to the next. In other words, the proportion of true score component in an obtained score varies from one person to the next.

Many factors contribute to errors of measurement. Some errors are random while others are systematic, reflecting *bias*. Common sources of measurement error include the following:

1. *Transient personal factors.* A person's score can be influenced by such personal states as fatigue or mood. In some cases, such factors directly affect the measurement, as when anxiety affects pulse rate measurement. In other cases, personal factors alter scores by influencing people's motivation to cooperate, act naturally, or do their best.
2. *Situational contaminants.* Scores can be affected by the conditions under which they are produced. A participant's awareness of an observer's presence (reactivity) is one source of bias. Environmental factors, such as temperature, lighting, and time of day, are potential sources of measurement error.
3. *Response set biases.* Relatively enduring characteristics of people can interfere with accurate measurements. Response sets such as social desirability or acquiescence are potential biases in self-report measures (Chapter 14).
4. *Administration variations.* Alterations in the methods of collecting data from one person to the next can result in score variations unrelated to variations in the target attribute. For example, if some physiologic measures are taken before a feeding and others are taken after a feeding, then measurement errors can potentially occur.
5. *Instrument clarity.* If the directions on an instrument are poorly understood, then scores may be affected. For example, questions in a self-report instrument may be interpreted differently by different respondents, leading to a distorted measurement of the variable.
6. *Item sampling.* Errors can be introduced as a result of the sampling of items used in the measure. For example, a nursing student's score on a 100-item test of critical care nursing knowledge will be influenced by *which* 100 questions are included. A person might get 94 questions correct on one test but 92 right on another similar test.

Major Types of Measures

Measurements can vary in a number of ways. For example, measurements can vary in terms of information source (i.e., self-reports, observation), complexity (e.g., a visual analog scale or a multidimensional scale with dozens of items), and type of scores they yield (e.g., continuous scores, categorical scores). Some measures are *generic*—that is, broadly applicable across different clinical or nonclinical populations; other measures are *specific*—that is, designed for use with specific groups of people. For example, there are self-efficacy scales that are generic, but there are many disease-specific self-efficacy scales (e.g., for diabetes or asthma).

Static and Adaptive Measures

Multi-item measures can be either static or adaptive. A **static measure** is administered in a comparable manner for everyone being measured. For a static composite scale, people complete an entire set of items and then are scored based on responses to all items. Most health-related measures are static. As an example, a widely used generic measure of depression is called the Center for Epidemiologic Studies Depression Scale, the CES-D (Radloff, 1977). Total scores on the full CES-D rely on responses to the same 20 questions for everyone. Static scales are used to illustrate many key measurement concepts in this book.

An **adaptive measure**, by contrast, involves using responses to early questions to guide the selection of subsequent questions. Dynamic adaptive measures are becoming popular as a way to obtain precise information about an attribute with minimum respondent burden. Adaptive testing has its origin in measurement advances from item response theory. *Item banks* with hundreds of items have been created for broad health topics, such as physical function, pain, and sleep disturbance. The most important example of item banking is PROMIS® (Patient-Reported Outcomes Measurement Information System), developed with support from the U.S. National Institutes of Health (Cella et al., 2007). An approach called **computerized adaptive testing (CAT)** uses these item banks to create measurements that are tailored to individuals. With such tailoring, the set of items used to measure a construct can be different for each person. Despite item differences, cross-person comparisons can be made because the testing places people along a dimension of interest.

Reflective Scales and Formative Indexes

An important distinction is whether a multi-item measure is formative or reflective, which concerns the nature of the relationship between a construct and the measure of the construct. Constructs are not directly observable—they must be inferred by the effects they have on observables, such as responses to items on a patient-reported outcome (PRO) or behaviors witnessed and recorded on an observational scale. Most health scales are **reflective scales**: the items are viewed as *reflections* of the construct. For example, on the CES-D, it is presumed that a person's underlying level of depression *causes* the person to respond in a certain way to the items about sleep disturbance, sadness, and on. The items on a reflective scale share a common cause—in this example, level of depression. Items on reflective scales are expected to be interrelated, because they all reflect (are caused by) the construct.

Not all multi-item instruments, however, are reflective. A multi-item measure can be conceptualized as having items that "cause" or define the attribute (rather than being the effect of the attribute). Such measures are called **formative measures**. Several writers advocate using the term *scale* for multi-item reflective measures, and the term **index** for multi-item formative measures (DeVellis & Thorpe, 2022; Streiner, 2003). A formative index involves constructs that are *formed* by its components, rather than causing them.

A good illustration of a formative index is the Holmes–Rahe Social Readjustment Scale, which is a measure of stress. Psychiatrists Holmes and Rahe studied whether stressful life events might cause illness and devised an index that asked patients to indicate which of 43 life events they had experienced in the previous year (Holmes & Rahe, 1967). Examples of life event items include death of a spouse, pregnancy, and change in residence. The life events are assigned different weights or "life change units" (e.g., 100 for death of a spouse, 20 for a change in residence), and the units are then added together. The sum of life change units defines the construct of stressful life events. The items are not the "effect" of the construct—for example, having high stress does not "cause" the death of a spouse or a residential move.

Because the items on an index are not *caused* by an underlying construct, they are not necessarily intercorrelated. In fact, items with modest correlations that capture different aspects of an attribute are desired in a formative index. Many screening tools are formative and are comprised of components that independently predict an outcome.

The development of reflective scales and formative indexes is necessarily different. For example, because the items on a formative index define the attribute, the specific items matter very much. If the item "I had crying spells" on the CES-D scale was removed, for example, the other 19 items could carry most of the burden of measuring depression. But if the item "Death of a spouse" was removed from the Holmes–Rahe index, the score would misrepresent the stress levels of people who had lost a spouse. Another consequence of having noncorrelated items on a formative index is that some of the standard assessment methods associated with CTT are not appropriate, as we explain later in this chapter.

> **TIP** Formative indexes are seldom created using standard psychometric approaches. Formative indexes are sometimes developed within the field of **clinimetrics**, which is devoted to the development of measures of clinical phenomena. Polit and Yang (2016) have written a chapter on clinimetrics in their measurement book.

MEASUREMENT PROPERTIES: AN OVERVIEW

In making decisions about measuring constructs, careful researchers select instruments that are known to be psychometrically sound—that is, ones that have good **measurement properties**. Psychometricians have traditionally focused on two measurement properties—reliability and validity. Measurement experts in health disciplines, however, have taken a broader view.

A Measurement Taxonomy

A working group based in the Netherlands used a Delphi-type approach with a panel of health measurement experts to identify key measurement properties and to develop a taxonomy and definitions of those properties. The result was the creation of **COSMIN**, the **Co**nsensus-based **S**tandards for the selection of health **M**easurement **In**struments (Mokkink et al., 2010a, 2010b; Terwee et al., 2012) (Information about COSMIN can be accessed at http://www.cosmin.nl). Polit and Yang (2016), building on the groundbreaking COSMIN work, made small modifications to the taxonomy to more clearly incorporate a time perspective. A graphic depiction of the Polit–Yang measurement taxonomy is shown in Figure 15.1.

In this taxonomy, there are four measurement property domains. Two are cross-sectional, addressing the quality of measurements at one point in time. These cross-sectional domains are *reliability* and *validity*, the properties used for decades by psychometricians. Two other domains in the taxonomy concern longitudinal measurement—the quality of measurements capturing changes over time. These two domains are called the *reliability of change scores* and *responsiveness*. New measures that are likely to be used to measure a construct at a single point *and* to measure how scores on the construct change over time ideally would be evaluated for all four measurement properties. The taxonomy also incorporates another concept—interpretability—that has relevance for both point-in-time scores and change scores.

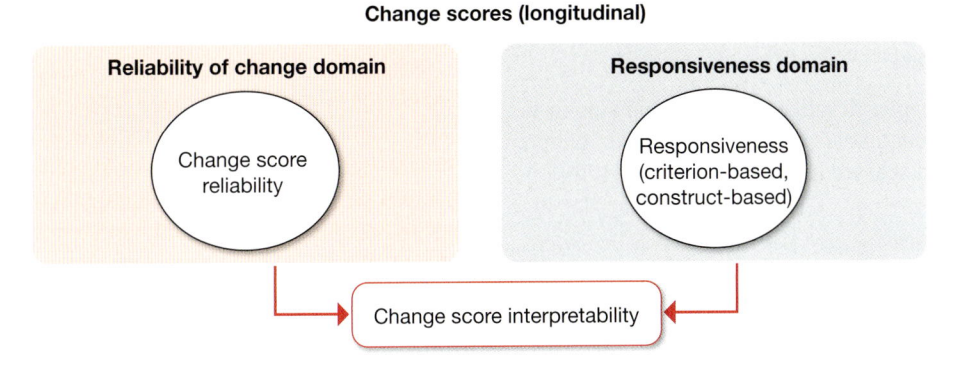

FIGURE 15.1 A taxonomy of measurement properties.

For each measurement property, researchers can estimate **measurement parameters** that quantify the degree to which scores on a measure have desirable attributes. These estimates are the means by which conclusions can be drawn about an instrument's quality, for a particular population and application.

The four measurement property domains and the two interpretability aspects correspond to six key measurement questions, which we illustrate with an example. Suppose we were testing the effects of a nurse-led support program for family caregivers of patients with dementia, and one of our outcome variables was depression. Suppose that we found that a caregiver in the intervention group had a score of 20 on the CES-D at baseline (high level of depression) and a score of 15 (less depression) at a 6-month follow-up. Six questions we could ask, corresponding to the elements in the measurement taxonomy, are as follows:

1. *Reliability:* Is the score of 20 at baseline the right score for this person—is it a dependable score value?
2. *Validity:* Is the scale truly measuring the construct depression, or is it measuring something else?
3. *Interpretation of a score:* What does a score of 20 *mean?* Is it high or low?
4. *Reliability of change:* Is the change from 20 to 15 a *real* change, or does it merely reflect random fluctuations in measurement?
5. *Responsiveness:* Does the change from 20 to 15 correspond to a commensurate improvement in degree of depression?
6. *Interpretation of a change score:* What does a 5-point improvement *mean?* Is the improvement large enough to be considered clinically significant?

This chapter describes the four domains in the measurement taxonomy. Issues relating to interpretation are discussed in Chapters 16 and 21.

TIP Nurse researchers have mainly followed standard psychometric approaches to assessing measurement properties, which means that most of their efforts have focused on reliability and validity. Longitudinal measurement properties have not been given much scrutiny, but changes are likely in light of the influential COSMIN work.

Measurement and Statistics

Assessments of measurement properties require some statistical knowledge. In this chapter, we mainly describe principles rather than statistical details. However, because several measurement properties rely on the calculation of a statistical index called a correlation coefficient, we must briefly explain this index before proceeding.

We have pointed out that researchers seek to detect and explain relationships among phenomena. For example, is there a relationship between patients' gastric acidity levels and their degree of stress? The **correlation coefficient** is a tool for quantitatively describing the magnitude and direction of a relationship between two variables. The most widely used correlation coefficient is called **Pearson's r**.

Two variables that are obviously related are people's height and weight. Tall people tend to be heavier than short people. We would say that there was a **perfect relationship** if the tallest person in a population were the heaviest, the second tallest person were the second heaviest, and so forth. Correlation coefficients summarize how perfect a relationship is. The possible values for a correlation coefficient range from -1.00 through 0.00 to $+1.00$. If height and weight were perfectly correlated, the correlation coefficient expressing this relationship would be $+1.00$. Because the relationship exists but is not perfect, the correlation coefficient is in the vicinity of $+0.50$ or $+0.60$ (which would typically be written as 0.50 and 0.60). The relationship between height and weight is a **positive relationship** because *increases* in height tend to be associated with *increases* in weight.

When two variables are totally unrelated, the correlation coefficient equals zero. One might expect that a female's height is unrelated to their intelligence. Tall females are as likely to perform well on IQ tests as short females. The correlation coefficient summarizing such a relationship would presumably be in the vicinity of 0.00.

Correlation coefficients running from 0.00 to -1.00 express **inverse** or **negative relationships**. When two variables are inversely related, increases in one variable are associated with *decreases* in the second variable. Suppose that there is an inverse relationship between people's age and the amount of sleep they get. This means that, on average, the older the person, the fewer the hours of sleep. If the relationship were perfect (e.g., if the oldest person in a population slept the fewest hours, and so on), the correlation coefficient would be −1.00. In actuality, the relationship between age and sleep is probably modest—in the vicinity of −0.15 or −0.20. A correlation coefficient of this magnitude describes a weak relationship: older people *tend* to sleep fewer hours and younger people *tend* to sleep more, but nevertheless some younger people sleep few hours, and some older people sleep a lot.

Correlation coefficients are important in evaluating the quality of measuring instruments.

RELIABILITY

The reliability of a quantitative measure is a major criterion for assessing its quality. **Reliability**, broadly speaking, is the extent to which scores are free from measurement error. However, from an operational perspective, an extended definition is more useful. Adapting slightly from COSMIN, we offer this definition:

- Reliability is the extent to which scores for people *who have not changed* are the same for repeated measurements, under several situations: repetition on different occasions, by different people, on different versions of a measure, or in the form of different items on a multi-item instrument (internal consistency).

In other words, reliability concerns consistency—the *absence* of variation—in measuring a stable attribute for a person. All types of reliability assessment involve a *replication* to evaluate the extent to which scores for a stable trait are the same. Assessments to evaluate consistency require a heterogeneous sample of people, because the role of a reliable measure is to allow people to be distinguished from one another.

In our taxonomy shown in Figure 15.1, as well as in the COSMIN taxonomy, the cross-sectional reliability domain encompasses three components: reliability, internal consistency, and measurement error. We briefly discuss each component and describe the measurement parameters corresponding to each component.

Reliability

The first component within the broad reliability domain is simply called reliability. It covers four different approaches to reliability assessment, including:

- **test–retest reliability:** administration of the same measure to the same people on two occasions (repetition over occasions),
- **interrater reliability:** measurements by two or more raters using the same instrument (repetition over people),
- **intrarater reliability:** measurements by the same rater on two or more occasions (repetition over occasions), and
- **parallel test reliability:** measurements of the same attribute using alternate versions of the same instrument, with the same people (repetition over versions).

Assessments of reliability involve the calculation of a statistic broadly called a **reliability coefficient**, sometimes symbolized as R. These coefficients, calculated from sample data, are estimates of how reliable the scores are. Different types of coefficients are used in different situations, but they typically range from a low of 0.00 (signifying no reliability) to a high of 1.00 and are thus like correlation coefficients, but not negative in value. The higher the coefficient, the more reliable the scores. Perfect reliability—a coefficient of 1.00—is virtually impossible to obtain, but it is the goal.

Test–Retest Reliability

In **test–retest reliability**, replication takes the form of administering a measure to the same people twice. The assumption is that for traits that have not changed, any differences in people's scores on the two tests reflect measurement error. When score differences across waves are small, reliability is high. This type of reliability is sometimes called *stability* or *reproducibility*—the extent to which scores can be reproduced on repeated administrations.

To illustrate, suppose we were interested in the test–retest reliability of a 16-item self-esteem scale. Self-esteem is a fairly stable attribute that does not fluctuate much from day to day; we would expect a reliable measure of it to yield consistent scores on two occasions. To assess the instrument's reliability, we administer the scale 2 weeks apart. Fictitious data for this example are shown in Table 15.1 for a sample of 10 people (in a real assessment, the sample would be larger). In general, differences in scores on the two tests are not large. The person who scored highest at time 1 (participant 3) also scored highest at time 2, for example.

When a measure yields continuous scores, as in this example, the preferred reliability parameter for test–retest reliability is the **intraclass correlation coefficient** or **ICC**. It is beyond the scope of this book to explain how the ICC is computed, but in our example, the value of the ICC is 0.95.[1] ICCs can be computed in major statistical software packages, such as the Statistical Software for the Social Sciences or SPSS.

> **TIP** Many nurse researchers compute a Pearson's *r* as the reliability estimate in retest situations. However, measurement experts consider Pearson's correlation inappropriate for estimating reliability (e.g., DeVet et al., 2011), even though the values of the ICC and *r* are usually close. In our example of self-esteem scores, the value of the Pearson's *r* coefficient is also 0.95.

Test–retest reliability can be assessed with virtually all measures, including biomarkers, observational measures, performance tests, 1-item measures (e.g., visual analog scales, single demographic questions), formative indexes, and reflective scales. Nevertheless, retest reliability assessment can be problematic. One issue is that many traits *do* change over time, independently of the measure's stability. Attitudes, knowledge, skills, and so on can be modified by experiences between tests—and true change would make a measure look less reliable than it actually is. For this reason, a major issue in retest reliability assessment is finding the right interval between tests.

TABLE 15.1 • Fictitious Data for 2-Week Test–Retest Reliability of Self-Esteem Scale

PARTICIPANT NUMBER	TIME 1	TIME 2	
1	55	57	
2	49	46	
3	78	74	
4	37	35	
5	44	46	
6	50	56	
7	58	55	
8	62	66	
9	48	50	
10	67	63	ICC = .95

ICC, intraclass coefficient.

Another issue is that people's responses on a second administration can be influenced by their memory of initial responses. Such memory interference, called a *carryover effect*, could result in spuriously high reliability coefficients. Another difficulty is that people may actually change *as a result of* the first administration. Finally, people may not be as careful using the same instrument a second time. If they find the process boring on the second occasion, then responses could be haphazard, resulting in a spuriously low estimate of reliability. Other complications relating to retest reliability assessments, and strategies to deal with them, have been described by Polit (2014).

The myriad problems of retest reliability assessment led some psychometricians to discourage using the test–retest approach (e.g., Nunnally & Bernstein, 1994). Healthcare researchers, however, have disagreed with this viewpoint and have emphasized retest reliability. Nurse researchers have often pursued standard psychometric methods, and so those who have developed new scales have not always estimated test–retest reliability; we hope this will change in the years ahead.

---

[1] ICCs can be computed using several different formulas. As explained more fully in Polit and Yang (2016), a main distinction is between what is called ICC for agreement vs. ICC for consistency. In our example in Table 15.1, the reliability estimate is 0.951 for $ICC_{Consistency}$ and 0.956 for $ICC_{Agreement}$. Researchers reporting the value of ICC should state which ICC was calculated.

Example of Test–Retest Reliability
Cabanas-Valdés et al. (2023) compared the 4-m walk test to the 10-m walk test in 36 people who were post stroke to compare the two measures of gait speed. A test-retest reliability and concurrent validity of the two measures indicated that each test had excellent test-retest reliability and concurrent validity with no significant difference in the means of the two measures ($p < .091$).

TIP Many reflective scales and formative indexes contain two or more **subscales**, each of which measures distinct but related concepts (e.g., a measure of fatigue might include subscales for mental and physical fatigue). The reliability of each subscale should be assessed. If subscale scores are summed for a total score, the scale's overall reliability is also computed.

Interrater and Intrarater Reliability

When observers make scoring judgments to measure a construct, a key source of measurement error can stem from the person making the measurements. This is a familiar situation for observational instruments (e.g., scales to measure agitation in nursing home residents), and for some biophysiologic measurements (e.g., skinfold measurement) and performance tests (balance tests). In such situations, it is important to evaluate how reliably the measurements reflect attributes of the person being rated rather than attributes of the raters. Developers of new observational measures need to know if their instruments are capable of yielding reliable scores with trained observers. And users of such measures need to know whether they can reliably apply the measure, and how much training is needed to achieve adequate reliability.

A typical approach is to undertake an **interrater** (or *interobserver*) **reliability** assessment, which involves having two or more observers independently applying the instrument with the same people. Then, the observers' scores are compared to see if the scores are consistent across raters.

A less frequently used approach—but one that is appropriate in many clinical situations—is an **intrarater reliability** assessment in which the *same* rater makes the measurements on two or more occasions, blinded to the ratings assigned previously. Intrarater reliability is an index of self-consistency. It is analogous to retest reliability, except that the focus in retest situations is the consistency of the person *being measured*, and intrarater reliability concerns the consistency of the person *making the measurements*. Like retest reliability, intrarater reliability assessments require a carefully selected interval between testings.

Estimates of inter- or intrarater reliability can be obtained by computing an ICC if the measurements yield continuous scores. In other situations, however, observers are asked to *classify* their observations into categories. When ratings are categorical, one procedure is to calculate the **proportion of agreement**, using the following equation:

$$\frac{\text{Number of agreements}}{\text{Number of agreements} + \text{disagreements}}$$

This formula unfortunately tends to overestimate agreements because it fails to account for agreement by chance. If a behavior were coded for absence vs. presence, observers would agree 50% of the time by chance alone. A widely used statistic in this situation is Cohen **kappa**, which adjusts for chance agreement. Values of kappa usually range from 0.00 to 1.00. Different standards have been proposed for acceptable levels of kappa, but there is some agreement that a value of 0.60 is minimally acceptable, and that values of 0.75 or higher are very good.

Example of Interrater Reliability
Do and colleagues (2023) tested the interrater reliability of surgical wound assessment tool (SWAT). Through convenience sampling, they recruited 260 postsurgical patients from one hospital in Viet Nam. Exploratory factor analysis was used to examine the construct validity of the surgical wound assessment tool. With an intraclass coefficient value of 0.79, the overall scale demonstrated excellent interrater reliability. The kappa value ranged from 0.5 to 1, reflecting almost perfect agreement on all items except pain.

Parallel Test Reliability

Multi-item *parallel tests* (or *alternative-form tests*) are not common in healthcare measurement, but there are a few examples. For instance, the latest version of the Mini-Mental State Examination (MMSE-2), a measure of cognitive impairment, has alternate forms (Folstein et al., 2010). Parallel tests can be created by randomly sampling two sets of items from an item pool. If the two tests are truly parallel, then they are replicates whose true scores are identical. Having measures that are parallel is useful when researchers expect to make measurements in a fairly short period of time and want to avoid carryover biases. Similar to test–retest reliability, **parallel test reliability** involves administration of the parallel tests to the same people and then estimating a reliability parameter, which would be the ICC.

Interpretation of Reliability Coefficients

Reliability coefficients are important indicators of an instrument's quality. Unreliable measures reduce statistical power and affect statistical conclusion validity. If data fail to support a hypothesis, one possibility is that the instruments were unreliable—not necessarily that the expected relationship does not exist.

For group-level comparisons, reliability coefficients in the vicinity of 0.70 may be adequate (especially for subscales), but coefficients of 0.80 or greater are desirable. By group-level comparisons, we mean when researchers compare scores of groups, such as males vs. females or experimental vs. control participants. The reliability coefficients for measures used for making decisions about individuals ideally should be 0.90 or better. For instance, if a score was used to make decisions about a patient's eligibility for a special intervention, then the test's reliability would be of critical importance.

Reliability coefficients have a special interpretation that relates to the decomposition of observed scores into error and true score components. Suppose we administered a scale that measures hopefulness to 50 patients with cancer. The scores would vary from one person to another—some people would be more hopeful than others. Some variability in scores is true variability, reflecting real individual differences in hopefulness; some variability, however, is measurement error. Thus,

$$V_O = V_T + V_E$$

where V_O = observed total variability in scores,

V_T = true variability,

V_E = variability owing to error

A reliability coefficient is directly associated with this equation. *Reliability is the proportion of true variability to the total obtained variability*, or

$$R = \frac{V_T}{V_O}$$

If, for example, the reliability coefficient were 0.85, then 85% of the variability in obtained scores would represent true individual differences, and 15% would reflect extraneous fluctuations. Looked at in this way, it should be clear why instruments with reliability lower than 0.70 are risky to use.

Factors Affecting Reliability

Several factors under researchers' control can affect the value of reliability coefficients. With observational scales, for example, reliability can be improved with greater clarity in explaining the underlying construct during observer training.

A measure's reliability is related to the heterogeneity of the sample with which it is tested. The more homogeneous the sample (i.e., the more similar their scores), the lower the reliability coefficient will be. This is because instruments are designed to measure differences among those being measured. If the sample is homogeneous, then it is more difficult for the instrument to discriminate reliably among those who possess varying degrees of the attribute. For example, suppose that the self-esteem scores shown in Table 15.1 were changed for two individuals. If participant 3 (the high scorer) had scores of 58 and 54 (rather than 78 and 74) and if participant 4 (the low scorer) had scores of 57 and 55 (rather than 37 and 35), the ICC would be 0.85 rather than 0.95 because now the range of scores is smaller (44–67 vs 37–78).

An important thing to keep in mind in computing or interpreting reliability coefficients within the CTT framework—or in selecting an instrument for use in a study—is that *reliability is not a fixed property of an instrument*. For a given measure, reliability will vary from one population to another or from one situation to another. It is better to think of reliability as a property of a particular set of scores than as a property of a measure itself. Users of an instrument need to consider how similar their population is to the population used to estimate reliability parameters. If the populations are similar, then the reliability estimate calculated by the scale developer is probably a reasonably good index of the instrument's accuracy in the new research. But if the population is very different, new estimates of reliability should be computed.

Internal Consistency

Another component within the reliability domain of the measurement taxonomy (Figure 15.1) is **internal consistency**. Our reliability definition supports including internal consistency within the reliability domain: Reliability is the extent to which scores for patients who have not changed are the same for repeated measurements. For internal consistency, replication involves people's responses to multiple items during a single administration. Whereas reliability estimates described in the previous section assess a measure's degree of consistency across time, raters, and versions of a measure, internal consistency captures consistency across items.

Single items are often inadequate for measuring a construct—indeed, the low reliability of single items is the reason for constructing multi-item scales. In responding to an item, people are influenced not only by the underlying construct but also by idiosyncratic reactions to the words. By sampling multiple items with various wordings, item irrelevancies are expected to cancel each other out. An instrument is said to be internally consistent to the extent that its items measure the same trait.

The most widely used statistic for evaluating internal consistency is **coefficient alpha** (or **Cronbach' alpha**). Coefficient alpha estimates the extent to which different subparts of an instrument (i.e., items) are reliably measuring the critical attribute, and greater internal consistency is obtained with a set of items that are highly intercorrelated. Coefficient alpha can be interpreted like other reliability coefficients: the normal range of values is between 0.00 and +1.00, and higher values reflect better internal consistency. Coefficients of 0.80 or higher are considered especially desirable. It is beyond the scope of this text to explain computations of coefficient alpha, but information is available in measurement textbooks (e.g., Polit & Yang, 2016). Most standard statistical software such as SPSS can be used to calculate alpha.

An important feature of internal consistency is that the value of coefficient alpha is partly a function of the scale's length. To improve internal consistency, more items tapping the same construct should be added.

Internal consistency has been the most widely reported aspect of reliability assessment among nurse researchers. Its popularity reflects the fact that it is economical (it requires only one administration) and is a means of assessing an important source of measurement error in psychosocial instruments, the sampling of items.

Internal consistency is a relevant measurement property only for multi-item reflective scales, however. It is *not* relevant for formative indexes, which are comprised of items that are not necessarily intercorrelated. For formative indexes, only retest reliability should be estimated. For most multi-item reflective scales (whether they are self-report scales or observational scales), both internal consistency and retest reliability should be assessed by the scale developer. Users of an existing scale should also compute coefficient alpha with data from their research sample.

Example of Internal Consistency Reliability
Qian and colleagues (2022) aimed to translate into Chinese, the Perinatal Bereavement Care Confidence Scale originally developed in Ireland. They tested its reliability and validity in a cohort of Chinese midwives and nurses. Four subscales were evaluated for internal consistency. The Cronbach alpha ranged from 0.835 to 0.901. The translated measure was found to be internally consistent.

> **TIP** Reliability estimates vary according to the procedures used to obtain them. A scale's test–retest reliability coefficient should not be expected to be the same or even similar in value to an internal consistency estimate (alpha).

Measurement Error

Measurement error is another component within the reliability domain of our taxonomy. The concepts of measurement error and reliability are inextricably connected: unless a reliability coefficient is 1.0 (which is virtually never the case), measurement error is present. Yet, measurement error statistics yield information that reliability coefficients do not provide. For example, measurement error statistics can be used to estimate the precision of a continuous score—that is, the range within which the true score probably lies.

The Standard Error of Measurement

The most widely used index of measurement error is the **standard error of measurement (SEM)**. The SEM can be thought of as quantifying "typical error" on a measure. It is an index that can be computed in connection with estimates of either reliability (e.g., test–retest reliability) or internal consistency.

Reliability coefficients, which typically range from 0.00 to 1.00, are not in the units of measurement associated with the actual measure. A reliability coefficient is a *relative* index that varies from sample to sample and across populations. SEMs, by contrast, are in the measurement units of the instrument. The SEM for a body weight would be in pounds (or grams), and the SEM for a scale such as the CES-D would be in the units of points on the CES-D scale. SEMs are more stable than reliability coefficients and not as affected by sample homogeneity.

The SEM can be estimated using one of several formulas. A popular and easy formula involves taking the square root of 1 minus the reliability coefficient (1 − R) and multiplying that value by an index of how variable the sample scores are.[2] (R could be either the ICC estimate from a test–retest analysis or alpha from an internal consistency analysis). Unfortunately, the SEM is not computed in many major software packages, which might explain why it is not more routinely reported in instrument development papers.

For the self-esteem scores shown in Table 15.1, the SEM is 2.65 at time 1 and 2.49 at time 2. Knowing the value of the SEM allows us to state the probability that a person's true score lies within a certain range. For example, participant 1 had a score of 55 at time 1. Knowing that the SEM is 2.65, we could state that there is a 95% probability that the participant's true score at time 1 was between about 50 and 60 (i.e., roughly twice the SEM on either side of the obtained score).

Limits of Agreement

An alternative index of measurement error is the **limits of agreement (LOA)**, derived from work done by Bland and Altman (1986). *Bland–Altman plots* are widely used by medical researchers to examine aspects of both the reliability and validity of measures but are seldom used by psychometricians or nurse researchers. A Bland–Altman plot is a useful device for visually interpreting and differentiating random measurement error and systematic error (bias) in retest or interrater assessments when scores are continuous.

Like the SEM, the LOA provides information about the precision of scores. LOA are easy to compute[3] but are not routinely calculated in standard statistical software packages such as SPSS. For the self-esteem scores in Table 15.1, the limits of agreement are about +7.0 around a difference score (i.e., the difference between time 1 and time 2 scores). This means that any difference in a person's score that is greater than 7 is beyond what we would expect for measurements of a stable trait. None of the score differences in Table 15.1 is greater than 7.

---

[2] Specifically, this formula for the SEM is: $SEM = SD\sqrt{1-R}$.

---

[3] Limits of agreement can be computed using output from a paired *t*-test analysis. For 95% confidence, the LOA is 1.96 times the standard deviation of difference between the test and retest scores.

> **Example of Measurement Error Information**
> Mazzotta et al. (2022) sought to translate a tool used to measure moral distress in nursing students. A sample of 282 students who had failed exams allowing them to progress in the nursing program were enrolled in the study. The tool was considered reliable and valid with a SEM that ranged from 1.064 to 4.659.

TIP Measurement error is routinely estimated for multi-item measures developed with item response theory (IRT) methods. Indeed, estimating measurement error typically replaces efforts to estimate internal consistency or reliability. One problem with measurement error in CTT measures is that the estimate is the same for everyone in a sample, whereas IRT models estimate measurement error for each person. In computer-adaptive tests, a "stopping rule" is established at a desired level of precision (i.e., for a maximum allowable amount of measurement error), and the stopping rule dictates how many items each respondent completes.

VALIDITY

A second domain in the taxonomy of measurement properties is validity. In measurement, **validity** is the degree to which an instrument is measuring the construct it purports to measure. When researchers develop a scale to measure *resilience*, they need to be sure that the resulting scores validly reflect this construct and not something else, such as self-efficacy, hope, or perseverance. Assessing the validity of abstract constructs requires a careful conceptualization of the construct—as well as conceptualization of what the construct is *not*.

Like reliability, validity has different aspects and assessment approaches. As shown in Figure 15.1, the three major components within the validity domain are content and face validity, criterion validity, and construct validity. Unlike reliability, however, an instrument's validity is difficult to gauge. There are no equations that can easily be applied to the scores of a resilience scale to estimate how good a job the scale is doing in measuring the critical variable. Validation is an evidence-building enterprise, in which the goal is to assemble sufficient evidence from which validity can be inferred. The greater the amount of evidence supporting validity, the more sound the inference.

TIP Reliability and validity are not totally independent properties of an instrument. A measuring device that is unreliable cannot be valid. An instrument cannot validly measure an attribute if it is inconsistent.

Content and Face Validity

Face validity refers to whether the instrument *looks* like it is measuring the target construct. Although face validity is not considered strong evidence of validity, it is helpful for a measure to have face validity if there is evidence of other types of validity. Face validity can be important if patients' resistance to being measured reflects the view that the scale is not relevant to their problems or situations. One reason for developing disease-specific measures, in fact, is that general measures sometimes lack face validity.

> **Example of Face Validity**
> In developing and testing the Emotional Intelligence and Health and Well-Being Scale (EQ-HWB), Brazier et al. (2022) achieved face validity by conducting qualitative interviews with a mix of 168 health and social care personnel, patients, caregivers and the general population across 6 countries (Argentina, Australia, China, Germany, United Kingdom, United States).

Content validity may be defined as the extent to which an instrument's content adequately captures the construct—that is, whether an instrument has an appropriate sample of items for the construct being measured. It is increasingly recognized that evaluating and enhancing a measure's content validity is a critical early step in enhancing the construct validity of an instrument. If the content of an instrument is a good reflection of a construct, then the instrument has a greater likelihood of achieving its measurement objectives.

Content validation typically involves consultations with a panel of experts. Three issues are pertinent: relevance, comprehensiveness, and balance.

- *Relevance.* An assessment for relevance involves feedback on the relevance of individual items and the overall set of items. For each item, one needs to know: Is this item relevant to the construct or to a specific dimension of the construct? Another consideration is whether the items have relevance for the target population.
- *Comprehensiveness.* The flip side of asking experts about the relevance of items is to ask them if there are notable omissions. To be content valid, a measure should encompass the full complexity of the construct.
- *Balance.* An instrument that is content valid represents the domains of the construct in a balanced manner. In a multi-item scale, a sufficient number of items are needed for each dimension to ensure high internal consistency of subscales.

Researchers designing a new instrument should begin with a thorough conceptualization of the construct. Such a conceptualization might be based on rich firsthand knowledge, an exhaustive literature review, consultation with experts, and in-depth conversations with members of the target population.

Example of Using Qualitative Data to Enhance Content Validity
The Integrated Palliative Care Outcome Scale for Dementia was developed by palliative care experts in England. It is a useful tool to comprehensively assess in people with advanced dementia their symptoms and concerns. Hodiamont and colleagues (2021) conducted qualitative interviews with 29 family caregivers and 6 people with dementia to determine the content validity of the measure for use in German cultures. While the tool was found to be comprehensive, cultural adaptation of the questionnaire was necessary.

An instrument's content validity is necessarily based on judgment. There are various approaches to assessing content validity using an expert panel, but nurse researchers have been in the forefront in developing an approach that involves the calculation of a **content validity index (CVI)**.

At the item level, a common procedure is to have experts rate items on a 4-point scale of relevance. There are several variations of labeling the 4 points, but the scale used most often is as follows: 1 = *not relevant*, 2 = *somewhat relevant*, 3 = *quite relevant*, and 4 = *highly relevant*. Then, for each item, the **item CVI (I-CVI)** is computed as the number of experts giving a rating of 3 or 4, divided by the number of experts—that is, the proportion in agreement about relevance. For example, an item rated as "quite" or "highly" relevant by 4 out of 5 experts would have an I-CVI of 0.80, which is considered an acceptable value. Items with an I-CVI below 0.78 should be carefully scrutinized and either revised or discarded.

There are two approaches to calculating **scale CVIs (S-CVIs)**, and unfortunately instrument development papers do not always indicate which approach was used (Polit & Beck, 2006). The approach we recommend is to compute the S-CVI by averaging all the I-CVIs. We suggest a value of 0.90 for the S-CVI/Averaging as the standard for establishing excellent content validity (Polit et al., 2007). Content validation should be done with at least three experts, but a larger group is preferable. Further guidance is offered in Chapter 16.

Example of Using a Content Validity Index
Barreiro and colleagues (2022) aimed to confirm the proposal for the nursing diagnosis of low self-efficacy in health by conducting a content validity. They convened a panel of 47 experts with interest in the nursing diagnosis to determine the relevance of the 16 clinical indicators and 18 etiological factors. A content validity index of 0.9 resulted in the 16 clinical indicators being reduced to 13 and the 18 etiological factors remaining.

Criterion Validity

Criterion validity is the extent to which the scores on an instrument are a good reflection of a "gold standard"—that is, a criterion considered an ideal measure of the construct. Not all measures can be validated using a criterion approach, because there is not always a gold standard to use.

One might reasonably ask: If there is an established criterion, why do we need the focal measure at all—why not simply use the gold standard? Reasons for creating a new measure include the following: (1) the expense of administering the gold standard measure is too high, (2) the criterion is burdensome, (3) there are risks or discomfort in using the gold standard, and (4) the criterion is not routinely available in a clinical setting.

A requirement for criterion validation is the availability of a reliable criterion with which measures on the focal instrument can be compared, which is not always the case. For example, it would be difficult to identify a criterion for such attributes as patients' satisfaction with care or quality of life. When a criterion is unavailable, construct validation approaches must be used.

Criterion validation involves testing an implicit hypothesis that the focal measure yields score information that is as good as that obtained from the criterion. This means that scores on the two are hypothesized to be correlated. When such a hypothesis is upheld through formal testing, users gain some assurance that the measure will support appropriate inferences regarding the attribute in question when used with the target population in a similar context.

One type of criterion validity, **concurrent validity**, is assessed when the measurements of the criterion and the new instrument occur at the same time. In such a situation, the implicit hypothesis is that the new measure is an adequate substitute for a contemporaneous criterion. In **predictive validity**, the focal measure is tested against a criterion that is measured in the future. Screening scales are often tested against some future criterion—the occurrence of the phenomenon for which a screening tool is sought.

A broad array of statistical procedures can be used to test whether the criterion validity hypothesis is supported by data from a relevant sample. The choice of statistics depends on whether the focal measure and the criterion are measured as a continuous score value or as categorical ones. Three situations are especially common.

Criterion Validity With a Continuous Measure and a Continuous Criterion

The first situation is when both the focal measure being tested and the criterion are continuous scores. For example, suppose we were assessing the criterion validity of a 2-minute walk test as a measure of functional performance, and we used the well-established 6-minute-walk test as the criterion. In this situation, we would obtain measures of both tests from a sample of patients and compute a Pearson's r (the correlation coefficient) between the two sets of scores. The higher the value of r, the better the evidence of criterion validity.

Example of Criterion Validity
Clover and colleagues (2022) examined the criterion validity of two patient-reported outcome anxiety measures for anxiety among oncology patients in Australia. A psychologist interviewed 132 oncology outpatients with a reported diagnosis of anxiety. Another member of the care team then administered the two anxiety measures. Findings support the criterion validity of the two measures relative to the psychologist's clinical assessment.

Criterion Validity With a Dichotomous Measure and a Dichotomous Criterion

When both the focal measure and the criterion are dichotomous, several statistical methods can be used but, most often, methods of assessing **diagnostic accuracy** are applied. **Sensitivity** is the ability of a measure to identify a "case" correctly, that is, to screen in or diagnosis a condition correctly. A measure's sensitivity is its rate of yielding "true positives." **Specificity** is the measure's ability to identify noncases correctly, that is, to screen *out* those without the condition. Specificity is an instrument's rate of yielding "true negatives." Of course, to evaluate an instrument's sensitivity and specificity, researchers need a reliable and valid criterion of "caseness" against which scores on the instrument can be assessed.

To illustrate, suppose we wanted to evaluate the validity of adolescents' self-reports about smoking, and we asked 100 teenagers whether they had smoked a cigarette in the previous 24 hours. The gold standard for nicotine consumption is cotinine levels in a body fluid, so we performed a urinary cotinine assay. We use the results to dichotomize the adolescents as positive (>200 ng/mL) or negative for smoking. Some fictitious data are shown in Table 15.2. Sensitivity is calculated as the proportion of teenagers who said they smoked *and* who had high concentrations of cotinine, divided by all

TABLE 15.2 • Example Illustrating Sensitivity, Specificity, and Likelihood Ratios

SELF-REPORTED SMOKING	URINARY COTININE LEVEL (CRITERION)		
	POSITIVE (>200 NG/ML)	NEGATIVE (<200 NG/ML)	TOTAL
Yes	Cell A: true positives 30	Cell B: false positives 5	35 (A + B)
No	Cell C: false negatives 10	Cell D: true negatives 55	65 (C + D)
Total	40 (A + C)	60 (B + D)	100 (A + B + C + D)
Sensitivity: A ÷ (A + C) = .75			
Specificity: D ÷ (B + D) = .92			
Positive predictive value (PPV): A ÷ (A + B) = .86			
Negative predictive value (NPV): D ÷ (C + D) = .85			
Likelihood ratio-positive (LR+): Sensitivity ÷ (1 − Specificity) = 9.04			
Likelihood ratio-negative (LR−): (1 − Sensitivity) ÷ Specificity = 0.27			

real smokers according to the urine test. Put another way, it is the true positives divided by all positives. In this example, smoking was underreported, so the sensitivity of the self-report was 0.75. Specificity is the proportion of teenagers who accurately reported they did not smoke: the true negatives divided by all negatives. In our example, specificity is 0.92. There was less overreporting of smoking ("faking bad") than underreporting ("faking good"). We would conclude that the sensitivity of the self-reports was moderate, but the specificity was good.

Other related indicators often are calculated with such data. **Predictive values** are posterior probabilities—the probability of an outcome after the results is known. A **positive predictive value** (or PPV) is the proportion of people with a positive result who have the target outcome. In our example, the PPV is the proportion of teens who said they smoke who actually *do* smoke, according to the cotinine test results. Thirty out of thirty-five of those who reported smoking had high concentrations of cotinine, and so PPV = 0.86. A **negative predictive value** (NPV) is the proportion of people who have a negative "score" on the focal measure who also have a negative result on the gold standard. As shown in Table 15.2, 55 out of the 65 teenagers who reported not smoking actually were nonsmokers, and so NPV in our example is 0.85.

Reporting **likelihood ratios** has come into favor because they summarize the relationship between specificity and sensitivity in a single number. The *positive likelihood ratio* (LR+) is the ratio of true positives to false positives. The formula for LR+ is sensitivity, divided by 1 minus specificity. For the data in Table 15.2, LR+ is 9.04: we are nine times more likely to find that a self-report of smoking really *is* for a true smoker than it is for a nonsmoker. The *negative likelihood ratio* (LR−) is the ratio of false-negative results to true-negative results. For the data in Table 15.2, the LR− is 0.27, indicating that we are substantially less likely to find that a self-report of nonsmoking is false than we are to find that it reflects a true nonsmoker.

These criterion validity indicators are often used when a *cutpoint* on a continuous focal measure is used to classify patients into two categories, which we discuss next.

TIP In Chapter 1, we discussed categories of evidence-based practice (EBP)-related questions, such as Therapy, Prognosis, and so on. One category concerns the accuracy of diagnostic or screening tests. The methods discussed in this section on criterion validity are especially important for providing evidence for this type of EBP question.

Criterion Validity With a Continuous Measure and a Dichotomous Criterion

When the measure being assessed is continuous and the criterion is dichotomous, criterion validation often uses an approach that involves plotting each score on the index measure against its specificity and sensitivity for correct classification based on the dichotomous criterion.

The indicators we calculated for the data in Table 15.2 are contingent upon the value that we established for cotinine concentration (200 ng/mL). Sensitivity and specificity would be different if we used 100 ng/mL as indicative of smoking status. There is almost invariably a tradeoff between the sensitivity and specificity of a measure. When sensitivity is increased to include more true positives, the proportion of true negatives declines. Therefore, a common task in developing new measures for which there is a continuous gold standard is to find an appropriate **cutoff point** (or *cutpoint*)—that is, a score to distinguish cases and noncases.

Researchers use a **receiver operating characteristic curve** (**ROC curve**) to identify the best cutoff point. In an ROC curve, the sensitivity of an instrument (i.e., the rate of correctly identifying a case vis-à-vis an established criterion) is plotted against the false-positive rate (i.e., the rate of incorrectly classifying someone as a case, which is the inverse of its specificity) over a range of different scores on the focal measure. The score (cutoff point) that yields the best balance between sensitivity and specificity can then be determined. The optimum cutoff is at or near the shoulder of the ROC curve.

Figure 15.2 presents an ROC curve from a study to assess the criterion validity of a brief cognitive screening instrument (the Montreal Cognitive Assessment, MoCA) for adolescents with congenital heart disease (Pike et al., 2017). The criterion

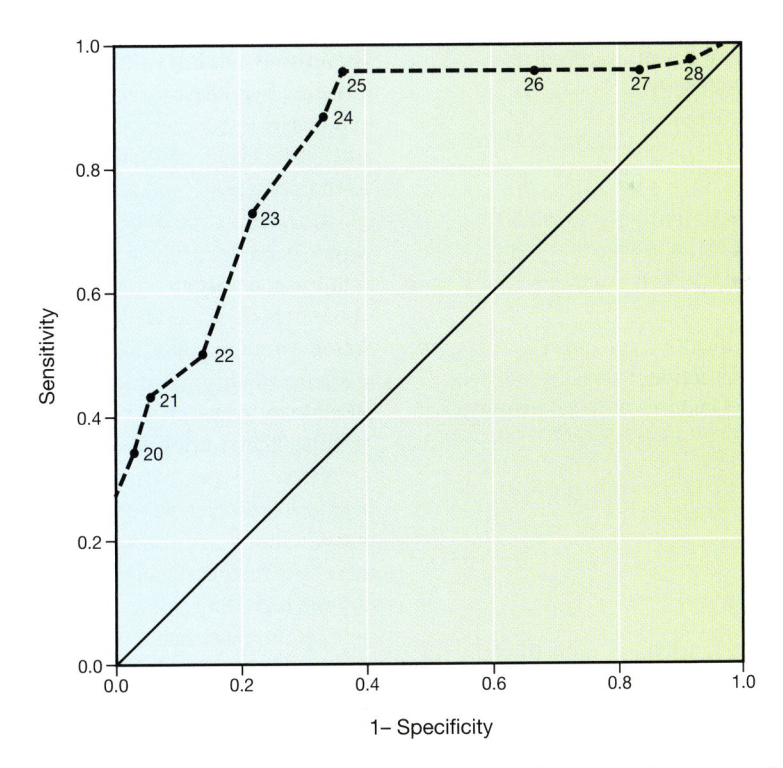

FIGURE 15.2 Receiver operating characteristic (ROC) curve for Montreal Cognitive Assessment Screener for Adolescents and Young Adults with Congenital Heart Disease. (Adapted with permission from Pike, N., Poulsen, M., & Woo, M. (2017). Validity of the Montreal Cognitive Assessment Screener for adolescents and young adults with and without congenital heart disease. *Nursing Research, 66*, 222–230.)

was a longer, widely accepted measure of cognition for this population—the General Memory Index (GMI). Scores on the GMI were dichotomized for "caseness" at 85. In this figure, sensitivity and 1 minus specificity are plotted for each MoCA score. The upper left corner represents sensitivity at its highest possible value (1.0) and false positives at its lowest possible value (0.00).

In ROC analyses, the **area under the curve** (**AUC**) can be used as a validity parameter. Desirable AUC values (close to 1.00) are found when the curve hugs close to the upper left corner. When the curve is close to the diagonal, the AUC value is 0.50, indicating that the measure cannot differentiate between those who are positive and negative on the criterion. Values of 0.70 are usually considered evidence of adequate validity. The AUC for the data portrayed in Figure 15.2 is 0.84. The cutoff score for the MoCA in this example was set at 26. At this cutoff value, sensitivity was 0.94 and specificity was 0.80; the PPV was 0.70 and NPV was 0.96.

Example of Sensitivity, Specificity, Predictive Values, and Likelihood Ratio
Flanagan and colleagues (2021) sought to develop a predictive model with intrinsic factors to identify older adults who, after an acute-care discharge to a skilled nursing facility, are more likely to be transferred to long-term care rather than be discharged to home. Using data from 23,662 people admitted from acute care facilities to skilled nursing facilities in Massachusetts, the explanatory model indicated there were 12 intrinsic predictors indicating admission to long-term care. The original logistic regression model reflected that the area under ROC was valid at 0.694. To classify patients at risk, with a threshold of 0.5, a second logistic regression predictive model indicated the specificity was very high 99.8% but the sensitivity at 1.6% was very low. However, the area under the ROC curve was 0.691, which suggests validity and generalizability.

Construct Validity

For many abstract attributes (constructs), no gold standard criterion exists, so other validation avenues must be pursued. The third component within the validity domain of our measurement taxonomy (Figure 15.1) is construct validity. The construct validity question is this: What attribute is *really* being measured? Borrowing from esteemed methodologists Shadish et al. (2002), we define **construct validity** as the degree to which evidence about a measure's scores in relation to other scores supports the inference that the construct has been appropriately represented.

Evidence for construct validity comes from tests of hypotheses about the nature of the construct and scores on the focal measure. The researcher must speculate: If my instrument is, in fact, really measuring construct X, then how would I expect the scores to perform? In a construct validation, the instrument developer must have a firm conceptualization not only of the construct itself (as in a content validity effort), but also a conceptualization of how the construct is related to other constructs. In other words, there needs to be an overarching conceptual model of processes and traits of relevance to the construct.

Construct validity encompasses three aspects: hypothesis-testing construct validity, structural validity, and cross-cultural validity.

Hypothesis-Testing Construct Validity

Hypothesis-testing validity involves testing to corroborate hypotheses about the focal measure. In hypothesis-testing construct validations, hypotheses are developed about relationships between scores on the focal measure and scores on measures of other constructs; data are collected to test the hypotheses with a sample from a specified population; and validity conclusions are reached based on results of the hypothesis tests. A successful construct validation effort requires ingenuity. Researchers must challenge themselves to develop diverse and complementary ways of testing whether their measure is, indeed, measuring the construct of interest.

Different types of evidence can be brought to bear on construct validity, leading to approaches that have been given different names. Unfortunately, there are inconsistencies in the measurement literature regarding some of those names. Because the terms associated with different validation approaches are often confusing, Table 15.3 presents a quick summary chart, which includes previously discussed validity terms as well.

Convergent Validity. Convergent validity is the degree to which scores on the focal measure are correlated with scores on measures of constructs

TABLE 15.3 • Types of Measurement-Related Validity

TYPE OF VALIDITY	EXPLANATION
Content and Face Validity	
Face validity	Concerns whether a measure "looks" as though it is measuring the relevant construct
Content validity	Concerns the adequacy of content for multicomponent measures
Criterion Validity	
Concurrent validity	Tests whether a measure is consistent with a criterion (a gold standard), measured at the same time
Predictive validity	Tests whether a measure is consistent with a criterion (a gold standard), measured at a future point in time
Construct Validity: Hypothesis Testing	
Convergent validity	In the absence of a gold standard, tests the correlation between the focal measure and a measure of a construct with which conceptual convergence is expected
Known-groups (discriminative) validity	Tests the degree to which a measure can discriminate between groups known to differ with regard to the focal construct
Divergent (discriminant) validity	Tests that the focal measure is not a measure of a different construct other than the one intended
Construct Validity: Other	
Structural validity	Tests whether a measure captures the hypothesized dimensionality of a construct
Cross-cultural validity	Concerns the extent to which a translated or adapted measure is equivalent to the original

with which there is a hypothesized relationship—that is, the degree of conceptual convergence. Sometimes the other measure is a different measure of the same construct (but not a measure that could be construed as a "gold standard"). For example, if we were developing a new, specific measure of fatigue in patients with cancer, we might predict that scores on our new scale would correlate fairly strongly and positively with patients' scores on a general measure of fatigue, such as the Piper Fatigue Scale.

From a broader perspective, convergent validity concerns the extent to which the focal measure correlates with variables in a manner consistent with an underlying theory or conceptual model. For example, we might hypothesize that inadequate social support is a factor contributing to postpartum depression (PPD). We could test the construct validity of a PPD scale by examining the correlation between scores on this scale with those on a measure of social support. In essence, researchers reason as follows:

- According to theory or prior evidence, construct X is positively related to construct Y.
- Instrument A is a measure of construct X; instrument B is a valid measure of construct Y.
- Scores on A and B are correlated positively, as predicted.
- Therefore, it is inferred that A is a valid measure of X.

This logical analysis does not offer proof of construct validity but yields supportive evidence. Construct validation is an ongoing evidence-building enterprise. With convergent validity, the validity parameter is typically the correlation coefficient between two measures—most often Pearson's *r*.

> **Example of Convergent Validity**
> De Oliveira Tavares et al. (2021) conducted a systematic review with a meta-analysis to examine the reliability and convergent validity of self-reported questionnaires to measure physical activity in people with psychiatric disorders. A total of nine studies that in total included a N of 1,344 participants were analyzed. Convergent validity was evaluated by examining self-report measures against objectives measures such as accelerometry. They concluded that the self-report measures were valid for assessing moderate physical activity.

Known-Groups Validity. **Known-groups validity**, which has also been called *discriminative validity*, tests hypotheses about a measure's ability to discriminate between two or more groups known (or expected) to differ on the construct of interest. For example, we might hypothesize that females who had planned their pregnancy would have more favorable scores on a PPD scale than females whose pregnancy was unwanted. If the scores on the PPD measure do not differ for the two groups, one might question the scale's validity, given the existing evidence that females whose pregnancies are wanted are less susceptible than other females to PPD. We would not necessarily expect large differences; some females in both groups would likely suffer from PPD. We would, however, hypothesize differences in *average* group scores. The known-groups approach is one of the most widely used methods of assessing construct validity.

A key difference between convergent validity and known-groups validity concerns how the validation variable is measured. Continuous scores on a comparator construct can be used to create "known" groups by dividing the sample into subgroups for known-groups validity, or the continuous scores can be used to test a correlation for convergent validity. It is best to divide sample members into subgroups for a known-groups validation when there is a well-established cutpoint for "caseness."

> **Example of the Known-Groups Technique**
> Li and colleagues (2022) developed and assessed the validity and reliability of the Short-Form Life Satisfaction Index (LSI-SF) among the older population. A total of 2,321 participants were included in the analysis from the Taiwan Longitudinal Study on Aging. Known groups' validity was determined from the difference between frailty stage and quality of life. Life satisfaction was highest in the nonfrailty stage and lowest in the frailty stage.

Divergent Validity. **Divergent validity** (which is often called *discriminant validity*) concerns evidence that a measure is *not* a measure of a different construct. We use the term *divergent* because it is a good contrast with *con*vergent validity and also because of possible confusion between the terms discriminant and discriminative (known-groups) validity.

In a divergent validation, researchers typically measure both the focal attribute and a similar—but distinct—attribute as a means of ensuring that the two are not really measures of the same construct but with different labels. Thus, in a divergent validation, the hypothesis is that the two measures are only weakly correlated.

Sometimes hypotheses for construct validations are stated in relative rather than absolute terms, especially when there are both convergent and divergent hypotheses. For example, an absolute hypothesis for a new PPD scale might predict that scores would correlate only modestly with scores on a measure of anxiety about maternal role performance, to distinguish the PPD construct from maternal anxiety. For a relative hypothesis, we might predict that scores on a PPD scale would correlate more strongly with scores on a general measure of depression (convergent validity) than with scores on the maternal anxiety scale (divergent validity).

The primary approach to divergent validation is to compute correlation coefficients. Researchers should stipulate in advance how "weak" a correlation would need to be as evidence of divergent validity, either in absolute or relative terms.

Example of Divergent Validity
Nakić Radoš and colleagues (2022) examined the divergent validity of the Birth Satisfaction Scale-Revised (BSS-R) with correlations to maternal age and time since birth. They found that the BSS-R demonstrated convergent validity with other measures of birth satisfaction. Further, the BSS-R was not related to maternal age and time since birth which demonstrated high divergent validity.

TIP An approach known as the **multitrait–multimethod matrix method** (**MTMM**) is a significant construct validation tool that involves tests of both convergent and divergent validity (Campbell & Fiske, 1959). Few nurse researchers have used an MTMM in its full form. The MTMM is explained more fully in Polit and Yang (2016).

Construct Validity Evidence. Most researchers identify multiple hypotheses for their construct validity work and include several different types of validation approaches in a single study. As a result, drawing conclusions about a measure's construct validity is typically more complex than interpreting results for other measurement properties, such as reliability. For many measurement parameters, only a single number needs to be interpreted. For example, when an ICC is computed with test–retest data, that value *is* the estimated reliability. However, there is seldom a single "validity coefficient" in construct validation, because typically several hypotheses are tested. Indeed, the more supporting evidence there is, the greater the confidence one can have about the measure's validity. An instrument does not possess or lack validity; it is a question of degree. An instrument's validity is not proved, established, or demonstrated but rather is supported to a greater or lesser extent by evidence. However, when there are multiple hypotheses, results may be "mixed"—some hypotheses are supported and others are not. This fact means that it is wise for researchers to establish a priori standards for how much confirmatory evidence is considered sufficient.

Structural Validity

Another aspect of construct validity is called structural validity. **Structural validity** refers to the extent to which the structure of a multi-item scale adequately reflects the hypothesized dimensionality of the construct being measured. Structural validity concerns which dimensions of a broader construct are captured by the instrument and whether the dimensions are consistent with theory. For example, we might conceptualize pain as having two dimensions: pain severity and pain interference. After developing a scale based on this conceptualization, we would want to test whether we were successful in capturing and distinguishing the two dimensions. Content validity work ideally paves the way for a good conceptualization of a construct's multiple dimensions.

Assessments of structural validity rely on a statistical procedure called factor analysis, which is computationally complex, but it is conceptually fairly simple. **Factor analysis** is a method for identifying clusters of related items—that is, dimensions underlying a broad construct. Each dimension, or **factor**, represents a relatively unitary attribute. The procedure is used to identify and group together different items measuring an underlying attribute. In effect, factor analysis constitutes another means of testing hypotheses about the interrelationships among variables and of formulating evidence of convergence and divergence at the item level.

As we discuss in the next chapter, there are two broad classes of factor analysis—exploratory and confirmatory. *Exploratory factor analysis* is an important tool in the development of multi-item scales. *Confirmatory factor analysis*, however, is the preferred method for testing structural validity hypotheses about the dimensionality of a scale.

It is important to note that information about a measure's structural validity does not constitute sufficient evidence of a measure's construct validity. Factor analysis can confirm a hypothesis that a complex construct has, for example, three underlying dimensions, but such an analysis does not in and of itself address the central construct validity question: Does this instrument really measure the construct it purports to measure?

Example of Structural Validation Using Factor Analysis

Breazeale and colleagues (2022) conducted an exploratory and confirmatory factor analysis to identify the factor structure underlying the somatic symptoms, sleep characteristics, and mood in a sample of 195 adult participants who had chronic heart failure and insomnia. They found that poor sleep was negatively associated with self-care maintenance, but not self-care confidence, whereas mood and somatic symptoms were negatively associated with self-care confidence.

TIP Structural validity is only relevant for multi-item reflective scales and not formative indexes. Factor analysis relies on items with strong intercorrelations.

Cross-Cultural Validity

A third type of construct validity is cross-cultural validity, which is relevant for measures that have been translated or adapted for use with a different cultural group than that for the original instrument. We define **cross-cultural validity** as the degree to which the components (e.g., items) of a translated or culturally adapted measure perform adequately and equivalently, individually and collectively, relative to their performance on the original instrument.

Developing a high-quality and cross-culturally valid instrument requires even more time and effort than starting from scratch with a new instrument. Yet, without such efforts, it would be impossible to understand health outcomes globally. If, for example, we want to learn whether health-related quality of life differs across countries, comparisons cannot be made with disparate instruments. Several coordinated multinational efforts have been undertaken to adapt widely used English-language health scales, such as the Mini-Mental State Examination and a quality-of-life scale called the SF-36. Also, many item banks of health outcomes have been translated for use in CAT as part of the PROMIS® initiative.

The methods used in cross-cultural validation are complex and multifaceted, and many of them require high levels of statistical sophistication. More detailed information is offered in Polit and Yang (2016).

RELIABILITY OF CHANGE SCORES

Two domains in our measurement taxonomy relate to measurements over time. Both of these domains concern change scores, so we briefly discuss the issue of measuring change.

Measuring Change

How does one measure whether a change in a construct has occurred? For some attributes, there is only one option: measuring it on two occasions and comparing the values—in other words, subtracting one value from the other to calculate a **change score** that represents the amount of change between two scores. If we want to learn, for example, whether a patient's blood pressure has decreased, we need to know what it was initially and what it is now and calculate the difference. For PROs, there are two other alternatives: asking patients directly whether a change has occurred and asking them to report retrospectively what their status was previously and then comparing it to their current status. Unfortunately, all three methods have potential problems.

In clinical trials, statisticians have argued against using change scores as the dependent variables in the analysis of treatment effects. When patients are randomized to groups, it is recommended that scores at the posttest be used as the outcome variables, rather than change scores. A major emphasis in randomized trials is on *difference scores* (the average difference between the randomized groups at posttest), rather than on *change scores*.

Yet, it is of inherent substantive interest to understand how much patients in all arms of a trial have changed. Some nonexperimental studies seek to describe outcomes over the course of an illness, which requires a direct examination of how scores have evolved. And, at the level of an individual patient, assessments of improvement, deterioration, or stability over time as measured by change scores may be the focus of clinical assessment and decision-making.

Change scores can be affected by several factors that can threaten their accuracy and validity. A major concern with change scores is the inevitability of measurement error. Change scores—the difference between an imperfectly reliable score at time 1 and another imperfectly reliable score at time 2—potentially can magnify a small change or mask a large one. The greater the degree of unreliability, the greater the risk that a change score will be misleading.

The reliability of change domain focuses on this issue: how do we know when a change score is "real" and not merely a random fluctuation? Except for measures created within an item response theory framework, reliable change has most often been assessed by computing one of two indexes: the smallest detectable change (SDC) or the reliable change index (RCI).

The Smallest Detectable Change

The usual approach to assessing the reliability of group-level change is to test the statistical significance of a group's change in scores from one point in time to another, using tests we describe in Chapter 18. From a measurement perspective, however, statistical significance may not be an informative way to understand change—and significance tells us nothing about whether a change was reliable for individuals.

Reliable change for continuous data often is estimated using an index called the **smallest detectable change (SDC)** or the *minimal detectable change (MDC)*.[4] An SDC can be defined as a change in scores that is beyond measurement error—a change of sufficient magnitude that the probability is low that it resulted from random error.

Operationally, the SDC is a change score that falls outside the LOA on a Bland–Altman plot. As noted earlier, the LOA can be estimated using test–retest data from a stable population. The LOA are an estimate of the probable range of score differences between a test and a retest, for a stable population over a specified interval. If a change score falls outside the LOA, there can be greater confidence that the change is reliable. High measurement error makes it more difficult to detect true change—underscoring the importance of using measures with high reliability.

Earlier we noted that the LOA for the self-esteem scores in Table 15.1 was about 7.0 (actually, 7.1). Suppose that we evaluated an intervention designed to improve the self-esteem and mental health of adolescents. The scores in Table 15.1 are from a test–retest administration of the scale but suppose that the time 2 scores were baseline values for a test of the intervention. Three months after the intervention, we would readminister the self-esteem scale (time 3). Based on the LOA, any improvement in self-esteem scores of 7 points or greater in a participant's score would be considered indicative of real (reliable) improvement in self-esteem.

> **Example of the Smallest Detectable Change**
> In a cross-sectional study, Bakhshandeh et al. (2022) aimed to develop and validate the Geriatrics Health Behavior Questionnaire (GHBQ) to assess the health behaviors of older adults. One of the measures to test the reliability of the tool was the minimal detectable change, which was 1.98 and indicated there was not a measurement error and that the GHBQ was reliable.

The Reliable Change Index

The SDC is similar to another index that is widely used in the field of psychotherapy. The **reliable change index (RCI)** was proposed by Jacobson and colleagues (1984), Jacobson and Truax (1991) as an element of a two-part process for assessing the clinical significance of patients' improvement as a result of psychotherapy. Jacobson argued that, to be clinically meaningful, a change score on psychotherapy outcomes must pass the test of being "real"—that is, a change beyond measurement error.

The RCI is calculated by using a formula that includes the amount of measurement error for the scale, as estimated by the SEM.[5] The cutoff values for reliable change are similar (but not identical) for the RCI and the SDC. In our example of the self-esteem scores in Table 15.1, the SDC is 7.10 and the RCI is 7.33.

---

[4] The term "minimal detectable change" is often used in the medical literature. We use "smallest detectable change" to be consistent with COSMIN. The SDC has also been called the "smallest detectable *difference*" or "minimal detectable *difference*," but, like the COSMIN group, we prefer "smallest detectable *change*" to emphasize the focus on *change* scores.

[5] For 95% confidence, the formula for the RCI is 1.96 times $\sqrt{2 \times SEM^2}$.

> **Example of the Reliable Change Index**
> Glendon and colleagues (2021) sought to establish the point at which the recovery of symptom burden occurred in college students who played rugby and had experienced concussions. The Reliable Change Index was used to compare to their individual baseline. They found that symptom burden was improved at 4 days and players returned to baseline at 8 days.

RESPONSIVENESS

The final domain in our measurement taxonomy also concerns measurements over time. We define the measurement property of **responsiveness** as the ability of a measure to detect change over time in a construct that has changed, commensurate with the amount of change that has occurred. Just as reliability can be extended to apply to change scores, responsiveness represents the extension of validity over time. Validity concerns whether a measure is truly capturing the intended construct, and responsiveness concerns whether a change score is truly capturing a real change in the construct.

> **TIP** Before COSMIN, there was no consensus about what responsiveness is or how to know when it has been achieved. Terwee and colleagues (2003), in a systematic review of the quality-of-life literature, found 25 definitions of responsiveness. The COSMIN group brought together health measurement experts who reached agreement in defining responsiveness as the validity of change scores.

Validity and responsiveness share many features, the main difference being the timeframe. The methods used to assess responsiveness overlap with methods used to assess validity. Validity and responsiveness are also both challenging to assess. Assessments require researchers to be creative in developing useful hypotheses. Furthermore, both responsiveness and validity rely on ongoing evidence building. The more evidence that can be brought to bear on a measure's responsiveness, the greater the confidence one has in the measure's capacity to capture true change in a construct. This evidence-building feature of both cross-sectional and longitudinal validity (responsiveness) means that there is no single number to quantify its value.

Psychometricians have not traditionally considered responsiveness as a measurement property. We agree with the COSMIN group, however, that responsiveness merits consideration. Change is critically important to healthcare professionals who hope to achieve improvements with clients.

Two broad approaches have been used in assessing responsiveness, similar to approaches used in validity testing: a criterion approach and a construct approach.

The Criterion Approach to Responsiveness

Like criterion validation, the criterion approach to responsiveness requires a gold standard—a well-established and reliable criterion that indicates that a change in the target construct has occurred. This approach to responsiveness assessment has also been called an **anchor-based approach**, with the criterion serving as the anchor.

A criterion-based assessment of responsiveness sometimes involves an examination of the relationship between changes on the target measure and changes on the criterion, which corresponds directly to a longitudinal assessment of criterion validity.

Another strategy for testing criterion-based responsiveness involves the use of a single-item **global rating scale** or **GRS** (also known as a **health transition rating**) as the criterion (DeVet et al., 2011). A GRS involves asking patients to rate directly the degree to which their status on the focal construct has changed over a time interval in which change is presumed to have occurred. Figure 15.3 provides an example of a 7-point GRS, which asks patients to rate changes in their ability to perform activities of daily living (ADLs). Such a GRS would be relevant for assessing the responsiveness of a physical function or ADL scale—for example, for measuring improvements in patients' physical function 3 months after a health promotion intervention.

Let us suppose we were assessing the responsiveness of a physical function scale, such as the Barthel Index (BI). We might administer the BI just prior to the intervention and then 3 months later. At the 3-month point, patients would also be asked to complete the GRS shown in Figure 15.3. Several statistical approaches could be used to test the BI's responsiveness. For example, the average BI change scores could be statistically compared for patients who said they had any improvement on the GRS (response options 1, 2, or 3) and patients who did not report improvements (options 4-7). Alternatively, change scores on the BI could be plotted on an ROC curve against the sensitivity and specificity for predicting the GRS criterion: improved vs. did not improve. The AUC would provide the estimate of responsiveness.

The Construct Approach to Responsiveness

The construct approach to evaluating a measure's responsiveness is analogous to a hypothesis-testing construct validation. Researchers develop and test hypotheses about changes on the focal measure in relation to other phenomena. Sometimes, the hypotheses concern an expected change on the construct resulting from a treatment of well-established efficacy (e.g., changes in quality of life after hip replacement). Alternatively, the hypotheses may concern the nature and magnitude of relationship between changes on the focal measure on the one hand and changes on measures of constructs that are theoretically linked to the focal construct on the other.

When hypotheses are developed about how changes in a focal measure are related to changes in other measures, a full array of strategies and analytic methods can be used, analogous to those described for hypothesis-testing construct validity. For example, some hypotheses are designed to support what might be called *convergent responsiveness*—the degree to which change scores on the focal measure are correlated with change scores on a measure of a construct with which a relationship is hypothesized. Similarly, it would be possible to hypothesize that changes on the focal construct, as captured in change scores on the focal measure, are *not* associated (or only weakly associated) with changes on another, unrelated measure (*divergent responsiveness*). Another option is *known-groups responsiveness*, the longitudinal extension of known-groups validity. In this approach, researchers test the hypothesis that changes on the focal measure are different for groups known (or hypothesized) to have different amounts of change.

Conceptually, construct-focused responsiveness assessment is an extension of construct validation, but procedurally there has been greater complexity in evaluating responsiveness. Polit and Yang (2016) provide more details about so-called responsiveness indexes and about **distribution-based approaches** to assessing responsiveness, which were given this label because they are based on change score distributions.

> **Example of Responsiveness Assessment**
> Guzelsoy et al. (2022) aimed to determine the similarity of three questionnaires that assessed lower urinary tract symptoms and to determine the relationship between education level and the responsiveness of the forms in terms of completion. With a sample of 224 patients in Turkey, the researchers found that the three tools were significantly correlated ($p = < 0.05$), education level did not impact the responsiveness rate, and overall, the incomplete response rate was 32.1%.

> Please rate the changes you have experienced in the past three months with regard to *your ability to perform regular activities of daily living*, such as standing up from a sitting position or taking a bath or shower:
>
> 1. Very much better
> 2. Much better
> 3. A little better
> 4. No change
> 5. A little worse
> 6. Much worse
> 7. Very much worse
>
> Shaded response options show one possible cut point on the criterion: Responses 1–3 (any improvement) versus 4–7 (no improvement)

FIGURE 15.3 Example of a global rating scale for a criterion-related assessment of responsiveness for an activities of daily living (ADL) scale.

TIP When you select an instrument to use in a study, you should seek evidence of its psychometric soundness by examining the instrument developers' report. The report ideally would provide evidence regarding all the measurement properties discussed in this chapter—but information about reliability of change scores and responsiveness may be absent. You should also consider evidence about the quality of the measure from others who have used it. Each time the scale "performs" as hypothesized, this constitutes supplementary evidence for its validity and possibly its responsiveness.

CRITICAL APPRAISAL OF DATA QUALITY IN QUANTITATIVE STUDIES

If data are seriously flawed, a study cannot contribute useful evidence. Therefore, in drawing conclusions about a study's evidence, you should consider whether researchers have taken appropriate steps to ensure high-quality measurements of key constructs. Research consumers need to ask: Can I trust the data in this study? Are the measurements of key constructs reliable and valid, and are change scores reliable and responsive?

Information about data quality should be provided in every quantitative research report. Reliability estimates are usually reported because they are easy to communicate. Ideally, for composite scales, the report should provide internal consistency reliability coefficients based on data from the study itself, not just from previous research. Interrater or interobserver reliability is especially crucial for coming to conclusions about data quality in observational studies. The values of the reliability coefficients should be sufficiently high to support confidence in the findings. In studies with nonsignificant findings, pay special attention to reliability information because the unreliability of measures can undermine statistical conclusion validity.

Validity is more difficult to document in a report than reliability. At a minimum, researchers should defend their choice of existing measures based on validity information from the developers, and they should cite the relevant publication. If a study involves the use of a screening or diagnostic measure, information should also be provided about its sensitivity and specificity.

Box 15.1 provides some guidelines for critically appraising aspects of the data quality of

---

BOX 15.1 Guidelines for Critically Appraising Measurement and Data Quality in Quantitative Studies

1. Was there congruence between the research variables as conceptualized (i.e., as discussed in the introduction of the report) and as operationalized (i.e., as described in the method section)?
2. If operational definitions (or scoring procedures) were specified, did they clearly indicate the rules of measurement? Do the rules seem sensible? Were data collected in such a way that measurement errors were minimized (e.g., training of data collectors)?
3. Did the report describe the measurement properties of the instruments used to measure key study constructs? Was the rationale for using the chosen instruments based on data quality issues (e.g., better measurement properties than alternative measures of the same construct)?
4. Did the report offer evidence of the reliability of the measures used in the study? Did the evidence come from the research sample itself, or was it based on other studies? If the latter, is it reasonable to conclude that data quality would be similar for the research sample as for the reliability sample (e.g., are sample characteristics similar)?
5. If reliability was reported, which estimation method was used? Was this method appropriate? Should an alternative or additional method of reliability appraisal have been used? Was the appropriate reliability coefficient computed (e.g., an ICC for test–retest reliability)? Is the reliability sufficiently high? Was measurement error reported?
6. Did the report offer evidence of the validity of the measures? Assuming validity evidence came from other studies, is it reasonable to believe that data quality would be similar for the research sample as for the validity sample (e.g., are the sample characteristics similar)?
7. If validity information was reported, which validity approach was used? Was this method appropriate? Does the validity of the instruments appear to be adequate?
8. If the study involved computing change scores, was information provided about the reliability of change scores? Was evidence about the responsiveness of change scores provided?
9. If there was information about the measurement properties of key instruments used in the study, what conclusion can you reach about the quality of the data in the study?
10. Were the research hypotheses supported? If not, might data quality have played a role in the failure to confirm the hypotheses?

quantitative measures. Francis and colleagues (2016) have also developed a checklist for evaluating PRO measures.

RESEARCH EXAMPLE

In this section, we describe a study that used a wide variety of measures to enhance data quality.

Study: Effects of a nurse-led eHealth cardiac rehabilitation program on health outcomes of patients with coronary heart disease: A randomized controlled trial (Su & Yu, 2021).

Aim: The aim of this study was to evaluate in people with coronary heart disease, the effect of a nurse-led electronically delivered video cardiac rehabilitation. Specific outcomes included health behaviors, cardiac self-efficacy, anxiety and depression, health-related quality of life, risk parameters, and unplanned use of care services for people with coronary heart disease.

Design: In this single-blinded randomized control design, 146 participants were assigned to either the electronically delivered video intervention or usual care, which did not include any follow-up care, but did include a 10-minute education session delivered by nurses on medication usage and lifestyle changes (e.g., physical activity, diet, and smoking cessation). The cardiac rehabilitation was a 6-week program that was initiated while the patient was hospitalized. During the initial session, the nurse met with patients to set their personal goals for self-care and cardiac risk factor modification, as well as to orient the patient to online platform. The video intervention was delivered electronically in small groups of 5–8 patients and ongoing support was provided by the nurses via the WeChat platform in groups of 12–16.

Instruments: Measures related to outcomes were taken at baseline, 6 and 12 weeks. The primary outcome focused on lifestyle changes, specifically physical activity as measured by a pedometer and health-promoting lifestyle habits and smoking cessation. The Health-Promoting Lifestyle Profile II is a 27-question measure capturing self-reported activity with acceptable test–retest reliability and intraclass correlation coefficients of 0.74 to 0.97. The translated Chinese version has a Cronbach's α coefficient of 0.63–0.81. Secondary outcomes included the following: (1) Cardiac Self-Efficacy Scale, a 5-point Likert scale that measured self-efficacy. The Chinese version of the scale had good internal consistency, with a Cronbach's alpha of 0.926; (2) the MacNew Heart Disease Health-related Quality of Life questionnaire, a 27-item measure to determine the impact of heart disease on a person's physical, emotional, and social well-being. The Chinese version of the MacNew questionnaire had intraclass correlation coefficients ranging from 0.88 to 0.93; 3) the translated Chinese version of the Depression Anxiety Stress Scale 21, which had good reliability and a Cronbach's alpha of ≥0.80). Other secondary outcomes were blood pressure, body mass index, waist circumference, and unplanned use of health services as captured by patient self-report.

Results: The primary outcomes at 6 weeks indicated the patients in the intervention group did demonstrate significant improvements in the number of steps per day, the number of minutes per week sitting, and their health-promoting lifestyle profile as compared to the control group. These changes were sustained at the 12-week endpoint. Secondary outcomes at 12 weeks showed no significant improvement in blood pressure, body mass index, and waist circumference, but there were improvements in self-efficacy and health-related quality of life as compared to the control group. The researchers suggest that consistent with other work, the changes in blood pressure, waist measurement, and body mass index may take a longer period of time for improvement. However, the video intervention did result in modification of behavioral risk factors and the improvement of health-related quality of life.

SUMMARY POINTS

- **Measurement** involves assigning numbers to objects to represent the amount of an attribute, according to rules. When researchers invent rules to capture a construct, they create a **measure** of the construct.
- **Psychometrics** is the branch of psychology concerned with the theory and methods of psychological measurement, and psychometrics have influenced health measurement. **Classical test theory (CTT)** is one major psychometric theory of measurement and **item response theory (ITT)** is another.

- Within CTT, **obtained scores** from a measure are conceptualized as having a **true score** component (the value that would be obtained for a hypothetical perfect measure of the attribute) and an error component, or **error of measurement**, that represents measurement inaccuracies. Sources of measurement error include situational contaminants, response set biases, and transient personal factors, such as fatigue.
- Measures can vary in several ways, including whether they are *generic* (broadly applicable) or *specific* to certain types of people, such as disease-specific measures. Measures can be **static** (the same instrument for everyone) or **adaptive**, with different questions from an *item bank* being administered to different people, usually using **computerized adaptive testing.**
- For multi-item measures, another distinction is important. In **reflective scales**, the items are viewed as being *caused by* the construct—responses are reflections of the underlying attribute. In a **formative index**, the items are viewed as defining the construct.
- A panel of health measurement experts defined key **measurement properties** in the **COSMIN** initiative. The taxonomy presented in this book modified the COSMIN taxonomy to include two cross-sectional measurement properties (reliability and validity) and two longitudinal measurement properties (reliability of change scores and responsiveness).
- Many measurement properties can be assessed by computing a statistic that estimates a **measurement parameter.** Several parameter estimates involve computing a **correlation coefficient** that indicates the magnitude and direction of a relationship between two variables. Correlation coefficients can range from −1.00 (a **perfect negative relationship**) through 0.00 to +1.00 (a **perfect positive relationship**).
- **Reliability** is the extent to which scores for people *who have not changed* are the same for repeated measurements, under several situations, including repetition on different occasions (test–retest and intrarater reliability), by different people (interrater reliability), on different versions of a measure (parallel test reliability), or with different items on a multi-item instrument (internal consistency).
- Assessments of **test–retest reliability** involve administering a measure twice to assess the stability of scores. When scores are continuous, the preferred index of test–retest reliability is the **intraclass correlation coefficient (ICC).** Reliability coefficients such as the ICC range from 0.00 to 1.00, with higher values reflecting greater reliability.
- **Interrater reliability** involves assessing the congruence of ratings or classifications of two or more independent observers. When observers make classifications, interrater agreement is usually assessed using the **kappa** statistic, which is an index of chance-adjusted **proportion of agreement.**
- **Internal consistency**, a component in the reliability domain, concerns the extent to which all the instrument's items are measuring the same attribute; it is usually assessed by **Cronbach alpha**. Internal consistency is not relevant for formative indexes.
- A third component in the reliability domain is measurement error, for which there are two indexes that indicate the precision of a score. The **standard error of measurement (SEM)**, which quantifies "typical error" on a measure, is in the units of measurement of the measure itself. Another index is called the **limits of agreement (LOA)** on a *Bland–Altman plot*. The LOA can be used to identify how much differences in scores in a retest study are reasonable if the attribute has in fact not changed.
- **Validity**, a second domain the measurement taxonomy, is the degree to which an instrument measures what it purports to measure. Validity has multiple components.
- **Face validity** refers to whether the instrument appears, on the face of it, to be measuring the appropriate construct.
- **Content validity** is the extent to which an instrument's content (its items) adequately captures the construct being measured. Expert ratings on the relevance of items can be used to compute **content validity index (CVI)** information. An **item CVI (I-CVI)** represents the proportion of

experts rating an item as relevant. A **scale CVI (S-CVI)** using the averaging method is the average of all I-CVI values for the set of items on the scale.
- **Criterion-related validity** (which includes both **predictive validity** and **concurrent validity**) is the extent to which scores on an instrument are an adequate reflection of a "gold standard" criterion. When both the focal measure and the criterion are continuous measures, correlation coefficients are used to estimate criterion validity.
- When both the focal measure and the criterion are dichotomous, criterion-related validity is assessed with indexes of **diagnostic accuracy**, namely sensitivity and specificity. **Sensitivity** is the instrument's ability to identify a case correctly (i.e., its rate of yielding true positives). **Specificity** is the instrument's ability to identify noncases correctly (i.e., its rate of yielding true negatives).
- Sensitivity is sometimes plotted against specificity in a **receiver operating characteristic curve (ROC curve)** to determine the optimum **cutoff point** for caseness with continuous measures. An ROC yields an index called the **area under the curve (AUC)** that can be used as an index of criterion validity.
- **Construct validity,** a third component in the validity domain, concerns what abstract construct an instrument is actually measuring. One aspect is **hypothesis-testing construct validity**: the extent to which hypotheses about what the instrument is measuring can be supported. Key approaches include **convergent validity**, the degree to which there is conceptual convergence between scores on the focal measure and another measure; **known-groups validity**, the extent to which hypotheses about groups expected to differ on a measure are supported; and **divergent validity**, the extent to which hypotheses about what an instrument does *not* measure are supported.
- Another aspect of construct validity is **structural validity**, which concerns the extent to which evidence supports hypotheses about the dimensionality of a complex construct. A statistical tool called **factor analysis** is used to assess structural validity.
- **Cross-cultural validity,** another aspect of construct validity, concerns the degree to which the items on a translated or culturally adapted scale perform adequately and equivalently in relation to their performance on the original instrument.
- Change is often measured by computing a **change score** that is the difference in value between two measurements. A major issue with change scores is that they tend to amplify measurement error, and hence a third domain in the taxonomy concerns the **reliability of a change score.**
- Two indexes summarize whether a change in a person's score over time is reliable or merely reflects random fluctuations. One is the **smallest detectable change (SDC)**, which is a value that is outside the LOA. The **reliable change index (RCI)** is a similar index that is based on a formula using the SEM.
- The final domain in the measurement taxonomy is **responsiveness**, which refers to the ability of a measure to detect change over time in a construct that has changed. Responsiveness, the longitudinal analog of validity, can be assessed by testing hypotheses about how changes in the focal measure are consistent with changes in other measures.
- Assessments of responsiveness, like validity, can involve a criterion approach or a construct approach. Some researchers used **health transition ratings** (also called **global rating scales**) as the criterion for change.

REFERENCES CITED IN CHAPTER 15

Bakhshandeh Bavarsad, M., Foroughan, M., Zanjari, N., Ghaedamini Harouni, G., & Jorjoran Shushtari, Z. (2022). Development and validation of the Geriatrics Health Behavior Questionnaire (GHBQ). *BMC Public Health*, *22*(1), 526. https://doi.org/10.1186/s12889-022-12927-1

Barreiro, R. G., & de Oliveira Lopes, M. V. (2023). Content validity of the nursing diagnosis low self-efficacy in health. *International Journal of Nursing Knowledge*, *34*(3), 216–225. https://doi.org/10.1111/2047-3095.12395

Bland, J. M., & Altman, D. G. (1986). Statistical methods for assessing agreement between two methods of clinical measurement. *Lancet*, *1*(8476), 307–310.

Brazier, J., Peasgood, T., Mukuria, C., Marten, O., Kreimeier, S., Luo, N., Mulhern, B., Pickard, A. S., Augustovski, F., Greiner, W., Engel, L., Belizan, M., Yang, Z., Monteiro, A., Kuharic, M., Gibbons, L., Ludwig, K., Carlton, J., Connell, J., ... Rejon-Parrilla, J. C. (2022). The EQ-HWB: Overview of the development of a measure of health and wellbeing and key results. *Value Health*, *25*(4), 482–491. https://doi.org/10.1016/j.jval.2022.01.009

Breazeale, S., Jeon, S., Hwang, Y., O'Connell, M., Nwanaji-Enwerem, U., Linsky, S., Yaggi, H. K., Jacoby, D. L., Conley, S., & Redeker, N. S. (2022). Sleep characteristics, mood, somatic symptoms, and self-care among people with heart failure and insomnia. *Nursing Research*, *71*(3), 189–199. https://doi.org/10.1097/NNR.0000000000000585

Cabanas-Valdés, R., García-Rueda, L., Salgueiro, C., Pérez-Bellmunt, A., Rodríguez-Sanz, J., & López-de-Celis, C. (2023). Assessment of the 4-meter walk test test-retest reliability and concurrent validity and its correlation with the five sit-to-stand test in chronic ambulatory stroke survivors. *Gait & Posture*, *101*, 8–13. https://doi.org/10.1016/j.gaitpost.2023.01.014

Campbell, D. T., & Fiske, D. W. (1959). Convergent and discriminant validation by the multitrait-multimethod matrix. *Psychological Bulletin*, *56*(2), 81–105.

Cella, D., Gershon, R., Lai, J., & Choi, S. (2007). The future of outcomes measurement: Item banking, tailored short-forms, and computerized adaptive assessment. *Quality of Life Research*, *16*(Suppl. 1), 133–141.

Clover, K., Lambert, S. D., Oldmeadow, C., Britton, B., Mitchell, A. J., Carter, G., & King, M. T. (2022). Convergent and criterion validity of PROMIS anxiety measures relative to six legacy measures and a structured diagnostic interview for anxiety in cancer patients. *Journal of Patient-Reported Outcomes*, *6*(1), 80. https://doi.org/10.1186/s41687-022-00477-4

De Oliveira Tavares, V. D., Galvão-Coelho, N. L., Firth, J., Rosenbaum, S., Stubbs, B., Smith, L., Vancampfort, D., & Schuch, F. B. (2021). Reliability and convergent validity of self-reported physical activity questionnaires for people with mental disorders: A systematic review and meta-analysis. *Journal of Physical Activity and Health*, *18*(1), 109–115. https://doi.org/10.1123/jpah.2020-0312

DeVellis, R. F., & Thorpe, C. T. (2022). *Scale development: Theory and application* (5th ed.). Sage Publications.

DeVet, H. C. W., Terwee, C., Mokkink, L. B., & Knol, D L. (2011). *Measurement in medicine: A practical guide*. Cambridge University Press.

Do, H. T. T., Edwards, H., & Finlayson, K. (2023). Surgical wound assessment tool: Construct validity and inter-rater reliability of a tool designed for nurses. *Journal of Clinical Nursing*, *32*(1–2), 83–95. https://doi.org/10.1111/jocn.16476

Flanagan, J., Boltz, M., & Ji, M. (2021). A predictive model of intrinsic factors associated with long-stay nursing home care after hospitalization. *Clinical Nursing Research*, *30*(5), 654–661. https://doi.org/10.1177/1054773820985276

Folstein, M., Folstein, S., White, T., & Messer, M. (2010). *MMSE-2: User's manual*. PAR.

Francis, D. O., McPheeters, M., Noud, M., Penson, D., & Feurer, I. (2016). Checklist to operationalize measurement characteristics of patient-reported outcome measures. *Systematic Review*, *5*(1), 129.

Glendon, K., Blenkinsop, G., Belli, A., & Pain, M. (2021). Prospective study with specific re-assessment time points to determine time to recovery following a sports-related concussion in university-aged student-athletes. *Physical Therapy in Sport*, *52*, 287–296. https://doi.org/10.1016/j.ptsp.2021.10.008

Guzelsoy, M., Erkan, A., Ozturk, M., Zengin, S., Coban, S., Turkoglu, A. R., Koc, A. (2022). Comparison of three questionnaire forms used in the diagnosis of lower urinary tract symptoms: A prospective study. *Prostate International*, *10*(4), 218–223. https://doi.org/10.1016/j.prnil.2022.06.001

Hodiamont, F., Hock, H., Ellis-Smith, C., Hock, H., Evans, C., Jünger, S., Diehl-Schmid, J., Burner-Fritsch, I., Bausewein, C., Burner-Fritsch, I., & Bausewein, C. (2021). Culture in the spotlight-cultural adaptation and content validity of the integrated palliative care outcome scale for dementia: A cognitive interview study. *Palliative Medicine*, *35*(5), 962–971. https://doi.org/10.1177/02692163211004403

Holmes, T. H., & Rahe, R. (1967). The social readjustment rating scale. *Journal of Psychosomatic Research*, *11*(2), 213–218.

Jacobson, N. S., Follette, W. C., & Revenstorf, D. (1984). Psychotherapy outcome research: Methods for reporting variability and evaluating clinical significance. *Behavior Therapy*, *15*, 336–352.

Jacobson, N. S., & Truax, P. (1991). Clinical significance: A statistical approach to defining meaningful change in psychotherapy research. *Journal of Consulting and Clinical Psychology*, *59*(1), 12–19.

Li, P. S., Hsieh, C. J., Tallutondok, E. B., Shih, Y. L., & Liu, C. Y. (2022). Development and assessment of the validity and reliability of the Short-Form Life Satisfaction Index (LSI-SF) among the elderly population. *Journal of Personalized Medicine*, *12*(5), 709. https://doi.org/10.3390/jpm12050709

Mazzotta, R., De Maria, M., Bove, D., Badolamenti, S., Saraiva Bordignon, S., Silveira, L. C. J., Vellone, E., Alvaro, R., & Bulfone, G. (2022). Moral distress in nursing students: Cultural adaptation and validation study. *Nursing Ethics*, *29*(2), 384–401. https://doi.org/10.1177/09697330211030671

Mokkink, L. B., Terwee, C., Patrick, D., Alonso, J., Stratford, P., Knol, D. L., Bouter, L. M., & de Vet, H. C. W. (2010a). The COSMIN study reached international consensus on taxonomy, terminology, and definitions of measurement properties for health-related patient-reported outcomes. *Journal of Clinical Epidemiology*, *63*(7), 737–745.

Mokkink, L. B., Terwee, C., Patrick, D., Alonso, J., Stratford, P., Knol, D. L., Bouter, L. M., & de Vet, H. C. W. (2010b). The COSMIN checklist for assessing the methodological quality of studies on measurement properties of health status measurement instruments: An international Delphi study. *Quality Life Research*, *19*(4), 539–549.

Nakić Radoš, S., Matijaš, M., Brekalo, M., Hollins Martin, C. J., & Martin, C. R. (2022). Further validation of the birth satisfaction scale-revised: Factor structure, validity, and reliability. *Current Psychology*, *42*, 1–10. https://doi.org/10.1007/s12144-021-02688-2

Nunnally, J., & Bernstein, I. H. (1994). *Psychometric theory* (3rd ed.). McGraw-Hill.

Pike, N., Poulsen, M., & Woo, M. (2017). Validity of the Montreal cognitive assessment screener in adolescents and young adults with and without congenital heart disease. *Nursing Research*, *66*(3), 222–230.

Polit, D. F. (2014). Getting serious about test-retest reliability: A critique of retest research and some recommendations. *Quality Life Research*, *23*(6), 1713–1720.

Polit, D. F., & Beck, C. T. (2006). The content validity index: Are you sure you know what is being reported? *Research in Nursing & Healthy*, *29*(5), 489–497.

Polit, D. F., Beck, C. T., & Owen, S. V. (2007). Is the CVI an acceptable indicator of content validity? Appraisal and recommendations. *Research in Nursing & Healthy*, *30*(4), 459–467.

Polit, D. F. & Yang, F. M. (2016). *Measurement and the measurement of change: A primer for health professionals.* Lippincott.

Qian, J., Wu, H., Sun, S., Wang, M., & Yu, X. (2022). Psychometric properties of the Chinese version of the Perinatal Bereavement Care Confidence Scale (C-PBCCS) in nursing practice. *PloS One*, *17*(1), e0262965. https://doi.org/10.1371/journal.pone.0262965

Radloff, L. S. (1977). The CES-D scale: A self-report depression scale for research in the general population. *Applied Psychological Measurement*, *1*, 385–401.

Shadish, W. R., Cook, T. D., & Campbell, D. T. (2002). *Experimental and quasi-experimental designs for generalized causal inference*. Houghton Mifflin Co.

Streiner, D. L. (2003). Being inconsistent about consistency: When coefficient alpha does and doesn't matter. *Journal of Personality Assessment*, *80*(3), 217–222.

Su, J. J., & Yu, D. S. (2021). Effects of a nurse-led eHealth cardiac rehabilitation programme on health outcomes of patients with coronary heart disease: A randomised controlled trial. *International Journal of Nursing Studies*, *122*, 104040. https://doi.org/10.1016/j.ijnurstu.2021.104040

Terwee, C. B., Dekker, F., Wiersinga, W., Prummel, M., & Bossuyt, P. (2003). On assessing responsiveness of health-related quality of life instruments: Guidelines for instrument evaluation. *Quality Life Research*, *12*(4), 349–362.

Terwee, C. B., Mokkink, L. B., Knol, D. L., Ostelo, R., Bouter, L. M., & DeVet, H. C. W. (2012). Rating the methodological quality in systematic reviews of studies on measurement properties: A scoring system for the COSMIN checklist. *Quality Life Research*, *21*(4), 651–657.

16 Developing and Testing Self-Report Scales

Learning Objectives

1. Understand the initial steps around instrument development.
2. Articulate the process for generating an item pool.
3. Distinguish the various types of item responses.
4. Recognize the importance of target audience and expert review of a measure.
5. Explicate the steps necessary for validating an instrument.

INTRODUCTION

Researchers sometimes are unable to find a suitable instrument to operationalize a construct. This may occur when the construct is new but often results from limitations of existing instruments. This chapter provides an overview of the steps involved in developing high-quality self-report scales. The scope of this chapter is fairly narrow. Specifically, we focus on multi-item reflective scales and, primarily, scales rooted in classical test theory (CTT).

TIP The development of high-quality scales is a lengthy, labor-intensive process that requires some statistical sophistication. We urge you to think carefully before embarking on a scale development endeavor and to consider involving a psychometric consultant if you proceed.

BEGINNING STEPS: CONCEPTUALIZATION AND ITEM GENERATION

Conceptualizing the Construct

A sound, insightful conceptualization of the construct to be measured is essential. You will not be able to quantify an attribute adequately if you do not thoroughly understand the **latent trait** (the underlying construct) you wish to capture. For reflective scales, the latent trait is the *cause* of people's responses to questions, which drives their scores on the measure. You cannot develop items to produce the right score if you are unclear about the construct. Thus, the first step in scale development is to become an *expert* on the construct.

Complex constructs have a number of different *dimensions*, and it is important to identify and understand each one. This is partly a content validity consideration: for the scale to be content valid, there must be items representing all facets of the construct. All scales—or subscales of a broader scale—need to be *unidimensional* (measuring a single construct or facet of a construct) and internally consistent.

During the early conceptualization, you also need to think about related constructs that should be differentiated from the target construct. If you are measuring, say, self-esteem, you have to be sure you can differentiate it from similar but distinct constructs, such as self-confidence. In thinking about the dimensions of the target construct, you should be certain that they are truly facets of the construct and not a different construct altogether.

You should also have an explicit conceptualization of the population for whom the scale is intended. For example, a general anxiety scale may not be suitable for measuring childbearing anxiety in pregnant females. There are arguments for developing patient-specific scales, particularly with respect to item relevance and face validity. On the other hand, a highly focused scale reduces the ability to make comparisons across populations. The point is that you should have a clear view of how and with whom the scale will be used. Without a good grasp of the population, it will be difficult to consider such issues as reading levels and cultural appropriateness in wording the items.

Deciding on the Type of Scale

Before items can be generated, you need to decide on the type of scale you wish to create, because item characteristics vary by scale type. Our focus is restricted to multi-item reflective scales, which are also featured in several books on scale development that can be consulted for more detail (DeVellis & Thorpe, 2022; Polit & Yang, 2016; Streiner et al., 2015). Two broad categories of scales fall into this category: traditional summated rating scales and latent trait scales.

Traditional summated rating scales (Chapter 14) are based in CTT. In CTT, items are presumed to be roughly comparable indicators of the underlying construct. The items gain strength in approximating a hypothetical true score through their aggregation. Traditional scales rely on items that are deliberately redundant, in the hope that multiple indicators of the construct will converge on the true score and balance out error.

Item response theory (IRT) is an alternative to CTT that is growing in popularity for scale development. IRT methods are complex and require statistical sophistication. We note a few characteristics of IRT here.

In CTT, traits are modeled at the level of the observed scale score, whereas in IRT, the models are at the level of observed item responses. The goal of IRT is to allow researchers to gain understanding of the characteristics of items independent of the people who complete them. *Latent trait scales* based on IRT models can use items like the ones used in CTT, such as items in a Likert-type format. In fact, a person completing a scale would likely not know whether it had been developed within the CTT or IRT framework. But a person *developing* a scale must decide which measurement theory is being used. Items on a CTT scale are designed to be similar to each other to tap the underlying construct in a comparable manner, but items on a latent trait IRT scale tap different levels of the attribute being measured.

As an example, suppose we were developing a scale to measure risk-taking behavior in adolescents. In a CTT scale, the items might include statements about risk-taking of similar intensity, to which respondents would respond with graded responses corresponding to frequency or strength of endorsement. The aggregate of responses would array respondents along a continuum indicating the propensity to take risks. In an IRT scale, the items themselves would be chosen to reflect different levels of risk-taking (e.g., not eating vegetables, smoking cigarettes, having unprotected sex, texting while driving). Each item could be described as having a different *difficulty*. It is "easier" to agree with or admit to lower-risk items than higher-risk items. Measurements based on an IRT model result in information about the *location* of both items and people on a trait continuum. If a pool of unidimensional items can readily be ordered into a hierarchy of difficulty, then a good IRT model fit is plausible.

Generating an Item Pool: Getting Started

An early step in scale construction is to develop a pool of possible items. Items—which collectively constitute the operational definition of the construct—need to be carefully crafted to reflect the latent variable they are designed to measure. This is often easier to do as a team because different people articulate an idea in diverse ways. Here are some possible sources for generating an **item pool**:

1. *Existing instruments.* Sometimes it is possible to adapt an existing scale rather than starting from scratch. Adaptations may involve adding,

deleting, or rewording items—for example, to simplify wording for a population with low reading skills. Permission from the author of the original scale should be sought because published scales are copyright-protected.
2. *The literature.* Ideas for item content often come from a thorough understanding of prior research.
3. *Concept analysis.* A related source of ideas is a concept analysis. Walker and Avant (2019) offer concept analysis strategies that could be used to develop items for a scale.
4. *In-depth qualitative research.* In-depth inquiry relating to the key construct is a rich source of items. A qualitative study can help you to understand the dimensions of a phenomenon and can give you actual phrases for items. If you are unable to undertake an in-depth study, pay attention to the verbatim quotes in published qualitative reports about your construct.
5. *Clinical observations.* Patients in clinical settings may be an excellent source of items. Ideas for items may come from direct observation of patients' behaviors in relevant situations or from listening to their comments.

Example of Sources of Items
Davis and colleagues (2021) developed a tool to measure women-centered care in midwives. The items were developed based on a review of the literature, expert external review, survey and psychometric testing.

DeVellis and Thorpe (2022) urged scale developers to start writing scale items without a lot of critical review in the early stages. Perhaps a good way to begin if you are struggling is to develop a simple statement with the key construct mentioned in it. For example, if the construct is test anxiety, you might start with, "I get anxious when I take a test." This could be followed by similar statements worded differently (e.g., "Taking tests makes me nervous").

Making Decisions About Item Features

In preparing to write items, you need to make decisions about such issues as the number of items to develop, the form of the response options, whether to include positively and negatively worded items, and how to deal with time.

Number of Items

In the CTT framework, a **domain sampling model** is assumed, which involves the random sampling of a homogeneous set of items from a hypothetical universe of items on the construct. Of course, sampling from a *universe* of all possible items does not happen in reality. The idea is to generate a fairly exhaustive set of item possibilities, given the construct's theoretical demands. For a traditional scale, redundancy (except for trivial word substitutions) is a good thing. The goal is to measure the construct with a set of items that capture its essence in slightly different ways so that irrelevant aspects of individual items cancel each other out.

There is no magic formula for how many items should be developed, but our advice is to generate a large pool of items. As you proceed, many items will be discarded. Longer scales tend to be more internally consistent, so starting with a large number of items promotes the likelihood of developing an internally consistent scale. DeVellis and Thorpe (2022) recommend starting with three to four times as many items as you will have in your final scale (e.g., 30–40 items for a 10-item scale), but the minimum should be 50% more (e.g., 15 items for a 10-item scale).

Response Options

Scale items involve both a *stem* (often a declarative statement) and *response options*. Traditional Likert scales involve response options on a continuum of agreement, but other continua are possible, such as frequency (never/always), importance (very important/unimportant), quality (excellent/very poor), and likelihood (definitely/definitely not).

How many response options should there be? There is no simple answer, but keep in mind the goal is to array people on a continuum, and so variability is essential. Variability can be enhanced by including a lot of items, numerous response options, or both. However, there is no merit in creating the illusion of precision when it does not exist. With 15 response options, for example, the difference between a score of 12 and 13 might not be meaningful. Moreover, too many options can be confusing.

Most scales have items with five to seven options, with verbal descriptors attached to each option and, often, numbers placed under the descriptors to further help respondents find an appropriate place on the continuum. An odd number of items give respondents an opportunity to be neutral or ambivalent (i.e., to choose a midpoint). Some scale developers prefer an even number (e.g., 4 or 6) to force even slight tendencies and to avoid equivocation. However, some respondents may actually *be* neutral or ambivalent, so a midpoint option allows them to express it. The midpoint can be labeled with such phrases as "neither agree nor disagree," "undecided," "agree and disagree equally," or simply "?".

> **TIP** Here are some frequently used words for response options, with midpoint terms not listed:
> - Strongly disagree, disagree, agree, strongly agree.
> - Never, almost never (or rarely), sometimes (or occasionally), often (or frequently), almost always (or always).
> - Very important, important, somewhat important, of little importance, unimportant.
> - Definitely not, probably not, possibly, probably, very probably, definitely.
> - With no trouble, with a little trouble, with some trouble, with a lot of trouble, not able to do.

Positive and Negative Stems

A generation ago, psychometricians advised scale developers to deliberately include both positively and negatively worded statements and to reverse-score negative items. As an example, consider these two items for a scale of depression: "I frequently feel blue," and "I rarely feel sad." The objective was to include items that would minimize the possibility of an acquiescence response set—the tendency to agree with statements regardless of their content.

Many experts currently advise against including negative and positive items on a scale. Some respondents are confused by reversing polarities. Responding to item with negative stems appears to be an especially difficult cognitive task for younger respondents. Some research suggests that acquiescence can be minimized by putting the most positive response options (e.g., strongly agree) at the end of the list rather than at the beginning.

Item Intensity

In a traditional summated rating scale, the intensity of the statements (stems) should be similar and fairly strongly worded. If items are worded such that almost anyone would agree with them, the scale will not be able to discriminate between people with different amounts of the underlying trait. For example, an item such as "Good health is important" would generate almost universal agreement. On the other hand, statements should not be so extremely worded as to result in universal rejection. For a latent trait scale, scale developers seek a range of item intensities. Yet, even on an IRT-based scale, there is no point in including items with which almost everyone would either agree or disagree.

Item Time Frames

Some items make an explicit reference to time (e.g., "In the past week I have had trouble falling asleep"), but others do not (e.g., "I have trouble falling asleep"). Sometimes instructions to a scale can designate a temporal frame of reference (e.g., "In answering the following questions, please indicate how you have felt in the past week"). And yet other scales ask respondents to respond in terms of a time frame: "In the past week, I have had trouble falling asleep: Every day, 5–6 days … Never."

A time frame should not emerge as a consequence of item development. You should decide in advance, based on your conceptual understanding of the construct and the needs for which the scale is being constructed, how to deal with time.

> **Example of Handling Time in a Scale**
> The Physical Activity Scale for the Elderly (PASE) asks respondents to rate their physical activity (PA) over the past 7 days as this time period is considered a good way to understand the average amount of PA over a week rather than possible daily fluctuations. Sia and colleagues (2023) used the PASE to determine average PA over the past 7 days in people with motor neuron disease to understand and describe personal and clinical characteristics that aligned with increased PA. They found that fatigue was the biggest barrier to PA participation in this population.

Wording the Items

In addition to the suggestions on question wording, we provided in Chapter 14, some additional tips specific to scale items are as follows:

1. *Clarity*. Scale developers should strive for clear, unambiguous items. Words should be chosen with the educational and reading level of the target population in mind. In most cases, this means developing a scale at about the seventh-grade reading level. You should use words that everyone understands and strive to have everyone reach the same conclusion about what the words mean.
2. *Length*. Avoid long sentences or phrases and eliminate unnecessary words. For example, "It is fair to say that in the scheme of things I do not get enough sleep," could more simply be worded, "I do not get enough sleep."
3. *Double negatives*. It is preferable to word things affirmatively ("I am usually happy" than negatively ("I am not usually sad"), but double negatives should always be avoided ("I am *not* usually *un*happy").
4. *Double-barreled items*. Avoid putting two or more ideas in a single item. For example, "I am afraid of insects and snakes" is a bad item because a person who is afraid of insects but not snakes (or vice versa) would not know how to respond.

TIP Here are some tips for scale developers who anticipate a translation into another language: (1) avoid metaphors, idioms, and colloquialisms; (2) use specific words rather than ones open to interpretation (e.g., "daily" rather than "frequently"); (3) avoid pronouns—repeat nouns to avoid ambiguity; (4) write in the present tense and avoid the subjunctive mode; and (5) use words with a Latin root if translation into a Romance language is expected (Hilton & Skrutkowski, 2002).

PRELIMINARY EVALUATION OF ITEMS

Internal Review

Once a large item pool has been generated, it is time for critical appraisal. Care should be devoted to such issues as whether individual items capture the construct, are grammatical, and are well worded. The initial review should also consider whether the items taken together adequately embrace the nuances of the construct.

It is imperative to assess the scale's **readability**, unless the scale is intended for a highly educated population. There are different approaches for assessing the reading level of written documents, but many methods require several hundreds of words of text and thus are not suited to evaluating scale items.

Many word processing programs provide some information about readability. In Microsoft Word, for example, you could type your items on a list and then get readability statistics for the items as a whole or for individual items, as described in Chapter 7. For example, take the following two sets of items for measuring fatigue:

Set A	Set B
I am frequently exhausted.	I am often tired.
I invariably get insufficient sleep.	I don't get enough sleep.

The Word software tells us that the items in set A have a *Flesch–Kincaid grade level* of 12.0 and a *Flesch reading ease score* of 4.8. (Reading ease scores rate text on a 100-point scale, with higher values associated with greater ease.) Set B, by contrast, has a grade level of 1.8 and a reading ease score of 89.4. Streiner et al. (2015) warn that word processing–based readability scores should be interpreted cautiously, but it is clear from the foregoing analysis that the second set of items would be superior for a population that includes people with limited education. A general principle is to avoid long sentences and words with four or more syllables.

Example of Assessing Readability
Sachdev et al. (2020) sought to develop and validate the 42-item Dental Nutrition Knowledge Competency Scale for low-income females. To assess the readability of the scale, the team had ten nutrition experts review the scale. Through that process, ten items were removed. To further test the readability, the team then conducted a focus group with six low-income females who suggested no changes to the scale. Further psychometric testing resulted in the elimination of eight additional items. The testing resulted in a 24-item reliable and valid measure.

Input From the Target Population

In the next step, the initial pool of items is pretested. In a conventional pretest, a small sample (20-40 people) representing the target population is invited to complete the items. Researchers then look for items with high rates of nonresponse, items with limited variability, items with numerous midpoint responses (fence-sitting), or items with the majority of responses at either extreme (*floor effects* or *ceiling effects*). Such items are candidates for deletion or revision.

Developments in cognitive science over the past 25 years have paved the way for a different approach to pretesting, often as a supplement to standard pretests. In **cognitive questioning**, people are asked to reflect upon their interpretation of the items and their answers so that the underlying process of response selection is better understood.

There are two basic approaches to cognitive interviewing. One is called the **think-aloud method**, wherein respondents are asked to explain step-by-step how they processed the question and arrived at an answer. A second approach is to conduct an interview in which the interviewer uses a series of targeted **probes** that encourage reflection about underlying cognitive processes.

Example of Cognitive Questioning
Camara and colleagues aimed to (2021) adapt a person-centered prenatal care scale for people of color. To assess the clarity, appropriateness, and relevance of the questions, members of the team conducted cognitive interviews with 15 females who were representative of potential respondents. Further psychometric testing in a sample of 293 females, 84% of whom were Black, indicated that the scale was reliable and valid in this population.

TIP When questioning pretest respondents about the clarity or meaning of the items, avoid using the word "item," which is research jargon (e.g., do not say, "Did any *items* confuse you?").

As an alternative or supplement to pretests, *focus groups* can also be used at this stage in scale development. Two or three groups can be convened to discuss whether, from the respondents' perspective, the items are understandable, linguistically and culturally appropriate, inoffensive, and relevant to the construct.

External Review by Experts

External review of the revised items by a panel of experts should be undertaken to assess the scale's **content validity**. It is advisable to undertake two rounds of review, if feasible—the first to refine or remove faulty items or to add new items and the second to formally assess the content validity of the items and scale. We discuss some procedures for such a two-step strategy.

Selecting and Recruiting the Experts

The panel of experts should include people with strong credentials regarding the construct being measured and the target population. In the first round, it is also desirable to include experts on scale construction.

In the initial phase of a two-part review, we advise having an expert panel of 8 to 12 members, with a good mix in terms of roles (e.g., clinicians, researchers) and disciplines. For example, for a scale designed to measure fear of dying in the elderly, the experts might include nurses, gerontologists, and psychiatrists. If the scale is intended for broad use, it might be advantageous to recruit experts from various regions because of possible regional variations in language. The second panel for formally assessing the content validity of a more refined set of items should consist of three to five experts in the content area.

Example of an Expert Panel
Conway and colleagues (2021) developed the scale Nursing Confidence in Managing Sedation Complications Scale to measure nurses' self-efficacy in managing complications related to sedative and analgesic medications administered during procedures. An expert panel of nurse clinicians in nurse-administered sedation reviewed the scale for content validity.

Experts are typically sent materials that include a cover letter, background information about the construct and target population, reviewer instructions, and a questionnaire soliciting their opinion. A critical component of the packet is a careful explanation of the construct's conceptualization, including an explication of the construct's dimensions that would be captured in subscales.

Preliminary Expert Review: Content Validation of Items

The experts' job is to evaluate individual items and the overall scale (and any subscales), using guidelines established by the scale developer. The first panel of experts is usually invited to rate each item along several dimensions, such as clarity of wording, relevance of the item to the construct, and appropriateness for the target population (e.g., developmental or cultural appropriateness). Experts can be asked to make judgments dichotomously (e.g., ambiguous/clear) or along a continuum. As noted in the previous chapter, relevance is most often rated as follows: 1 = *not relevant*, 2 = *somewhat relevant*, 3 = *quite relevant*, and 4 = *highly relevant*. Table 16.1 shows a possible format for a content validation assessment of relevance.

The questionnaire usually asks for detailed comments about items judged to be unclear, not relevant, or not appropriate, such as how wording might be improved, or why the item is deemed not to be relevant. In a first phase, experts are sometimes asked for overall recommendations—for example, retain the item exactly as worded, make major revisions to the item, make minor revisions to the item, and drop the item entirely.

In addition to evaluating each item, the initial expert panel should be asked whether the items taken together adequately cover the construct domain. Experts should be asked for specific guidance on items or subdomains that should be added. For scales constructed within an IRT framework, experts can also be asked whether the items span a continuum of difficulty.

TABLE 16.1 • Example of a Content Validation Form

The scale items shown below have been developed to measure one dimension of the construct of safe sexual behaviors among adolescents, namely **assertiveness**. Please read each item and score it for its relevance in representing this concept.

Assertiveness is defined as the use of verbal and interpersonal skills to negotiate protection during sexual activities.

ITEM	RELEVANCE RATING			
	NOT RELEVANT	SOMEWHAT RELEVANT	QUITE RELEVANT	HIGHLY RELEVANT
1. I ask my partner about their sexual history before having intercourse.	1	2	3	4
2. I don't have sex without asking the person if they have been tested for HIV/AIDS.	1	2	3	4
3. When I am having sex with someone for the first time, I insist that we use a condom.	1	2	3	4
4. I don't let my partner talk me into having sex without knowing something about how risky it would be.	1	2	3	4

Please comment on any of these items, including possible revisions or substitutions, or your thoughts about why an item is not relevant to the concept of assertiveness. Please suggest any additional items you feel would improve the measurement of assertiveness relating to adolescents' safe sexual behaviors.

The standard method for computing an item-level **content validity index** (I-CVI) is the number giving a rating of three or four on the 4-point relevance scale, divided by the number of experts. For example, if five experts rated an item as three and one rated the item as two, the I-CVI would be 0.83. Because of the risk of chance agreement, we recommend I-CVIs of 0.78 or higher (Polit et al., 2007). This means that when there are four or fewer experts, there must be 100% agreement. When there are five to eight experts, one rating of "not relevant" can be tolerated.

Items with lower-than-desired I-CVIs need careful scrutiny. If there are disagreements among the experts on individual items (or if there is agreement about lack of relevance), the items should be revised or dropped.

Content Validation of the Scale

In the second round of content validation, a smaller group of experts (3-5) can be used to evaluate the relevance of the revised set of items and to compute the scale content validity (S-CVI). Although it is possible to use a new group of experts, we recommend using a subset from the first panel—information from the first round can be used to select the most qualified judges. With information from round 1, for example, you can perhaps identify experts who did not understand the task, who were not as familiar with the construct as you thought, or who seemed biased. In other words, data from the first round can be analyzed with a view toward evaluating the performance of the experts, not just the items.

Here are a few considerations when selecting experts based on their ratings in the first round. First, experts who rated every item as "highly relevant" (or "not relevant") may not be sufficiently discriminating. Second, consider omitting an expert who gave high ratings to items that were judged by most others to not be relevant. Third, the proportion of items judged relevant should be computed for all judges. For example, if an expert rated 8 out of 10 items as relevant, the proportion for that judge would be 0.80. The pattern across experts can be examined for "outliers." If the average proportion across raters is, for example, 0.80, you might consider not inviting back experts whose average proportion was either very low (e.g., 0.50) or very high (e.g., 1.00). Useful qualitative feedback from an expert in round one might indicate both content capability and a commitment to the project. Finally, items known *not* to be relevant can be included in the first round to identify judges who wrongly say the items are relevant and so may not really be experts.

After ratings of relevance are obtained for a revised set of items, the S-CVI can be computed. There is more than one way to compute an S-CVI. We recommend the approach that averages across I-CVIs. On a 10-item scale, for example, if the I-CVIs for 5 items were 0.80 and the I-CVIs for the remaining 5 items were 1.00, then the S-CVI/Ave would be 0.90. An S-CVI/Ave of 0.90 or higher is desirable.

In summary, a scale can be judged to have excellent content validity if all its items have I-CVIs of 0.78 or higher and the scale has an S-CVI (using the averaging approach) of 0.90 or higher. This requires strong items, skillful experts, and clear instructions to the experts regarding the underlying constructs and the rating task.

> **TIP** When you describe content validation in a report, be specific about your criteria for accepting items (i.e., the cutoff value for your I-CVIs and the S-CVI). The report should indicate the range of obtained I-CVI values, and the method used to compute the S-CVI.

FIELD TESTING THE INSTRUMENT

At this point, you will have whittled down and refined your items based on your own and others' careful scrutiny. The next step is to undertake a quantitative assessment of the items, which requires that they be administered to a fairly large assessment sample. Testing a new instrument is a full study in and of itself, and care must be taken to design the study to yield useful evidence about the scale's worth. Important steps include the development of a sampling plan and data collection strategy.

Developing a Sampling Plan

The sample for testing the scale should be representative of the population for whom the scale is intended and should be large enough to support complex analyses. If it is not possible to administer the items to a random sample (as is typical), it is advantageous to recruit a sample from multiple sites to enhance representativeness and to assess geographic variation in responding to items. Other strategies to enhance representativeness should be sought, as well—for example, making sure that the sample includes older and younger respondents, males and females, people with varying educational and ethnic backgrounds, and so on, if these characteristics are relevant. You may also need to take steps to ensure that the sample includes the right subgroups of people for a "known-groups" validation.

How large is a "large" sample? There is neither consensus among experts nor hard-and-fast rules. Some suggest that 300 is an adequate number to support a factor analysis (Nunnally & Bernstein, 1994), whereas others offer guidance in terms of a ratio of items to respondents. Ten people per item are often recommended. That means that if you have 20 items, your sample should be at least 200. Having a sufficiently large sample is essential to ensure stability in estimating interitem relationships. For assessments of test–retest reliability, a smaller subsample of participants (e.g., 50–100) is usually sufficient.

You should make efforts to recruit a sample that is heterogeneous on the target attribute. Reliability and internal consistency estimates are dampened when the scores are not sufficiently diverse.

Developing a Data Collection Plan

A decision has to be made concerning how to administer the instrument (e.g., by mail, over the internet). You should choose an approach that best approximates how the scale typically would be administered after it is finalized.

The instrument should include the scale items and basic demographic information. If the intent is to estimate test–retest reliability, then contact information needs to be obtained for scheduling the second administration—and the same is true if the reliability of change scores and responsiveness are being assessed.

Thought also needs to be given to including other measures for validity assessments, if validation efforts are carried out with the development sample. Measures of constructs hypothesized to be correlated with the target construct usually should be included. If the data confirm a relationship predicted by theory or prior research, this would lend evidence to the new scale's validity.

TIP In deciding on what other measures to administer, keep in mind that respondents' willingness to cooperate may decline as the instrument gets longer.

Preparing for Data Collection

As with all data collection efforts, care should be taken to make the instrument attractive, professional-looking, and easy to understand. Instructions for completing the instrument should be clear and a readability assessment should be undertaken. Guidance in understanding the endpoints of response options might be needed if points along the continuum are not explicitly labeled. The instructions should encourage candor. Sometimes social desirability can be minimized by stating that there are no right or wrong answers.

One other consideration is how to sequence the items in the instrument. At issue is something that is called a *proximity effect*, the tendency to be influenced in responding to an item by the response given to the previous item. This effect would tend to artificially inflate estimates of internal consistency. One approach to deal with this is the random ordering of items. An alternative, for scales designed to measure several related dimensions, is to systematically alternate items that are expected to be scored into different subscales.

ANALYSIS OF SCALE DEVELOPMENT DATA

The analysis of data from multi-item scales is a topic about which entire books have been written. We provide only an overview. We assume that

Basic Item Analysis

Each item on the preliminary scale needs to be evaluated empirically in an **item analysis**. Within CTT, what is desired is an item that has a high correlation with the true score of the underlying construct. We cannot assess this directly, but if each item is a measure of that construct, then the items should correlate with one another.

The degree of **inter-item correlation** can be assessed by inspecting the *correlation matrix* of all the items. If there are items with substantial negative intercorrelations, some should perhaps be *reverse-scored*. Unless intentional, however, negative correlations are likely to reflect problems and may signal the need to remove items. For items on the same subscale, interitem correlations between 0.30 and 0.70 are recommended, with correlations lower than 0.30 suggesting little congruence with the underlying construct and ones higher than 0.70 suggesting over-redundancy. However, the evaluation depends on the number of items in the scale. An average interitem correlation of 0.57 is needed to achieve a coefficient alpha of 0.80 on a 3-item scale, but an average of only 0.29 is needed for a 10-item scale (DeVellis & Thorpe, 2022).

A next step is to compute preliminary total scale or subscale scores and then calculate correlations between items and total scores on the subscales they are intended to represent. If item scores do not correlate well with scale scores, the item is probably measuring something else and will lower the reliability of the scale. There are two types of **item-scale correlations**, one in which the total score includes the item under consideration (*uncorrected*) and another in which the item is removed in calculating the total scale score. The latter (*corrected*) approach is preferable because the inclusion of the item on the scale inflates the correlation coefficients. The standard advice is to eliminate items whose item-scale correlation is less than 0.30.

Descriptive information for each item should also be examined. Items should have good variability—without it, they will not correlate with the total scale and will dampen internal consistency. Means for the items that are close to the center of the range of possible scores are also desirable (e.g., a mean near 4 on a 7-point scale). Items with means near one extreme or the other tend not to discriminate well among respondents; also, such items may perform poorly if a goal is to assess changes because there may be no room for further improvement or deterioration (i.e., *floor* or *ceiling effects*).

> **Example of an Item Analysis**
> Zhang and colleagues (2021) performed an item analysis in their field testing of the Humanistic Practice Ability of Nursing Scale adapted for use in China. Their sample consisted of 430 clinical nurses in four hospitals. They conducted an item analysis using item-total correlation coefficients. All 29 items in five dimensions reached a level of significance, $p < .001$.

Exploratory Factor Analysis

A set of items is not necessarily a scale—the items form a scale only if they have a common underlying construct. **Factor analysis** disentangles complex interrelationships among items and identifies items that "go together" as unified concepts. This section deals with a type of factor analysis known as **exploratory factor analysis (EFA)**, which essentially assumes no a priori hypotheses about the dimensionality of a set of items.

Suppose we developed 50 items measuring females' attitudes toward menopause. We could form a scale by adding together scores from several individual items, but which items should be combined? Would it be reasonable to combine all 50 items? Probably not, because the 50 items are not all tapping the same thing—there are various *dimensions* to females' attitude toward menopause. One dimension may relate to aging and another to loss of reproductive ability. Other items may involve sexuality. These multiple dimensions to females' attitudes toward menopause should be measured on separate subscales. Females' attitude on one dimension may be independent of their attitude on another. Dimensions of a construct are usually identified during initial conceptualization and content validation. Preconceptions about dimensions, however, do not always "pan out" when tested against actual responses. Factor analysis offers an objective method of clarifying the underlying dimensionality of a set of items. Underlying dimensions in the analysis are called **factors**, which are weighted combinations of items.

> **TIP** Before undertaking an EFA, you should evaluate the *factorability* of your set of items. Procedures for a factorability assessment are described in Polit (2010) and Polit and Yang (2016).

Factor Extraction

EFA involves two phases. The first phase (**factor extraction**) condenses items into a smaller number of factors and is used to identify the number of underlying dimensions. The goal is to extract clusters of highly interrelated items from a correlation matrix. There are various methods of performing the first step, each of which uses different criteria for assigning weights to items. A widely used factor extraction method is **principal components analysis (PCA)** and another is **principal axis factor analysis**. Our discussion focuses mostly on PCA, although the two methods often lead to the same conclusion about dimensionality.

Factor extraction yields an *unrotated factor matrix*, which contains coefficients or *weights* for all original items on each extracted factor. Each extracted factor is a weighted linear combination of all the original items. For example, with three items, a factor would be item 1 (times a weight) + item 2 (times a weight) + item 3 (times a weight). In the PCA method, weights for the first factor are computed such that the average squared weight is maximized—this permits a maximum amount of variance to be extracted by that factor. The second factor, or linear weighted combination, is formed so that the highest possible amount of variance is extracted from what *remains* after the first factor. The factors thus represent independent sources of variation in the data matrix.

Factoring should continue until no further meaningful variance is left—a criterion must be applied to decide when to stop extraction. Several criteria can be described by illustrating information from a factor analysis. Table 16.2 presents fictitious values for eigenvalues, percentages of variance accounted for, and cumulative percentages of variance accounted for, for 10 factors. **Eigenvalues** are equal to the sum of the squared item weights for the factor. Many researchers establish as their cutoff point

TABLE 16.2 • Summary of Factor Extraction Results

FACTOR	EIGENVALUE	PERCENTAGE OF VARIANCE EXPLAINED	CUMULATIVE PERCENTAGE OF VARIANCE EXPLAINED
1	12.32	29.2	29.2
2	8.57	23.3	52.5
3	6.91	15.6	68.1
4	2.02	8.4	76.5
5	1.09	6.2	82.7
6	0.98	5.8	88.5
7	0.80	4.5	93.0
8	0.62	3.1	96.1
9	0.47	2.2	98.3
10	0.25	1.7	100.0

for extraction eigenvalues of 1.0 or greater. In our example, the first five factors meet this criterion. Another cutoff benchmark, called the *scree test,* is based on discontinuities: A sharp drop in the percentage of explained variance indicates a possible termination point. In Table 16.2, we might argue that there is considerable discontinuity between the third and fourth factors—that is, that three factors should be extracted. Another guideline concerns the amount of variance explained by the factors. Some advocate that the factors extracted should account for at least 60% of the total variance, and that for any factor to be meaningful it must account for at least 5% of the variance. In our table, the first three factors account for 68.1% of the total variance. Six factors contribute 5% or more to the total variance.

So, should we extract three, five, or six factors? One approach is to see whether there is any convergence among the criteria. In our example, two criteria (the scree test and total variance test) suggest three factors. Another approach is to see whether any of the rules yields a number consistent with our original conceptualization. In our example, if we had designed the items to represent three theoretically meaningful subscales, we might consider three factors to be the right number because the data provide sufficient support for that conclusion.

TIP Polit (2010) provides a "walk-through" demonstration of how decisions are made in undertaking an exploratory factor analysis.

Factor Rotation

The second phase of factor analysis—**factor rotation**—is performed on factors that have met extraction criteria, to make the factors more interpretable. The concept of rotation can be best explained graphically. Figure 16.1 shows two coordinate systems, marked by axes A1 and A2 and B1 and B2. The primary axes (A1 and A2) represent factors I and II, respectively, as defined *before* rotation. Points 1 through 6 represent six items. The weights for each item can be determined in reference to these axes. For instance, before rotation, item 1 has a weight of 0.80 on factor I and 0.85 on factor II, and item 6 has a weight of −0.45 on factor I and 0.90 on factor II.

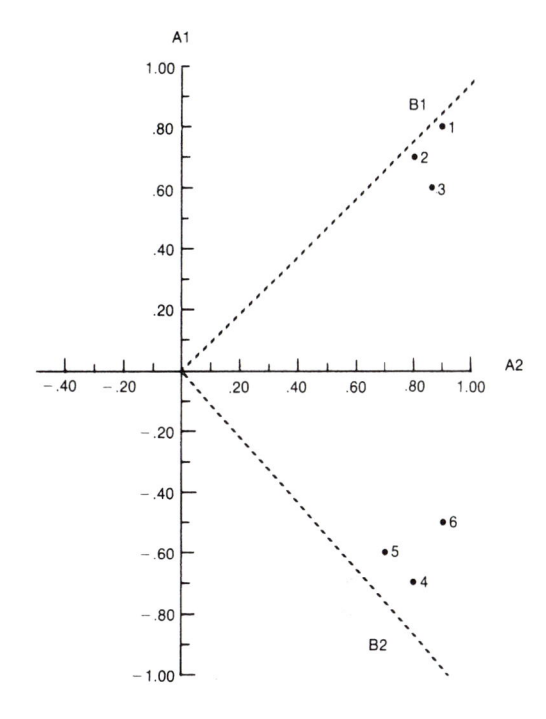

FIGURE 16.1 Illustration of factor rotation.

Unrotated axes account for a maximum amount of variance, but interpretability is enhanced by rotating the axes so that clusters of items are distinctly associated with a factor. In the figure, B1 and B2 represent rotated factors. After rotation, items 1, 2, and 3 have large weights on factor I and small weights on factor II, and the opposite is true for items 4, 5, and 6.

Researchers choose from two types of rotation. Figure 16.1 illustrates **orthogonal rotation**, in which factors are kept at right angles to one another. Orthogonal rotations maintain the independence of factors—that is, orthogonal factors are uncorrelated with one another. **Oblique rotations** permit rotated axes to depart from a 90° angle. In our figure, an oblique rotation would have put axis B1 between items 2 and 3 and axis B2 between items 5 and 6. This placement strengthens the clustering of items around an associated factor but results in correlated factors. Some writers argue that orthogonal rotation leads to greater theoretical clarity; others claim it is unrealistic. Advocates of oblique rotation point out that if the concepts *are* correlated, then the analysis should reflect this fact. In developing a scale with multiple dimensions, we likely would expect the dimensions to be correlated, and so oblique rotation might well be more meaningful. This can be assessed empirically: if an oblique rotation is specified, the correlation between factors is computed. If the correlations are low (e.g., less than 0.15 or 0.20), an orthogonal rotation may be preferred because it yields a simpler model.

Researchers work with a **rotated factor matrix** in interpreting the factor analysis. As an example, Table 16.3 shows factor analysis information for the final 12 items on the Uncivil Behavior in Clinical Nursing Education (UBCNE) scale (Anthony et al., 2014). The entries under each factor are the weights or **factor loadings**. For orthogonally rotated factors, factor loadings can range from −1.00 to +1.00 and can be interpreted like correlation coefficients—they express the correlation between items and factors. In this example, item 1 is highly correlated with factor 1, 0.83. By examining factor loadings, we can find which items "belong" to a factor. In this example, items 1, 2, 4, 7, 8, 11, and 12 had sizable loadings on factor 1. Loadings with an absolute value of 0.40 or higher often are used as cutoff values, but somewhat smaller values may be acceptable if it makes theoretical sense to do so. The underlying dimensionality of the items can then be interpreted. By inspecting the content of these seven items, we can search for a common theme that makes them "go together." The developers of the UBCNE called this first factor *Hostile/Mean/Dismissive*. Items 3, 5, 6, 9, and 10 had high loadings on factor 2, which they named *Exclusionary Behavior*. The naming of factors is a process of identifying underlying constructs—this naming often would have occurred during the conceptualization phase.

The results of the factor analysis can be used not only to identify the dimensionality of the

TABLE 16.3 • Factor Loadings: Uncivil Behavior in Clinical Nursing Education

HOW OFTEN HAVE YOU HAD A SITUATION WHERE A NURSE:	FACTOR 1	FACTOR 2
1. Embarrassed you …	**.83**[a]	.18
2. Rolled their eyes at you	**.73**	.30
3. Gave you an incomplete report	.02	**.70**
4. Used an inappropriate tone …	**.77**	.19
5. Avoided taking a report from you	.24	**.75**
6. Avoided giving you a report	.21	**.82**
7. Made snide remarks …	**.58**	.30
8. Raised their voice …	**.76**	.23
9. Did not involve you in a patient care decision …	.23	**.70**
10. Did not pass on patient information …	.18	**.78**
11. Told you that you were incompetent	**.82**	−.07
12. Refused to help you	**.77**	.18

Adapted from Table 6 and Appendix B of Anthony, M., Yastik, J., MacDonald, D., & Marshall, K. (2014). Development and validation of a tool to measure incivility in clinical nursing education. *Journal of Professional Nursing 30*, 48–55, with permission from Elsevier.
[a]High loadings are bolded; these are the ones used to name and interpret the factors. Factor 1 was named *Hostile/Mean/Dismissive* and factor 2 was named *Exclusionary Behavior*.

construct but also to make decisions about item retention and deletion. If items have low loadings on all factors, they likely are good candidates for deletion (or revision, if you can detect wording problems that may have caused different respondents to infer different meanings). Items with high loadings on multiple factors may also be candidates for deletion. In the development of the UBCNE, the researchers deleted six items that had high loadings on more than one factor (e.g., "Told you to go ask your instructor"). Items with marginal loadings (e.g., 0.35) but that had good content validity could be retained for the internal consistency analysis.

> **Example of an Exploratory Factor Analysis**
> Lee (2021) conducted an exploratory factor analysis of the Nursing Workaround Instrument translated from English to Korean. The tool captures nursing workarounds related to the electronic health record. The 20-item, four factor scale was tested in a sample of 104 nurses in Korea to determine which factors remained. While the four factors remained, the number of items in the scale was reduced from 20 to 12.

Internal Consistency Analysis

After a final set of items is selected based on the item and factor analysis results, an analysis should be undertaken to calculate coefficient alpha. Alpha, it may be recalled, provides an estimate of a key measurement property of multi-item scales: internal consistency reliability.

Most general-purpose statistical programs calculate the value of coefficient alpha for the full scale—and for a hypothetical scale when each individual item is removed. If the overall alpha is extremely high, it may be prudent to eliminate redundancy by deleting items that do not make a large contribution to alpha. (Sometimes removal of a faulty item actually *increases* alpha.) A modest reduction in reliability is sometimes worth the benefit of lowering respondent burden. Scale developers must consider the best trade-off between brevity and internal consistency.

Internal consistency estimates tend to capitalize on chance factors in a sample of respondents and may be lower in a new sample. Thus, you should aim for alphas that are a bit higher in the development sample than ones you would consider minimally acceptable so that if the alphas decay they will still be adequate. This is especially true if the development sample is small.

TIP If you have a very large sample, consider dividing the sample in half at random, running the factor analysis and internal consistency analysis with one subsample, and then rerunning them with the second one as a cross-validation.

Test–Retest Reliability Analysis

Although test–retest reliability analysis has not been a standard feature of psychometric assessment in nursing research, we urge developers of new scales to gather information about both internal consistency and test–retest reliability. The COSMIN group considers test–retest reliability a particularly important indicator of a scale's quality.

An issue of importance in a retest study is the timing of the retest relative to the initial administration. Timing decisions must balance the risks for different potential sources of error. When the time interval is too brief, carryover effects (the memory of answers on the previous measurement and the desire to be consistent) can lead to artificially high estimates of reliability. But other factors—including true change—could depress reliability coefficients. Some experts advise that the time interval between measurements should be in the vicinity of 1 to 2 weeks. Polit (2014) has offered several suggestions for strategies to improve decision-making about the retest interval and for basing decisions on evidence or theory about an attribute's stability, rather than assumptions. She also provides guidance on using test–retest results to identify items that may benefit from revision.

SCALE REFINEMENT AND VALIDATION

In some scale development efforts, the bulk of work is over at this point. For example, if you developed a scale as part of a larger substantive project because you were unable to identify a good measure of a key construct, you may be ready to pursue your substantive analyses. If, however, you are developing a scale for others to use, a few more steps are needed.

Revising the Scale

The analyses undertaken in the development study often suggest the need to revise or add items. For example, if subscale alpha coefficients are lower than 0.80 or so, consideration should be given to adding items for subsequent testing. In thinking about new items, a good strategy is to examine items that had high factor loadings because they may offer clues for good new items.

Before deciding that your scale is finalized, it is prudent to examine the content of the items in the scale. Sometimes alphas are inflated by items that have similar wording, so decisions about retaining or removing items are best made by also considering content validity information. It may be worthwhile to reexamine the I-CVIs of each item in making final decisions.

Scoring the Scale

Scoring a composite summated rating scale is easy: item scores are typically just added together (with reverse scoring of items, if appropriate) to form subscale scores. Subscale scores are sometimes added together to form total scale scores—although this is not always justifiable. Some scale developers create a total score that is the *average* across items so that the total score is on the same scale as the items. In either case, all items are weighted equally. Such scoring involves an implicit assumption that each item is equally important as a measure of the target construct.

> **TIP** It may sometimes be attractive to have differential weighting of items to reflect differences in the items' contribution to the measure—although weighting usually has been found to have little effect on a scale's measurement properties (Streiner et al., 2015). Thus, unitary weighting of items is typical for most composite scales.

Conducting a Validation Study

Scales designed for use by others require validity assessments. Scale developers who are not able to do a separate validation study should strive to undertake many of the activities described in this section with data from the original development sample. Designing a validation study entails much of the same issues (and advice) as designing a development study, in terms of sample composition, sample size, and data collection strategies. The exception is that if efforts will be made to assess longitudinal measurement properties, a longitudinal design is needed.

Confirmatory Factor Analysis

Confirmatory factor analysis (CFA) is playing an increasingly important role in validation studies. CFA is preferable to EFA as an approach to construct (structural) validity because CFA is a hypothesis-testing approach—testing the hypothesis that the items belong to specific factors, rather than having the dimensionality of a set of items emerge empirically, as in EFA.

CFA is a subset of an advanced class of statistical techniques known as **structural equation modeling** (SEM). CFA differs from EFA in a number of respects, many of which are technical. One concerns the estimation procedure. Many statistical procedures used by nurse researchers employ what is called *least-squares estimation*. In SEM, the estimation procedure is *maximum likelihood estimation*. Least-squares procedures have several stringent assumptions that are generally untenable—for example, the assumption that variables are measured without error. SEM can accommodate measurement error and avoid other restrictions.

CFA involves testing a **measurement model**, which specifies the hypothesized relationships among underlying constructs and the *manifest variables*—that is, the items. Loadings on the factors (the *latent variables*) provide a method for evaluating relationships between observed variables (the items) and unobserved variables (the construct's factors).

We illustrate with an example of a scale designed to measure two aspects of fatigue: physical fatigue and mental fatigue. In the example shown in Figure 16.2, both types of fatigue are captured by five items: items I1 to I5 for physical fatigue and items I6 to I10 for mental fatigue. According to the model, item responses are caused by respondents' level of physical and mental fatigue (the straight arrows indicate hypothesized causal paths) and are also affected by error (e_1 through e_{10}). It is expected that error terms are correlated, as indicated by the curved lines connecting the errors. Correlated measurement errors on items might arise from a person's desire to "look good"—a factor that would systematically affect all item scores. The two fatigue constructs also are hypothesized to be correlated.

The hypothesized measurement model would be tested against actual data. The analysis would yield loadings of observed variables on the latent variables, the correlation between the two latent variables, and correlations among the error terms. The analysis would also indicate whether the overall model fit is good, based on several *goodness-of-fit statistics*.

CFA is a complex topic, and we have described only basic characteristics. Further reading on the topic is imperative for those wishing to pursue it (e.g., Brown, 2015; Kline, 2016).

Example of Confirmatory Factor Analysis
Winquist and colleagues (2023) conducted an online survey with 489 nurses from 12 countries to confirm the factor structure of the Climate, Health, and Nursing Tool measure. A confirmatory factor analysis was conducted to determine whether the validity of the 22-item, five-factor demonstrated a good fit.

Bott and colleagues (2018) have written an article about free and accessible software (CBID) for performing confirmatory factor analyses and combining patient data with expert data from content validity assessments.

Other Validation Activities

A validation effort would be incomplete without undertaking additional activities, such as ones described in Chapter 15. The assessment of criterion or construct validity primarily relies on correlational evidence. In criterion-related validity, scores on the new scale are correlated with an external gold standard criterion. In construct validity, scores on the scale can, for example, be correlated with measures of constructs hypothesized to be related to the target construct; or supplementary measures of the same construct (convergent validity); or measures of a closely related but distinguishable construct (divergent validity). Validation

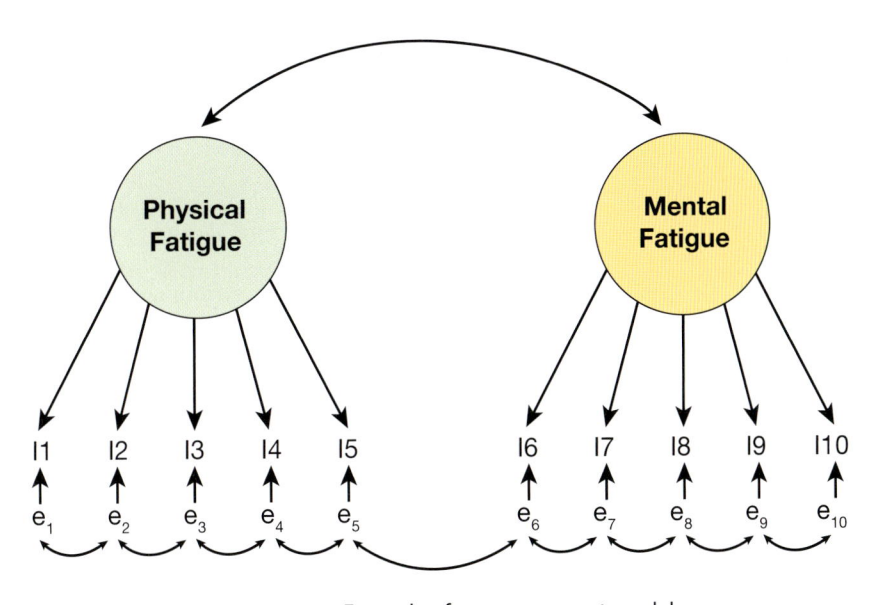

FIGURE 16.2 Example of a measurement model.

using a known-groups approach requires selecting people with membership in groups expected to be different, on average, on the scale. It is desirable to produce as much validity evidence as possible.

> **TIP** If a CFA is not possible, it is still advisable to undertake a "confirmatory" factor analysis using EFA with the validation sample. Comparisons between the original and new factor analyses can be made with respect to factor structure, loadings, variance explained, and so on. In the new analysis, the number of factors to be extracted and rotated can be prespecified, as this is now the working hypothesis about the underlying dimensionality of the construct.

Longitudinal Measurement Properties

In both clinical work and research, measurements of health outcomes are often made on two or more occasions to assess whether a change occurred. Scale developers who anticipate that their scales will be used to measure change should assess the reliability of change scores on the measure and its responsiveness (longitudinal construct validity).

Such assessments inherently require a longitudinal design so that measurements can be made twice. The study should be designed using a population in which change is expected to occur over a specified interval. This may be a population in which deterioration is anticipated (e.g., patients with a progressive disease) or a population receiving a treatment known to be effective. In terms of the time interval between measurements, enough time should have elapsed that one could reasonably expect change on the focal construct for a sizable subset of the sample. However, lengthy time periods may create several problems, including attrition.

Using our definition of responsiveness as longitudinal validity (Chapter 15), it follows that much of the advice we offered with regard to construct validation is relevant here. As with assessments of construct validity, multiple hypothesis tests are desirable for examining a measure's responsiveness—which typically means correlating change scores on the focal measure with change scores on other measures with which a relationship is expected. When a known-groups approach to responsiveness assessment is adopted, comparison groups whose change trajectories are expected to differ are needed. Further advice on testing responsiveness is offered in Polit and Yang (2016).

INTERPRETABILITY OF SCALE SCORES

In addition to the four measurement properties identified in our taxonomy (Figure 15.1), another important aspect of measurement concerns interpretability—that is, understanding what a score *means*. The COSMIN group defined **interpretability** as "the degree to which one can assign qualitative meaning—that is, clinical or commonly understood connotations—to an instrument's quantitative scores or change in scores" (Mokkink et al., 2010, p. 743).

A raw score on a scale is seldom directly interpretable. What does a score of 16 on the Center for Epidemiologic Studies Depression scale mean, for example? We briefly discuss some ways to enhance the interpretability of scale scores.

> **TIP** Ideally, if you expect the scale to be used by others, you should create a manual for its use. Guidelines for preparing manuals are published in *Standards for Educational and Psychological Testing* (AERA, APA, & NCME Joint Committee, 2014). Scale developers should consider registering a copyright, even if they do not plan to publish the scale commercially.

Percentiles

Raw score values from a scale can be made more interpretable by converting them to percentiles. A **percentile** indicates the percentage of people who score below a particular score. Percentiles provide information about how a person performs relative to others and are easily interpreted by most people. Percentiles can range from the 0th to the 99th percentile, and the 50th percentile corresponds to the median. Percentile values are most useful when they are determined with a large, representative sample.

Standard Scores

Standard scores transform raw scores into values that have been stripped of the original measurement metric. The transformation makes it possible to compare people on a measure along an easily interpretable scale, without needing to understand the raw score value. Standard scores also make it possible to compare a person's performance on multiple measures with different metrics (e.g., a 10-item fatigue scale and a 5-item pain scale).

Standard scores are expressed in terms of their relative distance from the mean, in standard deviation (*SD*) units. A standard score of 0.00 corresponds to a raw score at the scale's mean—regardless of what that mean is. A standard score of 1.0 corresponds to a score 1 *SD* above the mean, and a standard score of −1.0 corresponds to a score 1 *SD* below the mean. Standard scores can be readily calculated from raw scores once the mean and *SD* have been calculated (see Chapter 19).

It is often easier to work with score values that do not have negative values and decimal points. Standard scores can be transformed to have any desired mean and *SD*, and certain transformations are particularly common. In particular, standard scores with a mean of 50 and an *SD* of 10 are widely used and are called **T scores**. With T scores, a score of, say, 60 is immediately interpretable, even without knowing much about the scale—it is a score one SD above the mean.

Norms

In some cases, it might be desirable to standardize a new scale and establish norms. This typically occurs if it is expected that the scale will be widely used—and used by people who will rely on comparative information to help them evaluate scores. Norms are often established for key demographic subgroups.

A good sampling plan is critical in a norming effort. The sample should be geographically dispersed and representative of the population for whom the scale is intended. A large standardization sample is required so that subgroup values are stable.

Norms are often expressed in terms of percentiles. For example, an adult male with a score of 72 on the scale might be at the 80th percentile, but a female with the same score might be at the 85th percentile. Nunnally and Bernstein (1994) offer guidelines for norming instruments.

Cutoff Points

Interpretation of scores can often be facilitated if the instrument developer establishes *cutpoints* for classification purposes. Cutpoints are typically used as the basis for making decisions about needed treatments or further assessments. Sometimes cutpoints are defined in terms of percentiles. For example, for children's weights, those below the 5th percentile are considered underweight (or, in infants, "failure to thrive"), whereas those above the 95th percentile are considered overweight. In other cases, the cutpoints are designated with standard scores. For example, the World Health Organization defines osteoporosis as a standard score on a bone mineral density test at or below −2.5, which is 2½ *SD*s below the mean for female in their 30s. Cutpoints that are linked to the measure's distribution are considered *norm-referenced*.

Various methods—both empirical and subjective—have been developed for establishing cutoff points for raw scale scores. As described in Chapter 15, a frequently used method is the construction of receiver operating characteristic (ROC) curves to identify the cutpoint that maximizes and balances sensitivity and specificity. Scale developers who intend to develop ROC curves need to select highly reliable criteria for dividing people into groups (e.g., those with and those without the condition being screened), and the criteria must be independent of participants' responses on the scale.

> **TIP** It may be important to develop guidelines for interpreting *change scores*. If you are developing a scale that will be used to capture change (for example, as an outcome measure in an intervention study), then you should make an effort to establish the value of a *minimal important change* (Chapter 21) and the *smallest detectable change* (Chapter 15) for your scale.

CRITICAL APPRAISAL OF SCALE DEVELOPMENT STUDIES

Articles about scale development appear regularly in nursing journals. If you are planning to use a scale in a substantive study, carefully review the methods used to construct the scale and to evaluate its psychometric adequacy. Remember that you run the risk of undermining the statistical conclusion validity of your study (that is, of having insufficient power for testing your hypotheses) if you use a scale with weak reliability. And you can run the risk of poor construct validity in your study if your measures are not strong proxies for key constructs.

Box 16.1 provides broad guidelines for evaluating a research report on the development and validation of a scale. Additionally, many important evaluative questions with regard to reporting and study design for measurement studies have been incorporated into a series of checklists prepared by the COSMIN group (Terwee et al., 2012).

BOX 16.1 Guidelines for Critically Appraising Scale Development and Assessment Reports

1. Did the report offer a clear definition of the construct being measured? Did it provide sufficient context for the study through a summary of the literature and discussion of relevant theory? Is the population for whom the scale intended adequately described?
2. Did the report indicate how items were generated? Do the procedures seem sound? Was information provided about the reading level of scale items?
3. Did the report describe content validation efforts, and was the description thorough? Is there evidence of good content validity?
4. Were appropriate efforts made to refine the scale (e.g., through pretests, cognitive questioning, item analysis)?
5. Was the development/validation sample of participants appropriate in terms of representativeness, size, and diversity?
6. Was factor analysis used to evaluate or validate the scale's dimensionality? If yes, did the report offer evidence to support the factor structure and the naming of factors?
7. Were appropriate methods used to assess the scale's internal consistency and reliability? Were estimates of reliability and internal consistency sufficiently high?
8. Were appropriate methods used to assess the scale's criterion or construct validity? Is the evidence about the scale's validity persuasive? What other validation methods would have strengthened inferences about the scale's worthiness?
9. Were efforts made to assess the reliability of change scores and the responsiveness of the new measure?
10. Did the report provide information for scoring the scale and interpreting scale scores—for example, means and standard deviations, cutoff scores, norms?

RESEARCH EXAMPLE

In this section, we describe the development and testing of a widely used scale that was carefully created by one of this book's authors. This example demonstrates the depth of the work required to develop, test, and refine a measure. This tool continues to be an important measure for screening of perinatal depression.

Studies: Postpartum Depression Screening Scale: Development and psychometric testing (Beck & Gable, 2000); Further validation of the Postpartum Depression Screening Scale (Beck & Gable, 2001); Postpartum Depression Screening Scale: Spanish version (Beck & Gable, 2003).

Background: Beck studied postpartum depression (PPD) in a series of qualitative studies, using both phenomenologic and grounded theory approaches.

Based on her in-depth understanding of PPD, she sought to develop a scale that could be used to screen for PPD, the Postpartum Depression Screening Scale (PDSS). Beck and an expert psychometrician undertook methodologic studies to develop, refine, and validate the PDSS to screen females for PPD and to translate the scale into Spanish.

Scale development: The PDSS is a summated rating scale designed to tap seven dimensions, such as sleep disturbances, eating disturbances, and mental confusion. A 56-item pilot form of the PDSS was initially developed with 8 items per dimension, using a 5-point response option scale. Themes from Beck's qualitative research were used to craft the items for the seven dimensions. The reading level of the final PDSS was assessed to be at the third-grade level and the Flesch reading ease score was 92.7.

Content validity: Content validity was enhanced by using direct quotes from the qualitative studies as items on the scale (e.g., "I felt like I was losing my mind"). The pilot form was subjected to two content validations with a panel of five content experts. Feedback from these procedures led to some item revisions.

Construct validity: The PDSS was administered to a sample of 525 new mothers in six states (Beck & Gable, 2000). Preliminary item analyses resulted in the deletion of several items, based on item-total correlations. The PDSS was finalized as a 35-item scale with seven subscales, each with 5 items. This version of the PDSS was subjected to confirmatory factor analyses, which involved a validation of Beck's hypotheses about how individual items mapped onto underlying constructs, such as *mental confusion*. IRT analysis was also used and provided supporting evidence of the scale's construct validity. In a subsequent study, Beck and Gable (2001) administered the PDSS and two other depression scales to 150 new mothers and tested hypotheses about how scores on the PDSS would correlate with scores on other scales. The results indicated good convergent validity.

Internal consistency: In both studies, Beck and Gable evaluated the internal consistency of the PDSS and its subscales. Subscale alphas were high, ranging from 0.83 to 0.94 in the first study and from 0.80 to 0.91 in the second study. Figure 16.3 shows an internal consistency analysis printout (from the Statistical Package for the Social Sciences, or SPSS, Version 17.0) for the five items on the Mental Confusion subscale from the first study. In panel A, we see that Cronbach alpha for the 5-item subscale is high, 0.912. The first column of panel B (Item Statistics) identifies subscale items by number: Item 11, item 18, and so on. Item 11, for example, is the item "I felt like I was losing my mind." The item means and SDs for the 522 cases suggest adequate variability on each item. Panel C shows intercorrelations among the five items. The correlations are fairly high, ranging from 0.601 for item 25 with 53 to 0.814 for item 11 with 25. Panel D (Summary Item Statistics) presents descriptive item statistics. In panel E, the fourth column ("Corrected Item-Total Correlation") presents correlation coefficients for the relationship between females' score on an item and their score on the subscale, after removing the item from the scale. Item 11 has a corrected item-total correlation of 0.799, which is very high; all five items have excellent correlations with the total subscale score. The final column shows what the internal consistency would be if an item were deleted. If Item 11 were removed from the subscale and only 4 items remained, the reliability coefficient would be 0.888—less than the reliability for all 5 items (0.912). Deleting any of the items on the subscale would reduce its internal consistency but only by a rather small amount.

Criterion-related validity: In the second study, Beck and Gable correlated scores on the PDSS with an expert clinician's diagnosis of PPD for each female (the criterion). The coefficient was 0.70, which was higher than the correlations between the clinical diagnosis and scores on other depression scales, indicating its superiority as a screening instrument. Additionally, ROC curves were constructed to examine the sensitivity and specificity of the PDSS at different cutoff points, using the expert diagnosis to establish PPD caseness. In this sample, 46 of the 150 mothers had a diagnosis of major or minor depression. To illustrate the trade-offs the researchers made, the ROC curve (Figure 16.4) revealed that with a cutoff score of 95 on the PDSS, the sensitivity would be only 0.41, meaning that only 41% of the females actually diagnosed with PPD would be identified. A score of 95 has a specificity of 1.00, meaning that all cases *without* an actual PPD

A Reliability Statistics

Cronbach Alpha	Cronbach Alpha Based on Standardized Items	N of Items
.912	.912	5

B Item Statistics

	Mean	Std. Deviation	N
Item 11	2.36	1.424	522
Item 18	2.21	1.270	522
Item 25	2.21	1.374	522
Item 39	2.40	1.351	522
Item 53	2.28	1.349	522

C Interitem Correlation Matrix

	Item 11	Item 18	Item 25	Item 39	Item 53
Item 11	1.000	.654	.814	.646	.649
Item 18	.654	1.000	.603	.659	.751
Item 25	.814	.603	1.000	.652	.601
Item 39	.646	.659	.652	1.000	.724
Item 53	.649	.751	.601	.724	1.000

D Summary Item Statistics

	Mean	Minimum	Maximum	Range	Maximum / Minimum	Variance	N of Items
Item Means	2.292	2.205	2.399	.194	1.088	.008	5
Item Variances	1.835	1.612	2.029	.416	1.258	.023	5
Interitem Correlations	.675	.601	.814	.213	1.354	.006	5

E Item-Total Statistics

	Scale Mean if Item Deleted	Scale Variance if Item Deleted	Corrected Item-Total Correlation	Squared Multiple Correlation	Cronbach Alpha if Item Deleted
Item 11	9.09	21.371	.799	.715	.888
Item 18	9.24	23.006	.770	.623	.895
Item 25	9.25	22.097	.769	.691	.894
Item 39	9.06	22.290	.869	.610	.894
Item 53	9.18	22.176	.781	.666	.891

FIGURE 16.3 Statistical Package for the Social Sciences (SPSS) internal consistency analysis for the Mental Confusion subscale of the Postpartum Depression Screening Scale.

diagnosis would be accurately screened out. At the other extreme, a cutoff score of 45 would have 1.00 sensitivity but only 0.28 specificity (i.e., 72% false positive), an unacceptable rate of overdiagnosis. Beck and Gable recommended a cutoff score of 60, which would accurately screen in 91% of true PPD cases and would mistakenly screen in 28% who do not have PPD. Beck and Gable found that this cutoff point correctly classified 85% of their sample. In their ROC analysis, the area under the curve was excellent, 0.91.

Spanish translation: Beck collaborated with translation experts to develop a Spanish version of the PDSS. Eight bilingual translators from four backgrounds (Mexican, Puerto Rican, Cuban, and South American) translated and back-translated the items. The translators met as a committee to review each other's wordings and to arrive at a consensus. Both the English and Spanish versions were then administered, in random order, to a bilingual sample. Scores on the two versions correlated highly (e.g., 0.98 on the "Sleeping/Eating Disturbances" subscale). Coefficient alpha

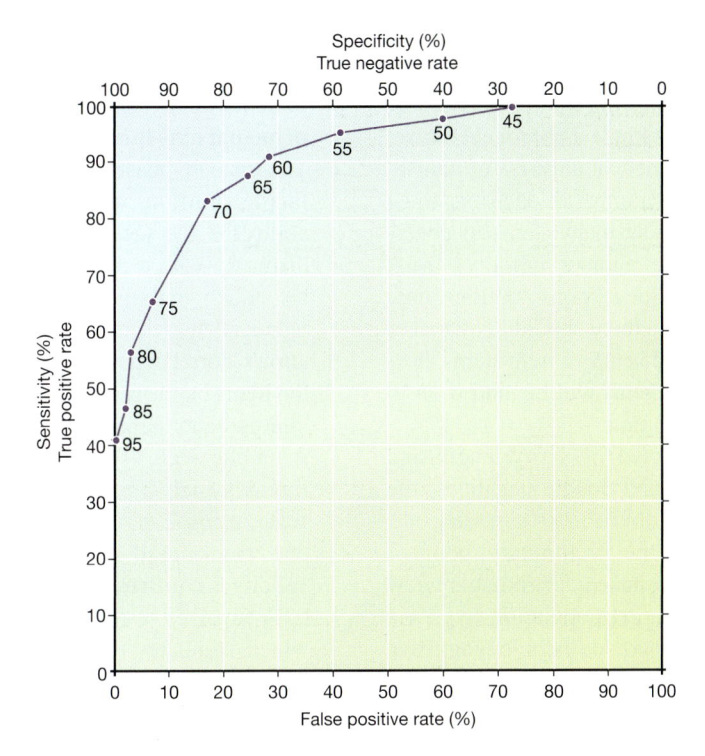

FIGURE 16.4 Receiver operating characteristic (ROC) curve for Postpartum Depression Screening Scale.

was 0.95 for the total scale and ranged from 0.76 to 0.90 for subscales. CFA yielded information that was judged to indicate an adequate fit with the hypothesized measurement model, and screening performance was found to be good (Beck & Gable, 2003, 2005). Another psychometric assessment of the Spanish version was undertaken by Lara and colleagues (2013) in Mexico, who found comparably good measurement properties.

Other translations: The PDSS has been translated into several other languages (e.g., Chinese, Portuguese, Turkish, Hungarian, Thai), and psychometric assessments in all cases suggest that the instrument has strong measurement properties. In the Turkish version of the PDSS, the 15-day test–retest reliability, which was not reported in other papers, was high, $r = 0.86$ (Karaçam & Kitiş, 2008). In the Hungarian version, the parallel forms reliability for the English and Hungarian versions was 0.97 (Hegedus & Beck, 2012).

Responsiveness: Responsiveness of the PDSS was not assessed by the scale developers. There is, however, evidence that PPD as measured by the PDSS is sensitive to interventions and to changes over time, suggesting good responsiveness of the scale. For example, in a study of the effects of kangaroo mother care in Brazil, scores on the PDSS dropped during the time the infants were in the NICU, consistent with the researchers' hypotheses (de Alencar et al., 2009). In an analysis of the effects of a psychoeducation intervention for pregnant females with abuse-related posttraumatic stress, Rowe et al. (2014) reported a significant decrease in PDSS scores. Zhao et al. (2018) examined how females' perinatal depression scores as measured on the PDSS changed across the perinatal period.

SUMMARY POINTS

- Scale development begins with a sound conceptualization of the construct (the **latent trait**) to be measured, including its *dimensionality*.
- An early step in scale construction is the generation of items. Common sources for items include existing instruments, the research literature,

- concept analyses, qualitative studies, and clinical observations.
- In CTT, a **domain sampling model** is assumed; the basic notion is to sample a homogeneous set of items from a hypothetical universe of items.
- In generating items, a number of decisions must be made, including how many items to generate (typically a large number initially), what continuum to use for the response options, how many response options there should be, whether to include positive and negative item stems, how intensely worded the items will be, and what to do about references to time.
- Items should be inspected for clarity, length, and avoidance of jargon and double negatives; the scale's **readability** should also be assessed.
- External review of the preliminary pool of items should be undertaken, including review by members of the target population (e.g., via a small pretest that could include **cognitive questioning**).
- **Content validity** should be built into the scale through careful efforts to conceptualize the construct and through content validation by a panel of experts—including the calculation of a quantitative index such as the CVI to summarize the experts' judgments of the relevance of scale items.
- Once content validity has been established at a satisfactory level, the scale must be administered to a development sample—typically 300 or more respondents who are representative of the target population.
- Data collected from the development sample are then analyzed using a number of techniques, including **item analysis** (e.g., a scrutiny of **interitem correlations** and **item-scale correlations**), **exploratory factor analysis (EFA)**, internal consistency analysis, and test–retest reliability analysis.
- EFA is used to reduce a large set of variables into a smaller set of underlying dimensions, called **factors**. Mathematically, each factor is a linear combination of variables in a data matrix.
- The first phase of EFA (**factor extraction**) identifies clusters of items that are strongly intercorrelated and helps to define the number of underlying dimensions in the items. A widely used factor extraction method is **principal components analysis (PCA)**; another method is **principal axis factor analysis.**
- The second phase of factor analysis involves **factor rotation**, which enhances the interpretability of the factors by aligning items more distinctly with a particular factor. Rotation can be either **orthogonal** (which maintains the independence of the factors) or **oblique** (which allows correlated factors). **Factor loadings** of the items on the rotated factor matrix are used to interpret and name the factors.
- After the scale is finalized based on the preliminary analyses, steps are taken to validate the scale, using a variety of validation techniques; one widely used approach to assess structural validity is **confirmatory factor analysis (CFA).**
- CFA involves tests of a **measurement model**, which stipulates the hypothesized relationship between latent traits and *manifest variables* (items). CFA is a subset of sophisticated statistical techniques called **structural equation modeling.**
- The **interpretability** of scale scores can be enhanced using such approaches as computing **percentiles**, converting raw scores to **standard scores** and developing **norms** and meaningful **cutoff points.**

REFERENCES CITED IN CHAPTER 16

AERA, APA, & NCME Joint Committee. (2014). *Standards for educational and psychological testing* (5th rev.). American Psychological Association.

Anthony, M., Yastik, J., MacDonald, D., & Marshall, K. (2014). Development and validation of a tool to measure incivility in clinical nursing education. *Journal of Professional Nursing, 30,* 48–55.

Beck, C. T., & Gable, R. K. (2000). Postpartum depression screening scale: Development and psychometric testing. *Nursing Research, 49,* 272–282.

Beck, C. T., & Gable, R. K. (2001). Further validation of the postpartum depression screening scale. *Nursing Research, 50,* 155–164.

Beck, C. T., & Gable, R. K. (2003). Postpartum depression screening scale: Spanish version. *Nursing Research, 52,* 296–306.

Beck, C. T., & Gable, R. K. (2005). Screening performance of the postpartum depression screening scale—Spanish version. *Journal of Transcultural Nursing, 16*, 331–338.

Bott, M., Karanevich, A., Garrard, L., Price, L., Mudaranthakam, D., & Gajewski, B. (2018). Confirmatory factor analysis alternative: Free, accessible CBID software. *Western Journal of Nursing Research, 40*, 257–269.

Brown, T. (2015). *Confirmatory factor analysis for applied research* (2nd ed.). Guilford Press.

Conway, A., Chang, K., Kamboj, N., & Sutherland, J. (2021). Development and validation of the Nursing Confidence in Managing Sedation Complications Scale. *Nursing Open, 8*(3), 1135–1144. https://doi.org/10.1002/nop2.725

Davis, D. L., Creedy, D. K., Bradfield, Z., Newnham, E., Atchan, M., Davie, L., McAra-Couper, J., Graham, K., Griffiths, C., Sweet, L., & Stulz, V. (2021). Development of the Woman-Centred Care Scale-Midwife Self Report (WCCS-MSR). *BMC Pregnancy and Childbirth, 21*(1), 523. https://doi.org/10.1186/s12884-021-03987-z

De Alencar, A., Arraes, L., de Albuquerque, E., & Alves, J. (2009). Effect of kangaroo mother care on postpartum depression. *Journal of Tropical Pediatrics, 55*, 36–38.

DeVellis, R. F. & Thorpe, C. T. (2022). *Scale development: Theory and application* (5th ed.). Sage Publications.

Hegedus, K. S., & Beck, C. T. (2012). Development and psychometric testing of the postpartum depression screening scale: Hungarian version. *International Journal for Human Caring, 16*, 54–58.

Hilton, A., & Skrutkowski, M. (2002). Translating instruments into other language: Development and testing processes. *Cancer Nursing, 25*, 1–7.

Karaçam, Z., & Kitiş, Y. (2008). The postpartum depression screening scale: Its reliability and validity for the Turkish population. *Türk Psikiyatri Dergesi, 19*, 187–196.

Kline, R. B. (2016). *Principles and practice of structural equation modeling* (4th ed.). The Guilford Press.

Lara, M., Navarette, L., Navarro, C., & Le, H. (2013). Evaluation of the psychometric measures for the postpartum depression screening scale—Spanish version for Mexican women. *Journal of Transcultural Nursing, 24*, 378–386.

Lee, S. (2021). Exploratory factor analysis for a Nursing Workaround Instrument in Korean and interpretations of statistical decision points. *Computers, Informatics, Nursing: CIN, 39*(6), 329–339. https://doi.org/10.1097/CIN.0000000000000693

Mokkink, L. B., Terwee, C., Patrick, D., Alonso, J., Stratford, P., Knol, D. L., … DeVet, H. (2010). The COSMIN study reached international consensus on taxonomy, terminology, and definitions of measurement properties for health-related patient-reported outcomes. *Journal of Clinical Epidemiology, 63*, 737–745.

Nunnally, J., & Bernstein, I. H. (1994). *Psychometric theory* (3rd ed.). McGraw-Hill.

Polit, D. F. (2010). *Statistics and data analysis for nursing research* (2nd ed.). Pearson.

Polit, D. F. (2014). Getting serious about test-retest reliability: A critique of retest research and some recommendations. *Quality of Life Research, 23*, 1713–1720.

Polit, D., Beck, C., & Owen, S. (2007). Is the CVI an acceptable indicator of content validity? Appraisal and recommendations. *Research in Nursing & Health, 30*, 459–467.

Polit, D. F., & Yang, F. M. (2016). *Measurement and the measurement of change: A primer for health professionals.* Lippincott.

Rowe, H., Sperlich, M., Cameron, H., & Seng, J. (2014). A quasi-experimental outcomes analysis of a psychoeducation intervention for pregnant women with abuse-related posttraumatic stress. *Journal of Obstetric, Gynecologic, and Neonatal Nursing, 43*, 282–293.

Sachdev, P., Freeland-Graves, J., & Babaei, M. (2020). Development and validation of the Dental Nutrition Knowledge Competency Scale for low-income women. *Public Health Nutrition, 23*(4), 691–700. https://doi.org/10.1017/S1368980019002714

Sia, T., Connors, K. A., & Morgan, P. (2023). Physical activity in people with motor neuron disease: Validity of the Physical Activity Scale for the elderly as a measuring tool. *Archives of Pphysical Medicine and Rehabilitation, 104*(1), 102–107. https://doi.org/10.1016/j.apmr.2022.09.007

Streiner, D. L., Norman, G. R., & Cairney, J. (2015). *Health measurement scales: A practical guide to their development and use* (5th ed.). Oxford University Press.

Terwee, C. B., Mokkink, L. B., Knol, D. L., Ostelo, R., Bouter, L. M., & DeVet, H. C. W. (2012). Rating the methodological quality in systematic reviews of studies on measurement properties: A scoring system for the COSMIN checklist. *Quality of Life Research, 21*, 651–657.

Walker, L. O., & Avant, K. C. (2019). *Strategies for theory construction in nursing* (6th ed.). Prentice Hall.

Winquist, A., Schenk, E. C., Cook, C., Demorest, S., & Burduli, E. (2023). Climate, Health, and Nursing Tool (CHANT): A confirmatory factor analysis. *Public Health Nursing (Boston, Mass.), 40*(2), 306–312. https://doi.org/10.1111/phn.13161

Zhang, J., Zhou, X., Wang, H., Luo, Y., & Li, W. (2021). Development and validation of the Humanistic Practice Ability of Nursing Scale. *Asian Nursing Research, 15*(2), 105–112. https://doi.org/10.1016/j.anr.2020.12.003

Zhao, Y., Munro-Kramer, M. L., Shi, S., Wang, J., & Luo, J. (2018). A longitudinal study of perinatal depression among Chinese high-risk pregnant women. *Women and Birth, 31*, e395–e402.

17 | Descriptive Statistics

Learning outcomes

1. Describe the various levels of measurement.
2. Understand the different types of descriptive statistics.
3. Identify various ways to display descriptive statistics.
4. Articulate the differences in risk predictions.

INTRODUCTION

Statistical analysis enables researchers to organize and communicate numeric information. Mathematic skill is not required to grasp basic statistics—only logical thinking ability is needed. In this book, we focus on explaining which statistics to use in different situations, and on how to understand what statistical results mean.

Statistics can be descriptive or inferential. **Descriptive statistics** are used to describe and synthesize data—for example, percentages are descriptive statistics. When a descriptive index is calculated from population data, it is a **parameter**. A descriptive index from a sample is a **statistic**. Research questions are about parameters, but researchers calculate statistics to estimate them and use **inferential statistics** to make inferences about the population. This chapter discusses descriptive statistics, and Chapter 18 focuses on inferential statistics. We first discuss levels of measurement because analytic options depend on how variables are measured.

LEVELS OF MEASUREMENT

Scientists have developed a system for classifying measures. The four **levels of measurement** are nominal, ordinal, interval, and ratio.

Nominal Measurement

The lowest level of measurement is **nominal measurement**, which involves assigning numbers to classify characteristics into categories. Examples of variables amenable to nominal measurement include gender, blood type, and marital status.

The numbers used in nominal measurement have no quantitative meaning. If we code married people as 1 and not married people as 2, the number 2 does not mean "more than" 1. The numbers are only symbols representing different values of marital status. We easily could use 1 for not married, 2 for married. Nominal measurement provides no information about an attribute except equivalence. If we were to "measure" the gender of Nate, Alan, Cathy, and Diane by assigning them the codes 1, 1, 2, and 2, respectively, this means Nate and Alan are equivalent on the gender attribute but are not equivalent to Cathy and Diane.

Nominal measures must have categories that are mutually exclusive and collectively exhaustive. For example, if we were measuring blood type, we might use these codes: 1 = A, 2 = B, and 3 = O. The requirement for collective exhaustiveness would not be met if there were people in a sample whose blood type was AB. Numbers in nominal measurement cannot be treated mathematically. It is not meaningful to calculate the average marital status of a sample, but we can compute percentages. In a sample of 50 patients with 30 not married and 20 married, we could say that 60% were not married and 40% were married.

Ordinal Measurement

Ordinal measurement involves sorting people based on their relative ranking on an attribute. This measurement level goes beyond categorization: Attributes are *ordered* according to some criterion. Ordinal measurement captures not only equivalence but also relative rank.

Consider this ordinal scheme for measuring ability to perform activities of daily living: (1) completely dependent, (2) needs another person's assistance, (3) needs mechanical assistance, and (4) completely independent. The numbers signify incremental ability to perform activities of daily living. People coded 4 are equivalent to each other with regard to functional ability *and*, relative to those in the other categories, have more of the attribute.

Ordinal measurement does not, however, tell us anything about how much greater one level is than another. We do not know if being completely independent is twice as good as needing mechanical assistance. Nor do we know if the difference between needing another person's assistance and needing mechanical assistance is the same as that between needing mechanical assistance and being completely independent. Ordinal measurement tells us only the relative ranking of the attribute's levels.

As with nominal measures, mathematic operations with ordinal-level data are restricted—for example, averages are usually meaningless. Frequency counts, percentages, and several other statistics to be discussed later are appropriate for ordinal-level data.

Interval Measurement

Interval measurement occurs when researchers can assume equivalent distance between rank-ordering on an attribute. The Fahrenheit temperature scale is an example: a temperature of 60°F is 10°F warmer than 50°F. A 10°F difference similarly separates 40°F and 30°F, and the two differences in temperature are equivalent. Interval-level measures are more informative than ordinal ones, but interval measures do not communicate absolute magnitude. For example, we cannot say that 60°F is twice as hot as 30°F. The Fahrenheit scale uses an arbitrary zero point: zero degrees does not signify an absence of heat. Most psychosocial scales are assumed to yield interval-level data.

Interval scales expand analytic possibilities—in particular, interval-level data can be averaged meaningfully. It is reasonable, for example, to compute an average daily body temperature for hospital patients.

Ratio Measurement

Ratio measurement provides information about ordering on the critical attribute, the intervals between objects, *and* the absolute magnitude of the attribute because there is a rational, meaningful zero. Many physical measures provide ratio-level data. A person's weight, for example, is measured on a ratio scale. We can say that someone who weighs 200 lb is twice as heavy as someone who weighs 100 lb.

Because ratio measures have an absolute zero, all arithmetic operations are permissible. Statistical procedures suitable for interval-level data are also appropriate for ratio-level data.

> **Example of Different Measurement Levels**
> Chen and colleagues (2022) conducted a randomized control trial to test the impact of a web-based self-care program to promote healthy lifestyles and control blood pressure in patients with primary hypertension. The presence vs. absence of comorbidities (e.g., diabetes, gout), marital status, living situation, and employment status were dichotomous nominal-level variables. Measures of the duration of having hypertension and number of medications to treat hypertension were captured as ordinal variables (e.g., 0, 1–4, 5–11, or 12+). The body mass index was a ratio-level variable.

TIP Nominal-level measures are often called *categorical*. Variables measured on an interval- or ratio-level scale are often called *continuous* variables.

Comparison of the Levels

The four levels of measurement form a hierarchy, with ratio scales at the top and nominal measurement at the base. Moving from a higher to a lower level of measurement results in an information loss. For example, if we measured a female's weight in pounds, this would be a ratio measure. If we categorized the weights into three groups (e.g., under 125, 125–175, and 176+), this would be an ordinal measure. With this scheme, we would not be able to differentiate a female who weighed 125 from one who weighed 175 lb—we have much less information with ordinal information. This example illustrates another point: With information at one level, it is possible to convert data to a lower level, but the converse is not true. If we were given only the ordinal measurements, we could not reconstruct actual weights.

It is not always easy to identify a variable's level of measurement. Nominal and ratio measures usually are discernible, but the distinction between ordinal and interval measures is more problematic. Some methodologists argue that most psychological measures that are treated as interval measures are really ordinal measures. Although instruments such as Likert scales produce data that are, strictly speaking, ordinal, many analysts believe that treating them as interval measures results in too few errors to warrant using less powerful statistical procedures.

TIP In operationalizing variables, it is best to use the highest measurement level possible because they are more powerful and precise. Sometimes, however, group membership is more informative than continuous scores, especially for clinicians who need "cutpoints" for making decisions. For example, for some purposes, it may be more relevant to designate infants as being of low vs. normal birth weight (nominal level) than to use actual birth weight values (ratio level). But it is best to *measure* at the higher level and then convert to a lower level if appropriate.

FREQUENCY DISTRIBUTIONS

When quantitative data are unanalyzed, it is difficult to discern even general trends. Consider the 60 numbers in Table 17.1, which are fictitious scores of 60 patients on a six-item anxiety scale—scores that we will consider as interval level. Inspection of the numbers does not help us understand patients' anxiety. A set of data can be described in terms of three characteristics: the shape of the distribution of values, central tendency, and variability. In this section, we focus on a distribution's shape.

Constructing Frequency Distributions

Frequency distributions are used to organize numeric data. A **frequency distribution** is a systematic arrangement of values from lowest to highest, together with a count of the number of times each value was obtained. Our 60 anxiety scores are shown in a frequency distribution in Table 17.2. We can readily see the highest and lowest scores, the most common score, where the bulk of scores clustered, and how many patients were in the sample (total sample size is typically depicted as *N*). None of this was apparent before we organized the data.

TABLE 17.1 • Patients' Anxiety Scores

22	27	25	19	24	25	23	29	24	20
26	16	20	26	17	22	24	18	26	28
15	24	23	22	21	24	20	25	18	27
24	23	16	25	30	29	27	21	23	24
26	18	30	21	17	25	22	24	29	28
20	25	26	24	23	19	27	28	25	26

CHAPTER 17 Descriptive Statistics • **365**

TABLE 17.2 • Frequency Distribution of Patients' Anxiety Scores

SCORE (X)	FREQUENCY (F)	PERCENTAGE (%)
15	1	1.7
16	2	3.3
17	2	3.3
18	3	5.0
19	2	3.3
20	4	6.7
21	3	5.0
22	4	6.7
23	5	8.3
24	9	15.0
25	7	11.7
26	6	10.0
27	4	6.7
28	3	5.0
29	3	5.0
30	2	3.3
	$N = 60 = \sum f$	$\sum\% = 100.0\%$

Frequency distributions consist of two parts: observed score values (the Xs) and the frequency of cases at each value (the fs). Scores are listed in order in one column, and corresponding frequencies are listed in another. The sum of numbers in the frequency column must equal the sample size. In less verbal terms, $\sum f = N$, which means the sum of (signified by Greek sigma, $\sum$) the frequencies (f) equals the sample size (N).

It is useful to display percentages for each value, as shown in column 3 of Table 17.2. Just as the sum of all frequencies should equal N, the sum of all percentages should equal 100.

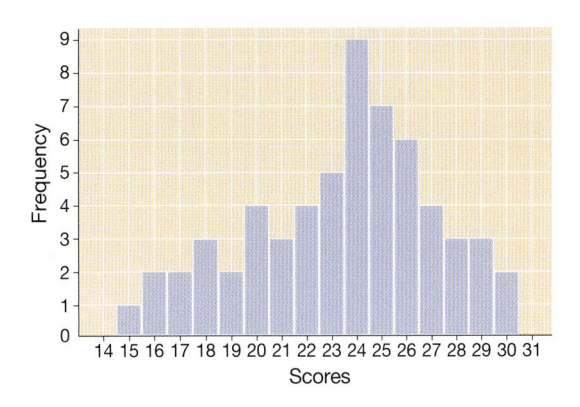

FIGURE 17.1 Histogram of patients' anxiety scores.

Frequency data can be displayed graphically. Graphs for displaying interval- and ratio-level data include **histograms** and **frequency polygons**, which are constructed in a similar fashion. First, score values are arrayed on a horizontal (X) axis, with the lowest value on the left, ascending to the highest value on the right. Frequencies or percentages are displayed vertically. A histogram is constructed by drawing bars above the score classes to the height corresponding to the frequency for that score. Figure 17.1 shows a histogram for the anxiety score data. Frequency polygons are similar, but dots corresponding to the frequencies are placed above each score (Figure 17.2). The dots are connected by straight lines and show the distribution's shape.

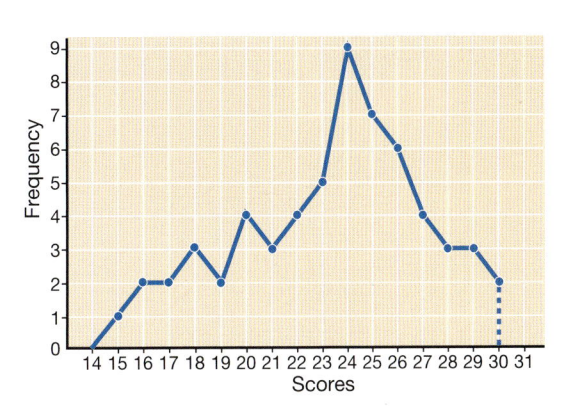

FIGURE 17.2 Frequency polygon of patients' anxiety scores.

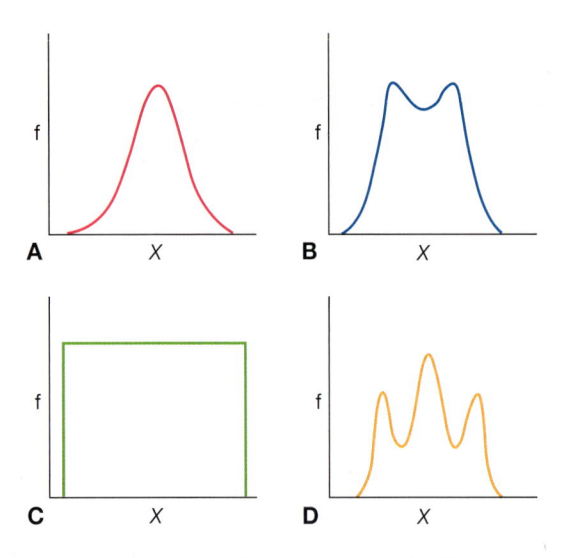

FIGURE 17.3 Examples of symmetric distributions.

Shapes of Distributions

A distribution is **symmetric** if, when folded over, the two halves are superimposed. All the distributions in Figure 17.3 are symmetric. With real data sets, distributions are rarely perfectly symmetric, but minor discrepancies are ignored in characterizing a distribution's shape.

In **skewed** (asymmetric) distributions, the peak is off center and one tail is longer than the other. When the longer tail points to the right, the distribution is **positively skewed** (Figure 17.4A). Personal income, for example, is positively skewed. Most people have low to moderate incomes, with relatively few high-income people in the tail. If the tail points to the left, the distribution is **negatively skewed** (Figure 17.4B). Age at death is negatively skewed: most people are at the upper end of the distribution, with relatively few dying at an early age. Patients' anxiety scores (Figure 17.2) were negatively skewed—high scores were more common than low ones.

Modality is a second aspect of a distribution's shape. A **unimodal distribution** has only one peak (i.e., a value with high frequency), whereas a **multimodal distribution** has two or more peaks. A distribution with two peaks is **bimodal**. Figure 17.3A is unimodal, and Figure 17.3B and D illustrate multimodal distributions. Symmetry and modality are independent: skewness is unrelated to how many peaks a distribution has.

Some distributions have special names. Of particular importance is the **normal distribution** (sometimes called a *Gaussian distribution* or *bell-shaped curve*). A normal distribution is symmetric, unimodal, and not too peaked (Figure 17.3A). Many human attributes (e.g., height, intelligence) approximate a normal distribution.

CENTRAL TENDENCY

Frequency distributions are a good way to clarify data patterns, but often a pattern is of less interest than an overall summary. Researchers ask such questions as, "What is the average body temperature of infants during bathing?" or "What is the average weight loss of patients with cancer?" Such questions

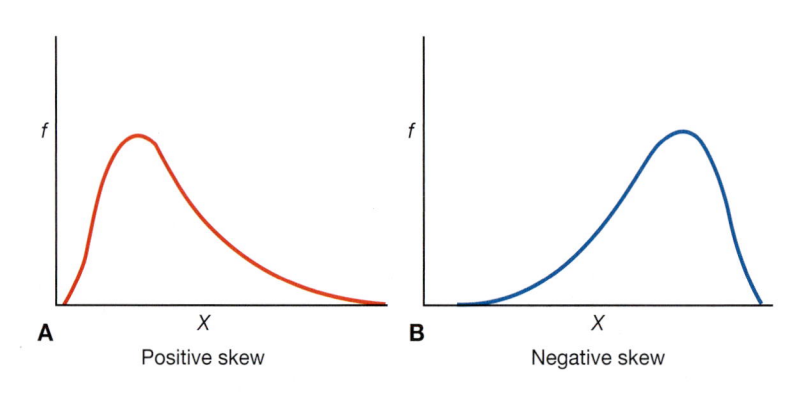

A Positive skew

B Negative skew

FIGURE 17.4 Examples of skewed distributions.

seek a single number to best represent a distribution. Because an index of typicalness is more likely to come from the center of a distribution than from an extreme, such indexes are called measures of **central tendency**. Lay people use the term *average* to designate central tendency. Researchers avoid this term because there are three indexes of central tendency: the mode, the median, and the mean.

The Mode

The **mode** is the most frequently occurring score value in a distribution. In the following distribution, the mode is 53:

50 51 51 52 53 53 53 53 54 55 56

The score of 53 occurred four times, a higher frequency than for any other score. The mode of patients' anxiety scores (Table 17.2) is 24. In multimodal distributions, there is more than one score value with high frequencies. Modes are a quick way to determine a "popular" score, but they are rather unstable. By *unstable*, we mean that modes tend to fluctuate from sample to sample drawn from the same population.

The Median

The **median** is the point in a distribution above and below which 50% of cases fall. As an example, consider the following set of values:

2 2 3 3 4 5 6 7 8 9

The value that divides the cases exactly in half is 4.5, the median for this set of numbers. The point that has 50% of the cases above and below it is halfway between 4 and 5. For the patient anxiety scores, the median is 24. An important characteristic of the median is that it does not take into account the quantitative values of scores—it is an index of average *position* in a distribution and is thus insensitive to extremes. In the above set of numbers, if the value of 9 were changed to 99, the median would remain 4.5. Because of this property, the median is often a preferred index of central tendency with skewed distributions. In research reports, the median may be abbreviated as **Md** or **Mdn**.

The Mean

The **mean,** often symbolized as M or $\overline{X}$, is the sum of all scores divided by the number of scores. The mean is what people usually refer to as the *average*. The mean of the patients' anxiety scores is 23.4 (1,405 ÷ 60). Let us compute the mean weight of eight people with the following weights: 85, 109, 120, 135, 158, 177, 181, and 195:

$$\overline{X} = \frac{85+109+120+135+158+177+181+195}{8} = 145$$

Unlike the median, the mean is affected by every score. If we were to exchange the 195-lb person in this example for one weighing 275 lb, the mean would increase from 145 to 155. Such a substitution would leave the median unchanged.

The mean is the most widely used measure of central tendency. When researchers work with interval-level or ratio-level measurements, the mean, rather than the median or mode, is usually the statistic reported.

Comparison of the Mode, Median, and Mean

The mean is the most stable index of central tendency. If repeated samples were drawn from a population, means would fluctuate less than modes or medians. Sometimes, however, the primary interest is to understand what is typical, in which case a median might be preferred. If we wanted to know about the economic well-being of U.S. citizens, for example, we would get a distorted impression by considering mean income, which would be inflated by the wealth of a minority. The median would better reflect how a typical person fares financially.

When a distribution is symmetric and unimodal, the three indexes of central tendency coincide. In skewed distributions, the values of the mode, median, and mean differ. The mean is always pulled in the direction of the long tail, as shown in Figure 17.5. A variable's level of measurement plays a role in determining the appropriate index of central tendency to use. In general, the mode is most suitable for nominal measures, the mode

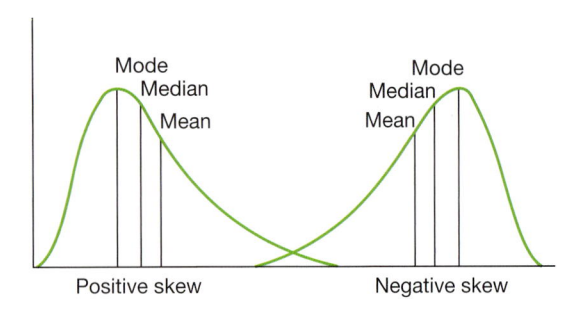

FIGURE 17.5 Relationships of central tendency indexes in skewed distributions.

or median is appropriate for ordinal measures, and the mean is appropriate for interval and ratio measures.

VARIABILITY

Two distributions with identical means could differ in **variability**—how spread out or dispersed the data are. Consider the two distributions in Figure 17.6, which represent fictitious scores for students from two schools on an IQ test. Both distributions have a mean of 100, but the score patterns differ. School A has a wide range of scores, from below 70 to above 130. In school B, by contrast, there are few low scores and few high scores. School A is more **heterogeneous** (i.e., more variable) than school B, and school B is more **homogeneous** than school A.

Researchers compute an index of variability to express the extent to which scores in a distribution differ from one another. Two common indexes are the range and standard deviation.

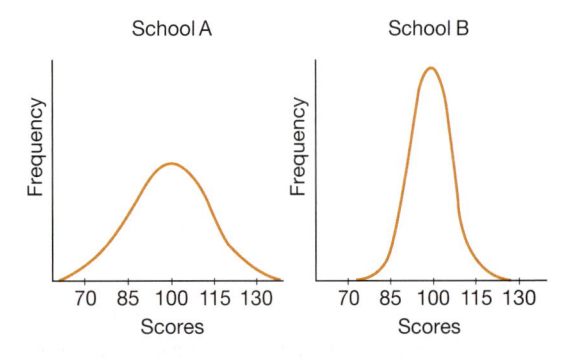

FIGURE 17.6 Two distributions of different variability.

The Range

The **range** is simply the highest score minus the lowest score in a distribution. In the example of patients' anxiety scores, the range is 15 (30 − 15). In the examples shown in Figure 17.6, the range for school A is about 80 (140 − 60), and the range for school B is about 50 (125 − 75).

The chief virtue of the range is computational ease, but, being based on only two scores, the range is unstable. From sample to sample from a population, the range tends to fluctuate widely. Another limitation is that the range ignores variations in scores between the two extremes. In school B of Figure 17.6, suppose one student obtained a score of 60 and another obtained a score of 140. The range of both schools would then be 80, despite clear differences in heterogeneity. For these reasons, the range is used mainly as a crude descriptive index.

> **TIP** Another index of variability is called the *interquartile range* (*IQR*), which is calculated based on *quartiles*. The IQR indicates the range of scores within which the middle 50% of score values lie. IQRs are infrequently reported but play a role in detecting extreme values (*outliers*).

The Standard Deviation

The most widely used measure of variability is the standard deviation. The **standard deviation** indicates the *average amount* of deviation of values from the mean and is calculated using every score. In research reports, the standard deviation is often abbreviated as **SD**.

A variability index needs to capture the degree to which scores deviate from one another. This concept of deviation is represented in the range by the minus sign, which produces an index of deviation, or difference, between two score points. The standard deviation is also based on score differences. In fact, the first step in calculating a standard deviation is to compute deviation scores for each score. A **deviation score** (symbolized as x) is the difference between an individual score and the mean. If a person weighed 150 lb and the sample mean were 140, then the person's deviation score would be +10.

Because we want an *average* deviation, you might think that a good variability index could be computed by summing all deviation scores and then dividing by the number of cases. The problem is that the sum of a set of deviation scores is always zero. Table 17.3 presents deviation scores for nine numbers. As shown in the second column, the sum of the xs is zero. Deviations above the mean always balance exactly deviations below the mean.

The standard deviation overcomes this problem by having each deviation score squared before summing. After dividing by the number of cases (minus 1), the square root is taken to bring the index back to the original unit of measurement. The formula for the standard deviation is:

$$SD = \sqrt{\frac{\sum x^2}{N-1}}$$

TIP For calculating the *SD* of a *population*, the formula has *N* rather than *N* − 1 in the denominator. Differences in the results from the two formulas are negligible unless the sample size is small. Statistical programs use *N* − 1 to compute *SD*s.

A standard deviation has been worked out for the data in Table 17.3. First, a deviation score is calculated for each of the nine raw scores by subtracting the mean ($\overline{X} = 7$) from them. Each deviation score is squared (column 3), converting all values to positive numbers. The squared deviation scores are summed ($\sum x^2 = 28$), divided by 8 ($N - 1$), and a square root taken to yield an *SD* of 1.87.

TIP The standard deviation often is shown in relation to the mean without a formal label. For example, patients' anxiety scores might be shown as $M = 23.4\ (3.7)$ or $M = 23.4 \pm 3.7$, where 23.4 is the mean and 3.7 is the standard deviation.

A related variability index is the **variance**, which is the value of the standard deviation before taking the square root. In other words, variance = SD^2. In our example, the variance is 1.87^2 or 3.50. The variance is rarely reported because it is not in the same unit of measurement as the original data, but it is important in statistical tests we discuss in Chapter 18.

A standard deviation is more difficult to interpret than other statistics, such as the mean. In our example, we calculated $SD = 1.87$. One might ask, 1.87 *what?* What does the number mean? First, the standard deviation is a variability index for a set of scores. If two distributions had a mean of 25.0, but one had an *SD* of 7.0 and the other had an *SD* of 3.0, we would know that the first sample was more heterogeneous.

Second, think of a standard deviation as an average of deviations from the mean. The mean tells us the single best value for summarizing a distribution; a standard deviation tells us how much, on average, scores deviate from that mean. A standard deviation can thus be interpreted as our degree of error when we use a mean to describe the entire sample.

TABLE 17.3 • Computation of a Standard Deviation

X	$x = X - \overline{X}$	$x^2 = (X - \overline{X})^2$
4	−3	9
5	−2	4
6	−1	1
7	0	0
7	0	0
7	0	0
8	1	1
9	2	4
10	3	9
$\sum X = 63$	$\sum x = 0$	$\sum x^2 = 28$
$\overline{X} = 7$		

$$SD = \sqrt{\frac{28}{8}} = \sqrt{3.50} = 1.87$$

The standard deviation can also be used to interpret individual scores in a distribution. Suppose we had weight data from a sample whose mean weight was 150 lb with $SD = 10$. The SD provides a *standard* of variability. Weights greater than 1 SD away from the mean (i.e., greater than 160 or less than 140 lb) are at a greater than the average "distance" from the mean.

In normal distributions, there are roughly 3 SDs above and 3 SDs below the mean. To illustrate, suppose we had normally distributed scores with a mean of 50 and an SD of 10 (Figure 17.7). In a normal distribution, a fixed percentage of cases falls within certain distances from the mean. Sixty-eight percent of cases fall within 1 SD of the mean (34% above and 34% below the mean). In our example, nearly 7 out of 10 scores fall between 40 and 60. Ninety-five percent of scores in a normal distribution fall within 2 SDs from the mean. Only a handful of cases—about 2% at each extreme—lie more than 2 SDs from the mean. In the figure, we can see that a person with a score of 70 had a higher score than about 98% of the sample.

In summary, the SD is a useful variability index for describing a distribution and interpreting individual scores. Like the mean, the standard deviation is a stable estimate of a parameter and is the preferred index of a distribution's variability.

TIP Descriptive statistics (e.g., percentages, means, standard deviations) are most often used to summarize sample characteristics, describe key research variables, and document methodologic features (e.g., response rates), rather than to answer research questions; inferential statistics (Chapter 18) are used for this purpose.

Example of Descriptive Statistics
Banister and colleagues (2022) studied the nursing documentation of patients hospitalized with COVID-19 to identify types and frequency of nurse-sensitive indicators, including social determinants of health. The authors provided descriptive information about the characteristics of the 94 patients in the sample. For example, their mean age was 58, 58.5% identified as an underrepresented racial group, 34.4% required interpreter services, and all but 3.2% were insured on public or private insurance.

BIVARIATE DESCRIPTIVE STATISTICS

The mean, mode, and standard deviation are **univariate** (one-variable) **descriptive statistics** that describe one variable at a time. Most research is about relationships between variables, and **bivariate** (two-variable) **descriptive statistics** describe such relationships, often through crosstabs tables and correlation indexes.

Crosstabs Tables

A **crosstabs table** (or *contingency table*) is a two-dimensional frequency distribution in which the frequencies of two variables are crosstabulated. Suppose we had data on patients' gender (male–female) and whether they were nonsmokers, light smokers (<1 pack of cigarettes a day), or heavy smokers (≥1 pack a day). The question is whether there is a tendency for males to smoke more heavily than females or vice versa (i.e., whether there is a relationship between smoking and gender).

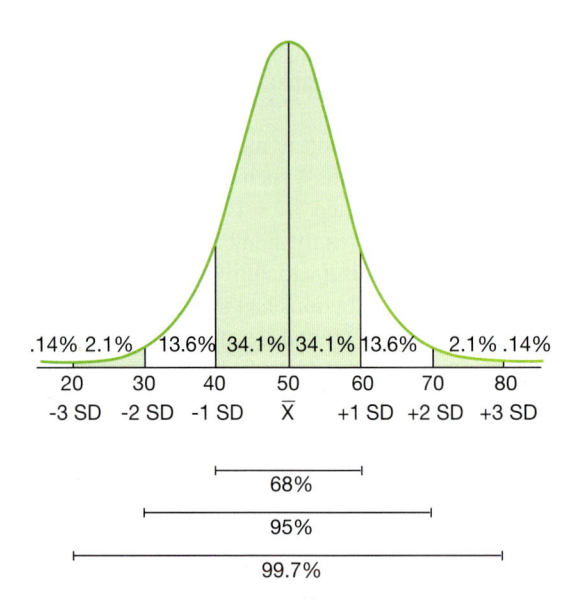

FIGURE 17.7 Standard deviations (SDs) in a normal distribution.

Fictitious data on these two variables are shown in Table 17.4. Six **cells** are created by placing one variable (gender) on one dimension and the other variable (smoking status) on the other. Each sample member is allocated to a cell based on their status on the two variables. For example, a female who does not smoke would be counted in the upper left of the six cells. After all participants are allocated to the appropriate cells, percentages are computed. The crosstab allows us to see that, in this sample, females were more likely than males to be nonsmokers (45.4% vs. 27.3%) and less likely to be heavy smokers (18.2% vs. 36.4%). Crosstabs tables are used with nominal data or ordinal data with few ranks. In the present example, gender is nominal, and smoking status, as defined, is ordinal.

Crosstabs tables are easy to construct by hand or by commands to a computer. A key issue is which variable to put in the rows and which in the columns. Crosstabs tables are often set up such that the percentages in a column add to 100%, as in Table 17.4. However, cell percentages can be computed based on either row totals or column totals. In Table 17.4, the number 10 in the first cell (nonsmoking females) was divided by the *column* total (i.e., total number of females—22) to arrive at the percentage of females who were nonsmokers (45.4%). This cell *could* have shown 62.5%—the percentage of nonsmokers who were females (10 ÷ 16). Thus, care must be taken in reading crosstabs tables.

Example of Crosstabulations
Skinner and Sogstad (2022) examined the different types of informal care provided by and caregivers in a Norwegian population across socio-demographic groups. Crosstabulations allowed them to examine the characteristics of the caregivers and the types of care provided. The types of care were personal care, keeping companionship, practical help, and companionship together and practical help only. They found that although females provided more personal care than males, there were no statistically significant differences between the type of care provided and gender.

Correlation

Relationships between two variables are usually described through **correlation** procedures. Correlation coefficients, briefly described in Chapter 15, can be computed with two variables measured on the ordinal, interval, or ratio scale. The correlation question is: To what extent are two variables related to each other? For example, to what degree are anxiety scores and blood pressure readings correlated?

Correlations between two variables can be graphed on a **scatter plot** (*scatter diagram*) using a coordinate graph. Values for one variable (*X*) are scaled on the horizontal axis, and values for the other variable (*Y*) are scaled vertically (Figure 17.8). This graph presents data for 10 people (a–j). For person a, the values for *X* and *Y* are 2 and 1, respectively. To graph person a's position, we go two units to the

TABLE 17.4 • Contingency Table for Gender and Smoking Status Relationship

SMOKING STATUS	N	FEMALES %	FEMALES N	MALES %	MALES N	TOTAL %
Nonsmoker	10	45.4	6	27.3	16	36.4
Light smoker	8	36.4	8	36.4	16	36.4
Heavy smoker	4	18.2	8	36.4	12	27.3
TOTAL	22	100.0	22	100.0	44	100.0

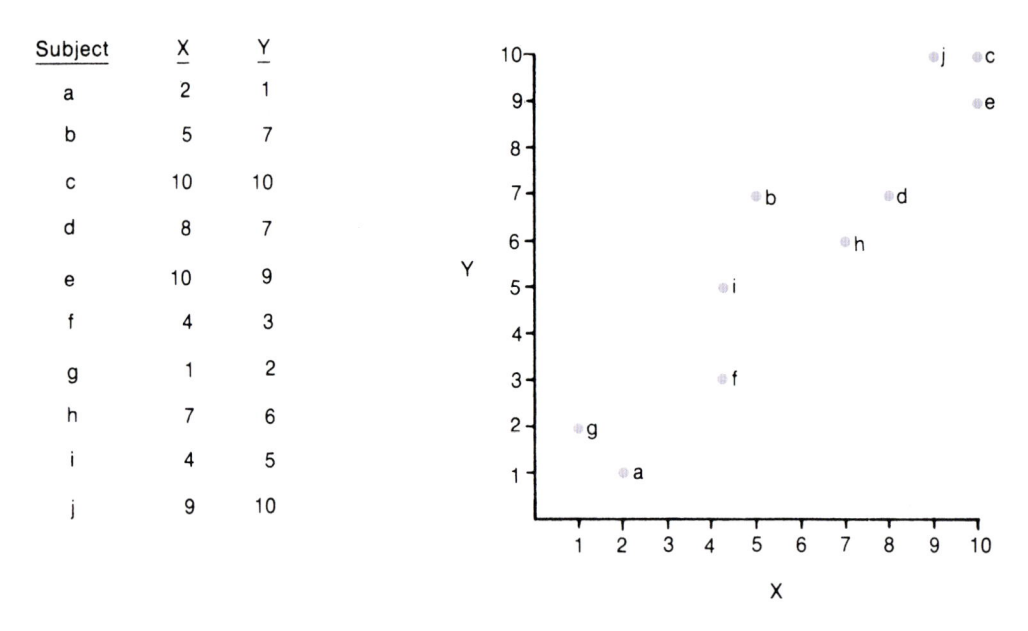

Subject	X	Y
a	2	1
b	5	7
c	10	10
d	8	7
e	10	9
f	4	3
g	1	2
h	7	6
i	4	5
j	9	10

FIGURE 17.8 Construction of a scatter plot.

right along the *X* axis and one unit up on the *Y* axis. The letters on the plot are shown to help identify individuals, but normally only dots appear.

In a scatter plot, the direction of the slope of points indicates the direction of the correlation. A positive correlation occurs when high values on one variable are associated with high values on a second variable. If the slope of points begins at the lower left corner and extends to the upper right corner, the relationship is positive. In the current example, *X* and *Y* are positively related. People with high scores on variable *X* tended to have high scores on variable *Y*, and low scorers on *X* tended to score low on *Y*.

A negative relationship is one in which high values on one variable are related to low values on the other. Negative relationships on a scatter plot are depicted by points that slope from the upper left corner to the lower right corner, as in Figure 17.9A and D.

When relationships are *perfect*, it is possible to predict perfectly the value of one variable by knowing the value of the second. For instance, if all people who were 6 feet 2 in tall weighed 180 lb, all people who were 6 feet 1 in tall weighed 175 lb, and so on, then weight and height would be perfectly, positively related. In such a situation, we would only need to know a person's height to know the person's weight. On a scatter plot, a perfect relationship is represented by a sloped straight line (Figure 17.9C). When a relationship is not perfect, as is usually the case, one can interpret the *degree* of correlation by seeing how closely the points cluster around a straight line. The closer the points are around a diagonal slope, the stronger the correlation. When the points are scattered all over the graph, the relationship is low or nonexistent. Various degrees and directions of relationships are shown in Figure 17.9.

It is more efficient to express relationships by computing a correlation coefficient, an index with values ranging from −1.00 for a perfect negative correlation, through zero for no relationship, to +1.00 for a perfect positive correlation. The higher the absolute value of the coefficient (i.e., the value disregarding the sign), the stronger the relationship. A correlation of −0.30, for instance, is stronger than a correlation of +0.20.

The most widely used correlation index is the **product-moment correlation coefficient**, also

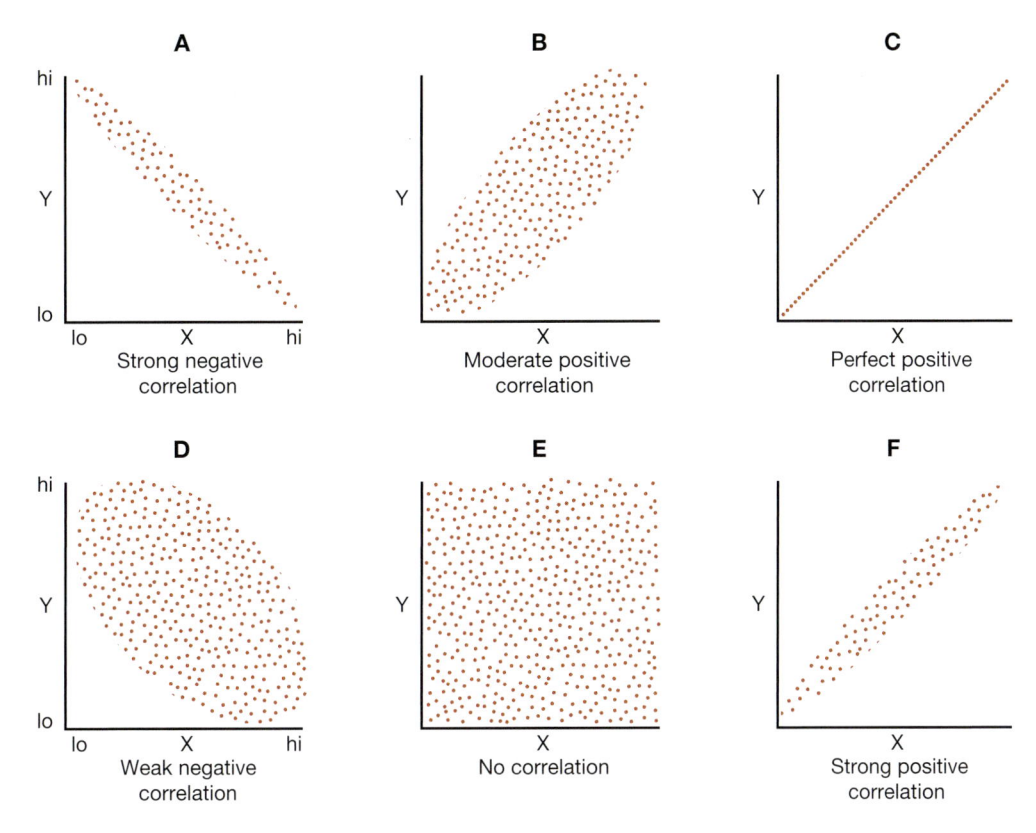

FIGURE 17.9 Various relationships graphed on scatter plots.

called **Pearson's** *r*. This coefficient is computed with variables measured on an interval or ratio scale. **Spearman's rho (ρ)** is a correlation index for ordinal-level data. The calculation of these correlation statistics is laborious and seldom performed by hand. (Computational formulas are available in statistics textbooks, such as that by Polit, 2010.)

It is difficult to offer guidelines on what to interpret as strong or weak relationships because it depends on the variables. If we measured patients' body temperatures orally and rectally, a correlation (*r*) of 0.70 between the two values would be low. For most psychosocial variables (e.g., stress and illness severity), an *r* of 0.70 is high; correlations between such variables are typically in the 0.30 to 0.40 range.

Correlation coefficients are sometimes displayed in a two-dimensional **correlation matrix**, in which every variable is displayed in both a row and a column and coefficients are displayed at the intersections. An example of a correlation matrix is presented at the end of this chapter.

RISK INDEXES

Several descriptive statistical indexes can be used to facilitate clinical decision-making. These indexes reflect the realization that risk and risk reduction must be interpreted within a context. If an intervention reduces the risk of an adverse event three times over, but the initial risk is miniscule, the intervention may be too costly to be practical. Both absolute and relative differences in risks are important in clinical decision-making.

TIP The indexes described in this section are often not reported in nursing journal articles but often can be calculated by readers. Further information about the use and interpretation of these indexes can be found in Guyatt et al. (2015) and Polit (2010).

We focus in this section on describing risk for dichotomous outcomes (e.g., alive/dead, had a fall/did not have a fall) in relation to exposure vs. nonexposure to a potentially beneficial treatment. This situation results in a 2 × 2 crosstabs table with four cells, as depicted in Table 17.5, which shows labels for the four cells so that computations can be explained. *Cell a* is the number with an undesirable outcome (e.g., death) in an intervention group; *cell b* is the number with a desirable outcome (e.g., survival) in an intervention group; and *cells c* and *d* are the two outcome possibilities for a nonexposed (control) group. We can now explain the meaning and calculation of several indexes of interest to clinicians.

TABLE 17.5 • Indexes of Risk and Association in a 2 × 2 Table

EXPOSURE	OUTCOME		TOTAL
	UNDESIRABLE OUTCOME	DESIRABLE OUTCOME	
Yes, exposed (E) to intervention—experimentals (or, NOT exposed to a risk factor)	a	b	$a+b$
No, not exposed (NE) to intervention—controls (or, exposed to a risk factor)	c	d	$c+d$
Total	$a+c$	$b+d$	$a+b+c+d$
Absolute risk, exposed group $(AR_E) = a/(a+b)$			
Absolute risk, nonexposed group $(AR_{NE}) = c/(c+d)$			
Absolute risk reduction $(ARR) = AR_{NE} - AR_E$			
Relative risk $(RR) = \dfrac{AR_E}{AR_{NE}}$			
Relative risk reduction $(RRR) = \dfrac{ARR}{AR_{NE}}$			
Odds, exposed group $(Odds_E) = a/b$			
Odds, nonexposed group $(Odds_{NE}) = c/d$			
Odds ratio $(OR) = \dfrac{Odds_E}{Odds_{NE}}$			
Number needed to treat $(NNT) = \dfrac{1}{ARR}$			

Absolute Risk

Absolute risk (AR) can be computed for those exposed to an intervention (or risk factor) and for those not exposed. **Absolute risk (AR)** is the proportion of people who experienced an undesirable outcome in each group. We illustrate this and other indexes with fictitious data from an intervention study in which 200 smokers were randomly assigned to a smoking cessation intervention or to a control group (Table 17.6). Smoking status 3 months after the intervention is the outcome variable. In this example, the AR of continued smoking was 0.50 in the intervention group and 0.80 in the control group. The risk of an undesirable outcome for a treatment group is sometimes called the *experimental event rate (EER)*, and the risk of an adverse outcome for untreated people is sometimes called the *baseline risk rate* or the *control event rate (CER)*. In the absence of the intervention, 20% of those in the experimental group might have stopped smoking anyway, but the intervention boosted the rate to 50%.

> **TIP** The computations shown in Table 17.5 specifically reflect risk indexes that assume that the intervention exposure will be beneficial, and that information for the *undesirable* outcome will be in cells a and c. If good outcomes rather than bad ones are put in cells a and c, formulas would have to be modified. For example, AR_E would then be b/(a + b), and so on. Similarly, if the research question involved the association between an adverse outcome and a hypothesized risk factor (e.g., the risk that smoking is associated with a cardiovascular accident), the group exposed to the risk factor (e.g., those who smoke) should be in the *bottom* row (cells c and d) and not the top row—or, again, the formulas would need to be adapted. As a general rule, to use the formulas shown in Table 17.6, the cell in the lower left corner (cell c) should be predicted to reflect the highest percentage of undesirable outcomes.

TABLE 17.6 • Hypothetical Data for Smoking Cessation Example Illustrating Risk Index Calculation

EXPOSURE TO SMOKING CESSATION INTERVENTION	OUTCOME CONTINUED SMOKING	OUTCOME STOPPED SMOKING	TOTAL
Yes, exposed: E (experimental group)	50 (*a*)	50 (*b*)	100
No, not exposed: NE (control group)	80 (*c*)	20 (*d*)	100
TOTAL	130	70	200
Absolute risk, exposed group (AR_E) = 50/100 = .50			
Absolute risk, nonexposed group (AR_{NE}) = 80/100 = .80			
Absolute risk reduction (ARR) = .80 − .50 = .30			
Relative risk (RR) = .50/.80 = .625			
Relative risk reduction (RRR) = .30/.80 = .375			
Odds ratio (OR) = $\left(\dfrac{50/50}{80/20}\right)$ = .25			
Number needed to treat = 1/.30 = 3.33			

Absolute Risk Reduction

The **absolute risk reduction (ARR)**, sometimes called the *risk difference* or *RD*, represents a comparison of the two risks. It is computed by subtracting the AR for the exposed group from the AR for the untreated group. This index indicates the estimated proportion of people who would be spared the undesirable outcome through exposure to the intervention. In our example, the value of ARR is 0.30: 30% of the control group participants would presumably have stopped smoking if they had received the intervention, over and above the 20% who stopped without it.

Relative Risk

Relative risk (RR), or the *risk ratio*, represents the estimated proportion of the original risk of an adverse outcome (in our example, continued smoking) that persists when people are exposed to the intervention. To compute an RR, the AR for exposed people is divided by the AR for nonexposed people. In our fictitious example, the RR is 0.625. This means that the risk of continued smoking after the smoking cessation intervention is estimated to be 62.5% of what it would have been in its absence.

Relative Risk Reduction

Relative risk reduction (RRR) is another useful index for evaluating the effectiveness of an intervention. RRR is the estimated proportion of untreated risk that is reduced through exposure to the intervention. This index is computed by dividing the ARR by the AR for the control group. In our example, RRR = 0.375. This means that the smoking cessation intervention decreased the RR of continued smoking by 37.5%, compared to not having had the intervention.

Odds Ratio

The **odds ratio (OR)** is a widely reported index, even though it is less intuitively meaningful than RR as an index of risk. The **odds**, in this context, is the proportion of people *with* the adverse outcome relative to those *without* it. In our example, the odds of continued smoking for the experimental group is 50 (the number who continued smoking) divided by 50 (the number who stopped), or 1. The odds for the control group is 80 divided by 20, or 4. The **odds ratio** is the ratio of these two odds, or 0.25 in our example. The estimated odds of continuing to smoke are one-fourth as high among those in the intervention group as among those in the control group. Turned around, we could say that the estimated odds of continued smoking are four times higher among smokers who did not get the intervention as among those who did.

TIP Odds ratios can be computed when the independent variable is not dichotomous, using a statistical procedure described in Chapter 19. For example, we could estimate the odds ratio for obesity among adults in four different income groups, using one of the groups as a reference.

Number Needed to Treat

A final index of interest is the **number needed to treat (NNT)**, which represents an estimate of how many people would need to receive a treatment or intervention to prevent one undesirable outcome. NNT is computed by dividing 1 by the value of the ARR. In our example, ARR = 0.30, and so NNT is 3.33. About three smokers would need to be exposed to the intervention to avoid one person's continued smoking. The NNT is inversely related to the RRR. An intervention that is twice as effective with regard to RRR will cut the NNT in half. The NNT is especially valuable for decision-makers because it can be integrated with monetary information to determine if an intervention is cost-effective.

Example of Relative Risk and Number Needed to Treat
Harrer and colleagues (2020) conducted a systematic review and meta-analysis to synthesize data on eating disorder interventions for university level students. They found that the relative risk of developing an eating disorder in this population was 0.62 (95% CI [0.44, 0.87] with a n of 8. The NNT was 26.08. These findings suggest that those students who were exposed to an intervention had a 38% decrease in incidence as compared to the control groups.

TIP Various tools on the internet facilitate the calculation of risk indexes.

BOX 17.1 Guidelines for Critically Appraising Descriptive Statistics

1. Did the report include descriptive statistics? Do these statistics sufficiently describe major characteristics of the sample?
2. Were descriptive statistics used appropriately—for example, were descriptive statistics used to describe sample characteristics, key variables, and methodologic features of the study, such as response rate or attrition rate? Were they used to answer research questions when inferential statistics would have been more appropriate?
3. Were the correct descriptive statistics used—for example, was a mean presented when percentages would have been more informative? If the median was used rather than the mean, was this appropriate?
4. Was the descriptive information presented in a useful format—for example, were tables used effectively? Is information in the text and the tables redundant? Is information in the text and tables consistent with each other? Were the tables clear, with a good title, carefully labeled headings, and good table notes?
5. Were any risk indexes computed? If not, would they have been useful?

CRITICAL APPRAISAL OF DESCRIPTIVE STATISTICS

Descriptive statistics help to set the stage for understanding quantitative evidence. Descriptive statistics are useful for communicating information about the study sample. Readers of reports cannot draw inferences about the study's applicability without understanding who the participants were with regard to key demographic characteristics and health-related attributes.

In addition to describing sample characteristics, descriptive statistics are useful in communicating information about the baseline values of key outcome variables in longitudinal or intervention studies, or correlations between a set of independent variables. Methodologic information about study quality also typically relies on descriptive statistics—for example, response rates and attrition rates are typically shown as percentages, and means are used to characterize such things as time elapsed between two interviews.

Descriptive statistics are sometimes used to directly address research questions in studies that are primarily descriptive. However, when only descriptive statistics are presented, readers should think about whether the inclusion of inferential statistics would have been preferable. If a research question is about a *population*, and not just about the particular people who participated in the research, inferential statistics are needed.

In critically appraising the researcher's use of descriptive statistics, readers can consider whether the information was adequate, whether the correct statistical indexes were used, and whether it was presented in a clear and efficient manner. Box 17.1 presents some guiding questions for a critical appraisal of the descriptive statistics presented in a research report.

RESEARCH EXAMPLE

We conclude this chapter with an example of a study that presented several of the descriptive statistics mentioned in this chapter.

Study: Physical function mediates the effects of sensory impairment on quality of life in older adults: Cross-sectional study using propensity-score weighting (Tseng et al., 2023).

Statement of purpose: This study had two aims. The first was to explore in older adults the impact of sensory impairment (SI) on quality of life (QoL). The second aim was to explore the possible mediating effect that physical function on SI and QoL.

Methods: The study used a cross-sectional design to recruit at minimum 600 older adults. The team captured demographic information and measures of hearing and vision, physical function (activities of daily living), and quality of life.

Analysis and findings: The researchers undertook numerous complex analyses that are not described here. In terms of descriptive statistics, they presented information about the 600 participants' demographic characteristics such as age, gender, and education level. For example, the mean age was 73.9 with a standard deviation (SD) of 6.4. the impact of SI on QOL, they described the demographics of the participants concerning sensory impairment by type: no sensory impairment, hearing impairment only, visual impairment only, or both hearing and vision impairment. While no sensory impairment was most common for married participants $n = 283$ or 75.6%, hearing loss was the most frequent sensory loss in this group, $n = 100$ (65. 3%). Next, the team considered the impact of the various types of sensory impairment on quality of life. Lastly, they conducted a mediation analysis to determine the direct and indirect effect of sensory impairment on quality of life as a result of physical function. Results indicated that in terms of sensory impairment, hearing ($n = 153$) had the least impact on quality of life whereas dual sensory loss ($n= 32$) had the most impact. Physical function had a statistically significant mediating effect on sensory impairment in the quality of life for older adults.

SUMMARY POINTS

- There are four **levels of measurement**: (1) **nominal measurement**—the classification of characteristics into mutually exclusive categories, (2) **ordinal measurement**—the ranking of objects based on their relative standing on an attribute, (3) **interval measurement**—indicating not only the ranking of objects but the amount of distance between them, and (4) **ratio measurement**—distinguished from interval measurement by having a rational zero point.
- **Descriptive statistics** enable researchers to summarize and describe quantitative data.
- **Frequency distributions** impose order on raw data. Numeric values are ordered from lowest to highest, accompanied by a count of the number (or percentage) of times each value was obtained.
- **Histograms** and **frequency polygons** are methods of displaying frequency information graphically.
- Data for a variable can be described in terms of the shape of the distribution, central tendency, and variability.
- A distribution is **symmetric** if its two halves are mirror images of each other. A **skewed** distribution is asymmetric, with one tail longer than the other.
- In **positively skewed distributions,** the long tail points to the right (e.g., personal income); in **negatively skewed distributions,** the tail points to the left (e.g., age at death).
- The **modality** of a distribution refers to the number of peaks: A **unimodal distribution** has one peak, and a **multimodal distribution** has more than one peak.
- A **normal distribution** (*bell-shaped curve*) is symmetric, unimodal, and not too peaked.
- Measures of **central tendency** are indexes that represent the average or typical value of a set of scores. The **mode** is the value that occurs most frequently in a distribution. The **median** is the point above which and below which 50% of the cases fall. The **mean** is the arithmetic average of all scores. The mean is a preferred index of central tendency because of its *stability* from sample to sample drawn from a population.
- Measures of **variability**—how spread out the data are—include the range and standard deviation. The **range** is the distance between the highest and lowest scores. The **standard deviation** (*SD*) indicates how much, on average, scores deviate from the mean.
- The *SD* is calculated by first computing **deviation scores**, which indicate the degree to which a person's score deviates from the mean. The **variance** is equal to the *SD* squared. In a normal distribution, 95% of scores fall within 2 *SD*s above and below the mean.
- **Bivariate descriptive statistics** describe relationships between two variables.
- A **crosstabs table** is a two-dimensional frequency distribution in which the frequencies of two nominal- or ordinal-level variables are crosstabulated.
- **Correlation coefficients** describe the direction and magnitude of a relationship between two variables. Researchers most often

compute the **product-moment correlation coefficient** (**Pearson's *r***), used with interval- or ratio-level variables. The **Spearman rho coefficient** is used to correlate ordinal-level variables.
- Graphically, the relationship between two continuous variables can be displayed on a **scatter plot**.
- Several risk indexes describe outcomes in relation to exposures (to interventions or risk factors) for a two-group (e.g., experimental vs. control) situation with dichotomous outcomes (e.g., alive/dead). These indexes are useful in clinical decision-making.
- **Absolute risk reduction (ARR)** expresses the estimated proportion of people who would be spared an adverse outcome through exposure to an intervention (or lack of exposure to a risk). **Relative risk (RR)** is the estimated proportion of the original risk of an adverse outcome that persists among people exposed to an intervention. **Relative risk reduction (RRR)** is the estimated proportion of untreated risk that is reduced through exposure to the intervention. The **odds ratio (OR)** is the ratio of the odds for the treated vs. untreated group, with the **odds** reflecting the proportion of people with the adverse outcome relative to those without it. The **number needed to treat (NNT)** is an estimate of how many people would need to receive the intervention to prevent one adverse outcome.

REFERENCES CITED IN CHAPTER 17

Banister, G., Carroll, D. L., Dickins, K., Flanagan, J., Jones, D., Looby, S. E., & Cahill, J. E. (2022). Nurse-sensitive indicators during COVID-19. *International Journal of Nursing Knowledge*, *33*(3), 234–244. https://doi.org/10.1111/2047-3095.12372

Chen, T. Y., Kao, C. W., Cheng, S. M., & Chang, Y. C. (2022). A web-based self-care program to promote healthy lifestyles and control blood pressure in patients with primary hypertension: A randomized controlled trial. *Journal of Nursing Scholarship*, *54*(6), 678–691. https://doi.org/10.1111/jnu.12792

Guyatt, G., Rennie, D., Meade, M., & Cook, D. (2015). *Users' guide to the medical literature: A manual for evidence-based clinical practice* (3rd ed.). McGraw Hill.

Harrer, M., Adam, S. H., Messner, E. M., Baumeister, H., Cuijpers, P., Bruffaerts, R., Auerbach, R. P., Kessler, R. C., Jacobi, C., Taylor, C. B., & Ebert, D. D. (2020). Prevention of eating disorders at universities: A systematic review and meta-analysis. *International Journal of Eating Disorders*, *53*(6), 813–833. https://doi.org/10.1002/eat.23224

Polit, D. F. (2010). *Statistics and data analysis for nursing research* (2nd ed.). Pearson.

Skinner, M. S., & Sogstad, M. (2022). Social and gender differences in informal caregiving for sick, disabled, or elderly persons: A cross-sectional study. *SAGE Open Nursing Journal*, *8*, 23779608221130585. https://doi.org/10.1177/23779608221130585

Tseng, Y. C., Gau, B. S., Hsieh, Y. S., Liu, T. C., Huang, G. S., & Lou, M. F. (2023). Physical function mediates the effects of sensory impairment on quality of life in older adults: Cross-sectional study using propensity-score weighting. *Journal of Advanced Nursing*, *79*(1), 101–112. https://doi.org/10.1111/jan.15423

18 Inferential Statistics

Learning Objectives

1. Understand the application of common inferential statistics in research studies.
2. Describe the difference between standard deviation and confidence interval.
3. Articulate the purpose of hypothesis testing and the level of significance.
4. Distinguish the difference between parametric and nonparametric testing.
5. Explain the importance of effect size estimates.

INTRODUCTION

Inferential statistics, based on the **laws of probability**, allow researchers to draw conclusions about a population, given data from a sample. Inferential statistics would help us with such questions as, "What can I infer about 1-minute Apgar scores of premature babies (the population) after calculating a mean Apgar score of 6.9 in a sample of 500 premature babies?" Inferential statistics provide a framework for making objective judgments about the reliability of sample statistics as estimates of population parameters. Different researchers applying inferential statistics to the same data are likely to draw the same conclusions.

SAMPLING DISTRIBUTIONS

To estimate population parameters, representative samples should be used, and probability sampling is the best way to get representative samples (Chapter 13). Inferential statistics assume random sampling from populations, an assumption that is widely violated. The validity of statistical calculations does depend, however, on the extent to which results from the sample are similar to what you would have obtained had you randomly selected people from the population.

Even when random sampling *is* used, sample characteristics are seldom identical to population characteristics. Suppose we had a population of 50,000 nursing school applicants whose mean score on a standardized entrance exam was 500.0 with a standard deviation (SD) of 100.0. Suppose we wanted to estimate the population mean from the scores of a random sample of 25 students. Would we expect a mean of *exactly* 500.0 for the sample? Obtaining the exact population value is unlikely. Let us say the sample mean is 505.1. If a new random sample were drawn, we might obtain a mean of, say, 497.8. The tendency for statistics to fluctuate from one sample to another reflects **sampling error**. The challenge is to decide whether sample values are good estimates of population parameters.

Researchers compute statistics with only *one* sample, but to understand inferential statistics we must perform a mental exercise. Consider drawing a sample of 25 students from the population of 50,000, calculating a mean, replacing the students, and drawing a new sample. Each mean is one datum. If we drew 100,000 such samples, we would have 100,000

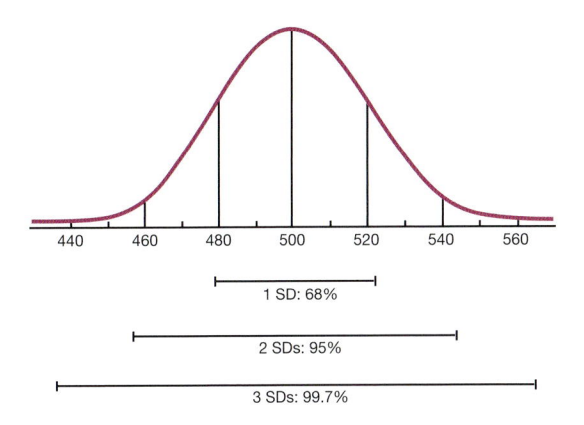

FIGURE 18.1 A sampling distribution of the mean.

means (data points) that could be used to construct a frequency polygon (Figure 18.1). This distribution is a **sampling distribution of the mean**. A sampling distribution is theoretical—in practice no one draws consecutive samples from a population and plots their means. Sampling distributions are the basis of inferential statistics.

Characteristics of Sampling Distributions

When an infinite number of samples are randomly drawn from a population, the sampling distribution of the mean has certain characteristics. (Our example of 100,000 samples is large enough to approximate these characteristics.) Sampling distributions of means are normally distributed, and the mean always equals the population mean. In the example shown in Figure 18.1, the mean of the sampling distribution is 500.0, the same as the population mean.

Remember that when data are normally distributed, 68% of values fall between ±1 SD from the mean. Because a sampling distribution of means is normally distributed, we can say that the probability is 68 out of 100 that any randomly drawn sample mean lies between +1 SD and −1 SD of the population mean. Thus, if we knew the standard deviation of the sampling distribution, we could interpret the accuracy of a sample mean.

Standard Error of the Mean

The standard deviation of a sampling distribution of the mean is called the **standard error of the mean (SEM)**. The word *error* signifies that the various means in the sampling distribution have some error as estimates of the population mean. The smaller the *SEM*—that is, the less variable the sample means—the more accurate is a single mean as an estimate of the population value.

No one actually constructs a sampling distribution, so how can its standard deviation be computed? Fortunately, there is a formula for estimating the *SEM* from a single sample, using two pieces of information: the sample's standard deviation and sample size. The equation for the SEM is $SD/\sqrt{N}$. In our example, if we use this formula to calculate the *SEM* for an *SD* of 100.0 with a sample of 25 students, we obtain

$$SEM = \frac{100.0}{\sqrt{25}} = 20.0$$

The standard deviation of the sampling distribution in our example is 20.0, as shown in Figure 18.1. This *SEM* is an estimate of how much sampling error there is from one sample mean to another when samples of 25 are randomly drawn and the *SD* is 100.0.

Given that a sampling distribution of means follows a normal curve, we can estimate the probability of drawing a sample with a certain mean. With a sample size of 25 and a population mean of 500.0, the chances are about 95 out of 100 that any sample mean will fall between 460 and 540 (i.e., 2 *SD*s above and below the mean). Only 5 times out of 100 would the mean of a randomly selected sample exceed 540 or be less than 460. Only 5 times out of 100 would we get a sample whose mean deviated from the population mean by more than 40 points.

Because the *SEM* is partly a function of sample size, we need only increase sample size to increase the accuracy of our estimate. If we used a sample of 100 applicants, rather than 25, the SEM would be 10 (i.e., $100/\sqrt{100} = 10.0$). In this situation, the chances are about 95 out of 100 that a sample mean will be between 480 and 520. The chances of drawing a sample with a mean very different from the population mean are reduced as sample size increases because large numbers promote the likelihood that extreme values will cancel each other out.

ESTIMATION OF PARAMETERS

Statistical inference consists of two techniques: (1) estimation of parameters and (2) hypothesis testing. Parameter estimates have not traditionally been presented in nursing research reports, but that situation is changing. The push for evidence-based practice (EBP) has heightened interest among practitioners in learning not only whether a hypothesis was supported (via hypothesis testing) but also the estimated value of a population parameter and the degree of accuracy of the estimate (via parameter estimation). Many medical research journals *require* that estimation information be reported because it is useful to clinicians. In this section, we present general concepts relating to parameter estimation and offer some examples based on one-variable descriptive statistics.

Confidence Intervals

Parameter estimation is used to estimate a parameter—for example, a mean, a proportion, or a mean difference between two groups (e.g., experimental and control group members). Estimation can take two forms: point estimation or interval estimation. **Point estimation** involves calculating a single statistic to estimate the population parameter. To continue with the earlier example, if we calculated the mean entrance exam score for a sample of 25 applicants and found that it was 510.0, then this would be the point estimate of the population mean.

Interval estimation is useful because it indicates a range of values within which the parameter has a specified probability of lying. With interval estimation, researchers construct a **confidence interval** (**CI**) around the estimate; the upper and lower limits are **confidence limits**. Constructing a CI around a sample mean establishes a range of values for the population value as well as the probability of being right—the estimate is made with a certain degree of confidence. By convention, researchers usually use either a 95% or a 99% CI.

Confidence Intervals Around a Mean

Calculating confidence limits around a mean involves using the *SEM*. In a normal distribution, 95% of the scores lie within about 2 *SD*s (more precisely, 1.96 *SD*s) from the mean. In our example, suppose the point estimate for mean entrance exam scores is 510.0, and the *SD* is 100.0. The *SEM* for a sample of 25 would be 20.0. We can build a 95% CI with the following formula:

$$\text{CI } 95\% = \left(\overline{X} \pm 1.96 \times SEM\right)$$

That is, confidence is 95% that the population mean lies between the values equal to 1.96 times the *SEM*, above and below the sample mean. In the example at hand, we would obtain the following:

$$\text{CI } 95\% = \left(510.0 \pm (1.96 \times 20.0)\right)$$
$$\text{CI } 95\% = \left(510.0 \pm (39.2)\right)$$
$$\text{CI } 95\% = \left(470.8 \leq \mu \leq 549.2\right)$$

The final statement may be read as follows: confidence is 95% that the population mean (symbolized by the Greek letter mu [μ] by convention) is between 470.8 and 549.2. This would be stated in a research report as 95% CI = 470.8 to 549.2, or 95% CI (470.8, 549.2).

CIs reflect the researchers' risk of being wrong. With a 95% CI, researchers accept the probability that they will be wrong five times out of 100. A 99% CI sets the risk at only 1% by allowing a wider range of possible values. The formula is as follows:

$$\text{CI } 99\% = \left(\overline{X} \pm 2.58 \times SEM\right)$$

The 2.58 reflects the fact that 99% of all cases in a normal distribution lie within ±2.58 *SD* units from the mean. In the example, the 99% CI would be as follows:

$$\text{CI } 99\% = \left(510.0 \pm (2.58 \times 20.0)\right)$$
$$\text{CI } 99\% = \left(510.0 \pm (51.6)\right)$$
$$\text{CI } 99\% = \left(458.4 \leq \mu \leq 561.6\right)$$

The price of having a reduced risk of being wrong is reduced *precision*. With 95% confidence, the range of the CI was about 80 points; with 99% confidence, the range is more than 100 points. The acceptable risk of error depends on the nature of the problem. In research with implications for the health of individual patients, a stringent 99% CI might be used; for most studies, a 95% CI usually is sufficient.

Confidence Intervals Around Proportions and Risk Indexes

Calculating CI around a proportion or percentage is important, especially with regard to risk estimates. Consider, for example, this question: "What proportion of people exposed to a certain hazard will contract a disease?" This question calls for an estimated proportion (an absolute risk index, as described in Chapter 17) that is more useful if it is reported within a 95% CI.

For proportions based on dichotomous variables, as in the above question (positive/negative for a disease), the theoretical distribution is a **binomial distribution**. A binomial distribution is the probability distribution of the number of "successes" (e.g., heads) in a sequence of independent yes/no trials (e.g., a coin toss), each of which yields "success" with a specified probability.

Building CIs around a proportion is computationally complex, and so we do not provide formulas here, but certain features of CIs around proportions are worth noting. First, the CI is rarely symmetric around a sample proportion. For example, if 3 out of 30 sample members were positive for an outcome (e.g., hospital readmission), the estimated population proportion would be 0.10 and the 95% CI would be from 0.021 to 0.265. Second, the width of the CI depends on both the sample size and the value of the proportion. The smaller the sample, the wider the CI. And the closer the sample proportion is to 0.50, the wider the CI. For example, with a sample size of 30, the range for a 95% CI for a proportion of 0.50 is 0.374 (0.313, 0.687), while the range for a proportion of 0.10 is only 0.188 (0.021, 0.265). Finally, the CI for a proportion never extends below 0 or above 1.0, but a CI can be constructed around an *obtained* proportion of 0 or 1.0. For example, if 0 out of our 30 participants were readmitted to the hospital, the estimated proportion would be 0.00 and the 95% CI would be from 0.00 to 0.116.

It is advisable to construct CIs around all the risk indexes described in the previous chapter, such as the ARR, RRR, OR, and NNT. The computed value of these indexes from study data represents a "best estimate" and CIs indicate the estimate's precision. Clearly, clinical inference is enhanced when information about a plausible range of values for risk indexes is presented. An easy method for constructing 95% CIs around major risk indexes is to use an online calculator, such as the one in the Evidence-Based Medicine Toolbox (https://ebm-tools.knowledgetranslation.net/calculator/prospective/).

Example of CIs Around Odds Ratios
Hamlin and colleagues (2021) aimed to compare birth outcomes of females cared for by Certified Nurse-Midwives (CNMs) vs. physicians in the Military Health System (MHS). While the team notes that physicians cared for more high-risk pregnancies (11.3%) than CNMs (7.6%), as compared to the physicians, the CNMs had a significantly higher odds of vaginal delivery and breastfeeding (odds ratio 2.5 with 95% CI [2.5, 2.6] and 1.5 with 95% CI [1.5, 1.6], respectively).

HYPOTHESIS TESTING

Statistical **hypothesis testing** provides objective criteria for deciding whether hypotheses are supported by data. Suppose we hypothesized that participation in a stress management program would reduce anxiety levels among patients with cancer. The sample is 25 control group patients who do not participate in the program and 25 patients who do. The mean posttreatment anxiety score for the intervention group is 15.8 and that for controls is 17.9. Should we conclude that the hypothesis is correct? Group differences are in the predicted direction, but the results might represent sampling error. With a new sample, group means might be nearly identical. Statistical hypothesis testing allows researchers to make objective decisions about whether study results likely reflect chance sample differences or true population differences.

The Null Hypothesis

Hypothesis testing is based on negative inference. In our example, patients participating in the intervention had lower mean anxiety scores than control group patients. There are two possible explanations: (1) the intervention was successful in reducing anxiety; or (2) the differences resulted from chance factors. The first explanation is our research hypothesis, and the second is the null hypothesis. The **null hypothesis**, it may be recalled, states that there is no relationship between variables. Statistical hypothesis testing is basically a process of rejection. It cannot be demonstrated directly that the research hypothesis is correct but, using theoretical sampling distributions, it can be shown that the null hypothesis has a high probability of being wrong. Researchers seek to reject the null hypothesis through various **statistical tests**.

The null hypothesis in our example can be stated formally as follows:

$$H_0: \mu_E = \mu_C$$

The null hypothesis (H_0) is that the mean population anxiety score for experimental group patients (μ_E) is the same as that for controls (μ_C). The **alternative**, or research, **hypothesis** (H_A) is that the means are *not* the same:

$$H_A: \mu_E \neq \mu_C$$

Null hypotheses are accepted or rejected based on sample data, but hypothesis testing is used to make inferences about the population.

Type I and Type II Errors

Researchers decide whether to accept or reject a null hypothesis by determining how *probable* it is that observed results are due to chance. Researchers cannot know with certainty whether a null hypothesis is or is not true based on data from a sample. They can only conclude that hypotheses are *probably* true or *probably* false, and there is always a risk of error.

Researchers can make two types of statistical error: rejecting a true null hypothesis or accepting a false null hypothesis. Figure 18.2 summarizes possible outcomes of researchers' decisions. Researchers make a **Type I error** by rejecting a null hypothesis that is, in fact, true. For instance, if we concluded that a drug was more effective than a placebo in reducing cholesterol, when in fact the observed differences in cholesterol levels resulted from sampling fluctuations, this would be a Type I error—a false-positive conclusion. Conversely, if we concluded that group differences in cholesterol resulted by chance, when in fact the drug *did* reduce cholesterol, this would be a **Type II error**—a false negative conclusion. In the context of drug testing, a good way to think about statistical error can be expressed as follows: A Type I error might allow an ineffective drug to come onto the market, but a Type II error might *prevent* an effective drug from coming onto the market.

Level of Significance

Researchers never know when they have made an error in statistical decision making. The validity of a null hypothesis could be known only by collecting data from the population. Researchers control the *risk* of a Type I error by selecting a **level of significance**, which signifies the probability of incorrectly rejecting a true null hypothesis.

The two most frequently used significance levels (referred to as **alpha** or α) are 0.05 and 0.01. With a 0.05 significance level, we accept the risk

		The actual situation is that the null hypothesis is:	
		True	False
The researcher calculates a test statistic and decides that the null hypothesis is:	True (Null accepted)	Correct decision	Type II error (False negative)
	False (Null rejected)	Type I error (False positive)	Correct decision

FIGURE 18.2 Outcomes of statistical decision-making.

that out of 100 samples drawn from a population, a true null hypothesis would be rejected 5 times. With a 0.01 significance level, the risk of a Type I error is *lower*: in only 1 sample out of 100 would we erroneously reject the null hypothesis. The minimum acceptable level for α usually is 0.05. A stricter level (e.g., 0.01 or 0.001) may be needed when the decision has important consequences.

> **TIP** A group of prominent researchers and statisticians have made a controversial proposal to "redefine statistical significance" by using a threshold of 0.005 rather than 0.05 for inferences of statistical significance (Benjamin et al., 2018). Their argument is based, in part, on the fact that many significant findings cannot be replicated. It remains to be seen if their viewpoint will predominate in the years ahead.

Naturally, researchers want to reduce the risk of committing both types of error, but unfortunately lowering the risk of a Type I error increases the risk of a Type II error. The stricter the criterion for rejecting a null hypothesis, the greater the probability of accepting a false null hypothesis. Researchers must deal with tradeoffs in establishing criteria for statistical decision making, but the simplest way of reducing the risk of a Type II error is to increase sample size. Type II errors are discussed later in this chapter.

Critical Regions

By selecting a significance level, researchers establish a decision rule. That rule is to reject the null hypothesis if the test statistic falls at or beyond the limits that establish a **critical region** on an applicable theoretical distribution, and to accept the null hypothesis otherwise. The critical region indicates whether the null hypothesis is *improbable*, given the results.

An example from our study of gender bias in nursing research (Polit & Beck, 2013) illustrates the statistical decision-making process. We examined whether males and females are equally represented as study participants in nursing studies—that is, whether the average percentage of females across studies in four leading nursing research journals was 50.0 as one would expect if there was no bias.

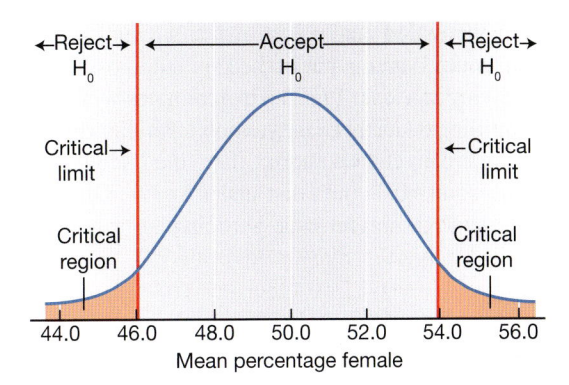

FIGURE 18.3 Critical regions in the sampling distribution for a two-tailed test: Gender bias example.

The null hypothesis is H_0: $\mu = 50.0$, and the alternate hypothesis is H_A: $\mu \neq 50.0$. We found, using a consecutive sample of 300 studies published over a 2-year period, that the mean percentage of female study participants was 74.1. Using statistical procedures, we tested the hypothesis that the mean of 74.1 was not merely a chance fluctuation from a population mean of 50.0.

In hypothesis testing, researchers assume the null hypothesis is true and then gather evidence to disprove it. Assuming a mean percentage of 50.0 for the population of nursing studies, a theoretical sampling distribution can be constructed. The *SEM* in this example is about 2.0, as shown in Figure 18.3.

Based on normal distribution characteristics,[1] we can determine *probable* and *improbable* values of sample means from the population of nursing studies. If, as is assumed in the null hypothesis, the population mean is 50.0, then 95% of all sample means would fall between 46.0 and 54.0, i.e., within 2 *SD*s above and below the mean of 50.0. The obtained sample mean of 74.1 is in the critical region considered *improbable* if the null hypothesis were true—in fact, any value greater than 54.0% female would be improbable with alpha = 0.05. In our study, the probability of obtaining an average of 74.1% female by chance alone was less than 1 in 10,000. We rejected the null hypothesis that the mean percentage of females in nursing studies was

---
[1] Strictly speaking, the appropriate theoretical distribution in this example is the *t* distribution, but with a large *N*, the *t* and normal distributions are highly similar.

50.0. We would not be justified in saying that we had *proved* our hypothesis because the possibility of having made a Type I error remains—but the possibility is, in this case, remote. We can *accept* the alternative hypothesis that the population mean is not 50.0—i.e., that males and females are not equally represented as participants in nursing studies.

> **TIP** Levels of significance are analogous to the CI values described earlier—an alpha of 0.05 is analogous to the 95% CI, and an alpha of 0.01 is analogous to the 99% CI. In our example of gender bias, the 95% CI around the mean percentage female of 74.1 was 71.1 to 77.1.

Statistical Tests

Researchers test hypotheses by computing **test statistics** with their data. For every test statistic, there is a related theoretical distribution. The value of the computed test statistic is compared to values of the critical limits for the relevant distribution.

When researchers calculate a test statistic that is beyond the critical limit, the results are said to be **statistically significant**. The word *significant* does not mean *important* or *clinically meaningful*. In statistics, *significant* means that obtained results are not likely to have been the result of chance, at a specified level of probability. A **nonsignificant result** means that an observed result could reflect chance fluctuations.

> **TIP** When the null hypothesis is retained (i.e., when results are nonsignificant), this is sometimes referred to as a *negative result*. Negative results are often disappointing to researchers and may lead to rejection of a manuscript by journal editors. Research reports with negative results are not rejected because editors are prejudiced against certain types of outcomes; they are rejected because negative results are inconclusive and difficult to interpret. A nonsignificant result indicates that the result *could* have occurred as a result of chance and provides no evidence that the research hypothesis is or is not correct.

One-Tailed and Two-Tailed Tests

In most hypothesis-testing situations, researchers use **two-tailed tests**. This means that both tails of the sampling distribution are used to determine improbable values. In Figure 18.3, for example, the critical region that contains 5% of the sampling distribution's area involves 2½% in one tail of the distribution and 2½% in the other. If the significance level were 0.01, the critical regions would involve ½% in each tail.

When researchers have a strong basis for a directional hypothesis, they sometimes use a **one-tailed test**. For example, if we did an RCT to test a program to improve prenatal practices among rural females, we would expect birth outcomes for the two groups not to just be *different*; we would expect program participants to *benefit*. It could be argued that it does not make sense to use the tail of the distribution signifying *worse* outcomes in the intervention group.

In one-tailed tests, the critical region of improbable values is in only one tail of the distribution—the tail corresponding to the direction of the hypothesis, as illustrated in Figure 18.4. Using our earlier gender bias example, the research hypothesis being tested might be that the population mean is *greater than* 50.0—i.e., that, on average, females are overrepresented in nursing studies. When a one-tailed test is used, the critical 5% area of "improbability" covers a bigger area of the specified tail, so one-tailed tests are less conservative. Thus, it is easier to reject the null hypothesis with a one-tailed test than

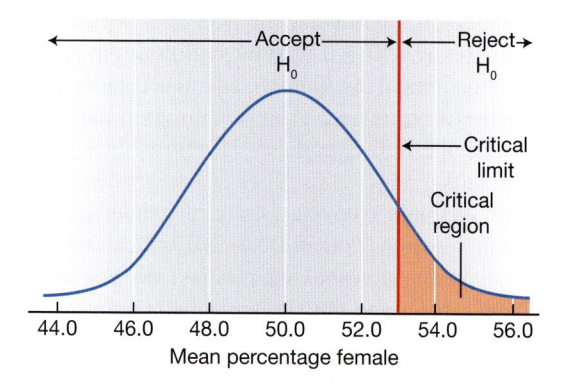

FIGURE 18.4 Critical region in the sampling distribution for a one-tailed test: Gender bias example.

with a two-tailed test. In our gender bias example, with an alpha of 0.05, a sample mean of 53.0 or greater would result in rejecting the null hypothesis for a one-tailed test, rather than 54.0 for a two-tailed test.

One-tailed tests are controversial. Most researchers use a two-tailed test even if they have a directional hypothesis. In reading research reports, one can assume that two-tailed tests were used unless one-tailed tests are specifically mentioned. When there is a strong theoretical reason for a directional hypothesis and for assuming that findings in the opposite direction are virtually impossible, however, a one-tailed test might be warranted. In the remainder of this chapter, the examples are for two-tailed tests.

> **TIP** You should choose a one-tailed test only if you state a directional hypothesis in advance of statistical testing. And you must be prepared to attribute any observed group differences in the "wrong" direction to chance, even if the group differences are large.

Parametric and Nonparametric Tests

There are two broad classes of statistical tests, parametric and nonparametric. **Parametric tests** involve estimation of a parameter, require measurements on at least an interval scale, and involve several assumptions, such as the assumption that the variables are normally distributed in the population. **Nonparametric tests**, by contrast, do not estimate parameters. They involve less restrictive assumptions about the shape of the variables' distribution than do parametric tests.

Parametric tests are more powerful than nonparametric tests and are usually preferred, but there is some disagreement. Purists insist that if the requirements of parametric tests are not met, they are inappropriate. Statistical studies have shown, however, that statistical decision-making is not affected when the assumptions for parametric tests are violated if sample sizes are large. Nonparametric tests are most useful when data cannot in any manner be construed as interval-level, when the distribution is markedly nonnormal, or when the sample size is very small.

> **TIP** Some statisticians advise that when N is 50 or greater, it may not be necessary to use nonparametric statistics, unless the population has a markedly unusual distribution. Such advice invokes the **central limit theorem**, which, briefly, concerns the fact that when samples are large, the theoretical distribution of sample *means* tends to follow a normal distribution—*even if* the variable itself is not normally distributed in the population. With small Ns, you cannot rely on the central limit theorem, so probability values could be wrong if a parametric test is used.

Between-Subjects Tests and Within-Subjects Tests

Another distinction in statistical tests concerns the nature of the comparisons. When comparisons involve different people (e.g., males vs. females), the study uses a between-subjects design, and the statistical test is a **test for independent groups**. Other designs involve a single group of people—for example, with a crossover design, participants are exposed to two or more treatments. In within-subjects designs, comparisons are not independent because the same people are used in all conditions, and the appropriate statistical tests are **tests for dependent groups**.

Overview of Hypothesis-Testing Procedures

This chapter describes several bivariate statistical tests. We have emphasized applications rather than computations, but urge you to consult other references (e.g., Dancey et al., 2012; Gravetter et al., 2018; Polit, 2010) for fuller explanations. In this research methods textbook, our goal is to provide an overview of the use and interpretation of some common statistical tests.

Each statistical test has a particular application, but the process of testing hypotheses is basically the same. The steps are as follows:

1. *Select an appropriate test statistic.* Figure 18.5 provides a quick reference guide for selecting many widely used bivariate statistical tests. (Multivariate tests are discussed in Chapter 19.)

Level of Measurement of Dependent Variable	Group Comparisons: Number of Groups (the Independent Variable)					Correlational Analyses (to Examine Relationship Strength)
	2 Groups		3+ Groups		
	Independent Groups Tests	Dependent Groups Tests	Independent Groups Tests	Dependent Groups Tests	
Nominal (categorical)	χ^2 (or Fisher exact test)	McNemar test	χ^2	Cochran's Q	Phi coefficient (dichotomous) or Cramér's V (not restricted to dichotomous)
Ordinal (rank)	Mann–Whitney U test**	Wilcoxon signed-rank test	Kruskal–Wallis H test	Friedman test	Spearman's rho (or Kendall's tau)
Interval or ratio (continuous)*	Independent group t-test	Paired t-test	ANOVA	RM-ANOVA	Pearson's r
	Multifactor ANOVA for 2+ independent variables				
	RM-ANOVA for 2+ groups x 2+ measurements over time				

*For distributions that are markedly nonnormal or samples that are small, the nonparametric tests in the row above may be needed.
**The Mann–Whitney U test is also known as the Wilcoxon rank-sum test.

FIGURE 18.5 Quick guide to bivariate statistical tests.

Researchers must consider such factors as which measurement levels were used, whether a parametric test is justified, whether a dependent groups test is appropriate, and whether the focus is correlations or group comparisons—and how many groups are being compared.

2. *Establish the level of significance.* Researchers establish the criterion for accepting or rejecting the null hypothesis. An α of 0.05 has been considered acceptable in most circumstances.
3. *Select a one-tailed or two-tailed test.* In most cases, a two-tailed test should be used.
4. *Compute a test statistic.* Using collected data, researchers calculate a test statistic.
5. *Determine the degrees of freedom* (symbolized as *df*). **Degrees of freedom** refers to the number of observations free to vary about a parameter. The concept is too complex for full elaboration, but *df* is easy to compute.
6. *Compare the test statistic with a tabled value.* Theoretical distributions for test statistics enable researchers to determine whether the test statistic (Step 4) is beyond the range of what is *probable* if the null hypothesis were true. Computed test statistic values are compared to values in a table. If the absolute value of the test statistic is larger than the tabled value, the results are statistically significant. If the computed value is smaller, the results are nonsignificant.

When analyses are done by a computer, as is usually the case, researchers follow only the first three steps and then give commands to the computer. The computer calculates the test statistic, degrees of freedom, and the *actual* probability that the null hypothesis is true. For example, the computer may show that the two-tailed probability (*p*) of an intervention group being different from a control group by chance alone is 0.025. This means that only 25 times out of 1,000 would a group difference as large as the one obtained reflect chance differences rather than true intervention effects. The computed probability can then be compared with the desired significance level (alpha). If the significance criterion were 0.05, then the results would be significant because 0.025 is more stringent than 0.05. By convention, any computed probability greater than 0.05 (e.g., 0.20) indicates nonsignificance (sometimes abbreviated *NS*)—that is, a result that could have occurred by chance in more than 5 out of 100 samples.

The reference guide in Figure 18.5 does not include every test you may need, but it does include bivariate tests most often used by nurse researchers. Many resources are available online to help you select an appropriate test, including interactive decision-tree tools.

In the sections that follow, several common bivariate statistical tests are described. It is important to note that our introduction to inferential statistics is simplified and neglects important issues such as specific assumptions underlying various tests. We urge readers to grasp statistical principles before undertaking quantitative analyses.

TESTING DIFFERENCES BETWEEN TWO GROUP MEANS

A common research situation involves comparing two groups of participants on a continuous outcome variable. For instance, we might compare an experimental and control group of patients with regard to their mean blood pressure. Or we might contrast males and females with regard to mean depression scores.

The parametric test for differences in two means is the *t*-test. A *t*-test can be used when there are two independent groups (e.g., experimental vs. control), and when the sample is dependent (e.g., mean pretreatment and posttreatment scores for the same people).

> **TIP** Suliman and colleagues (2020) studied nurses' perception of nurse managers' leadership styles in four hospitals in Jordan. One-**sample *t*-tests** were used to describe the respondents' mean scores of the study variables related to three leadership styles among the nurse managers. The transactional leadership style (mean = 2.35, standard deviation (SD) = 0.71) had the highest mean score, followed by the transformational (mean = 2.06, SD = 0.73) and the passive-avoidant (mean = 1.71, SD = 0.78) leadership styles.

t-Tests for Independent Groups

Suppose we wanted to test the effect of early discharge of maternity patients on perceived maternal competence. We administer a scale of perceived maternal competence at discharge to 20 primiparas who had a vaginal birth: 10 who remained in the hospital 25 to 48 hours (regular discharge group) and 10 who were discharged within 24 hours of giving birth (early discharge group). In Table 18.1, we see that mean scores for these two groups are 25.0 and 19.0, respectively. Are these differences *reliable* (i.e., would they be found in the population of early-discharge and later-discharge mothers?), or do group differences reflect chance factors?

Note that the 20 scores in Table 18.1—10 per group—vary from one person to another. Some variability reflects individual differences in perceived maternal competence. Some variability might be due to measurement error (e.g., the scale's imperfect reliability), some could result from participants' moods on a particular day, and so forth. The research question follows: Can a portion of the variability reliably be attributed to the independent

TABLE 18.1 • Fictitious Data for *t*-Test Example: Scores on a Perceived Maternal Competence Scale for Regular-Discharge and Early-Discharge Mothers

REGULAR-DISCHARGE MOTHERS	EARLY-DISCHARGE MOTHERS
30	23
27	17
25	22
20	18
24	20
32	26
17	16
18	13
28	21
29	14
Mean = 25.0	Mean = 19.0

$t = 2.86$; $df = 18$; $p = .011$.

variable—time of discharge from the hospital? The *t*-test allows us to answer this question objectively. The hypotheses are

$$H_0 : \mu_A = \mu_B \quad H_A : \mu_A \neq \mu_B$$

To test these hypotheses, we would compute a *t*-statistic. The formula for the *t* statistic uses group means, variability, and sample size to calculate a value for *t*. When the data from Table 18.1 are used in the formula, the value of *t* is 2.86. Next, degrees of freedom are calculated. In this situation, degrees of freedom equal the total sample size minus 2 (*df* = 20 − 2 = 18). A table of critical *t* values is shown in Table A.1, Appendix A. Degrees of freedom are listed in the left column, and different alpha values are shown in the top rows. The shaded column shows values for $\alpha = 0.05$ for a two-tailed test. We find in this column that for *df* = 18, the tabled value of *t* is 2.10. *This value establishes an upper limit to what is probable if the null hypothesis is true.* Thus, the calculated *t* of 2.86, which is larger than the tabled value of the statistic,[2] is improbable (i.e., statistically significant). We can now say that the primiparas discharged early had significantly lower perceptions of maternal competence than those who were not discharged early. The group difference in perceived maternal competence is sufficiently large that it is unlikely to reflect merely chance fluctuations. If a computer were used to analyze the data, the output would show the *exact* probability, which is 0.011. This means that in only 11 out of 1,000 samples would we expect a group difference in means of 6.0 points by chance alone.

Example of Independent *t*-Tests
Weston and Zauche (2021) studied the difference between an in-person pediatric clinical practicum and a virtual pediatric clinical practicum. Scores on the Assessment Technologies Institute Nursing Care of Children examination were compared using independent-samples *t* tests and they found that there were no significant differences in the student scores between the two pediatric practicum experiences (*p* = .485; 95% confidence interval, −2.24 to 4.71).

When multiple tests are run with the same data—that is, when there are multiple outcomes—the risk of a Type I error increases. One *t*-test with an $\alpha = 0.05$ has a 5% probability of a Type I error. Two *t*-tests with the same data set, however, have a probability of 9.75% of one spurious significant result, and with three tests, the risk goes up to 14.3%. Researchers sometimes apply a **Bonferroni correction** when they run multiple tests, to establish a more conservative alpha level. For example, if the desired α is 0.05, and there are three separate tests, the corrected alpha needed to reject the null hypothesis for *all* tests would be 0.017, not 0.05. The correction is computed by dividing the desired α by the number of tests—e.g., 0.05/3 = 0.017. If we concluded that mean group differences were significant for three tests at or below *p* = .017, there would be only a 5% probability of wrongly rejecting the null across all three comparisons. The Bonferroni correction can, however, be problematic in that it tends to increase the risk of a Type II error—incorrectly concluding there is no statistical association when in fact there is one.

Confidence Intervals for Mean Differences

CIs can be constructed around the difference between two means, and the results provide information about both statistical significance (i.e., whether the null hypothesis should be rejected) and precision of the estimated difference. Because CI information is more useful in clinical applications than *p* values, it is sometimes preferred—although nursing journals have not required it, as many medical journals have.

In the example in Table 18.1, the mean maternal competence scores were 25.0 in the regular discharge group and 19.0 in the early discharge group. Using a formula to compute the *standard error of the difference*, CIs can be constructed around the mean difference of 6.0. For a 95% CI, the confidence limits in our example are 1.6 and 10.4. This means that we can be 95% confident that the true difference in population means on the scores for early- and regular-discharge mothers lies somewhere between these limits.

In the *t*-test analysis, we obtained an estimate of mean group differences (6.0) and learned that

---

[2]The tabled *t* values should be compared to the absolute value of the calculated *t*. Thus, if the calculated *t* were −2.86, then the results would still be significant.

the group differences were probably not spurious ($p = .011$). The CI information tells us the range within which the mean difference probably lies. We can see from the CI that the mean difference is significant at the 0.05 level *because the range does not include 0*. Given that there is a 95% probability that the mean difference is not lower than 1.6, this means that there is less than a 5% probability that there is no difference at all—thus, the null hypothesis can be rejected.

Because the CI does not give exact probabilities about the plausibility of the null hypothesis, it is often useful to present both parameter estimation and hypothesis testing information. In the current example, the results could be reported as follows: "Mothers who were discharged early had significantly lower maternal competence scores (19.0) than mothers with a regular discharge (26.0) ($t = 2.86$, $df = 18$, $p = .011$). The mean difference of 6.0 had a 95% CI of 1.6 to 10.4." Such information is more conveniently displayed in tables when there are multiple outcomes.

Paired *t*-Tests

Researchers sometimes obtain two measurements from the same people, or from paired sets of participants (e.g., siblings). When means for two sets of scores are not independent, researchers should use a **paired *t*-test**—a *t*-test for dependent groups.

Suppose we were studying the effect of a special diet on the cholesterol level of older males. A sample of 50 males is selected, and their cholesterol levels are measured at baseline and then after 2 months on the special diet. The hypotheses being tested are

$$H_0 : \mu_{X1} = \mu_{X2} \quad H_A : \mu_{X1} \neq \mu_{X2}$$

where X_1 = pretreatment cholesterol levels

X_2 = posttreatment cholesterol levels

A *t*-statistic then would be computed from pretest and posttest data, using a different formula than for the independent groups *t*-test. The obtained *t* would be compared with tabled *t*-values. For this type of *t*-test, degrees of freedom equal the number of paired observations minus one ($df = N - 1$).

CIs can be constructed around mean differences for paired as well as independent means.

Example of Paired *t*-Test
Flanagan and colleagues (2022) conducted a study to determine the feasibility of a nurse-coached walking intervention using wireless pedometers for informal caregivers of people with dementia. Paired *t*-test analysis was conducted to determine if there was a change in the steps walked before and after the 8-week program. Findings indicated the intervention and control group each demonstrated a statistically significant increase in steps walked ($p = .01$ control; $p = .02$ intervention).

Nonparametric Two-Group Tests

In certain two-group situations, a nonparametric test may be needed—for example, if the outcome variable is on an ordinal scale, or if the distribution is markedly nonnormal. The **Mann–Whitney *U* test**, the nonparametric analogue of an independent groups *t*-test, involves assigning ranks to the two groups of scores. The sum of the ranks for the two groups can be compared by calculating the *U* statistic. (This test is sometimes referred to as the *Wilcoxon rank-sum test*.) When ordinal-level data are paired (dependent), the Wilcoxon signed-rank test can be used. The **Wilcoxon signed-rank test** involves taking the difference between paired scores and ranking the absolute difference.

TESTING MEAN DIFFERENCES WITH THREE OR MORE GROUPS

Analysis of variance (ANOVA) is the parametric procedure for testing differences between means when there are three or more groups. The statistic computed in ANOVA is the ***F*-ratio**. ANOVA decomposes total variability in an outcome variable into two parts: (1) variability attributable to the independent variable and (2) all other variability, such as individual differences, measurement error, and so on. Variation *between* groups is contrasted to variation *within* groups to get an *F*-ratio. When differences between groups are large relative to variation within groups, the probability is high that the independent variable is related to, or has caused, group differences.

One-Way ANOVA

Suppose we were comparing the effectiveness of alternative interventions to help people stop smoking. One group of smokers receives nurse counseling (group A); a second group receives peer counseling—i.e., from a former smoker (group B); and a third control group receives no special treatment (group C). The outcome variable is 1-day cigarette consumption measured 1 month after the intervention. Thirty smokers who wish to quit smoking are randomly assigned to one of the three conditions. **One-way ANOVA** tests the following hypotheses:

$$H_0 : \mu_A = \mu_B = \mu_C \quad H_A : \mu_A \neq \mu_B \neq \mu_C$$

The null hypothesis is that the population means for posttreatment cigarette smoking are the same for all three groups, and the alternative (research) hypothesis is inequality of means. Table 18.2 presents fictitious data for 30 participants. The mean numbers of posttreatment cigarettes smoked in 1 day are 16.6, 19.2, and 34.0 for groups A, B, and C, respectively. These means are different, but are they significantly different—or do differences reflect random fluctuations?

In calculating an *F*-statistic, total variability in the data is broken down into two sources. The portion of the variance due to group status (i.e., exposure to different treatments, the independent variable) is reflected in the **sum of squares between groups**, or SS_B. The SS_B is the sum of squared deviations of individual group means from the overall **grand mean** for all participants.

The second component is the **sum of squares within groups**, or SS_W. This index is the sum of the squared deviations of each individual score from its *own* group mean. SS_W indicates variability attributable to individual differences, measurement error, and so on.

Recall from Chapter 17 that the formula for calculating a sample variance is $\Sigma x^2 \div N - 1$. The two sums of squares are like the numerator of this variance equation: both SS_B and SS_W are sums of squared deviations from means. So, to compute variance within and variance between groups, we must divide the sums of squares by something similar to $N - 1$, namely degrees of freedom for each sum of squares. For between groups, $df_B = G - 1$ (number of groups minus 1). For within groups, df_W is the number of participants less 1, for each group.

In an ANOVA context, the variance is referred to as the **mean square** (MS). The formulas for the mean square between groups and the mean square within groups are

$$MS_B = \frac{SS_B}{df_B} \quad MS_W = \frac{SS_W}{df_W}$$

TABLE 18.2 • Fictitious Data for a One-Way ANOVA: Number of Cigarettes Smoked in 1 Day, 1 Month Postintervention in Three Treatment Groups

GROUP A NURSE COUNSELING		GROUP B PEER COUNSELING		GROUP C UNTREATED CONTROL	
28	19	0	27	33	35
0	24	31	0	54	0
17	0	26	3	19	43
20	21	30	24	40	39
35	2	24	27	41	36
$\bar{X}_A = 16.6$		$\bar{X}_B = 19.2$		$\bar{X}_C = 34.0$	

$F = 4.98$, $df = 2, 27$, $p = .01$.

TABLE 18.3 • ANOVA Summary Table for Example of Posttreatment Smoking After Intervention

SOURCE OF VARIANCE	SS	df	MEAN SQUARE	F	P
Between groups	1,761.9	2	880.9	4.98	.014
Within groups	4,772.0	27	176.7		
Total	6,533.9	29			

The F-ratio statistic is the ratio of these mean squares, or

$$F = \frac{MS_B}{MS_W}$$

The ANOVA summary table (Table 18.3) shows that the calculated F-statistic in our example is 4.98. For $df = 2$ and 27 and $\alpha = 0.05$, the tabled F value is 3.35 (see Table A.2 in Appendix A for values from the theoretical F distribution). Because our obtained F-value of 4.98 exceeds 3.35, we reject the null hypothesis that the population means are equal. The *actual* probability, calculated by computer, is 0.014. Mean group differences in the number of posttreatment cigarettes smoked in 1 day are beyond chance expectations. In only 14 samples out of 1,000 would differences this great be obtained by chance alone.

The data support the research hypothesis that different treatments were associated with different cigarette smoking, but we cannot tell from the test whether treatment A was significantly more effective than treatment B. Statistical analyses known as **multiple comparison procedures** (or **posthoc tests**) are needed. Their function is to isolate the differences between group means that are responsible for rejecting the overall ANOVA null hypothesis. Note that it is *not* appropriate to use a series of t-tests (group A vs. B, A vs. C, and B vs. C) because this would increase the risk of a Type I error. Multiple comparison methods are described in most intermediate statistical textbooks, such as that by Polit (2010).

Example of a One-Way ANOVA
Hwang and Sim (2021) used a one-way ANOVA to examine the association of living arrangements with happiness attributes among older adults in Korea. Findings from 14,687 older adults indicated that there was a significant difference in the happiness index among older adults living alone (6.22 ± 2.11), older adults living with their spouse (6.76 ± 1.99), and older adults living with their family (6.46 ± 1.94) (F = 88.69, p < .001).

Two-Way ANOVA

One-way ANOVA is used to test mean group differences for a single independent variable, such as participants in three different interventions. Data from studies with multiple factors, as in a factorial design, can be analyzed by *multifactor ANOVA*. In this section, we describe principles for **two-way ANOVA**.

Suppose we wanted to compare the effectiveness of two alternative smoking cessation modalities (in-person and by telephone) led by nurse counselors vs. peer counselors (ex-smokers). We randomly assign a sample of 40 smokers to one of the four treatment conditions. One month after the intervention, participants report the number of cigarettes they smoked the previous day. Fictitious data for this example are shown in Table 18.4.

With two independent variables, three hypotheses are tested. First, we are testing the effectiveness, for both modalities, of nurse counseling vs. peer counseling. Second, we are testing whether postintervention smoking differs for in-person counseling vs. telephone counseling, regardless of who does the counseling. These are tests for **main effects**. Third, we are testing **interaction effects**

TABLE 18.4 • Fictitious Data for a Two-Way (2 × 2) ANOVA: Number of Cigarettes Smoked in One Day, 1 month Postintervention for Type of Counselors and Counseling Modality Groups

FACTOR B—MODALITY	FACTOR A—TYPE OF COUNSELORS					TOTAL
	NURSES (1)		PEERS (2)		
In-Person (1)	24	25	27	23	In-Person
	28	38	0	18	$\bar{X}_{B1} = 21.0$
	2	21	45	20	
	19	0	29	12	
	27	36	22	4	
	$\bar{X}_{A1B1} = 22.0$		$\bar{X}_{A2B1} = 20.0$		
Telephone (2)	10	16	36	27	Telephone
	21	18	41	0	$\bar{X}_{B2} = 23.0$
	17	3	28	49	
	0	25	37	35	
	33	17	5	42	
	$\bar{X}_{A1B1} = 16.0$		$\bar{X}_{A2B2} = 30.0$		
Total	Nurse Counselors: $\bar{X}_{A1} = 19.0$				Peer Counselors: $\bar{X}_{A2} = 25.0$	$\bar{X}_T = 23.0$

(i.e., differential effects for the two counselor types in the two modalities). Interaction concerns whether the effect of one independent variable is consistent for all levels of a second independent variable.

The data in Table 18.4 reveal that participants in the Nurse Counseling group smoked less, on average, than those in the Peer Counseling group (19.0 vs. 25.0); that participants who got in-person counseling smoked less than those who got telephone counseling (21.0 vs. 23.0); and that those who got nurse counseling smoked less when exposed to telephone counseling, but those who got peer counseling smoked less when exposed to in-person counseling. By performing a two-way ANOVA on these data, we could learn whether the effects were statistically significant.

Multifactor ANOVA is not restricted to two-way analyses. In theory, any number of independent variables is possible, but in practice studies with more than two factors are rare. Other statistical techniques typically are used with three or more independent variables, as we discuss in Chapter 19.

Repeated-Measures ANOVA

Repeated-measures ANOVA (RM-ANOVA) is used in several situations, one of which is when there are three or more measures of the same outcome variable for each participant. For instance, in some studies, physiologic measures such as blood pressure or heart rate might be collected before, during, and after a medical procedure. In this situation, a one-way RM-ANOVA is an extension of a paired *t*-test. It can be used with a single group studied longitudinally, or in a crossover design with three or more different conditions. (In Chapter 19 we discuss RM-ANOVA for mixed designs.)

As an example, suppose we wanted to compare three interventions for preterm infants, with regard to effects on infants' feeding rates: (1) nonnutritive sucking; (2) nonnutritive sucking plus music; or (3) music alone. Using an experimental repeated measures crossover design, infants participating in the study are randomly assigned to different orderings of the three treatments. Bottle feeding rate, the outcome, is measured after the treatments. The null hypothesis for this study is that type of intervention is unrelated to feeding rate (i.e., $\mu_1 = \mu_2 = \mu_3$). The alternative hypothesis is that feeding rate and type of intervention are related (i.e., that the three population means are not equal).

We would find in such a study that there was variability in feeding rates both across infants within each condition, and across the three treatment conditions within infants. As was true with other ANOVA situations, total variability in the outcome is represented by the total sum of squares, which can be partitioned into contributing components. In RM-ANOVA, three sources of variation contribute to total variability:

$$SS_{total} = SS_{treatments} + SS_{subjects} + SS_{error}$$

Conceptually, *sum of squares-treatments* is analogous to sum of squares-between in regular ANOVA: it represents the effect of the independent variable. (When measurements are taken at multiple points without an intervention, it may be called *sum of squares-time*.) The *sum of squares-error* is similar to the sum of squares-within in regular ANOVA: both represent variations associated with random fluctuations. The third component, *sum of squares-subjects*, has no counterpart in a simple ANOVA, because those being compared in regular ANOVA are different people. The $SS_{subjects}$ term captures individual differences, the effects of which are consistent across conditions. That is, some infants tend to have high feeding rates and others tend to have low feeding rates, regardless of treatment. Because individual differences can be statistically isolated from the error term (random fluctuation), RM-ANOVA yields a more sensitive test of the relationship between the independent and dependent variables than between-subjects ANOVA. By statistical isolation, we mean that variability attributable to individual differences is removed from the denominator in computing the *F* statistic.

Example of RM-ANOVA
Lee and Ra (2021) examined the effects of olfactory stimulation with maternal breast milk on abnormal physiologic responses in preterm infants. Using a pretest-posttest design, 31 preterm infants were included in the study (13 in the experimental group, 18 in the control). The intervention was delivered three times per day for 5 days. Abnormal physiologic responses were assessed over 6 days. Using RM-ANOVA for the analysis, the experimental group demonstrated a significantly lower frequency of apnea than the control group did ($p = .021$).

Nonparametric "Analysis of Variance"

Nonparametric tests do not actually analyze variance, but there are nonparametric analogues to ANOVA when a parametric test is not appropriate. The **Kruskal–Wallis test** is a generalized version of the Mann-Whitney *U* test, based on assigning ranks to the scores of various groups. This test is used when the number of groups is greater than two and a one-way test for independent samples is desired. When multiple measures are obtained from the same subjects, the **Friedman test** for "analysis of variance" by ranks can be used. Both tests are described in Polit (2010) and other statistics textbooks.

TESTING DIFFERENCES IN PROPORTIONS

Tests discussed thus far involve continuous dependent variables, when group means are being compared. In this section, we examine tests of group differences when the outcome is on a nominal scale.

The Chi-Square Test

The **chi-square** (χ^2) **test** is used to test hypotheses about group differences in proportions, as when a crosstabs table has been created. Suppose we were studying the effect of nursing instruction on patients' compliance with a self-medication regimen. Nurses implement a new instructional strategy with 100 randomly assigned experimental patients, while 100 control group patients get the usual instruction. The research hypothesis is that a higher proportion of people in the intervention group than in the control group will be compliant.

The chi-square statistic is computed by comparing **observed frequencies** (i.e., values observed in the data) and expected frequencies. Observed frequencies for our example are shown in Table 18.5. As this table shows, 60 experimental participants (60%), but only 40 controls (40%), reported self-medication compliance after the intervention. The chi-square test enables us to decide whether a difference in proportions of this magnitude is likely to reflect a real treatment effect or only chance fluctuations. **Expected frequencies** are the cell frequencies that would be found if there were *no* relationship between the two variables. In this example, if there were no relationship between the two groups, the expected frequency would be 50 people per cell because, overall, exactly half the participants (100 out of 200) complied.

The chi-square statistic is computed by summarizing differences between observed and expected frequencies for each cell. Formulas and computations are not shown here, but in our example, $\chi^2 = 8.00$. For chi-square tests, *df* equals the number of rows minus 1 times number of columns minus 1. In the current case, $df = 1 \times 1 = 1$. With 1 *df*, the tabled value (Table A.3 of Appendix A) from a theoretical chi-square distribution that must be exceeded to establish significance at the 0.05 level is 3.84. The obtained value of 8.00 is much larger than would be expected by chance (actual $p = .005$). We can conclude that a significantly larger proportion of experimental patients than control patients were compliant.

Example of Chi-Square Test
Verd and colleagues (2021) conducted a secondary analysis of 691 children in Majorca, Spain, to examine if breastfeeding protected children from COVID-19. Using the Chi-square test they found that there was a higher prevalence of positive COVID-19 tests among children who were exclusively formula fed compared with those who were ever breastfed (OR 2.48; 95% CI 1.45, 3.51; $p = .036$).

Confidence Intervals for Differences in Proportion

As with means, it is possible to construct CIs around the difference between two proportions. To do this, we would need to calculate the *standard error of the difference of proportions*. In the example used to explain the chi square statistic (Table 18.5), the difference in proportions was 0.20 ($p < .01$), and the *SE* of the difference is 0.069. The 95% CI in this example is 0.06 to 0.34. We can be 95% confident that the true population difference in compliance rates between those exposed to the intervention and those not exposed is between 6% and 34%. This interval does not include 0%, indicating that we can be 95% confident that group differences are "real."

TABLE 18.5 • Observed Frequencies for Chi-Square Example: Patient Compliance in Two Treatment Groups

PATIENT COMPLIANCE	GROUP		TOTAL
	CONTROL	EXPERIMENTAL	
Compliant	40	60	100
Noncompliant	60	40	100
Total	100	100	200

$X^2 = 8.00$, $df = 1$, $p = .005$.

Other Tests of Proportions

Sometimes a chi-square test is not appropriate. When the total sample size is small (total N of 30 or fewer) or when there are cells with small frequencies (five or fewer), **Fisher exact test** should be used to test the significance of differences in proportions. When the proportions being compared are from two paired groups (e.g., when a pretest–posttest design is used to compare changes in proportions on a dichotomous variable), the appropriate test is **McNemar test**.

TESTING CORRELATIONS

The statistical tests discussed thus far are used to test *group* differences—they involve situations in which the independent variable is a nominal-level variable. In this section, we consider statistical tests used when both the independent variable and the outcome variable are ordinal, interval, or ratio.

Pearson's r

Pearson's r, the correlation coefficient calculated when two variables are measured on at least the interval scale, is both descriptive and inferential. Descriptively, the correlation coefficient summarizes the magnitude and direction of a relationship between two variables. As an inferential statistic, r is used to test hypotheses about population correlations, which are symbolized as ρ, the Greek letter rho. The null hypothesis is that there is no relationship between two variables; the alternate hypothesis is that a relationship exists in the population:

$$H_0 : \rho = 0 \quad H_A : \rho \neq 0$$

For instance, suppose we studied the relationship between patients' self-reported level of stress and the pH level of their saliva. In a sample of 50 people, we find that $r = -0.29$, indicating a modest tendency for people with high stress scores to have low pH levels. But does the coefficient of -0.29 reflect a random fluctuation, observable only for the people in our sample, or is the relationship likely to be true in the population? We can compare our computed r to a tabled value from a theoretical distribution for r. Degrees of freedom for r equal the number of participants minus 2, or $(N - 2)$. With $df = 48$, the tabled value for r for a two-tailed test with $\alpha = 0.05$ (Table A.4 in Appendix A) is 0.2803. Because the absolute value of the calculated r is 0.29, the null hypothesis can be rejected. We accept the research hypothesis that the correlation between stress and saliva acidity in the population is not zero.

Pearson's r can be used in both within-group and between-group situations. The example about the relationship between stress scores and the pH levels is a between-group situation: The question is whether people with high stress scores tend to have significantly lower pH levels than *different* people with low stress scores. If stress scores were obtained from the same people (e.g., before and after surgery), the correlation between the two scores would be a within-group situation.

> **Example of Pearson's r**
> In a study examining the impact of auditory feedback on walking balance in older adults, Cornwell and colleagues calculated a Pearson correlation to examine the changes in step length observed between the nonuse and use of ear plugs. They found a moderate negative relationship that approached significance (rho = −0.44; $p = .055$), which suggested that those with most difficulty with balance increased their step length the most with the ear plug use.

Other Tests of Bivariate Relationships

Pearson's r is a parametric statistic. When the assumptions for a parametric test are violated, or when the data are ordinal-level, then the appropriate coefficient of correlation is either **Spearman's rho** (r_S) or **Kendall's tau**. The values of these statistics range from −1.00 to +1.00, and their interpretation is similar to that of Pearson's r. Another correlation statistic that is used to correlate a dichotomous variable with a continuous one is called a **point-biserial correlation coefficient**. Interpretation of this statistic requires knowing how the dichotomous variable was coded (usually, it is 1 vs. 0).

Measures of the magnitude of relationships can also be computed with nominal-level data.

For example, the **phi coefficient** (Φ) is an index describing the relationship between two dichotomous variables. **Cramér's V** is an index of relationship applied to crosstabs tables larger than 2 × 2. Both statistics are based on the chi-square statistic and yield values that range between 0.00 and 1.00, with higher values indicating a stronger association between variables.

POWER ANALYSIS AND EFFECT SIZE

Many published nursing studies (and even more *un*published ones) have nonsignificant findings, and many of these could reflect Type II errors. As indicated earlier, researchers set the probability of committing a Type I error (a false positive) as the significance level, alpha (α). The probability of a Type II error (a false negative) is **beta** (β). The complement of beta ($1 - \beta$) is the *probability of detecting a true relationship or group difference* and is the **power** of a statistical test. Polit and Sherman (1990) found that many published nursing studies have insufficient power, placing them at risk for Type II errors—although a more recent study has found that, on average, power has improved in nursing studies, perhaps because of heightened awareness (Gaskin & Happell, 2014). Nevertheless, even in the more recent analysis, many studies were found to be **underpowered**.

Power analysis is used to reduce the risk of Type II errors and strengthen statistical conclusion validity by estimating in advance how big a sample is needed. There are four components in a power analysis, three of which must be known or estimated:

1. *The significance criterion*, α. Other things being equal, the more stringent this criterion, the lower the power.
2. *The sample size*, N. As sample size increases, power increases.
3. *The effect size* (ES). ES is an estimate of how wrong the null hypothesis is—that is, how strong the relationship between the independent variable and the outcome is in the population.
4. *Power, or $1 - \beta$*. This is the probability of rejecting a false null hypothesis.

Researchers typically use power analysis at the outset of a study to estimate the sample size needed to avoid a Type II error. To estimate needed sample size (N), researchers must specify α, ES, and $1 - \beta$. Researchers usually establish the risk of a Type I error (α) as 0.05. The conventional standard for $1 - \beta$ is 0.80. With power equal to 0.80, there is a 20% risk of committing a Type II error. Although this risk may seem high, a stricter criterion requires sample sizes larger than many researchers could afford.

With α and $1 - \beta$ specified, the information needed to solve for N is ES, the estimated population effect size. The **effect size** is the magnitude of the relationship between the research variables. When relationships (effects) are strong, they can be detected at significant levels even with small samples. With modest relationships, large sample sizes are needed to avoid Type II errors.

In using power analysis to estimate sample size needs, the population effect size is not *known*; if it were known, there would be no need for the new study. Effect size must be estimated using available evidence and theory. In essence, the effect size estimate represents the researcher's *hypothesis* about how strong relationships are. Researchers sometimes use findings from a pilot study as a basis for the estimate—although we explain in Chapter 29 why this is risky. More often an effect size is calculated based on findings from earlier studies on a similar problem. When there are *no* relevant earlier findings and when theory offers only broad guidance, researchers use conventions based on expectations of a *small*, *medium*, or *large* effect. Most nursing studies have modest (small-to-medium) effects.

TIP Researchers can usually find several studies from which the effect size can be estimated. In such a case, the estimate should be based on the one with the most reliable results. Researchers can also estimate effect size by combining information from multiple high-quality studies through averaging or weighted averaging.

Procedures for estimating effects and sample size needs vary from one statistical situation to another. We focus mainly on two-group mean-difference situations.

Sample Size Estimates for Testing Differences Between Two Means

Suppose we were testing the hypothesis that cranberry juice reduces the urinary pH of diet-controlled patients. We plan to assign some patients randomly to a control condition (no cranberry juice) and others to an experimental condition in which they will be given 300 mL of cranberry juice for 5 days. How large a sample is needed for this study, given a desired α of 0.05 and power of 0.80?

To answer this, we must first estimate ES. In a two-group situation in which mean differences are of interest, ES is usually designated as **Cohen's d**, the formula for which is as follows:

$$d = \frac{\mu_1 - \mu_2}{\sigma}$$

The effect size (d) is the difference between the two population means, divided by the population standard deviation (σ). These population values are never known but are estimated. For example, suppose we found an earlier nonexperimental study that compared the urinary pH of people who had or had not ingested cranberry juice in the previous 24 hours. The earlier study is a reasonable starting point. Suppose the results were as follows:

$$\bar{X}_1 \text{ (no cranberry juice)} = 5.70$$
$$\bar{X}_2 \text{ (cranberry juice)} = 5.50$$
$$SD = .50$$

The estimated value of d would be 0.40:

$$d = \frac{5.70 - 5.50}{.50} = .40$$

Table 18.6 presents approximate sample size requirements for various effect sizes and powers, for $\alpha = 0.05$ (for two-tailed tests), in a two-group mean-difference situation. We find in this table that the estimated n (number *per group*) to detect an effect size of 0.40 with power equal to 0.80 is 99 people. Assuming that the earlier study provided a good estimate of the population effect size, the total number of people needed in the new study would be about 200, with half assigned to the control group (no cranberry juice) and the other half assigned to the experimental group. With a sample size smaller than 200, there would be a greater than 20% chance of a false-negative conclusion, i.e., a Type II error. For example, a sample size of 128 (64 per group) would result in an estimated 40% chance of incorrect nonsignificant results.

TABLE 18.6 • Approximate Sample Sizes[a] per Group Needed to Achieve Selected Levels of Power as a Function of Estimated Effect Size for Test of Difference of Two Means, for $\alpha = 0.05$

Power	\multicolumn{11}{c	}{ESTIMATED EFFECT SIZE (d)[b]}
	0.10	0.15	0.20	0.25	0.30	0.35	0.40	0.50	0.60	0.70	0.80
0.60	979	435	245	157	109	80	62	40	28	20	16
0.70	1,233	548	309	198	137	101	78	50	35	26	20
0.80	1,576	701	394	253	176	129	99	64	44	33	25
0.90	2,103	935	526	337	234	172	132	85	59	43	33
0.95	2,594	1,154	649	416	289	213	163	105	73	53	41

[a]Sample size requirements for each group; total sample size would be twice the number shown.
[b]Estimated effect size (d) is the estimated population mean group difference divided by the estimated population standard deviation or $(\mu_1 - \mu_2)/s$.

If there is no prior research, researchers can, as a last resort, estimate whether the expected effect is small, medium, or large. By convention (Cohen, 1988), the value of *ES* in a two-group test of mean differences is estimated at 0.20 for small effects, 0.50 for medium effects, and 0.80 for large effects. With an α value of 0.05 and power of 0.80, the *n* (number of participants per group) for studies with expected small, medium, and large effects would be 394, 64, and 25, respectively. Most nursing studies cannot expect effect sizes in excess of 0.50; those in the range of 0.20 to 0.40 are most common. In Polit and Sherman's (1990) analysis of effect sizes for studies published in two nursing research journals, the average effect size for *t*-test situations was 0.35. A medium effect should be estimated only when the effect is so substantial that it can be detected by the naked eye (i.e., without formal research procedures).

> **TIP** Performing a power analysis based on estimates of an effect size is an *evidence-based* approach to designing a new study—that is, the new study uses evidence from earlier studies to estimate how many sample members will be needed to achieve an effect that seems plausible in light of what is already known. A useful supplementary approach is to ask, How big an effect would be needed to be clinically relevant? If effect-size estimates are both evidence-based and clinically meaningful, the study will be stronger.

Sample Size Estimates for Other Bivariate Tests

Power analysis can be undertaken for the other statistical tests described in this chapter. It is relatively easy to do a power analysis online. Here we discuss only a few basic features for situations in which ANOVA, Pearson's *r*, or a chi-square situation would be the basis for doing the power analysis.

There are alternative approaches to doing a power analysis in an ANOVA context. The simplest approach is to estimate **eta-squared** (η^2), which is an ES index indicating the proportion of variance explained in ANOVA. Eta-squared equals the sum of squares between (SS_B) divided by the total sum of squares (SS_T) and can be used directly as the estimate of effect size if sum of squares information is available. When eta-squared cannot be estimated, researchers can estimate whether effects are likely to be small, medium, or large. For ANOVA situations, the conventional estimates for small, medium, and large effects would be values of η^2 equal to 0.01, 0.06, and 0.14, respectively. Assuming $\alpha = 0.05$ and power = 0.80, this corresponds to sample size requirements of about 319, 53, or 22 subjects *per group* in a three-group study, and about 272, 44, and 19 *per group* in a four-group study,[3] (for the data in Table 18.2 and shown in an ANOVA summary table in Table 18.3, $\eta^2 = 0.27$, a large effect).

For Pearson correlations, the ES index is an estimate of ρ, the population correlation coefficient. Thus, the value of the correlation coefficient (*r*) from a relevant earlier study can be used directly as the estimated effect size. Table 18.7 shows sample size requirements for various effect sizes and powers when $\alpha = 0.05$ and the test statistic is Pearson's *r*. For example, if our estimated population correlation was 0.25, we would need a sample size of 123 for power = 0.80. With a sample this size, we can expect that we would wrongly reject a true null hypothesis 5 times out of 100 and wrongly retain a false null hypothesis 20 times out of 100. When prior estimates of effect size are unavailable, the conventional values of small, medium, and large effect sizes in a bivariate correlation situation are 0.10, 0.30, and 0.50, respectively (i.e., samples of 785, 85, and 29 for a power of 0.80 and a significance level of 0.05). In Polit and Sherman's (1990) study, the average correlation in nursing studies was found to be around 0.20.

Estimating sample size requirements for testing group differences in proportions is complex. The effect size for crosstabs tables is influenced not only by expected differences in proportions (e.g., 60% in one group vs. 40% in another, a 20% point difference), but also by the absolute values of the proportions. Effect sizes are *larger* (and thus sample size needs are *smaller*) at the extremes than near the midpoint. A 20% point difference is easier to detect if the percentages are 10% and 30% than if they are near the middle, such as 60% and 40%. Because of this

---
[3]Power tables are not provided here for ANOVA and chi-square situations.

TABLE 18.7 • Approximate Sample Sizes Necessary to Achieve Selected Levels of Power as a Function of Estimated Population Correlation, With $\alpha = 0.05$

	\multicolumn{11}{c}{ESTIMATED POPULATION CORRELATION COEFFICIENT (ρ)[a]}
Power	0.10	0.15	0.20	0.25	0.30	0.35	0.40	0.50	0.60	0.70	0.80
0.60	489	217	122	78	54	39	30	19	13	9	7
0.70	614	272	152	97	67	49	37	23	16	11	8
0.80	785	347	194	123	85	62	47	29	19	13	10
0.90	1,047	463	258	164	112	81	61	37	25	17	12
0.95	1,296	575	322	204	141	101	80	50	32	22	18

[a]Estimated effect size (r) is the estimated population correlation coefficient (ρ).

fact, it is difficult to offer information on values for small, medium, and large effects. We can, however, give *examples* of differences in proportions that conform to the conventions in a 2 × 2 situation:

Small: 0.05 vs. 0.10, 0.20 vs. 0.29, 0.40 vs. 0.50, 0.60 vs. 0.70, 0.80 vs. 0.87
Medium: 0.05 vs. 0.21, 0.20 vs. 0.43, 0.40 vs. 0.65, 0.60 vs. 0.82, 0.80 vs. 0.96
Large: 0.05 vs. 0.34, 0.20 vs. 0.58, 0.40 vs. 0.78, 0.60 vs. 0.92, 0.80 vs. 0.96

For example, if the expected proportion for a control group were 0.40, the researcher would need about 385, 70, and 24 per group if values higher than 0.40 were expected for the experimental group and the effect was expected to be small, medium, and large, respectively. As in other situations, researchers are encouraged to avoid using the conventions in favor of more precise estimates based on existing evidence. If the conventions cannot be avoided, conservative estimates should be used to minimize the risk of obtaining nonsignificant results.

Example of a Power Analysis
De Pinho and colleagues (2021) assessed the efficacy and feasibility of mental health nurses' provision of metacognitive training for patients with schizophrenia. A sample size of 36 with 18 participants in each group was established based on a power analysis that considered an expected attrition rate of 10%. Power was set to 0.80.

TIP Although power analysis is frequently used to estimate sample size needs, an alternative is to use *precision estimation*, which uses a confidence interval framework to estimate an appropriate sample size (Corty & Corty, 2011). Another approach is to consider benchmarks for *clinical significance* (Chapter 21) when estimating sample size needs.

Effect Size Calculations in Completed Studies

Power analysis concepts are sometimes used after analyses are completed to calculate estimated population effects based on *actual N*s. In this situation, power, alpha, and N are known, and so the task is to solve for ES. Effect sizes provide readers and clinicians with estimates about the magnitude of effects—an important issue in EBP. Effect size information can be crucial because, with large samples, even tiny effects can be statistically significant. p values tell you whether results are likely to be *real*, but effect sizes can suggest whether they are important. Effect size estimates are needed in doing meta-analyses (see Chapter 30), and so when these values are presented in a report, they are helpful to meta-analysts.

Example of Calculated Effect Size

Frigotto et al. (2023) aimed to verify if the functional capacity was different between institutionalized older adults who either survived or did not survive a COVID-19 infection. The functional capacity parameters reflected a small effect size and no significant differences between the groups for gait speed $p = .622$ (-8%; $d = 0.39$) or for the sit-to-stand test $p = .608$ (-9%; $d = 0.22$), but a moderate effect size was observed for handgrip strength, with lower values for the nonsurvivors' group $p = .371$ (-16%; $d = 0.53$).

CRITICAL APPRAISAL OF INFERENTIAL STATISTICAL ANALYSES

It is difficult to critically appraise researchers' data analysis decisions without good training in statistics. Nevertheless, there are certain things you can do to evaluate statistical analyses even if your background in statistics is modest.

You can begin by asking whether the report presents the results of statistical tests for all study hypotheses, and whether the researchers undertook analyses to address questions about the study's internal validity. For example, in a case-control study, was the comparability of the groups assessed (i.e., were analyses undertaken to test for selection biases)? Did groups differ with regard to attrition? As noted in Chapter 10, both analytic and design decisions can affect statistical conclusion validity. When sample size is small, when participation in an intervention is low, or when a weak statistical procedure is used in lieu of a more powerful one, then the risk of drawing the wrong conclusion about the research hypotheses is heightened. Threats to statistical conclusion validity should be considered when research hypotheses are not supported.

Other issues important in a thorough appraisal are whether the researcher used the right statistical tests, whether the statistical information reported is adequate to meet readers' information needs, and whether the results were presented in a clear and thoughtful manner, with a judicious combination of information reported in the text and in well laid-out tables. Box 18.1 presents

---

BOX 18.1 Guidelines for Critically Appraising Bivariate[a] Inferential Analyses

1. Did the report include any bivariate inferential statistics? Was a statistical test performed for each hypothesis or research question? If inferential statistics were not used, should they have been?
2. Were statistical tests used to strengthen inferences about the study's internal validity (e.g., to test for selection bias or attrition bias)? If not, should they have been?
3. Were the selected statistical tests appropriate, given the level of measurement of the variables and the nature of the hypotheses?
4. Were parametric tests used? Does it appear that the use of parametric tests was appropriate? If nonparametric tests were used, was a rationale provided, and does the rationale seem sound?
5. Was information provided about both hypothesis testing and estimation of parameters? Were effect sizes reported?
6. In general, did the report provide a rationale for the use of the selected statistical tests? Did the report contain sufficient information for you to judge whether appropriate statistics were used?
7. Were the results of any statistical tests significant? What do the tests tell you about the plausibility of the research hypotheses? Were effects sizable?
8. Were the results of any statistical tests nonsignificant? Is it plausible that these reflect Type II errors? What factors might have undermined the study's statistical conclusion validity?
9. Was an appropriate amount of statistical information reported? Are the findings clearly and logically organized?
10. Were tables or figures used judiciously to summarize large amounts of statistical information? Are the tables clearly presented, with good titles and carefully labeled column headings? Is the information in the text consistent with the information presented in the tables? Is the information totally redundant?

[a]Most of these questions are equally appropriate for critically appraising the multivariate statistics described in Chapter 19.

some guiding questions for critically appraising bivariate inferential statistics in a research report.

TIP You may find it helpful to consult the glossary of statistical symbols in the inside back cover if you find a symbol in a report that you do not recognize. Some symbols included in this glossary are not explained in this book; it may be necessary to refer to a statistics textbook for further information.

RESEARCH EXAMPLE

We conclude this chapter with an example of a study that used some of the statistical tests described in this chapter.

Study: Positive Mental Health and Self-Care in Patients with Chronic Physical Health Problems: Implications for Evidence-based Practice (Puig Llobet et al., 2020).

Statement of purpose: The purpose of this study was to determine the level of positive mental health (PMH) and self-care agency as well as the relations among sociodemographic variables in patients with chronic health conditions.

Methods: The research team conducted a descriptive, cross-sectional correlational study in a sample of 209 patients at a primary care center in Spain. Study measures included the following: sociodemographic variables including employment status, physical health variables, and the valid and reliable measures of the Positive Mental Health (PMH) Questionnaire and the Appraisal of Self-Care Agency (ASCA) scale.

Analysis and Findings: Descriptive statistics were used on the demographic variables including the employment status. Frequency distributions and percentages were used to present the demographic findings such 45% of the sample was more than 75 years of age. Means and standard deviations were calculated for each of the variables as appropriate. The t-test was used to describe the mean of the two measures: PMH and ASA scales. For example, the mean global PMH score was $X = 132$ ($SD = 13.0$), but the Pearson's test did not show a significant correlation between age and the PMH score. With a Cronbach's alpha of 0.88, the PMH was reliable. One way ANOVA indicated that there were significant differences in the correlations between four factors of the PMH scale. As for the ASA, the reliability scored a Cronbach's alpha of 0.80 and the mean score was 64.35 ($SD = 6.23$).

Student's t-test was used to compare the means of PMH scores and physical health conditions. The researchers found significant differences between the PMH scores and some illnesses such as COPD and osteoporosis, but not other health conditions such as hypertension, hypercholesterolemia, obesity, or osteoarthritis. The Spearman and Pearson correlation coefficients were used to examine PMH levels, and the number of chronic physical health conditions and this analysis suggested no significant correlation. The correlation between the ASA and PMH scores reflected a moderate, but significant correlation ($r = 0.46$; $p < .001$).

SUMMARY POINTS

- **Inferential statistics**, which are based on **laws of probability**, allow researchers to make inferences about a population based on data from a sample; it offers a framework for deciding whether **sampling error** resulting from sampling fluctuations is too high to provide reliable population estimates.
- The **sampling distribution of the mean** is a theoretical distribution of the means of an infinite number of samples drawn from a population. The sampling distribution of means is normally distributed, so the probability that a given sample value will be obtained can be ascertained.
- The **standard error of the mean (SEM)**—the standard deviation of this theoretical distribution—indicates the degree of average error of a sample mean; the smaller the SEM, the more accurate are the sample estimates of the population mean.
- Statistical inference consists of parameter estimation and hypothesis testing. **Parameter estimation** is used to estimate a population parameter from a sample statistic.
- **Point estimation** is a descriptive value of the population estimate (e.g., a mean or odds ratio). **Interval estimation** provides the upper and

- lower limits of a range of values—the **confidence interval (CI)**—between which the population value is expected to fall, at a specified probability. A 95% CI indicates a 95% probability that the true population value lies between the upper and lower **confidence limits.**
- **Hypothesis testing** through statistical procedures enables researchers to make objective decisions about the validity of their hypotheses.
- The **null hypothesis** states that there is no relationship between research variables, and that any observed relationship is due to chance. Rejection of the null hypothesis lends support to the research hypothesis.
- A **Type I error** occurs when a null hypothesis is incorrectly rejected (a false positive). A **Type II error** occurs when a null hypothesis is wrongly accepted (a false negative).
- Researchers control the risk of a Type I error by establishing a **level of significance** (or **alpha** [α] level), which is the probability that such an error will occur. The 0.05 level means that in only 5 out of 100 samples would the null hypothesis be rejected when it should have been accepted.
- In testing hypotheses, researchers compute a **test statistic** and then determine whether the statistic falls at or beyond the **critical region** on a relevant theoretical distribution. If the value of the test statistic indicates that the null hypothesis is "improbable," the result is **statistically significant** (i.e., obtained results are not likely to have occurred by chance, at the specified level of probability).
- Most hypothesis testing involves **two-tailed tests**, in which both ends of the sampling distribution are used to define the region of improbable values; a **one-tailed test** may be appropriate if there is a strong rationale for an a priori directional hypothesis.
- **Parametric tests** involve the estimation of at least one parameter, the use of interval- or ratio-level data, and the assumption of normally distributed variables; **nonparametric tests** are used when the data are nominal or ordinal or when a normal distribution cannot be assumed—especially when samples are small.
- **Tests for independent groups** compare different groups of people (between-subjects design), and **tests for dependent groups** compare the same group of people over time or conditions (within-subjects designs).
- Two common statistical tests are the *t*-**test** and **analysis of variance** (ANOVA), both of which are used to test the significance of the difference between group means; ANOVA is used when there are three or more groups (**one-way ANOVA**) or when there is more than one independent variable (e.g., **two-way ANOVA**). **Repeated measures ANOVA (RM-ANOVA)** is used when there are multiple means being compared over time.
- The **chi-square test** (χ^2) is used to test hypotheses about differences in proportions. For small samples or small cell sizes, **Fisher exact test** should be used.
- Statistical tests to measure the magnitude of bivariate relationships and to test whether the relationship is significantly different from zero include **Pearson's** *r* for interval-level data, **Spearman's rho** and **Kendall's tau** for ordinal-level data, and the **phi coefficient** and **Cramér's V** for nominal-level data. A **point-biserial correlation coefficient** can be computed when one variable is dichotomous and the other is continuous.
- Confidence intervals can be constructed around almost any computed statistic, including differences between means, differences between proportions, and correlation coefficients. CI information is valuable to clinical decision-makers, who need to know more than whether differences are probably real.
- **Power analysis** is a method of estimating either the likelihood of committing a Type II error or sample size requirements. Power analysis involves four components: desired significance level (α), **power** ($1 - \beta$), sample size (N), and estimated **effect size** (ES). Effect size estimates convey important information about the magnitude of effects in a study and are a useful supplement to *p* values and CI values. **Cohen's *d*** is a widely used effect size index summarizing mean-difference effects between two groups.

REFERENCES CITED IN CHAPTER 18

Benjamin, D. J., Berger, J. O., Johannesson, M., Nosek, B. A., Wagenmakers, E. J., Berk, R., Bollen, K. A., Brembs, B., Brown, L., Camerer, C., Cesarini, D., Chambers, C. D., Clyde, M., Cook, T. D., De Boeck, P., Dienes, Z., Dreber, A., Easwaran, K., Efferson, C., ... Johnson, V. E. (2018). Redefine statistical significance. *Nature Human Behaviour*, *2*(1), 6–10. https://doi-org.proxy.bc.edu/10.1038/s41562-017-0189-z

Cohen, J. (1988). *Statistical power analysis for the behavioral sciences* (2nd ed.). Lawrence Erlbaum Associates.

Corty, E. W., & Corty, R. (2011). Setting sample size to ensure narrow confidence intervals for precise estimation of population values. *Nursing Research*, *60*, 148–154.

Dancey, C., Reidy, J., & Rowe, R. (2012). *Statistics for the health sciences: A non-mathematical introduction*. Sage Publications.

De Pinho, L. M. G., Sequeira, C. A. D. C., Sampaio, F. M. C., Rocha, N. B., Ozaslan, Z., & Ferre-Grau, C. (2021). Assessing the efficacy and feasibility of providing metacognitive training for patients with schizophrenia by mental health nurses: A randomized controlled trial. *Journal of Advanced Nursing*, *77*(2), 999–1012. https://doi.org/10.1111/jan.14627

Flanagan, J., Post, K., Hill, R., & DiPalazzo, J. (2022). Feasibility of a nurse coached walking intervention for informal dementia caregivers. *Western Journal of Nursing Research*, *44*(5), 466–476. https://doi.org/10.1177/01939459211001395

Frigotto, M. F., Rodrigues, R., Rabello, R., & Pietta-Dias, C. (2023). COVID-19 in older adult residents in nursing homes: Factors associated with mortality and impact on functional capacity. *Sport Sciences for Health*, *19*, 1–9. https://doi.org/10.1007/s11332-022-01040-w

Gaskin, C., & Happell, B. (2014). Power, effects, confidence, and significance: An investigation of statistical practices in nursing research. *International Journal of Nursing Studies*, *51*, 795–806.

Gravetter, F., Wallnau, L., & Forzano, L. (2018). *Essentials of statistics for the behavioral sciences* (9th ed.). Wadsworth Publishing.

Hamlin, L., Grunwald, L., Sturdivant, R. X., & Koehlmoos, T. P. (2021). Comparison of nurse-midwife and physician birth outcomes in the military health system. *Policy, Politics & Nursing Practice*, *22*(2), 105–113. https://doi.org/10.1177/1527154421994071

Hwang, E. J., & Sim, I. O. (2021). Association of living arrangements with happiness attributes among older adults. *BMC Geriatrics*, *21*(1), 100. https://doi.org/10.1186/s12877-021-02017-z

Lee, W. A., & Ra, J. S. (2021). Olfactory stimulation of preterm infants with breast milk. *Clinical Nursing Research*, *30*(8), 1183–1192. https://doi.org/10.1177/10547738211018913

Polit, D. F. (2010). *Statistics and data analysis for nursing research* (2nd ed.). Pearson.

Polit, D. F., & Sherman, R. (1990). Statistical power in nursing research. *Nursing Research*, *39*, 365–369.

Polit, D., & Beck, C. (2013). Is there still gender bias in nursing research? An update. *Research in Nursing & Health*, *36*, 75–83.

Puig Llobet, M., Sánchez Ortega, M., Lluch-Canut, M., Moreno-Arroyo, M., Hidalgo Blanco, M. À., & Roldán-Merino, J. (2020). Positive mental health and self-care in patients with chronic physical health problems: Implications for evidence-based practice. *Worldviews on Evidence-Based Nursing*, *17*(4), 293–300. https://doi.org/10.1111/wvn.12453

Suliman, M., Aljezawi, M., Almansi, S., Musa, A., Alazam, M., & Ta'an, W. F. (2020). Effect of nurse managers' leadership styles on predicted nurse turnover. *Nursing Management (Harrow)*, *27*(5), 20–25. https://doi.org10.7748/nm.2020.e1956

Verd, S., Ramakers, J., Vinuela, I., Martin-Delgado, M. I., Prohens, A., & Díez, R. (2021). Does breastfeeding protect children from COVID-19? An observational study from pediatric services in Majorca, Spain. *International Breastfeeding Journal*, *16*(1), 83. https://doi.org/10.1186/s13006-021-00430-z

Weston, J., & Zauche, L. H. (2021). Comparison of virtual simulation to clinical practice for prelicensure nursing students in pediatrics. *Nurse Educator*, *46*(5), E95–E98. https://doi.org/10.1097/NNE.0000000000000946

19 | Multivariate Statistics

Learning Objectives

1. Explain the importance of multivariate statistics.
2. Articulate the differences in various types of regression analysis.
3. Recognize the usefulness of stepwise multiple regression.
4. Distinguish various ways to test logistic regression.
5. Understand the rationale for casual models.

INTRODUCTION

Scientists, in their efforts to explain or predict phenomena, have recognized that two-variable studies are often inadequate. The classic approach to data analysis, which involved studying the effect of a single independent variable on an outcome, is being replaced by sophisticated **multivariate**[1] **statistics**.

Multivariate statistics are computationally formidable. Our purpose is to provide a general understanding of how, when, and why multivariate statistics are used, without working out computations. Nevertheless, we must present more formulas than we did in the previous two chapters because, to read and create tables with results from multivariate procedures, you must understand underlying components. This chapter introduces a few frequently used multivariate techniques—although we acknowledge that many of the sophisticated analytic procedures that are coming increasingly into use—such as *generalized estimating equations (GEE)*—are not covered in this overview. Those needing more comprehensive coverage of multivariate statistics should consult books such as those by Tabachnick and Fidell (2018), Pituch and Stevens (2016), or Hair et al. (2019).

> **TIP** Multivariate statistics are never computed manually.

One widely used multivariate procedure is multiple regression analysis, which is used to analyze the relationship between two or more independent variables and a continuous dependent variable. The terms **multiple correlation** and **multiple regression** will be used almost interchangeably, consistent with the strong bond between correlation and regression. To comprehend this bond, we first explain simple (i.e., bivariate) regression.

SIMPLE LINEAR REGRESSION

Regression analysis is used to predict outcomes. In simple regression, one independent variable (X) is used to predict a dependent variable (Y). For instance, we could use simple regression to

---

[1] We use the term *multivariate* in this chapter to refer to analyses with at least three variables.

predict stress scores from noise levels. The higher the correlation between two variables, the more accurate the prediction. If the correlation between diastolic and systolic blood pressure (SBP) were perfect (i.e., if $r = 1.00$), we would need to measure only one to know the value of the other. Few variables are perfectly correlated, and so predictions made through regression analysis usually are imperfect.

The basic linear regression equation is

$$Y' = a + bX$$

where Y' = predicted value of dependent variable Y
a = intercept constant
b = regression coefficient
X = actual value of independent variable X

Regression analysis solves for a and b, and so a prediction about Y can be made for any value of X. You may remember from high school algebra that the preceding equation is the algebraic equation for a straight line. **Linear regression** is used to determine a straight-line fit to the data that minimizes deviations from the line.

As an illustration, consider the data in Table 19.1 for five people on two strongly correlated variables, X and Y ($r = 0.90$). If we used the five pairs of X and Y values to solve for a and b in a regression equation, we would be able to predict Y values for *any* person for whom we have information on variable X.

We do not show the formulas for computing the values of a and b here but suffice it to say they are straightforward calculations involving deviation scores from X and Y values. As shown at the bottom of Table 19.1, the solution to the regression equation is $Y' = 1.5 + .9X$. Now suppose that the X values in column 1 are the only data we have, and we want to predict values for Y. For the first person, $X = 1$, we would predict that $Y = 1.5 + (0.9)(1)$, or 2.4. Column 3 shows Y' values for each X. These numbers show that Y' does not equal Y, the *actual* values obtained (column 2). Most **errors of prediction** (e) are small, as shown in column 4. Errors of prediction occur because the correlation between X and Y is not perfect. Only when $r = 1.00$ or -1.00 does $Y' = Y$. The regression equation solves for a and b in a way that minimizes such errors. More precisely, the solution minimizes the sums of squares of prediction errors—standard regression analysis is said to use **least-squares estimation**, which is why it is sometimes called *ordinary least squares*, or *OLS, regression*. In column 5 of Table 19.1, the error terms—called **residuals**—have been squared and summed to yield a value of 7.60. Any values of a and b other than 1.5 and 0.9 would yield a larger sum of squared residuals.

TABLE 19.1 • Example of Simple Linear Regression

(1) X	(2) Y	(3) Y'	(4) E	(5) E²
1	2	2.4	−0.4	0.16
3	6	4.2	1.8	3.24
5	4	6.0	−2.0	4.00
7	8	7.8	0.2	0.04
9	10	9.6	0.4	0.16
$\overline{X} = 5.0$	$\overline{Y} = 6.0$		0.0	$\Sigma e^2 = 7.60$

$r = .90$
$Y' = a + bX = 1.5 + .9X$

Figure 19.1 shows the solution to this regression analysis graphically. Actual X and Y values are plotted with circles. The line running through these points represents the regression solution. The intercept (*a*) is the point at which the line crosses the Y axis, which is 1.5. The slope (*b*) is the angle of the line. With *b* = 0.90, the line slopes so that for every 4 units on the X axis, we must go up 3.6 units (0.9 × 4) on the Y axis. The line thus embodies the regression equation. To predict a value for Y, we would go to the point on the X axis for an obtained X value, go up to vertically to the point on the regression line directly above the X score, and then read the predicted Y′ value horizontally on the Y axis. For example, for an X value of 5, we would predict a Y′ of 6, indicated by the star.

Correlation coefficients express how variation in one variable is associated with variation in another. The square of *r* (r^2) tells us the proportion of variance in Y that is accounted for by X. In our example, *r* = 0.90, so r^2 = 0.81. This means that 81% of the variability in Y values can be understood in terms of variability in X values. The remaining 19% is variability due to other factors. Thus, the stronger the correlation, the better the prediction; the stronger the correlation, the greater the percentage of variance explained.

MULTIPLE LINEAR REGRESSION

The correlation between two variables is rarely perfect, and so researchers often try to improve predictions of Y by including multiple independent variables—which are called **predictor variables** in a multiple regression context.

Basic Concepts for Multiple Regression

Suppose we wanted to predict graduate nursing students' grade-point averages (GPAs). Not all applicants can be accepted, so we want to select those with the greatest likelihood of success. Suppose we had previously found that students with high scores on the verbal portion of an entrance exam (EE-V) tended to get better grades than those with lower EE-V scores. The correlation between EE-V and graduate GPAs is 0.50. With only 25% (0.50^2) of the variance of graduate GPA accounted for, there will be many errors of prediction: Many admitted students will not perform as well as expected, and many rejected applicants would have made good students. It may be possible, by adding information, to make more accurate predictions through multiple regression. The basic multiple regression equation is

$$Y' = a + b_1 X_1 + b_2 X_2 \ldots b_k X_k$$

where Y′ = predicted value for dependent variable Y
 a = intercept constant
 k = number of predictor (independent) variables
 b_1 to b_k = regression coefficients for the *k* variables
 X_1 to X_k = scores or values on the *k* independent variables

In our example of predicting graduate nursing students' GPAs, suppose we hypothesized that undergraduate GPA (GPA-U) and scores on the quantitative portion of the entrance exam (EE-Q) would improve the prediction of graduate GPA. Suppose the resulting equation were

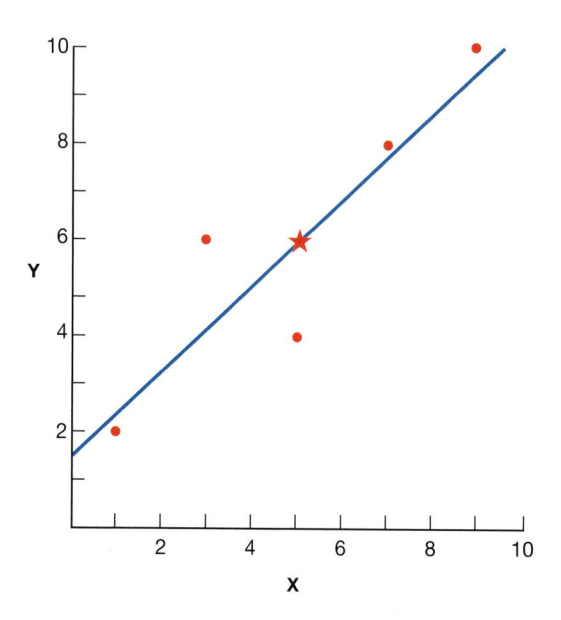

$$Y' = .4 + .05(\text{GPA-U}) + .003(\text{EE-Q}) + .002(\text{EE-V})$$

FIGURE 19.1 Example of simple linear regression.

For instance, suppose an applicant had an EE-V score of 600, an EE-Q score of 550, and a GPA-U of 3.2. The predicted graduate GPA would be

$$Y' = .4 + .05(3.2) + .003(550) + .002(600) = 3.41$$

We can assess the degree to which adding two predictor variables improved our ability to predict graduate school performance through the multiple correlation coefficient. In bivariate correlation, the index is Pearson's r. With two or more independent variables, the index is the **multiple correlation coefficient**, or R. Unlike r, R does not have negative values. R varies from 0.00 to 1.00, showing the *strength* of relationship between several independent variables and a dependent variable but not *direction*. R, when squared (R^2), indicates the proportion of variance in Y accounted for by the combined, simultaneous influence of the predictor variables.

R^2 provides a way to evaluate the accuracy of a prediction equation. Suppose that with the three predictors in the current example, the value of $R = 0.71$. This means that 50% ($.71^2$) of the variation in graduate GPA can be explained by the two EE scores and undergraduate grades. Adding two predictors doubled the variance accounted for by EE-V alone, from 0.25 to 0.50.

The multiple correlation coefficient is never less than the highest bivariate correlation between a predictor and the outcome variable. Table 19.2 presents a correlation matrix with the rs for all pairs of variables in this example. The predictor most strongly correlated with graduate grades is GPA-U, $r = 0.60$. The value of R could not be less than 0.60.

R is more readily increased when predictors have low correlations among themselves. In the current case, the correlations range from 0.40 (between EE-Q and GPA-U) to 0.70 (EE-Q and EE-V). All correlations are fairly substantial, which helps to explain why R is not much higher than the r between the GPA-GRAD and GPA-U alone (0.71 compared with 0.60). This somewhat puzzling phenomenon reflects redundancy of information among predictors. When correlations among independent variables are high, they add little predictive power to each other. With low correlations among predictors, each can contribute something unique to predicting an outcome. In our example, GPA-U predicts 36% of Y's variance ($.60^2$). The remaining two independent variables do not contribute as much as we would expect by considering their bivariate correlation with graduate GPA. Their *combined* added contribution is only 14% (0.50 − 0.36 = 0.14), which is small because the two test scores have redundant information with undergraduate grades.

As more predictors are added to the equation, increments to R tend to decline. It is rare to find predictor variables that correlate well with an outcome but negligibly with one another. Redundancy is difficult to avoid as more and more variables are added. The inclusion of predictor variables beyond the first three or four typically does little to improve the proportion of variance accounted for or the accuracy of prediction.

> **TIP** When predictors are too highly correlated, a problem called **multicollinearity** can occur, which can lead to unstable results. Most researchers assess the risk of multicollinearity before finalizing their regression model.

TABLE 19.2 • Correlation Matrix for Graduate Nursing Student Grade Example

	GPA-GRAD	GPA-U	EE-Q	EE-V
GPA-GRAD	1.00			
GPA-U	.60	1.00		
EE-Q	.55	.40	1.00	
EE-V	.50	.50	.70	1.00

EE, entrance examination; EE-Q, entrance examination quantitative score; EE-V, entrance examination verbal score; GPA, grade-point average; GPA-GRAD, graduate GPA; GPA-U, undergraduate GPA.

Dependent variables in multiple regression analysis, as in ANOVA, should be measured on an interval or ratio scale. Predictor variables, on the other hand, can either be interval- or ratio-level variables *or* categorical variables. Categorical variables usually are coded as dichotomous **dummy variables**, with the code of 1 designating the presence of an attribute and 0 designating its absence. For example, if females were coded 1 and males were coded 0, the code of 1 would represent "femaleness." A text such as that by Polit (2010) can be consulted for information on how to use and interpret dichotomous dummy variables.

Tests of Significance

Multiple regression analysis is not used solely (or even primarily) to develop prediction equations. Researchers typically test hypotheses about relationships among variables in the analysis. Several tests address different questions.

Tests of the Overall Equation and *R*

The basic null hypothesis in multiple regression is that the population multiple correlation coefficient equals zero. The test for the significance of *R* is based on principles analogous to those for ANOVA. With ANOVA, the *F*-ratio statistic is the ratio of the mean squares between, divided by mean squares within. In multiple regression, the form is similar:

$$F = \frac{SS_{\text{due to regression}} / df_{\text{regression}}}{SS_{\text{of residuals}} / df_{\text{residuals}}}$$

$$= \frac{\text{Mean Square}_{\text{due to regression}}}{\text{Mean Square}_{\text{of residuals}}}$$

As in ANOVA, variance from the independent variables is contrasted with variance attributable to other factors, or error. In our example of predicting graduate GPAs, suppose a multiple correlation coefficient of 0.71 ($R^2 = 0.50$) was calculated for a sample of 100 graduate students. The computed value of the *F*-statistic in this example is 32.05. The tabled value of *F* (with $df = 3$ and 96) for a significance level of 0.01 is about 4.00; thus, the probability that $R = 0.71$ resulted from chance fluctuations is considerably less than 0.01.

> **Example of Multiple Regression**
> In a cross-sectional study of 73 nursing homes in Belgium, Maenhout and colleagues (2020) used multiple linear regression to investigate which factors were significantly related to nursing home residents' quality of life. They found that mood, self-perceived health status, social satisfaction, and educational level were significant predictors ($p < .001$), explaining 38.1% of the variance.

Tests for Adding Predictors

Another question researchers may want to answer follows: Does *adding* X_k to the regression significantly improve the prediction of *Y* over that achieved with X_{k-1}? For example, does a third predictor increase our ability to predict *Y* after two predictors have been used? An *F*-statistic can be computed to answer this question.

In the current example, let us say that X_1 = GPA-U; X_2 = EE-Q; and X_3 = EE-V. We can then symbolize various correlation coefficients as follows:

$R_{y.1}$ = the correlation of *Y* with GPA-U = 0.60
$R_{y.12}$ = the correlation of *Y* with GPA-U *and* EE-Q = 0.71
$R_{y.123}$ = the correlation of *Y* with all three predictors = 0.71

We can see that EE-V scores made no independent contribution to the multiple correlation coefficient. The value of $R_{y.12}$ is identical to the value of $R_{y.123}$. We cannot tell at a glance, however, whether adding X_2 to X_1 *significantly* increased the prediction of *Y*. What we want to know is whether X_2 would improve predictions in the population, or if its added predictive power in this sample resulted from chance. In the current example, the value of the *F*-statistic for testing whether adding EE-Q scores significantly improves our prediction of *Y* is 27.16. If we consulted a table for the theoretical distribution of *F* with $df = 1$ and 97 and a significance level of 0.01, we would find that the critical value is about 6.90. Therefore, adding EE-Q to the regression equation with GPA-U significantly improved the accuracy of predicting graduate GPA, beyond the 0.01 level.

Tests of the Regression Coefficients

When a regression coefficient (*b*) is divided by its standard error, the result is a value for the *t* statistic, which can be used to assess the significance of individual predictors. A significant t indicates that the regression coefficient (b) is significantly different from zero.

In simple regression, the value of b indicates the amount of change in predicted values of Y for a specified rate of change in X. In multiple regression, the coefficients represent the number of units the dependent variable is predicted to change for each unit change in a predictor variable *when the effects of other predictors are held constant*. "Holding constant" other predictors means that they are statistically controlled, a feature that can enhance a study's internal validity. If a regression coefficient is significant when confounding variables are included in the regression equation, it means that the predictor associated with the coefficient contributed significantly to the regression, even after confounding variables are taken into account.

Strategies for Handling Predictors in Multiple Regression

Three alternative strategies for entering predictor variables into regression equations are simultaneous, hierarchical, and stepwise regressions.

Simultaneous Multiple Regression

The most basic strategy, **simultaneous multiple regression**, enters all predictor variables into the regression equation at the same time. One regression equation is developed, and statistical tests indicate the significance of R and of individual regression coefficients. This strategy is most appropriate when there is no basis for considering any particular predictor as causally prior to another, and when the predictors are of comparable importance to the research question.

Hierarchical Multiple Regression

Many researchers use **hierarchical multiple regression**, which involves entering predictors into the equation in a series of steps. Researchers control the order of entry, with the order typically based on theoretical considerations. For example, some predictors may be thought of as causally or temporally prior to others, in which case they could be entered in an early step. Another important reason for using hierarchical regression is to examine the effect of a key independent variable after first removing (controlling) the effect of confounding variables.

> **Example of Hierarchical Multiple Regression**
> In a secondary analysis, Aga et al. (2020) used a hierarchical linear regression analysis to assess whether greater diabetes self-care behaviors were associated with better glycemic control. They conducted five steps. At step one, they entered the demographic variables; at step two, the clinical variables; at step three, the comorbidity information; step four, the psychosocial variables; and at step five, the self-care behaviors were added. None of the variables entered in step one was a significant predictor of glycemic control, but as they progressed through the steps, predictors such as race, dyslipidemia, organ failure, and the number of medications began to emerge as predictors.

With hierarchical regression, researchers determine the number of steps and the number of predictors included in each step. When several variables are added as a block, as in the Aga example, the analysis is a simultaneous regression for those variables at that stage. Thus, hierarchical regression can be considered a controlled sequence of simultaneous regressions.

Stepwise Multiple Regression

Stepwise multiple regression involves *empirically* selecting the combination of independent variables with the most predictive power. In stepwise multiple regression, predictors enter the regression equation in the order that produces the greatest increments to R^2. The first step selects the single best predictor of the outcome variable, that is, the independent variable with the highest bivariate correlation with Y. The second variable to enter the equation is the one that produces the largest increase to R^2 when used simultaneously with the predictor selected in the first step. The procedure continues until no additional predictor significantly increases the value of R^2.

Figure 19.2 illustrates stepwise multiple regression. Suppose that the first variable (X_1) has a correlation of 0.60 with Y ($r^2 = 0.36$). Variable X_1 accounts for the portion of the variability of Y represented by the hatched area in step 1 of the figure. This hatched area is, in effect, removed from further consideration, because this portion of Y's

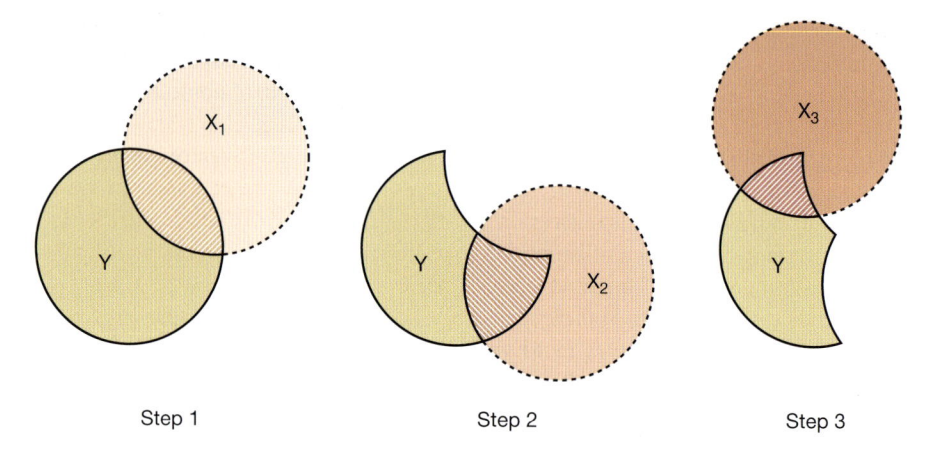

FIGURE 19.2 Visual representation of stepwise multiple regression analysis.

variability is explained. The variable chosen in step 2 is not always the X variable with the second largest correlation with Y. The selected predictor is the one that explains the largest portion of what *remains* of Y's variability after X_1 has been taken into account. Variable X_2, in turn, removes a second part of Y so that the independent variable selected in step 3 is the one that accounts for the most variability in Y after *both* X_1 and X_2 are removed.

Example of Stepwise Multiple Regression
Kim and Han (2020) conducted a stepwise multiple regression analysis to examine the factors related to self-care behaviors among patients with diabetic foot ulcers. The analysis indicated that perceived family support was significantly associated with diabetes management ($\beta = 0.32$ $p < .001$) and diabetes self-care education had the greatest effect on diabetic foot care behaviors ($\beta = 0.39$, $p = .001$).

TIP Stepwise regression is controversial because variables are entered into the regression equation based on statistical rather than theoretical criteria. If stepwise regression is used, cross-validation is recommended (e.g., by dividing the sample in half and running two independent series of regressions).

Relative Contribution of Predictors

Scientists want not only to predict phenomena, but to explain them. Predictions can be made in the absence of understanding. For instance, in our graduate school example, we could predict performance moderately well without explaining *why* the factors contributed to students' success. For practical applications, it may be sufficient to make accurate predictions, but researchers typically want to understand phenomena.

In multiple regression, one approach to understanding a phenomenon is to explore the relative importance of predictor variables. Unfortunately, determining the relative contributions of independent variables in predicting an outcome is a thorny issue. When predictor variables are correlated, as they usually are, there is no ideal way to disentangle the effects of variables in the equation.

It may appear that the solution is to compare the contributions of the Xs to R^2. In our graduate school example, GPA-U accounted for 36% of Y's variance; EE-Q explained an additional 14%. Should we conclude that undergraduate grades are more than twice as important as EE-Q scores in explaining graduate school grades? This conclusion would be inaccurate because the order of entry of variables in a regression equation affects their apparent contribution. If these two predictor variables were entered in reverse order (i.e., EE-Q first), R^2 would remain unchanged at 0.50; however, EE-Q's contribution would be 0.30 ($.55^2$), and GPA-U's contribution would be 0.20 (0.50 − 0.30). This is because whatever variance the independent variables have in common is attributed to the first variable entered in the analysis.

Another approach to assessing the relative importance of the predictors is to compare regression coefficients. Earlier, we presented an equation for multiple regression that included a (the constant), and bs (regression coefficients) for each predictor. The b values cannot be directly compared because they are in the units of original scores, which differ from one X to another. X_1 might be in milliliters, X_2 in degrees Fahrenheit, and so forth. The use of **standard scores** (or *z* scores) eliminates this problem by transforming all variables to scores with a mean of 0.0 and a standard deviation (SD) of 1.00 (Chapter 16). Transforming regular scores to *z* scores is easy—they are the difference between a score and the mean of that score divided by the SD, or

$$z_X = \frac{X - \bar{X}}{SD_X}$$

In standard score form, the regression equation uses standard scores (*z*s) instead of raw scores (*X*s), and the regression coefficients for each *z* are *standardized regression coefficients*, called **beta (β) weights**. With all the βs in the same measurement units, can their relative size shed light on the relative importance of predictors? Many researchers have interpreted beta weights in this fashion, but there are problems in doing so. These regression coefficients will be the same no matter what the order of entry of the variables. The difficulty, however, is that regression weights are unstable. Values of β tend to fluctuate from sample to sample. Moreover, when a variable is added to or subtracted from the equation, beta weights change. Because values of the regression coefficients fluctuate, it is difficult to attach theoretical importance to them.

One of the best solutions is to compare the **squared semipartial correlation coefficients** (sr^2) of the predictors. It is beyond the scope of this book to explain this index in detail, but we note that the sr^2 is useful because it indicates a predictor's unique contribution to variability in the dependent variable—that is, the contribution after other predictors are controlled.

Regression Results

There are no standard table formats for presenting regression results, and different formats are relevant depending on whether standard, hierarchical, or stepwise regression has been performed. The most frequently reported elements are β, R^2, and *p* values. We illustrate a table of regression results using a study of predictors of moral distress in a sample of critical care nurses in the United States (Hiler et al., 2018). The researchers hypothesized that nurses' moral distress could be predicted by perceptions of their practice environments. They used a two-step hierarchical regression in which they first entered scores on five self-reported measures of the nurses' perceptions of workplace plus an objective indicator—whether the ICU in which they worked had been recognized by a Beacon Award. In the second step, the researchers' entered predictors corresponding to participants' characteristics—their age and job satisfaction. Table 19.3 shows results for the final model in which all predictors were in the equation.

The first column shows the order of entry (in blocks) of the eight predictors, which are listed in the second column. The next column shows values for the standardized beta coefficients. The last column shows whether each predictor was statistically significant. For example, the nurses' perception of collegial nurse–physician relations (NPRs) was a highly significant predictor of the nurses' degree of moral distress. The negative coefficient for beta (−0.18) indicates that higher scores on the NPR scale were associated with lower scores on the moral distress scale. This is significant ($p = .001$): the probability is 1 in 1,000 that the relationship between NPR scores and moral distress scores is spurious. Also, older nurses have lower moral distress scores than younger ones ($p = .001$). The results suggest that certain aspects of the nurses' practice environment are significantly associated with moral distress even after controlling for the nurses' age and job satisfaction. Other factors (e.g., perceptions of nurse managers' leadership ability, Beacon award designation) were not significant independent predictors of moral distress.

At the bottom of the table, we see that the value of R^2 for the final model was 0.30, which is significant at $p < .001$. Adding age and job satisfaction in step 2 significantly increased the value

TABLE 19.3 • Multiple Regression Analysis Results: Predictors of Moral Distress in U.S. Critical Care Nurses (N = 328)

STEP[a]	PREDICTOR	BETA	P
1	Nurses' participation in hospital affairs	−.04	ns
1	Perceptions of nursing foundations for quality of care (patient safety)	−.12	ns
1	Nurse managers' ability, leadership, and support of nurses	−.00	ns
1	Staffing and resource adequacy	−.19	.003
1	Collegial nurse–physician relations (NPR scale)	−.18	.001
1	Beacon Award designation (1 = yes, 0 = no)	−.03	ns
2	Age	−.14	.001
2	Job satisfaction	−.22	<.001

For Step 1 regression: $R^2 = 0.25$, $F = 17.65$, $p < .001$.
For final regression: $R^2 = 0.30$, $F = 17.07$, $p < .001$.
Change in R^2 from Step 1 to Step 2: $F = 11.77$, $p < .001$.

[a]In this hierarchical regression, variables were entered in two steps, as designated. Parameter estimates for beta are shown for the step 2 results only.

Adapted from Table 3, Hiler, C., Hickman, R., Reimer, A., & Wilson, K. (2018). Predictors of moral distress in a U.S. sample of critical care nurses. *American Journal of Critical Care, 27*, 59–65.

of R^2, from 0.25 to 0.30 ($p < .001$). The remaining 70% of variation in levels of moral distress is explained by factors not included in the regression model.

Power Analysis for Multiple Regression

Small samples are especially problematic in multiple regression and other multivariate procedures. Inadequate sample size can lead to Type II errors and erratic regression coefficients.

One approach to estimating sample size needs concerns the ratio of predictor variables to total number of cases. Tabachnick and Fidell (2018) suggest this guideline: *N* should be greater than 50, plus eight times the number of predictors. So, with five predictors, the sample size should be greater than 90 (50 + [8 × 5]). Some experts recommend a ratio of 20 to 1 for simultaneous and hierarchical regression and a ratio of 40 to 1 for stepwise. More cases are needed for stepwise regression because this procedure capitalizes on the idiosyncrasies of a specific data set.

Another way to estimate sample size needs is to perform a power analysis. The number of participants needed to reject the null hypothesis that *R* equals zero is estimated based on effect size, number of predictors, desired power, and the significance criterion. In multiple regression, the estimated effect size is a function of the value of R^2. Researchers must either predict the value of R^2 on the basis of earlier research or use the convention that effect size will be small ($R^2 = 0.02$), moderate ($R^2 = 0.13$), or large ($R^2 = 0.30$).

Table 19.4 presents sample size estimates for 2 to 10 predictors and various values of R^2, for power = 0.80 and alpha = 0.05. As an example, suppose we were planning a study to predict functional ability in nursing home residents using five predictor variables. We estimate a moderate effect size ($R^2 = 0.13$) and want to achieve a power of 0.80 and $\alpha = 0.05$. A sample of about 92 nursing home residents is needed to detect a population R^2 of 0.13 with five predictors, with a 5% chance of a Type I error and a 20% chance of a Type II error.

TABLE 19.4 • Power Analysis Table for Multiple Regression: Sample Size Estimates to Test the Null Hypothesis That $R^2 = 0.00$, for Power = 0.80, and $\alpha = 0.05$ With 2-10 Predictor Variables

NO. OF PREDICTORS	ESTIMATED POPULATION R^2										
	.02	.04	.06	.08	.10	.13	.15	.20	.25	.30	.40
2	478	230	152	113	89	67	58	42	32	26	18
3	543	261	173	128	102	77	66	48	37	30	21
4	597	287	190	141	112	85	73	53	41	33	24
5	643	309	205	153	121	92	79	57	45	36	26
6	684	329	218	163	129	98	84	61	48	39	28
7	721	347	231	172	136	104	89	65	51	41	30
8	755	375	242	180	143	109	94	69	54	44	32
9	788	380	252	188	150	114	98	72	56	46	33
10	818	395	262	196	156	119	102	75	59	48	35

Shaded columns indicate conventions for small, medium, and large effect sizes.

TIP Several websites do instantaneous power calculations and sample size estimates for many multivariate procedures.

ANALYSIS OF COVARIANCE

Analysis of covariance (ANCOVA) has much in common with multiple regression, but it also has features of ANOVA. Like ANOVA, ANCOVA is used to compare the means of two or more groups, and the central question is the same: Are mean group differences likely to be *real* or spurious? Like multiple regression, ANCOVA allows researchers to control confounding variables statistically.

Uses of Analysis of Covariance

ANCOVA is especially useful in certain situations. For example, if a nonequivalent control group design is used to test an intervention, researchers must consider whether obtained results are influenced by preexisting group differences. When control through randomization is lacking, ANCOVA offers posthoc statistical control. Even in true experiments, ANCOVA can result in more precise estimates of group differences because, even with randomization, there are typically slight differences between groups. ANCOVA adjusts for initial differences so that the results more precisely illuminate the effect of an intervention.

Strictly speaking, ANCOVA should not be used with existing groups because randomization is an underlying assumption of ANCOVA. This assumption is often violated; however, when randomization is not feasible, ANCOVA can sometimes improve a study's internal validity.

ANCOVA Procedures

Suppose we were testing the effectiveness of biofeedback therapy on patients' anxiety. A group in one hospital is exposed to the treatment, and a comparison group in another hospital is not. Patients' anxiety levels are measured both before and after the intervention; thus, pretest anxiety scores can be statistically controlled through ANCOVA. In this situation, the outcome variable is the posttest anxiety scores, the independent variable is experimental/comparison group status, and the **covariate** is pretest anxiety scores. Covariates are usually continuous variables (e.g., anxiety scores), but can be dichotomous variables (male/female); the independent variable is a nominal-level variable.

ANCOVA tests the significance of differences between group means after adjusting scores on the outcome variable to remove the effect of covariates. In essence, the first step in ANCOVA is the same as the first step in hierarchical multiple regression. Variability in the outcome that can be explained by the covariate is removed from further consideration. ANOVA is performed on what remains of Y's variability to see whether, once the covariate is controlled, differences between group means are statistically significant.

Let us consider another example to explore further aspects of ANCOVA. Suppose we were testing the effectiveness of weight-loss diets, and we randomly assigned 30 people to one of three groups. ANCOVA, using pretreatment weight as the covariate, permits a more sensitive analysis of weight change than simple ANOVA. Some hypothetical data for such a study are shown in Table 19.5. Two aspects of the weight values in this table are discernible. First, despite random assignment to treatment groups, group means at baseline are different. Participants in diet B differ from those in diet C by an average of 10 lb (175 vs. 185 lb). This difference reflects chance fluctuations and is not significant ($F = 0.45$, $p = .64$). Second, posttreatment means are also different by a maximum of only 10 lb (160-170). However, the mean number of pounds *lost* ranged from 10 lb for diets A and B to 25 lb for diet C.

When we perform an ordinary ANOVA testing group differences in posttreatment weights, we get an F of 0.55, indicating nonsignificant mean group differences ($p = .58$). Based on ANOVA, we would conclude that all three diets had comparable effects on weight loss.

Now let us use ANCOVA to analyze the data. The first step breaks total variability in posttreatment weights into two components: (1) variability explained by the covariate (pretreatment weights) and (2) residual variability. The covariate accounts for a significant amount of variance, which is not surprising because there is a strong relationship between pretreatment and posttreatment weights: people who started out especially heavy tended to stay that way, relative to others in the sample. In the second step, residual variance is broken down to reflect between-group and within-group contributions. The resulting F of 17.54 ($df = 2, 26$) is significant beyond the 0.001 level. We can conclude that, after controlling for initial weight, there is a significant difference in weight loss in the different diet groups.

This fictitious example was contrived so that an ANOVA result of "no difference" would be altered by adding a covariate. Most actual results are less dramatic. Nonetheless, ANCOVA yields a more sensitive statistical test than ANOVA because the covariate reduces the error term (within-group variability), against which treatment effects are compared.

Theoretically, it is possible to use any number of covariates. It is seldom advisable, however, to use more than two or three. For one thing, a large number of covariates are often unnecessary because of the typically high degree of redundancy beyond the

TABLE 19.5 • **Fictitious Data for ANCOVA Example: Comparison of Pre- and Posttreatment Weights for Three Diet Interventions**

	DIET A	DIET B	DIET C	TOTAL
Pretreatment weight, mean (*SD*)	180.0 (23.5)	175.0 (22.5)	185.0 (24.6)	180.0 (23.1)
Posttreatment weight, mean (*SD*)	170.0 (21.7)	165.0 (22.0)	160.0 (20.3)	165.0 (20.0)
ANOVA $F(2, 27)$ for mean group differences in posttreatment weight = 0.55, $p = .58$			
ANCOVA $F(1, 26)$ for covariate (pretreatment weight) = 309.88, $p < .001$			
ANCOVA $F(2, 26)$ for mean group differences in posttreatment weight = 17.54, $p < .001$			

first few. Moreover, each covariate uses up a degree of freedom; fewer degrees of freedom means that a higher F is required for significance. For instance, with 2 and 26 df, an F of 5.53 is required for significance at the 0.01 level, but with 2 and 23 df (i.e., adding three covariates), an F of 5.66 is needed.

Selection of Covariates

Useful covariates are almost always available. Background characteristics, such as age and gender, are often good candidates. Background characteristics are especially important to control if they are predictors of the outcome and there are differences between the groups being compared. The literature is a good source of information about factors correlated with outcomes.

A baseline measure of the outcome is an excellent covariate, invariably strongly correlated with the final outcome. However, repeated-measures ANOVA (RM-ANOVA) is an alternative to ANCOVA when analyzing data from studies with pretest–posttest designs. *Propensity scores*, discussed briefly in Chapter 9, can be powerful covariates. Propensity scores capture group differences on a broad range of attributes because they represent an attempt to model group differences using available data. The use of propensity scores as covariates is described by Qin et al. (2008) and Schroeder et al. (2016).

In general, it is important to select covariates that have strong reliability. Measurement errors can lead to overadjustments or underadjustments of the mean and can contribute to type I or type II errors.

Adjusted Means

In our example of the three diets, the significant ANCOVA F test indicates that at least one of the three groups had a posttreatment weight that is significantly different from the overall grand mean, after adjusting for pretreatment weights. It sometimes is useful to examine **adjusted means**, that is, group means on the outcome variable after adjusting for (i.e., removing the effect of) covariates. In our example of posttreatment weights for participants in three diet interventions, the adjusted means for diets A, B, and C were 170.0, 169.4, and 155.6, respectively—values that clearly indicate differences among those exposed to the different diets.

When ANCOVA results in a significant group F test, researchers can reject the null hypothesis that the adjusted group means are equal. As with ANOVA, further analysis is needed to assess which pairs of adjusted group means are significantly different from one another. In our example, posthoc tests revealed that the mean weight for diet C is significantly different from that for both diets A and B, but diets A and B are not significantly different from each other.

> **TIP** For ANCOVA, an eta squared statistic can be computed to summarize the magnitude of the *adjusted* effect of the independent variable on the dependent variable. Estimates of eta squared can be used in a power analysis to estimate sample size needs when planning a study. In general, when ANCOVA is used with carefully selected covariates, the analysis of group differences is more powerful than with ANOVA because error variance is reduced. In our example of the three diets, the value of adjusted eta squared is 0.57.

Example of ANCOVA
Wang et al. (2022) aimed to evaluate the effectiveness of a 12-week Tai Chi training program on blood pressure and migraine-related trigger factors among Chinese females with a history of migraines. Participants were randomly assigned to either the Tai Chi group for 24 weeks or the wait list control group that maintained the usual lifestyle for 24 weeks. ANCOVA was used to test the difference of mean changes and the interaction effect between the time periods and groups across the baseline, at 12 weeks, and 24 weeks, respectively.

OTHER LEAST-SQUARES MULTIVARIATE TECHNIQUES

Many multivariate statistics discussed thus far are related. For example, ANOVA and multiple regression are similar. Both techniques analyze total variability in a continuous dependent measure, and contrast variability due to independent variables with that attributable to error. By tradition, experimental data typically are analyzed by ANOVA, and correlational data are analyzed by regression.

A broad class of statistical techniques are subsumed under the **general linear model (GLM)**, which include techniques that fit data to straight-line (linear) solutions. The GLM is the foundation for such procedures as the *t*-test, ANOVA, and multiple regression. The GLM is an important model because of its generality and applicability to numerous research situations, but a thorough understanding of the GLM requires advanced statistical training. In this section, other GLM methods are briefly introduced.

Repeated-Measures ANOVA for Mixed Designs

In Chapter 18, we discussed one-way RM-ANOVA, which is appropriate when one group of people is measured at multiple points. Many RCTs involve randomly assigning participants to different treatment groups, and then collecting postintervention data several times. When there are only two data collection points (e.g., a pretest and a posttest), ANCOVA is often used to test the null hypothesis that group means are equal, after removing the effect of pretest (baseline) scores. When data are collected three or more times, a **repeated-measures ANOVA for mixed designs** is often used.

As an example, suppose we collected heart rate data at 2 hours (T1), 4 hours (T2), and 6 hours (T3) postsurgery for people in an intervention and control group. Structurally, the ANOVA for analyzing these data would look similar to a 2 × 3 multifactor ANOVA, but calculations would differ in this mixed design—mixed because it involves both a within-subject factor and a between-subject factor. An *F*-statistic would be computed to test for a *between-subjects effect* (i.e., differences between experimentals and controls). This statistic would indicate whether, across all time periods, mean heart rate differed in the two groups. Another *F*-statistic would be computed to test for a *within-subjects effect* or time factor (i.e., differences at T1, T2, and T3). This statistic would indicate whether, for both groups, mean heart rates differed over time. Finally, an **interaction effect** would be tested to assess whether group differences varied across time. In mixed design RM-ANOVA, the interaction effect usually is of primary importance. When people are randomized to treatment groups, we would expect their mean values at baseline to be equivalent—but if there are treatment effects, group means would differ at subsequent points of data collection, thus resulting in a time × treatment interaction.

Tests within the GLM have several basic assumptions, all of which are fully described in statistics textbooks. Assumptions such as normality of the distributions and the equality of variances apply to most GLM procedures, but ANOVA and most of its variants are fairly **robust** to violation of assumptions (i.e., violations tend not to affect the accuracy of statistical decision-making). However, RM-ANOVA has some unique assumptions—the assumption of *sphericity* and the related assumption of *compound symmetry*, both of which are too complex to elaborate here. RM-ANOVA is not, unfortunately, robust to violations of these assumptions. Furthermore, there are different opinions about how to detect and address violations. Thus, RM-ANOVA tends to be more complex than many procedures discussed thus far. Polit (2010) and advanced statistical texts offer suggestions on using RM-ANOVA.

> **Example of a Mixed Design RM-ANOVA**
> In a quality improvement project, Pate and colleagues (2022) explored whether supplementing the existing education protocol in 25 patients with new ostomates with standardized education materials provided preoperatively would improve patient self-efficacy for management of their new ostomy. RM-ANOVA revealed that there was a statistically significant difference in the mean total summed scores ($F(2,48) = 45$, $P = .000$), indicating the standardized written education materials improved patients' stoma care self-efficacy.

Multivariate Analysis of Variance

Multivariate analysis of variance (MANOVA) is the extension of ANOVA to more than one outcome. MANOVA is used to test the significance of differences in group means for multiple dependent variables, considered simultaneously. For instance, if we wanted to test the effect of two methods of exercise on diastolic *and* SBP, MANOVA would be appropriate. Researchers often analyze such data by performing two separate ANOVAs. Strictly speaking, this practice is not appropriate. Separate ANOVAs imply that the outcomes were independent when, in fact, they were obtained from the same people and are correlated. MANOVA takes the intercorrelations of outcomes into account. ANOVA is, however, a more widely understood procedure than MANOVA, and thus its results may be more easily communicated to a broad audience.

MANOVA can be extended in ways analogous to ANOVA. For example, it is possible to perform **multivariate analysis of covariance (MANCOVA)**, which allows for the control of confounding variables (covariates) when there are two or more outcome variables.

TIP If you opt to use simpler analyses to enhance the accessibility of the evidence to clinical audiences (e.g., three separate ANOVAs rather than a MANOVA), you should run the analyses both ways. Then, you could present bivariate results (e.g., from ANOVAs) in the report and state whether the more complex analysis (e.g., MANOVA) yielded comparable results.

Example of MANOVA
Nanyonga et al. (2022) used MANOVA to assess the impact of a bundled nurse-led intervention on the biometric outcomes of BP and weight and the impact of these changes on lifestyle management. The overall mean reduction in systolic blood pressure was 9.5 mm Hg ($p = .001$) and the mean difference in weight was statistically significant at 7.7 kg (SD = 4.5; $p = .001$) and the biometric changes were associated with several lifestyle modification behaviors such as taking medicine as prescribed ($p = .008$) and controlling body weight ($p = .015$).

LOGISTIC REGRESSION

Logistic regression is a widely used multivariate technique. Like multiple regression, logistic regression analyzes the relationship between multiple independent variables and a dependent variable and yields a predictive equation. Logistic regression, however, relies on an estimation procedure that has less restrictive assumptions than multivariate procedures within the GLM and is used to predict categorical outcomes.

TIP A least-squares procedure for predicting categorical outcomes is called *discriminant analysis*. Although popular two decades ago, discriminant analysis is infrequently used and has been superseded by logistic regression.

Basic Concepts for Logistic Regression

Logistic regression uses **maximum likelihood estimation (MLE)**. Maximum likelihood estimators are ones that estimate the parameters most likely to have generated the observed data. Confirmatory factor analysis (CFA), discussed in Chapter 16, also uses MLE.

Logistic regression has few assumptions about the underlying distribution of variables. Logistic regression is well suited to many clinical questions because it models the probability of an outcome. For example, we might be interested in modeling the probability of engaging in breast self-examination, or the probability of a patient fall.

Logistic regression transforms the probability of an event occurring (e.g., that a patient will fall) into its odds. As discussed in Chapter 17, **odds** reflect the ratio of two probabilities: the probability of an event occurring and the probability that it will not occur. For example, if 10% of patients fall, the odds would be 0.10 divided by 0.90, or 0.111.

Probabilities, which range between zero and one, are then transformed into continuous variables that range between zero and infinity. Because this range is still restricted, a further transformation is performed, namely calculating the logarithm of the odds. The range of this new variable (the **logit**, short for *log*istic probability un*it*) is from minus to plus infinity. Using the continuous logit as the outcome variable, a maximum likelihood procedure estimates the coefficients of the independent variables.

The solution yields an equation that predicts the logit from a weighted combination of independent variables, plus a constant, much like a multiple regression equation. The interpretation, however, is different because the equation does not predict *actual* values of the dependent variable. In logistic regression, a regression coefficient (*b*) can be interpreted as the change in the log odds associated with a one-unit change in the associated predictor variable.

The Odds Ratio

A logistic regression equation is hard to interpret because we do not think in terms of log odds. The equation can, however, be transformed back to yield information in terms of odds rather than log odds. The factor by which the odds change is the *odds ratio* (*OR*), the risk index we discussed in Chapter 17.

For example, suppose that we used logistic regression to predict the probability of performing breast self-examination. One of the predictors might be whether the female has a family member (e.g., a sister) who had breast cancer. A logistic regression analysis might indicate that the *OR* was 12.1, with all other predictors in the equation held constant. (This is often called an *adjusted odds ratio*.) The odds ratio provides an estimate (around which confidence intervals can be built) of relative risk—the risk of an event occurring given one condition, vs. the risk of it occurring given a different condition. In our example, we would estimate that the "risk" of performing breast self-examination is about 12 times greater if a female has a family history of breast cancer than if they do not, with other factors controlled.

> **TIP** Just as there is simple regression with least-squares estimation—that is, the prediction of an outcome variable based on a single independent variable—*bivariate logistic regression* is also possible. This is often done to produce estimates of *unadjusted* (or *crude*) odds ratios—that is, odds ratios without controlling other variables.

Variables in Logistic Regression

The outcome variable in logistic regression is a dichotomous variable. The outcome is typically coded 1 to represent an event or a characteristic (e.g., had a fall, is obese), and 0 to represent the absence of the event or characteristic (no fall, not obese). Predictor variables can be continuous variables, categorical variables, or interaction terms. Although there are no strict limits to the number of predictors that can be included, it is best to achieve a parsimonious model with strong predictive power using a small set of good predictors.

When continuous variables are the predictors, the odds ratio is interpreted somewhat differently than with categorical variables. For example, suppose we were predicting whether a nursing home resident would have a fall, and one predictor variable was age. Suppose we found, for example, that the *OR* associated with age was 1.10. This means that for every additional year of age, the odds of falling increased by 10%, with everything else in the model held constant.

Dummy-coded variables are a common method of representing dichotomous predictors, such as smokes cigarettes (1) vs. does not smoke cigarettes (0). For variables with more than two categories, a series of dummy variables is needed. For example, if marital status were a predictor variable in a logistic regression for predicting breast self-examination, a bivariate logistic analysis could provide estimates of the relative risk of different marital statuses (e.g., never married, currently married, formerly married) on breast self-examination. In such an analysis, one group would be the **reference group**, with an *OR* of 1.0, and the other two groups would have *OR*s in relation to the reference group. As a hypothetical example, if the *OR* for a never-married reference group was 1.0 and the *OR* for currently married was 1.23, this means that married females were 23% more likely to perform breast self-examination than never-married females.

As with multiple regression, predictors in multiple regression can be entered into the equation if different ways. The options include simultaneous, hierarchical, and stepwise entry.

Significance Tests in Logistic Regression

Researchers usually want to assess the overall reliability of the model, that is, whether the set of predictors, taken as a whole, is significantly better than chance in predicting the probability of the outcome. Unfortunately, assessing the goodness of fit of a logistic regression model can be confusing because there are several different tests, and different authors use different names for the tests. Another potential source of confusion is that some tests indicate goodness of fit by a significant result, and others indicate goodness of fit by a *non*significant result. We briefly describe two approaches but recommend further reading in advanced textbooks such as Tabachnick and Fidell (2018) or Hosmer et al. (2013).

One statistic in logistic regression is the **likelihood index**, which is the probability of the observed results, given parameters estimated in the analysis. If the overall model fits the data perfectly, the likelihood index is 1.0. Because the likelihood index is typically a small decimal, it is usually transformed by multiplying it by −2 times the log of the likelihood. The transformed index (**−2LL**) is a small number when the fit is good; in a perfect fit, the value is zero. The chi-square statistic is then used to test the null hypothesis that all of the *b* regression coefficients are zero, in a **likelihood ratio test**. A **goodness-of-fit statistic**, which has a chi-squared distribution, is the analogue of the overall *F* test in multiple regression. This statistic is based on the residuals for all cases in the analysis—which is the difference between the observed probability of an event and the predicted probability. This statistic is thus a mechanism for evaluating the fit of the predictive model. The likelihood ratio test also can be used to evaluate the significance of *improvement* to −2LL with successive entry of predictors, when hierarchical or stepwise regression is performed.

An alternative approach to testing the overall model is the **Hosmer–Lemeshow test**, which compares the prediction model to a hypothetically "perfect" model. In brief, the perfect model is one that contains the exact set of predictors needed to duplicate the observed frequencies in the outcome. The full model can be tested against the perfect model by computing differences between observed frequencies and expected frequencies (i.e., those expected in the perfect model). With this test, a *nonsignificant* chi-square is desired. A nonsignificant result indicates that the model being tested is not reliably different from the perfect model. In other words, nonsignificance supports the inference that the model adequately duplicates the observed frequencies of the outcome.

> **TIP** There is no consensus on which approach for an overall model test is better, but logistic regression software programs can perform both tests, and some researchers present both results.

It is also possible to test the significance of individual predictors in the model—just as the *t* statistic is used in multiple regression. A frequently used statistic for this purpose is the **Wald statistic**, which is distributed as a chi-square. Significance can also be assessed by examining the confidence intervals around the odds ratios. If the 95% CI includes the value of 1.0, this indicates that the *OR* was not statistically significant at the 0.05 level.

Effect Size in Logistic Regression

Statisticians have worked on developing an effect size index for logistic regression that is analogous to R^2 in multiple regression. The main problem, however, is that R^2 in multiple regression can be interpreted as the percentage of variance in the outcome explained by the predictors, but this is more complex with a dichotomous outcome. Despite difficulties in achieving a good analog to least squares–based R^2, several **pseudo R^2** measures have been proposed for logistic regression. These indexes should be reported as approximations to an R^2 rather than as the percentage of variance explained. A statistic called the **Nagelkerke R^2** is the most frequently reported pseudo R^2 index.

> **Example of Logistic Regression**
> Lee and colleagues (2020) sought to identify factors associated with the job satisfaction and intention to leave in 113 perioperative nurses across a province in Canada. In their logistic regression analysis, they found that nurses who reported higher emotional exhaustion were more likely to report an intention to leave their current jobs in the next year than nurses who experienced lower levels of emotional exhaustion (OR = 1.75, 95% confidence interval = 1.25–2.11).

SURVIVAL AND EVENT HISTORY ANALYSIS

Some outcomes are time-related. **Survival analysis** is widely used by epidemiologists when the dependent variable is a time interval between an initial event (e.g., onset of a disease) and a terminal event (e.g., death). Survival analysis calculates a survival score, which compares survival time for one participant with that for others. When researchers are interested in group comparisons—for example, comparing the survival function of people in an intervention group vs. a control group—a statistic can be computed to test the null hypothesis that the groups are sampled from the same survival distribution.

Survival analysis can be applied to many situations unrelated to mortality. For example, survival analysis could be used to analyze such time-related phenomena as length of time in labor, length of stay in hospital, or length of time breastfeeding. Survival analysis can be used when time-related data are **censored**, that is, the observation period does not cover all possible events. As and example, if the outcome variable was hospital readmission and the data was collected two years after patients were released, the data would be considered censored because there may be readmissions beyond the two year period. Further information about survival analysis can be found in Hosmer et al. (2008).

Extensions of survival analysis have been developed that allow researchers to examine determinants of survival-type transitions in a multivariate framework. In these analyses, independent variables are used to model the risk (or hazard) of experiencing an event at a given point in time, given that one has not experienced the event before that time. The most common specification of the hazard is known as the *Cox proportional hazards model*. Further information about **Cox regression** may be found in O'Quigley (2008).

Example of Cox Regression
Brinati et al. (2021) aimed to identify the potential predictors of the number of days from an ICU admission to the development of unstable blood glucose. Using a multivariate Cox regression model, the team found that patients who received rigorous glucose control with regular insulin had a decrease of 0.19 in the odds of developing hyperglycemia (HR = 0.19; 95% CI, 0.05-0.70; p = .013). For each added day of the length of stay, the risk for developing hyperglycemia increased by 5% (HR = 1.05; 95% CI, 1.01-1.09; p = .004). Lastly, the risk of developing hypoglycemia was 9.02 times larger (95% CI, 1.17-69.19; p = .034) in patients on mechanical ventilation.

CAUSAL MODELING

Causal modeling involves testing a hypothesized causal explanation of a phenomenon, typically with data from nonexperimental (observational) studies.

In a causal model, researchers posit causal linkages among three or more variables, and then test whether hypothesized pathways from the causes to the effect are consistent with the data. Casual modeling is not a method for discovering causes; rather, it is a method applied to a prespecified model formulated based on prior knowledge and theory.

TIP Although causal modeling is most often performed with data from nonexperimental studies, it can also be used to test hypotheses about paths of mediation in randomized controlled trials.

Casual modeling is often referred to as **path analysis**. Until recently, nurse researchers performed path analysis primarily using ordinary least squares estimation. In fact, it is possible to conduct a path analysis with a series of multiple regression analyses. We begin our explanation of path analysis within an OLS framework.

Path analytic results are usually displayed in a **path diagram**, and we use such a diagram (Figure 19.3) to illustrate key concepts. This model postulates that the outcome variable, patients' functional ability (V4), is influenced by patients' capacity for self-care (V3); this, in turn, is affected by nursing actions (V1) and the severity of their illness (V2). The model in Figure 19.3 is a **recursive model**, which means that the causal flow is unidirectional. It is hypothesized that V2 is a cause of V3, but not that V3 is a cause of V2.

Path analysis distinguishes exogenous and endogenous variables. Determinants of an **exogenous variable** lie outside the model. In Figure 19.3, nursing actions (V1) and illness severity (V2) are exogenous; no attempt is made in the model to elucidate what causes different nursing actions or different degrees of illness. An **endogenous variable**, by contrast, is one whose variation is hypothesized to be affected by other variables in the model. In our example, self-care capacity (V3) and functional ability (V4) are endogenous.

Causal linkages are shown on a path diagram by arrows drawn from presumed causes to presumed effects. In our illustration, severity of illness is hypothesized to affect functional ability both directly (path p_{42}) and indirectly through the

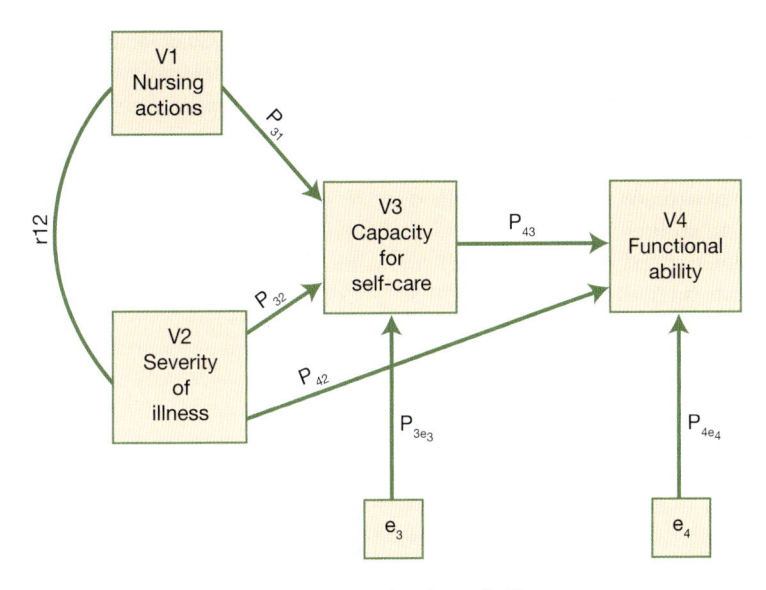

FIGURE 19.3 Example of a path diagram.

mediating variable self-care capacity (paths p_{32} and p_{43}). Correlated exogenous variables are indicated by curved lines, as shown by the curved line between nursing actions and illness severity.

Ideally, the model would totally explain the outcome, but this almost never happens because there are other determinants, which are **residual variables**. The two boxes labeled *e* in Figure 19.3 denote a composite of all determinants of self-care capacity (e_3) and functional ability (e_4) that are not in the model. If we could identify and measure additional causes and incorporate them into the theory, the model could be strengthened.

Path analysis solves for **path coefficients**, which are the weights representing the effect of one variable on another. In Figure 19.3, causal paths indicate that one variable (e.g., V3) is caused by another (e.g., V2), yielding a path labeled p_{32}. In research reports, path symbols would be replaced by actual path coefficients. Path coefficients are standardized partial regression slopes. For example, path p_{32} is equal to $\beta_{32.1}$—the beta weight between variables 2 and 3, holding variable 1 constant. Because path coefficients are in standard form, they indicate the proportion of an SD difference in the caused variable that is directly attributable to a 1 *SD* difference in the specified causal variable. Thus, path coefficients provide an indication about the relative importance of various determinants.

Structural equations modeling (SEM) using maximum likelihood estimation is a more powerful approach to path analysis that avoids several problems in OLS estimation, notably difficulties in meeting assumptions. Unlike an OLS approach, SEM can accommodate measurement errors, correlated residuals, and **nonrecursive models** that allow for reciprocal causation. Another attractive feature of SEM is that it can be used to analyze causal models involving one or more *latent variables*—a variable representing a construct that is not measured directly (Chapter 16). In SEM, latent variables are captured by two or more measured (manifest) variables that are indicators of the construct.

When there are latent variables, SEM proceeds in two phases. In the first phase, which corresponds to a CFA, a measurement model is tested (Chapter 16). When there is evidence of an adequate fit of the data to the hypothesized measurement model, the theoretical causal model is tested by structural equation modeling.

SEM yields information about the hypothesized causal parameters—that is, path coefficients that are presented as beta weights. The coefficients indicate the expected amount of change in the (latent) endogenous variable that is caused by a change in the (latent) causal variable. SEM programs yield information on the significance of individual paths. The overall fit of the model to the data can be tested by means of several statistics, such as the **goodness-of-fit index** (**GFI**) and **adjusted goodness-of-fit index** (**AGFI**). For both indexes, a value of 0.90 or greater indicates a good fit.

Path analysis using SEM has gained popularity among nurse researchers but is a complex procedure. Readers interested in further information can consult Loehlin and Beaujean (2017).

Example of a Path Analysis
Wojeck and colleagues (2021) conducted a prospective longitudinal study using data from the Scleroderma Patient-centered Intervention Network Cohort to determine whether changes in self-efficacy mediate changes in pain. Using path analysis, their model indicated that self-efficacy did not mediate the pain trajectories.

CRITICAL APPRAISAL OF MULTIVARIATE STATISTICS

As noted in the previous chapter, it is difficult to critically appraise researchers' statistical analysis without statistical skills. This caution is even more relevant when it comes to multivariate analyses.

As with bivariate statistics, one issue is whether the researcher selected the right tests. The selection of a multivariate procedure depends on several factors, including the nature of the research question and the measurement level of the variables. (It also depends on whether the data conformed to various assumptions underlying the tests—an issue we did not address in this brief chapter.) Table 19.6, which summarizes some of the major features of multivariate statistics discussed in this chapter, may help you assess the appropriateness of an analytic approach. It might also be noted that studies in which multivariate statistics were *not* used might well be critiqued in terms of whether they *should* have been used. As we illustrated, results from a bivariate test can sometimes be altered by controlling confounding variables. Conversely, some researchers apply multivariate statistics when their sample size is too small to justify their use.

No specific appraisal guidelines for multivariate statistics are presented in this chapter, but most of the questions presented in Box 18.1 are also relevant for researchers' use of complex statistics.

TIP The statistical analyses described in this chapter concern the analysis of data from individuals. Methods for analyzing dyadic/family data have been developed, some within a framework called the Actor–Partner Interdependence Model (Fitzpatrick et al., 2016; Kenny & Ledermann, 2010).

TABLE 19.6 • Guide to Selected Multivariate Analyses

TEST NAME	PURPOSE	MEASUREMENT LEVEL[a] OF VARIABLES[b]			NUMBER OF VARIABLES[b]		
		IV	DV	CV	IVS	DVS	CV
Multiple regression/ correlation	To test the relationship between 2+ IVs and 1 DV; to predict a DV from 2+ IVs	Nominal, continuous	Continuous	—	2+	1	—
Analysis of covariance (ANCOVA)	To test the difference between the means of 2+ groups while controlling for 1+ covariate	Nominal	Continuous	Nominal, continuous	1+	1	1+

(continued)

TABLE 19.6 • Guide to Selected Multivariate Analyses (Continued)

TEST NAME	PURPOSE	MEASUREMENT LEVEL[a] OF VARIABLES[b]			NUMBER OF VARIABLES[b]		
		IV	DV	CV	IVS	DVS	CV
Mixed design RM-ANOVA	To test mean differences for 2+ groups for outcomes measured multiple times	Nominal	Continuous	Nominal, continuous	1+	1	1+
Multivariate analysis of variance (MANOVA)	To test the difference between the means of 2+ groups for 2+ DVs simultaneously	Nominal	Continuous	—	1+	2+	—
Multivariate analysis of covariance (MANCOVA)	To test the difference between the means of 2+ groups for 2+ DVs simultaneously, while controlling for 1+ covariate	Nominal	Continuous	Nominal, continuous	1+	2+	1+
Logistic regression	To test the relationship between 2+ IVs and 1 DV; to predict the probability of an event; to estimate relative risk	Nominal, continuous	Nominal	—	2+	1	—

[a]Measurement levels: Continuous = interval-level or ratio-level.
[b]Variables: IV, independent variables; DV, dependent variable; CV, covariate.

RESEARCH EXAMPLE

We conclude with a summary of a study that used multivariate procedures.

Study: Depression and self-care in older adults with multiple chronic conditions: A multivariate analysis (Iovino, 2020).

Statement of purpose: The purpose of this study was to investigate the relationship between depression and self-care behaviors in older individuals with multimorbidity.

Methods: The study was a secondary analysis of data from a multicenter longitudinal study aimed at measuring self-care in patient with multimorbidity. The sample included 366 patients from the parent study. Data extracted included demographic variables, Montreal Cognitive Assessment Scale, the 9-Item Patient Health Questionnaire, the Self-Care of Chronic Illness Inventory with three subscales: self-care maintenance, self-care monitoring, and self-care management. The outcome variable was self-care behaviors.

Analysis and findings: The average age of the sample was 76.39 (*SD* 7.28) and 57% were female and 65%

were partnered. The three most common chronic conditions were diabetes (75%), followed by heart failure (34%) and COPD (14%). In addition to using means and standard deviations to describe the sample, the team used Chi square or independent sample t tests to describe the differences between two groups of participants: those who were depressed and those who were not. To explore the association between depression and the outcome variable of self-care, the team performed two sets of analyses. There was a significant difference in the ANOVA analysis between depression and self-care maintenance and monitoring but not with self-care management. A subsequent ANCOVA that controlled for variables such as demographics supported this same finding. The MANOVA analysis revealed a significant relationship between depression and the three scales of self-care and a MANCOVA that controlled for variables supported this finding.

SUMMARY POINTS

- **Multivariate statistics** are increasingly being used in nursing research to untangle complex relationships among three or more variables.
- Simple **linear regression** is used to predict the values of one variable based on values of a second variable. **Multiple regression** is a method of predicting a continuous dependent variable based on two or more independent (**predictor**) variables.
- **Multiple correlation coefficients** (R) can be squared (R^2) to estimate the proportion of variability in the outcome variable accounted for by the predictors. The F-statistic is used to test the overall regression model and changes to R^2 as new predictors are introduced.
- The regression equation yields **regression coefficients** (bs) for each predictor that, when raw scores are converted to **standard scores**, are called **beta weights** (βs).
- **Simultaneous multiple regression** enters all predictor variables into the regression equation at the same time. **Hierarchical multiple regression** enters predictors into the equation in a series of steps controlled by researchers.

- **Stepwise multiple regression** enters predictors in steps using a statistical criterion for order of entry.
- **Analysis of covariance (ANCOVA)**, an extension of ANOVA, removes the effect of confounding variables (**covariates**) before testing whether mean group differences on the outcome variable are statistically significant.
- **Mixed design RM-ANOVA** is used to test mean differences between groups (between-subjects factor) over time (within-subjects factor). In mixed design RM-ANOVAs, the interaction term (time × group) usually is of primary interest.
- **Multivariate analysis of variance (MANOVA)** is the extension of ANOVA to situations in which there is more than one outcome variable.
- The **general linear model (GLM)** encompasses a broad class of frequently used statistical techniques that fit data to straight-line (linear) solutions, including t-tests, ANOVA, ANCOVA, and multiple regression.
- **Least-squares estimation** used within GLM minimizes the square of **errors of prediction** (the **residuals**). An alternative is **maximum likelihood estimation** (**MLE**), which estimates the parameters most likely to have generated observed data.
- **Logistic regression**, which is based on MLE, is used to predict categorical outcomes. Logistic regression yields an **odds ratio** that is an index of relative risk for each predictor, that is, the risk of an outcome occurring given one condition vs. the risk of it occurring given a different condition, while controlling other predictors.
- The overall logistic regression model can be tested with a **likelihood ratio test** that uses a **goodness-of-fit chi-square** statistic. An alternative is the **Hosmer–Lemeshow** test, which tests how close the model is to a perfect model. Individual predictors can be tested with the **Wald statistic**. Several **pseudo R^2** indexes can be used to summarize overall effect size for logistic regression; the most widely reported is the **Nagelkerke R^2**.
- **Survival analysis** and other related event history methods, such as **Cox regression**, are used

when the dependent variable of interest is a time interval (e.g., length of time in hospital).
- **Causal modeling** involves the development and testing of a hypothesized causal explanation of a phenomenon.
- **Path analysis**, a method for testing causal models, involves the preparation of a **path diagram** that stipulates hypothesized causal links among variables. Path analysis can be performed using least-squares estimation, but currently is more likely to involve **structural equations modeling** (**SEM**), an MLE approach to causal modeling.

REFERENCES CITED IN CHAPTER 19

Aga, F., Dunbar, S. B., Kebede, T., Higgins, M. K., & Gary, R. (2020). Relationships of diabetes self-care behaviours to glycaemic control in adults with type 2 diabetes and comorbid heart failure. *Nursing Open*, *7*(5), 1453–1467. https://doi.org/10.1002/nop2.517

Brinati, L. M., de Fátima Januário, C., Balbino, P. C., Gonçalves Rezende Macieira, T., Cardoso, S. A., Moreira, T. R., & de Oliveira Salgado, P. (2021). Incidence and prediction of unstable blood glucose level among critically ill patients: A Cohort study. *International Journal of Nursing Knowledge*, *32*(2), 96–102. https://doi.org/10.1111/2047-3095.12299

Fitzpatrick, J., Gareau, A., Lafontaine, M., & Gaudreau, P. (2016). How to use the actor-partner Interdependence model (APIM) to estimate different dyadic patterns in MPLUS: A step-by-step tutorial. *Quantitative Methods for Psychology*, *12*, 74–86.

Hair, J. F., Black, W., Babin, B., & Anderson, R. (2019). *Multivariate data analysis* (8th ed.). Prentice-Hall.

Hiler, C., Hickman, R., Reimer, A., & Wilson, K. (2018). Predictors of moral distress in a US sample of critical care nurses. *American Journal of Critical Care*, *27*, 59–65.

Hosmer, D., Lemeshow, S., & May, S. (2008). *Applied survival analysis: Regression modeling of time to event data* (2nd ed.). New York: John Wiley.

Hosmer, D., Lemeshow, S., & Sturdivant, R. (2013). *Applied logistic regression* (3rd ed.). John Wiley & Sons.

Iovino, P., De Maria, M., Matarese, M., Vellone, E., Ausili, D., & Riegel, B. (2020). Depression and self-care in older adults with multiple chronic conditions: A multivariate analysis. *Journal of Advanced Nursing*, *76*(7), 1668–1678. https://doi.org/10.1111/jan.14285

Kenny, D. A., & Ledermann, T. (2010). Detecting, measuring, and testing dyadic patterns in the Actor-Partner Interdependence Model. *Journal of Family Psychology*, *24*, 359–366.

Kim, E. J., & Han, K. S. (2020). Factors related to self-care behaviours among patients with diabetic foot ulcers. *Journal of Clinical Nursing*, *29*(9–10), 1712–1722. https://doi.org/10.1111/jocn.15215

Lee, S. E., MacPhee, M., & Dahinten, V. S. (2020). Factors related to perioperative nurses' job satisfaction and intention to leave. *Japan Journal of Nursing Science: JJNS*, *17*(1), e12263. https://doi.org/10.1111/jjns.12263

Loehlin, J. C., & Beaujean, A. (2017). *Latent variable models: An introduction to factor, path, and structural equation analysis* (5th ed.). Routledge.

Maenhout, A., Cornelis, E., Van de Velde, D., Desmet, V., Gorus, E., Van Malderen, L., Vanbosseghem, R., & De Vriendt, P. (2020). The relationship between quality of life in a nursing home and personal, organizational, activity-related factors and social satisfaction: A cross-sectional study with multiple linear regression analyses. *Aging & Mental Health*, *24*(4), 649–658. https://doi.org/10.1080/13607863.2019.1571014

Nanyonga, R. C., Spies, L. A., & Nakaggwa, F. (2022). The effectiveness of nurse-led group interventions on hypertension lifestyle management: A mixed method study. *Journal of Nursing Scholarship: An Official Publication of Sigma Theta Tau International Honor Society of Nursing*, *54*(3), 286–295. https://doi.org/10.1111/jnu.12732

O'Quigley, J. (2008). *Proportional hazards regression*. Springer.

Pate, K., Powers, K., Coffman, M. J., & Morton, S. (2022). Improving self-efficacy of patients with a new ostomy with written education materials: A quality improvement project. *Journal of Perianesthesia Nursing: Official Journal of the American Society of PeriAnesthesia Nurses*, *37*(5), 620–625. https://doi.org/10.1016/j.jopan.2021.11.020

Pituch, K., & Stevens, J. (2016). *Applied multivariate statistics for the social sciences* (6th ed.). Routledge.

Polit, D. F. (2010). *Statistics and data analysis for nursing research* (2nd ed.). Pearson.

Qin, R., Titler, M., Shever, L., & Kim, T. (2008). Estimating effects of nursing intervention via propensity score analysis. *Nursing Research*, *57*, 444–452.

Schroeder, K., Jia, H., & Smaldone, A. (2016). Which propensity score method best reduces confounder imbalance? An example from a retrospective evaluation of a childhood obesity intervention. *Nursing Research*, *65*, 465–474.

Tabachnick, B. G., & Fidell, L. S. (2018). *Using multivariate statistics* (7th ed.). Pearson Education.

Wang, S., Tian, L., Ma, T., Wong, Y. T., Yan, L. J., Gao, Y., Zhang, D., Hui, S. S., & Xie, Y. J. (2022). Effectiveness of Tai chi on blood pressure, stress, fatigue, and sleep quality among Chinese women with episodic migraine: A randomised controlled trial. *Evidence-based Complementary and Alternative Medicine: eCAM*, *2022*, 2089139. https://doi.org/10.1155/2022/2089139

Wojeck, R. K., Silva, S. G., Bailey, D. E. Jr, Knisely, M. R., Kwakkenbos, L., Carrier, M. E., Nielson, W. R., Bartlett, S. J., Pope, J., & Thombs, B. D. (2021). Pain and self-efficacy among patients with systemic sclerosis: A Scleroderma Patient-Centered Intervention Network Cohort study. *Nursing Research*, *70*(5), 334–343. https://doi.org/10.1097/NNR.0000000000000528

20 Processes of Quantitative Data Analysis

Learning Outcomes

1. Recognize the importance of detailing an analysis plan when reporting quantitative research.
2. Articulate the elements to be included in the codebook.
3. Identify the steps needed for data cleaning.
4. Understand how to handle missing values.
5. Describe the steps needed to assure data quality.

INTRODUCTION

In this chapter, we offer an overview of the steps often taken to prepare for the analysis of quantitative data. Most of these activities would be undertaken *before* performing the statistical analyses described in the last few chapters, but we have positioned this chapter here because some of the material requires some familiarity with statistics.

Figure 20.1 shows what the flow of tasks in a quantitative analysis might look like, organized in phases. Progress in analyzing quantitative data is seldom as linear as this figure suggests, but it provides a framework for discussing key steps in the analytic process.

PREANALYSIS PHASE

The first phase of a quantitative analysis involves various clerical and administrative tasks, such as logging in forms, reviewing data for completeness and legibility, retrieving pieces of missing information, and assigning identification (ID) numbers. Another task involves selecting statistical software for doing the data analyses. Two widely used statistical software packages are the Statistical Package for the Social Sciences (SPSS) and the Statistical Analysis System, but there are many others. Next, researchers must code the data and enter them onto computer files to create a **dataset** (the total collection of data for all sample members).

Coding Quantitative Data

Coding is the process of transforming data into symbols—usually numbers. Certain variables are inherently quantitative (e.g., age, body temperature) and do not require coding, unless the data are gathered in categories (e.g., younger than 50 years of age vs. 50 or older). Even with "naturally" quantitative data, researchers need to inspect their data. All responses should be of the same form and precision. For example, for the variable *height* in the nonmetric system, researchers need to decide whether to record feet and inches as two separate "variables" or to convert the information entirely to inches. Whichever method is adopted, it must be used consistently for all participants. There must also be consistency in handling information reported by sample members with different degrees of precision (e.g., a decision about how to code a response such as 5 feet 2½ in).

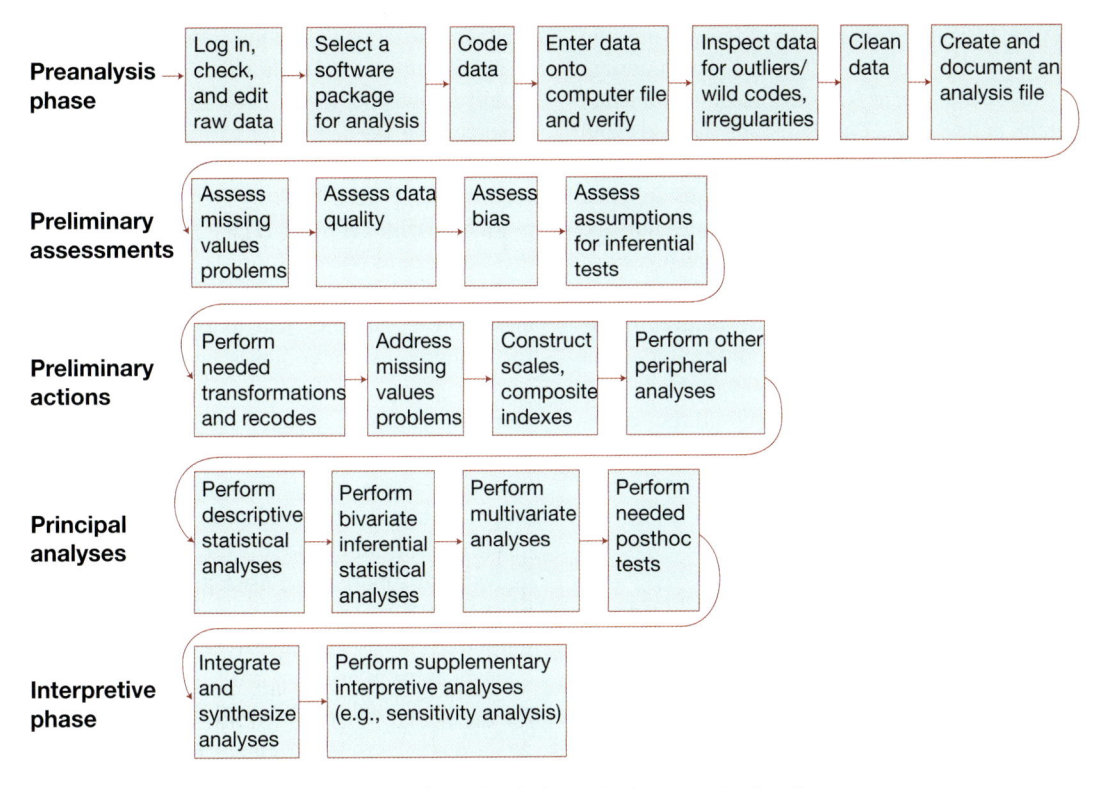

FIGURE 20.1 Flow of tasks in analyzing quantitative data.

Preanalysis phase: Log in, check, and edit raw data → Select a software package for analysis → Code data → Enter data onto computer file and verify → Inspect data for outliers/wild codes, irregularities → Clean data → Create and document an analysis file

Preliminary assessments: Assess missing values problems → Assess data quality → Assess bias → Assess assumptions for inferential tests

Preliminary actions: Perform needed transformations and recodes → Address missing values problems → Construct scales, composite indexes → Perform other peripheral analyses

Principal analyses: Perform descriptive statistical analyses → Perform bivariate inferential statistical analyses → Perform multivariate analyses → Perform needed posthoc tests

Interpretive phase: Integrate and synthesize analyses → Perform supplementary interpretive analyses (e.g., sensitivity analysis)

Most data from structured instruments can be precoded, with codes designated before data are collected. For example, questions with fixed response alternatives can be preassigned a numeric code and are sometimes printed on the data collection form, such as under age 50 = 1 and 50 and older = 2. Codes are often arbitrary, as in the case of the variable gender. Whether a female participant is coded 1 or 2 has no analytic importance so long as females are consistently assigned one code and males another code.

Respondents sometimes can check off more than one response to a question, as in the following question that might be used in a study about irritable bowel syndrome:

Which of the following symptoms have you experienced in the past week? (Check all that apply.)

Abdominal pain
Bloating
Constipation
Diarrhea
Flatulence

With questions of this type, responses must be coded as though there were five separate questions: "Did you experience abdominal pain?" "Did you experience bloating?" and so on. Each check is treated as a "yes." The question yields five variables, with one code (e.g., 1) signifying "yes" and another code (e.g., 0) signifying "no."

If data from open-ended questions are going to be used in quantitative analysis, they must be coded. Sometimes researchers can develop codes ahead of time, but unstructured data often are collected because responses cannot be anticipated. In such situations, researchers typically review a sizable portion of the data to understand content and then develop a coding scheme.

A code is needed for each variable for every sample member, even if there is no response. **Missing values** can be of various types. A person answering a question may be undecided, refuse to answer, or say, "Don't know." When skip patterns are used, there is missing information for questions that are irrelevant to some respondents. A single missing values code may suffice, but it may be important to distinguish different types of missing data using different codes (e.g., distinguishing refusals and *don't know*s).

The choice of what code to use for missing data is often arbitrary, but missing values codes must be ones that have not been used for actual pieces of information. Some researchers use blanks, periods, or negative values for missing information. Some use 9 as the missing code because this value is out of the range of real codes for many variables.

Precise coding instructions should be documented in a coding manual. Coders, like observers and interviewers, must be properly trained, and intercoder (or intracoder) reliability checks are recommended.

Entering, Verifying, and Cleaning Data

Coded data typically are transferred onto a data file via keyboard entry, but other options (e.g., scanning of forms, importing electronic health records information) are also available. Various programs can be used for data entry, including spreadsheets or databases. Major software packages for statistical analysis have data editors that make data entry fairly easy.

> **TIP** Sometimes sample members enter their own data directly onto a computer file—for example, when they complete an online questionnaire. This is clearly advantageous in terms of efficiency and costs.

Figure 20.2 shows a screenshot of a data file for the SPSS. This data file is very small: a 30 × 7 matrix, with 30 rows (1 for each participant) and 7 columns for the variables (i.e., one variable per column).

Each variable in a dataset has to be named. Usually the variable name is abbreviated—for example, in Figure 20.2, we can see that the variable names are all short (GROUP, BWEIGHT, etc.). The software allows users to enter a more detailed description of each variable. For example, for the variable BWEIGHT, the extended label is "Infant birthweight in ounces." This full name would appear on all output, rather than BWEIGHT.

Each participant's unique ID should be entered in the file along with their actual data, because this would allow you to go back to original sources if something needed to be verified. The ID number normally is entered as the first variable of the record, as in Figure 20.2.

The variables BWEIGHT, AGE, and PRIORS in this dataset are ones that are "naturally" quantitative (number of ounces, years, and prior pregnancies). Other variables had to be coded. GROUP, for example, uses a coding scheme of 1 for intervention group members and 2 for control group members. SMOKE is coded 1 for those who smoke and 0 for those who do not. We use a 1-2 code for GROUP because this coding would ensure that in output with statistical results the intervention group information would be first, which is the convention in research reports. We used a dummy 0-1 code for SMOKE to make regression results easier to interpret.

Data entry is prone to error, so it is essential to verify entries and correct mistakes. One method is to compare visually the numbers on a printout of the data file with codes on the original source, and another is to double-enter data. There are also special verifying programs designed to perform comparisons during direct data entry.

Even verified data need to be cleaned. **Data cleaning** involves two types of checks. The first is a check for outliers and wild codes. **Outliers** are values that lie outside the normal range. Outliers can be found by inspecting frequency distributions, paying special attention to the lowest and highest values. (Most researchers begin data analysis by constructing frequency distributions for all variables in their dataset.) Some outliers are true, legitimate values (e.g., an annual income of $1 million in a distribution where the mean is $50,000), but sometimes they result from data entry errors.

Another problem is **wild codes**—that is, codes that are not possible. For example, the variable gender might have these codes: 1 = female, 2 = male, 3 = other, and "blank" = missing. If someone were coded 5 for gender, there is an error. The computer could show the ID number of the faulty record, and the correct code could then be tracked down.

CHAPTER 20 Processes of Quantitative Data Analysis • **431**

| File Edit View Data Transform Analyze Direct Marketing Graphs Utilities Add-ons |

	ID	GROUP	AGE	PRIORS	SMOKE	BWEIGHT	REPEAT
1	1	1	17	1	1	107	1
2	2	1	14	0	0	101	0
3	3	1	21	3	0	119	0
4	4	1	20	2	0	128	1
5	5	1	15	1	1	89	0
6	6	1	19	0	1	99	0
7	7	1	19	1	0	111	0
8	8	1	18	1	1	117	1
9	9	1	17	0	0	102	1
10	10	1	20	0	0	120	0
11	11	1	13	0	1	76	0
12	12	1	18	0	1	116	0
13	13	1	16	0	0	100	1
14	14	1	18	0	0	115	0
15	15	1	21	2	1	113	0
16	16	2	19	0	0	111	1
17	17	2	21	1	0	108	0
18	18	2	19	2	1	95	0
19	19	2	17	0	1	99	0
20	20	2	19	0	0	103	1
21	21	2	15	0	1	94	0
22	22	2	17	1	0	101	1
23	23	2	21	2	0	114	0
24	24	2	20	1	0	97	0
25	25	2	18	0	1	99	1
26	26	2	18	0	1	113	0
27	27	2	19	1	0	89	0
28	28	2	20	0	0	98	0
29	29	2	17	0	0	102	0
30	30	2	19	1	1	105	0

Notes:

GROUP: Group status, 1 = Experimental group 2 = Control group
AGE: Mother's age in years
PRIORS: Number of prior pregnancies
SMOKE: Mother's smoking status, 1 = Smokes 0 = Does not smoke
BWEIGHT: Infant's birthweight, in ounces
REPEAT: Had repeat pregnancy within 18 months, 1 = Yes 0 = No

FIGURE 20.2 Fictitious dataset for intervention study with low-income pregnant adolescents (screenshot of an SPSS data file).

> **TIP** Such checks will never reveal all errors. If a male were incorrectly coded 1 for gender in the coding scheme just mentioned, the mistake might not be detected. Errors can have a big effect on the analysis and interpretation of data, so it is important to code, enter, verify, and clean data with care.

A second data-cleaning procedure involves **consistency checks**, which focus on internal data consistency. In this task, researchers check for errors by testing compatibility of data within a case. For example, one question in a survey might ask current marital status, and another might ask number of marriages. If the data were internally consistent, respondents who answered "Single, never married" to the first question should have a zero (or a missing values code) for the second. Researchers should search for opportunities to check the consistency of entered data.

Osborne (2013) has devoted an entire book to a discussion of data cleaning. Another very useful resource is a brief open-access paper on this topic by Van den Broeck and colleagues (2005). Dziadkowiec and colleagues (2016) offer advice on cleaning data extracted from electronic health records.

> **Example of Data Verification and Cleaning**
> Lyons and colleagues (2022) describe, through two case studies, the processes used to clean data from electronic health records. They point to the discrepancy of data in the health record used for clinical care as opposed to when data are retrieved for secondary analysis. They describe a theory-based process for evaluating data quality and cleaning data and provided examples of how this was completed for inclusion and exclusion data, demographic information, and clinical indicators.

Creating and Documenting the Analysis Files

The decisions that researchers make about coding and variable naming should be fully documented. Memory should not be trusted; several weeks after coding, researchers may no longer remember if males were coded 1 and female were coded 2, or vice versa. Moreover, colleagues may wish to borrow the data for a secondary analysis. Documentation should always be sufficiently thorough that someone unfamiliar with the original study could use the data.

Documentation usually involves preparing a codebook. A **codebook** is a listing of each variable together with information about placement in the file, codes associated with the values of the variable, and other basic information. Codebooks can be generated by statistical or data entry programs.

PRELIMINARY ASSESSMENTS AND ACTIONS

Researchers typically undertake several preanalytic activities before they test their hypotheses. Several preparatory activities are discussed next.

Assessing and Handling Missing Values Problems

Researchers strive to have data values for all participants on all key variables but usually find that their datasets have some **missing values**. An appropriate solution to a missing values problem depends on such factors as the extent of missing data, the importance of the variables with missing data, and the pattern of missingness.

There are three missing values patterns. The first, and most desirable, is **missing completely at random (MCAR)**, which occurs when cases with missing values are just a random subset of all cases. When data are MCAR, analyses remain unbiased—but missing values are seldom MCAR.

Data are considered **missing at random (MAR)** if missingness is related to variables in the dataset (e.g., gender)—but *not* related to the value of the variable that has the missing values. For example, if missing values for depression occur more frequently for males than for females—but not for people who are most or least depressed—the pattern of missingness may be MAR.

The third pattern is **missing not at random (MNAR)**, a pattern in which the value of the variable that is missing *is* related to its missingness (e.g., those declining to report their income tend to be rich). Missing values that are MAR or MNAR can result in biased results. Solutions are most readily accomplished when missing data are MAR and not MNAR—though it is difficult to know which of these two patterns applies.

A first step in analyzing missing data is to assess the extent of the problem by examining frequency distributions on a variable-by-variable basis. Another step is to examine the cumulative extent of missing values (e.g., what percentage of cases had no variables missing, one variable missing, and so on). Another task is to evaluate the randomness of missing values. A simple procedure is to divide the sample into two groups—those with and without missing data on a specified variable. The two groups can then be compared in terms of their characteristics to assess whether the two groups are comparable in terms of key demographic or clinical variables (e.g., Were males more likely than females to leave certain questions blank? Was the mean age of those with missing values different from that of people without missing values?).

Until recently, examining patterns of missingness was a tedious process, which may explain why some researchers simply ignore the problem of missing data (and therefore remain susceptible to the risk of bias that can be introduced). Now, however, programs in widely used statistical software have greatly simplified this important task. For example, the Missing Values Analysis (MVA) module within SPSS offers powerful means of detecting and handling missing values.

Once researchers have assessed the extent and patterning of missing values, they must address the problem. There are three basic types of solutions: deletions, imputations, and mixed modeling within longitudinal datasets. We discuss the first two here; sophisticated modeling solutions are discussed in Son et al. (2012).

Missing Data and Deletions

Listwise deletion (also called *complete case analysis*) is simply the analysis of those cases for which there are no missing data. Listwise deletion is based on an implicit assumption of MCAR. Researchers who use this method typically have not made a formal assessment of the extent to which MCAR is probable, but rather are simply disregarding the problem of missing data.

Perhaps the most widely used (but not the best) approach is to delete cases selectively, on a variable-by-variable basis by means of **pairwise deletion** (also called *available case analysis*). For example, in a test of an intervention to reduce patient anxiety, the outcomes might be blood pressure and self-reported anxiety. If 10 people from the sample 100 failed to complete the anxiety scale, we might base the analyses of anxiety data on the 90 people who completed the scale but use the full sample of 100 in the blood pressure analysis. If the number of cases fluctuates widely across outcomes, the results are difficult to interpret because the sample is essentially a "moving target."

> **TIP** Computer programs like SPSS use either listwise or pairwise deletion as the **default** (i.e., the option that will be used in the analysis unless there are specific instructions to the contrary).

Researchers sometimes use pairwise deletion in analyses involving a correlation matrix. From one pair of variables in the matrix to another, the number of cases can vary considerably. Although such correlation matrices may provide useful descriptive information, it is not wise to use pairwise deletion for correlation-based multivariate analyses such as multiple regression or factor analysis because the correlations are calculated on nonidentical subsets of people.

Another option is to delete a variable entirely. This option may be suitable when there are a lot of missing values for a variable that is not central to the analysis. Recommendations for how much missing data should drive this decision range from 15% to 40% of cases (Fox-Wasylyshyn & El-Masri, 2005).

Missing Data and Imputations

Preferred methods for addressing missing values involve **imputation**—that is, "filling in" missing data with values believed to be good estimates of what the values would have been, had they not been missing. An attractive feature of imputation is that it allows researchers to maintain full sample size, and thus statistical power is not compromised. The risk is that the imputations will be poor estimates of real values, leading to biases of unknown magnitude and direction.

The simplest procedure is mean substitution or median substitution, which involves using "typical" sample values to replace missing data that are continuous. For example, if a person's age were missing and if the average age of sample members were 45.2 years, we could substitute the value 45.2 in place of the missing values code. Mean substitution is, like listwise deletion, popular because of its simplicity. Yet, even though mean substitution increases sample size and leaves variable means unchanged, it is rarely the best approach. Regardless of what the underlying pattern of missingness is, mean imputation leads to underestimations of variance, and variance is what most statistical analyses are all about.

A refinement on mean substitution is to use the mean value for a relevant subgroup—called a **subgroup** (or *conditional*) **mean substitution**. The assumption is that a better estimate of the missing value can be obtained by making the substitution conditional on participants' characteristics. For example, rather than replacing a missing age value with 45.2, we could replace a male's missing value with males' mean age, and a female's mean value with females' mean age. This is a better option than mean substitution because the substituted values are presumably closer to the real values and because variance is not reduced as much. Nevertheless, conditional (subgroup) mean substitution is not a preferred approach, except when overall missingness is low.

When data are missing for items on a multi-item scale, it may be appropriate to replace a missing value with the mean of other similar items from the person with the missing value, an approach that assumes that people are "internally consistent" across similar questions. Such **case mean substitution**, which uses person-specific information to inform the estimate, has the advantage of not throwing out data altogether (listwise deletion) and not assuming that a person is similar to all others in a sample or subgroup (mean substitution). Case mean substitution has been found to be an acceptable method of imputation at the item level, even compared to more sophisticated methods.

Researchers are increasingly using imputation methods that make more extensive use of data in the dataset. One method uses regression analysis to "predict" the correct value of missing data. Suppose we found that participants' age was correlated with gender, education, and health status. Based on data from those with complete data, age could be regressed on these three variables to predict age for people with missing age data but whose values for the three other variables were not missing. Regression-based imputation is more accurate than previously discussed strategies, although variability remains underestimated.

Even more sophisticated solutions have been developed. Maximum likelihood estimation is useful because it uses all data points in a dataset to construct estimated replacement values. **Expectation maximization (EM)** involves using an iterative procedure with a maximum-likelihood–based algorithm to produce the best parameter estimates.

An approach called **multiple imputation (MI)** is currently considered the best method for addressing missing values problems. MI addresses a fundamental issue—the uncertainty of any given estimate—by imputing several (*m*) estimates of the missing data, and each estimate has an element of randomness introduced. Results from analyses across the *m* imputations are later pooled. MI has not often been used because of its complexity and the limited availability of appropriate software, but recent versions of the SPSS MVA module (version 17.0 and higher) do offer multiple imputation. Patrician (2002) has described multiple imputation in some detail.

> **Example of Handling Missing Values**
> In reporting the effectiveness of a rapid antigen test to triage patients to COVID-19 or non-COVID-19 hospital units in five German hospitals, Möckel and colleagues (2021) excluded 10 patients from an initial sample of 483 due to missing data.

It might be noted that the issue of missingness has been given a lot of attention in the analysis of data from randomized controlled trials (RCTs) because attrition in trials is common. The "gold standard" for analyzing data from RCTs is to use an **intention-to-treat (ITT) analysis**, which involves analyzing outcome data from all participants who were randomized, regardless of whether they dropped out of the study. A true ITT analysis is achieved only if there are no missing outcome data or if missing values are accounted for in the analysis, such as through imputation. A resource for advice on how to achieve ITT is offered in Polit and Gillespie (2010). Polit and Gillespie (2009) found, in their analysis of 124 nursing trials, that 75% of the RCTs had missing outcome data, and one out of four had 20% or more missing values. Only about 10% of the studies used imputation or mixed effects modeling in their ITT analyses. The approach most often used to impute values for missing outcome variables in these RCTs was a procedure called **last observation carried forward (LOCF)**, which imputes the missing outcome using the previous measurement of that same outcome. For example, if data were collected 1 month and 3 months after the intervention, but data for the 3-month outcome were missing for some participants, the 1-month value would replace the missing value. LOCF is no longer considered the best approach.

Procedures for dealing with missing data are discussed at greater length in McKnight and colleagues (2007), Enders (2010), and Molenberghs et al. (2015).

Assessing Data Quality

Assessing data quality is another preanalytic task. For example, when a composite scale is used, researchers should assess its internal consistency (Chapter 15). The distribution of data values for key variables also should be examined to assess any anomalies, such as limited variability, extreme skewness, or the presence of ceiling or floor effects. A **ceiling effect** occurs when values for a variable are restricted at the upper end of a continuum, and a **floor effect** occurs when values are restricted at the lower end. For example, a vocabulary test for 10-year-olds likely would yield a clustering of high scores in a sample of 11-year-olds, creating a ceiling effect that would reduce correlations between test scores and other characteristics of the children. Conversely, there likely would be a clustering of low scores on the same test with a sample of 9-year-olds, resulting in a floor effect with similar consequences. Floor and ceiling effects are of special concern when the goal is to measure change: if a measure has floor or ceiling effect, improvement (or deterioration) will not be adequately captured.

Earlier we discussed outliers in connection with efforts to clean a dataset to ensure data accuracy. Legitimate outliers—extreme scores that are true values—are a data quality issue. Outliers can distort study results and cause errors in statistical decision-making, and so outliers should be scrutinized. By convention, a value is considered an **extreme outlier** if it is greater than three times the *interquartile range (IQR)* above the third quartile or below the first quartile. The IQR, as noted briefly in Chapter 17, is an index of variability. Methods for detecting and addressing outlier problems are discussed in Polit (2010).

> **Example of Extreme Outliers**
> Edmonds and colleagues (2022) conducted a retrospective, cohort study of 6,970 births attended by 181 registered nurses in one hospital's maternity unit to examine the nurse-level cesarean birth rates. Although the authors were able to consistently identify extreme outliers using the three definitions, they found that the risk adjustment did not make a substantial difference in identifying high outliers among the nurses.

> **TIP** For those using the Statistical Package for the Social Sciences, the EXPLORE routine is invaluable in making assessments of data quality.

Assessing Bias

Researchers often undertake preliminary analyses to assess biases, including the following:

- *Nonresponse (volunteer) bias.* If possible, researchers should assess whether a biased subset of people participated in a study. If there is information about the characteristics of all people who were asked to participate (e.g., demographic information from hospital records), researchers should compare the characteristics of those who did and did not agree to participate to assess the nature of any biases.

- *Selection bias.* When nonrandomized comparison groups are used (e.g., in quasiexperimental studies), researchers should check for selection biases by comparing the groups' baseline characteristics. Detected differences should, if possible, be controlled—for example, through analysis of covariance—especially if a characteristic is a strong predictor of the dependent variable.
- *Attrition bias.* In studies with multiple points of data collection, it is important to check for attrition biases by comparing people who did and did not continue to participate in later waves of data collection, based on baseline characteristics.

In performing any of these analyses, significant group differences are often an indication of bias, and such bias must be taken into consideration in interpreting and discussing the results. To the extent possible, biases should be controlled in testing the principal hypotheses.

TIP It is not considered appropriate to test the significance of group differences on baseline variables in randomized controlled trials—even though this practice is adopted widely, and results are often reported in tables (Pocock et al., 2002). If randomization and allocation were done properly and the sample size is adequate, one would expect 5% of the group differences to be significant, when $\alpha = 0.05$—and this does not signify a bias. Experts advise that it is preferable to control for significant predictors of the outcome, even if group differences are not significant, than to control for a baseline variable with significant group differences but weakly related to the outcome.

Example of Assessing Bias
In a systematic review of socially disadvantaged females' children, Henwood and colleagues (2020) explored the effectiveness of home visiting programs on improving the children's language development. Eleven studies that met the inclusion criteria were assessed for their risk of bias through rating them as high, low, or unclear risk by one of the authors. A second author used the same process in a random sample of four studies. The agreement of the two raters was calculated as $\kappa = 0.69$; $n = 24$. However, when there were disagreements, the raters discussed the discrepancies and came to a consensus about the decision.

Testing Assumptions for Statistical Tests

Most statistical tests are based on several **assumptions**—conditions that are presumed to be true and, when violated, can lead to erroneous conclusions. For example, parametric tests assume that variables are distributed normally. Frequency distributions, scatter plots, and other assessment procedures provide researchers with information about whether underlying assumptions for statistical tests have been upheld.

Statistical indexes of skewness or peakedness are available to test whether the shape of the distribution is significantly skewed or peaked or flat. Many software programs include the *Kolmogorov–Smirnov test*, which tests that a distribution does not deviate significantly from a normal distribution.

Example of Testing Assumptions
Jourabch and colleagues (2020) used a pre-post-test design to examine the effect of relaxation on occupational stress in midwives working in a labor and delivery unit. To test the normality of the main variables and data distribution, the Kolmogorov–Smirnov goodness-of-fit test was used.

Performing Data Transformations

Raw data often need to be modified or transformed before hypotheses can be tested. Various **data transformations** can easily be handled through commands to the computer. For example, the scoring direction of some items on multi-item scales might need to be reversed before item scores can be summed. Guidance on *item reversals* was presented in Chapter 16.

Sometimes researchers want to create a variable that is a cumulative **count** of variables in the dataset. For example, suppose we asked people to indicate which types of illegal drug they had used in the past month, from a list of 10 options. Use of each drug would be answered independently as a yes (e.g., coded 1) or no (e.g., coded 0). We could create a new variable of number of different drugs used, representing a count of all the "1" codes for the 10 drug items. Other transformations involve **recodes** of original values. Recoding is often used to create *dummy variables* for multivariate analyses.

Transformations also can be undertaken to render data appropriate for statistical tests. For example, if a distribution is nonnormal, a transformation can sometimes help to make parametric procedures appropriate. A logarithmic transformation, for example, tends to normalize positively skewed distributions.

When you do transformations, it is important to check that they were done correctly by examining a sample of values for the original and transformed variables. This can be done by instructing the computer to list, for a sample of cases, the values of the newly created variables and the original variables used to create them.

> **Example of Transforming Variables**
> In a big data study, Park and colleagues (2020) sought to discover knowledge about hospital-acquired, catheter-associated urinary tract infections from multiple data sources to predict the patients at risk for the issue. In this work they described the steps of knowledge discovery and data mining (KDDM) using machine learning that was used. There are six steps in the KDDM approach one of which includes transforming the data.

Performing Additional Peripheral Analyses

Depending on the study, additional peripheral analyses may be needed before proceeding to substantive analyses. It is impossible to catalog all such analyses, but we offer a few examples to alert readers to the kinds of issues that need some thought.

Data Pooling

Researchers sometimes obtain data from more than one source—for example, when researchers recruit participants from multiple sites or when data are obtained from multiple cohorts. The risk is that participants from different sites/cohorts may not really be drawn from the same population, and so it is wise to evaluate whether **pooling** of data is warranted (Knapp & Brown, 2014). This type of evaluation involves comparing participants from the different sites or cohorts in terms of key research variables or comparing the extent to which correlations between key variables are similar across sites/cohorts.

> **Example of Testing for Pooling**
> Xu et al. (2023) conducted a systematic review and meta-analysis to examine the prevalence of ICU nurses' intention to leave their position worldwide. They reported that the pooled prevalence for turnover intention was 27.7% (95% confidence interval: 21.6%–34.3%).

Testing Ordering (Carryover) Effects

When a crossover design is used (i.e., people are randomly assigned to different orderings of treatments), researchers should assess whether outcomes are different for people in the different treatment-order groups. That is, did getting A before B yield different outcomes than getting B before A? In essence, such tests offer evidence that it is legitimate to pool the data from alternative orderings.

> **Example of Testing for Ordering Effects**
> Gronning et al. (2022) conducted a longitudinal study to examine the changes in self-management and health status in a group of patients from Norway 5 years after nurse-led patient education. They found that although there was a small deterioration in patients' physical function, the carry over effect indicated that the self-management skills of patients were improved at 5 years and that there were no changes in patient health status. Self-efficacy was positively associated with female gender, patient activation, less tiredness, and less psychological distress.

PRINCIPAL ANALYSES

At this point in the analysis process, researchers have a cleaned dataset, with missing data problems resolved and transformations completed; they also have some understanding of data quality and biases. They can now proceed with more substantive data analyses.

Planning the Substantive Data Analysis

In many studies, researchers collect data on dozens of variables. They cannot analyze every variable in relation to all others, and so a plan to guide data analysis must be developed. One approach is to prepare a list of the analyses to be undertaken, specifying both the variables and the statistical test to be used. Another approach is to develop table shells. **Table shells** are layouts of how researchers envision presenting their findings, without numbers filled in. Once a table shell is prepared, researchers can do the analyses needed to complete the table. Researchers do not need to adhere rigidly to table shells, but they provide a good mechanism for organizing the analysis of large amounts of data.

Substantive Analyses

Substantive analyses typically begin with descriptive analyses. Researchers usually develop a profile of the sample and may look descriptively at correlations among variables. These initial analyses may suggest further analyses or further data transformations that were not originally envisioned. They also give researchers an opportunity to become familiar with their data.

> **TIP** When you explore your data, resist the temptation of going on a "fishing expedition," that is, hunting for *any* significant relationships. The facility with which computers can generate statistics makes it easy to run analyses indiscriminately. The risk is that you will serendipitously find significant correlations between variables as a function of chance. For example, in a correlation matrix with 10 variables—which results in 45 nonredundant correlations—there are likely to be two to three *spurious* significant correlations when alpha = 0.05 (i.e., $0.05 \times 45 = 2.25$).

Researchers then perform statistical analyses to test their hypotheses. Researchers whose data analysis plan calls for multivariate analyses (e.g., MANOVA) often begin with bivariate analyses (e.g., a series of ANOVAs). The primary statistical analyses are complete when all research questions are addressed and when table shells have the applicable numbers in them.

Sensitivity Analyses

Sometimes supplementary analyses can facilitate interpretation of the results or strengthen conclusions. An important example is the use of **sensitivity analyses**, which are analyses that test research hypotheses using different assumptions or different strategies. One example is testing alternative strategies to address missing values problems. Some strategies are appropriate under varying conditions, so sensitivity analyses to understand how different strategies affect substantive results are valuable. Another example is running analyses with and without legitimate outliers to see if the results change. Thabane and colleagues (2013) offer a tutorial on sensitivity analyses.

> **Example of Sensitivity Analysis**
> Zhang and colleagues (2022) aimed to quantify the prevalence of lateral violence in nurses' workplaces. Although they originally identified 14 studies for the analysis, sensitivity analysis indicted the one study had an outsize impact of the overall result, so this study was excluded from the quantitative synthesis.

RESEARCH EXAMPLE

We conclude this chapter by describing a study that provided considerable detail about the data analyses. This study provides a useful overview of the steps the researchers took in their analyses.

Study: Relationships between Depressive Symptoms, Appetite, and Quality of Life in Heart Failure (De Martini et al., 2023).

Statement of purpose: The purpose of this study was to analyze the relationship between depressive symptoms, appetite, and quality of life in patients hospitalized with heart failure.

Method: The researchers used an observational, analytical, cross-sectional design to explore the relationship between the independent variable of quality of life and the dependent variables of depression and appetite. They used many covariates to describe the sample such as sociodemographic characteristics, clinical data such as BMI, time since diagnosis, and New York Heart Failure functional class. The study was conducted over 9 months in a hospital in Brazil.

Analyses: Categorical variables were summarized to provide the total and relative frequencies. The categorical variables were described by calculating the mean or median. Statistical tests used include the Student's *t*-test, Mann–Whitney *U*-test, Kruskal–Wallis test, ANOVA, Spearman correlation, and, as relevant, the Games–Howell and Duncan's posttests. To develop a model, multiple linear regression was used on all variables with a *p*-value less than or equal to 0.05 and with residuals following normality by the Shapiro–Wilk test. The reliability of the measures was evaluated by calculating Cronbach alpha.

Results: In this study, data were analyzed on 86 patients. The final linear regression model indicated that the factor associated with poor QoL was being dependent for four activities of daily living (estimate = 15.4, 95% CI = 0.23–30.64, p = .046). Minimal depressive symptoms as opposed to mild or moderate (estimate = –20.0, 95% CI = –28.3 to –11.73, p < .001) and not being at risk for weight loss (estimate = –11.08, 95% CI = –20.5 to –1.62, p = .022) were associated with better QoL. The final model explains 34.68% of the data variance.

SUMMARY POINTS

- Researchers who collect quantitative data typically progress through a series of steps in the analysis and interpretation of their data. Careful researchers lay out a data analysis plan in advance to guide that progress.
- Quantitative data typically must be **coded** into numerical values; codes need to be developed for legitimate data and for **missing values**. Decisions about coding and variable naming are documented in a **codebook**.
- **Data entry** is an error-prone process that requires verification and **data cleaning**. Cleaning involves checks for **outliers** (values that lie outside the normal range of values) and **wild codes** (codes that are not legitimate), as well as **consistency checks** (checks for internally consistent information).
- Decisions on handling missing values must be based on the amount of missing data and how missing data are patterned (i.e., the extent to which missingness is random). Addressing missing data is important for undertaking **intention-to-treat analyses.**
- The three missing values patterns are (1) **missing completely at random (MCAR)**, which occurs when cases with missing values are just a random subsample of all cases in the sample; (2) **missing at random (MAR)**, which occurs if missingness is related to other variables but is *not* related to the variable that has the missing values; and (3) **missing not at random (MNAR)**, a pattern in which the value of the variable that is missing is related to its missingness.
- Two basic missing values strategies involve **deletion** or **imputation**. Deletion strategies include deleting cases with missing values (i.e., **listwise deletion**), selective **pairwise deletion** of cases, or deleting variables with missing values. Imputation strategies include **mean substitution**, regression-based estimation of missing values, **expectation maximization (EM) imputation**, and **multiple imputation (MI)**, which is considered the best approach.
- Raw data often need to be transformed for analysis. Examples of **data transformations** include reversing the coding of items, recoding the values of a variable (e.g., for creating dummy variables), and transforming data to meet statistical assumptions (e.g., through logarithmic transformations to achieve normality).
- Researchers usually undertake additional steps to assess data quality, such as evaluating the internal consistency of scales, examining distributions for **extreme outliers** that are legitimate values and analyzing the magnitude and direction of any biases, such as nonresponse bias, selection bias, and attrition bias.
- Another assessment may involve a scrutiny for possible **ceiling effects** (which occurs when values for a variable are restricted at the upper end of a continuum) or **floor effects** (which occurs when values are restricted at the lower end).
- Sometimes peripheral analyses involve tests to determine whether **pooling** of participants is warranted in tests for **site/cohort effects** or **ordering effects.**
- Once the data are fully prepared for substantive analysis, researchers should develop a formal analysis plan, to reduce the temptation to go on a "fishing expedition." One approach is to develop **table shells** (i.e., fully laid-out tables without numbers in them).

- Supplementary statistical analyses can sometimes facilitate interpretation (e.g., doing **sensitivity analyses** that test whether results hold true under different assumptions or with different statistical procedures).

REFERENCES CITED IN CHAPTER 20

De Martini, G. D. A., Grisante, D. L., Gonçalves, A. L. P., D'Agostino, F., Lopes, J. d. L., Santos, V. B., & Lopes, C. T. (2023). Relationships between depressive symptoms, appetite, and quality of life in heart failure. *Western Journal of Nursing Research*, *45*(5), 416–424. https://doi.org/10.1177/01939459221142163

Dziadkowiec, O., Callahan, T., Ozkaynak, M., Reeder, B., & Welton, J. (2016). Using a data quality framework to clean data extracted from the electronic health record: A case study. *eGEMS*, *4*, 1201–1215.

Edmonds, J. K., Woodbury, S. R., Lipsitz, S. R., Weiseth, A., Farrell, M. E., Shah, N. T., Greene, N., & Gregory, K. D. (2022). Comparing methods of identifying outlying nurses in audits of low-risk cesarean delivery rates. *Journal of Nursing Care Quality*, *37*(2), 149–154. https://doi.org/10.1097/ncq.0000000000000588

Enders, C. K. (2010). *Applied missing data analysis*. The Guilford Press.

Fox-Wasylyshyn, S., & El-Masri, M. (2005). Handling missing data in self-report measures. *Research in Nursing & Health*, *28*(6), 488–495.

Grønning, K., Lim, S., & Bratås, O. (2022). A longitudinal study of educational needs among patients with inflammatory arthritis. *Musculoskeletal Care*, *20*(1), 151–157. https://doi.org/10.1002/msc.1575

Henwood, T., Channon, S., Penny, H., Robling, M., & Waters, C. S. (2020). Do home visiting programmes improve children's language development? A systematic review. *International Journal of Nursing Studies*, *109*, 103610. https://doi.org/10.1016/j.ijnurstu.2020.103610

Jourabchi, Z., Satari, E., Mafi, M., & Ranjkesh, F. (2020). Effects of Benson's relaxation technique on occupational stress in midwives. *Nursing*, *50*(9), 64–68. https://doi.org/10.1097/01.NURSE.0000694836.00028.28

Knapp, T. R., & Brown, J. (2014). Ten statistics commandments that almost never should be broken. *Research in Nursing & Health*, *37*(4), 347–351.

Lyons, A. M., Dimas, J., Richardson, S. J., & Sward, K. (2022). Assessing EHR data for use in clinical improvement and research. *American Journal of Nursing*, *122*(6), 32–41. https://doi.org/10.1097/01.NAJ.0000832728.09164.3f

McKnight, P., McKnight, K., Sidani, S., & Figueredo, A. (2007). *Missing data: A gentle introduction*. The Guilford Press.

Möckel, M., Corman, V. M., Stegemann, M. S., Hofmann, J., Stein, A., Jones, T. C., Gastmeier, P., Seybold, J., Offermann, R., Bachmann, U., Lindner, T., Bauer, W., Drosten, C., Rosen, A., & Somasundaram, R. (2021). SARS-CoV-2 antigen rapid immunoassay for diagnosis of COVID-19 in the emergency department. *Biomarkers*, *26*(3), 213–220. https://doi.org/10.1080/1354750X.2021.1876769

Molenberghs, G., Fitzmaurice, G., Kenward, M., Tsiatis, A., & Verbeke, G. (2015). *Handbook of missing data methodology*. Taylor & Francis.

Osborne, J. E. (2013). *Best practices in data cleaning: A complete guide to everything you need to do before and after collecting your data*. Sage Publications.

Park, J. I., Bliss, D. Z., Chi, C. L., Delaney, C. W., & Westra, B. L. (2020). Knowledge discovery with machine learning for hospital-acquired catheter-associated urinary tract infections. *CIN: Computers, Informatics, Nursing*, *38*(1), 28–35. https://doi.org/10.1097/CIN.0000000000000562

Patrician, P. A. (2002). Multiple imputation for missing data. *Reseach in Nursing & Health*, *25*(1), 76–84.

Pocock, S. J., Assmann, S., Enos, L., & Kasten, L. (2002). Subgroup analysis, covariate adjustment and baseline comparisons in clinical trial reporting: Current practice and problems. *Statistics in Medicine*, *21*(19), 2917–2930.

Polit, D. F. (2010). *Statistics and data analysis for nursing research* (2nd ed.). Pearson.

Polit, D. F., & Gillespie, B. (2009). The use of the intention-to-treat principle in nursing clinical trials. *Nursing Research*, *58*(6), 391–399.

Polit, D. F., & Gillespie, B. (2010). Intention-to-treat in randomized controlled trials: Recommendations for a total trial strategy. *Research in Nursing & Health*, *33*(4), 355–368.

Son, H., Friedmann, E., & Thomas, S. A. (2012). Application of pattern mixture models to address missing data in longitudinal data analysis using SPSS. *Nursing Research*, *61*(3), 195–203.

Thabane, L., Mbuagbaw, L., Zhang, S., Samaan, Z., Marcucci, M., Ye, C., Thabane, M., Giangregorio, L., Dennis, B., Kosa, D., Borg Debono, V., Dillenburg, R., Fruci, V., Bawor, M., Lee, J., Wells, G., Goldsmith, C. H., & Goldsmith, C. (2013). A tutorial on sensitivity analyses in clinical trials: The what, why, when, and how. *BMC Medical Research Methodology*, *13*, 92.

Van den Broeck, J., Cunningham, S., Eeckles, R., & Herbst, K. (2005). Data cleaning: Detecting, diagnosing, and editing data abnormalities. *PLoS Medicine*, *2*, 10.

Xu, G., Zeng, X., & Wu, X. (2023). Global prevalence of turnover intention among intensive care nurses: A meta-analysis. *Nursing in Critical Care*, *28*(2), 159–166. https://doi.org/10.1111/nicc.12679

Zhang, Y., Cai, J., Yin, R., Qin, S., Wang, H., Shi, X., & Mao, L. (2022). Prevalence of lateral violence in nurse workplace: A systematic review and meta-analysis. *BMJ Open*, *12*(3), e054014. https://doi.org/10.1136/bmjopen-2021-054014

21 | Clinical Significance and Interpretation of Quantitative Results

Learning Objectives

1. Describe the various ways to assess the credibility and accuracy of the results.
2. Identify various ways to estimate the magnitude of effects.
3. Discuss how to interpret the meaning of the results in light of causality.
4. Recognize the importance of the generalizability and applicability of the results.
5. Understand how to describe the implications of the results for practice and theory.

INTRODUCTION

In this chapter, we discuss the issue of interpreting statistical results. We begin with some general interpretive guidelines and then discuss an important emerging topic in health research: clinical significance.

INTERPRETATION OF QUANTITATIVE RESULTS

The analysis of research data provides the **results** of the study. These results need to be evaluated and interpreted, giving thought to the study's theoretical basis, existing research evidence, and limitations of the research methods used. Interpretation of statistical results forms the basis for the Discussion section of quantitative research reports.

Issues in Interpretation

The interpretive task is complex, requiring methodologic and substantive skills. Interpretation is difficult to teach, but we offer advice about ways of making sound inferences from study results.

The Interpretive Mindset

Evidence-based practice (EBP) encourages clinicians to make decisions based on a careful assessment of "best evidence." Thinking critically and demanding evidence are also part of a research interpreter's job. Just as clinicians must ask, "What *evidence* is there that this intervention or strategy will be beneficial?" so should research interpreters ask, "What *evidence* is there that the results are real, true, and important?" This is precisely why nurses need to develop skills in understanding research methods and appraising research reports. To be a good interpreter of your research results, it is appropriate to adopt a skeptical attitude, challenging the results until you are confident that the results are real and important.

> **TIP** You should ask such questions as: Is it *plausible* that my results were affected by selection biases? Is it *plausible* that if I had used a different instrument, or had gotten a larger sample, or had less attrition, my results would change? You hope that the answers to such questions are "no," but you should start with the working assumption that the answer is "maybe" until you have satisfied yourself that this is not true.

Aspects of Interpretation

Interpreting the results of a study involves attending to different but overlapping considerations:

- The credibility and accuracy of the results
- The precision of the estimate of effects
- The magnitude of effects and importance of the results
- The meaning of the results, especially regarding causality
- The generalizability and applicability of the results
- The implications of the results for practice, theory development, or further research

Credibility of Quantitative Results

One of the most important interpretive tasks is to assess whether the results are *correct*. This corresponds to the first EBP question we posed in Chapter 2 with regard to appraising research evidence: To what extent is the evidence valid? If the results are not credible, the remaining interpretive issues (meaning, magnitude, and so on) are not likely to matter.

Research findings are meant to reflect "truth in the real world." The findings are intended to be proxies for the true state of affairs in actual community or healthcare settings. Inference is the vehicle for linking results to the real world. Inferences about what is true in the real world are valid, however, to the extent that the researchers have made rigorous methodologic decisions. To come to a conclusion about whether the results closely approximate "truth in the real world," each aspect of the study—its design, procedures, sampling plan, measurements, and analytic approach—must be subjected to critical scrutiny.

There are various ways to assess credibility, including the use of the critical appraisal guidelines we have offered throughout this book. Here we share additional perspectives.

Proxies and Credibility

Researchers begin with abstract constructs and then devise ways to operationalize them. Constructs are linked to reality in a series of approximations, each of which affects interpretation because at each step there is potential for misrepresentation. The better the proxies, the more credible the results are likely to be. In this section, we illustrate successive proxies using sampling concepts, to highlight the potential for inferential challenges.

When researchers formulate research questions or hypotheses, the population is typically broad and abstract. Population specifications are delineated later, when eligibility criteria are defined. For example, suppose we wanted to test the effectiveness of an intervention to increase physical activity in low-income women. Figure 21.1 shows the series of steps between the abstract population construct (low-income women) and the *actual* women who participated in the study. Using data from the actual sample on the far right, the researcher would like to make inferences about the effectiveness of the intervention for a broader group, but each proxy along the way represents a potential problem for achieving the desired inference. In interpreting a study, readers must consider how *plausible* it is that the actual sample reflects the recruited sample, the accessible population, the target population, and then the population construct.

Table 21.1 presents a description of a hypothetical scenario in which the researchers moved from a population construct of low-income women to an actual sample of 161 women who participated in the study. The table shows some questions that a person trying to make inferences about the study

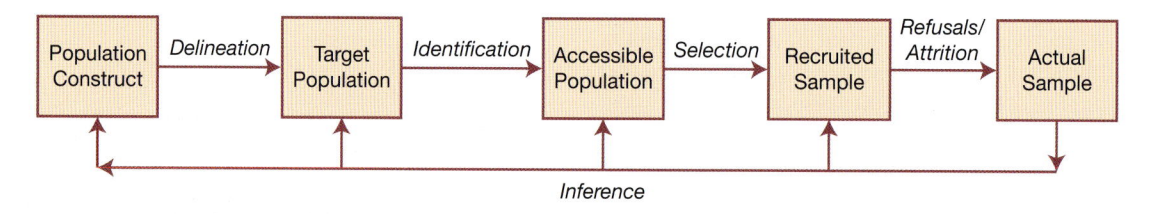

FIGURE 21.1 Inferences about populations: From the analysis sample to the population construct.

TABLE 21.1 • Successive Proxies in Sampling Example: From the Population Construct to the Analysis Sample

ELEMENT	DESCRIPTION	POSSIBLE INFERENTIAL CHALLENGES
Population construct	Low-income women	
Target population	All women who receive public assistance (cash welfare) in California	• Why only welfare recipients—why not people living below the poverty threshold? • Why California?
Accessible population	All women who receive public assistance in Los Angeles and who speak English or Spanish	• Why Los Angeles? • What about non-English/non-Spanish speakers?
Recruited sample	A consecutive sample of 300 female welfare recipients (English or Spanish speaking) who applied for benefits in January 2020 at two randomly selected welfare offices in Los Angeles	• Why only new applicants—what about women with long-term receipt? • Why only two offices? Are these representative? • Is January a typical month?
Actual sample	161 women from the recruited sample who fully participated in the study	• Who refused to participate (or was too ill, and so on) and why? • Who dropped out of the study, and why?

results might ask—these represent inferential challenges. Answers to these questions would affect the interpretation of whether the intervention *really* is effective with low-income women—or only with motivated, cooperative welfare recipients from two neighborhoods of Los Angeles who recently got approved for public assistance.

As Figure 21.1 suggests, researchers in our example made a series of methodologic decisions that affect inferences, and these decisions must be scrutinized in assessing study credibility. However, participant behavior and external circumstances also affect the results and need to be considered in the interpretation. In our example in Table 21.1, 300 women were recruited but only 161 provided useable data for analysis. The final sample of 161 almost surely would differ in important ways from the 139 who were not in the study, and these differences affect inferences about the value of the study evidence.

We illustrated how successive proxies in a study, from the abstract to the concrete, can affect inferences with regard to sampling, but we could focus on other aspects of the study. For example, Figure 21.2 considers successive proxies for an intervention for these women. As with our previous illustration, researchers move from an abstraction on the left (here, a theory about why an intervention might have beneficial outcomes), through the design of protocols that purport to operationalize the theory, to the actual implementation and use of the intervention on the right. Researchers want the right side to be a good proxy for the left side—and, in interpreting their results, they must assess the plausibility that they were successful in the transformation.

Credibility and Validity

Studies inherently involve making inferences. We *infer* that scores on a depression scale are, in fact, capturing the depression construct. We *infer* that a sample can tell us something about a population. We use inferential statistics to make inferences about parameters. Inference and validity are inextricably

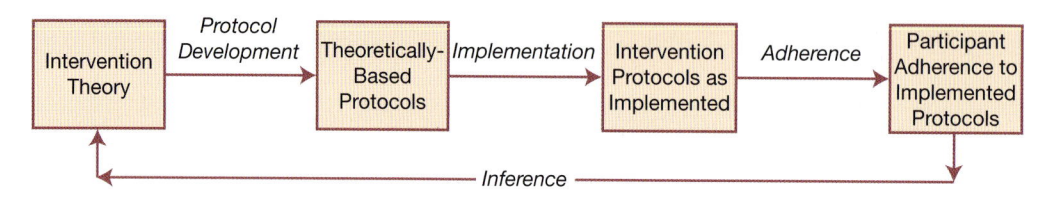

FIGURE 21.2 Inferences about interventions: From actual program operations to the intervention theory.

linked. Indeed, research experts Shadish et al. (2002) defined validity as "the approximate truth of an inference" (p. 34). To be careful interpreters, researchers must seek evidence within their study that desired inferences are, in fact, valid.

In Chapter 10, we discussed four types of validity that play a key role in assessing the credibility of quantitative results: statistical conclusion validity, internal validity, external validity, and construct validity. Let us use our sampling example (Figure 21.1 and Table 21.1) to demonstrate the relevance of methodologic decisions to all four types of validity—and hence to inferences about study results.

First, let us consider construct validity—a term that has relevance for many aspects of a study. In our example, the population construct was *low-income women*, which was the basis of the eligibility criteria stipulating public assistance recipients. There are, however, alternative operationalizations of the population construct—for example, women with incomes below the official poverty level. Construct validity, it may be recalled, involves inferences from the particulars of the study to higher-order constructs. So it is fair to ask this question: Do the specified eligibility criteria adequately capture the population construct of low-income women?

Statistical conclusion validity—the extent to which correct inferences can be made about whether relationships between key variables are "real"—is also affected by sampling decisions. Ideally, researchers would do a power analysis to estimate how large a sample is needed. In our example, let us say we estimated (based on previous research) a small-to-moderate effect size (ES) for the intervention, $d = 0.40$. For a power of 0.80, with risk of a type I error set at 0.05, we would need a sample of about 200 participants. The actual sample of 161 yields a nearly 30% risk of a Type II error (i.e., falsely concluding that the intervention was not successful).

External validity—the generalizability of the results—is also affected by sampling decisions. To whom would it be safe to generalize the results in this example—to the population construct of low-income women? to all welfare recipients in California? to all new welfare recipients in Los Angeles who speak English or Spanish? Inferences about the extent to which the study results correspond to "truth in the real world" must take sampling decisions and sampling problems (e.g., recruitment and retention difficulties) into account.

Finally, internal validity (the extent to which a causal connection between variables can be inferred) is also affected by sample composition. In particular (in this example), differential attrition would be a concern. Were those in the intervention group more likely (or less likely) than those in the control group to drop out of the study? If so, any observed differences in physical activity outcomes could be caused by individual differences in the two groups (for example, differences in motivation), rather than by the intervention itself.

Methodologic decisions and the careful implementation of those decisions—whether they be about sampling, intervention design, measurement, research design, or analysis—inevitably affect study validity and the interpretation of results.

Credibility and Bias

Part of a researcher's job in doing a study is to translate abstract constructs into plausible and meaningful proxies. Another job is to eliminate or reduce biases—or, as a last resort, to detect and understand them. In interpreting results, the risk for various biases should be assessed and taken into account when drawing conclusions.

Biases are factors that create distortions and undermine researchers' efforts to capture and reveal "truth in the real world." Biases are pervasive. It is not so much a question of whether there *are* biases in a study, so much as what types of bias are present, and how extensive and systematic the biases are. We have discussed many types of bias—some reflect design inadequacies (e.g., selection bias), others reflect recruitment or sampling problems (nonresponse bias), others are related to measurement (social desirability bias). To our knowledge, there is no comprehensive listing of biases that might arise in a study, but Table 21.2 presents a list of some of the biases and errors mentioned in this book. This list is not all-inclusive but is meant to serve as a reminder of potential problems to consider in interpreting study results.

TIP Different disciplines use different names for the same or similar biases, but the names are not especially important—what is important is to understand how different forces can distort the results and affect inferences.

Credibility and Corroboration

Yet another strategy for assessing credibility is to seek corroboration for results. Corroboration can come from both internal and external sources, and the concept of *replication* is an important one in both cases. Interpretations are aided by considering prior research on the topic, for example. Interpreters can examine whether the study results replicate (are congruent with) those of other studies. Consistency across studies supports the credibility of the findings.

Researchers can pursue opportunities for replication themselves. For example, in multisite studies, if results are similar across sites, this suggests that something "real" is occurring with some regularity. Triangulation can be another form of replication and sometimes can help to corroborate results. For example, if results are similar across different measures of an outcome, then there can be greater confidence that the results are "real" and do not reflect some peculiarity of an instrument. When mixed results occur, interpreters must dig deeper to uncover the reason.

Finally, we are strong advocates of mixed methods studies, a special type of triangulation (Chapter 27). When findings from the analysis of qualitative data are consistent with the results of statistical analyses, internal corroboration can be especially powerful and persuasive.

Precision of the Results

The results of statistical hypothesis testing indicate whether an observed relationship or group difference is probably real and replicable. A p value in hypothesis testing indicates how unlikely it is that

TABLE 21.2 • Selected List of Major Potential Biases or Errors in Quantitative Studies

RESEARCH DESIGN	SAMPLING	MEASUREMENT	ANALYSIS
Expectation bias	Sampling error	Social desirability bias	Type I error
Hawthorne effect	Volunteer bias	Acquiescence bias	Type II error
Performance bias	Nonresponse bias	Naysayers bias	
Detection bias		Extreme response set bias	
Contamination of treatments		Recall/memory bias	
Carryover (ordering) effects		Ceiling effects	
Noncompliance bias		Floor effects	
Selection bias/threat		Reactivity	
Attrition bias/threat		Observer biases	
History bias/threat			

the null hypothesis is true—it is not an estimate of a numeric value of direct relevance to clinicians. A *p* value offers information that is important, but incomplete.

Confidence intervals (CIs), by contrast, communicate how precise the study results are—that is, they indicate not only the estimate of an effect but also the range within which the actual effect probably lies. Dr. David Sackett, a founding father of the EBP movement, had this to say about CIs: "*p* values on their own are...not informative... By contrast, CIs indicate the strength of evidence about quantities of direct interest, such as treatment benefit. They are thus of particular relevance to practitioners of evidence-based medicine" (2000, p. 232). It is hoped nurse researchers will increasingly report CIs because of their value for interpreting study results and assessing their potential utility for nursing practice.

Magnitude of Effects and Importance

In quantitative studies, results that support the researcher's hypotheses are described as *significant*. A careful analysis of study results involves evaluating whether, in addition to being statistically significant, the effects are large and clinically important.

Attaining statistical significance does not necessarily mean that the results are meaningful to nurses and clients. Statistical significance indicates that the results are unlikely to be due to chance—not that they are necessarily valuable. With large samples, even modest relationships are statistically significant. For instance, with a sample of 500, a correlation coefficient of 0.10 is significant at the 0.05 level, but a relationship this weak may have little practical value. Estimating the magnitude and importance of effects is relevant to the issue of clinical significance, a topic we discus later in this chapter.

Meaning of the Results

In quantitative studies, standard statistical results are in the form of *p* values, ES, and CIs, to which researchers must attach meaning once they have concluded that these results are credible. Many questions about the meaning of statistical results reflect a desire to interpret causal connections.

Interpreting what results mean usually is not challenging in descriptive studies. For example, suppose we found that, among patients undergoing electroconvulsive therapy (ECT), the percentage who experience an ECT-induced headache is 59.4% (95% CI = 56.3, 63.1). This result is directly meaningful and interpretable. But if we found that headache prevalence is significantly lower for patients in a cryotherapy intervention group than for patients given acetaminophen, we would need to interpret what the results mean. In particular, we need to interpret whether it is plausible that cryotherapy *caused* reductions in headaches. Even if the results are deemed to be "real"—that is, statistically significant—interpretation involves coming to conclusions about internal validity when a causal inference is sought.

In this section, we discuss the interpretation of various research outcomes within a hypothesis-testing context, with an emphasis on causal interpretations. In thinking about causal interpretations, we encourage you to review the criteria for causal relationships (Chapter 9).

Interpreting Hypothesized Results

Interpreting statistical results is easiest when hypotheses are supported, that is, when there are *positive results*. In this situation, interpretations have been partly achieved beforehand because researchers have brought together prior findings, theory, and logic in developing hypotheses. This groundwork forms the context within which specific interpretations are made.

It is important to avoid the temptation of going beyond the data to explain what results mean, however. As an example, suppose we hypothesized that pregnant women's anxiety level about labor and delivery is correlated with the number of children they have borne. The data reveal a significant negative relationship between anxiety levels and parity ($r = -0.30$). We interpret this to mean that increased experience with childbirth results in decreased anxiety. Is this conclusion supported by the data? The conclusion seems logical, but in fact, there is nothing in the data that leads to this interpretation.

An important, indeed critical, research precept is *correlation does not prove causation*. The finding that two variables are related offers no evidence suggesting which of the two variables—if either—caused the other. In our example, perhaps causality runs in the opposite direction, that is, a woman's anxiety level influences how many children she bears. Or perhaps a third variable, such as the woman's relationship with her husband, influences both anxiety and number of children. Inferring causality is especially difficult in studies with a nonexperimental design.

TIP Froman and Owen (2014) have written a helpful paper about avoiding inappropriate causal language in research reports. They point out that researchers often use misleading "loaded words" that suggest a casual link even when the study design does not support a causal inference—words like *impact*, *effect*, and *determinant*.

Alternative explanations for the findings should always be considered. Researchers sometimes can test rival hypotheses directly. If competing interpretations can be ruled out, so much the better, but every angle should be examined to see if one's own explanation has been given adequate competition.

Empirical evidence supporting research hypotheses never constitutes *proof* of their veracity. Hypothesis testing is probabilistic. There is always a possibility that observed relationships resulted from chance—that is, that a Type I error occurred. Researchers must be tentative about their results and about interpretations of them. Even when the results are in line with expectations, researchers should draw conclusions with restraint and should give due consideration to limitations identified in assessing the credibility of the results.

Example of Corroboration of a Hypothesis
Bartzik and colleagues (2021) hypothesized nurses would report more perceived stress during the COVID-19 pandemic than before the pandemic. They found that nurses did report greater stress (t (173) = 3.14, p = .002, d_z = 0.24), emotional irritation (t (171) = 4.63, p < .001, d_z = 0.35), and more exhaustion (t (172) = 8.08, p < .001, d_z = 0.61) during the pandemic than prior to it, which supported their hypothesis.

TIP A mistake that many researchers make is to qualitatively interpret the *p* values in statistical tests. A *p* value of .0001 is not "more significant" than a *p* value of .05. The outcome of a significance test is dichotomous: the result either is or is not significant. Similarly, a *p* value of .08 is not "marginally significant"; if one has established alpha = 0.05, the result is not significant (Hayat, 2010). Mechanisms other than *p* values are needed to interpret magnitude and importance, as we discuss later in this chapter.

Interpreting Nonsignificant Results

Nonsignificant results pose interpretative problems because statistical tests are geared toward disconfirmation of the null hypothesis. Failure to reject a null hypothesis can occur for many reasons, and the real reason is usually difficult to discern. The null hypothesis *could* actually be true, for example: a nonsignificant result could accurately reflect the absence of a relationship among research variables. On the other hand, the null hypothesis could be false, in which case a Type II error has been committed. Nonsignificant results are inconclusive.

Retention of a false null hypothesis can result from several methodologic problems, such as poor internal validity, an anomalous sample, a weak statistical procedure, or unreliable measures. In particular, failure to reject null hypotheses is often a consequence of insufficient power resulting from too small a sample.

In any event, a retained null hypothesis should not be considered as proof of the *absence* of relationships among variables. *Nonsignificant results provide no evidence of the truth or the falsity of the hypothesis*. Interpreting nonsignificant results can, however, be aided by considering such factors as sample size and ES estimates.

Example of Nonsignificant Results
Flanagan, one of the authors of this textbook, and colleagues (2022) tested if pedometer use improved steps walked, perceived stress, or well-being in informal dementia caregivers. One group had nurse coaching, whereas the other group did not. While there was a statistical difference in the steps walked in each group, there was no statistical difference in well-being (p = .38 control; p = .08 intervention) or perceived stress (p = .56 control; p = .18 intervention).

Because statistical tests support the rejection of null hypotheses, they are not well-suited for testing *actual* research hypotheses about the absence of relationships or about group equivalence. Yet sometimes this is exactly what researchers want to do—and this is especially true in clinical situations in which the goal is to assess if one practice is as effective as another (an *equivalence trial*) or not less effective than another (a *noninferiority trial*). When the actual research hypothesis is null (i.e., a prediction of no group difference or no relationship), additional strategies must be used to provide supporting evidence. In particular, it is important to compute ES and CIs to show that the risk of a type II error was small. There may also be clinical standards that can be used to corroborate that nonsignificant—but predicted—results are plausible. In noninferiority and equivalence trials, clinical parameters must be stipulated for undertaking a power analysis (Tunes da Silva et al., 2009).

> **Example of Support for a Hypothesized Nonsignificant Result**
> Yıldırım and Gerçeker (2023) examined the effect of three different distraction methods on procedure-related fear and anxiety in children. Usual care, including talking to the children, was tested against virtual reality and cold vibration interventions. They found there were no statistical differences in the three approaches and concluded low-technology distraction techniques, such as talking, were as effective in reducing fear and anxiety as more technical approaches.

Interpreting Unhypothesized Significant Results

Unhypothesized significant results can occur in two situations. The first involves exploring relationships that were not anticipated during the design of the study. For example, in examining correlations among variables in the dataset, a researcher might notice that two variables that were not central to the research questions were nevertheless significantly correlated—and interesting. To interpret serendipitous findings, it is wise to consult the literature to see if similar relationships had been previously observed—and to recommend a replication.

> **Example of a Serendipitous Significant Finding**
> In a study examining nurse practitioners' vs. physicians' primary care of patients at high risk of hypoglycemia, Schuttner et al. (2023) found that patients assigned to a nurse practitioner had a 20.38 percentage-point lower average predicted probability (95% CI −37.92 to −2.83, $p = .02$) of having a $HgbA_1C < 7\%$ at 2 years than those being cared for by a physician. Incidental findings indicated that those being cared for by the nurse practitioners were older, non-Hispanic White, rural residents who lived ≥40 miles from the primary care clinic where they received care.

The second situation is more perplexing, and it does not happen often: obtaining results *opposite* to those hypothesized. For instance, a researcher might hypothesize that individualized teaching about AIDS risks is more effective than group instruction, but the results might indicate that group instruction was significantly better. Some researchers view such situations as awkward, but research should not be undertaken primarily to corroborate researchers' predictions but rather to arrive at truthful evidence. The interpretation of such findings should involve comparisons with other research, a consideration of alternative theories, and—if possible—in-depth interviews with a subsample of study participants.

> **Example of Significant Results Contrary to Hypotheses**
> Fulda and Miano (2023) studied periodic leg movements in children during sleep. They hypothesized that these leg movements would be more frequent in children with attention deficit hyperactivity disorder (ADHD) as compared to children without ADHD. In their case control matched study, they found there was no statistical difference in leg movement between children with ADHD and without, suggesting that these leg movements are a separate disorder requiring additional attention by providers.

Interpreting Mixed Results

Interpretation is often complicated by *mixed results*: some hypotheses are supported by the data, but others are not. Or a hypothesis may be accepted with one measure of the outcome but rejected with a different measure. When only some results run counter to a prediction, the research methods are the first aspect of the study deserving scrutiny. Differences in the validity and reliability of the various measures may account for such discrepancies, for example. Or the sample size might be sufficiently large when effects are large but insufficient for more modest effects. On the other hand, mixed results may suggest that a theory needs to be qualified or that certain constructs within the theory need to be reconceptualized. Mixed results sometimes present opportunities for conceptual advances because efforts to make sense of disparate pieces of evidence may lead to a breakthrough.

In summary, interpreting the meaning of research results is a demanding task but offers the possibility of intellectual rewards. Interpreters must play the role of scientific detectives, trying to make pieces of the puzzle fit together so that a coherent picture emerges.

TIP A major strength of mixed methods research is that it can prove invaluable in interpreting results, especially if the results are not consistent with expectations.

Generalizability and Applicability of the Results

Researchers are rarely interested in discovering relationships among variables for a specific sample of people at a specific point in time. If a new nursing intervention is found to be successful, others may want to adopt it. Thus, an important interpretive question is whether the intervention will "work" or whether relationships will "hold" in other settings, with other people. Part of the interpretive process involves asking, "To what groups, environments, and conditions can the results of the study reasonably be applied?" In interpreting the study results with regard to the generalizability, it is useful to consider our earlier discussion about proxies. For which higher-order constructs, which populations, which settings, or which versions of an intervention were the study operations good "stand-ins"? We discuss the issue of generalizability and applicability of research evidence at greater length in Chapter 31.

Implications of the Results

Once you have reached conclusions about the credibility, precision, importance, meaning, and generalizability of your results, you are ready to think about their implications. You might consider the implications with respect to future research (What should other researchers working in this area do? What is the right "next step"?) or theory development (What are the implications for nursing theory?). A key issue, though, is the implications of the evidence for nursing practice. Specific suggestions for implementing the results of the study in real nursing contexts are valuable.

TIP In interpreting your data, remember that others will be reviewing your interpretation with a critical and perhaps even a skeptical eye. The job of consumers is to make decisions about the credibility and utility of the evidence, which is likely to be affected by how much support you offer for the validity and meaning of your results.

CLINICAL SIGNIFICANCE

Attaining statistical significance does not indicate whether a finding is clinically meaningful or relevant. With a large enough sample, a trivial relationship can be statistically significant. Broadly speaking, we define **clinical significance** as the practical importance of research results in terms of whether they have genuine, palpable effects on the daily lives of patients or on the healthcare decisions made on their behalf.

More than 20 years ago, LeFort (1993) wrote, in a prominent nursing journal, about the "recent interest" in clinical significance—but that interest has had a bigger impact on fields other than nursing. Relatively few nurse researchers comment on the clinical significance of their findings when discussing their results. When nurse researchers mention clinical significance, they often use the phrase loosely and ambiguously, or sometimes they establish a criterion for clinical significance without offering a rationale (Bruner et al., 2012; Polit, 2017).

In fields other than nursing, notably in medicine and psychotherapy, a lot of attention has recently been paid to two key challenges relating to clinical significance: developing a conceptual definition of what it means and developing a way to operationalize it. Consensus has not been reached on either front, but a few conceptual and statistical solutions are used with considerable regularity. In this section, we briefly describe recent advances in defining and operationalizing clinical significance. Further information is available in Polit and Yang (2016).

In statistical hypothesis testing, a fair degree of consensus was reached decades ago that a p value of .05 would be the standard for statistical significance—although this criterion continues to be debated. It is unlikely that a uniform standard will ever be adopted with regard to clinical significance, however, in part because it is a more complex concept than statistical significance. For example, in some cases, *no change* over time could be clinically significant if it means that a group with a progressive disease has not experienced deterioration. In other cases, clinical significance is associated with improvements. Another issue concerns whose *perspective* on clinical significance is considered. Sometimes clinicians' perspective is paramount because of implications for health management (e.g., regarding blood pressure values), whereas for other outcomes the patient's view is what matters (e.g., about pain or quality of life). Two other issues concern whether clinical significance is for group-level findings or for individual patients and whether clinical significance is attached to point-in-time outcomes or to change scores. Most of the work that has been done to date, and therefore most of our discussion here, is about the clinical significance of *change scores* for individual patients. We begin, however, with a brief discussion of group-level clinical significance.

Clinical Significance at the Group Level

Many studies concern group-level comparisons. For example, one-group pretest–posttest designs involve comparing a group at two (or more) points in time, to test whether, on average, a change in outcomes has occurred. In randomized controlled trials and case–control studies, the comparisons are about average differences in outcomes for different groups of people. These comparisons are subjected to hypothesis-testing procedures, and statistical tests lead to decisions about rejecting the null hypothesis.

Group-level clinical significance (which is sometimes called *practical significance*) typically involves using statistical information other than p values to draw conclusions about the importance of the results. The most widely used statistics for this purpose are ES indexes, CIs, and number needed to treat (NNT). Many medical journals insist that information about CIs and ES be reported. Yet, it has been found that only a minority of articles in top nursing research journal report on CIs or ES (Gaskin & Happell, 2014; Polit, 2017).

ES indexes summarize the magnitude of a relationship or change score and thus provide insights into how a group, *on average*, might benefit from a treatment (or be spared a harm). A clinically significant finding at the group level means that the ES is sufficiently large to have relevance for the "average" patient.

CIs are espoused by several writers as useful tools for understanding clinical significance (e.g., Fethney, 2010). CIs provide the most plausible range of values, at a given level of confidence, for the unknown population parameter, such as means on an outcome after treatment. Fethney provided an example that illustrated how CIs were used in a study evaluating an intervention for premature infants. A weight gain value was established a priori as clinically significant by a panel of experts, and then a CI around the obtained mean weight gain was calculated to see if the CI encompassed the designated value.

NNTs are sometimes promoted as useful indicators of clinical significance in clinical trials because the information is in a format that is relatively easy to understand. For example, if the NNT for an important outcome is found to be 2.0, only two patients have to receive a treatment in order for one patient to benefit. If the NNT is 10.0, however, 9 patients out of 10 receiving the treatment would get no benefit.

When using any of the group-level indexes mentioned, researchers should designate in advance what would constitute clinical significance—just as they would establish an alpha value for statistical significance. For example, would an ES of 0.20 (for the d index described in Chapter 18) be considered clinically significant? A d of 0.20 was described by Cohen (1988) as a "small" effect, but sometimes small improvements can have clinical relevance. Claims about attainment of clinical significance for groups should be based on reasonable criteria. Table 21.3 presents some traditional guidelines for interpreting the strength of relationships for d, r, and the NNT, based on the work of Kraemer et al. (2003).

TIP In Chapter 18, we discussed using a power analysis to estimate sample size needs during the planning stage of the study based on a goal of detecting statistical significance. A compelling approach is to estimate sample size needs that will support goals for both clinical and statistical significance.

Clinical Significance at the Individual Level

Clinicians usually are not interested in what happens in a *group* of people—they are concerned with individual patients. A key goal in EBP is to personalize "best evidence" into decisions for a specific patient's needs, within a particular clinical context.

TABLE 21.3 • Traditional Guidelines for Interpreting Relationship Strength

SIZE OF THE EFFECT	EFFECT SIZE (*d*)	EFFECT SIZE (*r*)	NNT
Small	.20	.10	8.9
Moderate	.50	.30	3.6
Large	.80	.50	2.3
Very large	≥1.00	≥.70	≤1.9

NNT, number needed to treat.

Adapted from Kraemer, H., Morgan, G., Leech, N., Gliner, J., Vaske, J., & Harmon, R. (2003). Measures of clinical significance. *Journal of the American Academy of Child and Adolescent Psychiatry*, *42*, 1524–1529, Table 1, with permission from Elsevier.

Efforts to draw conclusions about clinical significance at the individual level can thus be directly linked to EBP goals.

Dozens of approaches to defining and operationalizing clinical significance at the individual level have been developed, but they share one thing in common: they involve establishing a **benchmark** (or *threshold*) that designates the value on a measure or a change score that would be considered clinically meaningful. When there is a benchmark for clinical significance, *each person in a study can be classified as to whether their score or change score is clinically significant*. Before looking at how the benchmarks have been established, we consider alternative definitions of clinical significance.

TIP The operationalization of clinical significance is linked to measurement interpretability, which is one of the elements in our measurement property taxonomy (Figure 15.1).

Conceptual Definitions of Clinical Significance

Dozens of definitions of clinical significance can be found in the health literature; most definitions concern changes in measures of patient outcomes. The various definitions fall mainly into one of four categories.

One definitional category is linked to statistical issues discussed in Chapter 15—whether a change score is statistically reliable. Some have reasoned that if a patient's improved score on an outcome is more than random error, the improvement has clinical significance.

Example of Defining Reliable Change as Clinical Significance

Cuijpers et al. (2023) conducted a meta-analysis of psychological treatments for depression in children and adolescents to examine reliable change in terms of deterioration or recovery as outcomes. They calculated a Reliable Change Index and Reliable Deterioration Index to determine significant change. They found clinically significant improvement in recovery for those who received therapy as compared to controls, but some in therapy (6%) experienced deterioration suggesting a need for other effective treatment strategies.

Reliable change also figures into a definition of clinical significance that appeared in the psychotherapy literature in the early 1990s. Jacobson and Truax (1991) proposed that a clinically significant change for patients undergoing a psychotherapeutic intervention would involve a reliable improvement *and* a return to "normal" functioning. They proposed several ways of deciding whether individual patients in a study had changed sufficiently to meet this criterion of normalcy. Their approach, sometimes referred to as the *J-T approach*, has been used for outcomes other than those used in psychotherapy research, such as in studies using measures of physical function (PF) as key outcomes (e.g., Mann et al., 2012).

Example of Using the J-T Approach
Marshall et al. (2020) describe a study protocol in which they aim to examine the effectiveness of five mobile apps in reducing symptoms of anxiety and/or depression. They plan to use the statistical approach proposed by Jacobson and Truax to determine the clinically significant changes in symptoms in individuals enrolled in the study.

TIP "Normalcy" sometimes can be defined as improvements that represent a return to a desirable value—especially for biophysiologic outcomes such as blood pressure or cholesterol levels. Thresholds for these outcomes are available in clinical guidelines.

A third way to conceptualize clinical significance is not linked to change scores explicitly. Tubach et al. (2006; 2007) argued that patients are more interested in "feeling good" than in simply "feeling better." In their view, a clinically significant state occurs when patients achieve an outcome that they perceive as important and meaningful. Tubach et al. called their benchmark the **patient acceptable symptom state (PASS)**. The PASS approach is discussed in greater detail in Polit and Yang (2016).

The fourth way of conceptualizing clinical significance dominates in medicine. In a paper cited hundreds of times in the medical literature, Jaeschke et al. (1989) offered the following definition: "The minimal clinically important difference (MCID) can be defined as the smallest difference in score in the domain of interest which patients perceive as beneficial and which would mandate, in the absence of troublesome side effects and excessive cost, a change in the patient's management" (p. 408). Although these researchers, and many after them, have referred to the threshold for clinical significance as a *minimal important difference* (MID) or *minimal clinically important difference* (MCID), we follow the COSMIN group in using the term **minimal important change (MIC)** (DeVet et al., 2011) because the focus is on individual *change* scores (not group *differences*). We focus on methods of operationalizing this benchmark.

Operationalizing Clinical Significance: Establishing the MIC Benchmark

To our knowledge, the definition of the MIC offered by Jaeschke et al. (1989) has never been fully operationalized. For example, side effects and costs are not typically taken into consideration in the thresholds, and input on how much change would trigger a change in patient management is seldom sought. Thus, although the Jaeschke et al.'s definition regarding change score benchmarks has been cited extensively, researchers have gone in many different directions in translating and quantifying it. Nevertheless, the focus on *patient input* to establish the MIC has had a profound effect on establishing benchmarks for patient-reported outcomes (PROs).

Benchmarks for clinically important change are usually the number of change score points on a PRO that an individual patient must achieve, but benchmarks sometimes are a percentage change. Two MICs are established for some measures: one MIC denoting the threshold for clinically significant improvement and a second MIC as the threshold for clinically significant deterioration.

Dozens of methods have been used to derive MICs for widely used healthcare measures—and the developers of many new multi-item scales now make efforts to estimate the MIC as part of the psychometric assessment of their instrument. Methods of establishing the MIC benchmark mainly fall into three categories.

A traditional approach to setting a benchmark for health outcomes is to obtain input from a panel of healthcare experts—often called a *consensus panel*. For example, the Initiative on Methods, Measurement, and Pain Assessment in Clinical Trials convened a special panel on clinical significance, and one recommendation of the consensus review was that a 30% improvement in self-reported pain intensity (e.g., on a visual analog scale) be considered the benchmark for moderately important clinical change and that a 50% decrease in pain be the benchmark for substantial change (Dworkin et al., 2008).

The COSMIN group has advocated a different approach. They defined the MIC as "the smallest change in score in the construct to be measured which patients perceive as important" (DeVet et al., 2011, p. 245). Even this definition has led to different interpretations: some researchers have emphasized the "smallest" aspect in looking at a change score, and others have emphasized the "important" aspect. This divergence can be best explained with an illustration.

A widely used method of establishing the MIC value is called an **anchor-based approach**. This approach requires administering the focal measure on two occasions to a sample of people in which change is expected, so that change scores can be computed. At the second administration, information about an "anchor" is also obtained. The anchor is a criterion for establishing the MIC benchmark on the focal scale. The anchor often is a single-item **global rating scale** (GRS), as we described in Chapter 15 in our discussion of the criterion approach to responsiveness.

Indeed, we can use the same example as the one shown in Figure 15.3, which illustrated a 7-point GRS for assessing the responsiveness of a PF scale. Figure 21.3 shows the mean scores on our PF scale for each response category on the GRS. If we wanted to operationalize the MIC for the PF scale in a manner that emphasized the *smallest* noticeable improvement in score ("a little better"), we might conclude that the MIC for the PF scale was 2.17. In this case, any change in a person's score of three or better would be interpreted as clinically significant. Other researchers, however, have argued that "minimal change" is an insufficient criterion. They would opt for using the GRS rating of "much better" as their anchor for establishing the MIC for the PF scale. In that case, the MIC in this example would be 3.89; a person's change would be deemed clinically significant only if their change score on the scale was 4 points or higher. Other statistical approaches can be used to establish an MIC using anchor-based methods, notably the use of a receiver operating characteristic curve analysis.

Please rate the changes you have experienced in the past 3 months with regard to *your ability to perform regular activities of daily living*, such as standing up from a sitting position or taking a bath or shower:

GRS Rating	Mean Change Score on Focal Physical Function Scale (Posttest − Baseline)
1. Very much better	5.50
2. Much better	3.89
3. A little better	2.17
4. No change	0.75
5. A little worse	−1.89
6. Much worse	−4.03
7. Very much worse	−5.98

Highlighted categories indicate possible MIC thresholds.

FIGURE 21.3 Example of a global rating scale anchor used to establish a minimal important change (MIC) for improvement on a physical function scale.

Note that despite the widespread endorsement of using patients' input in defining clinical significance for PROs, it is almost always the researcher, not the patient, who defines what is "minimally important." When reading about the MIC or when using a previously obtained MIC value in a study to assess clinical significance, it is crucial to understand how the researcher defined "minimally important."

> **TIP** The anchor used as the criterion for the MIC need not be based on patients' self-reported change on a GRS. For example, the anchor for a physical functioning scale could be based on performance tests.

Calculating an MIC using an anchor-based approach requires a lot of work, and it also requires a careful research design with a large sample of people whose changes over time are expected to vary. Using an anchor-based approach, an MIC must be established for every new scale; moreover, the MIC value is population-specific. The MIC on a measure of pain intensity might be different for a population experiencing chronic pain than for a population recovering from surgery—and in a group with chronic pain, a separate threshold might be needed for both improvement and deterioration.

These complexities have led to a third approach to defining the MIC—one that uses the distributional characteristics of a measure. **Distribution-based methods** rely on the statistical characteristics of a sample, and they express the MIC as a standardized metric. The most frequently used metric is based on Cohen's (1988) ES index, operationalized at the individual level as a fraction of the standard deviation (SD). Most often, the MIC using this approach is set to a threshold of 0.5—that is, one half an SD based on the distribution of baseline scores (Norman et al., 2003, 2004). Norman and colleagues found that there was "remarkable" consistency supporting a threshold equivalent to an SD of 0.5. They argued that this consistency was unlikely to be a coincidence and could be tied to theory and evidence on the psychology of human discrimination. They concluded that a change of 0.5 SD in baseline scores is a defensible benchmark for interpreting an individual's change score as important.

An MIC threshold value in change score units using this distribution approach can be easily computed. For example, if the baseline SD for a scale were 6.0, then the MIC using the 0.5 SD criterion would be 3.0. This value, like any MIC, can be used as the benchmark to classify individual patients as having or not having experienced clinically meaningful change.

An alternative distribution-based method is to establish the value of the MIC based on measurement error (see Chapter 15). A number of researchers have suggested using the standard error of measurement (SEM) to establish the threshold. Norman et al. (2003) pointed out that for measures with a test–retest reliability of 0.75, the 0.5 SD threshold is exactly equivalent to 1 SEM.

There is no consensus on which approach to calculating the MIC yields the most helpful benchmark of clinical significance, but many people agree that none is ideal. The anchor-based approach is preferred by the COSMIN group, but it adds more work to the burdensome effort of constructing and evaluating new scales. It has also been argued that a single GRS is a poor choice for the anchor, because a single item is unreliable and subject to recall bias.

MICs based on distribution approaches are appealing because they are easy to compute, but it is often difficult to communicate what such an MIC represents. A persistent criticism of distribution methods is that they yield values that are not linked to any clinical yardstick—they do not embody any notion of "meaningfulness" or "importance." Another problem with MICs based on SDs is that the value is dependent on the heterogeneity of the population under study. Those who have suggested distribution-based MICs often emphasize that they are a reasonable starting point or "an approximate rule of thumb in the absence of more specific information" (Norman et al., 2003, p. 590).

Triangulation of Methods for the MIC

Because there is no "gold standard" approach to setting the MIC, some experts argue that it is advantageous to triangulate information from more than one approach (e.g., Revicki et al., 2008). Many approaches to triangulation have been adopted. For example, some researchers have combined information from multiple anchors, including anchors reflecting both patients' and clinicians' perspectives. Most efforts at triangulation involve using both a distribution method, such as 1 SEM, plus an anchor-based method. This particular type of triangulation has the merit of enhancing the likelihood that a change score value is not only clinically meaningful but also reliable.

An example of triangulation comes from the field of respiratory medicine. Patel et al. (2013) sought to establish the MIC for King's Brief Interstitial Lung Disease Questionnaire (K-BILD). These researchers used two distribution methods (1 SEM and 0.3 *SD*), a clinical anchor (a forced vital capacity change of at least 7% from baseline) and patients' responses on four GRSs. Integrating all information, the researchers established the MIC on the K-BILD at eight points.

Example of Estimating MICs
Through qualitative interviews with informal caregivers and providers of those with Alzheimer Dementia (AD), Dubbelman et al. (2022) established the MIC in everyday functioning of those with AD. They then used these criteria to examine functional change in a longitudinal cohort study of patients in a memory care unit. They found that those with a dementia diagnosis and more atrophy of the medial temporal lobe had larger odds (odds ratio [OR] = 3.4, 95% CI [1.5–7.8] and OR = 5.0, 95% CI [1.2–20.0], respectively) of exceeding the MIC threshold representing decline than those with complaints of cognitive change but no atrophy.

Procedures for Clinical Significance Inquiries
Nurse researchers who wish to assess the clinical significance of their results for individual participants, using some of the procedures described in this chapter, should begin by coming to conclusions about how they wish to conceptualize clinical significance. This is most easily illustrated in the context of intervention research. Clinical significance can have many meanings, and so the researcher must be clear at the outset about treatment goals. Is the goal to have patients achieve *real change*? Return to *normal functioning*? Achieve a *favorable state*? Or experience change at a level that is *minimally important*?

If researchers decide in advance how they want to approach clinical significance, they will be in a better position to operationalize it when they plan their studies. For example, if "return to normal functioning" is the treatment goal, the researchers should investigate whether there are measures of key outcomes for which normative information is readily available. If depression, for instance, is an outcome, then a researcher interested in assessing clinically significant changes in depression should select a depression scale with published norms or recommended cutpoints. If, on the other hand, the treatment goal is for patients to achieve meaningful improvements, then researchers should search the literature for MIC values for their outcome measures. MIC values have been reported for many health scales. MIC values are population-specific, so it is important to identify MIC thresholds that are appropriate for study participants. By looking for MIC information before the study is underway, researchers may be able to select between alternative measures of a construct.

Example of Using MIC Values From Previous Research
Nie et al. (2023) examined the impact of body mass index on Patient-Reported Outcomes Measurement Information System (PROMIS) outcomes in patients undergoing lumbar decompression. They used several PROMIS measures including ones for physical function anxiety, pain interference, and sleep disturbance among others. Minimal clinically important differences were determined by previously established values.

Triangulation is sometimes adopted by those who wish to *use* existing benchmarks of clinical significance. For example, in a meta-analysis examining the effect of pain relief in those with osteoarthritis undergoing viscosupplementation injections, Pereira et al. (2022) reviewed 24 large, placebo-controlled trials. They noted the body of work in this area since 2009 and prior to their meta-analysis indicated that the existing benchmark of pain reduction was 5 mm on a 100 mm visual analogue scale. In their meta-analysis, they found pain intensity (injection vs. placebo) was reduced by −2.0 mm (95% CI −3.8 to −0.5) on a 100 mm visual analogue scale. Their findings indicate that while the injections were significantly associated with a small reduction in pain intensity (injection vs. placebo), this reduction was less than minimal clinically meaningful.

Many measures that are widely used by nurse researchers have not, however, been subjected to analysis for establishing an MIC—which suggests avenues for new research. When no MIC benchmark has been established for an outcome of interest, nurse researchers may have to adopt a distribution-based approach to estimating it.

Responder Analysis

A number of researchers (including nurse researchers) have used MIC values to interpret group-level findings. The MIC is, however, an index that concerns *individual* changes, not group differences. Experts have warned that it is not appropriate to interpret mean differences in relation to the MIC (Guyatt et al., 2002; Wyrwich et al., 2013). For example, if the MIC on an important outcome has been reported as 4.0 points, this value should not be used to interpret mean group differences for clinical significance. If the mean group difference were found to be 3.0, for instance, it would be inappropriate to conclude that the results were not clinically significant. A mean difference of 3.0 almost certainly implies that a sizable percentage of the participants achieved a meaningful benefit (i.e., an improvement of four points or more).

MIC thresholds can, however, be used to create new outcomes that facilitate the interpretation of group differences. Once the MIC is established, researchers can classify all people in the study in terms of their having attained or not attained the threshold. Study participants can be classified as *responders* or *nonresponders* (e.g., to an intervention) based on an established threshold of meaningful change. Then, researchers can undertake a **responder analysis** that compares the percentage of responders in the study groups (e.g., those in the intervention and those in the control group). A distinct advantage of a responder analysis is that it is easy to understand and can facilitate comparisons across trials or across different outcomes in a trial.

> **Example of a Responder Analysis**
> Justo-Henriques et al. (2022) used responder analysis in a 13-week randomized control trial examining positive and nonpositive predictors of responses to a reminiscent therapy. They found that the intervention had an impact on cognition and memory and that this impact was greatest on those with more executive dysfunction.

> **TIP** By classifying people as responders and nonresponders, researchers can go on to examine who did and did not respond at clinically significant levels and explore their characteristics and treatment experiences.

CRITICAL APPRAISAL OF INTERPRETATIONS

Researchers offer their interpretation of the findings and discuss what the findings might imply for nursing in the Discussion section of research reports. When critically appraising a study, your own interpretation and inferences can be contrasted against those of the researchers.

As a reviewer, you should be wary if a discussion section fails to point out any limitations. Researchers are in the best position to detect and assess the impact of sampling deficiencies, practical constraints, data quality problems, and so on, and it is a professional responsibility to alert readers to these difficulties. Moreover, when researchers note methodologic shortcomings, readers have some confidence that these limitations were considered in interpreting the results. Of course, researchers are unlikely to note all relevant shortcomings of their own work. The task of reviewer is to independently assess limitations and to challenge conclusions that do not appear to be warranted.

In addition to comparing your interpretation with that of the researchers, your appraisal should also draw conclusions about the stated implications of the study. Some researchers make grandiose claims or offer unfounded recommendations based on modest results.

We have discussed the issue of clinical significance at some length in this chapter. The conceptualization and operationalization of clinical significance have not received much attention in nursing (Polit, 2017). We hope that nurse researchers will pay more attention to this issue in the years ahead.

Some guidelines for evaluating researchers' interpretation and implications are offered in Box 21.1.

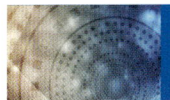

BOX 21.1 Guidelines for Critically Appraising Interpretations in Discussion Sections of Quantitative Research Reports

INTERPRETATION OF THE FINDINGS
1. Are all important results discussed?
2. Did the researchers discuss the limitations of the study and their possible effects on the credibility of the research evidence? In discussing limitations, were key threats to the study's validity and possible biases noted?
3. What types of evidence were offered in support of the researchers' interpretation, and was that evidence persuasive? If results were "mixed," were possible explanations offered? Were results interpreted in light of findings from other studies?
4. Did the researchers make any unwarranted causal inferences? Were alternative explanations for the findings considered? Were the rationales for rejecting these alternatives convincing?
5. Did the interpretation take into account the precision of the results and/or the magnitude of effects?
6. Did the researchers discuss the generalizability of the findings? Did they draw any unwarranted conclusions about generalizability?

IMPLICATIONS OF THE FINDINGS AND RECOMMENDATIONS
1. Did the researchers discuss the study's implications for clinical practice, nursing theory, or future nursing research? Did they make specific recommendations?
2. If yes, are the stated implications appropriate, given the study's limitations and the magnitude of the effects—as well as evidence from other studies? Are there important implications that the report neglected to include?

CLINICAL SIGNIFICANCE
1. Did the researchers mention clinical significance? Did they make a distinction between statistical and clinical significance? Did they identify explicit criteria for clinical significance?
2. If yes, was clinical significance interpreted in terms of group-level information (e.g., effect sizes) or individual-level results? If the latter, how was clinical significance operationalized?

RESEARCH EXAMPLE

We conclude this chapter with an example of a study that examined clinical significance.

Study: An Outpatient-Based Training Program Improves Family Caregivers' Preparedness in Caring for Persons with Mild Cognitive Impairment: A Randomized Controlled Trial (Tung et al., 2023)

Statement of purpose: The purpose of this study was to determine the impact of a caregiver training program on the primary outcome of perception of preparedness and the secondary outcomes of health-related quality of life and depressive symptoms in caregivers of older adults with mild cognitive impairment.

Method: Using a randomized control design, 54 family caregivers were enrolled: 28 to the experimental group and 26 to the control. The training program for the intervention group included topics such as information about the illness, strategies to promote function, and self-care management. The control group received written information about dementia. Outcomes measured were caregiver preparedness, health-related quality of life, and depressive symptoms, which were measured at baseline, 1, 3, and 6 months after completion of the program.

Analysis: Descriptive statistics were used to describe sample characteristics. Differences between groups were compared using the two-sample t test or chi-square test. Generalized estimating equations for repeated measures analysis were used to examine the outcomes of caregiver preparedness, health-related quality of life (HRQoL), and depressive symptoms,

Results: The sample characteristics of the care recipients were comparable between the two groups. However, the experimental group had significantly better cognitive function (Mini mental state examination (MMSE) = 23.96, SD = 3.50) than the control (MMSE = 19.15, SD = 6.60; $t = -3.311$, $p = .002$). The caregivers were also comparable except in the areas of preparedness and measures of mental health scores, each of which the experimental group performed significantly poorer than the control.

After the intervention, the experimental group demonstrated improvement in preparedness that was greater than the control group with statistical significance being achieved at 6 months ($p = .008$). Other noteworthy findings indicated that the intervention did not affect caregiver depressive symptoms over the time of the study: at 1 month ($b = -0.44, p = .483$), at 3 months ($\beta = -0.42$, $p = .601$) and at 6 months ($\beta = 0.43$, $p = .717$). The intervention did not impact overall caregiver HRQoL during the 6-month posttest period. However, the effect of time was critical for some aspects of HRQoL. In each group, the physical functioning (PF) declined significantly at 3 and 6 months ($\beta = -3.49$, $p = .041$, and $\beta = -5.01$, $p = .011$, respectively), as did the social functioning at 1 and 6 months ($\beta = -4.58$, $p = .028$, and $\beta = -5.37$, $p = .046$, respectively). Vitality in both groups declined significantly at 1 month ($\beta = -3.95$, $p = .027$) as did mental health at 1 month ($\beta = -3.33$, $p = .050$), but the mental component summary score in both groups improved significantly at 6 months ($\beta = 3.71$, $p < .001$).

Discussion: Findings from this study indicate that education aimed at preparing care givers individually over time with regular follow-up and telephone consultations, while providing professional resources and assisting with needed referrals as needed, improved caregiver preparation over time. Unlike many programs, this intervention included strategies to address caregivers' self-care, but the intervention did not significantly improve family caregivers' depressive symptoms or quality of life at 6 months. The researchers attributed this to the two groups having relatively positive scores on these measures at baseline, and therefore a ceiling effect would make statistical change and significance between the two groups on these measures difficult to identify. The authors did not include a discussion related to the findings of decreased vitality, social, or PF.

SUMMARY POINTS

- The interpretation of quantitative research **results** (the outcomes of the statistical analyses) typically involves consideration of the (1) credibility of the results; (2) precision of estimates of effects; (3) magnitude of effects; (4) underlying meaning of the results; (5) generalizability of results; and (6) implications for future research, theory development, and nursing practice.
- Inference is central to interpretation. Researchers' methodologic decisions affect the inferences that can be made about the correspondence between study results and "truth in the real world." A cautious outlook is appropriate in drawing conclusions about the credibility and meaning of study results.
- An assessment of a study's credibility can involve various approaches, one of which involves evaluating the degree of congruence between abstract constructs or idealized methods on the one hand and the proxies actually used on the other. Credibility assessments can also involve an analysis of validity threats and biases that could undermine the accuracy of the results. Corroboration (replication) of results is another approach in a credibility assessment.
- Broadly speaking, **clinical significance** refers to the practical importance of research results—whether the effects are genuine and palpable in the daily lives of patients or in the management of their health. Clinical significance has not received sufficient attention in nursing research.
- Clinical significance for group-level results is often inferred based on such statistics as ES indexes, CIs, and NNT. However, clinical significance is most often discussed in terms of effects for individual patients—especially, whether they have achieved a clinically meaningful change in outcomes.
- Definitions and operationalizations of clinical significance for individuals typically involve using a **benchmark** or threshold that designates the amount of change on an outcome that is meaningful. At the conceptual level, clinical significance has been defined in terms of whether a change in the attribute is real (reliable), whether

a patient in a dysfunctional state returns to normal functioning, whether a patient has achieved a symptom state that is acceptable to them, and whether the amount of change in an attribute can be considered minimally important.
- The efforts to operationalize clinical significance in medical fields have mostly focused on the last definition. The goal of such efforts is to establish a benchmark (change score value) on a health measure that can be considered a **minimal important change (MIC)**, also called a *minimal important difference (MID)* and *minimal clinically important difference* (MCID).
- The MIC benchmark is a value for the number of change score points that an individual patient must achieve to be counted as having a clinically important change.
- The primary methods of establishing the MIC for a measure are (1) through a consensus panel, (2) using an **anchor-based approach** that often involves linking changes on the focal measure to a criterion for meaningful change, and (3) using a **distribution-based method** that bases the MIC on the distributional characteristics of the sample (e.g., 0.5 *SD* of a baseline distribution or 1 SEM). Triangulation of approaches is increasingly common.
- MICs cannot legitimately be used to interpret group means or differences in means. However, the MIC can be used to ascertain whether each person in a sample has or has not achieved a change greater than the MIC, and then a **responder analysis** can be undertaken to compare the percentage of responders in different study groups.

REFERENCES CITED IN CHAPTER 21

Bartzik, M., Aust, F., & Peifer, C. (2021). Negative effects of the COVID-19 pandemic on nurses can be buffered by a sense of humor and appreciation. *BMC Nursing*, *20*(1), 257. https://doi.org/10.1186/s12912-021-00770-5

Bruner, S., Corbett, C., Gates, B., & Dupler, A. (2012). Clinical significance as it relates to evidence-based practice. *International Journal of Nursing Knowledge*, *23*(2), 62–74.

Cohen, J. (1988). *Statistical power analysis for the behavioral sciences* (2nd ed.). Routledge.

Cuijpers, P., Karyotaki, E., Ciharova, M., Miguel, C., Noma, H., Stikkelbroek, Y., Weisz, J. R., & Furukawa, T. A. (2023). The effects of psychological treatments of depression in children and adolescents on response, reliable change, and deterioration: A systematic review and meta-analysis. *European Child & Adolescent Psychiatry*, *32*(1), 177–192. https://doi.org/10.1007/s00787-021-01884-6

DeVet, H., Terwee, C., Mokkink, L., & Knol, D. (2011). *Measurement in medicine: A practical guide*. Cambridge University Press.

Dubbelman, M. A., Verrijp, M., Terwee, C. B., Jutten, R. J., Postema, M. C., Barkhof, F., Berckel, B. N. M., Gillissen, F., Teeuwen, V., Teunissen, C., van de Flier, W. M., Scheltens, P., & Sikkes, S. A. M. (2022). Determining the minimal important change of everyday functioning in dementia: Pursuing clinical meaningfulness. *Neurology*, *99*(9), e954–e964. https://doi.org/10.1212/WNL.0000000000200781

Dworkin, R., Turk, D., Wyrwich, K., Beaton, D., Cleeland, C. S., Farrar, J., Haythornthwaite, JA, Jensen, MP, Kerns, RD, Ader, DN, Brandenburg, N, Burke, LB, Cella, D, Chandler, J, Cowan, P, Dimitrova, R, Dionne, R, Hertz, S, Jadad, AR, ... Zavisic, S. (2008). Interpreting the clinical importance of treatment outcomes in chronic pain clinical trials: IMMPACT recommendations. *Journal of Pain*, *9*(2), 105–121.

Fethney, J. (2010). Statistical and clinical significance, and how to use confidence intervals to help interpret both. *Australian Critical Care*, *23*(2), 93–97.

Flanagan, J., Post, K., Hill, R., & DiPalazzo, J. (2022). Feasibility of a nurse coached walking intervention for informal dementia caregivers walking intervention for informal dementia caregivers. *Western Journal of Nursing Research*, *44*(5), 466–476. https://doi.org/10.1177/01939459211001395

Froman, R. D., & Owen, S. (2014). Why you want to avoid being a causist. *Research in Nursing Health*, *37*(3), 171–173.

Fulda, S., & Miano, S. (2023). Time to rest a hypothesis? Accumulating evidence that periodic leg movements during sleep are not increased in children with attention deficit hyperactivity disorder (ADHD): Results of a case-control study and a meta-analysis. *Sleep*, *46*(6), zsad046. Advance online publication. https://doi.org/10.1093/sleep/zsad046

Gaskin, C., & Happell, B. (2014). Power, effects, confidence, and significance: An investigation of statistical practices in nursing research. *International Journal of Nursing Studies*, *51*(5), 795–806.

Guyatt, G. H., Osoba, D., Wu, A., Wyrwich, K., Norman, G. R., & Clinical Significance Consensus Meeting Group. (2002). Methods to explain the clinical significance of health status measures. *Mayo Clinic Proceedings*, *77*(4), 371–383.

Hayat, M. J. (2010). Understanding statistical significance. *Nursing Research*, *59*(3), 219–223.

Jacobson, N. S., & Truax, P. (1991). Clinical significance: A statistical approach to defining meaningful change in psychotherapy research. *Journal of Consulting and Clinical Psychology*, *59*(1), 12–19.

Jaeschke, R., Singer, J., & Guyatt, G. H. (1989). Measurement of health status: Ascertaining the minimal clinically important difference. *Controlled Clinical Trials*, *10*(4), 407–415.

Justo-Henriques, S. I., Carvalho, J. O., Pérez-Sáez, E., Neves, H., Parola, V., & Alves-Apóstolo, J. L. (2022). Randomized trial of individual reminiscence therapy for older adults with cognitive impairment: A 3-month responder analysis. *Revue Neurologique, 74*(4), 107–116. https://doi.org/10.33588/rn.7404.2021322

Kraemer, H., Morgan, G., Leech, N., Gliner, J., Vaske, J., & Harmon, R. (2003). Measures of clinical significance. *Journal of American Academy of Child and Adolescent Psychiatry, 42*(12), 1524–1529.

LeFort, S. M. (1993). The statistical versus clinical significance debate. *Image Journal of Nursing Scholarship, 25*(1), 57–62.

Mann, B. J., Gosens, T., & Lyman, S. (2012). Quantifying clinically significant change: A brief review of methods and presentation of a hybrid approach. *The American Journal of Sports Medicine, 40*(10), 2385–2393.

Marshall, J. M., Dunstan, D. A., Bartik, W. (2020). Effectiveness of using mental health mobile apps as digital antidepressants for reducing anxiety and depression: Protocol for a multiple baseline across-individuals design. *JMIR Research Protocols, 9*(7), e17159. https://doi.org/10.2196/17159

Nie, J. W., Hartman, T. J., Zheng, E., Oyetayo, O. O., MacGregor, K. R., Federico, V. P., Massel, D. H., Sayari, A. J., & Singh, K. (2023). Impact of body mass index on PROMIS outcomes following lumbar decompression. *Acta Neurochirurgica, 165*(6), 1427, 1434. Advance online publication. https://doi.org/10.1007/s00701-023-05534-5

Norman, G. R., Sloan, J., & Wyrwich, K. W. (2003). Interpretation of changes in health-related quality of life: The remarkable universality of half a standard deviation. *Medical Care, 41*(5), 582–592.

Norman, G. R., Sloan, J., & Wyrwich, K. W. (2004). The truly remarkable universality of half a standard deviation: Confirmation through another look. *Expert Review of Pharmacoeconomics & Outcomes Research, 4*(5), 581–585.

Patel, A., Siegert, R., Keir, G., Bajwah, S., Barker, R., Maher, T., Renzoni, EA, Wells, AU, Higginson, IJ, Birring, SS, Birring, S. (2013). The minimal important difference of the King's Brief Interstitial Lung Disease Questionnaire (K-BILD) and forced vital capacity in interstitial lung disease. *Respiratory Medicine, 107*(9), 1438–1443.

Pereira, T. V., Jüni, P., Saadat, P., Xing, D., Yao, L., Bobos, P., Agarwal, A., Hincapié, C. A., & da Costa, B. R. (2022). Viscosupplementation for knee osteoarthritis: Systematic review and meta-analysis. *BMJ (Clinical Research ed.), 378*, e069722. https://doi.org/10.1136/bmj-2022-069722

Polit, D. F. (2017). Clinical significance in nursing research: A discussion and descriptive analysis. *International Journal of Nursing Studies, 73*, 17–23.

Polit, D. F. & Yang, F. M. (2016). *Measurement and the measurement of change: A primer for health professionals.* Lippincott.

Revicki, D., Hays, R., Cella, D., & Sloan, J. (2008). Recommended methods for determining responsiveness and minimally important differences for patient-reported outcomes. *Journal of Clinical Epidemiology, 61*(2), 102–109.

Sackett, D., Straus, S., Richardson, W., Rosenberg, W., & Haynes, R. (2000). *Evidence-based medicine.* (2nd ed.). Churchill Livingston.

Schuttner, L., Richardson, C., Parikh, T., Wong, E. (2023). "Low-value" glycemic outcomes among older adults with diabetes cared for by primary care nurse practitioners or physicians: A retrospective cohort study. *International Journal of Nursing Studies, 145*, 104532. https://doi.org/10.1016/j.ijnurstu.2023.104532

Shadish, W. R., Cook, T. D., & Campbell, D. T. (2002). *Experimental and quasi-experimental designs for generalized causal inference.* Houghton Mifflin.

Tubach, F., Dougados, M., Falissard, B., Baron, G., Logeart, I., & Ravaud, P. (2006). Feeling good rather than feeling better matters more to patients. *Arthritis & Rheumatology, 55*(4), 526–530.

Tubach, F., Ravaud, P., Beaton, D., Boers, M., Bombardier, C., Felson, D., van der Heijde, D, Wells, G, Dougados, M, Dougados, M. (2007). Minimal clinically important improvement and patient acceptable symptom state for subjective outcome measures in rheumatic disorders. *Journal of Rheumatology, 34*(5), 1188–1193.

Tunes da Silva, G. T., Logan, B., & Klein, J. (2009). Methods for equivalence and noninferiority testing. *Biology of Blood and Marrow Transplantation, 15*, 120–127.

Tung, Y. E., Kuo, L. M., Chen, M. C., Hsu, W. C., & Shyu, Y. I. L. (2023). An outpatient-based training program improves family caregivers' preparedness in caring for persons with mild cognitive impairment: A randomized controlled trial. *Journal of Nursing Research, 31*(1), e252. https://doi.org/10.1097/jnr.0000000000000541

Wyrwich, K. W., Norquist, J., Lenderking, W., Acaster, S., & Industry Advisory Committee of International Society for Quality of Life Research ISOQOL. (2013). Methods for interpreting change over time in patient-reported outcome measures. *Quality Life Research, 22*(3), 475–483.

Yıldırım, B. G., & Gerçeker, G. Ö. (2023). The effect of virtual reality and buzzy on first insertion success, procedure-related fear, anxiety, and pain in children during intravenous insertion in the pediatric emergency unit: A randomized controlled trial. *Journal of Emergency Nursing, 49*(1), 62–74. https://doi.org/10.1016/j.jen.2022.09.018

Part 4

DESIGNING AND CONDUCTING QUALITATIVE STUDIES TO GENERATE EVIDENCE FOR NURSING

Chapter 22 Qualitative Research Design and Approaches
Chapter 23 Sampling in Qualitative Research
Chapter 24 Data Collection in Qualitative Research
Chapter 25 Qualitative Data Analysis
Chapter 26 Trustworthiness and Rigor in Qualitative Research

22 Qualitative Research Design and Approaches

Learning objectives

1. Identify the major research traditions for qualitative research and describe the domain of inquiry of each.
2. Describe the main features and methods associated with ethnographic, phenomenological, and grounded theory studies.
3. Describe key characteristics of case studies, narrative analyses, and descriptive qualitative studies.
4. Discuss the goals and features of research with ideological perspectives using critical theory, feminist research, or participatory action research.
5. Describe guidelines for critically appraising qualitative designs.

THE DESIGN OF QUALITATIVE STUDIES

Quantitative researchers specify a research design before collecting their data and rarely depart from that design once the study is underway. In qualitative research, by contrast, the design typically evolves over the course of the study. Qualitative researchers use an **emergent design** that takes shape as they make ongoing decisions reflecting what they have already learned. An emergent design is a reflection of the researchers' desire to have the inquiry based on participants' realities and viewpoints, which are unknown at the outset (Lincoln & Guba, 1985).

Characteristics of Qualitative Research Design

Qualitative inquiry has been used in different disciplines, and each has developed methods for addressing particular types of questions. However, some characteristics of qualitative research design cut across disciplinary boundaries. In general, qualitative design:

- Is flexible, capable of adjusting to new information during data collection;
- Tends to be holistic, aimed at understanding the whole;
- Often involves merging various data collection strategies;
- Requires researchers to become intensely involved; and
- Relies on ongoing analysis of the data to formulate subsequent strategies and to determine when to stop collecting data.

Qualitative researchers often put together a complex array of data, derived from a variety of sources and using a variety of methods. This process has sometimes been described as **bricolage** and the qualitative researcher has been referred to as a *bricoleur*—a person who "is adept at performing diverse tasks, ranging from interviewing to intensive reflection and introspection" (Denzin & Lincoln, 2011, p. 5).

Qualitative Design and Planning

Although design decisions are not prespecified, qualitative researchers typically do advance planning to support an emergent design. Planning is especially useful with regard to the following:

- Selecting a broad inquiry framework or tradition (described in the next section) to guide design decisions
- Determining the maximum amount of time available for the study, given costs, and other constraints
- Developing a broad data collection strategy and identifying opportunities for enhancing trustworthiness (e.g., through triangulation)
- Collecting relevant site materials (e.g., maps, organizational charts, resource directories)
- Identifying the types of equipment needed for collecting data (e.g., audio recording equipment, computer tablets)
- Identifying personal biases, views, and presuppositions vis-à-vis the phenomenon, as well as ideological stances (reflexivity)

Thus, qualitative researchers need to plan for a variety of circumstances, but decisions about how to deal with them must be resolved when the social context is better understood. By allowing for and anticipating an evolution of strategies, qualitative researchers seek to make their research design responsive to the situation and to the phenomenon under study.

Qualitative Design Features

In Chapter 8, we discussed various features of research design, three of which are relevant to qualitative research—comparisons, settings, and timeframes. Here we briefly review these aspects of qualitative design.

Qualitative researchers seldom explicitly plan a comparative study (e.g., comparing children who have or do not have cancer). Nevertheless, patterns emerging in the data often suggest that certain comparisons are relevant and illuminating. Indeed, as Morse (2004) noted in an editorial in *Qualitative Health Research*, "All description requires comparisons" (p. 1323). Inevitably in categorizing qualitative information and evaluating whether categories are saturated, there is a need to compare "this" to "that." Morse pointed out that qualitative comparisons are often not dichotomous: "life is usually on a continuum" (p. 1324). Of course, comparisons sometimes *are* planned in qualitative studies (e.g., a comparison of nurses' and patients' perspectives about a phenomenon). Moreover, qualitative researchers can sometimes plan for the *possibility* of comparisons by selecting richly diverse people as participants.

Example of Comparisons in a Qualitative Study
Ahmed and colleagues (2023) conducted semistructured telephone interviews on the experiences of seven patients living with advanced colorectal cancer and five family caregivers who received early palliative care supports in a new program in Canada. The four main themes were then compared with the experiences of patients and caregivers prior to the program implementation.

In terms of research settings, qualitative researchers usually collect their data in real-world, naturalistic settings. And, whereas quantitative researchers usually strive to collect data in one type of setting to maintain constancy in environmental conditions (e.g., conducting all interviews in participants' homes), qualitative researchers may deliberately strive to study phenomena in a variety of natural contexts.

Regarding timeframes, qualitative research can be either cross-sectional, with one data collection point, or longitudinal, with multiple data collection points over an extended time period, to observe the evolution of some phenomenon. Sometimes qualitative researchers plan for a longitudinal design, but sometimes a decision to study a phenomenon longitudinally may be made after preliminary analysis of the data.

Example of a Longitudinal Qualitative Study
Lin and an interprofessional team (2022) conducted an in-depth longitudinal study to explore the experiences of stroke survivors and their family caregivers during hospital-to-home transitional care in China. Twenty-three stroke survivor/caregiver dyads were interviewed when stroke survivors were close to discharge and then 2 months postdischarge.

Causality and Qualitative Research

The issue of causality, which has been controversial throughout the history of science, is especially contentious in qualitative research. Some qualitative researchers think that causality is not an appropriate construct within the constructivist paradigm. Lincoln and Guba (1985) devoted a chapter of their book to a critique of causality and argued that it should be replaced with a concept they called *mutual shaping*. According to their view of mutual and simultaneous shaping, "Everything influences everything else, in the here and now. Many elements are implicated in any given action, and each element interacts with all of the others in ways that change them all while simultaneously resulting in something that we... label as outcomes or effects" (p. 151).

Others, however, believe that causal explanation is not only a legitimate pursuit in qualitative research, but also that qualitative methods are especially well suited to understanding causal relationships. For example, Maxwell (2012) argued that qualitative research is important for causal explanations, noting that they "depend on the in-depth understanding of meanings, contexts, and processes that qualitative research can provide" (p. 655).

In attempting to not only describe but to explain phenomena, qualitative researchers who undertake in-depth studies will inevitably reveal patterns and processes suggesting causal interpretations. These interpretations can be subjected to more systematic testing using more controlled methods of inquiry.

Overview of Qualitative Research Traditions

Despite some features common to many qualitative designs, a variety of approaches can be taken—but there is no agreed-upon classification system for these approaches. One system is to categorize qualitative research according to disciplinary traditions. These traditions (or *inquiry frameworks*) vary in their conceptualization of the types of questions that are important and the methods considered appropriate for answering them.

The research traditions and frameworks that have provided a theoretical underpinning for qualitative studies in healthcare fields come from such disciplines as anthropology, psychology, and sociology. As shown in Table 22.1, each discipline has focused on one or two broad domains of inquiry. Researchers in each tradition have developed methodologic strategies for the design and conduct of relevant studies. Thus, once a researcher has identified what aspect of the human experience is of greatest interest, there is typically a wealth of advice available about methods likely to be productive in designing and undertaking the study.

TIP Sometimes a research report identifies more than one tradition as the framework for a qualitative inquiry (e.g., a phenomenologic study using grounded theory methods). Such "method slurring" (Baker et al., 1992) has been criticized because each research tradition has different intellectual assumptions and methodologic guidelines. However, as noted by Nepal (2010), echoing some of the sentiments expressed in an editorial by Janice Morse (2009), mixed qualitative methods may be viable when "the researcher has ascertained, from the beginning…, that the research questions cannot be answered in their entirety unless and until there are two different qualitative methods used" (p. 281).

ETHNOGRAPHY

Ethnography, the research tradition of anthropologists, involves the description and interpretation of cultural behavior. Ethnographies are a blend of a process and a product—fieldwork and written text. Fieldwork is how the ethnographer comes to understand a culture, and the ethnographic text is how that culture is communicated and portrayed. Because *culture* is not visible or tangible, it must be constructed through ethnographic writing. Culture is inferred from the words, actions, and products of members of a group.

Ethnographic research is sometimes concerned with broadly defined cultures (e.g., a Nigerian village culture) in a **macroethnography.** Ethnographies often focus on more narrowly defined cultures in a **microethnography**

TABLE 22.1 • Overview of Qualitative Research Traditions

DISCIPLINE	DOMAIN	RESEARCH TRADITION/INQUIRY FRAMEWORK	AREA OF INQUIRY
Anthropology	Culture	Ethnography	Holistic view of culture
		Ethnoscience (cognitive anthropology)	Mapping of the cognitive world of a culture; a culture's shared meanings, semantic rules
Psychology/ philosophy	Lived experience	Phenomenology	Experiences of individuals within their lifeworld
		Hermeneutics	Interpretations and meanings of individuals' experiences
		Phenomenography	Differences in the ways in which people experience or think about a phenomenon
Psychology	Behavior	Ethology	Behavior observed over time in natural context
		Ecological psychology	Behavior as influenced by the environment
Sociology	Social settings and interactions	Grounded theory	Social structural processes within a social setting
		Ethnomethodology	Manner by which shared agreement is achieved in social settings
		Semiotics	Manner by which people make sense of social interactions
Sociolinguistics	Human communication	Discourse analysis	Forms and rules of conversation
History	Past behavior, events, and conditions	Historical research	Description and interpretation of historical events

or **focused ethnography** (Cruz & Higginbottom, 2013). Microethnographies are fine-grained studies of either small units in a group or culture (e.g., the culture of shelters for people who are homeless), or of specific activities in an organizational unit (e.g., how nurses communicate with children in an emergency department). An underlying assumption of the ethnographer is that every human group eventually evolves a culture that guides the members' view of the world and the way they structure their experiences.

Example of a Focused Ethnography
Wisnesky and colleagues (2022) conducted a focused ethnography to explore perceptions and experiences of mobility in a group of 23 Brazilian community-dwelling older individuals living with mobility challenges.

Ethnographers seek to learn from members of a cultural group—to understand their world view. Ethnographic researchers sometimes refer to "emic" and "etic" perspectives (terms from linguistics—phon*emic* vs. phon*etic*). An **emic perspective** is the way members of a culture envision their world—the insiders' view. The emic is the local language, concepts, or means of expression used by members of the group under study to characterize their experiences. The **etic perspective** is the outsiders' interpretation of the experiences of that culture; it is the language used by those doing the research to refer to the same phenomena. Ethnographers strive to acquire an emic perspective of a culture. Moreover, they strive to reveal **tacit knowledge** about the culture that is so deeply embedded in cultural experiences that members do not talk about it or may not even be consciously aware of it.

Ethnographic research typically is labor intensive, requiring long periods (months or even years) in the field. The study of a culture requires a certain level of intimacy with members of the cultural group, and such intimacy can only be developed over time. The concept of *researcher as instrument* is frequently used by anthropologists to describe the significant role ethnographers play in analyzing and interpreting a culture.

Three types of information usually are sought by ethnographers: cultural behavior (what members of the culture do), cultural artifacts (what people make and use), and cultural speech (what people say). This implies that ethnographers rely on a variety of data sources, including observations, in-depth interviews, records, and physical evidence such as photographs and diaries. Ethnographers often use a **participant observation** strategy in which they make observations of the culture while participating in its activities. Ethnographers observe people day after day in their natural environments to observe behavior in an array of circumstances. Ethnographers also enlist the help of **key informants** to help them understand and interpret the activities being observed.

Some ethnographers undertake an **egocentric network analysis**, which focuses on patterns of relationships and networks of individuals. Each person has their own network of relationships that are presumed to contribute to the person's behaviors and attitudes. In studying these networks, researchers develop lists of a person's network members (called *alters*) and seek to understand the scope and nature of interrelationships. Network data from such efforts are often quantified and analyzed statistically. Egocentric network analysis is used to understand features of personal networks and has been used to explain such phenomena as longevity, coping with crisis, and risk taking.

> **Example of an Egocentric Network Analysis**
> Using an egocentric network analysis, Prochnow and colleagues (2022) studied middle-school youth participation in an experiential sport program with 3- and 6-month follow-ups and summer care program networks. Four case studies of ethnically and racially diverse adolescents were presented.

The product of ethnographic research usually is a rich, holistic description and interpretation of the culture. Among healthcare researchers, ethnography provides access to the health beliefs and practices of a culture. Ethnographic inquiry can thus help to facilitate understanding of behaviors affecting health and illness.

In addition to written reports, ethnographers have recently used their research as the basis for performance ethnographies. **A performance ethnography** has been described as a scripted and staged reenactment of ethnographically derived notes that reflect an interpretation of the culture (Denzin, 2003).

A rich array of ethnographic methods has been developed and cannot be fully described in this general textbook. More information may be found in Fetterman (2020). Three variants of ethnographic research (ethnonursing research, institutional ethnography, and autoethnography) are described here, and a fourth (critical ethnography) is described later in this chapter.

Ethnonursing Research

Many nurse researchers have undertaken ethnographies. Leininger coined the phrase **ethnonursing research**, which she defined as "the study and analysis of the local or indigenous people's viewpoints, beliefs, and practices about nursing care behavior and processes of designated cultures" (1985, p. 38). In conducting an ethnonursing study, investigators use a broad theoretical framework to guide the research, such as Leininger's Theory of

Culture Care Diversity and Universality (Leininger & McFarland, 2006; McFarland & Wehbe-Alamah, 2015).

McFarland and Wehbe-Alamah (2015) described several enablers to support researchers' efforts in conducting ethnonursing research. *Enablers* are ways to discover complex phenomena like human care. Two of the enablers are the Stranger–Friend Model and the Observation–Participation–Reflection Model. The stranger–friend enabler guides researchers in mapping their progress and becoming aware of their feelings, behaviors, and responses as they transition from a stranger to trusted friend. The phases of Leininger's observation–participation–-reflection enabler go from (1) primary observation and active listening, (2) primary observation with limited participation, (3) primary participation with continuing observations, to (4) primary reflection and reconfirmation of results with informants.

Example of an Ethnonursing Study
Irie and colleagues (2022) conducted an ethnonursing study to explore cultural values and beliefs related to culturally congruent health activities among older adults in Japan's forest communities. Researchers used Leininger's qualitative ethnonursing research method to collect and analyze their data.

Institutional Ethnography

An ethnographic approach called **institutional ethnography** was pioneered by Dorothy Smith, a Canadian sociologist (1999). Institutional ethnography has been used in such fields as nursing, social work, and community health to study the organization of professional services, examined from the perspective of clients or frontline workers. Institutional ethnography seeks to understand the social determinants of people's everyday experiences in institutional settings. The focus is on social organization and institutional processes, and so research findings can play a role in organizational change.

In institutional ethnography, a person's actions in the social world are labeled as "social relations." Relations of *ruling* occur when social relations involve powerful coordination in people's lives and day-to-day activities. Where individuals are situated in the social location within an institution dictates relations of ruling.

Institutional ethnographers study the complexities of social and ruling relations. Rankin (2013) emphasized that an important step in an institutional ethnography is to decide on a standpoint within the organization of social relations. It is from that standpoint that the researcher studies how activities are socially organized. The research question focuses on "how does it happen?"

Example of Institutional Ethnography
Small et al. (2022) conducted an institutional ethnography to examine impacts of research texts and policy on midwives' and obstetricians' social organization of decision-making about intrapartum fetal monitoring in Australia.

TIP A relatively new approach, called **video-reflexive ethnography** (VRE), is gaining in popularity in healthcare settings. VRE is a collaborative visual method used by healthcare professionals to understand and interpret healthcare professionals' work practices and patient experiences (Carroll & Mesman, 2018).

Autoethnography

Ethnographers are often "outsiders" to the culture under study. A type of ethnography that involves self-scrutiny (including the study of groups or cultures to which researchers belong) is **autoethnography** (sometimes called *insider research* or *peer research*). Autoethnography offers numerous advantages, the most obvious being ease of access and recruitment and the ability to obtain candid, in-depth data based on pre-established trust and rapport. Another potential advantage is the researcher's ability to detect subtle nuances that an outsider might miss or take months to uncover. A potential limitation, however, is the researcher's inability to be objective about group (or self) processes, which can result in unsuspected myopia about important but sensitive issues. Autoethnography requires researchers to maintain consciousness of their role and monitor their internal state and their interactions with others during the study.

A type of autoethnography is evocative autoethnography. Bochner and Ellis (2016) define this type of autoethnography as writing that "displays multiple layers of consciousness, connecting the personal to the cultural" (p. 65). Evocative autoethnography can be presented in a variety of forms such as short stories, fiction, or poetry. Its text is full of emotion and embodiment.

Chang (2016) noted that successful autoethnographies need to provide not only a rich description of personal experiences but also a "sociocultural interpretation of such experiences" (p. 443). Chang recommends that autoethnographers ask themselves five evaluative questions, such as whether the autoethnography uses authentic data. Hughes and Pennington (2017) suggest methodologic strategies for autoethnographic work.

> **Example of an Autoethnography**
> Allan (2021) described an autoethnography that studied the effects on the patient experience of distanced nursing care during COVID-19 pandemic in the United Kingdom.

PHENOMENOLOGY

Phenomenology, rooted in a philosophical tradition developed by Husserl and Heidegger, is an approach to understanding people's everyday life experiences. Phenomenologic researchers ask: What is the *essence* of this phenomenon as experienced by these people and what does it *mean*? Phenomenologists assume there is an *essence*—an essential invariant structure—that can be understood, in much the same way that ethnographers assume that cultures exist. Essence is what makes a phenomenon what it is, and without which it would not be what it is. Phenomenologists investigate subjective phenomena in the belief that critical truths about reality are grounded in people's lived experiences. The phenomenologic approach is especially useful when a phenomenon has been poorly defined.

Phenomenologists believe that lived experience gives meaning to each person's perception of a phenomenon. The goal of phenomenologic inquiry is to understand lived experience and the perceptions to which it gives rise. Four aspects of lived experience of interest to phenomenologists are *lived space*, or spatiality; *lived body*, or corporeality; *lived time*, or temporality; and *lived human relation*, or relationality.

Phenomenologists view human existence as meaningful and interesting because of people's consciousness of that existence. The phrase **being-in-the-world** (or *embodiment*) is a concept that acknowledges people's physical ties to their world—they think, see, hear, feel, and are conscious through their bodies' interaction with the world.

In phenomenologic studies, in-depth conversations are the main data source, with researchers and informants as coparticipants. Through in-depth conversations, researchers strive to gain entrance into the informants' world, to have full access to their experiences as lived. Multiple interviews or conversations are sometimes needed. Typically, phenomenologic studies involve a small number of study participants—often fewer than 15. For some phenomenologic researchers, the inquiry includes not only gathering information from informants but also efforts to experience the phenomenon through participation, observation, and introspective reflection.

> **TIP** The notion that "insider research" can be a useful strategy in phenomenologic inquiries has emerged recently. Johnston and colleagues (2017) have described methodologic considerations relating to nurse researchers using their own experience of a phenomenon within a phenomenologic study.

Phenomenologists share their insights in rich, vivid reports. A phenomenologic text describing study results should help readers "see" something in a way that enriches their understanding of an experience. Van Manen (1997) warned that if a phenomenologic text is flat and boring, it "loses power to break through the taken-for-granted dimensions of everyday life" (p. 346). A wealth of resources on phenomenologic methods is available, including such classic sources as Giorgi (2009), Colaizzi (1973), or van Manen (1990) (2014).

There are several variants and methodologic interpretations of phenomenology. The two main schools of thought are descriptive phenomenology and interpretive phenomenology (hermeneutics). Matua and Van der Wal (2015) provide useful discussions about the need to differentiate the two in nursing.

Descriptive Phenomenology

Descriptive phenomenology was developed by Husserl (1962), who was primarily interested in the question: What do we know as people? His philosophy emphasized descriptions of human experience. Descriptive phenomenologists insist on the careful description of ordinary conscious experience of everyday life—a description of "things" as people experience them. These "things" include hearing, seeing, believing, feeling, remembering, deciding, evaluating, and acting. Two acts are key to Husserl's philosophical approach: bracketing (also called *epoché*) and reduction. **Bracketing** is the process of identifying and holding in abeyance preconceived beliefs and opinions about the phenomenon under study. Bracketing helps to remove influences that can block access to the meaning of a phenomenon. Phenomenologic **reduction** is a meditative and liberating practice wherein the phenomenologist attains a more attentive openness by constantly questioning the meaning of an experience.

Descriptive phenomenologic studies often involve the following four general steps: bracketing, intuiting, analyzing, and describing. Bracketing can never be achieved totally, but researchers strive to bracket out the world and any presuppositions in an effort to confront the data in pure form. Bracketing is an iterative process that involves preparing, evaluating, and providing systematic ongoing feedback about the effectiveness of the bracketing. Phenomenologic researchers (as well as other qualitative researchers) often maintain a **reflexive journal** in their efforts to bracket. Ahern (1999) provided 10 tips to help qualitative researchers with bracketing through notes in a reflexive journal:

1. Make note of interests that, as a researcher, you may take for granted.
2. Clarify your personal values and identify areas in which you know you are biased.
3. Identify areas of possible role conflict.
4. Recognize gatekeepers' interest and make note of the degree to which they are favorably or unfavorably disposed toward your research.
5. Identify any feelings you have that may indicate a lack of neutrality.
6. Describe new or surprising findings in collecting and analyzing data.
7. Reflect on and profit from methodologic problems that occur during your research.
8. Even after data analysis is complete, reflect on how you write up your findings.
9. Reflect on whether the literature review is truly supporting your findings or whether it is expressing the similar cultural background that you have.
10. Consider whether you can address any bias in your data collection or analysis by interviewing a participant a second time or reanalyzing the transcript in question.

Intuiting, the second step in descriptive phenomenology, occurs when researchers remain open to the meanings attributed to the phenomenon by those who have experienced it. Phenomenologic researchers then proceed to the analysis phase (i.e., extracting significant statements, categorizing, and making sense of the essential meanings of the phenomenon), as we describe in Chapter 25. Finally, the descriptive phase occurs when researchers come to understand and define the phenomenon.

TIP Descriptive phenomenology is often called the *Duquesne School* of phenomenology, named for three psychology professors who developed descriptive phenomenologic methods at Duquesne University—Colaizzi, Giorgi, and van Kaam.

Example of a Descriptive Phenomenologic Study
Zohn (2022) used a descriptive phenomenological approach to study the experiences of nursing students while caring for patients at risk for suicide.

Interpretive Phenomenology and Hermeneutics

Nurse researchers have also used methods that can be described as interpretive phenomenology, which encompasses several approaches to inquiry.

Heideggerian Hermeneutics

Heidegger, a student of Husserl, moved away from his professor's philosophy into **interpretive phenomenology** (**hermeneutics**). To Heidegger (1962), the critical question is: What is *being*? He stressed interpreting and understanding—not just describing—human experience. His premise is that the lived experience is inherently an interpretive process. Heidegger argued that hermeneutics is a basic characteristic of human existence. Indeed, the term hermeneutics refers to the art and philosophy of interpreting the meaning of an object (such as a *text*, work of art, and so on). The goals of interpretive phenomenologic research are to enter another's world and to discover the practical wisdom, possibilities, and understandings found there.

Gadamer (1976), another influential phenomenologist, described the interpretive process as a circular relationship known as the **hermeneutic circle** where one understands the whole of a text (for example, a transcribed interview) in terms of its parts and the parts in terms of the whole. In his view, researchers enter into a dialogue with the text and continually question its meaning.

Interpretive phenomenologists, like descriptive phenomenologists, rely primarily on in-depth interviews with individuals who have experienced the phenomenon of interest, but they may go beyond a traditional approach to gathering and analyzing data. For example, interpretive phenomenologists sometimes augment their understandings of the phenomenon through an analysis of supplementary texts, such as novels, poetry, or other artistic expressions—or they use such materials in their conversations with study participants.

In an interpretive phenomenologic study, bracketing does not necessarily occur. For Heidegger, it was impossible to bracket one's being-in-the-world. Hermeneutics presupposes prior understanding on the part of the researcher. Gearing (2004) described *reflexive bracketing*—in which researchers attempt to identify internal suppositions to facilitate greater transparency, but without bracketing them out—as a tool for hermeneutical inquiry. Interpretive phenomenologists ideally approach each interview text with openness—they must be open to hearing what the text is saying. As Heidegger (1971) stated, "We never come to thoughts. They come to us" (p. 6). Guidance in undertaking a hermeneutic phenomenologic nursing study is offered by Cohen and colleagues (2000); analytic methods for hermeneutic inquiry that were developed by nurse researchers (Benner, 1994; Diekelmann et al., 1989) are described in Chapter 25.

> **Example of a Hermeneutic Study**
> Mutsonziwa and colleagues (2022) conducted a hermeneutic phenomenological study that examined and interpreted the experience of physical isolation of patients infected with multidrug resistant organisms in Australia.

The Utrecht School of Phenomenology

Another approach comes from the *Utrecht School* in the Netherlands. The Utrecht School incorporates components of both descriptive and interpretive phenomenology. Influenced by the Utrecht school, van Manen (1990) noted that "Hermeneutic phenomenology tries to be attentive to both terms of its methodology: it is a descriptive (phenomenologic) methodology because it wants to be attentive to how things appear, it wants to let things speak for themselves; it is an interpretive (hermeneutic) methodology because (of) its claim that there are no such things as uninterpreted phenomena" (p. 180). For Van Manen (2017), phenomenology is a science of examples: examples are reflected on to discover exemplary aspects of the meaning of a phenomenon. We discuss van Manen's methods in greater detail in Chapter 25.

Interpretive Phenomenologic Analysis

In some recent studies, nurse researchers have cited the work of a group of psychological phenomenologists, who have described an approach called **interpretive phenomenologic analysis** or **IPA** (Smith et al., 2009). The focus of IPA is on the subjective experiences of people—their *lifeworld*. Studying individuals' experiences requires interpretation on the part of the researcher and the participant because it is not possible to directly access a person's lifeworld. There are three key principles to IPA: (1) it investigates the phenomenon of experience of a person, (2) it requires intense interpretation and engagement with the data obtained from the person, and (3) it is examined in detail.

Example of Interpretive Phenomenologic Analysis
Traboulssi et al. (2022) used interpretive phenomenological analysis (IPA) to study the experiences of Arab men following their wives' diagnosis and treatment for breast cancer in Bahrain.

Reflective Lifeworld Research

A nurse researcher and colleagues in Sweden (Dahlberg et al., 2008) have created another approach that combines descriptive and interpretive phenomenology, called **reflective lifeworld research** (RLR). Lifeworlds can be reached through an open attitude, which requires sensitivity toward the things being studied. Dahlberg and colleagues use the term *bridling* rather than *bracketing* to describe having an open and respectful attitude that permits the phenomenon being studied to present itself. Their view is that *bracketing* points backwards, as the researcher's energy is focused on restraining preunderstanding. A goal of RLR is to enable a reflection on taken-for-granted assumptions so that the phenomenon being studied can show itself more fully. "The understanding process is. . . slowed down in order to let new and surprising meanings arise that otherwise might have been clouded by the researcher's own preunderstandings or established meanings of the phenomenon" (Dahlberg et al., 2016, pp. 3–4).

Example of Reflective Lifeworld Research
In their study of parents' experiences with public health nursing during the postpartum period in Norway, Hogmo and colleagues (2022) were guided by the reflective lifeworld approach.

The Parse Phenomenologic-Hermeneutic Research Method

Some nurse researchers use approaches that have been formulated by Rosemarie Rizzo Parse (2014), based on her Humanbecoming Paradigm. Parse's methods have been evolving. Most recently, she has proposed two modes of inquiry under this paradigm: humanbecoming hermeneutic sciencing (Parse, 2016a) and Parsesciencing (2016b).

In **humanbecoming hermeneutic sciencing**, the researcher's aim is to uncover emergent meanings of universal living experiences that are expressed in published texts and artforms. It consists of three phases: discoursing with penetrating engaging, interpreting with quiescent beholding, and understanding with inspiring envisaging. Parse acknowledges that "yet there remains a knowing that the vessel of inquiry can never be filled. There is always the veil of mystery, the barely seen" (Parse, 2016a, p. 129).

Parse's (2016b) second mode of inquiry is **Parsesciencing**, which she describes as "coming to know the meanings of universal humanuniverse living experiences" (p. 271). Parsesciencing consists of dialoging-engaging, distilling-fusing, and heuristic interpreting. Using these three phases, the researcher's purpose is to discover universal humanuniverse living experiences through descriptions from "historians"—the individuals who agree to describe their experiences. Data are gathered in the first phase through dialoging-engaging, which are not interviews per se, but rather unique dialogues in which the researcher is a true presence with participants who are asked to talk about the experience being studied. In the next phases, the researcher dwells with the descriptions and strives to attain higher levels of abstraction.

Example of Parse's Phenomenologic Method
Reding (2022) used Parse's method to investigate the living experience of feeling peaceful. Through engagement with 10 participants from the American Indian population, the researcher identified the structure: feeling peaceful is serene contemplation surfacing with gratifying engagements while enduring hardship.

Phenomenography

Phenomenography is another approach to studying how phenomena are conceived and understood. An important assumption in phenomenography is that people differ in terms of how they experience the world, but differences can be described and understood by others. Phenomenographers distinguish between first-order perspectives—what the essence of something really is, that is, the actual phenomenon—and second-order perspectives—how a phenomenon is perceived and conceptualized. The second-order perspective is the focus of phenomenography. In a phenomenographic study, researchers strive to understand the qualitatively different ways in which people experience a phenomenon or think about it. In analyzing their data, phenomenographers sort perceptions emerging from the data into categories of description. The categories, which are logically related to one another, become the phenomenographic essence of the phenomenon. A good resource for learning more about phenomenography is the book by Marton and Booth (1997).

> **Example of a Phenomenographic Study**
> Larsson et al. (2022) undertook a phenomenographic study to describe older adults' experiences of how participating in a senior summer camp in Sweden affected their lives. The researchers interviewed 19 older adults and identified 3 descriptive categories: mitigating loneliness, developing as a person, and gaining inspiration.

GROUNDED THEORY

Grounded theory has contributed to the development of many middle-range nursing theories. Grounded theory was formulated in the 1960s as a systematic method of qualitative inquiry by two sociologists, Glaser and Strauss (1967).

Grounded theory tries to account for actions in a substantive area from the perspective of those involved. Grounded theory researchers seek to understand actions by focusing on the main concern or problem that the individuals' behavior is designed to address (Glaser, 1998). The manner in which people resolve this main concern is called the **core variable**. One type of core variable is called a **basic social process (BSP).** The goal of grounded theory is to discover this main concern and the BSP that explains how people continually resolve it. The main concern must be discovered from the data.

Conceptualization is a key aspect of grounded theory (Glaser, 2003). Grounded theory researchers generate conceptual categories and their properties and integrate them into a substantive theory grounded in the data. Through this conceptual process, the generated grounded theory represents an abstraction based on participants' actions and their meanings. The grounded theorist uncovers and names latent patterns (categories) from the participants' accounts. Glaser emphasized that concepts transcend time, place, and person: "In grounded theory, behavior is a pattern that a person engages in; it is not the person. People are not categorized, behavior is" (p. 53).

Grounded theory methods constitute an entire approach to the conduct of field research. For example, a study that follows Glaser and Strauss's method does not begin with a focused research problem; the problem emerges from the data. In a grounded theory study, both the problem and the process used to resolve it are discovered.

A fundamental feature of grounded theory research is that data collection, data analysis, and sampling of participants occur simultaneously. The grounded theory process is recursive: researchers collect data, categorize them, describe the emerging central phenomenon, and then recycle earlier steps. In-depth interviews and observation are the most common data sources in grounded theory studies, but other data sources such as documents may also be used.

A procedure called **constant comparison** is used to develop and refine theoretically relevant categories. Categories elicited from the data are constantly compared with data obtained earlier so that commonalities and variations can be determined. As data collection proceeds, the inquiry becomes increasingly focused on emerging theoretical concerns.

CHAPTER 22 Qualitative Research Design and Approaches • 473

Example of a Glaser and Strauss Grounded Theory Study

Reyes (2022) used Glaser and Strauss's grounded theory method to study the process of how 23 college-student military veterans with PTSD symptoms learn mindfulness and acceptance through the use of a mobile app based on acceptance and commitment therapy. The core category discovered was mindful scaffolding which involved the process of how student veterans coped with interruptions and intrusions while learning mindfulness and acceptance.

Like most theories, a grounded theory is modifiable as the researcher (or other researchers) collects new data. Modification is an ongoing process and is the method by which theoretical completeness is enhanced (Glaser, 2001). As more data are found and more qualitative studies are published in the substantive area, the grounded theory can be modified to accommodate new or different dimensions.

Example of a Modification of a Grounded Theory Study

Beck (2023), one of the authors of this textbook, modified her 1993 original grounded theory of postpartum depression, "Teetering on the edge," for the third time. In this third modification, Beck focused on postpartum depression in immigrant and refugee women. She included data from 13 qualitative studies that focused on this vulnerable population. Maximizing differences among comparative groups is a powerful method for enhancing theoretical properties and extending the theory.

TIP Glaser and Strauss (1967) distinguished two types of grounded theory: substantive and formal. **Substantive theory** is grounded in data on a specific substantive area, such as postpartum depression. It can serve as a springboard for **formal grounded theory**, which is at a higher level of conceptualization and is abstract of time, place, and people. The goal of formal grounded theory is not to discover a new core variable but to develop a theory that goes beyond the substantive grounded theory and extends the general implications of the core variable.

Alternate Views of Grounded Theory: Strauss and Corbin

In 1990, Strauss and Corbin published what was to become a controversial book, *Basics of Qualitative Research: Grounded Theory Procedures and Techniques*. The authors stated that the book's purpose was to provide beginning grounded theory researchers with basic procedures involved for building theory at the substantive level.

Glaser, however, disagreed with some of the procedures advocated by Strauss (his original coauthor) and Corbin (a nurse researcher). Glaser published a rebuttal in 1992, *Emergence vs. Forcing: Basics of Grounded Theory Analysis*. Glaser believed that Strauss and Corbin developed a method that is not grounded theory but rather what he called "full conceptual description." According to Glaser, the purpose of grounded theory is to generate concepts and theories about their relationships that explain, account for, and interpret variation in behavior in the substantive area under study. *Conceptual description*, in contrast, is aimed at describing the full range of behavior of what is occurring in the substantive area, "irrespective of relevance and accounting for variation in behavior" (Glaser, 1992, p. 19). In their latest edition, Corbin and Strauss (2015) stated that their method reflects Strauss's approach to doing grounded theory, which is based on the philosophies of pragmatism and interactionism.

Nurse researchers have conducted grounded theory studies using both the original Glaser and Strauss and the Strauss and Corbin approaches. Heath and Cowley (2004) provide a comparison of the two approaches. We describe analytic differences in Chapter 25.

Example of Strauss and Corbin's Grounded Theory Methods

Barreto and colleagues (2022) used Corbin and Strauss's grounded theory method to examine the experiences of patients, relatives, and health professionals regarding family presence during emergency care in Brazil.

Constructivist Grounded Theory: Charmaz

Strauss and Glaser had different training and backgrounds. Strauss, trained at the University of

Chicago, had a background in symbolic interaction and pragmatist philosophy. Glaser, by contrast, came from a tradition of positivism and quantitative methods at Columbia University. In one of Glaser's (2005) later publications, in which he discussed the takeover of grounded theory by symbolic interaction, he argued that "grounded theory is a general inductive method possessed by no discipline or theoretical perspective or data type" (p. 141).

In recent years, an approach called **constructivist grounded theory** has emerged. A leading advocate is sociologist Kathy Charmaz, who has sought to bring the Chicago School antecedents of grounded theory into the forefront again. She has called for returning to the pragmatist foundation which "assumes that interaction is inherently dynamic and interpretive and addresses how people create, enact, and change meanings and actions" (Charmaz, 2014, p. 9). Charmaz views Glaser and Strauss's (and Strauss and Corbin's) versions of grounded theory as being based in the positivist tradition. Her position is that what is missing from their objective grounded theory method is the researcher's influence on the data collected and analyzed, and interactions between the researcher and participants.

Charmaz uses the term "constructivist" "to acknowledge subjectivity and the researcher's involvement in the construction and interpretation of data" (2014, p. 14). In her approach, the developed grounded theory is seen as an interpretation. The analyzed data are acknowledged to be constructed from shared experiences and relationships between the researcher and the participants. Charmaz's view is that "we start with the assumption that social reality is multiple, processual, and constructed, then we must take the researcher's position, privileges, perspective, and interactions into account as an inherent part of the research reality (p. 13). Reflexivity of both the researcher's own interpretations and the interpretations of the participants is important. Higginbottom and Lauridsen (2014) have described how Charmaz's approach is similar to and different from original grounded theory.

Example of a Constructivist Grounded Theory
Buechel et al. (2022) undertook constructivist ground theory methods to understand how active-duty service members and their partners navigate their infertility care process within the Military Health System while managing a military career.

TIP Beginning qualitative researchers should be aware that a grounded theory study is a lengthier and more complex process than a phenomenologic study. This may be important to consider if there are constraints in the amount of time you can devote to a study.

OTHER TYPES OF QUALITATIVE RESEARCH

Qualitative studies often can be characterized in terms of the disciplinary research traditions discussed in the previous section. However, several other important types of qualitative research also deserve mention. This section discusses qualitative research that is not associated with any particular discipline.

Case Studies

Case studies are in-depth investigations of a single entity (or small number of entities), which could be an individual, family, institution, community, or other social unit. In a case study, researchers obtain a wealth of descriptive information and may examine relationships among different phenomena or may examine trends over time. Case study researchers attempt to analyze and understand issues that are important to the history, development, or circumstances of the entity under study.

One way to think of a case study is to consider what is at center stage. In most studies, whether qualitative or quantitative, a certain phenomenon or variable (or set of variables) is the core of the inquiry. In a case study, the *case* itself is central. As befits an intensive analysis, the focus of case studies is typically on understanding *why* a person thinks, behaves, or develops in a particular manner rather than on *what* a person's status, progress, or actions are. It is not unusual for probing research of this type to require detailed study over a considerable period. Data are often collected that relate not only to the person's present state but also to past experiences and situational factors relevant to the problem being examined.

Yin (2018) has described several designs for case studies. A **single case study** is an appropriate design when (1) it is a critical case in testing a well-formulated theory, (2) it represents an extreme or unique case, (3) it is a representative or typical case, (4) it is a revelatory case, or (5) it is a longitudinal case. A **multiple case design** is a study that involves more than one case. Single and multiple case studies can be either holistic or embedded. In a **holistic design**, the global nature of a case—be it a person, community, or organization—is examined. An **embedded design** involves multiple units of analysis. A wide variety of data can be used in case studies, including data from interviews, observations, documents, and artifacts.

A distinction is sometimes drawn between an intrinsic and instrumental case study. In an *intrinsic case study*, researchers do not have to select the case. For instance, a process evaluation of implementing an innovation is often a case study of a particular program or institution; the "case" is a given. In an *instrumental case study*, researchers begin with a research question or problem and seek a case that offers illumination. The aim is to use the case to understand a phenomenon of interest. In such a situation, a case is usually selected not because it is typical but rather because it can maximize what can be learned about the phenomenon.

Although understanding a particular case is the central concern of case studies, they are sometimes a useful way to explore phenomena that have not been rigorously researched. The information obtained in case studies can be used to develop hypotheses to be tested more rigorously in subsequent research. The intensive probing that characterizes case studies often leads to insights concerning previously unsuspected relationships. Furthermore, case studies may serve the important role of clarifying concepts or of elucidating ways to capture them.

TIP Case study research is not a distinct methodology (Sandelowski, 2011). Many ethnographies focus on a specific "case," as do many historical studies. Although case studies typically involve the collection of in-depth qualitative information, some case studies are quantitative and use statistical methods to analyze data. And some case studies used mixed methods (i.e., both qualitative and quantitative approaches).

The greatest strength of case studies is the depth that is possible when a limited number of individuals, institutions, or groups are being investigated. Case studies provide researchers with opportunities of having an intimate knowledge of a person's condition, thoughts, actions (past and present), intentions, and environment. On the other hand, this same strength is a potential weakness because researchers' familiarity with the person or group may make objectivity difficult. Perhaps the biggest concern about case studies is generalizability: If researchers discover important relationships, it is difficult to know whether the same relationships would occur with others. However, case studies can play a role in challenging generalizations based on other types of research.

It is important to recognize that case study *research* is not simply anecdotal descriptions of a particular incident or patient, such as a case report. Case study research is a disciplined process and typically requires a long period of data collection. The writings of Yin (2018) and Baxter and Jack (2008) are good resources for learning more about case study research.

Example of a Case Study
Whiteing and colleagues (2022) used a multiple case study to investigate RN practice in rural, remote, or very remote locations in Australia.

Narrative Analyses

Narrative analysis focuses on *story* as the object of inquiry, to examine how individuals make sense of events in their lives. Narratives are viewed as a type of "cultural envelope" into which people pour their experiences (Riessman, 1991). What distinguishes narrative analysis from other types of qualitative research designs is its focus on the broad contours of a narrative; stories are not fractured and dissected. The broad underlying premise of narrative research is that people most effectively make sense of their world—and communicate these meanings—by constructing, reconstructing, and narrating stories. Individuals construct stories when they wish to understand specific events and situations that require linking an inner world of desire and motive to an external world of observable actions. Narrative analysts explore *form* as well as content, asking "Why was the story told that way?" (Riessman, 2008).

A number of approaches can be used to examine stories. One approach is Burke's (1969) **pentadic dramatism**. For Burke, there are five key elements of a story: act, scene, agent, agency, and purpose. Analysis of a story "will offer some kind of answers to these five questions: what was done (act), when or where it was done (scene), who did it (agent), how he did it (agency), and why (purpose)" (p. xv). The five terms of Burke's pentad are meant to be understood paired together as ratios such as, act: agent, act: scene, agent: agency, and purpose: agent. The analysis focuses on the internal relationships and tensions of these five terms to each other. Each pairing in the pentad provides a different way of directing the researcher's attention. What drives the narrative analysis is not just the interaction of the pentadic terms but an imbalance between two or more terms. Bruner (1991) modified Burke's pentad with the addition of a sixth term that he called Trouble. Bruner included this sixth element to provide more focus in narrative analysis on Burke's imbalance between the terms in his pentad.

Example of a Narrative Analysis Using Burke's Approach
Lewis et al. (2021) undertook a narrative analysis of birth stories of 16 women on the autism spectrum. Burke's pentad of terms was used to analyze these narratives and revealed numerous accounts of act: agency and agent: scene tensions. Highlighted in their narratives included participants feeling their concerns were minimized during labor and delivery, and their sensory sensitivities impaired their ability to communicate with providers and to participate in the birth.

Another approach is that of Riessman (1993, 2008), whose method of thematic narrative analysis involves protecting each story as a whole and not fragmenting them. Each story is analyzed separately for themes. Then all the stories are compared to identify common themes for a *mega story*. The researcher can choose specific stories to illustrate common themes. The narrative analyst remains focused on the content of the stories rather than how or why the stories are told. Riessman (1993) described five levels of experience in the research process for narrative analysts:

1. Attending: participants create personal meaning by actively thinking about reality in new ways. Participants reflect and remember their experiences; they compose their own realities.
2. Telling: participants "re-present" the events of an experience. They share the event by recounting characters, significant events, and their interpretation of the experience. The interviewer takes part in the narrative by listening to the story and asking questions (to clarify/further understand the story). As participants tell their story, they are also creating a vision of themselves.
3. Transcribing: participants' stories are typically captured through video or audio recording. The analyst then creates a written narrative representing the conversation.
4. Analyzing: the researcher analyzes each individual transcript. Similarities are noted and a "mega story" is created by defining critical moments within narratives and making meaning out of each story. The analyst also makes decisions about form, order, and style of presentation of the narratives.
5. Reading: the final level of experience in the research process is reading. Drafts are commonly shared with colleagues. The researcher frequently incorporates this editorial feedback into a final report that reflects the researcher's interpretation of the narrative.

Example of a Narrative Analysis Using Riessman's Approach
Nkamabule and colleagues (2021) used Riessman's narrative analysis to understand the insulin treated diabetes illness experience among people in rural Malawi. The study involved the analysis of the stories told by 10 participants, whose narratives identified the struggles living with insulin treated diabetes in the context of low resources.

Descriptive Qualitative Studies

Many qualitative studies have a link to one of the research traditions discussed in this chapter. Many other qualitative studies, however, claim no particular disciplinary or methodologic roots. The researchers may simply indicate that they have conducted a qualitative study or a naturalistic inquiry, or they may say that they have done a *content analysis* or a *thematic analysis* of their qualitative data (i.e., an analysis of themes and patterns that emerge in the narrative content). We refer to the many qualitative studies that do not have a formal name as **descriptive qualitative studies**, although they are sometimes called *generic qualitative inquiries* (Patton, 2015).

Sandelowski (2000), in a widely read article, noted that in doing descriptive qualitative studies, researchers tend not to penetrate their data in any interpretive depth. These studies present comprehensive summaries of a phenomenon or of events. Qualitative descriptive designs tend to be eclectic, and they often borrow or adapt methodologic techniques from other qualitative traditions, such as constant comparison.

In a more recent article, Sandelowski (2010) warned researchers not to call their studies *qualitative description* "after the fact to give a name to poorly conceived and conducted studies" (p. 80). She noted that qualitative descriptive studies produce findings closer to the data ("data-near") than studies within such traditions as phenomenology or grounded theory, but that good qualitative descriptions are still interpretive products. She recognized that her article from 2000 had provided justification for studies that primarily reproduce raw data and stated that she "never intended to communicate... that qualitative description removes the researcher's obligation to do any analyzing or interpreting at all" (p. 79). Rather than being a distinct methodologic classification, qualitative description is perhaps viewed as a "distributed residual category" (p. 82) that signals a "confederacy" of diverse groups of qualitative researchers.

> **Example of a Descriptive Qualitative Study**
> Liow et al. (2022) undertook a descriptive qualitative study to explore the experiences of Asian women with gestational breast cancer in Singapore.

Sally Thorne (2008) expanded qualitative description into a realm she called **interpretive description**. Her book outlined an approach that extends "beyond mere description and into the domain of the 'so what' that drives all applied disciplines" (p. 33) such as nursing. While acknowledging that her approach is neither novel nor distinctive, Thorne emphasizes the importance of having a disciplinary conceptual frame (such as nursing): "Interpretive description becomes a conceptual maneuver whereby a solid and substantive logic derived from the disciplinary orientation justifies the application of specific techniques and procedures outside of their conventional context" (p. 35). An important thrust of her approach is that it requires integrity of purpose from an actual practice goal and seeks to generate new insights that can help shape applications of qualitative evidence to practice.

Thorne (2013) has acknowledged that she developed interpretive description to free qualitative nurse researchers from the constraints of qualitative methodologies. She noted that "the nursing disciplinary mind never truly accepts standardization; it always seeks to ensure that there is room for necessary variation" (p. 296). Interpretive description holds no attachment to any one qualitative method, but rather it uses the wealth of research techniques available. Thorne offered examples of typical research questions for interpretive description, such as, "What are the common ways in which patients' experience...?" (p. 298).

> **Example of an Interpretive Description Study**
> Oliffe and colleagues (2022) used interpretive description in a Canadian study that explored 47 men's help-seeking for mental health after an intimate partner relationship break-up.

RESEARCH WITH IDEOLOGICAL PERSPECTIVES

Some qualitative researchers conduct inquiries within an ideological framework, to focus attention on the problems or needs of certain groups and to effect change. These approaches, which are sometimes described as being within a **transformative paradigm** (Mertens, 2007), are briefly described in this section.

Critical Theory

Critical theory originated with a group of Marxist-oriented German scholars in the 1920s, referred to as the Frankfurt School. A critical researcher is concerned with a critique of society and with envisioning new possibilities.

Critical social science is typically action oriented. Its broad aim is to integrate theory and practice such that people become aware of disparities and become inspired to change them. Critical researchers reject the idea of an objective, disinterested inquirer and pursue a transformation process. An important feature of critical theory is that it calls for inquiries that foster enlightened self-knowledge and sociopolitical action. Critical theory also involves a self-reflective aspect. To prevent a critical theory of society from becoming yet another self-serving ideology, critical theorists must account for their own transformative effects.

A critical inquiry often begins with a thorough analysis of aspects of a problem. For example, critical researchers might analyze and critique taken-for-granted assumptions that underlie the problem, the language used to depict the situation, or the biases of prior researchers studying the problem. Critical researchers often triangulate multiple methodologies and emphasize multiple perspectives on problems (e.g., alternative racial or social class perspectives). They typically interact with study participants in ways that emphasize participants' expertise. Some of the features that distinguish more traditional qualitative research and critical research are summarized in Table 22.2.

Critical theory has played an especially important role in ethnography. **Critical ethnography** focuses on raising consciousness and aiding emancipatory goals in the hope of effecting social change. Critical ethnographers address the historical, social, political, and economic dimensions of cultures and their value-laden agendas. An assumption in critical ethnographic research is that actions and thoughts are mediated by power relationships. Critical ethnographers attempt to increase the political dimensions of cultural research and undermine oppressive systems—there is an explicit political purpose. Cook (2005) has argued that critical ethnography is especially well-suited to health promotion research because both are concerned with enabling people to take control of their own situation.

TABLE 22.2 • Comparison of Traditional Qualitative Research and Critical Research

ISSUE	TRADITIONAL QUALITATIVE RESEARCH	CRITICAL RESEARCH
Research aims	Understanding; reconstruction of multiple constructions	Critique; transformation; consciousness-raising; advocacy
View of knowledge	Transactional/subjective; knowledge is created in interaction between investigator and participants	Transactional/subjective; value-mediated and value-dependent; importance of historical insights
Methods	Dialectic: truth is arrived at logically through conversations	Dialectic and didactic: dialogue designed to transform naivety and misinformation
Evaluative criteria for inquiry quality	Authenticity; trustworthiness	Historical situatedness of the inquiry; erosion of ignorance; stimulus for change
Researcher's role	Facilitator of multivoice reconstruction	Transformative agent; advocate; activist

Carspecken (1996) developed a five-stage approach to critical ethnography that has been found useful in nursing studies (e.g. (Bidabadi et al., 2019)) and in health promotion research. Madison (2020) also provides guidance about critical theory methods.

> **Example of a Critical Ethnography**
> Acosta and Morris McEwen (2023) conducted a critical ethnography to study postrape experiences of six undocumented immigrant women of Mexican origin living in the U.S.–Mexico border region. They found that marginalization of these survivors and the intersections of cultural and sociopolitical context of the border region detrimentally impacted their experiences.

Feminist Research

In **feminist research,** the focus is on gender domination and discrimination within patriarchal societies. Like critical researchers, feminist researchers seek to establish collaborative and nonexploitative relationships with their informants, to avoid objectification, and to conduct research that is transformative.

Gender is the organizing construct in feminist research, and investigators seek to understand how gender and a gendered social order have shaped women's lives and their consciousness. The aim is to ameliorate the "invisibility and distortion of female experience in ways relevant to ending women's unequal social position" (Lather, 1991, p. 71).

Although feminist researchers agree on the importance of focusing on women's diverse situations and the relationships that frame those situations, there are many variants of feminist inquiry. Three broad models (within each of which there is diversity) have been identified: (1) *feminist empiricism*, whose adherents usually work within fairly standard norms of qualitative inquiry but who seek to portray more accurate pictures of the social realities of women's lives; (2) *feminist standpoint research*, which holds that inquiry ought to begin in and be tested against the lived everyday sociopolitical experiences of women, and that women's views are particular and privileged; and (3) *feminist postmodernism*, which stresses that "truth" is a destructive illusion and views the world as endless stories, texts, and narratives. In nursing and healthcare, feminist empiricism and feminist standpoint research have been most prevalent.

> **TIP** An emerging construct is *intersectionality*, a term used to designate overlapping or intersecting social identities (e.g., gender and race) and related systems of oppression or discrimination. Intersectionality emphasizes that multiple social identities intersect to create a whole that differs from its components. Caiola and colleagues (2017), for example, studied how African American mothers with HIV describe their situation at the intersection of gender, race, and social inequality.

The scope of feminist research ranges from studies of the subjective views of individual women to studies of social movements, structures, and broad policies that affect (and often exclude) women. Feminist research methods typically include in-depth, interactive, and collaborative individual or group interviews that offer the possibility of reciprocally educational encounters. Feminists usually seek to negotiate the meanings of the results with those participating in the study and to be self-reflective about what they themselves are experiencing and learning.

Feminist research, like other research that has an ideological perspective, has raised the bar for the conduct of ethical research. With the emphasis on trust, empathy, and nonexploitative relationships, proponents of these newer modes of inquiry view any type of deception or manipulation as abhorrent. Those interested in feminist methodologies may wish to consult the writings of Hesse-Biber (2014) or Brisolara et al. (2014).

> **Example of Feminist Research**
> Jefferies et al. (2022) used Black feminist theory to guide their study of African Nova Scotian nurses' perceptions and experiences of leadership.

Participatory Action Research

A type of research known as participatory action research (PAR) is closely allied to both critical research and feminist research. **Participatory action research (PAR)**, one of several types of *action research* that originated in the 1940s with social psychologist Kurt Lewin, is based on a recognition that the production of knowledge can be political and can be used to exert power. Action researchers typically work with groups or communities that are vulnerable to the control or oppression of a dominant group or culture.

In PAR, researchers and study participants collaborate in defining the problem, selecting research methods, analyzing the data, and deciding on the use to which findings are put. The aim of PAR is to produce not only knowledge but also action and consciousness-raising. Researchers seek to empower people through the process of constructing and using knowledge. The PAR tradition has as its starting point a concern for the powerlessness of the group under study. Thus, a key objective is to produce an impetus that is directly used to make improvements through education and sociopolitical action.

In PAR, research methods take second place to processes of collaboration that can motivate, increase self-esteem, and generate community solidarity. "Data-gathering" strategies are not only the traditional methods of interview and observation (including both qualitative and quantitative approaches) but may include storytelling, sociodrama, drawing and painting, plays and skits, and other activities designed to encourage people to find creative ways to explore their lives, tell their stories, and recognize their own strengths. Chevalier and Buckles (2019) offer a useful resource for learning more about PAR and its theory and methods.

Example of PAR
Blanchfield and O'Connor (2022) undertook a participatory action research study to inform an alternative combined type 2 diabetes and chronic kidney disease care provided in the context of advanced practice nursing. The project involved cocreated knowledge between patients and healthcare teams to address gaps in care provision.

CRITICAL APPRAISAL OF QUALITATIVE DESIGNS

Evaluating a qualitative design is often difficult. Qualitative researchers do not always document design decisions and seldom describe the process by which such decisions were made. Researchers often do, however, indicate whether the study was conducted within a specific qualitative tradition, and this information can be used to come to some conclusions. For example, if a report indicated that the researcher conducted 2 months of fieldwork for an ethnographic study, there would be reason to suspect that insufficient time had been spent in the field to obtain an emic perspective of the culture under study. Ethnographic studies may also be suspect if their only source of information was from interviews, rather than from a broader range of data sources, particularly observations.

In a grounded theory study, look for evidence about when the data were collected and analyzed. If all the data were collected before analysis, you might question whether constant comparison was used correctly. Glaser and Strauss (1967) offered four properties on which a grounded theory should be evaluated: fitness, understanding, generality, and control. The theory should fit the substantive area for which the data were collected. A grounded theory should increase the understanding of people working in that substantive area. Also, the categories in the grounded theory should be abstract enough to allow the theory to be a general guide to changing situations—but not so abstract to decrease their sensitizing features. Lastly, the substantive theory must be sufficiently flexible that people who want to apply the grounded theory in practice can modify and control it if necessary.

In appraising a phenomenologic study, you should first determine if the study is descriptive or interpretive. This will help you to assess how closely the researcher kept to the basic tenets of that qualitative research tradition. For example, in a descriptive phenomenologic study, did the researcher bracket? When critically appraising phenomenologic studies, in addition to evaluating the methods, you should look at their power to demonstrate the meaning of the phenomena being studied. Van Manen (1997) called for phenomenologic researchers to address five textual features in their reports: lived thoroughness (placing the phenomenon concretely in the lifeworld), evocation (vividly bringing the phenomenon into presence), intensification (giving key phrases their full value), tone

CHAPTER 22 Qualitative Research Design and Approaches • 481

> **BOX 22.1** Guidelines for Critically Appraising Qualitative Designs
>
> 1. Was a research tradition for the qualitative study identified? If none was identified, can one be inferred? If more than one was identified, is this justifiable or does it suggest "method slurring"?
> 2. Is the research question congruent with a qualitative approach and with the specific research tradition (i.e., is the domain of inquiry for the study congruent with the domain encompassed by the tradition)? Are the data sources, research methods, and analytic approach congruent with the research tradition?
> 3. How well is the research design described? Are design decisions explained and justified? Does it appear that the researcher made all design decisions up-front, or did the design emerge during data collection, allowing researchers to capitalize on early information?
> 4. Is the design appropriate, given the research question? Does the design lend itself to a thorough, in-depth, intensive examination of the phenomenon of interest? What design elements, if any, might have strengthened the study (e.g., a longitudinal perspective rather than a cross-sectional one)?
> 5. Did the researcher spend a sufficient amount of time doing fieldwork or collecting the research data?
> 6. Was there evidence of reflexivity in the design?
> 7. Was the study undertaken with an ideological perspective? If so, is there evidence that ideological methods and goals were achieved? (e.g., was there evidence of full collaboration between researchers and participants? Did the research have the power to be transformative, or is there evidence that a transformative process occurred?)

(letting the text speak to the reader), and epiphany (suddenly grasping the meaning).

The guidelines in Box 22.1 are designed to assist you in critically appraising the designs of qualitative studies.

RESEARCH EXAMPLES

Nurse researchers have conducted studies in all of the qualitative research traditions described in this chapter, and several actual examples have been cited. In the following sections, we present more detailed descriptions of three qualitative nursing studies.

Research Example of an Ethnographic Study

Study: Holistic health practices of rural Thai homebound older adults: A focused ethnographic study (Detthippornpong et al., 2022)

Statement of Purpose: The purpose of this ethnographic study was to explore the self-care practices of rural Thai homebound older adults to maintain Bai Lod or total health.

Setting: The research was conducted in Suratthani Providence in Southern Thailand, which is a rural community of about 5,000 people.

Method: A focused ethnographic approach was used with field work conducted over an 8-month period. Data were collected using participant observation through interviews with increasing participation in daily activities of the homebound older adults. Researchers kept field notes on the environment, participants' attitudes and behaviors, interaction with family members, and special events attended. Semistructured interviews were also conducted lasting between 45 and 60 minutes. A group interview which health professionals led was held at a local hospital to gain knowledge of the health services offered to these rural older adults.

Key findings: The daily health practices of housebound older rural adults included three patterns: (1) self-care to stay health, (2) sharing life with community and society in a positive way, and (3) incorporating both folk and modern medicines to maintain health, such as herbs planted around the home to make herbal juice and tea and Ya Pickle (a traditional Thai medicine).

Research Example of a Phenomenologic Study

Study: Effects of fourth-degree perineal lacerations on women's physical and mental health conducted by one of the authors of this textbook (Beck, 2021).

Statement of purpose: The purpose of this descriptive phenomenologic study was to describe the physical and emotional effects of fourth-degree perineal lacerations that occur during childbirth.

Sample: Study participants were 18 women who had sustained a fourth-degree perineal tear during childbirth. Women were recruited via a notice placed on the Facebook support group Mothers with Fourth Degree Tears.

Method: Interviews were conducted over the internet. Women were asked to write in as much detail as they wished their experiences of the physical and emotional impact of their fourth-degree perineal tears that occurred during childbirth on their daily lives. Women sent their descriptions on attachment to the researcher's university email address. Data were collected for 6 months until saturation was achieved and then analyzed using Colaizzi's phenomenological method.

Key findings: Seven themes were identified: (1) Why wasn't I informed I had this injury? (2) The unthinkable: Fecal incontinence and so much more, (3) It has cost me so much, (4) Seeking relief: Enduring surgery after surgery, (5) Why didn't anyone ask me about my mental health? (6) To have more children: that is the question, and (7) Are there any positives in all of this?

Research Example of a Grounded Theory Study

Study: Navigating asthma-the immigrant child in a tug-of-war: A constructivist grounded theory (Sudarsan et al., 2022)

Statement of purpose: The aim of this study was to explore the beliefs, practices, and experiences of asthma among Indian immigrant children and their family caregivers by means of a constructivist grounded theory design.

Setting: New Zealand

Method: The researchers used a constructivist grounded theory approach to understand Indian immigrant children's experiences with asthma. Data were collected through in-depth interviews with 10 family caregivers and nine Indian immigrant children ages 8 to 17. To help facilitate interviews with the children younger than 14 years of age, drawing and photography were used. Data collection and analysis occurred concurrently and data collection continued until theoretical saturation occurred.

Key findings: The metaphor of tug of war was used to describe the basic social process that occurred due to the clash between Indian and New Zealand cultures. The tug of war consisted of three main categories: being fearful, seeking support, and clashing cultures.

SUMMARY POINTS

- Qualitative research involves an **emergent design**—a design that emerges in the field as the study unfolds. Although qualitative design is flexible, qualitative researchers plan for broad contingencies that pose decision opportunities for study design in the field.
- As *bricoleurs*, qualitative researchers tend to be creative and intuitive, putting together an array of data drawn from many sources to develop a holistic understanding of a phenomenon.
- Qualitative research traditions have their roots in anthropology (e.g., ethnography and *ethnoscience*); philosophy (phenomenology, hermeneutics, and phenomenography); psychology (*ethology* and *ecological psychology*); sociology (grounded theory, *ethnomethodology*, and *semiotics*); sociolinguistics (*discourse analysis*); and history (*historical research*).
- **Ethnography** focuses on the culture of a group of people and relies on extensive fieldwork that usually includes **participant observation** and in-depth interviews with **key informants.** Ethnographers strive to acquire an **emic** (insider's) perspective of a culture rather than an **etic** (outsider's) perspective.
- Ethnographers use the concept of *researcher as instrument* to describe the researcher's significant role in analyzing and interpreting a culture. The product of ethnographic research is typically a holistic description of the culture, but sometimes the products are **performance ethnographies** (interpretive scripts that can be performed).
- Nurses sometimes refer to their ethnographic studies as **ethnonursing research.** Other types of ethnographic work include **institutional ethnographies** (which focus on the organization of professional services from the perspective of the frontline workers or clients) and

- **autoethnographies** or *insider research* (which focuses on the group or culture to which the researcher belongs).
- **Phenomenology** seeks to discover the *essence* and *meaning* of a phenomenon as it is experienced by people, mainly through in-depth interviews with people who have had the relevant experience.
- In **descriptive phenomenology**, which seeks to describe lived experiences, researchers strive to **bracket** out preconceived views and to **intuit** the essence of the phenomenon by remaining open to meanings attributed to it by those who have experienced it. **Interpretive phenomenology (hermeneutics)** focuses on interpreting the meaning of experiences, rather than just describing them. Various approaches to interpretive phenomenology have been developed, including **interpretive phenomenologic analysis (IPA)**, **reflective lifeworld research (RLR)**, and Parse's research methods (**humanbecoming hermeneutic sciencing** and **Parsesciencing**).
- **Phenomenography** involves gaining an understanding of the different ways in which people experience or think about a phenomenon.
- **Grounded theory** aims to discover theoretical precepts grounded in the data. Grounded theory researchers try to account for people's actions by focusing on the main concern that the behavior is designed to resolve. The manner in which people resolve this main concern is the **core variable**. The goal of grounded theory is to discover this main concern and the **basic social process (BSP)** that explains how people resolve it.
- Grounded theory uses **constant comparison**: categories elicited from the data are constantly compared with data obtained earlier.
- A controversy among grounded theory researchers concerns whether to follow the original Glaser and Strauss procedures or to use the adapted procedures of Strauss and Corbin; Glaser argued that the latter approach does not result in *grounded theories* but rather in *conceptual descriptions.*
- More recently, Charmaz's **constructivist grounded theory** has emerged as a method to emphasize interpretive aspects in which the grounded theory is constructed from shared experiences and relationships between the researcher and study participants.
- **Case studies** are intensive investigations of a single entity or a small number of entities, such as individuals, groups, organizations, or communities; such studies usually involve collecting data over an extended period. Case study designs can be **single** or **multiple**, and **holistic** or **embedded.**
- **Narrative analysis** focuses on *story* in studies in which the purpose is to explore how people make sense of events in their lives. Several different structural approaches can be used to analyze narrative data, including, for example, Burke's **pentadic dramatism.**
- **Descriptive qualitative studies** are "generic" qualitative inquiries that do not fit into any disciplinary tradition but that aim at rich description of a phenomenon. Qualitative description has been expanded into a realm called **interpretive description,** which emphasizes the importance of having a disciplinary conceptual frame, such as nursing.
- Research is sometimes conducted within an ideological perspective, and such research tends to rely primarily on qualitative research.
- **Critical theory** entails a critique of existing social structures; critical researchers strive to conduct inquiries that involve collaboration with participants and foster enlightened self-knowledge and transformation. **Critical ethnography** applies the principles of critical theory to the study of cultures.
- **Feminist research**, like critical research, is designed to be transformative; the focus is on how gender domination and discrimination shape women's lives and their consciousness.
- **Participatory action research (PAR)** produces knowledge through close collaboration with groups or communities that are vulnerable to control or oppression by a dominant social group; in PAR research, methods take second place to emergent processes that can motivate people and generate community solidarity.

REFERENCES CITED IN CHAPTER 22

Acosta, L. A., Morris McEwen, M. (2023). Post-rape experiences of undocumented Mexican women in the U.S.-Mexico border region: A critical ethnography. *Hispanic Health Care International*, *21*(1), 30–37. https://doi.org/10.1177/15404153221102797

Ahern, K. J. (1999). Ten tips for reflexive bracketing. *Qualitative Health Research*, *9*, 407–411.

Ahmed, S., Naqvi, S. F., Sinnarajah, A., McGhan, G., Simon, J., & Santana, M. J. (2023). Patient and caregiver experiences: Qualitative study comparison before and after implementation of early palliative care for advanced colorectal cancer. *Canadian Journal of Nursing Research*, *51*(1), 110125. https://doi.org/10.1177/08445621221079534

Allan, H. T. (2023). An auto-ethnographic reflection on the nature of nursing in the UK during the Covid-19 pandemic. *Health*. *27*(5), 756–769. https://doi.org/10.1177/13634593211064122

Baker, C., Wuest, J., & Stern, P. N. (1992). Method slurring: The grounded theory/phenomenology example. *Journal of Advance Nursing*, *17*(11), 1355–1360.

Barreto, M. d. S., Garcia-Vivar, C., da Silva, T. P., & Girardon-Perlini, N. M. O., & Marcon, S. S. (2022). A Corbin and Strauss grounded theory on the experiences of patients, relatives, and health professionals about the family presence during emergency care. *ANS Advances in Nursing Science*, *45*(1), E1–E14. https://doi.org/10.1097/ANS.0000000000000390

Baxter, P., & Jack, S. (2008). Qualitative case study methodology: Study design and implementation for novice researchers. *The Qualitative Report*, *13*, 544–559.

Beck, C. T. (2021). Effects of fourth-degree perineal lacerations on women's physical and mental health. *Journal of Obstetric, Gynecologic, & Neonatal Nursing*, *50*(2), 133–142. https://doi.org/10.1016/j.jogn.2020.10.009

Beck, C. T. (2023). Teetering on the edge: A third grounded theory modification of postpartum depression. *ANS Advances in Nursing Science*, *46*(1), 14–27. https://doi:10.1097/ANS.0000000000000432

Benner, P. (1994). The tradition and skill of interpretive phenomenology in studying health, illness, and caring practices. In Benner, P. (Ed.). *Interpretive phenomenology* (pp. 99–127). Sage.

Bidababi, F., Yazdannik, A., & Zargham-Boroujeni, A. (2019). Patient's dignity in intensive care unit: A critical ethnography. *Nursing Ethics*, *26*(3), 738–752.

Blanchfield, D., & O'Connor, L. (2022). A participatory action research study to inform combined type 2 diabetes and chronic kidney disease care provided in the context of advanced practice nursing. *Journal of Advanced Nursing*, *78*(10), 3427–3443. https://doi.org/10.1111/jan.15362

Bochner, A. P., & Ellis, C. (2016). *Evocative autoethnography: Writing lives and telling stories*. Routledge.

Brisolara, S., Seigart, S., & SenGupta, S. (Eds.). (2014). *Feminist evaluation and research: Theory and practice*. Guilford Press.

Bruner, J. (1991). *Acts of meaning*. Harvard University Press.

Buechel, J., Spalding, C. N., Brock, W.W., Dye, J. L., Todd, N., Wilson, C., & Fry-Bowers, E. K. (2024). A grounded theory approach to navigating infertility care during U.S. Military service. *Military Medicine*, *189*(1–2), 352–360. https://doi.org/10.1093/milmed/usac174

Burke, K. (1969). *A grammar of motives*. University of California Press.

Caiola, C., Barroso, J., & Docherty, S. (2017). Capturing the social location of African American mothers living with HIV: An inquiry into how social determinants of health are framed. *Nursing Research*, *66*(3), 209–221.

Carroll, K., & Mesman, J. (2018). Multiple researcher roles in video-reflexive ethnography. *Qual Health Res*, *28*(7), 1145–1156.

Carspecken, P. F. (1996). *Critical ethnography in educational research*. Routledge.

Chang, H. (2016). Autoethnography in health research: Growing pains? *Qualitative Health Research*, *26*(4), 443–451.

Charmaz, K. (2014). *Constructing grounded theory: A practical guide through qualitative analysis* (2nd ed.). Sage Publications.

Chevalier, J. M., & Buckles, D. J. (2019). *Participatory action research: Theory and methods for engaged inquiry*. Routldege.

Cohen, M. Z., Kahn, D., & Steeves, R. (2000). *Hermeneutic phenomenological research: A practical guide for nurse researchers*. Sage.

Colaizzi, P. F. (1973). *Reflection and research in psychology*. Kendall/Hunt Publishing Co.

Cook, K. E. (2005). Using critical ethnography to explore issues in health promotion. *Qualitative Health Research*, *15*(1), 129–138.

Corbin, J., & Strauss, A. (2015). *Basics of qualitative research: Techniques and procedures for developing grounded theory* (4th ed.). Sage Publications.

Cruz, E. V., & Higginbottom, G. (2013). The use of focused ethnography in nursing research. *Nursing Research*, *20*(4), 36–43.

Dahlberg, K., Dahlberg, H., & Nyström, M. (2008). *Reflective lifeworld research*. Studentlitteratur.

Dahlberg, H., Ranheim, A., & Dahlberg, K. (2016). Ecological caring: Revisiting the original ideas of caring science. *International Journal of Qualitative Studies on Health and Well-Being*, *11*, 33344.

Denzin, N. K. (2003). *Performance ethnography: Critical pedagogy and the politics of culture*. Sage.

Denzin, N. K., & Lincoln, Y. S. (Eds.). (2011). *Handbook of qualitative research* (4th ed.). Sage.

Detthippornpong, S., Songwathana, P., & Bourbonnais, A. (2022). Holistic health practices of rural Thai homebound older adults: A focused ethnographic study. *Journal of Transcultural Nursing*, *33*(4), 521–528. https://doi.org/10.1177/10436596221090270

Diekelmann, N. L., Allen, D., & Tanner, C. (1989). *The NLN criteria for appraisal of baccalaureate programs: A critical hermeneutic analysis*. NLN Press.

Fetterman, D. M. (2020). *Ethnography: Step by step* (4th ed.). Sage.

Gadamer, H. G. (1976). *Philosophical hermeneutics* (D. E. Linge, Ed. & Trans.). University of California Press.

Gearing, R. E. (2004). Bracketing in research: A typology. *Qualitative Health Research, 14*(10), 1429–1452.

Giorgi, A. (2009). *The descriptive phenomenological method in psychology: A modified Husserlian approach*. Duquesne University Press.

Glaser, B. (1992). *Emergence versus forcing: Basics of grounded theory analysis*. Sociology Press.

Glaser, B. (1998). *Doing grounded theory: Issues and discussions*. Sociology Press.

Glaser, B. (2001). *The grounded theory perspective: Conceptualization contrasted with description*. Sociology Press.

Glaser, B. (2003). *The grounded theory perspective II: Description's remodeling of grounded theory methodology*. Sociology Press.

Glaser, B. (2005). *The grounded theory perspective III: Theoretical coding*. Sociology Press.

Glaser, B. G., & Strauss, A. (1967). *The discovery of grounded theory: Strategies for qualitative research*. Aldine de Gruyter.

Heath, H., & Cowley, S. (2004). Developing a grounded theory approach: A comparison of Glaser and Strauss. *International Journal of Nursing Studies, 41*(2), 141–150.

Heidegger, M. (1962). *Being and time*. Harper & Row.

Heidegger, M. (1971). *Poetry, language, thought*. Harper & Row.

Hesse-Biber, S. (Ed.). (2014). *Feminist research practice: A primer* (2nd ed.). Sage Publications.

Higginbottom, G., & Lauridsen, E. (2014). The roots and development of constructivist grounded theory. *Nurse Researcher, 21*(5), 8–13.

Hogmo, B. K., Bondas, T., & Alstveit, M. (2022). Patients' experiences with public health nursing during the postnatal period: A reflective lifeworld research study. *Scandinavian Journal of Caring Science, 37*(2), 373–383. https://doi.org/10.1111/scs.13117

Hughes, S. A., & Pennington, J. L. (2017). *Autoethnography: Process, product, and possibility for critical social research*. Sage.

Husserl, E. (1962). *Ideas: General introduction to pure phenomenology*. Macmillan.

Irie, Y., Hohashi, N., Suto, S., Fujimoto, Y. (2022). Culturally congruent health activities for the prevention of functional disabilities among older adults in Japan's forest communities. *Journal of Transcultural Nursing, 33*(1), 16–25. https://doi.org/10.1177/10436596211042072

Jefferies, K., Martin-Misener, R., Murphy, G. T., Gahagan, J., & Bernard, W. T. (2022). African Nova Scotian nurses' perceptions and experiences of leadership: A qualitative study informed by Black feminist theory. *CMAJ, 194*(42), E1437–E1447. https://doi.org/10.1503/cmaj.220019

Johnston, C., Wallis, M., Oprescu, F., & Gray, M. (2017). Methodological considerations related to nurse researchers using their own experience of a phenomenon within phenomenology. *Journal of Advanced Nursing, 73*(3), 574–584.

Larsson, K., Wallroth, V., & Schröder, A. (2023). Older adults' experiences of how participating in a senior summer camp has affected their lives—a phenomenographic study. *Journal of Gerontological Social Work, 66*(3), 321–338. https://doi.org/10.1080/01634372.2022.2103763

Lather, P. (1991). *Getting smart: Feminist research and pedagogy with/in the postmodern*. Routledge.

Leininger, M. M. (Ed.). (1985). *Qualitative research methods in nursing*. Grune and Stratton.

Leininger, M. M., & McFarland, M. (2006). *Culture care diversity and universality: A worldwide nursing theory* (2nd ed.). Jones & Bartlett.

Lewis, L. F., Schirling, H., Beaudoin, E., Scheibner, H., & Cestrone, A. (2021). Exploring the birth stories of women on the autism spectrum. *Journal of Obstetric, Gynecologic, & Neonatal Nursing, 50*(6), 679–690. https://doi.org/10.1016/j.jogn.2021.08.099

Lin, S., Wang, C., Wang, Q., Xie, S., Tu, Q., Zhang, H., Peng, M., Zhou, J., & Redfern, J. (2022). The experience of stroke survivors and caregivers during hospital-to-home transitional care: A qualitative longitudinal study. *International Journal of Nursing Studies, 130*, 104213. https://doi.org/10.1016/j.ijnurstu.2022.104213

Lincoln, Y. S., & Guba, E. G. (1985). *Naturalistic inquiry*. Sage.

Liow, K. H., Ng, T. R. P., Choo, C. H., Koh, S. S. L., & Shorey, S. (2022). The experiences and support needs of women with gestational breast cancer in Singapore: A descriptive qualitative study. *Cancer Nursing, 45*(1), E263–E269. https://doi.org/10.1097/NCC.0000000000000912

Madison, D. S. (2020). *Critical ethnography: Methods, ethics, and performance* (3rd ed.). Sage.

Marton, F., & Booth, S. (1997). *Learning and awareness*. Erlbaum.

Matua, G., & Van der Wal, D. (2015). Differentiating between descriptive and interpretive phenomenological research approaches. *Nurse Researcher, 22*(6), 22–27.

Maxwell, J. (2012). The importance of qualitative research for causal explanation in education. *Qualitative Inquiry, 18*, 655–661.

McFarland, M. R., & Wehbe-Alamah, H. B. (2015). *Leininger's culture care and diversity and puniversality: A worldwide nursing theory*. Jones & Bartlett Learning.

Mertens, D. M. (2007). Transformative paradigm: Mixed methods and social justice. *Journal of Mixed Methods Research, 1*, 212–225.

Morse, J. M. (2004). Qualitative comparison: Appropriateness, equivalence, and fit. *Qualitative Health Research, 14*(10), 1323–1325.

Morse, J. M. (2009). Mixing qualitative methods. *Qualitative Health Research, 19*(11), 1523–1524.

Mutsonziwa, G. A., Green, J., & Blundell, J. (2022). A phenomenological exploration of source isolation in patients infected with multi-drug resistant organisms. *Journal of Advanced Nursing, 78*(1), 211–223. https://doi.org/10.1111/jan.15014

Nepal, V. (2010). On mixing qualitative methods. *Qualitative Health Research, 20*(2), 281.

Nkambule, E., Msosa, A., Wella, K., & Msiska, G. (2021). "This disease would suit better those who have money": Insulin-treated diabetes illness experience in rural Malawi. *Malawi Medical Journal, 33*(Postgraduate Supplementary Iss), 16–22.

Oliffe, J. L., Kelly, M. T., Gonzalez Montaner, G., Seidler, Z. E., Kealy, D., Ogrodniczuk, J. S., & Rice, S. M. (2022). Mapping men's mental health help-seeking after an intimate partner relationship break-up. *Qualitative Health Research, 32*(10), 1464–1476. https://doi.org/10.1177/10497323221110974

Parse, R. R. (2014). *The humanbecoming paradigm: A transformational worldview*. Discovery International Publication.

Parse, R. R. (2016a). Humanbecoming hermeneutic sciencing: Reverence, awe, betrayal, and shame in the lives of others. *Nursing Science Quarterly, 29*(2), 128–135.

Parse, R. R. (2016b). Parsesciencing: A basic science mode of inquiry. *Nursing Science Quarterly, 29*(4), 271–274.

Patton, M. Q. (2015). *Qualitative research & evaluation methods* (4th ed.). Sage.

Prochnow, T., Patterson, M., Umstattd Meyer, M. R., Lightner, J., Gomez, L., & Sharkey, J (2022). Conducting physical activity research on racially and ethnically diverse adolescents using social network analysis: Case studies for practical use. *International Journal of Environmental Research and Public Health, 19*(18), 11545. https://doi.org/10.3390/ijerph191811545

Rankin, J. M. (2013). Institutional ethnography. In Beck, C.T. (Ed.). *Routledge international handbook of qualitative nursing research* (pp. 242–255). Routledge.

Reding, N. (2022). The living experience of feeling peaceful. *Nursing Science Quarterly, 35*(4), 464–474. https://doi.org/10.1177/08943184221115133

Reyes, A. T. (2022). The process of learning mindfulness and acceptance through the use of a mobile app based on acceptance and commitment therapy: A grounded theory analysis. *Issues in Mental Health Nursing, 43*(1), 3–12. https://doi.org/10.1080/01612840.2021.1953652

Riessman, C. K. (1991). Beyond reductionism: Narrative genres in divorce accounts. *Journal of Narrative and Life History, 1*, 41–68.

Riessman, C. K. (1993). *Narrative analysis*. Sage Publications.

Riessman, C. K. (2008). *Narrative methods for the human sciences*. Sage.

Sandelowski, M. (2000). Whatever happened to qualitative description? *Research in Nursing & Health, 23*(4), 334–340.

Sandelowski, M. (2010). What's in a name? Qualitative description revisited. *Research in Nursing & Health, 33*(1), 77–84.

Sandelowski, M. (2011). "Casing" the research case study. *Research in Nursing & Health, 34*(2), 153–159.

Small, K.A., Sidebotham, M., Fenwick, J., & Gamble, J. (2023). The social organisation of decision-making about intrapartum fetal monitoring: An institutional ethnography. *Women Birth, 36*(3), 281–289. https://doi.org/10.1016/j.wombi.2022.09.004

Smith, D. E. (1999). *Writing the social: Critique, theory, and investigation*. University of Toronto Press.

Smith, J. A., Flowers, P., & Larkin, M. (2009). *Interpretive phenomenological analysis: Theory, method and research*. Sage Publications.

Sudarsan, I., Hoare, K., Sheridan, N., & Roberts, J. (2023). Navigating asthma-the immigrant child in a tug-of-war: A constructivist grounded theory. *Journal of Clinical Nursing, 32*(13–14), 4009–4023. https://doi.org/10.1111/jocn.16521

Thorne, S. (2008). *Interpretive description*. Left Coast Press.

Thorne, S. (2013). Interpretive description. In Beck, C. T. (Ed.). *Routledge international handbook of qualitative nursing research* (pp. 295–306). Routledge.

Traboulssi, M., Pidgeon, M., & Weathers, E. (2022). My wife has breast cancer: The lived experience of Arab men. *Seminars in Oncology Nursing, 38*(4), 151307. https://doi.org/10.1016/j.soncn.2022.151307

Van Manen, M. (1990). *Researching lived experience*. SUNY Press.

Van Manen, M. (1997). From meaning to method. *Qualitative Health Research, 7*, 345–369.

Van Manen, M. (2014). *Phenomenology of practice: Meaning-giving methods in phenomenological research and writing*. Left Coast Press.

Van Manen, M. (2017). Phenomenology in its original sense. *Qualitative & Health Research, 27*(6), 810–825.

Whiteing, N., Barr, J., & Rossi, D.M. (2022). The practice of rural and remote nurses in Australia: A case study. *Journal of Clinical Nursing, 31*(11–12), 1502–1518. https://doi.org/10.1111/jocn.16002

Wisnesky, U. D., Paul, P., Olson, J., & Dahlke, S. (2022). Perceptions and experiences of functional mobility for community-dwelling older people A focused ethnography. *International Journal of Older People Nursing, 17*(5), e12464. https://doi.org/10.1111/opn.12464

Yin, R. (2018). *Case study research: Design and methods* (6th ed.). Sage.

Zohn, J. H. (2022). The experiences of nursing students while caring for patients at risk for suicide: A descriptive phenomenology. *Nursing Education Perspectives, 43*(6), E91–E93. https://doi.org/10.1097/01.nep.0000000000000950

23 | Sampling in Qualitative Research

Learning objectives

1. Describe the logic of sampling for qualitative studies.
2. Identify and describe several types of sampling approaches in qualitative studies.
3. Compare and contrast sampling in ethnography, phenomenology, and grounded theory.
4. Describe guidelines for critically appraising qualitative sampling designs.

INTRODUCTION

In Chapter 13, we presented concepts relating to sampling in quantitative research. Sampling in qualitative studies is quite different. Qualitative studies almost always use small, nonrandom samples. This does not mean that qualitative researchers are unconcerned with the quality of their samples, but rather that they use different considerations in selecting participants who will strengthen their findings. Indeed, as Patton (2015) has noted in his widely read book on qualitative methods, "What you sample is what you have something to say about in the end" (p. 244). This chapter describes sampling approaches used by qualitative researchers.

THE LOGIC OF QUALITATIVE SAMPLING

Quantitative researchers measure attributes and study relationships in a population. A representative sample is desired in quantitative studies to enhance the likelihood that the measurements accurately reflect and can be generalized to the population. The aim of most qualitative studies, by contrast, is to discover *meaning* and to uncover multiple realities, not to generalize to a population.

Qualitative researchers begin with the following types of sampling question in mind: Who would be an information-rich data source for my study? Whom should I talk to or observe to maximize my understanding of the phenomenon? A critical first step in qualitative sampling is selecting settings with potential for information richness. As the study progresses, new sampling questions emerge: Who can confirm my understandings? Challenge my understandings? Enrich my understandings? Thus, as with the overall design in qualitative studies, sampling often is emergent and capitalizes on early findings to guide subsequent direction.

TIP Individuals are not always the *unit of analysis* in qualitative studies. Glaser and Strauss (1967) have noted that "incidents" or experiences are sometimes the basis for analysis. An information-rich informant may contribute dozens of incidents (e.g., stressful life events), and so even a small number of informants can generate a large sample for analysis.

Qualitative researchers do not articulate an explicit population to whom results are intended to be generalized, but they do establish the kinds of people who are eligible to participate in their research. A prime criterion is whether a person has experienced the phenomenon, culture, or process that is under study. Practical issues, such as costs, accessibility, and health constraints also affect who can be included in the sample.

> **Example of Eligibility Criteria in a Qualitative Study**
> In their qualitative descriptive study of perceived facilitators and barriers to sleep health among young adults with type 1 diabetes during the COVID-19 pandemic, Griggs and colleagues (2022) used the following criteria for sample inclusion: Being between the ages of 18 to 25 years, diagnosed with type 1 diabetes for at least 6 months, no other self-reported major health problems, English speaking, and not currently participating in intervention studies.

TYPES OF QUALITATIVE SAMPLING

Several different approaches to sampling in qualitative research are reviewed in this section. Despite differences, however, a few key features that characterize most sampling strategies have been distilled from an analysis of the qualitative literature (Curtis et al., 2000).

- Participants are not selected randomly. A random sample is not considered the best method of selecting people who will make good informants, that is, people who are knowledgeable, articulate, reflective, and willing to talk at length with researchers.
- Samples tend to be small and studied intensively, with each participant provided a wealth of data. Typically, qualitative studies involve fewer (and sometimes much fewer) than 50 participants.
- Sample members are not prespecified; their selection is emergent.
- Sample selection is driven largely by conceptual requirements rather than by a desire for representativeness.

Convenience Sampling

Qualitative researchers often begin with a convenience sample, which is sometimes called a *volunteer sample*. Volunteer samples are especially likely to be used when researchers need to have participants come forward and identify themselves. For example, if we wanted to study the experiences of people with frequent nightmares, we might recruit sample members by placing a notice on a bulletin board or on Internet sites, requesting people with frequent nightmares to contact us. In this situation, we would be less interested in obtaining a representative sample of people with nightmares, than in obtaining a diverse group representing various experiences with nightmares.

Sampling by convenience is easy, but it is not a preferred sampling approach, even in qualitative studies. The goal in qualitative studies is to extract the greatest possible information from the few cases in the sample, and a convenience sample may not provide the most information-rich sources. However, a convenience sample may be an economical way to begin the sampling process, relying on other strategies later.

Convenience sampling may also work well with participants who need to be recruited from a particular clinical setting or from a specific organization. Thorne (2008), however, has advised that in such situations the researcher should carefully reflect on and understand any peculiarities of the study context. In essence, researchers must consider whether participants' narrations reflect the experience of the healthcare or organizational setting to a greater extent than the experience of the phenomenon under study.

> **Example of a Convenience Sample**
> Ma and colleagues (2022) undertook a qualitative descriptive study to capture inpatients' psychological experiences with acute pancreatitis. A convenience sample of 28 patients was recruited from two tertiary hospitals in Eastern China.

Snowball Sampling

Qualitative researchers, like quantitative researchers, sometimes use snowball (or *chain*) sampling, asking early informants to refer other study participants. Snowball sampling has advantages over convenience sampling from a broad population. The first is that it may be more cost-efficient. Researchers may spend less time screening people to determine if they are appropriate for the study, for example. Furthermore, with an introduction from the referring person, researchers may have an easier time establishing a trusting relationship with new participants. Finally, researchers can more readily specify the characteristics that they want new participants to have. For example, in the study of people with nightmares, we could ask early respondents if they knew anyone else who had the same problem *and* who was verbally expressive. We could also ask for referrals to people who would add new dimensions to the sample, such as people who vary in age, race, socioeconomic status, and so on.

A weakness of this approach is that the eventual sample might be restricted to a rather small network of acquaintances. Moreover, the quality of the referrals may be affected by whether the referring sample members trusted the researcher and truly wanted to cooperate.

TIP Researchers should be careful about protecting the rights of the individuals who are referred. It is wise to suggest that early informants first check with the potential referrals to make sure they are interested in participating before their names are shared with the researcher. This is especially true if the study focuses on sensitive issues (e.g., suicide attempts).

Example of Snowball Sampling
Beagan et al. (2022) conducted a critical interpretive qualitative study on how interpersonal, institutional, and structural racism intersect in the professional experiences of racialized nurses in Canada. The sample of 13 self-identified racialized nurses was recruited primarily by snowball sampling.

Purposive Sampling

Qualitative sampling may begin with volunteer informants and may be supplemented with new participants through snowballing, but many qualitative studies eventually evolve to a purposive (or *purposeful*) sampling strategy—that is, selecting specific cases that will most benefit the study.

More than a dozen purposive sampling strategies have been identified (Patton, 2015). We briefly describe several strategies to illustrate the diverse approaches qualitative researchers have used to meet their conceptual and substantive needs—although researchers themselves do not necessarily use these labels for their sampling plans. As an organizing structure, we have adapted the typology of purposive sampling proposed by Tashakkori et al. (2021).

TIP Some qualitative researchers appear to call their sample *purposive* simply because they "purposely" selected people who have experienced the phenomenon of interest. However, exposure to the phenomenon is an eligibility criterion—the group of interest comprises people with that exposure. If the researcher then recruits *any* person with the desired experience, the sample is selected by convenience, not purposively. Purposive sampling implies an intent to choose *particular* exemplars or *types* of people who can best enhance the researcher's understanding of the phenomenon.

Example of a purposive sample
Castaldo et al. (2022) studied factors contributing to medication errors in Italian nursing students. Views of the nursing students on factors that potentially facilitated or discouraged medication error reporting were explored. A purposive sample was used to recruit 37 third-year nursing students in their final year of their bachelor's program.

Sampling for Representativeness or Comparative Value

The first broad category of purposive sampling involves two general goals: (1) sampling to find examples that are typical or representative of a broader group on a dimension of interest or (2) sampling to set up the possibility of comparisons across different types of cases on a dimension of interest.

Maximum variation sampling is the most widely used method of purposive sampling. It involves purposefully selecting people (or settings) with variation on dimensions of interest. By selecting participants with diverse backgrounds, researchers invite enrichments of and challenges to emerging conceptualizations. Maximum variation sampling might involve ensuring that people with diverse backgrounds are represented in the sample (ensuring that there are males and females, low-income, and affluent people, and so on). It might also involve deliberate attempts to include people with different viewpoints about the phenomenon under study. For example, researchers might use snowballing to ask early participants for referrals to people who hold different points of view. One major advantage of maximum variation sampling is that any common patterns emerging despite the diversity of the sample are likely to be capturing core experiences.

Maximum variation sampling is often an emergent approach: Information from initial participants helps to guide the subsequent selection of a diverse group of participants. However, there may be an advantage to having some upfront insights into the dimensions of variation that will likely prove productive. The factors that affect the health or wellness experience under scrutiny can often be anticipated or identified in advance, and having a mental list of such factors can be useful in ensuring sufficient diversity in the sample.

Example of Maximum Variation Sampling
Li and Luo (2022) undertook a qualitative study to identify the influencing factors of clinical nurses' problem-solving dilemma. A sample of 14 nurses from a tertiary hospital in China was recruited. Using maximum variation sampling, the researchers selected nurses who varied with regard to gender, education level, professional title, marital status, seniority, and administrative office.

Although maximum variation sampling is one of the most popular approaches to sampling in qualitative research, other types of purposive sampling include the following:

- **Homogeneous sampling** deliberately reduces variation and permits a more focused inquiry; researchers may use this approach if they wish to understand a particular group of people especially well.
- **Typical case sampling** involves selecting cases that illustrate or highlight what is typical, average, normal, or representative. Identifying typical cases can help the researcher understand key aspects of a phenomenon as they are manifested under ordinary circumstances.
- **Stratified purposive sampling** involves selecting participants in distinct subgroups along a single dimension (e.g., pain levels above average, average, or below average). In this approach, each "stratum" would comprise a fairly homogeneous sample.
- **Extreme (deviant) case sampling** (also called *outlier sampling*) provides opportunities for learning from the most unusual and extreme informants—cases that at least on the surface seem like "exceptions to the rule" (e.g., outstanding successes and notable failures). Most often, this approach is a supplement to other sampling strategies—extreme cases are sought to develop a richer or more nuanced understanding of the phenomenon under study.
- **Intensity sampling** is similar to extreme case sampling but with less emphasis on the extremes. Intensity samples involve information-rich cases that manifest the phenomenon of interest intensely but not as extreme or potentially distorting manifestations. The goal in intensity sampling is to select rich cases that offer *strong* examples of the phenomenon.
- **Reputational case sampling** involves selecting cases based on a recommendation of an expert or key informant. This approach, most often used in ethnographies, is useful when researchers have little information about how best to proceed with sampling and must rely on recommendations from others.

Many of these sampling strategies require that researchers have some knowledge about the study context. For example, to choose extreme cases, typical cases, or homogenous cases, researchers must have information about the range of variation of the phenomenon and how it manifests itself. Early participants may be helpful in pursuing these sampling strategies.

Sampling Special or Unique Cases

The second broad category of purposive sampling involves selecting special or unique cases. In these approaches, individual cases or a specific group of cases are the focus of the investigation. Several of these approaches are especially likely to be used in case study research.

Criterion sampling involves selecting cases that meet a predetermined criterion of importance. For example, in studying patient satisfaction with nursing care, researchers might sample only those patients whose responses to questions upon discharge expressed a complaint about nursing care. Criterion sampling has the potential for identifying and understanding cases that are fertile with experiential information on the phenomenon of interest.

Example of Criterion Sampling
Savas and colleagues (2021) explored the origin of the pain beliefs of chronic headache. The researchers used criterion sampling to obtain their sample of six chronic headache patients in Turkey.

Yin (2018), whose work on case study research is widely cited, described **revelatory case sampling.** This approach involves identifying and gaining access to a single case representing a phenomenon that was previously inaccessible to research scrutiny.

A final type of special-case sampling is **sampling of politically important cases.** This approach is used to select or search for politically sensitive cases (or sites) for analysis. Sometimes, politically salient cases or sites can enhance the visibility of a study or increase the likelihood that it has an impact. The approach sometimes is used to select *out* politically sensitive locales or individuals, to avoid attracting unwanted attention.

Sampling Sequentially

Several of the purposive strategies already described can be combined in a single study. For example, extreme case sampling could occur after an initial strategy such as maximum variation sampling. The strategies in this third broad category of purposive sampling involve a gradual, and often planned, sequence of sampling. One such strategy, theory-based or theoretical sampling, is discussed separately in the next section.

Opportunistic sampling (or *emergent sampling*) involves adding new cases to a sample based on changes in research circumstances as data are being collected or in response to new leads and opportunities that may develop in the field. As the researcher gains greater knowledge of a setting or a phenomenon, on-the-spot sampling decisions can take advantage of unfolding events. This approach, although seldom labeled as opportunistic sampling, is used often in qualitative research because of its flexible and emergent nature.

Sampling confirming and disconfirming cases tends to be used toward the end of data collection. This approach involves testing ideas and assessing the viability of emergent findings and conceptualizations with new data. **Confirming cases** are additional cases that fit researchers' conceptualizations and offer enhanced credibility, richness, and depth to the analysis and conclusions. **Disconfirming cases** (or **negative cases**) are examples that do not fit and serve to challenge researchers' interpretations. These negative cases may simply be "exceptions that prove the rule," but they may be exceptions that disconfirm earlier insights and suggest rival explanations about the phenomenon. These cases can bring to light how the original conceptualization needs to be revised or expanded.

Theoretical Sampling

Although Patton (2015) categorized theoretical sampling as a type of purposive sampling, we devote a separate section to this sampling strategy because of its importance in grounded theory. Glaser (1978) defined theoretical sampling as "the process of data collection for generating theory whereby the analyst jointly collects, codes, and analyzes his data and decides what data to collect next and where to find them, in order to develop his theory as it emerges" (p. 36). The process of sampling theoretically is guided by the developing grounded theory. Theoretical sampling is not envisioned as a single, unidirectional line. This complex sampling technique requires researchers to be involved with multiple lines and directions as they go back and forth between data and categories in the emerging theory. Theoretical sampling supports the constant comparative method that is a key feature of grounded theory research.

In Glaser's view, theoretical sampling is not the same as purposive sampling. The purpose of theoretical sampling is to discover categories and their properties and to offer interrelationships that occur in the substantive theory. "The basic question in theoretical sampling is: what groups or subgroups does one turn to next in data collection?" (Glaser, 1978, p. 36). These groups are not chosen before the research begins but only as they are needed for their theoretical relevance for developing emerging categories.

Most reports on grounded theory studies state that theoretical sampling was used. However, as noted by McCrae and Purssell (2016), many grounded theory studies do not demonstrate the use of theoretical sampling. The following example provides insights into an effective theoretical sampling strategy.

> **Example of a Theoretical Sampling**
> In their grounded theory study of disorienting grief responses among young adults with advanced cancer, Currin-McCulloch et al. (2022) used theoretical sampling to recruit 13 young adults, ages 23 to 38 years, and diagnosed with stage 3 or 4 cancer. Theoretical sampling guided the recruitment of new comparison groups that would fulfill further exploring of the physical, social, or psychological factors needed to elaborate the theory.

> **TIP** No matter what type of qualitative sampling you use, you should keep a journal or notebook to jot down ideas and reminders regarding the sampling. Memos to yourself will help you remember valuable ideas about your sample.

SAMPLE SIZE IN QUALITATIVE RESEARCH

In qualitative studies, sample size should be based on informational needs. One guiding principle that is often used is **data saturation**—that is, sampling to the point at which no new information is obtained and redundancy is achieved. The goal is to generate enough in-depth data to illuminate the patterns, categories, and dimensions of the phenomenon under study. Redundancy, and hence sample size, can be affected by the type of sampling strategy used. For example, a larger sample is likely to be needed with maximum variation sampling than with typical case sampling.

Morse (2000) noted that the number of participants needed to reach saturation depends on several factors. One factor concerns the scope of the research question: the broader the scope, the more participants likely will be needed. A broader scope may mean not only more interviews with people who have experienced the phenomenon but also a search for supplementary data sources.

Data quality can also affect sample size. If participants are good informants who can reflect on their experiences and communicate effectively, saturation can be achieved with a relatively small sample. For this reason, convenience sampling may require more cases to achieve saturation than purposive or theoretical sampling.

> **TIP** Malterud and colleagues (2016) have argued that sample size in qualitative studies should be guided by *information power* rather than saturation: the more *information* a sample holds, the fewer participants are needed. In their view, information power depends on such factors as the study aim, the use of established theory, and the quality of the data. Saunders et al. (2018) and Thorne (2020) offer that saturation may not even be the goal of all qualitative research and saturation is dependent upon the question, method, or the theory guiding the study.

Another issue that can affect sample size is the sensitivity of the phenomenon being studied. If the topic is one that is deeply personal, participants may be more reluctant to fully share their thoughts. Thus, to obtain sufficient data for a deep understanding of sensitive or controversial phenomena, more participants may be needed.

Greater amounts of data can be created by increasing the sample size, but sometimes depth and richness in the data can be achieved by longer, more intense interviews (or observations) or by going back to the same participants more than once. Multiple interviews often have the advantage of not only generating more data but also yielding better-quality data if participants are more forthcoming in later sessions because of increased trust.

Morse (2000) noted that sample size can be affected by the availability of what she called *shadowed data*. These are data from participants who are able to discuss not only their own experiences but also the experiences of others. Morse noted that shadowed data can provide researchers "with some idea of the range of experiences and the domain of the phenomena beyond the single participant's personal experience" (p. 4). Shadowed data can help inform decisions relevant to purposive and theoretical sampling.

The skills and experience of the researcher also can affect sample size. Researchers with strong interviewing or observational skills often require fewer participants because they are more successful in putting participants at ease, encouraging candor, and soliciting important revelations. Thus, students who are just starting out on a qualitative project are likely to require a larger sample size to achieve data saturation than their more experienced mentors.

One final suggestion that may be especially important for beginning researchers is to "test" whether data saturation has been achieved. Essentially, this involves adding one or two cases after achieving informational redundancy to ensure that no new information emerges.

Example of Data Saturation
Chien and Huang (2022) studied the self-care experience of advanced prostate cancer survivors who underwent androgen deprivation therapy in Taiwan. Data were collected from 13 prostate cancer survivors by face-to-face interviews. Interviews were conducted with two additional participants to confirm data saturation.

TIP Sample size estimation can create practical dilemmas if you are seeking approval or funding for a project. Patton (2015) recommended that, in a proposal, researchers should specify *minimum* samples that would reasonably be adequate for understanding the phenomenon. Additional cases can then be added, as necessary, to achieve saturation.

SAMPLING IN THE THREE MAIN QUALITATIVE TRADITIONS

There are similarities among the various qualitative traditions with regard to sampling: samples are small, probability sampling is not used, and final sampling decisions usually take place during data collection. However, there are some differences as well.

Sampling in Ethnography

Ethnographers may begin by adopting a "big net" approach—that is, mingling with and having conversations with as many members of the culture under study as possible. Although they may converse with many people, they often rely heavily on a smaller number of key informants. **Key informants** (or *cultural consultants*) are individuals who are highly knowledgeable about the culture or organization and who develop ongoing relationships with the researcher. These key informants are often the researcher's main link to the "inside."

Key informants are chosen purposively, guided by the ethnographer's informed judgments. Developing a pool of potential key informants often depends on ethnographers' prior knowledge to construct a relevant framework. For example, an ethnographer might make decisions about different types of key informants to seek out based on roles (e.g., physicians, nurse practitioners) or on some other substantively meaningful distinction. Once a pool of potential key informants is developed, the primary considerations for final selection are the informants' level of knowledge about the culture and their willingness to collaborate with the ethnographer in revealing and interpreting the culture.

TIP It is prudent not to choose key informants too quickly. The first participants who volunteer to be key informants may be atypical members of the culture being studied. If ethnographers align themselves with marginal members of the culture, this may prevent gaining access to other valuable informants (Bernard, 2018).

Sampling in ethnography typically involves more than selecting informants because observation and other means of data collection play an important role in helping researchers understand a culture. Ethnographers have to decide not only *whom* to sample but *what* to sample as well. For example, ethnographers need to make decisions about observing *events* and *activities*, about examining *records* and *artifacts*, and about exploring *places* that provide clues about the culture. Key informants can play an important role in helping ethnographers decide what to sample.

Sampling in Phenomenologic Studies

Phenomenologists tend to rely on very small samples—typically 10 to 15 participants. One key principle guides sample selection for a phenomenologic study: all participants must have experienced the phenomenon and must be able to articulate what it is like to have lived that experience. Although phenomenologic researchers seek participants who have had the targeted experiences, they also want to explore diversity of individual experiences. Thus, they may specifically look for people with demographic or other differences who have shared a common experience.

> **Example of a Sample in a Phenomenologic Study**
> Sun and colleagues (2022) conducted a descriptive phenomenological study to explore parents' perspectives on hospitals' care and management of the remains of their stillborn babies. The researchers used purposive sampling to recruit 20 couples of stillborn infants.

Sampling in Grounded Theory Studies

Grounded theory research is typically done with samples of about 20 to 30 people, using theoretical sampling. The goal in a grounded theory study is to select informants who can best contribute to the evolving theory. Sampling, data collection, data analysis, and theory construction occur concurrently. Study participants are selected serially and contingently (i.e., contingent on the emerging conceptualization). Sampling might evolve as follows:

1. The researcher begins with a general notion of where and with whom to start. The first few cases may be solicited purposively, by convenience, or through snowballing.
2. In the early part of the study, a strategy such as maximum variation sampling might be used, to gain insights into the range and complexity of the phenomenon under study.
3. The sample is adjusted in an ongoing fashion. Emerging conceptualizations help to inform the theoretical sampling process.
4. Sampling continues until saturation is achieved.
5. Final sampling may include a search for confirming and disconfirming cases to test, refine, and strengthen the theory.

> **Example of a Sample in a Grounded Theory Study**
> Avilés and colleagues (2022) studied families' experiences in Chile when being approached for organ donation authorization after brainstem death. The participants included 71 families and healthcare professionals. At first purposive sampling was used and then the researchers changed to theoretical sampling to compare experiences and practices in a second hospital.

TRANSFERABILITY

Qualitative researchers seldom worry explicitly about generalizability. The goal of most qualitative studies is to provide a contextualized understanding of human experience through the intensive study of a few cases. Sampling decisions are not guided by a desire to generalize to a target population.

Yet, in our evidence-based practice environment, the issue of applying research findings beyond the particular people who took part in a study is important. Indeed, Groleau and colleagues (2009), in discussing generalizability, have argued that an important goal of qualitative studies is to shape the opinion of decision-makers whose actions affect people's health and well-being. They noted that "it is not qualitative data itself that must have a direct impact on decision makers but the insights they foster in relation to the problem under investigation" (p. 418). Many scholars who have written about generalizability in qualitative research attempt to find a balance between the generalizable and the particular through *reasonable extrapolation*.

Firestone (1993) developed a useful typology depicting three models of generalizability. The first model is extrapolating from a sample to a population, the model on which sampling in quantitative research is based, as discussed in Chapter 13. The second model is analytic or conceptual generalization, and the third is case-to-case translation, which is more often referred to as transferability—both of which have relevance for qualitative research. In **analytic generalization**, the goal is to generalize from the particulars to a broader theory. Case-to-case translation (**transferability**) involves judgments about whether findings from an inquiry can be extrapolated to a different setting or group of people. **Thick description**—richly thorough depictions of research settings and the sample of study participants (or events)—is needed in qualitative reports to support transferability.

CRITICAL APPRAISAL OF QUALITATIVE SAMPLING PLANS

Qualitative researchers do not always fully describe their method of identifying, recruiting, and selecting participants. Yet, readers will have difficulty drawing conclusions about the study findings without understanding researchers' sampling strategies. Indeed, there have been increased demands for making sampling decisions and processes in qualitative research more "public" (Onwuegbuzie & Leech, 2007). To facilitate transferability, qualitative reports should ideally describe the following:

- The type of sampling approach used (e.g., snowball, purposive, theoretical), together with an indication of how variation was dealt with (for example, in maximum variation sampling, the dimensions chosen for diversification);
- Eligibility criteria for inclusion in the study;
- The nature of the setting or community;
- The time period during which data were collected;
- The number of participants, and a rationale for the sample size, such as an explicit statement that data saturation was achieved; and
- The main characteristics of participants (e.g., age, gender, length of illness, and so forth).

Inadequate description of the sampling strategy can undermine assessments of the strategy's success. Moreover, if the description is vague, it will be difficult for readers to reach conclusions about whether the evidence can be applied in their clinical practice. In appraising a report, you should evaluate whether the researcher provided an adequately rich description of the sample and the context in which the study was carried out so that someone interested in transferring the findings could make an informed decision.

Various writers have proposed criteria for evaluating sampling in qualitative studies. Morse (1991), for example, advocated two criteria: adequacy and appropriateness. *Adequacy* refers to the sufficiency and quality of the data the sample yielded. An adequate sample provides data without "thin" spots. When the researcher has truly obtained data saturation, the resulting description or theory is richly textured and complete.

Appropriateness concerns the methods used to select a sample. An appropriate sample is one resulting from the identification and use of participants who can best supply information according to the conceptual requirements of the study. Researchers should use a strategy that yields the fullest possible understanding of the phenomenon of interest. A sampling approach that excludes negative cases or that fails to include participants with unusual experiences may not meet the information needs of the study.

Curtis and colleagues (2000) proposed six criteria for evaluating qualitative sampling strategies. These criteria are as relevant for a self-evaluation by qualitative researchers as for an appraisal by readers. First, the sampling strategy should be relevant to the tradition, conceptual framework, and research question addressed by the research. Second, the sample should yield rich information on the phenomenon under study. Third, the sample should enhance the analytic generalizability of the findings. Fourth, the sample should produce believable descriptions, in the sense of being true to real life. Fifth, the strategy should be ethical. Finally, the sampling plan should be feasible in terms of resources, time, and researcher's skills—and the researcher's or participants' ability to cope with the data collection process.

Some specific questions that can be used to critically appraise sampling in a qualitative study are presented in Box 23.1.

BOX 23.1 Guidelines for Critically Appraising Qualitative Sampling Designs

1. Is the setting or context adequately described? Is the setting appropriate for the research question? Is there an explanation of why the setting was chosen?
2. Are the sample selection procedures clearly delineated? What type of sampling strategy was used?
3. Were the eligibility criteria for the study specified? How were participants recruited into the study? Did the recruitment strategy yield information-rich participants?
4. Given the information needs of the study—and, if applicable, its qualitative tradition—was the sampling approach appropriate? Are dimensions of the phenomenon under study adequately represented?
5. Is the sample size adequate and appropriate for the qualitative tradition of the study? Did the researcher indicate that saturation had been achieved?
6. Do the findings suggest a richly textured and comprehensive set of data without any apparent "holes" or thin areas? Did the sample contribute sufficiently to analytic generalization?
7. Are key characteristics of the sample described (e.g., age, gender)? Is a rich description of participants and context provided, allowing for an assessment of the transferability of the findings?

RESEARCH EXAMPLE

Examples of various approaches to sampling in qualitative research have been presented throughout this chapter. In this section, we describe more fully the sampling plan used in an ethnographic study.

Study: Care and rearing of institutionalized girls in Arequipa, Peru: An ethnographic approach (Sánchez-Luque et al., 2022)

Purpose: The researchers sought to understand the care and upbringing of institutionalized girls in a Catholic childcare organization in Peru.

Method: The researchers used an ethnographic approach to obtain a comprehensive understanding of the care and upbringing of institutionalized girls. Data were collected mainly through participant observation and semistructured interviews during a 2-month period.

Sampling Strategy: The main participants of the study were 27 girls between 5 and 17 years of age. The researchers' sampling included two female professional caregivers in their forties who had been hired by the institution for supervision, assistance with meals, and taking the girls to and from school. Also included in the sample were two young women (supporters) who were former institutionalized girls themselves and whose role was for general assistance. Lastly, the sampling included two volunteers who arrived at the institution during data collection.

Key Findings: Five main themes were identified: (1) The little house (foster home) is better than my house, (2) They take care of me—even when I am sick, (3) But... the care of the volunteers had an expiration date, (4) What I have lived is what I am, and (5) Happiness fits in the casita.

SUMMARY POINTS

- Qualitative researchers use the conceptual demands of the study to select articulate and reflective informants with certain types of experience in an emergent way, typically capitalizing on early learning to guide subsequent sampling decisions. Qualitative samples tend to be small, nonrandom, and intensively studied.
- Sampling in qualitative inquiry may begin with a convenience (or *volunteer*) sample. Snowball (*chain*) sampling may also be used.
- Qualitative researchers often use **purposive sampling** to select data sources that enhance information richness. Various purposive sampling strategies have been used by qualitative researchers and can be loosely categorized as (1) sampling for representativeness or comparative value; (2) sampling special or unique cases; or (3) sampling sequentially.

- An important purposive strategy in the first category is **maximum variation sampling,** which entails purposely selecting cases with a range of variation. Other strategies used for comparative purposes include **homogeneous sampling** (deliberately reducing variation), **typical case sampling** (selecting cases that illustrate what is typical), **extreme case sampling** (selecting the most unusual or extreme cases), **intensity sampling** (selecting cases that are intense but not extreme), **stratified purposeful sampling** (selecting cases within defined strata), and **reputational case sampling** (selecting cases based on a recommendation of an expert or key informant).
- Purposive sampling in the "special cases" category includes **criterion sampling** (studying cases that meet a predetermined criterion of importance), **revelatory case sampling** (identifying and gaining access to a case representing a phenomenon that was previously inaccessible to research scrutiny), and **sampling politically important cases** (searching for and selecting or deselecting politically sensitive cases or sites).
- Although many qualitative sampling strategies unfold while in the field, purposive sampling in the "sequential" category involves deliberative emergent efforts and includes **theoretical sampling** (selecting cases based on their contribution to important constructs) and **opportunistic sampling** (adding new cases based on changes in research circumstances or in response to new leads that develop in the field). Another important sequential strategy is **sampling confirming and disconfirming cases**—that is, selecting cases that enrich or challenge the researchers' conceptualizations.
- A guiding sample size principle is **data saturation**—sampling to the point at which no new information is obtained and redundancy is achieved. Factors affecting sample size include data quality, researcher skills and experience, and scope and sensitivity of the problem.
- Ethnographers make numerous sampling decisions, including not only *whom* to sample but *what* to sample (e.g., activities, events, documents, artifacts); **key informants,** who serve as guides and interpreters of the culture, often assist with sampling decisions.
- Phenomenologists typically work with a small sample of people (15 or fewer) who meet the criterion of having lived the experience under study.
- Grounded theory researchers typically use *theoretical sampling* in which sampling decisions are guided in an ongoing manner by the emerging theory. Samples of about 20 to 30 people are typical in grounded theory studies.
- Two models of generalizability have relevance for qualitative research. In **analytic generalization**, researchers strive to generalize from particulars to broader conceptualizations and theories. **Transferability** involves judgments about whether findings from an inquiry can be extrapolated to a different setting or group of people. **Thick description**—richly thorough depictions of research settings and participants—is needed in qualitative reports to support transferability.

REFERENCES CITED IN CHAPTER 23

Avilés, L., Kean, S., & Tocher, J. (2023). Ambiguous loss in organ donor families: A constructivist grounded theory. *Journal of Clinical Nursing, 32*(17–18), 6504–6518. https://doi.org/10.1111/jocn.16574

Babadağ Savaş, B., Balcı Alparslan, G., & Gülec, S. (2021). Pain beliefs of chronic headache patients. *Agri, 33*(2),103–115. https://doi.org/10.14744/agri.2020.02212

Beagan, B. L., Bizzeth, S. R., & Etowa, J. (2023). Interpersonal, institutional, and structural racism in Canadian nursing: A culture of silence. *Canadian Journal of Nursing Research, 55*(2), 195–205. https://doi.org/10.1177/08445621221110140

Bernard, H. R. (2018). *Research methods in anthropology: Qualitative and quantitative approaches* (6th ed.). AltaMira Press.

Castaldo, A., Ferrentino, M., Ferrario, E., Papini, M., & Lusignani, M. (2022). Factors contributing to medication errors: A descriptive qualitative study of Italian nursing students. *Nurse Education Today, 118,* 105511. https://doi.org/10.1016/j.nedt.2022.105511

Chien, C. H., & Huang, X. Y. (2022). Self-care experiences of advanced prostate cancer survivors who underwent androgen deprivation therapy. *Cancer Nursing, 45*(3), 190–200. https://doi.org/10.1097/ncc.0000000000000933

Currin-McCulloch, J., Kaushik, S., & Jones, B. (2022). "When will I feel normal?" *Cancer Nursing*, *45*(2), E355–E363. https://doi.org/10.1097/ncc.0000000000000977

Curtis, S., Gesler, W., Smith, G., & Washburn, S. (2000). Approaches to sampling and case selection in qualitative research: Examples in the geography of health. *Social Science & Medicine*, *50*(7–8), 1001–1014.

Firestone, W. A. (1993). Alternative arguments for generalizing from data as applied to qualitative research. *Educational Researcher*, *22*, 16–23.

Glaser, B. (1978). *Theoretical sensitivity*. The Sociology Press.

Glaser, B. G., & Strauss, A. (1967). *The discovery of grounded theory: Strategies for qualitative research*. Aldine de Gruyter.

Griggs, S., Harper, A., Pignatiello, G., & Hickman, R. L. (2022). "Feeling anxious about catching COVID": Facilitators and barriers of sleep health among young adults with type 1 diabetes. *Behavioral Sleep Medicine*, *20*(3), 357–367. https://doi.org/10.1080/15402002.2022.2032711

Groleau, D., Zelkowitz, P., & Cabral, I. (2009). Enhancing generalizability: Moving from an intimate to a political voice. *Qualitative Health Research*, *19*(3), 416–426.

Li, Y. M., & Luo, Y. F. (2022). The influencing factors of clinical nurses' problem solving dilemma: A qualitative study. *International Journal of Qualitatives Studies on Health and Well-being*, *17*(1), 2122138. https://doi.org/10.1080/17482631.2022.2122138

Ma, S., Yang, X., He, H., Gao, Y., Chen, Y., Qin, J., Zhang, C., Lu, G., Gong, W., Chen, W., & Ren, Y. (2022). Psychological experience of inpatients with acute pancreatitis: A qualitative study. *BMJ*, *12*(6), e060107. https://doi.org/10.1136/bmjopen-2021-060107

McCrae, N., & Purssell, E. (2016). Is it really theoretical? A review of sampling in grounded theory studies in nursing journals. *Journal of Advanced Nursing*, *72*(10), 2284–2293.

Morse, J. M. (1991). Strategies for sampling. In Morse, J. M., (Ed.), *Qualitative nursing research: A contemporary dialogue*. Sage.

Morse, J. M. (2000). Determining sample size. *Qualitative Health Research*, *10*, 3–5.

Onwuegbuzie, A., & Leech, N. (2007). Sampling designs in qualitative research: Making the sampling process more public. *The Qualitative Report*, *12*, 238–254.

Patton, M. Q. (2015). *Qualitative research and evaluation methods* (4th ed.). Sage.

Sánchez-Luque, B., Martìnez-Angulo, P., Cantón-Habas, V., & Ventura-Puertos, P. E. (2022). Care and rearing of institutionalized girls in Arequipa, Peru: An ethnographic approach. *Journal of Transcultural Nursing*, *33*(2), 190–198. https://doi.org/10.1177/10436596211057898

Saunders, B., Sim, J., Kingstone, T., Baker, S., Waterfield, J., Bartlam, B., Burroughs, H., & Jinks, C. (2018). Saturation in qualitative research: Exploring its conceptualization and operationalization. *Quality & Quantity*, *52*(4), 1893–1907. https://doi.org/10.1007/s11135-017-0574-8

Sun, J.C., Rei, W., Chang, M. Y., & Sheu, S. J. (2022). Care and management of stillborn babies from the parents' perspective: A phenomenological study. *Journal of Clinical Nursing*, *31*(7–8), 860-868. https://doi.org/10.1111/jocn.15936

Tashakkori, A., Johnson, R. B., & Teddlie, C (2021). *Foundations of mixed methods research* (2nd ed.). Sage Publications.

Thorne, S. (2008). *Interpretive description*. Left Coast Press.

Thorne, S. (2020). The great saturation debate: What the "S Word" means and doesn't mean in qualitative research reporting. *The Canadian Journal of Nursing Research*, *52*(1), 3–5. https://doi.org/10.1177/0844562119898554

Yin, R. (2018). *Case study research and application: Design and methods* (6th ed.). Sage.

24 Data Collection in Qualitative Research

Learning objectives

1. Describe some data collection issues in qualitative studies.
2. Compare and contrast data collection in ethnography, phenomenology, and grounded theory.
3. Identify and describe methods of collecting and recording unstructured self-report data.
4. Identify and describe methods of collecting and recording unstructured observational data.
5. Describe guidelines for critically appraising unstructured data collection methods.

INTRODUCTION

This chapter provides an overview of data collection approaches used in qualitative research, with a focus on self-reports and observations.

DATA COLLECTION ISSUES IN QUALITATIVE STUDIES

In qualitative studies, data collection usually is more fluid than in quantitative research; decisions about types of information to collect evolve in the field. For example, as researchers gather and digest their data, they may realize that it would be fruitful to pursue a new line of questioning. Even while allowing for and profiting from this flexibility, however, qualitative researchers make several up-front decisions about data collection, and need to be prepared for problematic situations that may arise in the field.

Types of Data for Qualitative Studies

Qualitative researchers typically begin a study knowing the most likely sources of data, while not ruling out other possible sources that might come to light as data collection progresses. The primary method of collecting qualitative data is by interviewing study participants. Observation is used in many qualitative studies as well. Physiologic data are rarely collected in a constructivist inquiry, except perhaps to describe participants' characteristics or to ascertain eligibility for the study.

Table 24.1 compares the types of data used by researchers in the three main qualitative traditions, as well as other aspects of the data collection process for each tradition. Ethnographers typically collect a wide array of data, with observation and interviews being the primary methods. Ethnographers also examine products of the culture under study, such as documents, artifacts, photographs, and so on. Phenomenologists and grounded theory researchers rely primarily on in-depth interviews, although observation and documents may also play a role in grounded theory studies.

Field Issues in Qualitative Studies

Collecting qualitative data often gives rise to several important concerns, which are particularly salient

TABLE 24.1 • Comparison of Data Collection Issues in Three Qualitative Traditions

ISSUE	ETHNOGRAPHY	PHENOMENOLOGY	GROUNDED THEORY
Types of data	Primarily observation and interviews, plus artifacts, documents, photographs, genealogies, maps, social network diagrams	Primarily in-depth interviews, sometimes diaries, other written materials	Primarily individual interviews, sometimes group interviews, observation, participant journals, documents
Unit of data collection	Cultural systems	Individuals	Individuals
Data collection points	Mainly longitudinal	Mainly cross-sectional	Cross-sectional or longitudinal
Length of time for data collection	Typically long, many months or years	Typically moderate	Typically moderate
Data recording	Field notes, logs, interview notes/recordings	Interview notes/recordings	Interview notes/recordings, memoing, observational notes
Salient field issues	Gaining entrée, reactivity, determining a role, learning how to participate, encouraging candor and other interview logistics, loss of objectivity, premature exit, reflexivity	Bracketing one's views, building rapport, encouraging candor, listening while preparing what to ask next, keeping "on track," handling emotionality	Building rapport, encouraging candor, listening while preparing what to ask next, keeping "on track," handling emotionality

in ethnographies. Ethnographic researchers must deal with such issues as gaining entrée, negotiating for space and privacy for interviewing and recording data, deciding on an appropriate role (i.e., the extent to which they will participate in the culture's activities), and taking care not to exit from the field prematurely. Ethnographers also need to be able to cope with culture shock and should have a high tolerance for uncertainty and ambiguity. Other field issues apply to most qualitative research.

Gaining Trust

Qualitative researchers must gain and maintain a high level of trust with participants and strive to achieve *empathic neutrality*. This may be a delicate balancing act: researchers must try to "be like" the people being studied while at the same time keeping a certain distance. "Being like" participants means that researchers should be sensitive to such issues as styles of dress, modes of speech, and customs. In ethnographic research, it is important not to take sides on any controversial issue and not to appear strongly affiliated with a particular subgroup of the culture—especially with leaders or prominent members of the culture. It is often impossible to gain the trust of the larger group if researchers appear close to those in power.

Preparing for the Intensity of Data Collection

In qualitative studies, data collection can be an intense and exhausting experience, especially if the phenomenon being studied is an illness experience or other stressful life event (e.g., domestic violence). Petty (2017) has written about "emotion work" in qualitative inquiry, referring to qualitative researchers' emotional responses in exploring difficult experiences. Collecting high-grade qualitative data requires deep concentration and energy. The process can be an emotional strain for which researchers need to prepare—Petty refers to this as cultivating "emotional intelligence." One way to deal with this is to collect data at a pace that minimizes stress (e.g., one interview a day) and to engage in emotionally releasing activities (e.g., exercising) between interviews. It may also be helpful to debrief about any feelings of distress with a coresearcher, colleague, or advisor.

Emotional Involvement With Participants

Qualitative researchers need to guard against getting too emotionally involved with participants, a pitfall that has been called "**going native**." Researchers who get too close to participants run several risks, including compromising their ability to collect meaningful and trustworthy data, and becoming overwhelmed with participants' suffering. It is important, of course, to be supportive and to listen carefully to people's concerns, but it usually is not advisable to try to solve participants' problems or to share personal problems with them. If participants need help, it is better to give advice about where they can get it than to give it directly.

Reflexivity

As noted in Chapter 8, reflexivity is an important concept in qualitative data collection. Reflexivity refers to researchers' awareness of themselves as part of the data they are collecting. Researchers need to be conscious of the part they play in their own study and reflect on how their own experiences can affect the data they obtain. McNair and colleagues (2008) have discussed how reflexivity can be used to enhance in-depth interviewing skills.

> **Example of Reflexivity**
> Hantke and colleagues (2022) undertook a qualitative study to increase understanding of how whiteness gets performed by nursing faculty and poses antiracism education as a necessary tool to address systemic racism in Canadian healthcare. The first author is a white settler cisgender woman. She worked under the supervision of the other two authors who were Indigenous scholars. The first author used reflexivity to examine her judgments and preconceptions under the mentorship of the Indigenous scholars to mitigate the risks of perpetuating settler colonialism.

Recording and Storing Qualitative Data

In addition to thinking about the types of data to be gathered, qualitative researchers need to plan for how data will be recorded and stored. To ensure that interview data are participants' actual verbatim responses, qualitative interviews should be recorded and subsequently transcribed rather than relying on interviewer notes. Notes tend to be incomplete and may be affected by the interviewer's personal views or by memory lapses. Moreover, note-taking can distract interviewers, whose main job is to listen intently and direct the flow of questioning based on what has already been said.

> **TIP** In addition to traditional audio-recording equipment, new technologies are emerging to facilitate recording in the field. For example, digital voice recorders with transcription capabilities allow researchers to record and transfer voice data to a personal computer using a USB interface or Bluetooth connectivity. Some digital voice recorders come bundled with voice recognition software. A recent innovation is the *smartpen*—a ballpoint pen with an embedded computer and digital audio recorder—that can record up to 200 hours of audio. When used with *digital paper*, the smartpen records written material for uploading to a computer and synchronizes the notes with any material that was audio-recorded. There are smartpens that can integrate with the cloud, enabling the automatic upload of notes to cloud-based storage systems.

Environmental distractions are a common pitfall in recording interviews. A quiet setting without disruptions is ideal but is not always possible. The second author of this book (Beck) has conducted many challenging interviews. As an example, a mother of three children was interviewed in her home about her experience with postpartum depression. The interview was scheduled during the toddlers' normal naptime, but when Beck arrived, the toddlers had already taken their nap. The television was on to occupy the toddlers, but they kept trying to play with the audio recorder. The 6-week-old baby was fussy, crying through most of the interview. The background noise level on the recording made accurate transcription difficult.

> **TIP** Many researchers use their smartphones to record interviews, which requires special precautions to ensure the security of the interviews. There are special cell phone apps that can encrypt the interview data. Without special encryption, the interviews should be transferred from a cell phone to a secure device as soon as possible and deleted from the cell phone.

When observations are made, detailed observational notes must be maintained, unless it is possible to video-record. Observational notes should be made shortly after an observational session, usually onto a computer file. Whatever method is used to record observations, researchers need to go into the field with the equipment or supplies needed to record their data and to be sure that the equipment is functioning properly.

Grounded theory (and other) researchers write **analytic memos** that document researchers' ideas about their analyses (e.g., how some categories are interrelated). These memos can vary in length from a sentence to multiple pages. Charmaz (2014) offers guidance on preparing grounded theory notes and memos.

If assistants are used to conduct interviews, qualitative researchers need to hire appropriate staff and train them to elicit rich and vivid descriptions. Qualitative interviewers need to be good listeners; they need to hear all that is being said, rather than trying to anticipate what is coming next. A good data collector must be self-aware and attentive to participants (e.g., paying attention to nonverbal behavior). Qualitative data collectors must be able to create an atmosphere that safely allows for the sharing of experiences and feelings. Respect and authentic caring for participants are critical.

> **TIP** In qualitative studies, data are sometimes collected by a single researcher working alone. In such cases, self-training and self-preparation are important. When a team of researchers works together on a qualitative study, attention needs to be paid to team issues related to fieldwork and to group decision-making.

QUALITATIVE SELF-REPORT TECHNIQUES

Unstructured or loosely structured self-report methods provide narrative data for qualitative analysis. Most qualitative self-report data are collected through interviews rather than by self-administered questionnaires.

Types of Qualitative Self-Reports

Researchers use various approaches in collecting qualitative self-report data. The main methods are described here.

Unstructured Interviews

Researchers who do not have preconceived views of the content or flow of information to be gathered may conduct completely **unstructured interviews**. Unstructured interviews are conversational and are the mode of choice when researchers do not have a clear idea of what it is they do not know. Researchers using unstructured interviews do not have a set of prepared questions because they do not yet know what to ask or even where to begin—they let participants tell their stories, with little interruption. Phenomenologic, grounded theory, and ethnographic studies may involve unstructured interviews, especially at the outset.

Researchers using a completely unstructured approach often begin by informally asking a broad question (a **grand tour question**) relating to the research topic, such as, "What happened when you first learned you had AIDS?" Subsequent questions are more focused, guided by responses to the broad question. Some respondents may request direction after the initial question is posed, perhaps asking, "Where should I begin?" Respondents should be encouraged to begin wherever they wish.

Van Manen (1990) provided suggestions for guiding a phenomenologic interview in a manner likely to produce rich descriptions of the experience under study:

- "Describe the experience from the inside, as it were; almost like a state of mind: the feelings, the mood, the emotions, etc.

- Focus on a particular example or incident of the object of experience: describe specific events, an adventure, a happening, a particular experience.
- Try to focus on an example of the experience which stands out for its vividness, or as it was the first time.
- Attend to how the body feels, how things smell(ed), how they sound(ed), etc." (pp. 64–65).

Kahn (2000), discussing unstructured interviews in hermeneutic studies, recommended interviews that resemble conversations. If the experience under study is an ongoing one, Kahn suggested obtaining as much detail as possible about the participant's daily life. For example, a question that can be used is, "Pick a normal day for you and tell me what happened" (p. 62). If the experience being studied is primarily in the past, then Kahn advocated beginning with a general question such as, "What does this experience mean to you?" (p. 63) and then probing for more detail until the experience is thoroughly described.

Example of Unstructured Interviews
Pourgholam and colleagues (2022) studied the experiences of paternalistic care behavior with seven patients who had been hospitalized in hospitals. The data were collected over an 8-month period using unstructured interviews. Each interview started with a general question, "What is your experience of nursing care?" and followed with other open-ended questions. In these in-depth interviews researchers asked follow-up questions such as, "May you explain more about this?"

In grounded theory, questioning changes as the theory is developed. At the outset, interviews are similar to open-ended conversations using unstructured interviews. Glaser and Strauss (1967) suggested researchers initially should just sit back and listen to participants' stories. Later, as the theory emerges, researchers ask more direct questions related to categories in the grounded theory. The more direct questions can be answered rather quickly, and so the interviews tend to get shorter as the grounded theory develops.

Ethnographic interviews are also unstructured. Spradley (1979) describes three types of questions used to guide interviews: descriptive, structural, and contrast questions. *Descriptive questions* ask participants to describe their experiences in their own language and are the backbone of ethnographic interviews. *Structural questions* are more focused and help to develop the range of terms in a category or domain. Last are *contrast questions*, which are asked to distinguish differences in the meaning of terms and symbols.

Example of Ethnographic Interviewing
Farzi and colleagues (2022) conducted an ethnographic study to gain an understanding of the communication culture in nursing care of patients with cancer. The study was based on Spradley's ethnographic method that included descriptive, structural, and contrast questions in sequence when interviewing.

Semistructured Interviews

Researchers sometimes want to be sure that a specific set of topics is covered in their qualitative interviews. They know what they want to ask but cannot predict what the answers will be. Their role in the process is somewhat structured, whereas the participants' is not. In such **focused** or **semistructured interviews**, researchers prepare a written **topic guide**, which is a list of areas or questions to be covered with each participant. The interviewer's job is to encourage participants to talk freely about all the topics on the guide and to tell stories in their own words. This technique ensures that researchers will obtain all the information required and yet gives people the freedom to provide as many illustrations and explanations as they wish.

In preparing a topic guide, questions should be ordered in a logical sequence—perhaps chronologically or perhaps from the general to the specific. Interviewers need to be attentive, however, because respondents often volunteer information about questions that are later on the list. The topic guide might include suggestions for *probes* designed to elicit more detailed information. Examples of such probes include, "What happened next?" and "When that happened, how did you feel?" Questions that require one- or two-word responses, such as "yes" or "no," should be avoided. Questions should give people an opportunity to provide rich, detailed information about the phenomenon under study.

McIntosh and Morse (2015) have described different types of semistructured interviews.

> **Example of Semistructured Interviews**
> Choi and colleagues (2022) conducted a qualitative interpretive study to understand what matters most to older adults in Canada. Eleven older adults were interviewed using a semistructured interview guide of seven open-ended questions such as "If you had a magic wand, is there anything you would want to change in your life?" and "What are things that you do every day that are important to you?"

Focus Group Interviews

Focus group interviews have become popular in the study of health problems. In a focus group interview, a group of people (usually five or more) is assembled for a discussion, although some focus group discussions are conducted online. The interviewer (or **moderator**) guides the discussion according to a written set of questions or topics to be covered, as in a semistructured interview. Focus group sessions are carefully planned discussions that take advantage of group dynamics and synergies for accessing rich information in an economical manner.

Typically, the people selected are fairly homogeneous, to promote a comfortable group dynamic. People usually feel more at ease expressing their views when they share a similar background with other group members. Thus, if the overall sample is diverse, it is best to organize focus groups for people with similar characteristics (e.g., in terms of age or gender). Several writers have suggested that the optimal group size for focus groups is 6 to 12 people, but some have advised even smaller groups when the topic is emotionally charged or sensitive.

> **TIP** In recruiting group members, it is usually wise to recruit one or two more people than is considered optimal, because of the risk of no-shows. Monetary incentives can help reduce this risk. It is also important to call recruits the night before the session to confirm attendance.

Moderators play a critical role in the success of focus group interviews. At the start of a session, moderators establish some ground rules with the participants. For example, they might advise participants to please speak one at a time, to be respectful of each other, and to maintain the confidentiality of what is said in the group. Moderators must take care to solicit input from all group members and not let a few vocal people dominate the discussion. Researchers other than the moderator should be present to take detailed observational notes about each session.

A major advantage of a group format is that it is efficient—researchers obtain the viewpoints of many people in a short time. Moreover, focus groups capitalize on the fact that members react to what is being said by others, thereby potentially leading to deeper expressions of opinion. Focus group interviews are also usually stimulating to respondents, but one problem is that some people are uncomfortable about communicating their views in front of a group. Another concern is that the dynamics of the session may foster a group culture that could inhibit individual expression as "group think" takes hold. Studies of focus groups suggest that they are similar to individual interviews in terms of number and quality of ideas generated (Kidd & Parshall, 2000), but some critics have worried about whether data from focus groups are as "natural" as data obtained from individual interviews (Morgan, 2001).

The researcher's *questioning route*—the series of questions used to guide the interview—is key to effective focus group sessions. A typical 2-hour focus group session should include about 12 questions. Krueger and Casey (2015) provided these guidelines for developing a good questioning route:

1. Brainstorm.
2. Sequence the questioning. Arrange general questions first and then more specific questions. Ask positive questions before negative ones.
3. Phrase the questions. Use open-ended questions. Ask participants to think back and reflect on their personal experiences. Avoid asking "why" questions. Keep questions simple and make your questions sound conversational. Be careful about giving examples.
4. Estimate the time for each question. Consider the following when estimating time: the complexity of the questions, the category of questions, level

of participant's expertise, the size of the focus group, and the amount of discussion you want related to the question.
5. Obtain feedback from others.
6. Revise the questions.
7. Test the questions.

Rothwell and colleagues (2016) have proposed a *deliberative discussion* approach to certain types of focus group studies. In such studies, researchers develop methods of educating and informing participants about the focal topic prior to the group interview. They argue that this approach can "promote more quality data from informed opinions" (p. 734).

Focus groups have been used by researchers in many qualitative research traditions and can play a role in feminist, critical theory, and participatory action research. Nurse researchers have offered excellent guidance on studies with focus groups (e.g., Carey, 2016; Côté-Arsenault, 2013), and books on how to do focus group research are available (e.g., Krueger & Casey, 2015).

Example of Focus Group Interviews
Agénor and an interprofessional team (2022) studied the specific and unique sexual and reproductive healthcare experiences of transmasculine young adults of color. They conducted five focus groups with 19 Black, Latinx, Asian, Native, and other transmasculine people of color. The focus group discussion guide included the following topics: sources of sexual and reproductive health information, sexual and reproductive health beliefs and risk perceptions, and sexual and reproductive healthcare attitudes, needs, preferences, and experiences.

Joint Interviews
Nurse researchers are sometimes interested in phenomena that involve interpersonal relationships. For example, the phenomenon might be the grief that mothers *and* fathers experience on losing a child, or the experiences of patients with AIDS *and* their caretakers. In such cases, it can be productive to conduct **joint (dyadic) interviews** in which two or more people are simultaneously questioned, using either an unstructured or semistructured format. Unlike focus group interviews, which typically involve group members who do not know each other, joint interviews involve respondents who are intimately related.

Joint interviews usually supplement rather than replace individual interviews, because there are things that cannot readily be discussed in front of the other party (e.g., criticisms of the other person's behavior). Joint interviews can be especially helpful, however, when researchers want to *observe* the dynamics between two key actors. Voltelen and colleagues (2018) and Zarhin (2018) have described ethical issues to consider when conducting joint interviews with couples or close relatives.

Example of Joint Interviews
Ikander et al. (2022) conducted joint interviews with patients and family caregivers in end-of-life decisions during palliative chemotherapy in Denmark. The researchers explored their decisions during the cancer trajectory, daily life with cancer, and end-of-life discussions at the outpatient clinic and at home.

Diaries and Journals
Personal **diaries** have long been used as a source of data in historical research. It is also possible to generate new data for a study by asking study participants to maintain a diary or journal over a specified period—or by asking them to share a diary they wrote. Diaries can be useful in providing an intimate and detailed description of a person's everyday life.

The diaries may be completely unstructured; for example, individuals who have undergone organ transplantation could be asked to spend 10 to 15 minutes a day jotting down their thoughts and feelings. Frequently, however, participants are requested to make entries into a diary regarding a specific aspect of their experience, sometimes in a semistructured format (e.g., about their appetite or sleeping). Nurse researchers have used health diaries to collect information about how people prevent illness, maintain health, experience morbidity, and treat health problems.

Although diaries are a useful means of learning about ongoing experiences, one limitation is that they can be used only by people with adequate literacy skills, although there are examples of studies in which diary entries were audio-recorded rather than written out. Diaries also require a high level of participant cooperation.

Example of Diaries
Negro and colleagues (2022) studied the contents of ICU patient diaries filled in by their family caregivers in Italy. Thirty-two diaries were analyzed, and seven themes identified, such as future plans and memories, the love surrounding the patient, clinical progression of the patient, and communication/reflection on the likely death of the patient.

Photo Elicitation and Photovoice

Photo elicitation involves an interview stimulated and guided by photographic images. This procedure, most often used in ethnographies, is a method that can break down barriers between researchers and study participants and promote a collaborative discussion (Frith & Harcourt, 2007). The photographs sometimes are ones that researchers have made of the participants' world, through which researchers can gain insights into the new culture. Participants may need to be continually reassured that their taken-for-granted explanations of the photos are providing useful information. Photo elicitation can also be used with photos that participants have in their homes, although in such case, researchers have less time to frame useful questions and no opportunity to select the photos that will be the stimulus for discussion.

Researchers are also using an increasingly popular technique of asking participants to take photographs themselves and then interpret them, a method called **photovoice**. Photovoice can be used as a strategy to promote empowerment and give voice to participants in addressing social and political change and thus is often used in participatory action research (Liebenberg, 2018). Oliffe and colleagues (2008) offered useful suggestions for a four-part strategy of analyzing participant-produced photographs, and Jaiswal and colleagues (2016) offered 12 tips to facilitate a photovoice project. Photovoice can be an empowering data collection strategy, but ethical challenges may emerge because people not involved in the research are often photographed (Caiola et al., 2018; Creighton et al., 2018).

Example of a Study With Photovoice
Al-Hamad et al. (2022) explored undergraduate nursing and medical students' perceptions of food security and access to healthy food in Qatar. The 16 participants were asked to take photographs of their environment and the places linked to the purpose of the study, such as home, university, grocery shops, markets, and parks.

Video-Stimulated Recall Interviews

A related technique is called a **stimulated recall interview**, which is used to explore how people approach social interactions. The researcher video-records study participants engaging in various activities in social situations. Then, in follow-up interviews, the researcher discusses aspects of the participants' behavior with them. For example, the interviewer might probe how the person chose from various options in deciding how to react to the behavior and actions of others. Stimulated recall interviews are considered a valuable tool for investigating cognitive processes in connection with specific events. Stimulated recall has most often been used in ethnographic research (Dempsey, 2010).

TIP **Digital storytelling** is an emergent method for collecting short first-person accounts in an electronic format. Digital stories are usually 3 to 5 minutes long and can include a person's photographs or drawings, video segments, and audio recording in the person's own voice. It is being used in community-based participatory research to address health inequities in vulnerable, underrepresented populations. Briant and colleagues (2016) have described the power of digital storytelling as a culturally relevant tool in health promotion projects.

Self-Report Narratives on the Internet

In addition to the possibility of soliciting narrative data on the internet through structured or semi-structured "interview" methods (as we describe in the next section), a potentially rich data source for qualitative researchers involves narrative self-reports available directly on the internet. For example, researchers can enter into long conversations with other users in a chat room.

Some data that can be analyzed qualitatively are simply "out there," as when a researcher enters a chat room, blog site, or online forum and analyzes the content of existing, unsolicited messages. As pointed out by Keim-Malpass et al. (2014), the internet is a rich source of interactive and socially mediated data, giving rise to "*Internet ethnography.*" Interest has focused, in particular, on illness blogs as a means of studying illness experiences.

Example of Blog Analysis
Beck (2022), one of the authors of this textbook, conducted a qualitative study to describe women's experiences of perinatal obsessive-compulsive disorder as written in their blogs. Forty-three different posts from women in the United Kingdom, United States, Australia, and South Africa were analyzed. Five themes were identified: (1) Starting to tighten the grip during pregnancy, (2) Keeping horrific secrets all to themselves, (3) Tortured with terrifying images and thoughts, (4) Driven to compulsive behaviors to protect their infants, and (5) Long difficult road to recovery but so worth it.

Using the internet to access narrative data has obvious advantages. This approach is economical and allows researchers to obtain information from geographically dispersed and perhaps remote internet users. However, a number of ethical concerns have been raised, and authenticity and other methodologic challenges need to be considered (Smith et al., 2017).

Example of an Analysis of Facebook Posts
Kelly et al. (2022) explored the use of a Facebook-based support group for caregivers of children and youth with complex care needs in Canada. A total of 108 caregivers joined the closed Facebook group. Content analysis of 93 posts revealed that informational and emotional posts were the most common.

Other Unstructured Self-Reports

We have described the primary means of collecting in-depth self-report, but other forms of unstructured self-reports have been developed. Examples include the following:

- **Life history interviews**, which are individual interviews directed at documenting a person's life story or an aspect of it that has developed over the life course;
- **Oral histories**, a method often used by historical researchers to gather personal recollections about events or issues;
- The **critical incidents technique**, a method of gathering in-depth information about specific incidents experienced by participants; and
- The **think-aloud method**, which involves obtaining real-time narrative data about how a person solves a problem or makes a decision.

Gathering Qualitative Self-Report Data Through Interviews

The purpose of gathering narrative self-report data is to enable researchers to construct reality in a way that is consistent with the constructions of the people being studied. This goal requires researchers to take steps to overcome communication barriers and to enhance the flow of meaning. Asking good questions and eliciting good narrative data are more difficult than you might think. This section offers some suggestions about gathering qualitative self-report data through in-depth interviews. Further advice is offered by Rubin and Rubin (2012) and Brinkman and Kvale (2015).

Locating the Interview
Researchers must decide where the interviews will take place. For one-on-one interviews, in-home interviews are often preferred because interviewers can then observe the participants' world and take observational notes. When in-home interviews are not desired by participants (e.g., if they prefer more privacy), it is wise to identify alternatives, such as an office, coffee shop, and so on. The important thing is to select places that offer privacy, that protect against interruptions insofar as possible, and that are suitable for recording purposes. It is sometimes useful to let participants select the setting, but the setting may be dictated by circumstances, as when interviews take place while participants are hospitalized.

Settings for focus group sessions should be selected carefully and, ideally, should be neutral. Churches, hospitals, or other settings that are strongly identified with particular values or expected behaviors may not be suitable, depending on the topic. The location should be comfortable, accessible, easy to find, and acoustically amenable to audio recording.

Most qualitative interviews are conducted in person, but new technologies have opened up other options. For example, videoconferencing makes it possible to conduct face-to-face interviews with participants remotely (Irani, 2019). Videoconferencing is advantageous from the perspective of having both a visual and auditory record of the interview.

> **Example of Videoconferencing Interviews**
> Ferguson et al. (2022) in Australia undertook a qualitative study to understand the educational and self-management needs of adults living with atrial fibrillation. A total of 34 participants were interviewed one-to-one by videoconference or phone. The sample included 8 patients, 13 clinicians, and 13 expert key stakeholders.

Another option is to conduct interviews using Zoom, Facebook, or other synchronous online services, which have become widely available. Such technologies are especially useful for gathering data from geographically dispersed participants or from people living in rural areas. Virtual focus groups open the door for including people who are unable or unwilling to participate in traditional focus groups that meet physically in a room.

Liamputtong (2011) has described the advantages of virtual focus groups. For example, in addition to being relatively inexpensive, participants' inhibitions are often lessened, anonymity can be enhanced, and pressures to conform can be reduced. The potential disadvantages of online focus groups include limits to group interaction, comments that are short and direct, and limited opportunity for the moderator to drive in-depth conversations (Carey, 2016). However, Woodyatt and colleagues (2016), in their comparison of data from in-person and online focus groups on a sensitive topic, found less sharing of in-depth stories in the in-person groups, but noted that "the content of the data generated is remarkably similar" (p. 741).

Study participants can also be "interviewed" asynchronously (not in real time) via emails or on social media platforms. A distinct advantage of online interviewing is that participants' narratives are already typed, thus avoiding the expense of transcribing recorded interviews. Fritz and Vandermause (2018) have offered advice about internet interviewing. Asynchronous methods have also been used with focus groups (e.g., Biedermann, 2018).

> **Example of Internet Interviewing**
> Beck, one of the authors of this textbook, and Twomey (2023) conducted a qualitative study via the internet about women's experiences of posttraumatic growth following postpartum psychosis. They recruited participants from postings on three Facebook groups for postpartum psychosis. Women who were interested in participating contacted Beck at her university email address. Participants were asked to respond to the following statement: "Please describe in as much detail as you can remember your experiences of any positive changes in your beliefs or life as a result of your having had postpartum psychosis." Women sent their narratives to the researchers on attachment via email.

TIP In an internet environment, researchers need to devote time and effort to crafting individual email responses to make sure all participants feel valued and understand that their narratives made important contributions to the study.

Preparing for In-Depth Interviews

Although qualitative interviews are conversational, this does not mean that they are entered into casually. The conversations are purposeful and require advance preparation. For example, careful thought should be given to the wording of questions. To the extent possible, the wording should make sense to respondents and reflect their world view. Researchers and respondents should, for example, have a common vocabulary. If the researcher is studying a culture or a group that uses distinctive terms or slang, efforts should be made before data collection begins to understand those terms and their nuances.

Researchers usually prepare for the interview by developing, mentally or in writing, the broad questions to be asked (or the initial questions, in unstructured interviews). Sometimes it is useful to do a practice interview with a stand-in respondent.

It is a good idea to ask any sensitive questions late in the interview after rapport has been established.

TIP Memorize key questions if you have written them out, so that you will be able to maintain eye contact with participants.

It is important to decide in advance how to present yourself—as a researcher, a nurse, an ordinary person like participants, a humble "learner," and so on. An advantage of assuming the nurse role is that people often trust nurses. Yet, people may be overly deferent if nurses are perceived as better educated or more knowledgeable than they are. Moreover, participants may use the interview as an opportunity to ask health questions or to solicit opinions about health practitioners.

For interviews done in the field, researchers must anticipate needs for equipment and supplies. Preparing a checklist of all such items is helpful. The checklist typically would include recording equipment, laptop computers or tablets, batteries or chargers, consent and demographic forms, notepads, and pens. Other possibilities include incentive payments, cookies or donuts to help break the ice, and distracting toys or books if children will be home. It may be necessary to bring proper identification to assure participants of the legitimacy of the visit. And, if the topic under study is likely to elicit emotional narratives, tissues should be readily at hand.

Conducting the Interview

Qualitative interviews are typically long, sometimes lasting hours. Researchers often find that the respondents' construction of their experience begins to emerge after lengthy, in-depth dialogues. Interviewers must prepare respondents for the interview by putting them at ease. Part of this process involves sharing pertinent information about the study (e.g., about confidentiality), and another part is using the first few minutes for icebreaking exchanges of conversation before actual questioning begins. Up-front "small talk" can help to overcome stage fright, which can occur for both interviewers and respondents. Participants may be particularly nervous when interviews are being recorded. They typically forget about the recorder after the interview is underway, so the first few minutes should be used to help both parties "settle in."

Participants will not share much information with interviewers they do not trust. Close rapport with respondents provides access to richer information and to intimate details of their stories. Interviewer personality plays a role in developing rapport: Good interviewers are usually congenial people who are able to see the situation from the respondent's perspective. Nonverbal communication can be critical in conveying concern and interest. Facial expressions, nods, and so on help to set the tone for the interview.

A critical skill for in-depth interviewers is being a good listener. It is especially important not to interrupt respondents, to "lead" them, to offer advice or opinions, or to counsel them. The interviewer's job is to listen intently to the respondents' stories. Only by attending carefully to what respondents are saying can interviewers develop appropriate follow-up questions. Even when a topic guide is used, interviewers must not let the flow of dialogue be bound by those questions.

TIP In-depth interviewers must be comfortable with pauses and silences and should let participants set the pace. Interviewers can encourage respondents with nonspecific prompts, such as "Mmhm."

Interviewers need to be prepared for strong emotions, such as anger, fear, or grief, to surface. Narrative disclosures can "bring it all back" for respondents, which can be a cathartic or therapeutic experience if interviewers create an atmosphere of concern and caring—but it can also be stressful.

Interviewers may need to manage potential crises during the interviews. One problem is a flawed recording of the interview. Thus, even when interviews are recorded, notes should be taken immediately after the interview to ensure the highest possible reliability of data and to prevent total information loss. Interruptions (usually the telephone) and other distractions are other common problems when interviewing in participants' homes. If respondents are willing, telephones can be controlled by unplugging them or turning them off. Interruptions by personal intrusions of friends or family members may be more difficult to manage. In some cases, the interview may need to be terminated and rescheduled—for example, when a woman is discussing domestic violence and the perpetrator enters and stays in the room.

Interviewers should strive for positive closure to interviews. The last questions in in-depth interviews should usually be along these lines: "Is there anything else you would like to tell me?" or "Are there any other questions that you think I should have asked you?" Such probes can often elicit a wealth of important information. In closing, interviewers normally ask respondents whether they would mind being contacted again, in the event that additional questions come to mind after reflecting on the information, or in case interpretations of the information need to be verified.

TIP It is usually unwise to schedule back-to-back interviews. You should not cut short the first interview to be on time for a next one, and you may be too emotionally drained for another interview. It is also important to have an opportunity to write out notes, impressions, and analytic ideas, and it is best to do this when an interview is fresh in your mind.

Postinterview Procedures

Recorded interviews should be listened to and checked for audibility and completeness soon after the interview is over. If there have been problems with the recording, the interview should be reconstructed in as much detail as possible. Listening to the interview may also suggest possible follow-up questions that could be asked if respondents are recontacted.

Steps also need to be taken to ensure that interview transcriptions are done with rigor. Transcriptionists, like interviewers, can be affected by hearing heart-wrenching interviews. Researchers may need to warn transcriptionists about upcoming interviews that are particularly stressful and allow transcribers the opportunity to talk about their reaction to interviews (Hennessy et al., 2022).

TIP Transcriptions can be the most expensive part of a study. It generally takes about 4 to 5 hours of transcription time for every hour of interviewing. New and improved voice recognition computer software may help with transcribing interviews. Transcription features built into conferencing and collaboration platforms have a wide range of availability and functionality. An automated speech recognition system is affected by a variety of factors, including audio quality, background noise, and speech patterns. In selecting a program, it is important to take into account factors such as language support, accuracy, and customization capabilities.

Evaluation of Qualitative Self-Report Approaches

In-depth interviews are a flexible approach to gathering data and offer distinct advantages. In clinical situations, for example, it is often appropriate to let people talk freely about their problems and concerns, allowing them to take much of the initiative in directing the flow of information. Unstructured self-reports may allow investigators to ascertain what the basic issues or problems are, how sensitive or controversial the topic is, how individuals conceptualize and talk about the problems, and what range of opinions or behaviors exists relevant to the topic. In-depth interviews may also help elucidate the underlying meaning of a pattern or relationship repeatedly observed in more structured research. On the other hand, qualitative self-reports are extremely time-consuming and demand strong skills for gathering high-quality data.

UNSTRUCTURED OBSERVATION

Qualitative researchers sometimes collect loosely structured observational data, often as a supplement to self-report data. The aim is to understand the behaviors and experiences of people as they actually occur in naturalistic settings.

Unstructured observational data are most often gathered in field settings through **participant observation**. Participant observers participate in the functioning of the social group under investigation and strive to observe, ask questions, and record information within the contexts and structures that are relevant to group members. Participant observation is characterized by prolonged periods of social interaction between researchers and participants, in the participants' sociopolitical and cultural milieu.

> **Example of Participant Observation**
> In their focused ethnographic study, Ohueri and colleagues (2022) sought to understand how participants self-manage and cope with their two chronic conditions of diabetes and HIV. The researchers collected data by semi-structured interviews and participant observation with 22 participants over a 9-month period. Participant observations included visits to the local grocery store, observing medication-taking routines, and attending a lunch with two of the participants who were part of the same HIV support group.

Not all qualitative observational research is *participant* observation (i.e., with observations occurring from *within* the group under study). Some unstructured observations involve watching and recording behaviors without participating in activities.

Nevertheless, if a key research objective is to learn how group interactions and activities give meaning to human behaviors and experiences, then participant observation is an appropriate method. The members of any group or culture are influenced by assumptions they take for granted, and observers can, through active participation as members, hope to gain access to these assumptions. Participant observation is most often used by ethnographers, but it is also used by grounded theory researchers and researchers with ideological perspectives.

The Observer–Participant Role in Participant Observation

The role that observers play in the groups under study is important because the observers' social position determines what they are likely to see. That is, the behaviors that are likely to be available for observation depend on observers' position in a network of relations.

McFarland and Wehbe-Alamah (2015), in describing Leininger's methods, depicted a participant observer's role as evolving through a four-phase sequence:

1. Primarily observation and active listening
2. Primarily observation with limited participation
3. Primarily participation with continued observation
4. Primary reflection and reconfirmation of findings with informants

In the initial phase, researchers observe and listen to those under study to obtain a broad view of the situation. This phase allows both observers and the observed to "size up" each other, to become acquainted, and to become comfortable interacting. In the next phase, observation is enhanced by a modest degree of participation. By participating in the group's activities, researchers can study people's behaviors as well as people's reactions. In phase 3, researchers become more active participants, learning by the actual experience of doing rather than just by watching and listening. In phase 4, researchers reflect on what transpired and how people interacted with and reacted to them.

Junker (1960) described a somewhat different continuum that does not assume an evolving process: complete participant, participant as observer, observer as participant, and complete observer. Complete participants conceal their identity as researchers, entering the group ostensibly as regular members. For example, a nurse researcher might accept a job as a clinical nurse with the express intent of studying, in a concealed fashion, some aspect of the clinical environment. At the other extreme, complete observers do not attempt participation in the group's activities, but rather make observations as outsiders. At both extremes, observers may have difficulty asking probing questions: complete participants may arouse suspicion if they make inquiries not congruent with a participant role, and complete observers may not have personal access to, or the trust of, those being observed. Most observational fieldwork lies in between these two extremes.

> **Example of Participant–Observer Roles**
> Thomann et al. (2022) undertook a qualitative study to describe daily restraint practices and the factors which influence their use. Unstructured participant observation was conducted at a department of geriatrics and department of intensive care in an acute care hospital in Switzerland. A total of 67 hours of observation occurred. The observer was a nurse with professional experience in acute psychiatry and outpatient care. Each observation period consisted of the observer, as an outsider, shadowing a nurse during their shift. To prepare, the observation process was defined in detail together with an expert in qualitative research. The nurse's role was to observe the following aspects: behavior, communication, and involvement.

> **TIP** Being a fully participating member of a group does not *necessarily* offer the best perspective for studying a phenomenon—just as being an actor in a play does not offer the most advantageous view of the performance.

> **Example of a Windshield Survey**
> Jin and colleagues (2022) undertook a community needs assessment in Seattle to examine factors in a partnership between a public university and a regional food bank aimed to promote health in food insecure communities. The researchers did a windshield survey to identify the community's priorities.

Getting Started

Observers must overcome two initial hurdles: gaining entrée into the social group or culture under study and establishing rapport and developing trust within the social group. Without gaining entrée, the study cannot proceed; but without the group's trust, researchers could be restricted to "frontstage" knowledge (Leininger, 1985), that is, information distorted by the group's protective facades. The observer's goal is to "get backstage"—to learn about the realities of the group's experiences and behaviors. This section discusses some practical and interpersonal aspects of getting started in the field.

Gaining an Overview

In the earliest stage of observational fieldwork, it is often useful to gather some written or pictorial descriptive material that provides an overview of the site. In an institutional setting, for example, it is helpful to obtain a floor plan, an organizational chart, an annual report, and so on. Then, a preliminary personal tour should be undertaken to gain familiarity with its ambiance and to note major activities, social groupings, and transactions.

In community studies, ethnographers sometimes conduct a **windshield survey** (or *windshield tour*), which involves an intensive exploration (sometimes in an automobile, and hence the name) to "map" important features of the community. Such community mapping can document community resources (e.g., churches, businesses, public transportation, community centers), community liabilities (e.g., vacant lots, empty stores, dilapidated buildings), and social and environmental characteristics (e.g., condition of streets and buildings, traffic patterns, types of signs, children playing in public places).

Establishing Rapport

After gaining entrée into a setting and obtaining permissions and suggestions from gatekeepers, the next step is to enter the field. It may be possible just to "blend in" or ease into a social group, but often researchers walk into a "head-turning" situation in which they stand out as strangers. Participant observers often find that, for their own comfort level and for that of participants, it is best to have a brief, simple explanation about their presence. Except in rare cases, deception is neither necessary nor recommended, but vagueness has many advantages. People rarely want to know *exactly* what researchers are studying, they simply want an introduction and enough information to satisfy their curiosity and erase suspicions about the researchers' ulterior motives.

After initial introductions with members of the group, it is usually best to keep a low profile. At the beginning, researchers are not yet familiar with the customs, language, and norms of the group, and it is critical to learn these things. Politeness and friendliness are essential, but ardent socializing is not appropriate at the early stages of fieldwork. As rapport is developed and trust is established, researchers can play a more active participatory role and collect observational data in earnest.

> **TIP** Your initial job is to listen intently and learn what it takes to fit into the group, that is, what you need to do to become accepted as a member. To the extent possible, you should downplay any expertise you might have. Your goal is to gain people's trust and to move relationships to a deeper level.

Gathering Unstructured Observational Data

Participant observers typically place few restrictions on the nature of the data collected, in keeping with the goal of minimizing observer-imposed meanings and structure. Nevertheless, participant observers often have a broad plan for the types of information to be gathered. Among aspects likely to be considered relevant are the following:

1. *The physical setting.* What are key features of the setting? What is the context within which human behavior unfolds? What behaviors are promoted (or constrained) by the physical environment?
2. *The participants.* What are the characteristics of the people being observed? How many people are there? What are their roles? Who is given free access to the setting—who "belongs"? What brings these people together?
3. *Activities and interactions.* What are people doing and saying? Is there a discernible progression of activities? How do people interact with one another? How—and how often—do they communicate? What type of emotions do they show during their interactions? How are participants interconnected to one another or to activities underway?
4. *Frequency and duration.* When did the activity or event begin, and when is it scheduled to end? How much time has elapsed? Is the activity a recurring one, and if so, how regularly does it recur? How typical of such activities is the one that is under observation?
5. *Precipitating factors.* Why is the event or interaction happening? What contributes to how the event or interaction unfolds?
6. *Organization.* How is the event or interaction organized? How are relationships structured? What norms or rules are in operation?
7. *Intangible factors.* What did *not* happen (especially if it ought to have happened)? Are participants saying one thing verbally but communicating different messages nonverbally? What types of things were disruptive to the activity or situation?

Clearly, this is far more information than can be absorbed in a single session (and not all categories may be relevant to the research question). However, this framework provides a starting point for thinking about observational possibilities while in the field.

TIP When we enter a social setting in our everyday lives, we unconsciously process many of the questions on this list. Usually, however, we do not consciously *attend* to our observations and impressions in any systematic way and are not careful about making note of the details that contribute to our impressions. This is precisely what participant observers must learn to do.

Spradley (1980) distinguished three levels of observation that typically occur during fieldwork. The first level, **descriptive observation**, tends to be broad and helps observers figure out what is going on. During descriptive observations, researchers attempt to observe as much as possible. Later in the inquiry, observers do **focused observations** of carefully selected events and interactions. Based on the research aims and on what has been learned from descriptive observations, participant observers begin to focus more sharply on key aspects of the setting. From these focused observations, they may develop a system for organizing observations, such as a taxonomy or category system. **Selective observations** are the most highly focused and are undertaken to facilitate comparisons between categories or activities. Spradley describes these levels as analogous to a funnel, with an increasingly narrow and more systematic focus.

While in the field, participant observers need to decide how to sample observations and select observational locations. **Single positioning** means staying in a single location for a period to observe behaviors and transactions in that location. **Multiple positioning** involves moving around the site to observe behaviors from different locations. **Mobile positioning** involves following a person throughout a given activity or period. It is usually useful to use a combination of positioning approaches.

Because participant observers cannot spend a lifetime in one site and cannot be in more than one place at a time, observation is almost always supplemented with information from unstructured interviews or conversations. For example, key informants may be asked to describe what went on in a meeting that the observer was unable to attend or to describe events that occurred before the observer entered the field. In such a case, the informant functions as the observer's observer.

Recording Observations

Participant observers may be tempted to put more emphasis on the *participation* and *observation* parts of their research than on the recording of those activities. Without systematic recording of observational data, however, the project can flounder. Observational information cannot be trusted to memory; it must be diligently recorded as soon after the observations as possible.

Types of Observational Records

The most common forms of record-keeping in participant observation are logs and field notes, but photographs and video recordings may also be used. A **log** (or **field diary**) is a daily record of events and conversations in the field. A log is a chronological listing of how researchers have spent their time and can be used for planning, for keeping track of expenses, and for reviewing what work has already been completed. Box 24.1 presents an example of a log entry from one of the authors of this textbook's grounded theory study of mothers of twins (Beck, 2002).

Field notes are broader, more analytic, and more interpretive than a simple listing of occurrences. Field notes represent the observer's efforts to record information and to synthesize and understand the data. Phillippi and Lauderdale (2018) have written an excellent guide to preparing field notes in qualitative research.

TIP Field notes are valuable in many types of qualitative studies, not just in studies involving participant observation. Field notes are an important means of documenting contextual information and should be maintained even when the only data source is from interviews.

The Content of Field Notes

Participant observers' field notes contain a narrative account of what is happening in the field; they

---

BOX 24.1 Example of a Log Entry: Mothering Multiples Grounded Theory Study

Log entry for Mothers of Multiples Support Group Meeting.
    July 15, 1999 10–11:30 a.m.

   This is my fourth meeting that I have attended. Nine mothers came this morning with their twins. One other woman attended. She was pregnant with twins. She came to the support group for advice from the other mothers regarding such issues as what type of stroller to buy, etc. All the moms sat on the floor with their infants placed on blankets on the floor next to them. Toddlers and older children played together off to the side with a box of toys. I sat next to a mom new to the group with her twin 4-month-old girls. I helped her hold and feed one of the twins. On my other side was a mom who had signed up at the last meeting to participate in my study. I hadn't called her yet to set up an appointment. She asked how my research was going. We then set up an appointment for next Thursday at 10 a.m. at her home for me to interview her. The new mother that I sat next to also was eager to participate in the study. In fact, she said we could do the interview right after the meeting ends today, but I couldn't due to another meeting. We scheduled an interview appointment for next Thursday at 1 p.m. I also set up a third appointment for an interview for next week with I.K. for Monday at 1 p.m. She had participated in an earlier study of mine. She came right over to me this morning at the support group meeting.

From the author's records for the study reported in the following paper: Beck, C. T. (2002). Releasing the pause button: Mothering twins during the first year of life. *Qualitative Health Research, 12,* 593–608.

serve as the data for analysis. Most "field" notes are not written while observers are literally in the field but rather are written after an observational session in the field has been completed.

Field notes are usually lengthy and time consuming to prepare. Observers need to discipline themselves to provide a wealth of detail, the meaning and importance of which may not emerge for weeks. Descriptions of what has transpired must include enough contextual information about time, place, and actors to portray the situation fully. *Thick description* is the goal for participation observers' field notes (as it is in describing a completed qualitative study).

TIP Especially in the early stages of fieldwork, a general rule of thumb is this: When in doubt, write it down.

Field notes are both descriptive and reflective. **Descriptive notes** (or **observational notes**) are objective descriptions of observed events and conversations. Information about actions, dialogue, and context is recorded as completely and objectively as possible.

Reflective notes, which document the researcher's personal experiences, reflections, and progress while in the field, can serve several purposes:

- **Methodologic notes** are reflections about observational strategies. Sometimes observers do things that do not "work," and methodologic notes document thoughts about new approaches or about why a strategy was especially effective. Methodologic notes also can provide instructions or reminders about how subsequent observations will be made.
- **Analytic notes** (or **theoretical notes**) document researchers' thoughts about how to make sense of what is going on. These notes serve as a starting point for subsequent analysis.
- **Personal notes** are comments about researchers' own feelings in the field. Almost inevitably, field experiences give rise to emotions and challenge researchers' assumptions. It is essential to reflect on such feelings, because there is no other way to know whether they are influencing

what is being observed. Personal notes can also contain reflections relating to ethical dilemmas.

Box 24.2 presents examples of various types of field notes from Beck's (2002) study of mothering twins.

Reflective notes are typically not integrated into the descriptive notes but are kept separate as parallel notes; they may be maintained in a journal or a series of self-memos. Strauss and Corbin (1990) argue that reflective memos help researchers to achieve analytic distance from the actual data and play a critical role in the project's success.

TIP Personal notes should begin even before entering the field. By recording your feelings and expectations, you will have a baseline against which to compare feelings and experiences that emerge in the field.

The Process of Writing Field Notes

The success of participant observation depends on the quality of the field notes, and timing is important to quality. Field notes should be written as soon as possible after an observation is made. The longer the interval between an observation and field note preparation, the greater the risk of forgetting or distorting the data. With long delays, details will be forgotten and memory of what was observed may be biased by things that happened subsequently.

TIP Be sure not to talk to anyone about your observation before you have had a chance to write up the observational notes. Such discussions could color what you record.

Participant observers cannot usually write their field notes while they are in the field, in part because this would distract them from their job of being keen observers, and because it would undermine their role as ordinary members. Researchers must develop the skill of making detailed mental notes that can later be committed to a permanent record. Observers often try to jot down unobtrusively a phrase or sentence that will later serve as a reminder of an event, conversation, or

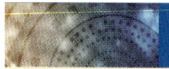

> **BOX 24.2** Example of Field Notes: Mothering Multiples Grounded Theory Study
>
> **Observational notes:** O.L. attended the mothers of multiples support group again this month but she looked worn out today. She was not as bubbly as she had been at the March meeting. She explained why she was not doing as well this month. She and her husband had just found out that their house has lead-based paint in it. Both twins do have increased lead levels. She and her husband are in the process of buying a new home.
>
> **Analytic notes:** So far, all the mothers have stressed the need for routine in order to survive the first year of caring for twins. Mothers, however, have varying definitions of routine. I.R. had the firmest routine with her twins. B.L. is more flexible with her routine, i.e., the twins are always fed at the same time but are not put down for naps or bed at night at the same time. Whenever one of the twins wants to go to sleep is fine with her. B.L. does have a daily routine in regards to housework. For example, when the twins are down in the morning for a nap, she makes their bottles up for the day (14 bottles total).
>
> **Methodologic notes:** The first sign-up sheet I passed around at the Mothers of Multiples Support Group for women to sign up to participate in interviews for my grounded theory study only consisted of two columns: one for the mother's name and one for her telephone number. I need to revise this sign-up sheet to include extra columns for the age of the multiples, the town where the mother lives, and older siblings and their ages. My plan is to start interviewing mothers with multiples around 1 year of age so that the moms can reflect back over the process of mothering their infants for the first 12 months of their lives.
>
> Right now, I have no idea of the ages of the infants of the mothers who signed up to be interviewed. I will need to call the nurse in charge of this support group to find out the ages.
>
> **Personal notes:** Today was an especially challenging interview. The mom had picked the early afternoon for me to come to her home to interview her because that is the time her 2-year-old son would be napping. When I arrived at her house, her 2-year-old ran up to me and said hi. The mom explained that he had taken an earlier nap that day and that he would be up during the interview. So in the living room with us during our interview were her two twin daughters (3 months old) swinging in the swings and her 2-year-old son. One of the twins was quite cranky for the first half hour of the interview. During the interview, the 2-year-old sat on my lap and looked at the two books I had brought as a little present. If I did not keep him occupied with the books, he would keep trying to reach for the microphone of the tape recorder.
>
> From the author's records for the study reported in the following paper: Beck, C. T. (2002). Releasing the pause button: Mothering twins during the first year of life. *Qualitative Health Research, 12,* 593–608.

impression. Many experienced field-workers use the tactic of frequent trips to the bathroom to record these **jottings**, either in a small notebook or onto a recording device. With the widespread use of cell phones, researchers can also excuse themselves to make a call, and "phone in" their jottings. Observers use jottings to develop more extensive field notes.

> **TIP** It is important to schedule enough time to record field notes after an observation. An hour of observation can take three to 4 hours to record. Try to find a quiet place for writing up field notes, preferably a location where you can work undisturbed for several hours.

Observational field notes should be as detailed as possible. This means that hundreds of pages of field notes typically will be created, and so systems need to be developed for managing them. For example, each entry should have the date and time the observation was made, the location, and the name of the observer (if several are working as a team). It is useful to give observational sessions a name that will trigger a memory (e.g., "Emotional Outburst by a Patient with Ovarian Cancer").

Thought also needs to be given to how to record participants' dialogue. The goal is to record conversations as accurately as possible, but it is not always possible to make verbatim recordings if researchers are trying to maintain a stance as regular group members.

Procedures are needed to distinguish different levels of accuracy in recording dialogue (e.g., by using quotation marks and italics for true verbatim recordings, and a different designation for paraphrasings).

TIP Observation, participation, and record-keeping are exhausting, labor-intensive activities. It is important to establish the proper pace of these activities to ensure the highest possible quality notes for analysis.

Evaluation of Participant Observation

Participant observation can provide a deeper and richer understanding of human behaviors and social situations than is possible with structured observation. Participant observation is particularly valuable for its ability to "get inside" a situation and provide understanding of its complexities. Furthermore, this approach is inherently flexible and gives observers the freedom to reconceptualize problems after becoming more familiar with the situation. Participant observation is a good method for answering questions about phenomena that are difficult for insiders to explain because these phenomena are taken for granted.

Like all research methods, however, participant observation faces potential problems. Observer bias and observer influence are prominent risks. Observers may lose objectivity in viewing and recording observations; they may also inappropriately sample events and situations to be observed. Once researchers begin to participate in a group's activities, the possibility of emotional involvement becomes a salient concern. Researchers in their member role may fail to attend to research-relevant aspects of the situation or may develop a myopic view on issues of importance to the group. Participant observation may thus be unsuitable when the risk of identification is strong. Another important issue concerns the ethical dilemmas that often emerge in participant observation studies. Finally, the success of participant observation depends on the observer's observational and interpersonal skills—skills that may be difficult to cultivate.

On the whole, participant observation and other unstructured observational methods are extremely profitable for in-depth research in which researchers wish to develop a comprehensive description and conceptualization of phenomena within a social setting or culture.

TIP Although this chapter emphasized the two most frequently used methods of collecting unstructured data (self-reports and observation), we encourage you to think about other data sources, such as documents.

CRITICAL APPRAISAL OF DATA COLLECTION IN QUALITATIVE RESEARCH

It is usually not easy to appraise the decisions that researchers have made in collecting qualitative data because details about those decisions are seldom spelled out in research reports. In particular, there is often scant information about participant observation. It is not uncommon for a report to simply say that the researcher undertook participant observation, without descriptions of how much time was spent in the field, what exactly was observed, how observations were recorded, and what level of participation was involved. In fact, we suspect that many projects described as having used a participant observation approach were unstructured observations with little actual participation. Thus, an appraisal may focus on how much information the research report provided about the data collection methods used. Even though space constraints in journals make it impossible for researchers to fully elaborate their methods, researchers have a responsibility to communicate basic information about their approach so that readers can assess the quality of evidence that the study yields. Researchers should provide examples of questions asked and types of observations made.

As we discuss in Chapter 26, *triangulation* of multiple data collection methods provides opportunities for qualitative researchers to enhance the quality of their data. Thus, an important issue to consider in evaluating unstructured data is whether the types and amount of data collected are sufficiently rich to support an in-depth, holistic understanding of the phenomena under study. Box 24.3 provides guidelines for critically appraising the collection of unstructured data.

BOX 24.3 Guidelines for Critically Appraising Unstructured Data Collection Methods

1. Was the collection of unstructured data appropriate to the study aims?
2. Given the research question and the characteristics of study participants, did the researcher use the best method of capturing study phenomena (i.e., self-reports, observation)? Should supplementary data collection methods have been used to enrich the data available for analysis?
3. If self-report methods were used, did the researcher make good decisions about the specific method used to solicit information (e.g., focus group interviews, semistructured interviews, and so on)? Was the modality of obtaining the data appropriate (e.g., in-person interviews, telephone interviews, Internet questioning, etc.)?
4. If a topic guide was used, did the report present examples of specific questions? Were the questions appropriate and thorough? Did the wording encourage full and rich responses?
5. Were interviews recorded and transcribed? If interviews were not recorded, what steps were taken to ensure the accuracy of the data?
6. Were self-report data gathered in a manner that promoted high-quality responses (e.g., in terms of privacy, efforts to put respondents at ease, etc.)? Who collected the data, and were they adequately prepared for the task?
7. If observational methods were used, did the report adequately describe what the observations entailed? What did the researcher actually observe, in what types of settings did the observations occur, and how often and over how long a period were observations made? Were decisions about positioning described?
8. What role did the researcher assume in terms of being an observer and a participant? Was this role appropriate?
9. How were observational data recorded? Did the recording method maximize data quality?

RESEARCH EXAMPLE

This section provides an example of a qualitative study that collected a rich variety of unstructured data.

Study: Female genital mutilation as a social norm: Examining the beliefs and attitudes of women in this diaspora (Gutiérrez-Garcìa et al., 2022)

Statement of purpose: The aim of this study was to identify the beliefs, values, and attitudes of women in the sub-Saharan diaspora regarding female genital mutilation and how the processes involved in migration had influenced these women's perspectives.

Design: The researchers used an ethnographic approach that involved the use of multiple data collection methods. A convenience sample of 10 women was recruited in the Valencian community of Spain, which has the fourth highest population of immigrants originating in countries where female genital mutilation occurs.

Data collection: Life histories and lifelines were used. Researchers created life histories from interviews with the participants. Interviews were divided into three sessions: (1) origin and experiences of childhood and adolescence, (2) marriage and sex life (female genital mutilation, pregnancies, and children), and (3) situation at the time of the interview. Interviews were conducted out in the participants' homes or at the facilities of the associations they used. Interviews were audiotaped and the participants' gestures and expressions were noted. Each interview session lasted between 1 and 1 ½ hours. In addition, lifelines were created where participants pointed out major events that had been turning points in their life stories. Participants annotated these lifelines with drawings or an explanatory phrase.

Key findings: The researchers used the data to learn that women in this study believed that the main motivation for female genital mutilation was control of female sexuality and its relationship with male polygamy. The taboo permeating this mutilation remains intact even outside of Africa. The link between female genital mutilation and marriage has lost its relevance in the diaspora because it is no longer a required condition for marriage.

SUMMARY POINTS

- Qualitative researchers typically adopt flexible data collection plans that evolve as the study progresses. Self-reports are the most frequently used type of data in qualitative studies, followed by observation. Ethnographers are likely to combine these two data sources with other sources such as the products of the culture (e.g., photographs, documents, artifacts).
- Qualitative researchers often confront such fieldwork issues as gaining participants' trust, pacing data collection to avoid being overwhelmed by the intensity of data, avoiding emotional involvement with participants ("**going native**"), and maintaining reflexivity (awareness of the part they play in the study and possible effects on their data).
- Qualitative researchers need to plan for how their data will be recorded and stored. If technical equipment is used (e.g., audio recorders, video recorders), care must be taken to select equipment that functions properly in the field.
- Unstructured and loosely structured self-reports, which offer respondents and interviewers latitude in their questions and answers, yield rich narrative data for qualitative analysis.
- Methods of collecting qualitative self-report data include: (1) **unstructured interviews**, which are conversational discussions on the topic of interest; (2) **semistructured** (or **focused**) **interviews**, in which interviewers are guided by a **topic guide** listing broad questions to be asked; (3) **focus group interviews**, which involve discussions with small, homogeneous groups; (4) **joint interviews**, which involve simultaneously talking with members of a dyad; (5) **diaries** and journals, in which participants maintain ongoing records about some aspects of their lives; (6) **photo elicitation interviews**, which are stimulated and guided by photographic images and **photovoice**, which involves having participants take photos themselves; (7) **stimulated recall interviews** that involve video recordings of participants in social interactions, followed by interviews; and (8) narrative materials available on the internet. Additional methods include **life histories, oral histories, critical incident interviews,** and **think-aloud methods.**
- In preparing for in-depth interviews, researchers learn about the language and customs of participants, formulate broad questions, make decisions about how to present themselves, develop ideas about interview settings, and take stock of equipment needs.
- Most qualitative interviews take place in face-to-face situations, but technological advances are making remote synchronous interviewing possible (e.g., via Skype).
- Conducting good in-depth interviews requires considerable skill in putting people at ease, developing trust, listening intently, and managing possible crises in the field.
- Ethnographers (and other qualitative researchers) also collect unstructured observational data, often through **participant observation.** Participant observers obtain information about the dynamics of social groups or cultures within members' own frame of reference.
- In the initial phase of participant observation studies, researchers are primarily observers gaining an understanding of the site, sometimes including *windshield surveys* to get a "lay of the land." Researchers later become more active participants.
- Observations tend to become more focused over time, ranging from **descriptive observation** (broad observations) to **focused observation** of more carefully selected events or interactions, and then to **selective observations** designed to facilitate comparisons.
- Participant observers usually select events to be observed through a combination of **single positioning** (observing from a fixed location), **multiple positioning** (moving around the site to observe in different locations), and **mobile positioning** (following a person around a site).
- **Logs** of daily events and **field notes** are the major methods of recording unstructured observational data. Field notes are both descriptive and reflective.
- Descriptive notes (or **observational notes**) are detailed, objective accounts of what transpired

in an observational session. Observers strive for detailed, thick description.
- **Reflective notes** include **methodologic notes** that document observers' thoughts about their strategies; **analytic notes** (or **theoretical notes**) that represent ongoing efforts to make sense of the data; and **personal notes** that document observers' feelings and experiences.
- In-depth unstructured data collection methods tend to yield data of considerable richness and are useful in gaining an understanding about little-researched phenomena, but they are time-consuming and yield a volume of data that are challenging to analyze.

REFERENCES CITED IN CHAPTER 24

Agénor, M., Zubizarreta, D., Geffen, S., Ramanayake, N., Giraldo, S., McGuirk, A., Caballero, M., & Bond, K. (2022). "Making a way out of no way": Understanding the sexual and reproductive health care experiences of transmasculine young adults of color in the United States. *Qualitative Health Research*, *32*(1), 121–134. https://doi.org/10.1177/10497323211050051

Al-Hamad, A., MacNevin, S., & Daher-Nashif, S. (2022). Undergraduate nursing and medical students' perceptions of food security and access to healthy food in Qatar: A photovoice study. *Journal of Nutritional Science*, *11*, e32. https://doi.org/10.1017/jns.2022.28

Beck, C. T. (2002). Releasing the pause button: Mothering twins during the first year of life. *Qualitative Health Research*, *12*(5), 593–608.

Beck, C. T. (2022). Narrating perinatal obsessive-compulsive disorder through blogs. *MCN American Journal of Maternal Child Nursing*, *47*(5), 273–280. https://doi.org/10.1097/nmc.0000000000000842

Beck, C. T., & Twomey, T. (2023). Posttraumatic growth after postpartum psychosis. *MCN: American Journal of Maternal Child Nursing*, *48*(6), 303-311. https://doi.org/10.1097/nmc.0000000000000954

Biedermann, N. (2018). The use of Facebook for virtual asynchronous focus groups in qualitative research. *Contemporary Nurse*, *54*(1), 26–34.

Briant, K., Halter, A., Marchello, N., Escareno, M., & Thompson, B. (2016). The power of digital storytelling as a culturally relevant health promotion tool. *Health Promotion Practice*, *17*(6), 793–801.

Brinkman, S., & Kvale, S. (2015). *InterViews: Learning the craft of qualitative research interviewing* (3rd ed.). Sage.

Caiola, C., Barroso, J., & Docherty, S. (2018). Black mothers living with HIV picture the social determinants of health. *Journal of the Association of Nurses in AIDS Care*, *29*(2), 204–219.

Carey, M. A. (2016). Focus groups—what is the same, what is new, what is next? *Qualittive Health Research*, *26*(6), 731–733.

Charmaz, K. (2014). *Constructing grounded theory*. Sage.

Choi, L. L. S., Jung, P., Harder, M., & Zhang, K. (2022). What matters most to older Chinese adults. *Journal of Transcultural Nursing*, *33*(2), 169–177. https://doi.org/10.1177/10436596211053655

Côté-Arsenault, D. (2013). Focus groups. In Beck, C. T. (Ed.), *Routledge handbook of qualitative nursing research* (pp. 307–318). Routledge.

Creighton, G., Oliffe, J., Ferlatte, O., Bottorff, J., Broom, A., & Jenkins, E. (2018). Photovoice ethics: Critical reflections from men's mental health research. *Qualitative Health Research*, *28*(3), 446–455.

Dempsey, N. (2010). Stimulated recall interviews in ethnography. *Qualitative Sociology*, *33*, 349–367.

Farzi, S., Taleghani, F., Yazdannik, A., & Esfahani, M. S. (2022). Communication culture in cancer nursing care: An ethnographic study. *Support Care Cancer*, *30*(1), 615–623. https://doi.org/10.1007/s00520-021-06388-2

Ferguson, C., Hickman, L. D., Lombardo, L., Downie, A., Bajorek, B., Ivynian, S., Inglis, S. C., & Wynne, R. (2022). Educational needs of people living with atrial fibrillation: A qualitative study. *Journal of American Heart Association*, *11*(15), e025293. https://doi.org/10.1161/jaha.122.025293

Frith, H., & Harcourt, D. (2007). Using photographs to capture women's experiences of chemotherapy: Reflecting on the method. *Qualitative Health Research*, *17*(10), 1340–1350.

Fritz, R., & Vandermause, R. (2018). Data collection via in-depth email interviewing: Lessons from the field. *Qualitative Health Research*, *28*(10), 1640–1649.

Glaser, B. G., & Strauss, A. (1967). *The discovery of grounded theory: Strategies for qualitative research*. Aldine de Gruyter.

Gutiérrez-Garcìa, A. I., Solano-Ruiz, C., Perpiñá-Galvañ, J., & Siles-González, J., Jimenez-Ruiz, I. (2022). Female genital mutilation as a social norm: Examining the beliefs and attitudes of women in this diaspora. *Qualittive Health Research*, *32*(7), 1153–1166. https://doi.org/10.1177/10497323221097885

Hantke, S., St Denis, V., & Graham, H. (2022). Racism and antiracism in nursing education: Confronting the problem of whiteness. *BMC Nursing*, *21*(1), 146. https://doi.org/10.1186/s12912-022-00929-8

Hennessy, M., Dennehy, R., Doherty, J., & O'Donoghue, K. (2022). Outsourcing transcription: Extending ethical considerations in qualitative research. *Qualitative Health Research*, *32*(7),1197–1204. https://doi.org/10.1177/10497323221101709

Ikander, T., Dieperink, K. B., Hansen, O., & Raunkiaer, M. (2022). Patient, family caregiver, and nurse involvement in end-of-life discussions during palliative chemotherapy: A phenomenological hermeneutic study. *Journal of Family Nursing*, *28*(1), 31–42. https://doi.org/10.1177/10748407211046308

Irani, E. (2019). The use of videoconferencing for qualitative interviewing: Opportunities, challenges, and considerations. *Clinical Nursing Research*, *28*(1), 3–8.

Jaiswal, D., To, M. J., Hunter, H., Lane, C., States, C., Cameron, B., Clarke, S. K., Cox, C., MacLeod, A., & MacLeod, A.

(2016). Twelve tips for medical students to facilitate a photovoice project. *Medical Teacher*, *38*(10), 981–986.

Jin, X., Ezeonwu, M., Ayad, A., & Bowman, K. (2022). Using a food bank as a platform for educating communities during the COVID-19 pandemic. *Journal of Community Health Nursing*, *39*(1), 50–57. https://doi.org/10.1080/07370016.2022.2037052

Junker, B. H. (1960). *Field work: An introduction to the social sciences*. University of Chicago Press.

Kahn, D. L. (2000). How to conduct research. In Cohen, M. Z., Kahn, D. L., & Steeves, R. H. (Eds.), *Hermeneutic phenomenological research* (pp. 57–70). Sage.

Keim-Malpass, J., Steeves, R., & Kennedy, C. (2014). Internet ethnography: A review of methodological considerations for studying online illness blogs. *International Journal of Nursing Studies*, *51*(12), 1686–1692.

Kelly, K.J., Doucet, S., Luke, A., Azar, R., & Montelpare, W. (2022). Exploring the use of a Facebook-based support group for caregivers of children and youth with complex care needs: Qualitative descriptive study. *JMIR Pediatrics and Parenting*, *5*(2), e33170. https://doi.org/10.2196/33170

Kidd, P. S., & Parshall, M. B. (2000). Getting the focus and the group: Enhancing analytical rigor in focus group research. *Qualitative Health Research*, *10*(3), 293–308.

Krueger, R., & Casey, M. (2015) *Focus groups: A practical guide for applied research* (5th ed.). Sage.

Leininger, M. (Ed.). (1985). *Qualitative research methods in nursing*. Grune and Stratton.

Liamputtong, P. (2011). *Focus group methodology: Principles and practice*. Sage Publications.

Liebenberg, L. (2018). Thinking critically about photovoice: Achieving empowerment and social change. *International Journal of Qualitative Methods*, *17*, 1–9.

McFarland, M. R., & Wehbe-Alamah, H. B. (2015). *Leininger's culture care diversity and universality: A worldwide nursing theory*. Jones & Bartlett Learning.

McIntosh, M., & Morse, J. M. (2015). Situating and constructing diversity in semi-structured interviews. *Global Qualitative Nursing Research*, *2*, 2333393615597674.

McNair, R., Taft, A., & Hegarty, K. (2008). Using reflexivity to enhance in-depth interviewing skills for the clinician researcher. *BMC Medical Research Methodology*, *8*, 73.

Morgan, D. L. (2001). Focus group interviewing. In Gubrium, J. F., & Holstein, J. A. (Eds.), *Handbook of interview research: Context and method* (2nd ed., pp. 141–159). Sage.

Negro, A., Villa, G., Zangrillo, A., Rosa, D., & Manara, D. F. (2022). Diaries in intensive care units: An Italian qualitative study. *Nursing in Critical Care*, *27*(1), 36–44. https://doi.org/10.1111/nicc.12668

Ohueri, C. W., Garcia, A. A., & Zuniga, J. A. (2022). Counting, coping, and navigating the flux: A focused ethnographic study of HIV and diabetes self-management. *Qualitative Health Research*, *32*(3), 399–412. https://doi.org/10.1177/10497323211064231

Oliffe, J., Bottorff, J., Kelly, M., & Halpin, M. (2008). Analyzing participant-produced photographs from an ethnographic study of fatherhood and smoking. *Research in Nursing & Health*, *31*(5), 529–539.

Petty, J. (2017). Emotion work in qualitative research: Interviewing parents about neonatal care. *Nurse Researcher*, *25*(3), 26–30.

Phillippi, J., & Lauderdale, J. (2018). A guide to field notes for qualitative research: Context and conversation. *Qualitative Health Research*, *28*(3), 381–388.

Pourgholam, N., Shoghi, M., & Borimnejad, L. (2022). Patients' lived experiences of the paternalistic care behavior: A qualitative study. *Journal of Caring Science*, *11*(3), 163–171. https://doi.org/10.34172/jcs.2022.10

Rothwell, E., Anderson, R., & Botkin, J. (2016). Deliberative discussion focus groups. *Qualitative Health Reserch*, *26*(6), 734–740.

Rubin, H., & Rubin, I. S. (2012). *Qualitative interviewing: The art of hearing data* (3rd ed.). Sage.

Smith, H., Bulbul, A., & Jones, C. (2017). Can online discussion sites generate quality data for research purposes? *Frontiers in Public Health*, *5*, 156.

Spradley, J. (1979). *The ethnographic interview*. Holt Rinehart & Winston.

Spradley, J. P. (1980). *Participant observation*. Holt, Rinehart & Wilson.

Strauss, A., & Corbin, J. (1990). *Basics of qualitative research: Grounded theory procedures and techniques*. Sage.

Thomann, S., Zwakhalen, S., Siegrist-Dreier, S., & Hahn, S. (2023). Restraint practice in the somatic acute care hospital: A participant observation study. *Journal of Clinical Nursing*, *32*(11–12), 2603–2615. https://doi.org/10.1111/jocn.16322

Van Manen, M. (1990). *Researching lived experience: Human science for an action sensitive pedagogy*. Althouse Press.

Voltelen, B., Konradsen, H., & Østergaard, B. (2018). Ethical considerations when conducting joint interviews with close relatives or family: An integrative review. *Scandinavian Journal of Caring Science*, *32*(2), 515–526.

Woodyatt, C., Finneran, C., & Stephenson, R. (2016). In-person versus online focus group discussions: A comparative analysis of data quality. *Qualitative Health Research*, *26*(6), 741–749.

Zarhin, D. (2018). Conducting joint interviews with couples: Ethical and methodological challenges. *Qualitative Health Research*, *28*(5), 844–854.

25 Qualitative Data Analysis

Learning Objectives

1. Describe activities that qualitative researchers perform to manage and organize their data.
2. Discuss the general procedures used to analyze qualitative data.
3. Discuss the procedures used to analyze qualitative data used in ethnographic, phenomenological, grounded theory, and qualitative descriptive research.
4. Describe guidelines for critically appraising qualitative analyses and interpretations.

INTRODUCTION

Qualitative data come from a variety of sources, such as verbatim interview transcripts, observational field notes, and diaries kept by study participants. This chapter describes methods for analyzing such narrative data.

INTRODUCTION TO QUALITATIVE ANALYSIS

The purpose of data analysis is to organize, provide structure to, and elicit meaning from data. In qualitative studies, data collection and data analysis often occur concurrently, rather than after all data are collected. When the person collecting the data is the person who analyzes the data, the search for important concepts and patterns begins as data collection is underway.

Qualitative analysis is a labor-intensive activity that requires creativity, conceptual sensitivity, and sheer hard work. We begin by discussing some general issues.

Qualitative Analysis Challenges

Qualitative data analysis is very challenging. There are no universal rules for analyzing qualitative data, and the absence of standard procedures makes it hard to explain how to do such analyses. It is also difficult for researchers to describe their analytic process at length in a report and to present findings in a way that their validity is apparent.

A second challenge of qualitative analysis is the enormous amount of work required. In most studies, hundreds of pages (and sometimes thousands of pages) of transcribed interviews and field notes have to be read, reread, coded and recoded, analyzed, and interpreted.

Another challenge comes in reducing data for reporting purposes. Quantitative results can often be summarized in a few tables. Qualitative researchers, by contrast, must balance the need to be concise with the need to maintain the richness and evidentiary value of their data.

Decisions in Qualitative Analysis

Qualitative researchers make numerous decisions that affect the analytic process. Not all decisions are independent—that is, one decision may affect another decision. In this section, we discuss some key decisions for qualitative analysts.

Who Will Do the Analysis?

Many qualitative studies are undertaken by a single researcher who designs the study, selects participants, collects the data, and then analyzes the data. In some studies, however, two to three researchers work collaboratively on analytic tasks. Increasingly, qualitative analysis is being undertaken by interprofessional teams that include both clinicians and researchers from different disciplines—and may even include lay people.

Who Will Do the Transcriptions?

Audio-recorded interviews and field notes are major data sources in qualitative studies. Verbatim transcription of the recordings is a critical step in preparing for data analysis. Without accurate transcriptions, the data available for analysis could be flawed. Some have argued that the person who leads the analysis should do the transcriptions, as a way to get immersed in the data. Others, however, urge transcriptions by professionals as a means of enhancing consistency and accuracy.

Will Coding and Analysis Be Inductive or Deductive?

An early step in most qualitative analyses is the coding and indexing of data so that relevant segments can be retrieved for analysis. In most cases, the codes will be inductive—that is, driven by the data themselves. With an *inductive* (or "bottoms-up") *approach*, analysts identify meaningful concepts that appear with some regularity in the data. In a so-called *deductive* (or "top-down") *approach*, researchers begin with an a priori framework that typically is based on an existing theory, prior research, or personal conceptualization. In such an approach, the researcher codes the data into a preexisting coding frame (sometimes called a *template*), although modifications may be necessary to accommodate the data. Critics worry that researchers who use an existing coding frame risk premature analytic closure, but a deductive approach can be productive when the inquiry is guided by an existing theory. Sometimes a so-called *abductive approach* is used, which combines induction and deduction.

> **Example of Using an Existing Framework**
> Ou and colleagues (2022) conducted a qualitative study to explore maternal anger after childbirth. They used Relational Autonomy Theory as their theoretical framework.

Will the Focus of the Analysis Be Description or Interpretation?

Some qualitative researchers have as a central aim a rich and thorough description of a phenomenon. Others seek to describe *and* to interpret the meaning of the phenomenon. A distinction is sometimes made between an analysis of the manifest content vs. the latent content of the narrative material. The *manifest content* is the actual words and actions of study participants; analyses of manifest content are primarily descriptive in nature, with modest interpretation. Analyses of *latent content* involve a search for underlying ideas and conceptualizations. Efforts are made to understand the broader meanings that underpin what is articulated in the data. Description may be an important and worthwhile goal in some studies, but cultivating the full potential of the data requires efforts to interpret what the data mean.

What Will Be the Final Product?

Relatedly, researchers should have a sense of what their final product will be. If the focus of the research is primarily description, the final product may take the form of a list of categories or a *taxonomy*—that is, an orderly system of classification. Morgan (2018) has noted that most qualitative results are reported as theories, models, or themes—with themes being the most typical format. *Themes* are meaningful patterns in the data and can be descriptive or interpretive. Morgan describes *models* as "low-level theories" that connect themes and are often presented in graphic form. *Theories* specify links between a set of themes *and* they explain why they are related in a specified manner. Grounded theory research is explicitly geared toward theory development. Researchers should decide upfront whether they will pursue a theory-building analysis.

Will Computer Software Be Used in the Analysis?

Software to facilitate the management and analysis of qualitative data is used with growing regularity. Some experts have advised beginning researchers—or those whose dataset is small—to use primarily manual (paper-and-pencil) methods. The rationale for this advice is that manual methods allow researchers to get closer to their data, and that the time spent learning the software may reduce the time available for actual analysis. Qualitative software does, however, offer many advantages.

The Qualitative Analysis Process

The analysis of qualitative data is a complex and creative process that is fundamentally iterative and nonlinear. This means that analysts move forward and backward between various analytic tasks in their effort to discern the meaning of the data.

Broad processes of qualitative data analysis are shown in Figure 25.1, but there are some caveats. Some qualitative analyses do not involve all activities in this figure. For example, *coding* is commonly used as a preliminary data management and analysis step in many—but not all—studies. Relatively few qualitative studies involve the development of a theory. Also, Figure 25.1 suggests a more linear set of activities than is ever the case. Nevertheless, the figure offers a broad overview of common sequences in the analysis of qualitative data and illustrates that qualitative researchers move from a massive amount of particulars (the data) to smaller, more general units of understanding.

One activity in the figure is, however, universal. First and foremost, analysts must totally immerse themselves in their data. A good analysis requires researchers to scrutinize their data carefully and deliberatively, reading transcriptions over and over (and relistening to recordings) in search of understanding. Insights cannot occur until researchers "live" their data. Relatedly, conscientious analysts get into the habit of writing down their thoughts and observations in the margins of the transcripts and in **analytic memos** as they read through the data and reflect upon their meaning and importance.

Analysis and interpretation often rely on the development of a coding system that allows the researchers to index and retrieve segments for closer scrutiny. **Precoding** typically occurs during data collection, as researchers read interview transcripts or field notes to help them hone their questioning and select new participants. Precoding typically involves circling, underlining, or highlighting passages or concepts that strike the analyst as significant or noteworthy. Without precoding (at least mentally if not in writing), researchers would not be able to discern when their data are saturated.

When data collection is complete, analysts usually develop a more formal coding scheme and then apply the codes to segments of the data—and then

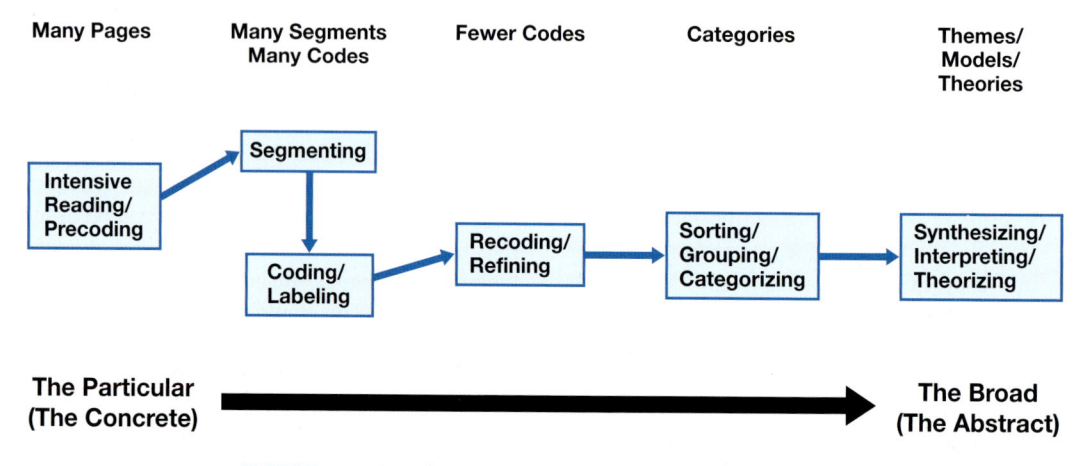

FIGURE 25.1 Broad overview of qualitative analysis processes.

refine the codes as they seek to "dig deeper" or to verify the coding. Coding is an important mechanism for organizing the data and is also a process that stimulates insights.

The actual analysis of the data may involve multiple iterations of reading the entire dataset, developing new higher-order codes, looking for patterns, grouping codes into categories, identifying relationships among the categories, forming and reforming conceptualizations, exploring the properties and dimensions of categories and themes, and continually testing the formulations against the data.

CODING AND QUALITATIVE DATA MANAGEMENT

Qualitative analysis often begins with efforts to organize and manage the mass of narrative data, while at the same time developing ideas about what is going on in the data. In the next few sections, we discuss the widely used strategy of *coding* the data.

Developing a Coding Scheme

In qualitative analysis, a **code** is used to identify (in a data segment, such as a phrase, sentence, or paragraph) an interesting, salient, evocative, or essential feature of the data in relation to the phenomenon under investigation. Most coding schemes in qualitative analyses are data-driven and developed through induction as analysts read and reread their data.

> **TIP** Many qualitative researchers move from initial codes to higher-order analytic procedures, such as grouping codes into categories or clustering categories into themes. However, in some research traditions, notably grounded theory, there are *multiple* cycles of coding. Our discussion in this section focuses on initial coding.

Developing a high-quality inductive coding scheme requires a careful reading of the data, with an eye to identifying underlying concepts. Even if computer software will be used to *apply* codes to the data, most coding schemes are *developed* using paper-and-pencil methods—that is, by using printed copies of transcripts or field notes and writing preliminary codes next to the relevant segment. Typically, this process involves formatting the pages with two columns—one for the data and the other for the codes.

Codes can take many forms. Saldaña (2021) recommends that the codes be entire words or phrases, such as those shown in the right column of Table 25.1, which shows an excerpt from Beck's (2023a) study, one of the authors of this textbook, study about women's experiences of hyperemesis gravidarum. Depending on the nature of the coding, the codes can be nouns ("immobility," "fatigue"), adjectives ("powerless," "fearful"), verb phrases ("gained a lot of weight"), gerund-based phrases ("losing hope"), or even questions ("What went wrong?").

In developing preliminary codes, it is useful to select a mix of cases, to maximize opportunities for diverse content. One strategy is to deliberately select materials that vary along key dimensions, such as participant characteristics (e.g., males vs. females), role (patient vs. caretaker), or time-related factors (e.g., patients with different time elapsed since a diagnosis). A substantial sample of the data should be read before the scheme is applied to the dataset.

> **TIP** Saldaña (2021) has identified several skills and characteristics that promote excellence in coding. These include good organizational skills, flexibility, creativity, perseverance, and the capacity to deal with ambiguity. He also noted that having an extensive vocabulary is a desirable attribute, because word choices matter. He recommended using tools such as a thesaurus and dictionary while coding.

There are no straightforward or easy guidelines for the task of developing codes—and no magic number for how many codes are needed. Sometimes researchers develop 100 or more codes in a study, although "code proliferation" can complicate subsequent analytic work. Some methodologists advocate "lean coding" using a small number of codes. When the analytic segments being coded are phrases or sentences, many codes are needed to capture the detailed information. Fewer codes are needed if the "chunks" being coded are entire paragraphs. Table 25.1 shows an example of fairly detailed coding.

TABLE 25.1 • Example of a Coded Excerpt

DATA EXTRACT	CODES
"**From this point on I did 1–2 week stays** on the maternity ward with occasional days at home here and there to break it up. I remember those days at home so well, my husband would go to work, and **I'd lay in bed with a bucket and vomit 5–6 times every 20–30 minutes the entire day**. **Sleeping** was the only way it seemed to slow down. I couldn't watch TV or read or even talk. I would lay there in a dark room staring at the walls **crying a lot. I didn't even have the energy to sit up while vomiting** and would often choke. I started **vomiting blood due to a tear in my esophagus.** Time dragged on and I remember **wanting to give up so many times**. I have never **felt so unwell in my entire life. Almost everything set me off.** The smell of absolutely anything. Loud noises, the sight of food, perfumes, moisturizers, walking, car trips, and specifically showering.	Frequent hospital stays Almost continuous vomiting Sleeping to slow vomiting Crying a lot No energy Vomiting blood Wanting to give up Feeling so unwell Triggers to vomiting

From the author's (unpublished) coding scheme for the study reported in the following paper: Beck, C. T. (2023a). Survivors' experiences of hyperemesis gravidarum. *Journal of Infusion Nursing, 46*(6), 338–346.

Saldaña (2021) has identified 30 different types of "first-cycle" coding approaches that vary along several dimensions, such as amount of detail and level of abstraction. Here are some examples, with coded excerpts from a study of hunger and food insecurity in low-income families (Polit et al., 2000):

- **Descriptive coding** uses mainly nouns as codes and is often the method of choice of beginning qualitative researchers; it does not, however, provide much insight into meaning.
  - *Excerpt:* "The other day, we ran out of everything and we had to go to a church and get food"
  - *Code:* Food pantry use
- **Process coding** often involves using gerunds as codes to connote action and observable activity (including conceptual action) in the data.
  - *Excerpt:* "The other day, we ran out of everything and we had to go to a church and get food"
  - *Code:* Running out of food (or, using community resources)
- **Concept coding** involves using a word or phrase to represent symbolically a broad meaning beyond observable facts or behaviors; the codes are usually nouns or gerunds.
  - *Excerpt:* "The other day, we ran out of everything and we had to go to a church and get food"
  - *Code:* Coping with the risk of hunger
- **In vivo coding** (also called "literal" or "verbatim" coding) involves using participant-generated words and phrases; it is used as initial coding in many grounded theory studies but is also applied in other types of qualitative research.
  - *Excerpt:* "The other day, we <u>ran out of everything</u> and we <u>had to go to a church and get food</u>"
  - *Codes:* Ran out of everything; had to go to a church and get food

- **Holistic coding** involves using codes to grasp broad ideas in large "chunks" of data, rather than coding smaller segments.
  - *Excerpt:* "I buy on deals. I learned how to, you know, what to buy and what not to buy. Where to shop, where to look for sales. I'll go to all the stores. And I clip coupons from the paper and stuff. But sometimes that's not enough. The other day, we ran out of everything and we had to go to a church and get food."
  - *Code:* Food management strategies

Saldaña (2021) acknowledges that some researchers, especially those doing phenomenologic research, label and analyze portions of the data with an extended thematic statement rather than a shorter code. He refers to this type of "coding" as theming the data.

As these examples show, the same excerpt can be coded in various ways—there is no single "right" way to code data, and two people are unlikely to develop identical codes for the same data. Sometimes researchers explore alternative ways of coding their data until they achieve a desirable solution. When working in teams, the team should reach a decision about the type of coding to use; team members should independently develop codes and then collaboratively work toward achieving a consensus.

> **Example of a Descriptive Coding Scheme**
> Karahan and colleagues (2022) studied the experiences of six nurses who cared for burn patients. Data were collected by semistructured face-to-face interviews. Initial codes were generated across the dataset. The relationships between the codes were evaluated and themes determined.

> **TIP** While coding, it is inevitable that you will notice important patterns in the data. Your evolving ideas and observations should be faithfully maintained in analytic memos.

Coding Qualitative Data

When a coding scheme has been developed, it should be reviewed and pilot-tested with a sample of texts. It is sometimes recommended that a single person apply the codes to the entire dataset, to ensure the highest possible coding consistency across interviews or observations, but team coding is recommended by others. It is often prudent to have at least a portion of the texts coded by two or more people early in the coding process, to evaluate and enhance reliability.

Researchers often create two products at this point. One is a master list of codes or *index*, usually in alphabetical order or in some hierarchical arrangement. The second is a *codebook*, which is a compilation of the codes with good descriptions and one or more excerpts that typify content for that code.

Once a coding scheme has been developed, the data are read in their entirety and coded for correspondence to the codes. Researchers may have difficulty deciding the most appropriate code or may not fully comprehend the underlying meaning of some data segments. It may take several readings of the data to grasp its nuances.

Researchers often discover during coding that the initial codes were incomplete. Concepts frequently emerge during coding that were not initially identified. When this happens, it is risky to assume that the concept was absent in materials that have already been coded. A concept might not be identified as salient until it has emerged several times. In such a case, it would be necessary to reread all previously coded material to ensure that the code is applied in a comprehensive fashion.

Another issue is that narrative materials seldom are linear. For example, paragraphs from transcribed interviews may contain elements relating to three or four different codes, embedded in a complex fashion. Table 25.1 provides an example of a paragraph with multiple codes.

Qualitative Data Management

Coding is an important early step in analyzing data in most qualitative studies, and it also plays an important role in data organization. Researchers must be able to gain access to parts of the data, without having repeatedly to reread the dataset in its entirety. Coding converts the data into smaller, more manageable units that can be retrieved and reviewed. Coding the data can be done manually using paper-and-pencil methods, followed by manual methods of data organization. Increasingly, however, special software is being used to code and manage the data.

Manual Methods of Managing Qualitative Data

Before the advent of computer software for managing qualitative data, a typical procedure was to develop **conceptual files**. In this approach, researchers begin with printed copies of the data with the codes in the margins. They create a physical file folder for each code and insert material relating to that code into the file by cutting up excerpts from the data. All of the content for a particular code can be retrieved by going to the applicable file folder.

Researchers must also provide enough context that the cut-up material can be understood, including material preceding or following the directly relevant materials. Finally, researchers must usually include pertinent administrative information. For example, for interview data, each excerpt would need to include the participant's ID number so that researchers could, if necessary, obtain additional information from the master copy of the transcript.

> **TIP** Other methods of manual organization include the use of file cards that can be sorted into piles, or post-it notes that can be arrayed on a large surface. For small datasets with few codes, researchers sometimes use different colored fonts for excerpts with different codes.

Computer Software for Managing Qualitative Data

Computer-assisted qualitative data analysis software (**CAQDAS**) removes the work of cutting up pages of narrative material. These programs allow researchers to enter and store the entire data file on a computer, code each portion of the narrative, and then retrieve and display text tagged with specified codes for analytic reflection. Most software allows researchers to write analytic memos, and some offer transcription services. The software can also be used to examine relationships between codes. Software cannot, however, *do* the coding, and it cannot tell researchers how to analyze the data. Researchers must continue to be analysts and critical thinkers.

Dozens of CAQDAS have been developed. The main types of available packages include software for text retrieval, coding and retrieval, theory building, concept mapping, and data conversion/collection. Tutorials on the mechanics of using various software packages are widely available on YouTube.

A popular option is sophisticated *theory-building software,* which permits researchers to examine relationships between concepts, develop hierarchies of codes, construct diagrams, and generate hyperlinks to create nonhierarchical networks. Examples of theory-building packages include NVivo, ATLAS.ti, HyperRESEARCH, MAXQDA, Quirkos, and QDA Miner, most of which are available in Mac and PC versions. As with any product, each has its own set of features, interfaces, and pricing structure. When choosing the most appropriate software for the management of qualitative data, researchers must take into account their specific needs and preferences.

> **TIP** Transana is an example of specialty software that enables the coding of large digital audio and video files. Dedoose is cloud-based software known for its ability to work well in mixed methods studies with both qualitative and quantitative data. Several qualitative data analysis software packages are available using cloud-based platforms, enabling users to access and analyze qualitative data via web browsers and cloud-based applications. For example, ATLAS.ti Web can be accessed on any computer with internet access, allowing teams to collaborate in real time. NVIVO works with a browser extension called NCapture that allows users to import web pages, online content, and social media data such as Facebook or Twitter content captured as datasets and imported directly from a web browser into the NVIVO software program. Several qualitative data analysis software programs incorporate Artificial Intelligence (AI) analysis features to enhance data analysis and interpretation. The field of Artificial Intelligence (AI) varies across different versions or editions of software and the field of AI is constantly evolving.

Software for concept mapping permits researchers to construct more sophisticated diagrams than theory-building software. Concept maps are a means for organizing and representing knowledge. Cmap Tools, an example of concept mapping software, is available at no cost (Cmap Tools Free). Most qualitative data analysis packages offer limited support for concept mapping functionality, but many allow users to export data and work on concept maps in external applications.

Data conversion and collection software, such as voice recognition software, converts audio into text. Such software may be attractive because of the time and expense needed to transcribe audio-recorded interviews. Voice recognition software is designed for both single user and multiuser scenarios, making it important to consider the specific needs and requirements of the researcher when using voice recognition software. The software must be "trained" to recognize the voice of the user, typically an *oral transcriptionist*. In multiuser scenarios, the software features options for handling user profiles in multiuser scenarios. As cloud-based services continue gaining popularity, users can access cloud-based voice recognition through web browsers or dedicated applications, creating flexibility and enabling user collaboration.

The performance of voice recognition software is variable and depends on such factors as computer capabilities, the quality of the microphone, and the amount of background noise. One disadvantage is the inability of voice recognition software to automatically punctuate. The oral transcriptionist must specifically state the punctuation, such as "period" and "comma." Oral transcriptionists also need to edit the text to correct errors. For instance, voice recognition programs often misinterpret common homonyms like "to," "too," and "two." Thus, the time-saving advantages in using voice recognition software may be modest.

Computer programs offer many advantages for managing qualitative data, but some people prefer manual methods as a means of getting closer to the data. Others have raised objections to having a process that is basically cognitive turned into an activity that is mechanical. Another disadvantage is that a considerable amount of time is typically needed to learn the software—but, once learned, the skills can be used for future projects. Despite concerns, many researchers have switched to computerized data management. Proponents insist that it frees up their time and permits them to pay greater attention to important conceptual issues.

Example of Using Computers to Manage Qualitative Data
Modula (2022) explored the support needs provided to families raising children with intellectual disability in South Africa. In depth interviews and focus groups were conducted with 26 families. Transcripts were uploaded to Atlas.ti qualitative data analysis software for coding and analysis.

OVERVIEW OF ANALYTIC PROCEDURES

Data coding and *management* in qualitative research are reductionist in nature: They involve converting masses of data into smaller, manageable segments. By contrast, qualitative data *analysis* is constructionist: segments are put together into meaningful conceptual patterns. Qualitative analysis involves discovering pervasive ideas and searching for general concepts (*analytic generalization*) through an inductive process. Although there are various approaches to qualitative data analysis, some features are common to several of them.

The analysis of qualitative materials often begins with the identification of broad **categories**, which are clusters of codes that are connected conceptually. In Table 25.1, which shows a coded excerpt from Beck's (2023a) study of survivors of hyperemesis gravidarum two of the codes ("inability to keep fluids down" and "vomiting so violently") were clustered with other codes to form the category "Physical symptoms." Ideas for categories usually begin to emerge during coding or precoding and would likely be documented in analytic memos.

In many qualitative studies, the next phase involves the identification of themes. In their thorough review of how the term *theme* is used among qualitative researchers, DeSantis and Ugarriza (2000) offered this often-cited definition: "A **theme** is an abstract entity that brings meaning and identity to a current experience and its variant manifestations. As such, a theme captures and unifies the nature or basis of the experience into a meaningful whole" (p. 362).

The analysis of themes involves not only discovering commonalities across participants, but also seeking natural variation. Themes are never universal. Researchers must attend not only to what themes arise but also to how they are patterned. Does the theme apply only to certain types of people? In certain contexts? At certain periods? What are the conditions that precede the observed phenomenon, and what are the apparent consequences of it? In other words, the qualitative analyst must be sensitive to *relationships* in the data.

Researchers' search for themes and patterns sometimes can be facilitated by charting devices that enable them to summarize the evolution of behaviors, events, and processes. For example, for qualitative studies that focus on dynamic experiences—such as decision-making—it is sometimes useful to develop flowcharts or timelines that highlight time sequences, major decision points and events, and factors affecting the decisions. Another device that depicts the clustering of codes and categories is called a **dendrogram**, which is a tree diagram that illustrates the arrangement of clusters in a hierarchically ordered system (Krippendorff, 2019). Figure 25.2 is a dendrogram from Beck's (2023a) study of survivors' experiences of hyperemesis gravidarum. Codes were clustered to create categories and these categories were the basis of the theme.

Two-dimensional matrices are another method of displaying thematic material (Miles et al., 2020). Traditionally, each row of a matrix represents individual participants, and columns are used for codes or themes. The entries at the intersection are the raw data or summaries. Matrices can be constructed by hand, but computer spreadsheets enhance opportunities for sorting the data.

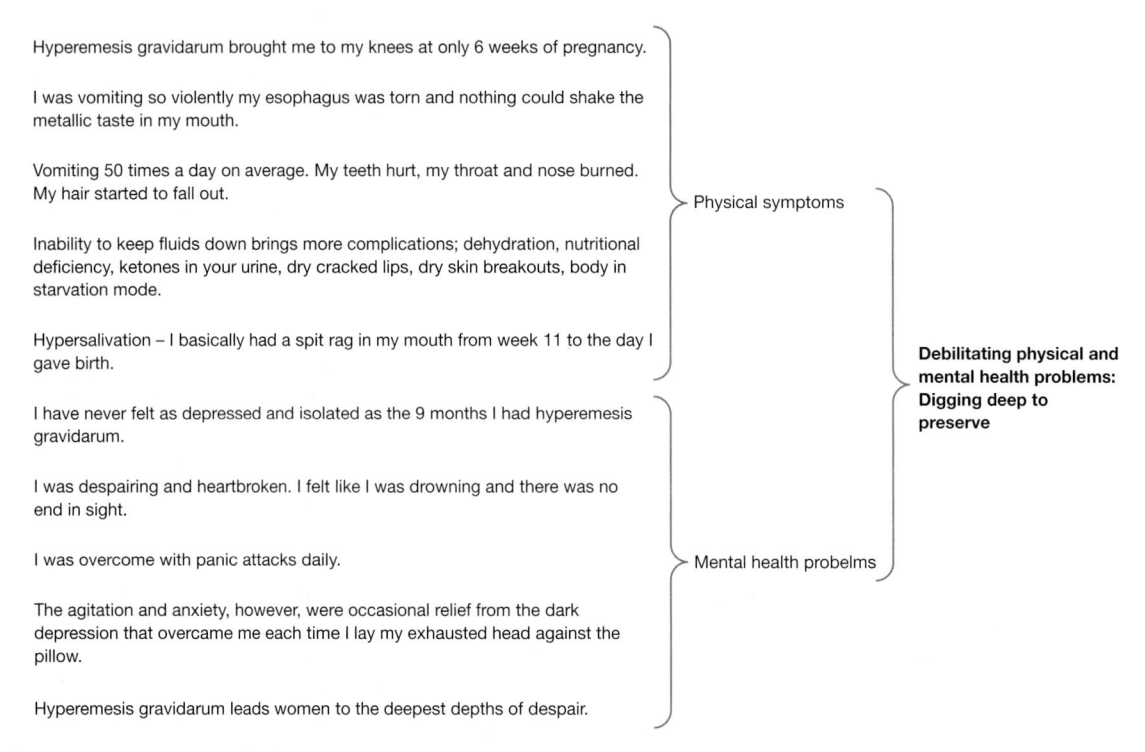

FIGURE 25.2 Codes and categories shown in a dendrogram for theme 1: Debilitating physical and mental health problems: Digging deep to persevere. (Reprinted from Beck C. T., & Gable R. (2012). A mixed methods study of secondary traumatic stress in labor and delivery nurses. *Journal of Obstetric, Gynecologic, & Neonatal Nursing, 41*, 747–760, with permiission of Elsevier.)

Some qualitative researchers—especially phenomenologists—use metaphors as an analytic strategy. A metaphor is a symbolic comparison, using figurative language to evoke a visual analogy. Metaphors can be a powerfully expressive tool for qualitative analysts. As a literary device, metaphors can permit greater insight and understanding in qualitative analysis and can help link together parts to the whole. Thorne and Darbyshire (2005), however, expressed concern about overusing metaphors. In their view, metaphoric allusions can be a compelling approach to depicting human experience but can run the risk of "supplanting creative insight with hackneyed cliché masquerading as profundity" (p. 1111). Carpenter (2008) also warned that when researchers mix metaphors, fail to follow through with metaphors, or use metaphors that do not fit, they can misrepresent their data. It is also possible to do an analysis of the metaphors that study participants themselves use.

Example of a Metaphor
Beck (2022a) conducted a metaphorical analysis of the impact of traumatic birth on mothers' breastfeeding experiences. Some of the metaphors used by the mothers to describe their experiences included an empty affair, head in a vise, mechanical, true grit, and a form of forgiveness.

Identifying key categories and themes is seldom a tidy, linear process. Researchers derive themes from the narrative materials, go back to the materials with the themes in mind to see if the materials really do fit, and then refine the themes as necessary. Sometimes apparent insights early in the analysis need to be abandoned.

Some level of interpretation is essential in analyzing narrative materials, with interpretation and analysis occurring virtually simultaneously and iteratively. Interpretation is a challenging activity in qualitative analysis—and the most difficult to explain in a manner that makes clear how to achieve it. Although it is hard to provide guidance on interpretation, there is considerable agreement that the ability to "make meaning" from qualitative texts depends on researchers' immersion in and closeness to the data. **Incubation** is the process of *living* the data, a process in which researchers must try to understand the data's meanings, find their essential patterns, and draw legitimate, insightful conclusions. Another key ingredient in interpretation and meaning-making is researchers' self-awareness and the ability to reflect on their own world view and perspectives—that is, reflexivity.

Creativity also plays an important role in uncovering meaning in the data. Hunter and colleagues (2002) have written about the role of creativity in qualitative analysis and offer insights designed to "shed light on the magic of understanding the mysteries within data" (p. 388). Chandler, in writing about the transition from *saturation* to *illumination*, wrote that "Strategies for creativity take time and require incubation for new ideas to percolate" (Chandler in Hunter et al., p. 396). Researchers need to give themselves sufficient time to achieve the *aha* that comes with making meaning beyond the facts.

Researchers strive to weave thematic pieces together into an integrated whole. The various themes or categories need to be interrelated to provide an overall structure (such as an integrated description, model, or theory) to the data. The integration task is difficult because it demands ingenuity and intellectual rigor. In drawing conclusions, qualitative researchers are increasingly considering the transferability of the findings and the potential uses to which the qualitative evidence can be put. Like quantitative researchers, qualitative researchers need to give thought to the implications of their study findings for future research and for nursing practice.

Braun and Clarke's (2022) reflexive thematic analysis is a popular method for identifying themes in descriptive qualitative studies. Their method involves a six-phase process. Braun and Clarke state that their method of thematic analysis is differentiated from other thematic analyses by their emphasis on reflexivity of the researcher. Phase 1 entails the researchers familiarizing themselves with their dataset. Coding, which is a process of interpretation, occurs in phase 2 and can be inductive or deductive. Coding can range from semantic, which is descriptive, and participant driven to latent, which is conceptual and researcher driven. In phase 3, the researcher generates initial themes from clusters of codes. The researcher next develops and reviews themes in phase 4. Refining, defining, and naming themes occur in phase 5. The sixth and final phase focuses on writing up the results of the reflexive thematic analysis.

> **Example of Braun and Clarke's Reflexive Thematic Analysis**
> In Sweden, Lillieskold and colleagues (2022) studied parents' experiences of immediate skin-to-skin contact after the birth of their very preterm neonates. The researchers analyzed interviews with six parent couples using Braun and Clarke's reflexive thematic analysis. Three themes were identified: a pathway to connectedness, just being in a vulnerable state, and creating a safe haven in an unknown terrain.

QUALITATIVE ANALYSIS WITHIN RESEARCH TRADITIONS

In this section, we provide an overview of analytic approaches that have been advocated by researchers within the three main research traditions described in this book—ethnography, phenomenology, and grounded theory. These overviews are not sufficiently detailed to provide guidance on how to actually do an analysis; references are provided for further assistance.

Ethnographic Analysis

Analysis begins from the moment ethnographers set foot in the field. Ethnographers are continually looking for *patterns* in the behavior of participants, comparing one pattern against another, and analyzing many patterns simultaneously (Fetterman, 2020). As they become immersed in the everyday lives of participants, ethnographers acquire a deeper understanding of the culture being studied. Maps, flowcharts, and organizational charts are useful tools that help to crystallize and illustrate the data. Matrices (two-dimensional displays) can also help to highlight a comparison graphically, to cross-reference categories, and to discover emerging patterns.

Spradley's (1979) research sequence is sometimes used to analyze ethnographic data. His method is based on the premise that language is the primary means that relates cultural meaning in a culture. His sequence of 12 steps, which includes data collection and data analysis, is as follows:

1. Locating an informant
2. Interviewing an informant
3. Making an ethnographic record
4. Asking descriptive questions
5. Analyzing ethnographic interviews
6. Making a domain analysis
7. Asking structural questions
8. Making a taxonomic analysis
9. Asking contrast questions
10. Making a componential analysis
11. Discovering cultural themes
12. Writing the ethnography

Spradley's method involves four levels of data analysis, the first of which is **domain analysis**. Domains, which are units of cultural knowledge, are broad categories that encompass smaller ones. During this first level of data analysis, ethnographers identify relational patterns among terms in the domains that are used by members of the culture. The ethnographer focuses on the cultural meaning of terms and symbols (objects and events) used in a culture and their interrelationships.

In **taxonomic analysis**, the second level of data analysis, ethnographers decide how many domains the analysis will encompass. Will only one or two domains be analyzed in depth, or will several domains be studied less intensively? After making this decision, a **taxonomy**—a system of classifying and organizing terms—is developed to illustrate the internal organization of a domain and the relationship among the subcategories of the domain. In **componential analysis**, the ethnographer analyzes data for similarities and differences among cultural terms in a domain. Finally, in **theme analysis**, cultural themes are uncovered. Domains are connected in cultural themes, which help to provide a holistic view of the culture being studied. The discovery of cultural meaning is the outcome.

> **Example Using Spradley's Method**
> Hwang et al. (2024) followed Spradley's analytic sequence in an ethnographic study on cultivating a positive research culture in clinical practice. The researchers conducted ethnographic interviews with six registered nurses working in a medical–surgical unit in a Korean tertiary hospital. Participant observation also was done both within the actual clinical environment of that hospital and in web-based spaces during video research conferences.

Other approaches to ethnographic analysis have been developed. For example, in Leininger's ethnonursing research method, as described in McFarland and Wehbe-Alamah (2015), ethnographers follow a four-phase ethnonursing data analysis guide. In the first phase, ethnographers collect, describe, and record data. The second phase involves identifying and categorizing descriptors. In phase 3, data are analyzed to discover repetitive patterns in their context. The fourth and final phase involves abstracting major themes and presenting findings.

Example Using Leininger's Method
Burkett and colleagues (2022) explored promotores' (community health workers) perspectives on recruiting Latino(a) immigrant community members for an intervention study on autism spectrum disorders. Focus group interviews were analyzed using Leininger's data analysis enabler.

Phenomenologic Analysis

Many qualitative analysts use what might be called "fracturing" strategies that break down the data and rearrange them into categories. Phenomenologists tend to prefer holistic, "contextualizing" strategies that involve interpreting the narrative data within the context of a "whole text." We look briefly at three broad approaches to phenomenologic analysis.

Descriptive Phenomenology

Three frequently used methods for descriptive phenomenology are the methods of Colaizzi (1978), Giorgi (1985), and van Kaam (1966). All three are from the Duquesne School of phenomenology, based on Husserl's philosophy.

Phenomenologic analysis using these methods involves a search for common patterns, but there are differences among these approaches, as summarized in Table 25.2. The basic outcome of all three methods is the description of the meaning of an experience, often through the identification of essential themes. Colaizzi's method, however, is the only one that calls for a validation of results by returning to study participants. Giorgi's analysis relies solely on researchers. His view was that it is inappropriate to return to participants to validate findings or to use external judges to review the analysis. Van Kaam's method requires that intersubjective agreement be reached with other expert judges.

Example of a Study Using Colaizzi's Method
Park et al. (2022) studied 40 South Korean's experiences of death and a funeral in a hospital setting. Colaizzi's data analysis steps were followed. Three major findings included vagueness of funeral culture, distortion of meaning in funeral culture, and the need to prepare for death and the process of grief.

The Utrecht School of Phenomenology

Another approach to phenomenology is the Utrecht School, which combines characteristics of descriptive and interpretive phenomenology. Van Manen's (1990) method is an example of this approach, in which researchers try to grasp the essential meaning of the experience being studied. According to van Manen, thematic aspects of experience can be uncovered from participants' descriptions of the experience by three methods: (1) the holistic approach, (2) the selective (highlighting) approach, and (3) the detailed (line-by-line) approach. In the **holistic approach**, researchers view the text as a whole and try to capture its meanings. In the **selective approach**, researchers highlight or pull out statements or phrases that seem essential to the experience under study. In the **detailed approach**, researchers analyze every sentence. Once themes have been identified, they become the objects of reflection and interpretation through follow-up interviews with participants. Through this process, essential themes are discovered.

Van Manen (2006) emphasized that this phenomenologic method cannot be separated from the practice of writing. Writing up the results of qualitative analysis is an active struggle to understand and recognize the lived meanings of the phenomena studied. The text written by a phenomenologic researcher must lead readers to a "questioning wonder." Van Manen (2017) has recently asserted that "the outcomes of phenomenologic research are full-fledged reflective texts that induce the reader into a wondering engagement with certain questions that may be explored through the identification, critical examination, and eloquent elaboration of themes

TABLE 25.2 • Comparison of Three Phenomenologic Analytic Methods

COLAIZZI (1978)	GIORGI (1985)	VAN KAAM (1966)
1. Read all protocols to acquire a feeling for them.	1. Read the entire set of protocols to get a sense of the whole.	1. List and group preliminarily the descriptive expressions that must be agreed upon by expert judges. Final listing presents percentages of these categories in that particular sample.
2. Review each protocol and extract significant statements.	2. Discriminate units from participants' description of phenomenon being studied.	2. Reduce the concrete, vague, and overlapping expressions of the participants to more descriptive terms. (Intersubjective agreement among judges needed.)
3. Spell out the meaning of each significant statement (i.e., formulate meanings).	3. Articulate the psychological insight in each of the meaning units.	3. Eliminate elements not inherent in the phenomenon being studied or that represent blending of two related phenomena.

4. Organize the formulated meanings into clusters of themes.
  a. Refer these clusters back to the original protocols to validate them.
  b. Note discrepancies among or between the various clusters, avoiding the temptation of ignoring data or themes that do not fit.
	4. Synthesize all of the transformed meaning units into a consistent statement regarding participants' experiences (referred to as the "structure of the experience"); can be expressed on a specific or general level.	4. Write a hypothetical identification and description of the phenomenon being studied.

5. Integrate results into an exhaustive description of the phenomenon under study.		5. Apply hypothetical description to randomly selected cases from the sample. If necessary, revise the hypothesized description, which must then be tested again on a new random sample.
6. Formulate an exhaustive description of the phenomenon under study in as unequivocal a statement of identification as possible.		6. Consider the hypothesized identification as a valid identification and description once preceding operations have been carried out successfully.
7. Ask participants about the findings thus far as a final validating step.		

that help the reader recognize the meaningfulness of certain human experiences and events" (p. 777).

> **Example of a Study Using van Manen's Method**
> Dolan and colleagues (2022) studied the experience of being at risk for falling in the hospital among nine older adults. Interview data were analyzed using van Manen's interpretive phenomenological method. Five themes were identified: relying on myself, managing balance problems in unfamiliar environment, struggling to maintain identify, following hospital rules, and maintaining dignity in relationships with nursing staff.

In addition to identifying themes from participants' words, van Manen also called for gleaning thematic descriptions from artistic sources. Van Manen urged qualitative researchers to keep in mind that literature, music, painting, and other art forms can provide experiential information that can increase insights as the phenomenologist tries to grasp the essential meaning of the experience being studied. Experiential descriptions in literature and art help challenge and stretch phenomenologists' interpretive sensibilities.

Interpretive Phenomenology and Hermeneutics

A third broad category of phenomenology is interpretive phenomenology (hermeneutics). As noted in Chapter 22, a key concept in a hermeneutic study is the *hermeneutic circle*. The circle signifies a methodologic process in which, to reach understanding, there is continual movement between the parts and the whole of the text being analyzed. Gadamer (1975) stressed that, to interpret a text, researchers cannot separate themselves from the meanings of the text and must strive to understand possibilities that the text can reveal. Ricoeur (1981) broadened this notion of text to include not just the written text but any human action or situation.

Diekelmann et al. (1989) proposed a seven-stage process of data analysis in hermeneutics that involves collaboration by a team of researchers:

1. All the interviews or texts are read for an overall understanding.
2. Interpretive summaries of each interview are written.
3. A team of researchers analyzes selected transcribed interviews or texts.
4. Any disagreements on interpretation are resolved by going back to the text.
5. Common meanings are identified by comparing and contrasting the text.
6. Relationships among themes emerge.
7. A draft of the themes with exemplars from texts is presented to the team. Responses or suggestions are incorporated into the final draft.

According to Diekelmann and colleagues, the discovery in step 6 of a **constitutive pattern**—a pattern that expresses the relationships among relational themes and is present in all the interviews or texts—is the highest level of hermeneutic analysis. A situation is constitutive when it gives actual content to a person's self-understanding or to a person's way of being in the world.

> **Example of a Diekelmann's Hermeneutic Analysis**
> The purpose of Chatreewatanakul and colleagues' (2022) hermeneutic phenomenological study was to understand the experiences of symptom recognition and to explain the pattern of symptom management successfully among exacerbation COPD patients. Using Diekelmann's approach, the research team identified two constitutive patterns: symptom recognition and symptom management.

Benner (1994) offered another analytic approach for hermeneutics. Her interpretive analysis consists of three interrelated processes: the search for paradigm cases, thematic analysis, and the analysis of exemplars. **Paradigm cases** are "strong instances of concerns or ways of being in the world" (p. 113). Paradigm cases are used early in the analytic process as a strategy for gaining understanding. Thematic analysis is done to compare and contrast similarities across cases. Paradigm cases and thematic analysis can be enhanced by identifying **exemplars** that illuminate aspects of a paradigm case or theme. The presentation of paradigm cases and exemplars in reports allows readers to play a role in consensual validation of the results by deciding whether the cases support the researchers' conclusions.

Example Using Benner's Hermeneutic Analysis

Létourneau and colleagues (2022) studied nursing students and nurses' recommendations that can foster the development of humanistic caring in Canada. Data from individual interviews with 26 participants were analyzed using Benner's phenomenological method. The researchers identified five themes: pedagogical strategies, educators' approach, considerations in teaching humanistic caring, work overload, and volunteerism and externship.

Parse's (2016) Parsesciencing is another hermeneutic approach. Parse's second phase of inquiry, distilling-fusing, involves the researcher dwelling with transcribed interviews and audio recordings. A story is constructed that captures the central ideas about the phenomenon from each "historian's" (participant's) dialogue. These central ideas are labeled *essences*. Essences, written in the historian's language, are brought to a higher abstraction using the researcher's language. Next, the essences are fused and lead to a language art for each historian. A discerning extant moment of the universal human universe living experience is created. In the final phase, heuristic interpreting entails transmogrifying, transsubstantiating, metaphorical emergings, and artistic expressions. In *transmogrifying*, language is shifted to a new level of abstraction. Then in *transsubstantiating*, the language is shaped into the core language of humanbecoming. The statements shared by the historians that are described in symbolic language are the *metaphorical emergings*. Lastly, the researcher's own personal choice for the art form to present the results of their Parsesciencing is the focus of artistic expression.

TIP Another approach mentioned in Chapter 22 is *reflective lifeworld research* (RLR). Dahlberg and colleagues (2008) presented steps for the analysis of data in both descriptive phenomenologic RLR studies and hermeneutic RLR studies. Beck, one of the authors of this textbook, and Watson (2019) used the RLR approach in their phenomenological study of women's experiences interacting with their infants after traumatic childbirth.

Grounded Theory Analysis

Grounded theory methods emerged in the 1960s in connection with Glaser and Strauss's (1967) research program on dying in hospitals. The two co-originators eventually split and developed divergent schools of thought, which have been called the "Glaserian" and "Straussian" versions of grounded theory. A third grounded theory approach—constructivist grounded theory—has emerged more recently. The differences among these approaches mainly concern the analysis of the data (see Table 25.3).

Glaser and Strauss's Grounded Theory Method

Constant comparison is a core feature in all grounded theory analyses and in many other qualitative analyses. This method involves a comparison of elements present in one data source (e.g., in one interview) with those in another to determine if they are similar. The process continues until the content of each source has been compared to the content in all sources. In this fashion, commonalities are identified.

The concept of fit is a key element in Glaserian grounded theory analysis. By **fit,** Glaser meant that the developing categories of the substantive theory must fit the data. Fit enables the researcher to determine if data can be placed in the same category or if they can be related to one another. However, Glaser (1992) warned qualitative researchers not to force an analytic fit, noting that "if you torture data enough it will give up!" (p. 123). Forcing a fit hinders the development of a viable theory. *Fit* is also an important issue when a grounded theory is applied in new contexts: the theory must closely "fit" the substantive area where it will be used (Glaser & Strauss, 1967).

In the classic Glaserian approach, the substance of the data is conceptualized through *substantive codes*, while *theoretical codes* provide insights into how substantive codes relate to each other. Substantive coding includes both open coding and selective coding. **Open coding,** used in the first stage of the constant comparative analysis, captures what is going on in the data. Through open coding, data are broken down into incidents and their similarities and differences are examined.

TABLE 25.3 • Comparison of Alternative Grounded Theory Approaches

	GLASER	**CORBIN AND STRAUSS**	**CHARMAZ**
Initial data analysis	Breaking down and conceptualizing data, with comparisons so that patterns emerge	Breaking down and conceptualizing data, which include taking apart a single sentence, observation, or incident	Creating link between collecting data and developing emergent theory; defining what is occurring in data and beginning to analyze what it means
Types of coding	Open, selective, theoretical	Open, axial, and selective	Initial, focused
Connections between categories: strategies	18 coding families plus theoretical codes from different disciplines	Paradigm (conditions, actions–interactions, and consequences or outcomes) and the conditional/consequential matrix	Analytic strategies are emergent rather than procedural application; categories, subcategories, and links
Outcome	Emergent theory (discovery)	Conceptual description (verification)	An interpretive theory constructed through researcher's past and present involvement with people, perspectives, and research practices

There are three levels of open coding, with increasing degrees of abstraction. **Level I codes** (or *in vivo codes*) are derived directly from the participants' words and have vivid imagery. Table 25.4 presents five level I codes from Beck's (2002) grounded theory study on mothering twins and interview excerpts associated with those codes. Researchers constantly compare new level I codes to previously identified ones and then condense them into broader **level II codes** (categories). For example, in Table 25.4, Beck's five level I codes were collapsed into the level II category, "Reaping the Blessings." **Level III codes** (or theoretical constructs) are the most abstract. These constructs "add scope beyond local meanings" (Glaser, 1978, p. 70) to the generated theory. Collapsing level II codes aids in identifying constructs. In Beck's study, the level II code of "Reaping the Blessings" was collapsed with another level II code ("Becoming manageable") into the level III code "Resuming Own Life."

Open coding ends when the core category is discovered and then selective coding begins. The **core category** is a pattern of behavior that is relevant for participants. The primary function of a core category is to integrate the theory and make it dense and saturated. The core category in Glaserian grounded theory earns its prominence by accounting for most of the variation in processing the participants' main concern that has emerged as the study focus and by explaining the latent pattern of behavior that accounts for its resolution (Holton, 2010). In **selective coding**, researchers code only those data that relate to the core variable. One kind of core variable is a **basic social process (BSP)** that evolves over time in two or more phases. All BSPs are core variables, but not all core variables have to be BSPs. In Beck's

TABLE 25.4 • Collapsing Level I Codes Into the Level II Code *"Reaping the Blessings"* (Beck, 2002)

QUOTE	LEVEL I CODE
I enjoy just watching the twins interact so much. Especially now that they are mobile. They are not walking yet but they are crawling. I will tell you they are already playing. Like one will go around the corner and kind of peek around and they play hide and seek. They crawl after each other.	Enjoying Twins
With twins it's amazing. She was sick and she had a fever. He was the one acting sick. She didn't seem like she was sick at all. He was. We watched him for like 6–8 hours. We gave her the medicine and he started calming down. Like WOW! That is so weird. Cause you read about it but it's like, Oh come on! You know that doesn't really happen and it does. It's really neat to see.	Amazing
These days it's really neat cause you go to the store or you go out and people are like "Oh, they are twins, how nice." And I say, "Yeah they are. Look, look at my kids."	Getting Attention
I just feel blessed to have two. I just feel like I am twice as lucky as a mom who has one baby. I mean that's the best part. It's just that instead of having one baby to watch grow and change and develop and become a toddler and school-age child you have two.	Feeling Blessed
It's very exciting. It's interesting and it's fun to see them and how the twin bond really is. There really is a twin bond. You read about it and you hear about it but until you experience it, you just don't understand. One time they were both crying and they were fed. They were changed and burped. There was nothing wrong. I couldn't figure out what was wrong. So I said to myself, "I am just going to put them together and close the door." I put them in my bed together and they patty-caked their hands and put their noses together and just looked at each other and went right to sleep.	Twin Bonding

From data for the study reported in the following paper: Beck, C. T. (2002). Releasing the pause button: Mothering twins during the first year of life. *Qualitative Health Research 12*, 593–608.

(2002) study, the core category—a BSP—was "Releasing the Pause Button."

Glaser (1978) provided nine criteria to help researchers decide on a core category:

1. It must be central, meaning that it is related to many categories.
2. It must reoccur frequently in the data.
3. It takes more time to saturate than other categories.
4. It relates meaningfully and easily to other categories.
5. It has clear and grabbing implications for formal theory.
6. It has considerable carry-through.
7. It is completely variable.
8. It is a dimension of the problem.
9. It can be any kind of a theoretical code.

Theoretical coding, which typically begins while selective coding is still in progress, helps grounded theorists to weave the broken pieces of data back together. Theoretical codes connect the categories and constructs that relate to the core category. Theoretical codes have the power "to grab," which Glaser (2005) called "theoretical code capture" (p. 74). Theoretical codes provide a grounded theory with greater explanatory power because they enhance the abstract meaning of the relationships among categories. Glaser (1978) first proposed 18 "families" of theoretical codes that researchers can use to conceptualize how substantive codes relate to each other (Box 25.1). Glaser (2005) later identified many new possibilities for theoretical codes, offering examples from biochemistry (bias random walk), economics (amplifying causal looping),

CHAPTER 25 Qualitative Data Analysis • 539

> **BOX 25.1   Families of Theoretical Codes for Grounded Theory Analysis**
>
> 1. The six Cs: causes, contexts, contingencies, consequences, covariances, and conditions
> 2. Process: stages, phases, passages, transitions
> 3. Degree: intensity, range, grades, continuum
> 4. Dimension: elements, parts, sections
> 5. Type: kinds, styles, forms
> 6. Strategy: tactics, techniques, maneuverings
> 7. Interaction: mutual effects, interdependence, reciprocity
> 8. Identity–self: self-image, self-worth, self-concept
> 9. Cutting point: boundaries, critical junctures, turning points
> 10. Means–goal: purpose, end products
> 11. Cultural: social values, beliefs
> 12. Consensus: agreements, uniformities, conformity
> 13. Mainline: socialization, recruiting, social order
> 14. Theoretical: density, integration, clarity, fit, relevance
> 15. Ordering/elaboration: structural ordering, temporal ordering, conceptual ordering
> 16. Unit: group, organization, collective
> 17. Reading: hypotheses, concepts, problems
> 18. Models: pictorial models of a theory
>
> Adapted from Glaser, B. G. (1978). *Theoretical sensitivity*. Mill Valley, CA: Sociological Press. https://sociologypress.com/book.htm

and political science (conjectural causation). Glaser believed that the large array of theoretical codes available reduces a researcher's tendency to force a pet or favorite theoretical code on the developing theory.

Throughout coding and analysis, grounded theory analysts document their ideas about the data, categories, and emerging conceptual scheme in *memos*. Memos preserve ideas that may initially not seem productive but may later prove valuable once further developed. Memos also encourage researchers to reflect on and describe patterns in the data, relationships between categories, and emergent conceptualizations.

> **TIP** Glaser (1978) offered guidelines for preparing effective memos to generate substantive theory, including the following:
> - Keep memos separate from data.
> - Stop coding when an idea for a memo occurs, so as not to lose the thought.
> - A memo can be brought on by forcing it, by beginning to write about a code.
> - Memos can be modified as growth and realizations occur.
> - In writing memos, do not focus on people; talk conceptually about substantive codes.
> - When you have two ideas, write each idea up as a separate memo to prevent confusion.
> - Always remain flexible with memoing approaches.

Glaser's grounded theory method is concerned with the *generation* of categories and hypotheses rather than testing them. The product of the typical grounded theory analysis is a model that endeavors to generate "a theory of continually resolving the main concern, which explains most of the behavior in an area of interest" (Glaser, 2001, p. 103). Once a problem or central concern emerges, the grounded theorist goes on to discover the process these participants experience in coping with or resolving the problem.

Example of Glaser and Strauss Grounded Theory Analysis

Figure 25.3 presents Beck's, one of the authors of this textbook (2002), model from a grounded theory study. "Releasing the Pause Button," the core category, was conceptualized as the process through which mothers of twins progressed as they attempted to resume their lives after giving birth. According to this model, the process involves four phases: Draining Power, Pausing Own Life, Striving to Reset, and Resuming Own Life. Beck used 10 coding families in her theoretical coding for the Releasing the Pause Button process. The bottom of Figure 25.3 shows the theoretical codes for the phases of her grounded theory: Conditions, Consequences, Strategies, and Consequences. Another theoretical code was the family *cutting point*. Three months seemed to be the turning point for mothers, when life started to become more manageable. Here is an excerpt that Beck coded as a cutting point: "Three months came around and the twins sort of slept through the night and it made a huge, huge difference."

Although Glaser cautioned against consulting the literature before a theory is stabilized, he also viewed grounded theory as an "ever-modifying process" (Glaser, 1978, p. 5) that could benefit from scrutiny of other work. Glaser discussed the evolution of grounded theories through the process of **emergent fit**, to prevent individual substantive theories from being "respected little islands of knowledge" (p. 148). Glaser pointed out that generating grounded theory does not necessarily require discovering all new categories or ignoring ones previously identified in the literature. Through constant comparison, researchers can compare concepts emerging from the data with similar concepts from existing theory or prior studies to assess which parts have emergent fit with the theory being generated.

In Glaser's (2001) view, grounded theory modification is an ongoing process. As data from new studies become available, the grounded theory can be modified to accommodate varying conditions, in an effort to increase the theory's power and completeness. Constantly comparing data from new research to the existing theory can illuminate new properties of the categories. When a grounded theory is continually modified, it is brought to a higher level of theoretical completeness.

Corbin and Strauss Approach

The Corbin and Strauss (2015) approach to grounded theory analysis (the "Straussian" approach) differs from the original Glaser and Strauss method with regard to method, process, and outcomes, as summarized in Table 25.3.

Glaser believed that to generate a grounded theory, the basic problem must emerge from the

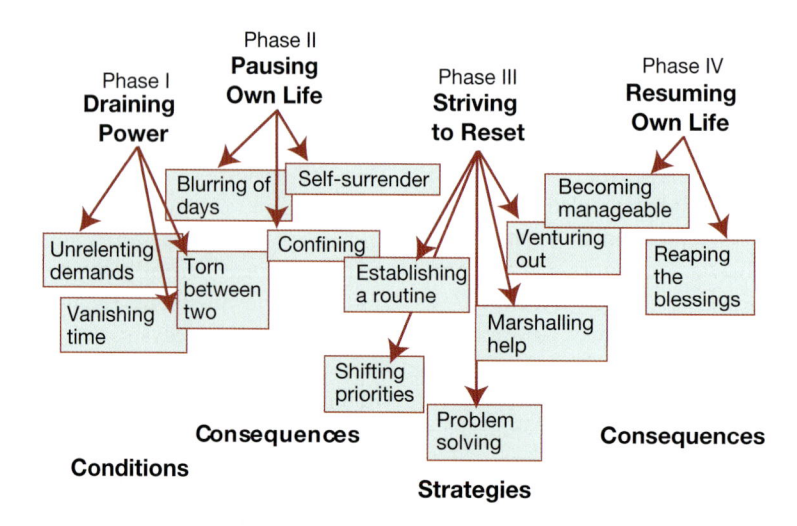

FIGURE 25.3 Beck's (2002) model of mothering twins. (Reprinted with permission from Beck, C. T. (2002). Releasing the pause button: Mothering twins during the first year of life. *Qualitative Health Research, 12*, 593–608.)

data—it must be discovered. The theory is grounded in the data, rather than starting with a preconceived problem. Corbin and Strauss, however, argued that the research itself is only one possible source of a problem. Research problems can, for example, come from the literature, a researcher's personal and professional experience, an advisor or mentor, or a pilot project.

The Corbin and Strauss method involves three types of coding: open, axial, and selective coding. In **open coding**, data are broken down into parts and concepts identified for interpreted meaning of the raw data. In **axial coding**, the analyst groups the open codes according to conceptual categories that reflect commonalities among the codes. The term *axial coding* reflects the idea of clustering the open codes around "axes" or points of intersection. In axial coding, the analyst is "locating and linking action–interaction within a framework of subconcepts that give it meaning and enable it to explain what interactions are occurring, and why and what consequences real or anticipated are happening" (Corbin & Strauss, 2015, p. 156). **Selective coding** involves the process of integrating and refining the theory.

In the Corbin and Strauss approach, the *paradigm* is used as an analytic strategy to help integrate structure and process. The basic components of the paradigm include conditions, actions–interactions, and consequences or outcomes. Corbin and Strauss suggested the conditional/consequential matrix as an analytic strategy for considering the range of possible conditions and consequences that can enter into the context.

The first step in integrating the findings is to decide on the **central category** (also called the *core category*), which is the main theme of the research. Recommended techniques to facilitate identification of the central category are writing the storyline, using diagrams, and reviewing and organizing memos. The outcome of the Corbin and Strauss approach is, as Glaser (1992) termed it, a full conceptual description. The original Glaserian grounded theory method, by contrast, generates a theory that explains how a basic social problem that emerged from the data is processed in a social setting.

Example of Corbin and Strauss Grounded Theory Analysis
In Australia Townsend and colleagues (2023) explored 25 women's experiences negotiating water immersion for labor and birth after a previous cesarean birth. Interview data were analyzed using Corbin and Strauss's analytic process. Taking the reins was the core category explaining women's experiences of assuming authority over their birth.

Constructivist Grounded Theory Approach

The constructivist approach to grounded theory is not dissimilar to a Glaserian approach. Charmaz's approach, however, puts more emphasis on interpretation and on the researcher's influence in data analysis. According to Charmaz (2014), in constructivist grounded theory, the "coding generates the bones of your analysis. Theoretical centrality and integration will assemble these bones into a working skeleton" (p. 113).

Charmaz distinguishes initial coding and focused coding. In **initial coding**, the pieces of data (e.g., words, lines, segments, incidents) are coded as the researcher begins to learn what participants view as problematic. Charmaz advises grounded analysts to "keep your initial codes short, simple, spontaneous—and analytic. The rest will fall in place" (p. 161).

In **focused coding** the analysis is directed toward using the most significant and frequent codes from the initial coding to help sort, integrate, and organize large chunks of data. The researcher decides which codes are most important for further analysis, which are then theoretically coded. Focused codes are more conceptual than initial codes and advance the direction of the developing theory. Charmaz encourages the use of theoretical sensitivity to aid in analyzing the data. *Theoretical sensitivity* is "the ability to understand and define phenomena in abstract terms and to demonstrate abstract relationships between studied phenomena" (p. 161).

Charmaz's method also involves a crucial step of memo writing where researchers stop, weigh, and analyze categories and their relationship to each other. Charmaz views *writing* as a strategy for developing a grounded theory. Use of prewriting exercises such as *clustering* helps to foster creativity and to organize analytic findings. Clustering produces a tentative map or chart: analysts make a circle for their main category and then use spokes from the circle to smaller circles to help illustrate properties and relationships. Charmaz advocates a writing style that is both literary and scientific—that is, analytic but also evocative of the participants' experiences. Her work provides guidance on making meaning from the data and rendering participants' words into accessible theoretical interpretations. She advocates for maintaining the participants' presence throughout the analysis and write-up.

> **Example of a Constructivist Grounded Theory Analysis**
> In Italy, Cilluffo et al. (2022) designed a qualitative study to develop a conceptual framework for the process of mutuality between nurses and patients. A sample of 33 patients with one or more chronic diseases and 35 nurses was interviewed. Their analysis was guided by Charmaz's constructivism. The mutuality process included three dimensions: developing and going beyond, being a reference, and deciding and sharing care.

QUALITATIVE ANALYSIS NOT LINKED TO A RESEARCH TRADITION

Broad guidelines for analyzing data from "generic" qualitative inquiries have been emerging to facilitate the analytic process and to make it less opaque and intimidating. Examples of analytic guidelines that have been used by nurse researchers include guides for qualitative content analysis (Krippendorff, 2019; Kyngäs et al., 2020), and thematic analysis (Braun & Clarke, 2022).

Qualitative Content Analysis

Content analysis is a family of analytic approaches ranging from intuitive and impressionistic analyses to strict systematic textual analyses. Indeed, quantitative researchers sometimes perform a content analysis—for example by counting words or phrases and formally testing hypotheses.

Qualitative content analysis is the analysis of the content of narrative data to identify prominent themes and patterns among the themes and is often used in descriptive qualitative studies. Patton (2015) defined qualitative content analysis as "any qualitative data reduction and sense-making effort that takes a volume of qualitative material and attempts to identify core consistencies and meaning" (p. 541).

Qualitative content analysis involves breaking down data into smaller units. The literature on content analysis often includes references to **meaning units**. In their widely cited paper on content analysis, Graneheim and Lundman (2004) defined a meaning unit as "words, sentences or paragraphs containing aspects related to each other through their content and context" (p. 106). A meaning unit, essentially, is the smallest segment of a text that contains a recognizable piece of information.

The labels attached to meaning units are the codes (sometimes called *tags*). Codes are heuristic devices; "labeling a condensed meaning unit with a code allows the data to be thought about in new and different ways" (Graneheim & Lundman, 2004, p. 107). The success of a content analysis depends on the integrity of the coding process. Codes are, in turn, the basis for developing categories. In what is sometimes referred to as "secondary coding," the creation of categories involves gathering meaning units together that capture the substance of a topic and fit into a cluster (Krippendorff, 2019).

In descriptive studies, qualitative researchers may decide to focus mainly on summarizing the data's manifest content (what the text actually says). Many content analysts also analyze what the text talks *about,* which involves interpretation of the meaning of its latent content. Interpretations vary in depth and level of abstraction and are usually the basis for themes.

Kyngäs et al. (2020) developed a method for qualitative content analysis. Their content analysis can be inductive or deductive. A researcher would use inductive content analysis if the purpose is to create concepts, categories, and themes from the qualitative data. In deductive content analysis, on the other hand, the researcher would apply either a structured or semistructured matrix of analysis to the data. Researchers should choose deductive content analysis when the starting point of their study is prior theoretical knowledge.

Example of Kyngäs and Colleagues' Inductive Content Analysis

Renbarger and an interdisciplinary team (2023) conducted a qualitative study to explore perspectives of women in the lay public in Indiana about the topic of maternal mortality. Interviews with 20 participants were analyzed using Kyngäs and colleagues' inductive content analysis. Three main themes were identified: (1) Women are not worried about mortality until they experience pregnancy complications; (2) Women have limited information on maternal mortality; and (3) Women often feel dismissed during maternity care.

Example of Krippendorff's Content Analysis

Using Krippendorff's content analysis, Beck (2023b), one of the authors of this textbook, analyzed 25 stories of postpartum preeclampsia that were posted on the internet. Five themes were developed: (1) not even on my radar as a new mom; (2) bombarded with physical and emotional symptoms; (3) life-threatening situation: dismissed or misdiagnosed; (4) heartbroken: separation from my newborn; and (5) trust your instincts and advocate for yourself.

Analysis of Focus Group Data

Focus group interviews yield rich and complex data that pose special analytic challenges. Indeed, there is little consensus about analyzing data from focus groups, despite their widespread use.

A controversial issue in the analysis of focus group data is whether the unit of analysis is the group or individual participants. Analysis of group-level data involves a scrutiny of themes, interactions, and sequences within and between groups. Others, however, have argued that analysis should occur at both the group and individual level. Those who insist on only group-level analysis argue that what individuals say in focus groups cannot be treated as personal disclosures because they are inevitably influenced by the dynamics of the group. However, even in personal interviews, individual responses are shaped by social processes, and analysis of individual-level data (independent of group) is thought by some analysts to add important insights. Carey and Smith advocated a third level of analysis—namely, the analysis of individual responses *in relation* to group context (e.g., whether a participant's view is in accord with or in contrast to majority opinion).

For those who wish to analyze data from individual participants, it is essential to maintain information about what each person said—a task that is not possible if researchers rely solely on audio recordings. Video recordings, as supplements to audio recordings, are sometimes used to identify who said what in focus group sessions. More frequently, however, researchers have members of the research team in attendance at the sessions, and their job is to take detailed field notes about the order of speakers and about significant nonverbal behavior, such as pounding or clenching of fists, crying, aggressive body language, and so on.

Because of group dynamics, focus group analysts must be sensitive to both the thematic content of these interviews and to how, when, and why themes are developed. Some issues that could be central to focus group analysis include the following:

- Does an issue raised in a focus group constitute a *theme* or merely a strongly held viewpoint of one or two members?
- Do the same issues or themes arise in more than one group?
- If there are group differences, why might this be the case—were participants different in characteristics and experiences, or did group processes affect the discussions?
- Are some issues sufficiently salient that not only are they discussed in response to specific questions posed by the moderator but also emerge spontaneously at multiple points in the session?

Some focus group analysts use quantitative methods as adjuncts to their qualitative analysis. Using CAQDAS, they conduct such analyses as assessing similarities and differences between groups, determining coding frequencies to aid pattern detection, examining codes in relation to participant characteristics, and examining how much dialogue individual members contributed. They use such methods not so that interpretation can be based on frequencies, but so that they can better understand context and identify issues that require further critical scrutiny and interpretation.

> **Secondary Qualitative Data Analysis**
> Like quantitative researchers, qualitative researchers have come to recognize the value of **secondary qualitative analysis** of existing datasets (Beck, 2019). In some cases, secondary analysis of a qualitative dataset is undertaken by the same researcher who conducted the original study; in other cases, the data are used by new researchers.

Thorne (2013) identified five types of qualitative secondary analyses. She stressed these five types are not mutually exclusive:

- Analytic expansion occurs when a researcher goes back to an original dataset to ask new questions that were not envisioned with the primary study.
- Retrospective interpretation is a type of analytic expansion that involves a temporal aspect. The analysis occurs long after the results of the primary study were published. The researcher looks back on the original data to further examine issues or findings that were only superficially dealt with the first time around.
- Armchair induction is undertaken by theoretical scholars who have not conducted any fieldwork themselves. They are removed from the field but analyze existing qualitative datasets to develop different types of results than the primary researcher.
- Cross-validation involves use of multiple datasets from different researchers to confirm or challenge the original interpretations.
- Amplified sampling enhances transferability of an original dataset by analyzing different qualitative datasets across populations and contexts.

Thorne (2013) warned of potential problems in qualitative secondary analysis. One of the main issues focuses on ethical complications that need to be worked out. Most important is the issue of informed consent: Did the original informed consent include consent for reuse of the data? Another ethical issue concerns confidentiality. This can occur if someone other than the original researcher is undertaking the qualitative secondary analysis. This researcher doing the secondary data analysis may unintentionally violate shared understanding of the boundaries of confidentiality that were clearly understood by the primary researcher.

The suitability of the available dataset for new research questions is another issue that researchers contemplating qualitative secondary data analysis need to consider. If researchers have permission to use another researcher's primary dataset, how much of it will they have access to: transcribed interviews, original recording, or both? While secondary analysis of a qualitative dataset is appealing because it can be efficient, these important issues must be resolved.

Qualitative datasets are becoming increasing available for further analysis. In the United States, there are a few qualitative archives. One useful repository is maintained at the Qualitative Data Repository at Syracuse University. The Henry A. Murray Research Archive, an endowed repository of qualitative and quantitative research, is available at the Radcliffe College at Harvard University. Its emphasis is on longitudinal studies on human development and social change, with special focus on the lives of American women. A third repository is the Inter-University Consortium for Political and Social Research at the Institute for Social Research at the University of Michigan which began archiving qualitative datasets in 2011. The National Institute of Health has a data sharing policy where researchers are expected to submit a data sharing plan with their grant application of $500K or more in direct support in any given year. In the United Kingdom, an important resource is the UK Data.

> **Example of a Qualitative Secondary Data Analysis**
> Beck (2022b), one of the authors of this textbook, conducted a secondary qualitative analysis combining data from three of her primary studies to investigate the presence of symptoms of moral injury in obstetric and neonatal nurses. Beck answered a new research question that was not part of her original studies. The three primary datasets that she combined included descriptions of secondary traumatic stress by 75 labor and delivery nurses, 75 nurse-midwives, and 22 NICU nurses. Using content analysis, Beck categorized segments of the nurses' descriptions according to 10 symptoms of moral injury that the Moral Injury Symptoms Scale-Health Professionals Version measures. Beck reported the top three most frequently cited symptoms of nurses' moral injury were moral concern, guilt, and self-condemnation.

CRITICAL APPRAISAL OF QUALITATIVE ANALYSIS

It is not easy to evaluate a qualitative analysis as described in a report. Readers do not have access to the information they need to confirm that researchers exercised good judgment and insight in coding the narrative materials, developing a thoughtful analysis, and integrating materials into a meaningful whole. Researchers are seldom able to include more than a handful of examples of actual data in a journal article. Moreover, the process they used to abstract meaning from the data is difficult to describe and illustrate.

The report should provide information about the approach used to analyze the data. For example, a report for a grounded theory study should indicate whether the researchers used the Glaser, Corbin, and Strauss, or constructivist method. It would, however, be inappropriate to criticize a grounded theory analysis for following Charmaz's approach rather than Glaser's approach. Both are respected methods of conducting a grounded theory study—although researchers themselves may have cogent reasons for preferring one approach over the other.

One aspect of a qualitative analysis that *can* be appraised, however, is whether the researchers documented that they have used one approach consistently and have been faithful to the integrity of its procedures. Thus, for example, if researchers say they are using the Glaserian approach to grounded theory analysis, they should not mention axial coding from the Corbin and Strauss method. An even more serious problem occurs when, as sometimes happens, the researchers "muddle" traditions. For example, researchers who describe their study as a grounded theory study should not present *themes*, because grounded theory analysis does not yield themes.

Some guidelines that may be helpful in evaluating qualitative analysis are presented in Box 25.2.

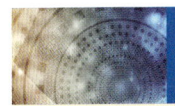

BOX 25.2 Guidelines for Critically Appraising Qualitative Analyses and Interpretations

1. Was the data analysis approach appropriate for the research design, the qualitative tradition, and nature of the data?
2. Were major analytic decisions communicated in the report (e.g., who did the analysis and transcription)? Were the decisions reasonable ones?
3. Were the coding process and coding scheme described? If so, does the process seem reasonable? Does the scheme appear logical and complete? Does there seem to be unnecessary overlap or redundancy in the codes?
4. Were manual methods used to index and organize the data, or was computer software used?
5. Does the report adequately describe the process by which the actual analysis was performed? If codes were collapsed into categories, does the resulting set of categories make sense?
6. Does the report indicate whose approach to data analysis was used (e.g., in grounded theory studies, Glaserian, Straussian, or constructivist)? Was this method consistently and appropriately applied?
7. What major themes or processes were gleaned from the data? If excerpts from the data were provided, do the themes appear to capture the meaning of the narratives—that is, does it appear that the researcher adequately interpreted the data and conceptualized the themes or categories? Is the analysis parsimonious—could two or more themes be collapsed into a broader conceptualization?
8. What evidence does the report provide that the analysis is accurate and appropriate? Were data shared in a manner that allows you to verify the researcher's conclusions?
9. Was a conceptual map, model, or diagram presented? Did it illuminate important processes, patterns, or relationships?
10. Was a metaphor used to communicate key elements of the analysis? Did the metaphor offer an insightful view of the findings, or did it seem contrived?
11. Was the context of the phenomenon adequately described? Does the report give you a clear picture of the social or emotional world of study participants?
12. Did the analysis yield a meaningful and insightful picture of the phenomenon under study—or is the resulting theory or description trivial and obvious?

RESEARCH EXAMPLES

We have illustrated different analytic approaches through examples of studies throughout this chapter. Here we present more detailed descriptions of two qualitative nursing studies.

Example of a Phenomenologic Analysis

Study: When fear surrounding childbirth leads women to request a planned cesarean birth (Bryanton et al., 2022).

Statement of purpose: The purpose of this study was to explore primiparous and multiparous women's experiences of fear surrounding childbirth in relation to their decision to request a planned cesarean birth.

Method: In this descriptive phenomenologic study, the researchers conducted in-depth interviews with 16 women living in Canada. Most of the interviews were conducted in person with a few conducted on Skype or the telephone. Interviews lasted between ½ to 1 ¾ hours. Women were asked to describe their thoughts and feelings about the fear they experienced surrounding their childbirth. Women also shared their blogs and journals they had written.

Analysis: Colaizzi's method was used to analyze (manually) the data from the mothers' transcribed interviews. First all the significant statements from the transcripts were extracted, and their meanings were formulated. Here is an example:

Significant statement: "Like it's just all-consuming and you can't do anything but experience it. You can't get away from it, it's just like a, I don't know. It's just intense (p. 647).

Formulated meaning: "The fear is all consuming. She can't get away from it and must just experience it and it is intense" (p. 647).

Next, the researchers organized all the formulated meanings into clusters of themes and integrated them into an exhaustive description of the phenomenon. No modifications to their analysis were necessary based on feedback from some participants.

Key findings: The analysis of participants' accounts of their fear surrounding childbirth that led them to request a planned cesarean birth yielded five themes: (1) setting the stage: antecedents of fear, (2) so many fears: not always easily disclosed, (3) living with fear: the looming monster, (4) coping strategies: taking control of the uncontrolled, and (5) resolution: beginning the healing process.

Example of a Grounded Theory Analysis

Study: Stabilizing life: A grounded theory of surviving critical illness (Vogel et al., 2021).

Statement of purpose: The purpose of this study was to develop an exploratory theory of patients' pattern of behaviors from becoming critically ill until recovery at home.

Method: This study used classic (Glaserian) grounded theory methods. The researchers conducted formal interviews with 13 participants in Sweden who had been cared for in an ICU. Observations of seven awake conscious patients were conducted in two ICUs. Each interview lasted about 1 to 1 ½ hours. Each observation lasted between 4 and 6 hours. Theoretical sampling was used to choose patients with different demographic characteristics and reasons for admission and time in the ICU.

Analysis: The data for the study included interview transcripts, field notes, and memos that documented the researchers' analytic insights. Data were analyzed using Glaser's constant comparative method. The analysis began with line-by-line open coding where patterns of behavior were identified. Once the core category was discovered, then selective coding began. Theoretical coding was performed based on memos that had been written throughout the analysis.

Key findings: Being out of control emerged as the basic problem for patients during the process from being critically ill to recovery at home. Stabilizing life was the core category which described a process that included three categories: recapturing life, recoding life, and emotional balancing.

SUMMARY POINTS

- Qualitative analysis is a challenging, labor-intensive activity, with few standardized rules—although guidelines have begun to appear to make the process less mystifying.

- Researchers make many decisions in analyzing qualitative data, including who will do the analysis and transcription; whether coding (if any) will be inductive or deductive; whether the focus will be on description or interpretation; whether both *manifest content* and *latent content* will be analyzed; whether computer software will be used to manage and organize the data; and whether the analysis will follow a formal guideline—and, if so, which one.
- Although there are no universal qualitative analytic methods, several broad and iterative processes are typical, including immersing oneself in the data; segmenting and coding the data; collapsing codes into broader and (usually) more interpretive categories; and then integrating and developing themes, models, or theories.
- Qualitative analysis usually begins with efforts to understand and manage the mass of narrative data by developing a *coding scheme*. Analysts use **codes** to identify (in a data segment, such as a sentence or paragraph) an interesting, salient, or essential feature of the data in relation to the phenomenon of interest. Data segments can be coded in different ways, depending on the goals of the research.
- Once a coding scheme is devised, researchers apply the codes to data segments, a process that allows analysts to retrieve data segments easily.
- Traditionally, researchers organized their data by developing **conceptual files**—physical files in which excerpts of data relevant to specific codes are placed. Computer-assisted qualitative data analysis software (**CAQDAS**) is now widely used to index the data and to facilitate analysis.
- The analysis of qualitative materials often involves a search for broad **categories**, which are clusters of codes that are connected conceptually. In many qualitative studies, the next phase involves the identification of themes. A **theme**, which often cuts across several categories, is a recurring regularity that captures meaningful patterns in the data. Identifying themes involves the discovery not only of commonalities across participants but also of natural variation and patterns in the data.
- Some qualitative analysts use **metaphors** or figurative comparisons to evoke a visual and symbolic analogy. Analysts also use various graphic or charting devices, such as timelines and **dendrograms** (tree diagrams illustrating hierarchically ordered codes and categories).
- Interpreting qualitative data in efforts to make meaning from the data typically requires total immersion in the data and a period of **incubation** and creative reflection.
- In ethnographies, analysis begins as the researcher enters the field. Ethnographers continually search for *patterns* in the behavior and expressions of study participants.
- One approach to analyzing ethnographic data is Spradley's method, which involves four levels of data analysis: **domain analysis** (identifying *domains* or units of cultural knowledge), **taxonomic analysis** (selecting key domains and constructing **taxonomies** or systems of classification), **componential analysis** (comparing and contrasting cultural terms in a domain), and a **theme analysis** (uncovering cultural themes).
- Leininger's ethnonursing method involves four phases: collecting and recording data; categorizing descriptors; searching for repetitive patterns; and abstracting major themes.
- There are numerous approaches to phenomenologic analysis, including the descriptive methods of the Duquesne School. Colaizzi, Giorgi, and Van Kaam recommend somewhat different procedures, but a common goal is to find recurrent patterns of experiences relating to a phenomenon of interest.
- In van Manen's approach, which involves efforts to grasp the essential meaning of the experience being studied, researchers search for themes, using either a **holistic approach** (viewing text as a whole); **selective approach** (pulling out key statements and phrases); or **detailed approach** (analyzing every sentence). Van Manen's approach is within the Utrecht school of phenomenology.
- Central to analyzing data in an interpretive phenomenologic (hermeneutic) study is the notion of the **hermeneutic circle**, which signifies a methodologic process in which there is

- continual movement between the parts and the whole of the text under analysis.
- There are several choices for hermeneutic data analysis, including the methods of Parse, Diekelmann, and Benner. Diekelmann's team approach calls for the discovery of a **constitutive pattern** that expresses the relationships among themes. Benner's approach consists of three processes: searching for **paradigm cases**, thematic analysis, and analysis of **exemplars**.
- Grounded theory researchers (as well as others) use the **constant comparative** method of analysis, which involves identifying characteristics in one piece of data and comparing them with those of others to assess similarity.
- One approach to grounded theory is the Glaser and Strauss (Glaserian) method, in which there are two broad types of codes: *substantive codes* (in which the empirical substance of the topic is conceptualized) and *theoretical codes* (in which higher-order relationships are conceptualized).
- Substantive coding involves **open coding** to capture what is going on in the data. Open codes begin with **level I (in vivo) codes**, which are collapsed into a higher level of abstraction in **level II codes** (categories). Level II codes are then used to formulate **level III codes**, which are theoretical constructs. **Selective coding** can then proceed, in which only data relating to a core category are coded. The **core category** is a behavior pattern that has relevance for participants and can be used to integrate the theory; a **basic social process (BSP)** is one example of a core category. **Theoretical coding** helps weave the coded pieces of data back together.
- In Corbin and Strauss approach, an alternative grounded theory method, the outcome is a full conceptual description. Their method involves three types of coding: **open** (in which categories are generated), **axial coding** (where categories are linked with subcategories and integrated), and **selective coding** (which involves the process of integrating and refining the theory).
- In Charmaz's constructivist grounded theory approach, coding can be word-by-word, line-by-line, or incident-by-incident. Such **initial coding** leads to **focused coding.** Her approach puts special emphasis on interpretation and on the researcher's influence in data analysis.
- Several systems have been developed to guide qualitative researchers who are not conducting a study within a disciplinary tradition. For example, researchers whose focus is qualitative description may use content analysis as their analytic method. **Qualitative content analysis** is an analysis of the content of narrative data to identify prominent themes or patterns. Content analysts using an inductive approach strive to identify **meaning units** that are then coded (tagged); the codes are the basis for developing categories.
- **Secondary qualitative analysis** of existing data sets can be used to answer new research questions that were not envisioned in the primary study or were only superficially dealt with the first time around.

REFERENCES CITED IN CHAPTER 25

Beck, C. T. (2002). Releasing the pause button: Mothering twins during the first year of life. *Qualitative Health Research*, *12*, 593–608.

Beck, C. T. (2019). *Secondary qualitative data analysis for the health and social sciences*. Routledge.

Beck, C. T. (2022a). The impact of traumatic childbirth on women's breastfeeding experiences: A metaphor analysis. *Clinical Lactation*, *13*(1), 54–59.

Beck, C. T. (2022b). Secondary qualitative analysis of moral injury in obstetric and neonatal nurses. *Journal of Obstetric, Gynecologic, and Neonatal Nursing*, *51*(2), 166–172. https://doi.org/10.1016/j.jogn.2021.12.003

Beck, C. T. (2023a). Survivors' experiences of hyperemesis gravidarum. *Journal of Infusion Nursing*, *46*(6), 338–346. https://doi.org/10.1097/NAN.0000000000000520

Beck, C. T. (2023b). Postpartum preeclampsia: What can stories posted on the Internet tell us? *Advanced Emergency Nursing Journal*, *45*(2):154–163. https://doi.org10.1097/TME.0000000000000457

Beck, C. T., & Watson, S. (2019). Mothers' experiences interacting with their infants after traumatic childbirth. MCN: *American Journal of Maternal Child Nursing*, *44*(6), 338–344. https://doi.org/10.1097/nmc.0000000000000565

Benner, P. (1994). The tradition and skill of interpretive phenomenology in studying health, illness, and caring practices. In Benner, P. (Ed.), *Interpretive phenomenology* (pp. 99–127). Sage Publications.

Braun, V., & Clarke, V. (2022). *Thematic analysis: A practical guide.* Sage.

Bryanton, J., Beck, C. T., & Morrison, S. (2022). When fear surrounding childbirth leads women to request a planned cesarean birth. *Western Journal of Nursing Research, 44*(7), 643–652.

Burkett, K., Kamimura-Nishimura, K. I., Suarez-Cano, G., Ferreira-Corso, L., Jacquez, F., & Vaughn, L. M. (2022). Latino-to-Latino" Promotores' beliefs on engaging Latino participants in autism research. *Journal of Racial and Ethnic Health Disparities, 9*(4), 1125–1134. https://doi.org/10.1007/s40615-021-01053-0

Carpenter, J. (2008). Metaphors in qualitative research: Shedding light or casting shadows? *Research in Nursing & Health, 31*, 274–282.

Charmaz, K. (2014). *Constructing grounded theory* (2nd ed.). Sage Publications.

Chatreewatanakul, B., Othaganont, P., & Hickman, R. L. (2022). Early symptom recognition and symptom management among exacerbation COPD patients: A qualitative study. *Applied Nursing Research, 63*, 151522. https://doi.org/10.1016/j.apnr.2021.151522

Cilluffo, S., Bassola, B., Pucciarelli, G., Vellone, E., & Lusignani, M. (2022). Mutuality in nursing: A conceptual framework on the relationship between patient and nurse. *Journal of Advanced Nursing, 78*(6), 1718–1730. https://doi.org/10.1111/jan.15129

Colaizzi, P. F. (1978). Psychological research as the phenomenologist views it. In Valle, R., & King, M. (Eds.), *Existential phenomenological alternatives for psychology.* Oxford University Press.

Corbin, J., & Strauss, A. (2015). *Basics of qualitative research: Techniques and procedures for developing grounded theory.* Sage Publications.

Dahlberg, K., Dahlberg, H., & Nyström, M. (2008). *Reflective lifeworld research.* Studentlitteratur.

DeSantis, L., & Ugarriza, D. (2000). The concept of theme as used in qualitative nursing research. *Western Journal of Nursing Research, 22*, 351–372.

Diekelmann, N. L., Allen, D., & Tanner, C. (1989). *The NLN criteria for appraisal of baccalaureate programs: A critical hermeneutic analysis.* NLN Press.

Dolan, H., Rishel, C., Rainbow, J. G., & Taylor-Piliae, R. (2022). Relying on myself: The lived experience of being at risk for falling in the hospital among older adults. *Geriatric Nursing, 47*, 116–124. https://doi.org/10.1016/j.gerinurse.2022.06.016

Fetterman, D. M. (2020). *Ethnography: Step by step* (4th ed.). Sage Publications.

Gadamer, H. G. (1975). *Truth and method.* G. Borden & J. Cumming (trans). Sheed and Ward.

Giorgi, A. (1985). *Phenomenology and psychological research.* Duquesne University Press.

Glaser, B. (1978). *Theoretical sensitivity.* The Sociology Press.

Glaser, B. (1992). *Emergence versus forcing: Basics of grounded theory analysis.* Sociology Press.

Glaser, B. (2001). *The grounded theory perspective: Conceptualization contrasted with description.* Sociology Press.

Glaser, B. (2005). *The grounded theory perspective III: Theoretical coding.* Sociology Press.

Glaser, B. G., & Strauss, A. (1967). *The discovery of grounded theory: Strategies for qualitative research.* Aldine de Gruyter.

Graneheim, U., & Lundman, B. (2004). Qualitative content analysis in nursing research: Concepts, procedures and measures to achieve trustworthiness. *Nurse Education Today, 24*, 105–112.

Holton, J. A. (2010). The coding process and its challenges. *Grounded Theory Review: An International Journal, 9*, 1.

Hunter, A., Lusardi, P., Zucker, D., Jacelon, C., & Chandler, G. (2002). Making meaning: The creative component in qualitative research. *Qualitative Health Research, 12*, 388–398.

Hwang, H., DeGagne, J. C., Yoo, L., Lee, M., Jo, H. K., & Kim, J.E. (2024). Exploring nursing research culture in clinical practice: Qualitative ethnographic study. *Asian/Pacific Island Nursing Journal, 8*, e50703 https://doi.org/10.2196/50703

Karahan, S., Erbas, A., & Tuncbilek, Z. (2022), Experiences, difficulties, and coping methods of burn nurses: An exploratory-descriptive qualitative study. *Journal of Burn Care & Research, 43*(6), 1277–1285. https://doi.org/10.1093/jbcr/irac019

Krippendorff, K. (2019). *Content analysis: An introduction to its methodology* (4th ed.). Sage Publications.

Kyngäs, H., Mikkonen, K., & Kääriäinen, M. (eds). (2020). *The application of content analysis in nursing science research.* Springer.

Létourneau, D., Goudreau, J., & Cara, C. (2022). Nursing students and nurses' recommendations aiming at improving the development of the humanistic caring competency. *Canadian Journal of Nursing Research, 54*(3), 292–303. https://doi.org/10.1177/08445621211048987

Lillieskold, S., Zwedberg, S., Linnér, A., & Jonas, W. (2022). Parents' experiences of immediate skin-to-skin contact after the birth of their very preterm neonates. *Journal of Obstetric, Gynecologic, and Neonatal Nursing, 51*(1), 53–64. https://doi.org/10.1016/j.jogn.2021.10.002

McFarland, M. R., & Wehbe-Alamah, H. B. (2015). *Leininger's culture care diversity and universality: A worldwide nursing theory.* Jones & Bartlett Learning.

Miles, M., Huberman, M., & Saldaña, J. (2020). *Qualitative data analysis: A methods sourcebook* (4th ed.). Sage Publications.

Modula, M. J. (2022). The support needs of families raising children with intellectual disability. *African Journal of Disability, 11*(0), a952. https://doi.org/10.4102/ajod.v11i0.952

Morgan, D. L. (2018). Themes, theories, and models. *Qualitative Health Research, 28*, 339–345.

Ou, C. H. K., Hall, W. A., Rodney, P., & Stremler, R. (2022). Seeing red: Grounded theory study of women's anger after childbirth. *Qualitative Health Research, 32*(12), 1780–1794. https://doi.org/10.1177/10497323221120173

Park, S., Jang, M. K., Seo, Y. J., & Doorenbos, A. Z. (2022). Funeral experience in South Korea: A phenomenological study. *OMEGA-Journal of Death and Dying, 84*(4), 1025–1044. https://doi.org/10.1177/0030222820921586

Parse, R. R. (2016). Parsesciencing: A basic science mode of inquiry. *Nursing Science Quarterly, 29*, 271–274.

Patton, M. Q. (2015). *Qualitative research and evaluation methods* (4th ed.). Sage Publications.

Polit, D. F., London, A., & Martinez, J. (2000). *Food insecurity and hunger in poor, mother-headed families in four U.S. cities*. MDRC.

Renbarger, K., Place, J.M., Twibell, R., Trainor, K., & McIntire, E. (2023). Perspectives of maternal morbidity among women who live in Indiana. *Journal of Obstetric, Gynecologic, and Neonatal Nursing, 52*(1), 62–71. https://doi.org/10.1016/j.jogn.2022.09.006

Ricoeur, P. (1981). *Hermeneutics and the social sciences* (J. Thompson, trans. & ed.). Cambridge University Press.

Saldaña, J. (2021). *The coding manual for qualitative researchers* (4th ed.). Sage Publications.

Spradley, J. (1979). *The ethnographic interview*. Holt Rinehart & Winston.

Thorne, S. (2013). Secondary qualitative data analysis. In Beck, C. T. (Ed.), *Routledge international handbook of qualitative research* (pp. 393–404). Routledge.

Thorne, S. & Darbyshire, P. (2005). Land mines in the field: A modest proposal for improving the craft of qualitative health research. *Qualitative Health Research, 15*, 1105–1113.

Townsend, B., Fenwick, J., McInnes, R., & Sidebotham, M. (2023). Taking the reins: A grounded theory study of women's experiences of negotiating water immersion for labour and birth after a previous caesarean section. *Women and Birth, 36*(2), e227–e326. https://doi.org/10.1016/j.wombi.2022.07.171

Van Kaam, A. (1966). *Existential foundations of psychology*. Duquesne University Press.

Van Manen, M. (1990). *Researching lived experience: Human science for an action sensitive pedagogy*. Althouse Press.

Van Manen, M. (2006). Writing qualitatively or the demands of writing. *Qualitative Health Research, 16*, 713–722.

Van Manen, M. (2017). But is it phenomenology? *Qualitative Health Research, 27*, 775–779.

Vogel, G., Joelsson-Alm, E., Forinder, U., Svensen, C., & Sandgren, A. (2021). Stabilizing life: A grounded theory of surviving critical illness. *Intensive Critical Care Nursing, 67*, 103096. https://doi.org/10.1016/j.iccn.2021.103096

26 Trustworthiness and Rigor in Qualitative Research

Learning Objectives

1. Discuss some controversies relating to the issue of quality and integrity in qualitative research.
2. Identify the criteria proposed in a major framework for evaluating qualitative research.
3. Discuss quality-enhancement strategies in qualitative research during data collection and analysis.
4. Describe guidelines for critically appraising quality and integrity in qualitative studies.

INTRODUCTION

Integrity in qualitative research is an all-encompassing concern that begins as questions are formulated and continues through writing the report. This is an important chapter for those learning to do qualitative research.

> **TIP** In thinking about quality enhancement in qualitative inquiry, attention needs to be paid to both "art" and "science." Creativity and insightfulness need to be encouraged and sustained but not at the expense of functional excellence—and the quest for rigor cannot sacrifice inspiration and elegant abstractions, or else the results are likely to be "perfectly healthy but dead" (Morse, 2006, p. 6). Good qualitative work is both descriptively sound and interpretively rich and innovative.

PERSPECTIVES ON QUALITY IN QUALITATIVE RESEARCH

Qualitative researchers agree on the importance of doing high-quality research, yet few issues in qualitative inquiry have generated more controversy than efforts to define what is meant by "high-quality." We provide an overview of some aspects of this debate to help you identify a position that is compatible with your philosophical and methodologic views.

Debates About Rigor and Validity

One contentious issue in the debate about quality concerns the use of terms such as *rigor* and *validity*. These terms are opposed by some critics because of their association with positivism—rigor and validity are not seen as suitable goals for the constructivist or critical paradigms. These critics argue that the philosophical underpinnings are fundamentally different from the positivist paradigm and require distinctive terminology. In their view, the concept of rigor does not fit into an interpretive approach that values insight and creativity (e.g., Denzin & Lincoln, 2000). As Sandelowski (1993a) put it, "We can preserve or kill the spirit of qualitative work; we can soften our notion of rigor to include the… soulfulness (and) imagination…we associate with more artistic endeavors, or we can further harden it by the uncritical application of rules. The choice is ours: rigor or rigor mortis" (p. 8).

Some qualitative researchers, however, argue for using the term rigor (e.g., Cypress, 2017; Morse, 2015). Others defend using the term *validity*. Whittemore and colleagues (2001), for example, argued that validity is an appropriate term in all paradigms, noting that the dictionary definition of validity (the quality of being sound, just, and well-founded) lends itself equally to qualitative and quantitative research. Morse and colleagues (2002) posited that the "concepts of reliability and validity can be applied to all research because the goal of finding plausible and credible outcome explanations is central to all research" (p. 3). A pragmatic argument favoring the use of "mainstream" terms like validity and rigor is precisely that they *are* mainstream. In the scientific community, whose criteria are used to make funding decisions, it may be useful to use recognizable terms and criteria.

Sparkes (2001) contended that there are four possible perspectives on the issue of validity. The first, which he called the *replication perspective*, is that validity is an appropriate criterion for assessing quality in both qualitative and quantitative studies, although qualitative researchers use different procedures to achieve it (e.g., Morse, 2015). Those who adopt a *parallel perspective* maintain that a separate set of evaluative criteria are needed for qualitative inquiry. This perspective resulted in the development of standards for the **trustworthiness** of qualitative research that parallel the standards of reliability and validity in quantitative research (Lincoln & Guba, 1985). The third perspective in Sparke's typology is the *diversification of meanings perspective*, which is characterized by efforts to establish new forms of validity that do not have reference points in quantitative research. As an example, Lather (1986) discussed *catalytic validity* in critical and feminist research as the degree to which the research process energizes study participants and alters their consciousness. The final perspective in Sparke's typology was what he called the *letting-go-of-validity perspective*, which involves a total abandonment of the concept of validity. Wolcott (1994), an ethnographer, represented this perspective in his discussion of the absurdity of validity. Yet, as Wolcott (1995) himself noted, validity can be dismissed, but the issue itself will not go away: "Qualitative researchers need to understand what the debate is about and *have* a position; they do not have to resolve the issue itself" (p. 170).

Generic vs. Specific Standards

Another controversial issue concerns whether there should be a generic set of standards or specific standards for different types of study—for example, for ethnographers or grounded theory researchers. Many writers have endorsed the notion that research conducted within different traditions must attend to different concerns, and that techniques for enhancing and demonstrating research integrity vary.

Some writers believe, however, that certain quality criteria are universal within the constructivist paradigm. For example, in their synthesis of criteria for developing evidence of validity in qualitative studies, Whittemore and associates (2001) proposed four primary criteria that they viewed as essential to all qualitative inquiry.

Standards for Conduct vs. Appraisal of Qualitative Research

Yet another issue concerns whose point of view is being considered in the quality standards. Morse and colleagues (2002) contended that many of the established standards are relevant for *assessment* by readers rather than as guides to conducting high-quality qualitative research. They believe that Lincoln and Guba's criteria—often considered the gold standard—are best described as *posthoc* tools that reviewers can use to evaluate trustworthiness of a completed study: "While strategies of trustworthiness may be useful in attempting to *evaluate* rigor, they do not in themselves *ensure* rigor" (p. 9).

As an example of favoring the viewpoint of evaluators, one suggested indicator of integrity is **researcher credibility**—that is, the faith that can be put in the researcher (Patton, 1999, 2015). Such a criterion might affect readers' confidence in the integrity of the inquiry, but it clearly is not a *strategy* that researchers can adopt to make their study more rigorous.

Morse and colleagues (2002) emphasized the importance of verification strategies that researchers can use throughout the inquiry "so that reliability and validity are actively attained, rather than proclaimed by external reviewers on the completion of the project" (p. 9). In their view, responsibility for ensuring rigor should rest with researchers, not with external judges. They advocated a proactive stance involving self-scrutiny and verification. Morse (2006) noted that "good qualitative inquiry must be verified reflexively in each step of the analysis. This means that it is self-correcting" (p. 6).

From the point of view of qualitative researchers, the ongoing question must be: How can I be confident that my account is an accurate and insightful representation? From the point of view of a critical reader, the question is: How can I trust that the researcher has offered an accurate and insightful representation?

Terminology Proliferation and Confusion

The result of all these controversies is that there is no common vocabulary for quality criteria in qualitative research—nor, for that matter, for quality goals. Terms such as *goodness, integrity, truth value, rigor,* and *trustworthiness* abound, and for each proposed descriptor, several critics assert that the term is inappropriate.

Establishing a consensus on what the quality criteria for qualitative inquiry should be, and what they should be named, remains elusive. Some feel that the ongoing debate is healthy, but others feel that "the situation is confusing and has resulted in a deteriorating ability to actually discern rigor" (Morse et al., 2002, p. 5).

Given the lack of consensus and the heated arguments supporting and contesting various frameworks, it is difficult to offer definitive guidance. We present information about *criteria* from a widely used framework in the section that follows and then describe *strategies* for minimizing threats to integrity in qualitative research. We recommend that these strategies be viewed as points of departure for explorations on how to make a qualitative study as rigorous/trustworthy/insightful/valid as possible.

THE LINCOLN–GUBA FRAMEWORK

Although not without critics, the quality criteria most often cited by qualitative researchers are those proposed by Lincoln and Guba, who in their original work (1985) proposed four criteria for enhancing the **trustworthiness** of a qualitative inquiry: credibility, dependability, confirmability, and transferability. These four criteria represent parallels to the positivists' criteria of internal validity, reliability, objectivity, and external validity, respectively. This framework provided the platform on which much of the current controversy on rigor emerged. Responding to numerous criticisms and to their own evolving conceptualizations, a fifth criterion that is more distinctively within the constructivist paradigm was added: authenticity (Guba & Lincoln, 1994).

Credibility

Credibility is viewed by Lincoln and Guba as an overriding goal of qualitative research, and is a criterion identified in several qualitative frameworks. **Credibility** refers to confidence in the truth of the data and interpretations of them. Qualitative researchers must strive to establish confidence in the truth of the findings for the particular participants and contexts in the research. Lincoln and Guba pointed out that credibility involves two aspects: first, carrying out the study in a way that enhances the believability of the findings and second, taking steps to *demonstrate* credibility in research reports.

Dependability

Dependability, the second criterion in the Lincoln–Guba framework, refers to the stability or reliability of data over time and conditions. The dependability question is: Would the findings of an inquiry be repeated if it were replicated with the same (or similar) participants in the same (or similar) context? Credibility cannot be attained in the absence of dependability.

Confirmability

Confirmability refers to objectivity, that is, the potential for congruence between two or more independent people about the data's accuracy, relevance, or meaning. Confirmability is enhanced by efforts to establish that the data represent participants' viewpoints, and that the interpretations of those data are not invented by the inquirer. For this criterion to be achieved, findings must reflect the participants' voice and the conditions of the inquiry and not the researcher's biases or perspectives.

Transferability

Transferability refers to the potential for extrapolation, that is, the extent to which findings can be transferred to or have applicability in other settings or groups. Lincoln and Guba noted that investigators have a responsibility to provide sufficient descriptive data so that consumers can evaluate the relevance of the data to other contexts: "Thus the naturalist cannot specify the external validity of an inquiry; he or she can provide only the thick description necessary to enable someone interested in making a transfer to reach a conclusion about whether transfer can be contemplated as a possibility" (p. 316).

> **TIP** You may run across the term *fittingness*, a term Guba and Lincoln used earlier to refer to the degree to which research findings have meaning to others in similar situations. In later work, however, they used the term *transferability*. Similarly, they used the term *auditability*, a concept that was later refined and called *dependability*.

Authenticity

Authenticity refers to the extent to which researchers fairly and faithfully show a range of realities. Authenticity emerges in a report when it conveys the feeling tone of participants' lives as they are lived. A text has authenticity if it invites readers into a vicarious experience of the lives being described and enables readers to develop a heightened sensitivity to the issues being depicted. When a text achieves authenticity, readers are better able to understand the lives being portrayed "in the round," with some sense of the mood, feeling, experience, language, and context of those lives.

> **TIP** Whittemore et al. (2001), who are nurse researchers, synthesized quality criteria from 10 prominent frameworks. In their view, four primary criteria are essential to all qualitative inquiry (credibility, authenticity, integrity, and criticality) and six secondary criteria provide supplementary benchmarks that are not relevant to every study. Researchers decide, based on the goals of their research, the optimal weight to give each criterion.

STRATEGIES TO ENHANCE QUALITY IN QUALITATIVE INQUIRY

The criteria for establishing integrity in a qualitative study pose challenges. Various strategies have been proposed to address these challenges, and this section describes many of them.

Quality-enhancing strategies often address multiple criteria simultaneously. For this reason, we have not organized strategies according to quality criteria. Instead, we have organized strategies according to the different phases of an inquiry, namely data collection, coding and analysis, and report preparation. This organization is imperfect, due to the nonlinear and iterative nature of tasks in qualitative studies, and so we acknowledge that some activities described under one aspect of a study are likely to have relevance under another.

Quality-Enhancement Strategies in Collecting Data

Several strategies that qualitative researchers use to enrich and strengthen their studies have been mentioned in previous chapters and will not be elaborated here. For example, sampling an adequate number of information-rich and theoretically relevant data sources, intensive listening during an interview, careful probing to obtain rich and comprehensive data, audio-recording interviews for transcription, and monitoring transcription accuracy are all strategies to enhance data quality, as are methods to gain people's trust during fieldwork (Chapter 24). In this section, we focus on additional strategies used during the collection of qualitative data.

Prolonged Engagement and Persistent Observation

An important step in establishing credibility is **prolonged engagement** (Lincoln & Guba, 1985)—the investment of sufficient time collecting data to have an in-depth understanding of the people under study, to test for misinformation and distortions, and to ensure saturation of key categories. Prolonged engagement is also essential for building trust and rapport with informants, which in turn makes it more likely that rich, detailed information will be obtained. In planning a qualitative study, researchers must ensure that they have adequate time and resources to stay engaged in fieldwork for a sufficiently long period.

TIP *Premature closure* can undermine data quality (Thorne & Darbyshire, 2005). Without a commitment to prolonged engagement, researchers may make a claim of saturation simply because they have reached a convenient stopping point. In arguing against the checklists that are used to assure quality, Thorne (2020) questions if saturation is actually a goal of qualitative research and instead suggests that the goal should be new insights and a greater and more meaningful understanding of a phenomenon.

Example of Prolonged Engagement
In Poland, Baranowska et al. (2022) explored women's pathways to free birth without midwifery and medical assistance. The study took place over 2 years with the researchers, two of whom were midwives, who participated in various events in which the topic of free birth was discussed with maternity users and providers.

High-quality data collection in qualitative inquiries also involves **persistent observation**, which concerns the salience of the data being gathered and recorded. Persistent observation refers to the researchers' focus on the characteristics or aspects of a situation or a conversation that are relevant to the phenomena being studied. As Lincoln and Guba (1985) noted, "If prolonged engagement provides scope, persistent observation provides depth" (p. 304).

Example of Persistent Observation
Nepali and colleagues (2022) undertook an ethnographic study to examine the everyday workplace practices in the NICU to gain insight into how nurses made sense of the social and power relations between themselves and senior colleagues in Australia. Observations occurred mostly in 2-hour time slots that covered 24 hours a day, 7 days a week, to capture different scenes and events occurring at various times of the day and months of the year over 18 months. Data included fieldnotes of 100 hours of observation.

Reflexivity Strategies

As noted in Chapter 8, reflexivity involves attending systematically and continually to the context of knowledge construction—and, in particular, to the researcher's effect on the collection, analysis, and interpretation of data. Reflexivity involves awareness that the researcher brings to the inquiry a unique personal background and set of values that can affect the research process.

The most widely used strategy for maintaining reflexivity and delimiting subjectivity is to maintain a reflexive journal or diary. Reflexive notes can be used to record, from the outset of the study and in an ongoing fashion, thoughts about the impact of previous life experiences and previous readings about the phenomenon on the inquiry. Through self-interrogation and reflection, researchers seek to be well-positioned to probe deeply and to grasp the experience, process, or culture under study through the lens of participants.

Other reflexive strategies can be used. For example, researchers sometimes begin a study by being interviewed themselves regarding the phenomenon under study—an approach that only makes sense if the researcher has experienced that phenomenon. Other researchers ask a colleague to conduct a "bracketing interview." In such an interview, a person who is knowledgeable about reflexivity and about the study phenomenon queries the researcher about their a priori assumptions and perspectives.

Example of a Reflexive Interview
Using reflexive thematic analysis, Rost et al. (2023) studied advancing and limiting factors of autonomy in birth as perceived by 15 perinatal care practitioners in Switzerland. The researchers critically reflected on their own underlying assumptions and positionalities. They acknowledged that their interpretation of the data was linked to their positions, experiences, and theoretical background.

Researchers often state in their reports that reflexivity was used or that bracketing was undertaken. Some researchers, however, provide a stronger description of addressing their initial perspectives or biases.

> **Example of Communicating "Preunderstandings"**
> Pape and an interdisciplinary team (2022) investigated the experiences and needs of partners as informal caregivers of patients with major low anterior resection syndrome in Belgium. One of the researchers had experience in counseling patients with low anterior resection syndrome and their informal caregivers. She wrote out her frame of reference and preunderstanding to increase reflexivity. Throughout data analysis, all the researchers continuously reflected on their individual and professional experiences.

Data and Method Triangulation

Triangulation refers to the use of multiple referents to draw conclusions about what constitutes truth; it has been compared to convergent validation. The aim of triangulation is to "overcome the intrinsic bias that comes from single-method, single-observer, and single-theory studies" (Denzin, 1989, p. 313). Patton (1999) also encouraged triangulation, arguing that "no single method ever adequately solves the problem of rival explanation" (p. 1192). Triangulation can also help to capture a more complete and contextualized portrait of key phenomena. Denzin identified four types of triangulation (data triangulation, method triangulation, investigator triangulation, and theory triangulation), the first two of which we describe here because they relate to data collection.

Data triangulation involves the use of multiple data sources for the purpose of validating conclusions and can take several forms: triangulation over time, space, and people. **Time triangulation** involves collecting data on the same phenomenon multiple times. Time triangulation can involve gathering data at different times of the day or at different times in the year. This concept is similar to test–retest reliability assessment—the point is not to study a phenomenon longitudinally to evaluate change but to assess congruence of the phenomenon over time. **Space triangulation** involves collecting data on the same phenomenon in multiple sites, to test for cross-site consistency. Finally, **person triangulation** involves collecting data from different types or levels of people (e.g., individuals, their family members, clinical staff), with the aim of validating data through multiple perspectives on the phenomenon.

> **Example of Person and Space Triangulation**
> In Thailand, Chodjdjah and colleagues (2022) explored psychosocial problems experienced by families of early adolescents with leukemia. The researchers gathered data from mothers, fathers, and siblings in the hospital and in the homes.

Method triangulation involves using multiple methods of data collection about the same phenomenon. In qualitative studies, researchers often use a rich blend of unstructured data collection methods (e.g., interviews, observations, documents) to develop a comprehensive understanding of a phenomenon. Multiple data collection methods provide an opportunity to evaluate the extent to which a consistent and coherent picture of a phenomenon or process emerges.

> **Example of Method Triangulation**
> In Norway, Nyhagen and an interdisciplinary team (2023) conducted a qualitative study to uncover communication challenges between patients, family members, and nurses in the intensive care unit. The researchers collected data through participant observation and interviews with six patients, six family members, and nine healthcare professionals.

Comprehensive and Vivid Recording of Information

In addition to taking steps to record interview data accurately, researchers need to prepare thoughtful field notes that are rich with descriptions of what transpired in the field. Even if interviews are the primary data source, researchers should maintain notes about the participants' demeanor and behaviors during the interactions and should thoroughly describe the interview context. Other record-keeping activities are also important. A log of decisions needs to be kept, reflexive journals should be maintained regularly with rich detail, and analytic memos are needed to facilitate a thoughtful analysis.

Researchers sometimes specifically develop an **audit trail**, that is, a systematic collection of materials and documentation that would allow an independent auditor (or other team members) to come to conclusions about the data. Types of records that are useful in creating an adequate audit trail include the following: (1) the raw data (e.g., interview transcripts); (2) data reduction and analysis products (e.g., annotated transcripts, codebooks, analytic memos); (3) materials relating to researchers' disposition (e.g., reflexive notes); and (4) data reconstruction products (e.g., charting matrices, drafts of the final report).

> **TIP** Diligent documentation does not in and of itself ensure the validity of the inquiry. Morse and colleagues (2002) pointed out that "audit trails may be kept as proof of the decisions made throughout the project, but they do not identify the quality of those decisions, the rationale behind those decisions, or the responsiveness and sensitivity of the investigator to data" (pp. 6–7).

Example of an Audit Trail
Tanner and colleagues (2022) explored the experience of attending school as an adolescent with psychogenic nonepileptic seizures. The researchers maintained an audit trail during data analysis to capture potential explanations, conclusions, inferences, and meanings.

Member Checking

Lincoln and Guba considered member checking a particularly important technique for establishing the credibility of qualitative data. In a **member check**, researchers provide feedback to participants about the study—including emerging interpretations—and elicit participants' reactions. The argument is that if researchers' understandings and interpretations are good representations of participants' realities, participants should be able to confirm their legitimacy.

Member checking can be carried out in an ongoing way as data are being collected (for example, through deliberate probing to ensure that participants' meanings were understood) and more formally after data have been processed or analyzed. Birt and colleagues (2016) identified five approaches to member checking:

- having participants review transcribed verbatim transcripts, to confirm accuracy;
- conducting a member checking interview with individual participants, using their transcribed interview as an opportunity to coconstruct the participants' meaning;
- conducting a member checking interview with individual participants, based on a preliminary interpretation of the original interview, to verify researcher's interpretation;
- conducting a member check focus group interview to review preliminary analyses of the data set; and
- conducting member checks (in writing or in person) with individual participants, using a synthesis of the analyzed data to confirm the interpretation.

Member checks are sometimes done in writing. For example, researchers can ask participants to review and comment on interpretive notes or thematic summaries. Member checks are often done in face-to-face discussions with individual participants.

Birt and colleagues (2016) developed a systematic approach to member checking, which they called *Synthesized Member Checking* (SMC). Their approach involves the preparation of a preliminary synthesis based on themes identified in the analysis, with interview excerpts included to illustrate the themes. The summary is sent to participants, with explicit questions, such as "Does this match your experience?" and "Do you want to change anything or add anything?" Their approach also includes careful documentation and analysis of participants who responded, so that readers can make judgments about the thoroughness of the validation. Participants' responses to the member check are considered a new data source and are coded and integrated with other data in the final interpretation.

> **TIP** If member checking is used as a validation strategy, participants should be encouraged to provide critical feedback about errors or interpretive deficiencies. In writing about the study, it is important to be explicit about how member checking was done and what role it played as a validation strategy. Readers cannot develop much confidence in the study simply by learning that "member checking was done."

Despite the potential contribution that member checking can make to a study's credibility, several issues need to be kept in mind. First, not all participants are willing to engage in this process. Some—especially if the topic is emotionally charged—may feel they have attained closure once they have shared their experiences. Birt and colleagues (2016) have described several possible ethical concerns in member checking, especially in situations when member checking does not occur in face-to-face situations.

Another issue is that member checks can lead to misleading conclusions of trustworthiness if participants "share some common myth or front or conspire to mislead or cover up" (Lincoln & Guba, 1985, p. 315). Also, some participants might agree with researchers' interpretations either out of politeness or in the belief that researchers are "smarter" or more knowledgeable than they themselves are. Thorne and Darbyshire (2005), in fact, caution against what they irreverently called *Adulatory Validity*, which they described as "the epistemological pat on the back for a job well done, or just possibly it might be part of a mutual stroking ritual that satisfies the agendas of both researcher and researched" (p. 1110). They noted that member checking tends to privilege interpretations that place study participants in the most favorable light.

Thorne and Darbyshire are not alone in their concerns about member checking as a validation strategy. Indeed, few strategies for enhancing data quality are as controversial as member checking. Morse (1999, 2015), for example, disputed the idea that participants have more analytic and interpretive authority than the researcher. Morse and colleagues (2002), as well as Sandelowski (1993b), have worried that because study results have been synthesized, decontextualized, and abstracted across various participants, individual participants may not recognize their own experiences or perspectives in a member check. Even more scathingly, some critics view member checking as antithetical to the epistemology of qualitative inquiry. Smith (1993) criticized the philosophical contradictions inherent in this strategy, arguing that it is inconsistent with inquiry that purports to reveal multiple realities and multiple ways of knowing.

Example of Member Checking
Cooley and colleagues (2022) undertook a qualitative study to determine nurses' perceptions of narcotic administration in patients with subarachnoid hemorrhage. Interviews were conducted with nine nurses. A member check was done with the nurses through a phone call, email, or by an in-person meeting to discuss the major themes.

TIP For focus group studies, member checking often occurs in situ. That is, moderators develop a summary of major themes or viewpoints in real time and present that summary to focus group participants at the end of the session for their feedback. Rich data often emerge from participants' reactions to those summaries.

Quality-Enhancement Strategies Relating to Coding and Analysis

Excellent qualitative inquiry is likely to involve the concurrent collection and analysis of data, and so several strategies described in the preceding section are also relevant to promoting analytic integrity. Also, we discussed in Chapter 25 some strategies for analytic rigor (e.g., intensive and multiple readings of texts, preparing analytic memos). In this section, we introduce a few other strategies that relate to the coding, analysis, and interpretation of qualitative data.

Investigator and Theory Triangulation

The overall purpose of triangulation is to converge on the truth. Triangulation offers opportunities to discover the "truth" in the data through the use of multiple perspectives. Several types of triangulation are pertinent during analysis. **Investigator triangulation** refers to the use of two or more researchers to make coding, analysis, and interpretation decisions. The premise is that investigators can reduce the risk of biased judgments and idiosyncratic interpretations through collaboration.

Investigator triangulation, conceptually similar to interrater reliability in quantitative studies, is often used in coding qualitative data. Coding consistency depends on having clear codes and decision rules that are documented in a codebook. Researchers sometimes formally compare two or more independent coding schemes or a subset of independent coding decisions.

Example of Independent Coding
In Singapore Rusli et al. (2022) described home-based care nurses' practice experiences. Interviews with 17 nurses from four service providers were completed. Two researchers independently analyzed and coded the transcripts to increase credibility.

Collaboration is also often used at the analysis stage. If investigators bring to the analysis task a complementary blend of methodologic, disciplinary, and clinical expertise, the analysis and interpretation can potentially benefit from divergent perspectives. As noted in Chapter 25, some approaches to qualitative data analysis are explicitly designed for work in teams (e.g., Diekelmann's approach to hermeneutics).

TIP In focus group studies, immediate post-session debriefings are recommended. In such debriefings—which should be audio-recorded—team members who were present during the session meet to discuss issues and themes. They also should share their views about group dynamics, such as coercive group members, censoring of controversial opinions, individual conformity to group viewpoints, and discrepancies between verbal and nonverbal behavior.

With **theory triangulation**, researchers use competing theories or hypotheses in analyzing and interpreting the data. Qualitative researchers who develop alternative hypotheses while still in the field can test the validity of each because the flexible design of qualitative studies provides ongoing opportunities to direct the inquiry. Theory triangulation can help researchers to rule out rival hypotheses and to prevent premature conceptualizations.

Although Denzin's (1989) seminal work discussed four types of triangulation, other types have been suggested. For example, Kimchi and colleagues (1991) described **analysis triangulation** (i.e., using two or more analytic techniques to analyze the same set of data). This approach offers another opportunity to validate the meanings inherent in a qualitative data set. Analysis triangulation can also involve using multiple units of analysis (e.g., individuals, dyads, families). Renz and colleagues (2018), for example, described an intramethod analytic approach to triangulation in a study in which two different strategies of qualitative content analysis were used.

Search for Confirming Evidence

Member checking with participants, as already noted, is one approach to validating the findings. Another verification strategy is to seek external evidence from other studies or from sources such as literary representations of the phenomenon. This is analogous to a strategy of seeking corroborating evidence to enhance credibility in quantitative studies (Chapter 21). Another possibility, and one that has implications for transferability, is to have people from other sites, or other disciplines, review preliminary findings.

Example of Confirming Evidence
Jack et al. (2022) studied 29 young mothers' experiences with mental healthcare services in Ontario, Canada. Among the young mothers' decisions to seek professional mental health support were their hesitancy due to past negative experiences or fears of being judged, being medicated, or experiencing child protection involvement. The researchers noted a strength of their study was that the findings confirmed those of previous studies.

Search for Disconfirming Evidence and Competing Explanations

A powerful verification procedure that occurs at the intersection of data collection and data analysis involves a systematic search for data that will challenge an emerging categorization or explanation. The search for disconfirming cases can occur through purposive or theoretical sampling methods, as described in Chapter 23. Clearly, this strategy depends on concurrent data collection and data analysis: researchers cannot look for disconfirming data unless they have a sense of what they need to know.

Member checking can also provide opportunities for soliciting disconfirming evidence.

If participants are encouraged to give totally honest feedback, disconfirming voices can enrich the final analysis and interpretation.

> **Example of Disconfirming Evidence**
> Zhu and colleagues and an interdisciplinary team (2023) investigated the barriers and facilitators to selecting active surveillance among patients with low-risk papillary thyroid carcinoma in China. Thirty-nine participants diagnosed with this type of cancer participated in semistructured interviews. Inductive content analysis was used to analyze the interview data and themes were identified for both barriers and facilitators that were involved in patients choosing active surveillance of their cancer. Member checks were performed with all 39 participants, and all but three confirmed that the results resonated with their perspectives.

Lincoln and Guba (1985) discussed the related activity of **negative case analysis.** This strategy is a process by which researchers search for cases (or data segments) that appear to disconfirm earlier hypotheses and then revise their interpretations as necessary. The goal of this procedure is to continuously refine a hypothesis or theory. Morse (2015) pointed out that negative cases may provide the key to understanding "the norm"—that is, the most commonly occurring cases. She argued that data from negative cases should also be saturated.

> **Example of a Negative Case Analysis**
> Jahner et al. (2023) examined how RNs in rural practice deal with psychologically traumatic events when living and working in the same rural community. Interviews were conducted with 19 RNs from six rural acute care hospitals. Theoretical sampling in their constructivist grounded theory helped to identify four negative or contrasting cases from the analysis of data from the full sample. All four cases reported they found it difficult to manage to move forward from prior traumatic events.

Patton (1999) similarly encouraged a systematic exploration for rival themes and explanations during the analysis: "Failure to find strong supporting evidence for alternative ways of presenting the data or contrary explanations helps increase confidence in the original, principal explanation generated by the analyst" (p. 1191). This strategy can be addressed both inductively and logically. Inductively, the strategy involves seeking other ways of organizing the data that might lead to different conclusions and interpretations. Logically, it means conceptualizing other logical possibilities and then searching for evidence that could support those competing explanations.

Peer Review and Debriefing

External review is another quality-enhancement strategy. **Peer debriefing** involves sessions with peers to review and explore various aspects of the inquiry. Peer debriefing exposes researchers to the searching questions of others who are experienced in either the methods of qualitative inquiry, the phenomenon being studied, or both.

In a peer debriefing session, researchers might present written or oral summaries of the data, emergent categories and themes, and interpretations of the data. In some cases, recorded interviews might be played or transcripts might be shared with reviewers. Peer reviewers might be asked to address questions such as the following:

- Is there evidence of researcher bias? Have the researchers been sufficiently reflexive?
- Do the data adequately portray the phenomenon?
- Are there any apparent errors of fact?
- Are there possible errors of interpretation? Are there competing interpretations? More comprehensive or parsimonious interpretations?
- Have all important themes or patterns been identified?
- Are the themes and interpretations knit together into a cogent and creative conceptualization of the phenomenon?

> **TIP** Morse (2015) expressed some concern about the use of peer review as a validation strategy. She recommended that researchers listen to alternative points of view, but that they need to take "final responsibility for the results, and its implications and applications" (p. 1215).

Example of Peer Debriefing
Etowa and colleagues (2022) used descriptive qualitative methods in their community-based participatory research in Canada. The purpose of their study was to generate knowledge to guide effective HIV responses with African, Caribbean, and Black (ACB) men and to identify the individual and structural factors that enable resilience and decrease HIV-related vulnerabilities among heterosexual ACB men and youth. The research team engaged in peer debriefing during data analysis to discuss the emerging themes.

Inquiry Audits
A similar, but more formal, approach is to undertake an **inquiry audit**, which involves scrutiny of the data and supporting documents by an external reviewer. Such an audit requires careful documentation of all aspects of the inquiry, as previously discussed. Once the audit trail materials are assembled, the inquiry auditor proceeds to audit, in a fashion analogous to a financial audit, the trustworthiness of the data and the meanings attached to them. Although such auditing is complex, it can serve as a tool for persuading others that qualitative findings are worthy of confidence. Relatively few comprehensive inquiry audits have been reported in the literature, but some studies report partial audits. Rodgers and Cowles (1993) and Erwin and colleagues (2005) provide useful information about inquiry audits.

Example of an External Audit
Johanna and colleagues (2022) studied nurses' experiences of encountering patients with mental illness in prehospital emergency care in Sweden. Seventeen nurses participated in in-depth interviews. The analysis and formulated sub-themes and themes were presented at a critical research seminar with junior and senior researchers outside the research group at the Centre of Interprofessional Collaboration with Emergency Care before the final themes were agreed upon.

TIP In validating and refining themes, some researchers introduce **quasistatistics**—a tabulation of the frequency with which certain themes or insights are supported by the data. The frequencies cannot be interpreted like frequencies in quantitative studies, but, as Becker (1970) pointed out, "Quasi-statistics may allow the investigator to dispose of certain troublesome null hypotheses. A simple frequency count of the number of times a given phenomenon appears may make untenable the null hypothesis that the phenomenon is infrequent" (p. 81).

Quality-Enhancement Strategies Relating to Presentation
The strategies discussed thus far are steps that researchers can undertake to convince *themselves* that their study has integrity and credibility. This section describes some issues relating to convincing *others* of the high quality of the inquiry.

Disclosure of Quality-Enhancement Strategies
A large part of demonstrating integrity to others involves providing a description of the quality-enhancement activities that were undertaken. Many research reports fail to include information that would give readers confidence in the integrity of the research. Some qualitative reports do not address the subject of validity or trustworthiness at all, while others pay lip service to such concerns, simply noting that, for example, member checking was undertaken. Just as clinicians seek *evidence* supporting healthcare decisions, readers of reports need *evidence* that the findings are credible. Readers can draw sensible conclusions about study quality only if they are provided with meaningful information about quality-enhancement strategies.

TIP Avoid stating—as many researchers do—that your quality-enhancement strategies *assured* or *ensured* rigor or trustworthiness. Strategies are used to *enhance* or *promote* rigor, but nothing ensures it.

Thick and Contextualized Description
Thick description, as noted in previous chapters, refers to a rich, thorough, and vivid description of the research context, the people who participated in the study, and the experiences and processes

observed during the inquiry. Transferability cannot occur unless investigators provide detailed information to permit judgments about contextual similarity. Lucid and textured descriptions, with the judicious inclusion of verbatim quotes from study participants, also contribute to the authenticity and vividness of a qualitative study.

TIP Sandelowski (2004) cautioned that "…the phrase *thick description* likely ought not to appear in write-ups of qualitative research at all, as it is among those qualitative research words that should be seen but not written" (p. 215).

In high-quality studies, descriptions typically need to go beyond a faithful and thorough rendering of information. Powerful description often has an evocative quality and the capacity for emotional impact. Qualitative researchers must be careful, however, not to misrepresent their findings by sharing only the most dramatic or poignant stories. Thorne and Darbyshire (2005) cautioned against "lachrymal validity," a criterion for evaluating research based on the extent to which the report can bring tears from its readers. At the same time, they noted that the opposite problem with some reports is that they are "bloodless." Bloodless findings are characterized by a tendency of some researchers to "play it safe in writing up the research, reporting the obvious…, failing to apply any inductive analytic spin to the sequence, structure, or form of the findings" (p. 1109).

Researcher Credibility

In qualitative studies, researchers *are* the data collecting instruments—as well as creators of the analytic process. Therefore, researcher qualifications, experience, and reflexivity are relevant in establishing confidence in the findings. Patton (2015) argued that trustworthiness is enhanced if the report contains information about the researchers and their credentials. In addition, the report may need to make clear the personal connections researchers had to the people, topic, or community under study. For example, it is relevant for a reader of a report on AIDS patients' coping to know that the researcher is HIV positive. Patton recommended that researchers report "any personal and professional information that may have affected data collection, analysis, and interpretation—either negatively or positively…" (p. 700).

Example of Researcher Credibility
Nthenge and colleagues (2022) explored the experience of women of short stature during the perinatal period. Nine women of short stature, including five with dwarfism and four with osteogenesis imperfecta comprised the sample. The researchers used Braun and Clarke's six-phase reflexive thematic analysis to identify patterns of meaning. Participants expressed concerns regarding lack of clinicians' knowledge and experience in administering epidural anesthesia to women of short stature. Two of the researchers were women who had a physical disability.

TIP Janice Morse (2015), an influential qualitative nurse researcher, disagrees with some aspects of the Lincoln and Guba framework. For example, she believes that member checking should never be done and that certain strategies described in this chapter are sometimes inappropriate. For instance, she believes that assessments of coder consistency are not suitable when the data are from unstructured interviews, and that prolonged engagement is a useful strategy only with observational research.

DEVELOPING A QUALITY-MINDED OUTLOOK

Conducting high-quality qualitative research is not just about what researchers *do*. It is also about who the researchers *are*—their outlook, self-demands, and ingenuity. As Morse and colleagues (2002) succinctly put it, "Research is only as good as the investigator" (p. 10). Attributes that good qualitative researchers must possess are difficult to teach, but it is important to know what those attributes are so they can be cultivated. We express several important attributes as *commitments* to which researchers should aspire.

1. **Commitment to Transparency.** Good qualitative inquiry cannot be a secretive enterprise that masks decisions, biases, and limitations from outside scrutiny. Conscientious qualitative researchers maintain the records needed to document and justify decisions. A commitment to transparency also means making efforts to

have decisions reviewed by others. To the extent possible, researchers should seek opportunities to demonstrate transparency in their writing, including showing how themes and categories were formulated from the initial data.

2. **Commitment to Thoroughness and Diligence.** Meticulousness is essential to high-quality research. Researchers who are not thorough run the risk of having thin, unsaturated data that thwart rich description of phenomena. The concept of *replication* within the study is crucial: there must be sufficient, and redundant, data to account for all the aspects of the phenomenon (Morse et al., 2002). In good qualitative research, investigators must commit to reading and rereading their data, returning repeatedly to check whether their interpretations are true to their data. Thoroughness also implies that researchers will seek opportunities to challenge early conceptualizations and to find sources of corroborating evidence both internally (i.e., within the study data) and externally (e.g., in the literature).

3. **Commitment to Verification.** Confidence in the data, and in the analysis and interpretation of those data, is possible only when researchers are committed to instituting verification and self-correcting procedures throughout the study. Morse and colleagues (2002) wrote at length about the importance of verification, noting that verification is "the process of checking, confirming, making sure, and being certain" (p. 9). A commitment to verification strengthens methodologic coherence and helps to promote the likelihood that errors and missteps are corrected before they undermine the enterprise.

4. **Commitment to Reflexivity.** While there is not always agreement about the forms that self-reflection will assume, there is widespread agreement that qualitative researchers need to devote time and energy to analyzing and documenting their presuppositions, biases, and ongoing emotions. Reflexivity involves a continuous self-scrutiny and asking: How might my previous experiences, values, background, and prejudices be shaping my methods, my analysis, and my interpretations?

5. **Commitment to Participant-Driven Inquiry.** In good qualitative research, the inquiry is driven forward by the participants, not the researcher. Researchers must continuously remain responsive to the flow and content of interactions with, and observations of, their informants. Participants shape the scope and breadth of questioning, and they help to guide sampling decisions. The analysis and interpretation must give voice to those who participated in the inquiry.

6. **Commitment to Insightful Interpretation.** Morse (2006) has written that *insight* is a major process in qualitative inquiry but has been neglected and overlooked in the literature—perhaps because it is not easily acquired. Morse argued that researchers must be *ready* for insight—they must have considerable knowledge about their data and be able to link them meaningfully to relevant literature. Immersion in one's own data and having good-quality data are essential. Morse also noted, however, that qualitative researchers need to give themselves "*permission* to use insight and the confidence to do it well" (p. 3). Relatedly, Morse and colleagues (2002) urged researchers to *think theoretically*, which "requires macro-micro perspectives, inching forward without making cognitive leaps, constantly checking and rechecking, and building a solid foundation" (p. 13).

CRITICAL APPRAISAL OF QUALITY IN QUALITATIVE STUDIES

For qualitative research to be judged trustworthy, investigators must *earn* their readers' trust. Many qualitative reports do not provide much information about the researchers' efforts to enhance trustworthiness. In a world that is very conscious about the quality of research evidence, qualitative researchers need to be proactive in doing high-quality research and sharing their quality-enhancement efforts with readers.

Part of the difficulty that qualitative researchers face in demonstrating trustworthiness and authenticity is that page constraints in journals impose conflicting demands. It takes a precious amount of space to report quality-enhancement strategies adequately and convincingly. Using space for such documentation means that there is less space for

> **BOX 26.1** Guidelines for Critically Appraising Quality and Integrity in Qualitative Studies
>
> 1. Did the report discuss efforts to enhance or monitor the quality of the data and the overall inquiry? If so, was the description sufficiently detailed and clear? If not, was there other information that allowed you to draw inferences about the quality of the data, the analysis, and the interpretations?
> 2. Which specific techniques (if any) did the researcher use to enhance the trustworthiness and integrity of the inquiry? What quality-enhancement strategies were *not* used? Would additional strategies have strengthened your confidence in the study and its evidence?
> 3. Did the researcher adequately represent the multiple realities of those being studied? Do the findings seem *authentic*?
> 4. Were results interpreted in light of findings from other studies?
> 5. Did the report discuss any study limitations and their possible effects on the credibility of the results or on interpretations of the data?
> 6. Given the efforts to enhance data quality, what can you conclude about the study's validity/rigor/trustworthiness?
> 7. Did the researchers discuss the study's implications for clinical practice or future research? Were the implications well-grounded in the study evidence?

the thick description of context and the rich verbatim accounts that are also necessary in high-quality qualitative research. As Pyett (2003) has noted, qualitative research is often characterized by the need for critical compromises, which should be kept in mind when reading qualitative research reports.

RESEARCH EXAMPLE

Examples of various quality-enhancement strategies used by qualitative nurse researchers have been noted throughout this chapter. In this section, we describe more fully the strategies used by one team of researchers.

Study: Managing safety in perioperative settings: Strategies of meso level nurse leaders (Brooks & Nelson-Brantley, 2023).

Statement of purpose: The purpose of this study was to describe the experiences of middle (meso) nurse leaders in creating a culture of safety in perioperative settings.

Method: In this qualitative descriptive study, the researchers interviewed 17 middle level nurse leaders in perioperative settings. Inductive thematic analysis was used to analyze the content from the interviews.

Quality-enhancement strategies: The report included a section on their efforts to demonstrate trustworthiness in their research. Researchers used peer debriefing to enhance the credibility. Dependability was assessed by means of an audit trail of research activities and field notes. The researchers engaged in reflexivity, critically examining how their personal values and experiences influenced data collection, analysis, and interpretation. Transferability was supported by including thick description of the data and balanced interpretation. Authenticity was enhanced by including multiple middle level nurse leader roles from a variety of perioperative service lines.

Key findings: The researchers identified four strategies that the middle level nurse leaders used to foster safety: (1) Recognizing the unique perioperative management environment, (2) Learning not to take interactions personally, (3) Developing super meso-level nurse leaders skills, and (4) Appealing to policies and patient safety.

SUMMARY POINTS

- Several controversies surround the issue of *quality* in qualitative studies, one of which involves terminology. Some have argued that terms such as *rigor* and *validity* are quantitative terms that are unsuitable goals in qualitative inquiry, but others think these terms are appropriate.

- Other controversies involve what criteria to use as indicators of integrity, whether there should be generic or tradition-specific criteria, and what strategies to use to address the quality criteria.
- The most-often used framework of quality criteria is that of Lincoln and Guba, who identified five criteria for evaluating the **trustworthiness** of the inquiry: credibility, dependability, confirmability, transferability, and authenticity.
- **Credibility**, which refers to confidence in the truth value of the findings, is sometimes said to be the qualitative equivalent of internal validity. **Dependability** refers to the stability of data over time and conditions and is somewhat analogous to reliability in quantitative studies. **Confirmability** refers to the objectivity or neutrality of the data. **Transferability**, the analog of external validity, is the extent to which findings from the data can be transferred to other settings or groups. **Authenticity** refers to the extent to which researchers fairly and faithfully show a range of different realities and convey the feeling tone of lives as they are lived.
- Strategies for enhancing the quality of qualitative data as they are being collected include **prolonged engagement**, which strives for adequate scope of data coverage; **persistent observation**, which is aimed at achieving adequate depth; reflexivity; comprehensive and vivid recording of information (including maintenance of an **audit trail** of key decisions and products); triangulation, and member checking.
- **Triangulation** is the process of using multiple referents to draw conclusions about what constitutes the truth. During data collection, key forms of triangulation include **data triangulation** (using multiple data sources to validate conclusions) and **method triangulation** (using multiple methods, such as interviews and observations, to collect data about the same phenomenon).
- **Member checks** involve asking participants to review and react to study data and emerging themes and conceptualizations. A procedure called *Synthesized Member Checking* (SMC) is an effort to make member checking more systematic. Member checking is among the most controversial methods of addressing quality issues in qualitative inquiry.
- Strategies for enhancing quality during the coding and analysis of qualitative data include **investigator triangulation** (independent coding and analysis of at least a portion of the data by two or more researchers); **theory triangulation** (use of competing theories or hypotheses in the analysis and interpretation of data); searching for confirming and disconfirming evidence; searching for rival explanations and undertaking a **negative case analysis** (revising interpretations to account for cases that appear to disconfirm early conclusions); external validation through **peer debriefings** (exposing the inquiry to the searching questions of peers); and launching a formal **inquiry audit** (a formal scrutiny of audit trail documents by an independent external auditor).
- Strategies to convince qualitative report readers of high quality include disclosure of key quality-enhancement strategies; using *thick description* to vividly portray contextualized information about participants and the central phenomenon; and making efforts to be transparent about researcher credentials and reflexivity so that **researcher credibility** can be assessed.
- Doing high-quality qualitative research is not just about *method* and what the researchers *do*—it is also about who they *are*. To become an outstanding qualitative researcher, there must be a commitment to transparency, thoroughness, verification, reflexivity, participant-driven inquiry, and insightful and artful interpretation.

REFERENCES CITED IN CHAPTER 26

Baranowska, B., Wegrzynowska, M., Tataj-Puzyna, U., & Crowther, S. (2022), "I knew there has to be a better way": Women's pathways to free birth in Poland. *Women and Birth*, *35*(4), e328–e336. https://doi.org/10.1016/j.wombi.2021.07.008

Becker, H. S. (1970). *Sociological work*. Aldine.

Birt, L., Scott, S., Cavers, D., Campbell, C., & Walter, F. (2016). Member checking: A tool to enhance trustworthiness or merely a nod to validation? *Qualitative Health Research*, *26*(13), 1802–1811.

Brooks, J. V., & Nelson-Brantley, H. (2023). Managing safety in perioperative settings: Strategies of meso-level nurse leaders. *Health Care Management Review Journal*, 48(2), 175–184. https://doi.org/10.1097/HMR.0000000000000364

Chodidjah, S., Kongvattananon, P., & Liaw, J. J. (2022). "Changed our lives": Psychosocial issues experienced by families of early adolescents with leukemia. *European Journal of Oncology Nursing*, 56, 102077. https://doi.org/10.1016/j.ejon.2021.102077

Cooley, R., Venkatachalam, A. M., Aguilera, V., Olson, D. M., & Stutzman, S. E. (2022). A qualitative study of nurses' perceptions of narcotic administration after subarachnoid hemorrhage. *Pain Management Nursing*, 23(2), 151–157. https://doi.org/10.1016/j.pmn.2021.03.008

Cypress, B. S. (2017). Rigor or reliability and validity in qualitative research: Perspectives, strategies, reconceptualization, and recommendations. *Dimensions in Critical Care Nursing*, 36(4), 253–263.

Denzin, N. K., & Lincoln, Y. S. (Eds.). (2000). *Handbook of qualitative research* (2nd ed.). Sage Publications.

Denzin, N. K. (1989). *The research act* (3rd ed.). McGraw-Hill.

Erwin, E., Meyer, A., & McClain, N. (2005). Use of an audit in violence prevention research. *Qualitative Health Research*, 15(5), 707–718.

Etowa, J., Kakuru, D. M., Gebremeskel, A., Etowa, E. B., & Kohoun, B. (2022). De-problematizing masculinity among heterosexual African, Caribbean, and Black male youth and men. *Canadian Journal of Public Health*, 113(4), 611–621. https://doi.org/10.17269/s41997-021-00596-3

Guba, E., & Lincoln, Y. (1994). Competing paradigms in qualitative research. In Denzin, N., & Lincoln, Y. (Eds.), *Handbook of qualitative research* (pp. 105–117). Sage Publications.

Jack, S.M., Duku, E., Whitty, H., Van Lieshout, R.J., Niccols, A., Georgiades, K., & Lipman, E. L. (2022). Young mothers' use of and experiences with mental health care services in Ontario, Canada: A qualitative descriptive study. *BMC Women's Health*, 22(1), 214. https://doi.org/10.1186/s12905-022-01804-z

Jahner, S., Penz, K., Stewart, N.J., Morgan, D., & Kulig, J. (2023). "Staying strong": A constructivist grounded theory of how registered nurses deal with the impact of trauma-related events in rural acute care practice. *Journal of Clinical Nursing*, 32(5–6), 879–893. https://doi.org/10.1111/jocn.16459

Johanna, Z., Elin, V., Mats, H., Henrik, A., & Jonas, A. (2022). Nurses' experiences of encountering patients with mental illness in prehospital emergency care-a qualitative interview study. *BMC Nursing*, 21(1), 89. https://doi.org/10.1186/s12912-022-00868-4

Kimchi, J., Polivka, B., & Stevenson, J. S. (1991). Triangulation: Operational definitions. *Nursing Research*, 40(6), 364–366.

Lincoln, Y. S., & Guba, E. G. (1985). *Naturalistic inquiry*. Sage Publications.

Morse, J. M. (1999). Myth # 93: Reliability and validity are not relevant to qualitative inquiry. *Qualitative Health Research*, 9, 717–718.

Morse, J. M. (2006). Insight, inference, evidence, and verification: Creating a legitimate discipline. *International Journal of Qualitative Methods*, 5(1), Article 8.

Morse, J. M. (2015). Critical analysis of strategies for determining rigor in qualitative inquiry. *Qualitative Health Research*, 25(9), 1212–1222.

Morse, J. M., Barrett, M., Mayan, M., Olson, K., & Spiers, J. (2002). Verification strategies for establishing reliability and validity in qualitative research. *International Journal of Qualitative Methods*, 1(2), Article 2.

Nepali, S., Einboden, R., & Rudge, T. (2023). Control of resources in the nursing workplace: Power and patronage relations. *Nursing Inquiry*, 30(2), e12523. https://doi.org/10.1111/nin.12523

Nthenge, S., Smith, L., Ho, S., & Mitra, M. (2022). Experiences of women of short stature during the perinatal period. *Journal of Obstetric, Gynecologic, and Neonatal Nursing*, 51(4), 418–427. https://doi.org/10.1016/j.jogn.2022.03.006

Nyhagen, R., Egerod, I., Rustøen, T., Lerdal, A., & Kirkevold, M. (2023). Unidentified communication challenges in the intensive care unit: A qualitative study using multiple triangulations, *Australian Critical Care*, 36(2), 215–222. https://doi.org/10.1016/j.aucc.2022.01.006

Pape, E., Decoene, E., Debrauwere, M., Van Nieuwenhove, Y., Pattyn, P., Feryn, T., Pattyn, P.R.L., Verhaeghe, S., Van Hecke, A., Belgian LARS collaborative group. (2022). Experiences and needs of partners as informal caregivers of patients with major low anterior resection syndrome: A qualitative study. *European Journal of Oncology Nursing*, 58: 102143. https://doi.org/10.1016/j.ejon.2022.102143

Patton, M. (1999). Enhancing the quality and credibility of qualitative analysis. *Health Services Research*, 34(5 pt 2), 1189–1208.

Patton, M. Q. (2015). *Qualitative research and evaluation methods* (4th ed.). Sage Publications.

Pyett, P. M. (2003). Validation of qualitative research "in the real world". *Qualitative Health Research*, 13(8), 1170–1179.

Renz, S., Carrington, J., & Badger, T. (2018). Two strategies for qualitative content analysis: An intramethod approach to triangulation. *Qualitative Health Research*, 28(5), 824–831.

Rodgers, B. L., & Cowles, K. V. (1993). The qualitative research audit trail: A complex collection of documentation. *Research in Nursing and Health*, 16(3), 219–226.

Rost, M., Stuerner, Z., Niles, P., & Arnold, L. (2023). Between "a lot of room for it" and "it doesn't exist"- Advancing and limiting factors of autonomy in birth as perceived by perinatal care practitioners: An interview study in Switzerland. *Birth*, 50(4), 1068–1080. https://doi.org10.1111/birt.12757

Rusli, K.D., Ong, S.F., Speed, S., Seah, B., McKenna, L., Lau, Y., & Liaw, S. Y. (2022). Home-based care nurses' lived experiences and perceived competency needs: A phenomenological study. *Journal of Nursing Management*, 30(7), 2992–3004.https://doi.org/10.1111/jonm.13694

Sandelowski, M. (1993a). Rigor or rigor mortis: The problem of rigor in qualitative research revisited. *Advances in Nursing Science*, 16(2), 1–8.

Sandelowski, M. (1993b). Theory unmasked: The uses and guises of theory in qualitative research. *Research in Nursing & Health*, *16*(3), 213–218.

Sandelowski, M. (2004). Counting cats in zanzibar. *Research in Nursing & Health*, *27*(4), 215–216.

Smith, J. (1993). *After the demise of empiricism: The problem of judging social and educational inquiry*. Ablex.

Sparkes, A. (2001). Myth 94: Qualitative health researchers will agree about validity. *Qualitative Health Research*, *11*(4), 538–552.

Tanner, A. L., von Gaudecker, J. R., Buelow, J. M., Oruche, U. M., & Miller, W. R. (2022). "It's hard!": Adolescents' experience attending school with psychogenic nonepileptic seizures. *Epilepsy & Behavior*, *132*, 108724. https://doi.org/10.1016/j.yebeh.2022.108724

Thorne, S. (2020). The great saturation debate: What the "S word" means and doesn't mean in qualitative research reporting. *The Canadian Journal of Nursing Research = Revue canadienne de recherche en sciences infirmieres*, *52*(1), 3–5. https://doi.org/10.1177/0844562119898554

Thorne, S., & Darbyshire, P. (2005). Land mines in the field: A modest proposal for improving the craft of qualitative health research. *Qualitative Health Research*, *15*(8), 1105–1113.

Whittemore, R., Chase, S. K., & Mandle, C. L. (2001). Validity in qualitative research. *Qualitative Health Research*, *11*(4), 522–537.

Wolcott, H. (1994). *Transforming qualitative data*. Sage Publications.

Wolcott, H. (1995). *The art of fieldwork*. Sage Publications.

Zhu, P., Zhang, Q., Wu, Q., Shi, G., Wang, W., Xu, H., Zhang, L., Qian, M., & Hegarty, J. (2023). Barriers and facilitators to the choice of active surveillance for low-risk papillary thyroid cancer in China. A qualitative study examining patient perspectives. *Thyroid*, *33*(7), 826–834. https://doi.org/10.1089/thy.2022.0347

Part 5

DESIGNING AND CONDUCTING MIXED METHODS STUDIES TO GENERATE EVIDENCE FOR NURSING

Chapter 27 Basics of Mixed Methods Research
Chapter 28 Developing Complex Nursing Interventions Using Mixed Methods Research
Chapter 29 Feasibility and Pilot Studies of Interventions Using Mixed Methods

27 Basics of Mixed Methods Research

Learning Objectives

1. Understand the importance of using mixed methods research in the development and testing of instruments, interventions, and programs.
2. Articulate quantitative, qualitative, and integrative questions a researcher may ask in high-quality mixed methods research.
3. Identify the core designs of mixed methods research and the rationale for each.
4. Describe the key decisions necessary when considering sequencing the components of a study.
5. Explain the various types of sampling strategies used in mixed methods research.
6. Explicate the methods used to integrate the data in mixed methods studies.

OVERVIEW OF MIXED METHODS RESEARCH

A methodologic trend that has been gaining momentum in health research is the planned integration of qualitative and quantitative data within single studies or a coordinated series of studies. **Mixed methods research** in the health sciences has been called "a quiet revolution" (O'Cathain, 2009). Two decades ago, there was little guidance on conducting mixed methods research. Now there are abundant resources in the form of handbooks and textbooks (e.g., Creamer, 2018; Creswell et al., 2011; Creswell & Plano Clark, 2018; Morse, 2017; Plano Clark & Ivankova, 2016; Tashakkori et al., 2020) and many examples of mixed methods studies in the nursing and healthcare literature. New resources are becoming available continuously in this rapidly evolving field.

This chapter presents basic information about mixed methods research in nursing, and the next discusses the use of mixed methods in developing and testing nursing interventions. To streamline these chapters, we use the acronym MM to refer to mixed methods research.

Definition of Mixed Methods Research

The concept of combining qualitative and quantitative data in a study is straightforward, but definitions of MM research are not. This is partly because, in some sense, most studies could be considered MM if the definition is too broad. For example, if a grounded theory researcher asks structured demographic questions about age and education at the end of an in-depth interview, does that count as mixed methods? Or, if a survey asks a broad open-ended question at the end of a questionnaire (e.g., "Is there anything else you would like to add?"), is that MM research? We do not consider such inquiries as MM research.

We use the definition offered in the first issue of *Journal of Mixed Methods Research*, which is that MM research is "research in which the investigator collects and analyzes data, *integrates* the findings, and *draws inferences* using both qualitative and quantitative approaches or methods in a single study or program of inquiry" (Tashakkori & Creswell, 2007, p. 4, emphasis added). MM research involves not just collecting qualitative and quantitative data, but also *integrating* the two at multiple points in the research process, giving rise to meta-inferences. A **meta-inference** is a conclusion generated by integrating inferences from the results of the qualitative and quantitative strands of an MM study.

Rationale for Mixed Methods Studies

The dichotomy between quantitative and qualitative data represents a key methodologic distinction in the behavioral and health sciences. Some have argued that the paradigms that underpin qualitative and quantitative research are fundamentally incompatible. Many people now believe, however, that health research can be enriched through the judicious integration of qualitative and quantitative data. The advantages and "added value" of mixed methods include the following:

- *Complementarity.* Qualitative and quantitative approaches are complementary—words and numbers are the two fundamental languages of human communication. By using mixed methods, researchers can allow each to do what it does best.
- *Practicality.* Given the complexity of phenomena, it is practical to not have one's hands tied by rigid adherence to one methodology. MM researchers often ask questions that cannot be answered with a single approach.
- *Enhanced validity.* When a hypothesis, model, or description is supported by complementary types of data, researchers can be more confident about the validity of their results. The integration of methods can provide opportunities for testing alternative interpretations, for obtaining corroboration, and for assessing whether context helped to shape the results.

Paradigm Issues and Mixed Method Studies

Although MM research has been around for decades, broad acceptance is recent. Mixed methods research emerged from the ashes of the so-called *paradigm wars* involving debates between the positivist and constructivist camps that erupted during the 1970 and 1980s. MM research gained momentum at the turn of the 21st century.

Discussions about an appropriate paradigmatic stance for MM research abound. Viewpoints range from those claiming the irrelevance of paradigms, to those advocating multiple paradigms. The paradigm called **pragmatism** is often associated with MM research—a paradigm that some consider offers an "umbrella worldview" for a study (Creswell & Plano Clark, 2018, p. 69). Pragmatist researchers consider that it is the *research question* that should drive the inquiry and the methods used. They reject a forced choice between the traditional positivists' and constructivists' modes of inquiry. In the pragmatist paradigm, both induction and deduction are important, theory generation and theory verification can be accomplished, and a pluralistic view is encouraged. Pragmatism is practical: whatever works best to arrive at good evidence is appropriate.

> **TIP** The qualitative component of most MM studies is often "generic qualitative" (i.e., not allied with a research tradition). However, some have discussed incorporating phenomenologic (Mayoh & Onwuegbuzie, 2015) and grounded theory (Guetterman et al., 2019) components into MM research.

Applications of Mixed Methods Research

Creswell and Plano Clark (2018) identified seven broad types of research situations that are especially well suited to MM research:

1. Neither a qualitative nor a quantitative approach, by itself, is adequate in addressing the complexity of the research problem;
2. The findings from one approach can be greatly enhanced with a second source of data that has explanatory power;
3. The phenomenon needs to be explored in-depth before formal instruments can be developed and administered;

4. Quantitative results from an intervention study require qualitative data to help to explain and interpret the results;
5. Different types of cases need to be described and compared;
6. An effort is being made to involve study participants in the study; and
7. A program needs to be developed, implemented, and evaluated.

As this list suggests, mixed methods research can be used in various situations. Some specific applications are noteworthy because MM research has made important contributions in these areas in health disciplines.

Confirmation and Explication

Mixed methods studies are sometimes undertaken as a confirmatory strategy—that is, to converge on the truth. Additionally, some researchers deliberately collect qualitative data to explicate the *meaning* of quantitative findings. Quantitative methods can demonstrate that variables are systematically related but may fail to provide insights about *why* they are related. Such explications can corroborate statistical findings and guide the interpretation of results. Qualitative data can provide more global, dynamic, and contextualized views of the phenomena under study.

Example of Confirming and Explicating With Mixed Methods
Forde and colleagues (2020) used a parallel mixed method convergent design to study the structures, processes, and content of nurse-to-nurse handover at the change of shift in an acute setting in Ireland. Guided by the British Medical Association's Safe Handover—Safe Patients framework, researchers used a bedside handover tool to measure the quantitative data of 30 episodes of bedside handovers. Thirty audio recordings of the nurse-to-nurse reports were also collected and qualitatively analyzed using content analysis. The findings provided insights both positive and for areas in need of improvement in the structure, process, and content or nurse-to-nurse handover.

Instrumentation

Researchers sometimes collect qualitative data as a basis for developing structured instruments for research or clinical applications. Questions for a formal instrument are sometimes derived from clinical experience or prior research. When a construct is new, however, these mechanisms may be inadequate to capture its nuances. Thus, researchers sometimes gather qualitative data as the basis for generating items for quantitative instruments that are then rigorously tested, as described in Chapter 16.

Example of MM in Instrumentation
Lippe and Davis (2023) used a sequential, exploratory, mixed methods study design. The study involved three phases: development, preparation, and confirmation. After conducting a literature review to develop the model and assessment tool, the team brought together 24 participants with expertise in palliative care to engage in focus groups. The researchers used a semi-structured interview guide to qualitatively explore the experts' opinion of the completeness, clarity, and utility of the model and assessment tool. Quantitative data included an online survey to validate the competencies identified in the model and assessment tool.

Intervention Development

Qualitative research is playing an increasingly important role in the development of promising nursing interventions. There is growing recognition that the development of effective interventions must take clients' perspective into account. Intervention research is increasingly likely to be MM research, a topic we address in the next chapter.

Example of MM in Intervention Development Research
Logsdon and colleagues (2020) conducted a mixed methods design and an iterative process to develop a mobile app aimed at helping new mothers monitor their own health after childbirth. Participants provided qualitative data about their preferences for the delivery of education and their opinion of a prototype mobile app. Quantitative data included a scale that asked mothers to rate the features of the mobile app. The team concluded that these findings provide the requisite information needed for a clinical trial to test the app.

Intervention and Program Evaluation

Program evaluations have a long history of using MM approaches (see Patton, 2015). As described in Chapter 11, impact analyses that evaluate the effectiveness of a program typically rely on quantitative data, but process evaluations that examine how a program *works* involve the integration of qualitative and quantitative information. *Realist evaluations* almost always used mixed methods approaches to program evaluation.

> **Example of Mixed Methods in Program Evaluation**
> Gore and colleagues (2022) conducted a mixed methods study to evaluate a program that was developed to support Black churches in becoming dementia-friendly communities. They collected quantitative data from church partner ambassadors and conducted two qualitative focus group interviews. Their findings provided insights into areas requiring modifications to improve the program and important insights into how to sustain the program.

The Issue of Integration in Mixed Method Studies

Integration is often considered a central feature of MM research—a centerpiece that sets it apart from other methodologies. Meaningful integration in MM research allows researchers to "produce a whole…that is greater than the sum of the individual qualitative and quantitative parts" (Fetters & Freshwater, 2015, p. 115). Mixed methods research can only achieve its full potential for providing enhanced insights when integration occurs.

Integration is a topic that has been given considerable recent attention. Leading thinkers have encouraged "divesting" from the term *triangulation* in MM research, using the newer language of *integration* of qualitative and quantitative methods (Fetters & Molina-Azorin, 2017a).

Some MM experts have provided guidance about the *when* and the *how* of integration. In all three editions of their widely used textbook on MM research, Creswell and Plano Clark (2018) have described options for integration at the analysis and interpretation stage, using broad analytic strategies such as mixing, merging, and connecting. For example, the data types can be *mixed* during the interpretation of the qualitative and quantitative findings. *Merging* can occur during data analysis, through a combined analysis. Integration also can occur during data collection by using a strategy of *connecting* in which the results from one strand influence data collection in a subsequent strand.

Creamer (2018), however, has advocated for fully integrated MM research in which there is an intention to mix or integrate throughout the planning and conduct of the study. She advocates for deliberative integration during these five stages: planning and design, data collection, sampling, analysis, and inference development.

Similarly, the editors of the *Journal of Mixed Methods Research* recently wrote a lengthy editorial in which they suggest integration across 15 dimensions that encompass the entire range of activities in an MM study (Fetters & Molina-Azorin, 2017b). They defined integration as "the linking of qualitative and quantitative approaches and dimensions together to create a new whole or a more holistic understanding than achieved by either alone" (p. 293). They sought to identify integration approaches "at the philosophical, methodologic, and methods levels to inform an all-encompassing mixed methods research approach" (p. 293). Thus, MM researchers are urged to consider the issue of integration for every decision they make throughout the research process, including putting together a team, undertaking a literature review, and framing research questions.

Practical Issues: Skills and Resources for Mixed Methods

Mixed methods studies have become attractive to both new and seasoned researchers, but the decision to pursue such a study should not be made lightly. The researcher's skills should be critically evaluated in deciding whether to undertake an MM study because the researcher must have some level of competence in both qualitative and quantitative methods. Many courses are now available to teach mixed methods skills, and NIH offers mixed methods training programs. Also, a computer application (app) has been developed to help novice researchers plan a MM project (Luo & Creswell, 2016).

A team approach to MM research is often advocated. A research team provides opportunity for collaboration between qualitative and quantitative researchers working on similar problems. Although a team approach is a useful way to proceed because experts in both approaches can make contributions, all team members should be methodologically bilingual and have basic understanding of varied approaches. Increasingly, mixed methods collaboration involves teams of professionals in diverse disciplines (Hesse-Biber, 2016). Fetters and Molina-Azorin (2017c) noted that when working in teams MM researchers "need to understand the culture associated with disciplines that have been traditionally mono-method" (p. 428).

> **TIP** In dissertation MM research, the judicious selection of advisers with a mix of methodologic skills is imperative. Keep in mind, however, that advisers from different backgrounds may have conflicting views about the merit of your strategies and the emphasis given to different aspects of your study. Frels and colleagues (2015) have written about the important role of mentoring in MM research.

Mixed methods research can be expensive. Although funding agencies increasingly are looking favorably on MM studies, it is obviously costly to collect, analyze, and integrate two or more types of data. Relatedly, mixed methods studies are often time consuming. It is wise to develop a realistic timeline before embarking on an MM inquiry.

GETTING STARTED ON A MIXED METHODS STUDY

In this chapter, we discuss many aspects of mixed methods research, with emphasis on research design and the analysis of MM data. We begin, however, by considering the intent of an MM study and the kinds of questions that lend themselves to MM research.

The Purpose/Intent of a Mixed Methods Study

In an article in which several key scholars discussed current challenges of mixed methods research, one expert (Tashakkori) advised new researchers to use mixed methods only if MM is *required* (Fetters & Molina-Azorin, 2017c, p. 427). This implies that researchers need to develop and state a justifiable mixed methods purpose, as expressed in a purpose statement.

In writing mixed methods purpose statements, researchers should communicate the purpose of both the quantitative and qualitative components. They should also articulate a mixed methods purpose that states the overall **intent** of integrating the two approaches. The study's MM intent is what drives the study design, and so it is important to clarify what that intent is (e.g., To explore? To explicate or explain? To confirm? To compare?). Creswell and Plano Clark's (2018) book offers useful "scripts" for writing MM purpose statements.

> **Example of a Mixed Methods Purpose Statement**
> Macedo and colleagues (2022) conducted a mixed methods study to examine self-care in patients in rural areas of Brazil who had not achieved optimal diabetes management. The purpose of their study was to assess the self-care practices in these patients and to understand the positive and negative experiences associated with poor diabetes control. Qualitatively they explored the patients' experiences through focus group interviews. Quantitatively, they conducted surveys exploring sociodemographic characteristics and diabetes self-care activities.

Research Questions for Mixed Methods Research

In mixed methods studies, the research questions are the driving force behind the scope of the inquiry. Investigators in MM studies typically pose questions that can *only* be addressed (or that can *best* be addressed) with more than one type of data.

In mixed methods research, there are inevitably at least two research questions, each of which requires a different approach. For example, MM researchers may simultaneously ask exploratory (qualitative) questions and confirmatory (quantitative) questions. MM researchers can examine causal *effects* in a quantitative component but can also shed light on causal *mechanisms* in a qualitative component.

In addition to mono-method questions, MM studies should ask a specific MM question relating to the integration of qualitative and quantitative data, and that makes explicit what will be answered through such integration. Examples include such questions as, "To what extent do the two types of data confirm each other?" and "How does one type of data help to explain the results from the other type?"

Creswell and Plano Clark's (2018) book includes a table with a series of mixed methods questions (pp. 169–170).

> **Example of a Mixed Methods Research Question**
> Bocquier and colleagues (2023) conducted a concurrent mixed method to understand school personnel's knowledge of HPV, HPV vaccination, and perceptions of the school's role in promoting HPV vaccination. To answer their question, they combined quantitative data of online surveys with qualitative data obtained from three focus groups to identify the barriers, facilitators, and needs of the school personnel in developing and implementing interventions to promote HPV vaccination in French middle schools.

MIXED METHODS DESIGNS

Mixed methods designs are continuing to evolve as greater thought is given to fruitful approaches—and as greater experience in conducting MM research occurs. Over a dozen design typologies have been developed by mixed methods scholars, so it is challenging to discuss this important topic. We begin by noting some key design issues, then present methods of portraying designs through a notation system and diagrams, and finally describe the design typology offered by Creswell and Plano Clark (2018).

Key Decisions in Mixed Methods Designs

In designing an MM study, researchers make several important decisions, which we briefly review in this section.

Fixed vs. Emergent Designs

One issue concerns whether to establish a design at the outset. In some cases, the research intent will lead to a certain type of MM research design. Novice researchers are especially likely to benefit by having a "roadmap" to follow. Experienced researchers may, however, prefer the flexibility of allowing answers from an initial **strand** (e.g., the qualitative component) guide them in subsequent strands (e.g., the quantitative component). Emergent MM designs may result from issues that develop during a mono-method study—for example, an inadequacy in fully understanding the construct or phenomenon of interest.

As noted by Creswell and Plano Clark (2018), "fixed" and "emergent" designs are probably best understood as endpoints on a continuum rather than as a dichotomy. No typology of designs encompasses every possible MM design, because a hallmark of the MM approach is that it permits creativity and paths to deeper understanding. Typologies and nomenclatures for designs are useful primarily because of their role in communicating an approach to others in proposals, IRB applications, and research articles. The designs we describe in this chapter are ones that have been adopted in many studies, but other possibilities exist for structuring an MM study, and the possibilities may emerge during a study that initially had a fixed design.

Sequencing in Mixed Methods Designs

There are three options for sequencing the strands of a mixed methods study: qualitative data are collected first, quantitative data are collected first, or both types are collected simultaneously (or at approximately the same time). When the two types of data are not collected at the same time, the approach is called **sequential**. When the data are collected at the same time, the approach is called **concurrent** (or *simultaneous*). Concurrent designs occur in a single phase, whereas sequential designs unfold in two or more phases. In well-conceived sequential designs, the analysis and interpretation in one phase informs the collection and analysis of data in the second. Another possibility is *multiphase timing*, which occurs when researchers launch a multiphase project that includes several sequential and/or concurrent substudies over a program of study. In an analysis of 294 MM studies in nursing, Beck, one of the authors of this textbook, and Harrison (2016) found that slightly more than half (53%) used a concurrent design.

Prioritization in Mixed Methods Designs

Researchers may decide whether one strand will be given greater weight or emphasis. One option is that the two components are given equal, or roughly equal, weight. Often, however, one strand is given **priority**. The distinction is sometimes referred to as *equal status* vs. *dominant status*.

The overall intent of the study usually affects the priority decision, as we discuss later in this section. The researcher's worldview is another influence. Researchers' philosophical orientation (positivist or constructivist) leads them to tackle research problems for which one approach is dominant, and the other is viewed as a useful supplementary data source. Practical considerations also may influence the weighting decision. If resources are limited, or if the researcher's skills are stronger in qualitative or quantitative methods, these issues will probably result in an MM study in which one approach has dominant status.

The issue of priority, however, has become somewhat controversial. Some experts worry about designating a priority based on relatively superficial criteria such as the amount of data rather than the information value of different strands (Fetters & Molina-Azorin, 2017c). Nevertheless, design notation continues to be used to represent prioritization decisions—although in Beck and Harrison's (2016) review of MM nursing studies, only a minority of researchers specified priority.

Notation and Diagramming in Mixed Methods Designs

Morse (1991), a prominent nurse researcher, made a crucial contribution to the MM literature by proposing a notation system that has been adopted across disciplines. Her notation system concerns the sequencing and prioritization decisions and is thus useful in quickly summarizing major features of an MM design.

In Morse's system, priority is designated by upper case and lower-case letters: QUAL/quan designate a mixed methods study in which the dominant approach is qualitative, while QUAN/qual designates the reverse. If neither approach is dominant (i.e., both are equal), the notation stipulates QUAL/QUAN. Sequencing is indicated by the symbols + or →. The arrow designates a sequential approach. For example, QUAN → qual is the notation for a primarily quantitative MM study in which qualitative data collection occurs in phase II. When both approaches occur concurrently, a plus sign is used (e.g., QUAL + quan).

TIP Other notations symbols have been suggested (e.g., parentheses, brackets, double-sided arrows), but the notations for sequence and priority are the ones most frequently used.

In addition to the notation system, MM designs can be visually diagrammed. Such diagrams can be useful in illustrating processes to reviewers and can also provide guidance to researchers themselves. Figure 27.1 illustrates a basic diagram for a QUAN + QUAL study. Additional information can be added under the boxes in the diagram to provide richer detail. For example, under the first box (Quantitative data collection and analysis), there might be a notation such as "Administered survey to 281 patients," and under the second box for the qualitative strand, there might be another notation (e.g., "Conducted focus group interviews with 24 patients").

TIP Creswell and Plano Clark (2018) offer ten guidelines for drawing visual diagrams of MM studies (Figure 3.2, p. 64). Their book also includes dozens of such visual diagrams that can serve as models.

Core Mixed Methods Designs

Although numerous design typologies have been developed by different MM methodologists, we focus on the one proposed by Creswell and Plano Clark (2018), two leading experts on MM research. They identified three designs that they call *core MM designs*, which we briefly describe in this section. Notations for these three designs are shown in Table 27.1. It should be noted that many published MM nursing studies do not fall exactly into the current Creswell-Plano Clark typology.

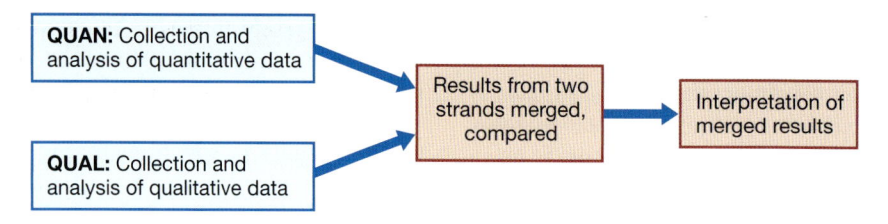

FIGURE 27.1 Diagram of a mixed methods convergent design.

Convergent Design

The purpose of the **convergent design** is to obtain different, but complementary, data about the central phenomenon under study. In this design, qualitative and quantitative data are collected simultaneously and, most often, with equal priority. The notation for a typical convergent design is QUAN + QUAL. The diagram in Figure 27.1 illustrates this design.

The convergent design is appropriate if the researcher wants to (1) compare the QUAL and QUAN results with the goal of obtaining a more complete understanding of a problem, (2) validate findings from one strand with those from another, (3) illustrate quantitative results with qualitative findings or vice versa, or (4) contrast people's answers to structured and unstructured questions. The overall goal of this design is to converge on "the truth" about a problem or phenomenon.

With the convergent design, researchers analyze the two datasets separately. They then use various strategies to merge and compare the datasets. For example, they may seek to identify the similarities and differences within one set of results based on dimensions that are prominent in the other set.

The convergent design has several variants. The most conventional is the *parallel databases variant* (Creswell & Plano Clark, 2018). In this variant, QUAN data are collected and analyzed in parallel with the collection and analysis of QUAL data. The results of the two separate analyses are brought together for an overall interpretation of results. The goal is to develop internally confirmed conclusions about a single phenomenon.

Another variant is called the *data transformation variant*. This design also involves the separate but concurrent collection of QUAL and QUAN data, followed by QUAL and QUAN analysis. A novel step in this variant involves transforming the QUAL data into quan data (or the QUAN data into qual data) and then comparing and interrelating the datasets. Data transformations are described later in this chapter.

A third variant is the *questionnaire variant* in which both closed-ended questions and probing open-ended questions are included on a questionnaire. The open-ended questions are analyzed thematically and used to confirm or validate the quantitative results. Such a variant might in some cases be notated as QUAN + qual if the main use of the qualitative data is to illustrate the quantitative findings with interesting quotes.

A major advantage of convergent designs is that they are efficient: both types of data are collected concurrently. A major drawback, however, is that these designs, which usually give equal weight to QUAL and QUAN strands, may be difficult for a single researcher working alone to do. Another potential problem can arise if the data from the two strands are not congruent.

TABLE 27.1 • Core Mixed Methods Designs

DESIGN NAME[a]	NOTATION AND PROCESS
Convergent	QUAN + QUAL → Results merged → Interpretation
Explanatory Sequential	QUAN → qual (QUAN results explained by qual) → Interpretation OR quan → QUAL (quan results explained by QUAL) → Interpretation
Exploratory Sequential	QUAL → Development (e.g., qual + quan) → QUAN (Testing) → Interpretation

[a]Design names are based on Creswell and Plano Clark (2018).

> **Example of a Convergent Design**
> Durante et al. (2022) conducted a multicenter convergent mixed methods study in Italy, Spain, and the Netherlands. The study aim was to understand the perception of resilience and associated factors in informal caregivers of persons with heart failure. The quantitative data included measures of resilience, caregiver burden, anxiety, and depression in a sample of 195 caregivers. A subset or nested sample of 50 caregivers were qualitatively interviewed. The data were first analyzed separately. A subsequent mixed analysis confirmed the findings that depression reduced these caregivers' resilience.

Explanatory Sequential Designs

Explanatory designs are sequential designs with quantitative data collected in the first phase, followed by qualitative data collected in the second phase. Either the qualitative or the quantitative data can be given a stronger priority in explanatory designs. That is, the design can be either QUAN → qual or quan → QUAL; the former sequence is more typical.

In explanatory designs, data from the second phase are used to build on or explain data from the initial phase. A QUAN → qual design is especially suitable when the quantitative results are surprising (for example, significant serendipitous results), when results are complicated and tricky to interpret, or when the sample has numerous outliers that are difficult to explain. Thus, this design is used to inform data collection for the second stage after the first-stage data have been analyzed. In reporting the use of this design, specific QUAN/quan results that were followed up should be identified.

Creswell and Plano Clark (2018) described two variants of the explanatory design. In the *follow-up explanations variant*, the researcher collects qual data that can best help to explain the initial QUAN findings. The primary emphasis is on the quantitative aspects of the study, and the analysis involves connecting data between the two phases. This model is one that is often attractive to researchers who are primarily quantitative, but who recognize that their study can be enriched by adding a follow-up qualitative component.

The second variant is the *case selection variant* in which first-stage quan data are in service of the second-phase QUAL component. In this model, information about the characteristics of a large group, as identified in the first phase, is used to purposefully select cases in the second dominant phase—for example, using extreme case sampling or stratified purposive sampling (Chapter 22).

> **TIP** In describing a design in a proposal or a report, it is probably best to combine words and notation. A citation should be provided for specifically named designs. For example, a design might be summarized as follows: "A sequential, qualitative-dominant (quan → QUAL) explanatory design (Creswell & Plano Clark, 2018), will be adopted in the proposed research." A visual diagram is a good supplement if space allows.

Advantages of explanatory designs are that they are straightforward, are easy to describe, and can be done by a single researcher. Another attractive feature, given page constraints in journals, is that the results can often be summarized in two separate papers. On the other hand, explanatory designs can be time consuming—the second phase cannot begin until data from the first phase are analyzed. Also, it may be difficult to secure upfront approval from funders or ethical review boards because details of the phase II design are seldom known in advance.

> **Example of an Explanatory Sequential Design**
> Bults and colleagues (2022) used an explanatory sequential (QUAN → qual) design to study the use, barriers, and enhancers of using diabetes-related mobile health apps in patients with T2DM in the Netherlands. An online survey captured actual use, barriers, and drivers of app use in 103 responders. This was followed by semistructured qualitative interviews in a subset of 16 participants. Their findings suggested that health provider support of app use and insurance coverage for the app were areas that may improve app use.

> **TIP** Creswell and Plano Clark's explanatory sequential design requires analysis of the QUAN data, with results serving as the springboard for making decisions for the qual strand. Many studies, however, have a sequential approach that does not involve a preliminary analysis of the QUAN data—the qual component is completed in a second phase, but the intent is to compare and contrast results (rather than to explain the QUAN findings), and is thus more like a convergent design.

Exploratory Sequential Designs

The **exploratory sequential design** is a three-phase MM design in which qualitative data are collected first. The design has as its central premise the need for initial in-depth exploration of a phenomenon, often to better understand contextual or cultural issues relevant to a phenomenon. Its intent is to use rich contextualized information to inform the development of a quantitative feature, such as a new measure, survey, intervention, or digital tool such as a website or app.

Findings from the initial qualitative phase are used to develop (phase II) and test (phase III) an innovation. The development phase can involve gathering additional quan or qual data (e.g., qual in a "think aloud" cognitive interview, quan in a pilot test). The final phase is a QUAN evaluation of the new product. For example, in instrument development studies, the researchers would undertake a psychometric assessment of the measure in phase III. The notation for this design might be QUAL → quan + qual → QUAN, but alternative decisions about prioritization might make sense. Creswell and Plano Clark (2018) described several variants of an exploratory design, such as the *new variable development variant*, the *survey (instrument) development variant*, and the *intervention-development variant*.

Example of an Exploratory Sequential Design
Ocak et al. (2023) used an exploratory sequential, mixed-method (QUAL → quan → QUAN) research design to develop a scale to measure screen fatigue in adolescents. They completed a literature search and qualitative interviews to develop the initial 56-item pool. They then conducted an exploratory factor analysis in 365 students and a subsequent confirmatory factor analysis in 417 students. These analyses resulted in a 24-item scale with four factors of screen fatigue: behavioral, physical, affective, and cognitive.

The advantages and disadvantages of an explanatory MM design also apply to exploratory MM designs. Separate phases make the inquiry easy to explain, implement, and report. A major challenge is that this design is time consuming and almost inevitably requires two or more rounds of sampling.

TIP In an earlier edition of their MM textbook, Creswell and Plano Clark described a design called the *embedded design*. An embedded design is one in which a second type of data is totally subservient to the other type of data. Creswell and Plano Clark (2018) now see embedding as an analytic strategy rather than as a design type.

Other Mixed Methods Designs

In some projects, core designs do not adequately characterize the complex series and sequences of mixing qualitative and quantitative data. Many advanced MM design options exist, including ones that are multiphase (progressing in multiple phases with various quan/qual combinations in each phase) and ones that are multilevels (gathering different combinations of qual/quan data from multiple tiers of an organizational system). Thus, although the core categories are a useful way to begin thinking about an MM study—especially for novice MM researchers—the typologies should not be used to force what should be a fluid and creative process into oversimplified boxes.

Creswell and Plano Clark (2018) described several *complex MM designs* that involve intersecting the core designs with other research approaches or frameworks. One is the *mixed methods experimental/intervention design*, using multiple methods and intricately related components that unfold over time. This type of MM research is described in the next chapter. *Participatory-social justice designs* are MM designs within a critical framework. A third complex design is the *mixed methods case study design*, which involves the use of one of the core designs within the framework of case study research. The fourth complex design is the *mixed methods evaluation design*, some features of which we described in Chapter 11.

TIP Mixed methods research is considered one category of *multimethod research* (Fetters & Molina-Azorin, 2017a). Other categories include quantitative studies with two or more approaches and qualitative studies with two or more approaches. Morse (2012; 2017), for example, has argued that a qualitative–qualitative study is a legitimate form of inquiry, using either a concurrent or sequential design. One of the qualitative methods is a "complete" method (e.g., grounded theory, phenomenology), and the other is supplemental (e.g., QUAL + qual or qual → QUAL). The supplementary strategy is not sufficiently complete to stand on its own.

Example of a Qualitative–Qualitative Mixed Methods Design
Odberg and colleagues (2019) conducted a QUAL-qual mixed methods study to increase the understanding of the nurse role during medication administration in the context of nursing homes in Norway. The nurse researchers collected data using participant observation and semistructured interviews. Inductive content analysis was used to analyze qualitative data. Three main categories were identified: Compensating, Flexible, and Adaptable.

Selecting a Mixed Methods Design

The most critical issue in selecting a design is its appropriateness for the research questions. The *design* should correspond to the study *intent*. Having a name for a design is less important than having a strong rationale for structuring a study in a certain way.

Practical issues are also relevant in designing a study. For example, few researchers are equally skillful in qualitative and quantitative methods. This suggests three options: (1) selecting a design in which your methodologic strengths are dominant; (2) working as a team with researchers whose strengths are complementary; or (3) strengthening your skills in your nondominant area. The first option is likely to be most realistic for many students. Practical concerns such as resource availability and time constraints also play a role in choosing a design. Concurrent designs often require shorter time commitments, and dominant designs can often be less resource-intensive.

It is advisable to learn the details of a particular MM design before making a selection. In addition to reading methodologic writings of MM scholars, it is useful to examine the methods section of reports that have used a design you are considering. Teddlie and Tashakkori (2009) also advised that "you should look for the most appropriate or single best available research design, rather than the 'perfect fit.' You may have to combine existing designs, or create new designs, for your study" (p. 163).

TIP MM designs are often portrayed as cross-sectional, even when they are sequential—that is, the goal in sequential designs usually is not to understand how a phenomenon unfolds over time. Plano Clark and colleagues (2015) have presented a conceptualization of longitudinal mixed methods designs.

SAMPLING AND DATA COLLECTION IN MIXED METHODS STUDIES

When a study design has been selected, an MM researcher can then plan how best to collect the needed data. Sampling and data collection in MM studies are often a blend of approaches that we described in earlier chapters. A few special sampling and data collection issues for an MM study merit brief discussion.

Sampling in a Mixed Methods Study

Mixed methods researchers can combine sampling designs in various creative ways. The quantitative component is likely to rely on a sampling strategy that enhances the researcher's ability to generalize to a broader population. As noted in Chapter 13, probability samples are well suited to selecting a representative sample of participants, but nurse researchers often must compromise, using such designs as consecutive samples or quota samples to enhance representativeness. For the qualitative strand of the study, MM researchers usually adopt purposive sampling methods (Chapter 23) to select information-rich cases.

Sample sizes are often different in the qualitative and quantitative components, in predictable ways—that is, larger samples for the quantitative strand. Ideally, MM researchers should use power analyses to guide sample size decisions for the quantitative component, to diminish the risk of type II errors in statistical analyses. In the qualitative sample, saturation is the principle often used to decide when to stop sampling.

A unique sampling issue in MM studies concerns whether the same people will be in both the qualitative and quantitative strands. The best strategy depends on the study purpose and the research design, but using overlapping samples can be advantageous. Having the same people in both parts of an MM study offers opportunities for convergence and for comparison between the two datasets.

Onwuegbuzie and Collins (2007) categorized mixed methods sampling designs according to the *relationship* between the qualitative and quantitative components. The four relationships are identical, parallel, nested, or multilevel. An **identical** relationship occurs when the same people are in both strands of the study—a situation that is especially likely in convergent designs. This approach might occur if everyone in a survey or intervention study was asked a series of probing, open-ended questions—or if everyone in a primarily QUAL study was administered a formal instrument, such as a self-efficacy scale.

Example of Identical Sampling
Piil and colleagues (2022) used identical sampling in their mixed methods convergent design study that examined health related quality of life and the daily life perspectives of long-term brain cancer survivors and their caregivers. Quantitative measures included self-reported surveys on anxiety, depression, functional assessment of brain cancer, and leisure-time activity. Additionally, they conducted telephone interviews with patients who had the diagnosis for greater than 3 years and their caregivers.

In a **parallel** relationship, the samples in the two strands are completely different, although they are usually drawn from the same population. Like identical sampling, parallel sampling can occur in either concurrent or sequential designs, and with any prioritization scheme. Parallel sampling is especially common in exploratory sequential designs: a phenomenon is explored with a relatively small sample of participants, and different samples are used to develop and test a new QUAN feature.

Example of Parallel Sampling
In a convergent parallel mixed methods study, Prompahakul and colleagues (2021) aimed to describe the experience of moral distress and related factors among nurses in Southern province of Thailand. The team collected the quantitative and qualitative data in parallel. The analysis of the quantitative and qualitative data was conducted separately and then integrated.

In a **nested** relationship, participants in the qualitative strand are a subset of the participants in the quantitative strand. Nested sampling is especially common in studies with an explanatory design as is highlighted in the example above by Durante and colleagues (2022). Indeed, as discussed in the previous section, a variant of an explanatory design is geared to participant selection from the QUAN phase for in-depth scrutiny in the qual phase, to help explain the QUAN results. Examples of the kinds of nested sampling strategies include the sampling of participants who are "typical," who are "outliers," or who differ in their scores on significant predictors in the QUAN analysis. If the intent of a qualitative component is to offer detail and elaboration about phenomena and relationships captured quantitatively, then a nested sample is likely to enrich the researcher's understanding.

Finally, a **multilevel** relationship involves selecting samples from different levels of a hierarchy. Usually this means sampling from different but related populations (e.g., hospital administrators, clinical staff, and patients).

Example of Multilevel Sampling
Cullinen and colleagues (2021) utilized multilevel multisite sampling to explore evidence-based interventions aimed at improving sexually transmitted infection screening and testing of those at risk for HIV across nine sites in the United States. Quantitative data included needs assessment data that were evaluated in light of semistructured interviews. The qualitative data were triangulated with quantitative findings to provide a more depth understanding of the issues related to screening/testing and to identify future interventions for improvement.

The overall mixed method sampling plan should generate thorough datasets about the phenomenon under study and should be consistent with the intent of the mixed methods design.

Data Collection in a Mixed Methods Study

All data collection methods discussed in Chapters 14 (structured methods) and 24 (unstructured methods) can be creatively combined in a mixed method study. Thus, possible sources of data for MM studies include group and individual interviews, psychosocial scales, observations, biomarkers, records, diaries, performance tests, Internet postings, photographs, and physical artifacts. Mixed methods studies can involve both *intramethod mixing* (for example, structured and unstructured self-reports), and *intermethod mixing* (for example, biomarkers and in-depth interviews). Moreover, mixed methods researchers can use secondary analysis of an existing dataset (Watkins, 2023).

> **Example of Mixed Methods With a Secondary Analysis**
> Powell and colleagues (2021) conducted an exploratory mixed methods study to understand if and to what extent nursing homes had the capability for data sharing. They conducted a secondary analysis of data from a national survey representing every state in the United States. The sample included 815 nursing home leaders. Then they sampled 12 administrators who had varying data sharing capabilities and conducted semi-structured interviews to gain a greater understanding of their experiences of the challenges and benefits of data sharing.

In selecting data sources for each strand of an MM study, a goal should be to use each method to address the research questions in a manner that enhances overall understanding of the problem. An important consideration concerns the methods' complementarity—that is, having the limitations of one method be offset by the strengths of the other.

Another consideration concerns the focus of the data being collected. For example, if the intent of the study is to compare or contrast results in the two strands, then common constructs/phenomena should be included in both datasets.

TIP Self-reports are the most common data source in both qualitative and quantitative nursing studies, and blending unstructured and structured self-report data is the most common approach in MM research as well (Beck & Harrison, 2016).

In concurrent designs, data collection decisions are made upfront. In sequential designs, however, MM researchers may have an emergent approach, with the types of data to be collected in the second phase shaped to some extent by findings in the first phase. Sequential designs thus have rich potential for incremental findings that build on one another.

In planning a data collection strategy, MM researchers may need to consider whether one method could introduce bias in the other method. For example, do closed-ended questions about a phenomenon affect how participants think about the phenomenon when asked in an unstructured fashion (or vice versa)? In other words, researchers should give some thought to whether one of the methods is an "intervention" that could influence people's behavior or responses.

One final issue concerns the possible need for additional data at the analysis and interpretation stage. If findings from the qualitative and quantitative strands conflict, it is sometimes useful to collect supplementary data to shed light on and possibly resolve contradictions or inconsistencies.

ANALYSIS OF MIXED METHODS DATA

Mixed methods data analysis involves analytic techniques applied to both the quantitative and qualitative datasets—and the integration of the two strands—to answer mixed methods questions. MM data analysis is one of the greatest challenges in doing mixed methods research. It is not uncommon, unfortunately, for the two strands of data to be analyzed and reported separately, without any integration of the findings. Beck and Harrison (2016), for example, found that nearly half of the 294 MM nursing studies they reviewed had no analytic or interpretive integration.

Integration is the central feature of a high-quality MM data analysis. The real benefits of MM research cannot be realized if there is no attempt to merge or connect results from the two strands, and to develop interpretations based on integrated understandings. As eloquently observed by Sandelowski (2003), a high-quality MM analysis merges measurement with meaning, graphs with graphical accounts, and tables with tableaux. Some MM researchers acknowledge that analytic integration "was the key to unfolding the complex relationships in the topic of the study" (Bazely, 2009b, p. 205).

Students often want specific guidance about how to analyze their data, but there are no rules for MM data analysis and integration. Decisions about how to blend the datasets hinge on several factors. Research design, especially sequencing of strands, strongly affects analytic choices. Sampling is another important factor. Several analytic techniques are appropriate only for identical and nested samples (i.e., for sampling plans with both qualitative and quantitative data obtained from the same people).

This section describes a few analytics considerations in MM studies, but our presentation is far from comprehensive. Additional resources should be consulted, such as the works of Bazely (2009a, 2009b, 2012) and Creswell and Plano Clark (2018).

Decisions in Analyzing Mixed Methods Data

Before pursuing a specific analytic strategy, MM researchers often make several preliminary decisions that will affect how they proceed. Our list is not exhaustive but is meant to encourage preanalytic thinking about several issues.

1. *What will be the unit of analysis?* The unit usually is individual participants, but other options include events (Happ et al., 2006) or subgroups of people. If the MM design is multilevel, the levels are usually the unit of primary interest.
2. *Will either type of data be converted or transformed?* Sometimes researchers convert their qualitative data into quantitative data, and vice versa.
3. *Will direct comparisons be made between the qualitative and quantitative data—and, if so, at what level will the comparisons be made?* In nested and identical sampling designs, comparisons can be made at the individual level—for example, comparing each participant's score on a health promotion scale with how they described lifestyle and activities in in-depth interviews. Comparisons can also be made between subgroups—for example, how high scorers on the health promotion scale differ from low scorers in terms of themes that emerge in the qualitative analysis. Finally, overall comparisons are possible—for example, is the picture of the salience of health promotion consistent in the qualitative and quantitative datasets? Comparisons are a major feature of convergent designs but are sometimes used in other MM designs.
4. *Will integration involve the use of specialized software*? Tremendous advances have been made regarding software for analytic integration in MM studies. Leading software include Dedoose, QDA Miner, and MAXQDA. Statistical packages such as SPSS now have text analyses software than can categorize text responses and combine them with other quantitative variables. Even if specialized software for combining qualitative and quantitative data is not used, MM researchers can use basic spreadsheets to good advantage.

Integration Intent in Mixed Methods Data Analysis

The intent of analytic integration in MM studies reflects the researcher's analytic goal. As discussed earlier, intent is a key issue in selecting an MM design, and the design affects the analytic procedures that are feasible and productive. In QUAL + QUAL convergent designs, the integration intent is to *merge* the results, and to develop integrated mixed methods results and interpretations that are comprehensive and confirmatory and that expand understanding.

In explanatory sequential designs, the intent is to *connect* the results in a sequential integration. The connected results are used to provide a strong explanation (from the qual strand) of specific results from the QUAN strand. The analytic goal is to shed light on particular quantitative findings with rich, insightful, and nuanced information—not to compare or contrast findings from the two strands. The integrated interpretation should reveal the added value of the qualitative component.

Sequential integration is also a feature in exploratory designs, in which the intent is to *build* (generate) a contextually appropriate quantitative feature (e.g., an intervention or measure) based on an in-depth exploration in the initial phase. Integrated interpretations are designed to reveal how the quantitative results support the integrity and contextual specificity of the newly developed feature.

In developing an analytic plan, it is also important to consider intent in terms of evidence-based practice goals: how can the data best be analyzed and integrated to yield high-quality evidence for practicing nurses?

TIP Uprichard and Dawney (2019) have observed that while data integration is a sensible *goal*, it is not always successfully achieved. They challenge "the presupposition that it is necessarily the optimal *outcome* of mixed methods research" (p. 19). They offered suggestions for how to use a strategy they call *diffraction* as an approach that supports instances where the data strands do not integrate or "cohere."

Data Analysis Procedures in Mixed Methods Research

This section describes some specific MM analytic procedures, many of which are especially common in convergent designs. In such designs, quantitative data are analyzed using statistical techniques and qualitative data are analyzed using qualitative analysis methods (often via content or framework analysis), both according to standards of excellence for each method. Findings from the two separate analyses are then drawn together to answer the mixed methods question.

In convergent designs, the focus of the MM analysis is on *comparing* and *contrasting* the two sets of findings. The two sets of results for a given construct are compared to explore ways in which they confirm, disconfirm, qualify, or expand each other. One approach to facilitate the comparison is to create matrices, and another strategy is to transform the data. Both methods are described later in this section.

Some researchers formally "audit" the extent to which there is congruence. For example, Tonkin-Crine and colleagues (2016) used a "triangulation protocol" to compare four sets of data in a multinational trial of the effectiveness of physician training in communication skills. The protocol was used to classify pairwise findings from two strands (QUAL and QUAN) and two perspectives (physicians and patients) into one of four categories: agreement, partial agreement, dissonance, or "silence" (i.e., an instance in which only one dataset of the two being compared contained data on a particular finding).

Example of Analytic Integration in a Convergent Design
Dickson, Jun, and Melkus (2021) used a convergent mixed methods design to describe the self-care practices in older adult workers with cardiovascular disease. Quantitative data on 108 participants included measures of self-care, clinical factors, and work and job characteristics. Forty participants contributed to qualitative findings around self-care and working. Data were integrated in the final analytic phase contributing to a greater understanding of the impact of work on self-care.

Analytic integration can also occur in sequential designs—although such integration is often what Bazely (2009a) called "integration 'on the way'" (p. 92) rather than formal integration at the end of the study. That is, the analysis of one data strand is interpreted and used to inform the design and analysis of the second strand. An overall integration of the two strands should also occur to address the MM question, but sometimes such integration does not occur.

Bazely (2009a) has described what she called *iterative analysis*, which involves ongoing interpretive feedback loops. Iterative analysis involves "taking what is learned in one stage of a project into a further stage to inform that data collection or analysis, and then on again for refinement or development through one or more subsequent iterations" (p. 109). She offered as an example a study in which a researcher developed a formal instrument based on themes from in-depth phenomenologic interviews. The factor analytic results from psychometric testing of the scale were then taken back to the phenomenologic data for further thematic exploration. Similarly, Mendlinger and Cwikel (2008) provided a useful illustration of how "spiraling" between qualitative and quantitative data contributed to an integration of their data strands—a strategy that has been used by nurse researchers trying to resolve problems with the Japanese translation of a widely used measure of depression (St. Arnaud et al., 2016).

Constructing Meta-Matrices

One approach to analytic integration in MM studies involves the use of matrices, a method that can be used to identify patterns and make comparisons across data sources if identical or nested sampling was used. Matrices are a method that has been advocated for qualitative data analysis (Miles et al., 2020) and are an explicit feature of framework analysis, which we described in Chapter 25 (Gale et al., 2013). The concept has gained popularity among MM researchers.

In a meta-matrix, researchers array information from qualitative and quantitative data sources. In a typical case-by-variable meta-matrix, the rows correspond to cases—to individual participants. Then, for each participant, data from multiple data sources are entered in the columns, so that the analyst can see at a glance such information as demographic information, scores on psychosocial measures, responses to probing open-ended questions (e.g., verbatim narratives), hospital record data (e.g., biomarker data), and observational field notes. A third dimension can be added if, for example, there are multiple sources of data relating to multiple constructs (e.g., depression, pain). A third dimension can also be used if the qualitative and quantitative data have been collected longitudinally.

Patterns of regularities, as well as anomalies, often come to light through detailed inspection of meta-matrices. Their key advantage is that they allow for fuller exploration of all data sources simultaneously. The construction of a meta-matrix also allows researchers to explore whether statistical conclusions are supported by the qualitative data for individual study participants, and vice versa.

A simplified example of a meta-matrix for a study of sleep problems is presented in Figure 27.2. This example shows only five cases and a handful of variables/constructs, but it illustrates how

Case	Pseudonym	Age	Sex	Average Hours of Sleep Daily	Current Fatigue Level Rating[a]	Use of Sleep Medication[b]	Fatigue Narrative
1	Anna	57	F	6.0	9	1	I *never* sleep through the night. I usually don't have much trouble falling asleep, but I just can't *stay* asleep. There is never a day when I don't wake up exhausted.
2	Jonathan	45	M	5.5	5	1	I've never really needed all that much sleep. Ever since I was in college, I get by with just a few hours and I feel just fine.
3	Claire	49	F	8.0	2	1	I'm a good sleeper, I can fall asleep anywhere, anytime. So, I get what I need.
4	Rosalind	51	F	7.0	7	2	I sleep just fine, but my husband is an insomniac, and a pain in my neck. When he's awake, he wants me awake, too!
5	Michael	54	M	7.5	6	3	I like my shut-eye. I can't concentrate if I don't get enough. I do what I have to, which usually means going to bed before anyone else and taking sleeping pills.

[a]Rating scale anchors: 0 = extremely energetic, 10 = totally exhausted
[b]Use of medication codes: 1 = Never, 2 = Occasionally, 3 = Regularly

FIGURE 27.2 Fictitious example of a meta-matrix with raw qualitative data.

diverse information can be displayed to facilitate inferences about patterns and relationships. It also suggests, however, that such meta-matrices may be unwieldy with large samples—although one strategy is to have separate matrices for distinct subgroups within a large sample (e.g., in our example, those with high vs. low levels of fatigue). Meta-matrix data such as those portrayed in Figure 27.2 can easily be entered in spreadsheet software and several analytic software packages. Software has important advantages over manual methods—in particular, the ability to sort and resort the data to identify patterns.

> **Example of a Study Using a Meta-Matrix**
>
> Valenta and colleagues (2021) conducted a convergent-parallel, mixed-method randomized control trial to explore the learning processes of a pain self-management intervention for cancer outpatients from three Swiss university hospitals. They collected quantitative data, including data related to pain management knowledge and self-efficacy and qualitative data on patient and family caregivers' learning experiences. They integrated the data using case-level comparisons and a meta-matrix.

Transforming Quantitative and Qualitative Data

A technique that can be used in analytic and interpretive integration in mixed methods research involves converting data of one type into data of another type. Qualitative data are sometimes converted into numeric codes that can be analyzed quantitatively (**quantitizing**). It is also possible to transform quantitative data into qualitative information (**qualitizing**). Such transformed data can be included in meta-matrices.

Although some qualitative researchers believe that quantitizing is inappropriate, Sandelowski (2001) argued that some amount of quantitizing occurs regularly. She noted that every time qualitative researchers use terms such as *a few, many,* or *most,* they are implicitly conveying quantitative information about the frequency of occurrence of a theme or pattern. Quantification of qualitative data can sometimes offer benefits. Sandelowski described how this strategy can be used to achieve two important goals:

- *Generating meaning from qualitative data.* If qualitative data are displayed in a quantitative fashion (e.g., by displaying frequencies of certain phenomena), *patterns* sometimes emerge with greater clarity than they might have had the researchers simply relied on their impressions.
- *Documenting and confirming conclusions.* The use of numbers can assure people that researchers' conclusions are valid. Researchers can be more confident that the data are fully accounted for if they document the extent to which emerging patterns were observed—or *not* observed. Sandelowski noted that quantitizing can address some pitfalls of qualitative analysis, which include giving too much weight to dramatic or vivid accounts, giving too little weight to disconfirming cases, and smoothing out variation to clean up some of the "messiness" of human experience.

In a more recent article, Sandelowski and her colleagues (2009) noted that quantitizing can also serve the critical function of encouraging researchers to think about and interact with their data. They noted that quantitizing, "when used creatively, critically, and reflexively, can show the complexity of qualitative data and, thereby the 'multivariate nature' of the experiential worlds researchers seek to understand" (p. 219). Such higher-level understanding of a phenomenon is an overarching goal of many MM studies.

Presenting Integrated Mixed Methods Results: Joint Displays

Integrated mixed methods results are often reported in a narrative fashion. In convergent designs, narrative presentations often take the form of direct comparisons of the QUAN and QUAL findings, or QUAL data are used to illustrate the statistical findings using direct quotes. Narrative presentations are often supplemented with tables or figures that highlight features of the integrated results. A **joint display** has been defined as a way "to integrate the data by bringing the data together through a visual means to draw out new insights beyond the information gained from the separate quantitative and qualitative results" (Fetters et al., 2013, p. 2143).

Guetterman and colleagues (2015) have written about the importance of joint displays in helping readers understand how mixed methods contribute new insights and enriched understanding. Their paper provides example of joint displays for all three Creswell and Plano Clark's (2018) core designs from the health literature.

Although there are no "rules" or standard formats for joint MM displays, certain types are especially common. One is a two-dimensional *statistics-by-theme* display, a kind of cross-tabulation table that can be used when some (or all) participants are in both strands of a convergent or explanatory MM study. For example, for our fictitious sleep problem study (Figure 27.2), we could create a joint display that summarizes key themes from the QUAL data for subgroups defined by responses to a structured question on the use of sleep medication, as shown in Figure 27.3. Another statistics-by-theme possibility, again for our fictitious sleep study, would be to divide the sample into subgroups based on a QUAN measure (e.g., high scorers vs. low scorers on the fatigue measure), and then include actual quotes from the QUAL strand in the display.

Another type of joint display is what Guetterman and colleagues (2015) refer to as a *side-by-side joint display*. Such displays typically put statistical results in one column and relevant qualitative results or data in another column. Side-by-side displays can be presented in tables or in figures.

Happ and colleagues' (2006) article is another useful resource for thinking about joint MM displays. Their paper included examples of using bar charts to show frequencies of quantitized qualitative data. Another type of joint display is a *modified stem leaf plot*. In their example from a study of health locus of control in lung transplant recipients, behaviors that were considered "internality behaviors" from unstructured data sources were listed on one side, and the identification numbers of the lung transplant recipients who exhibited those behaviors were listed on the right. The result was a re-presentation of the qualitative data in a quantitative manner that "provided a visual sense of the proportion of recipients who exhibited the internality behaviors" (p. S46). The display prompted further analyses about commonalities and differences among recipients' behaviors.

Another clever use of visualization in the Happ et al. (2006) paper involved the construction of a scatterplot. The values along the vertical axis were internality scores, those along the horizontal axis were externality scores. The scatterplot space was divided into quadrants (e.g., high internality, high

Use of Sleep Medication	Themes from In-Depth Interviews		
	The Role of Others	**Health Issues**	**Patterns of Sleep**
Never (n = 18, 45%)	• No one in household with sleeping problems • No pets in household	• No special health problems • Avoids *all* medication	• Never a problem falling asleep • Lifelong history of being good sleeper • Despite problems, averse to sleeping aids
Occasionally (n = 16, 40%)	• Spouse sleeping problems • Teens coming home late • Pet disturbances	• Stressful job • On a diet causing jitters • Anxiety about upcoming medical procedures/tests	• Problem staying asleep, not falling asleep • Sleeping only a problem if under stress • Frequent napping
Regularly (n = 6, 15%)	• Spouse works late or irregular shift • Infant in household • Severely ill family member	• Recent hospitalization • Diagnosed with life-threatening illness • Severely depressed	• Problems arise if medications not taken • Daily battles with insomnia

FIGURE 27.3 Fictitious example of a summary meta-matrix.

externality) that corresponded to four profiles of health locus of control beliefs. The identification numbers of participants were then plotted in the two-dimensional space. This visual display allowed the researchers to more clearly identify clusterings and "outliers" that were difficult to identify from quantitative analysis alone.

Although most joint displays are for studies in which the QUAN and QUAL samples are identical or nested, joint displays from studies using parallel samples can sometimes be created. For example, Guetterman and colleagues (2015) showed a joint display for an instrument development MM study (exploratory), in which information from the QUAL strand was shown in one column and corresponding items from the QUAN strand in another.

Innovative ideas for joint displays appear regularly in mixed methods papers. For example, Johnson and colleagues (2019) described a technique they called the "Pillar Integration Process," which is an approach for building a "pillar" to integrate QUAN data and QUAL codes. Clearly, data analysis in mixed methods research is ripe with opportunities for creative blending and juxtaposition of data visually. Further advice regarding joint displays of information from mixed methods analyses is provided by Dickson and Page (2021), Younas and Durante (2023), and Creswell and Plano Clark (2018).

> **Example of an MM Study With Joint Displays**
> Othman and colleagues (2021) used a sequential explanatory mixed methods approach to develop and evaluate the impact of a healthy eating education workshop/webinar for midwives in South Australia. They tested 44 midwives' level of knowledge and confidence in teaching healthy eating information during pregnancy prior to the education program, immediately following, and at 6 to 8 weeks post the program. Quantitative data included demographic characteristics and a questionnaire that assessed midwives' level of knowledge and confidence related to healthy eating education. At 6 to 8 weeks post the intervention, they used a qualitative descriptive design to interview a subset (nested) sample of seven participants to gain in-depth knowledge of the midwives' views and experiences of the education intervention. After analyzing the quantitative and qualitative data separately, the team integrated the data to provide a comprehensive understanding of the findings. They used joint displays for each of the main study findings: knowledge and confidence.

Meta-Inferences in Mixed Methods Research

It has been argued that the most important step in mixed methods studies is when the integrated findings from the qualitative and quantitative components are incorporated into an overall conceptualization that effectively answers the overarching mixed methods question. To achieve this, *active* interpretation and exploration of the results are required.

In convergent designs, interpretations focus on making sense of the degree to which the findings converge. Most researchers consider that an ideal situation occurs when findings from each strand are consistent and shed complementary perspectives on the phenomenon of interest. Yet, many MM scholars have noted the critical role that divergent results can play in advancing knowledge because they may yield opportunities for further generative work.

Moffatt and colleagues (2006) suggested possible steps to take when MM findings conflict. Their study involved quantitative data from 126 participants in a clinical trial and in-depth data from a purposive nested sample of 25 of them. The quantitative results suggested that the intervention (which was designed to improve health and social outcomes for older people) was not successful, yet the qualitative data suggested wide-ranging improvements. The researchers suggested six ways of further exploring the discrepancy: (1) treating the methods as fundamentally different; (2) examining rigor in the respective strands; (3) exploring dataset comparability; (4) collecting additional data; (5) exploring intervention processes; and (6) exploring whether the outcomes of the two components were really matched. Creswell and Plano Clark (2018) suggest that perhaps the easiest way to address discordant results is to return to the databases to look for clues and ways to resolve the discrepancy.

Although many MM scholars discuss convergence-divergence of results as a dichotomy, in fact, it is often the case that interpretive integration leads to a nuanced portrayal of the phenomenon because results are neither precisely convergent nor divergent. Thus, although the MM research question being addressed may be, "To what extent do the quantitative and qualitative data converge?", another important question might be, "How do the findings from one strand qualify, delimit, or temper findings from the other?"

An example comes from an MM study of one of this book's authors, whose convergent design involved a survey of nearly 4,000 women who had low incomes and in-depth interviews with 67 women from a parallel sample (Polit et al., 2000). The analyses focused on hunger and food insecurity, and in both samples, about half the women had food insecurity—results that appeared convergent. Yet, the in-depth interviews revealed that the term "food secure" in low-income urban families may be misleading: Mothers in the qualitative sample had to *struggle* enormously to be food secure, piecing together with great effort numerous strategies to provide an adequate amount of food for themselves and their children. This led the authors to hypothesize that *food security* is experienced differently in low-income vs. middle-class families—and is perhaps a totally different phenomenon.

In explanatory designs, interpretations are typically geared to understanding how the qualitative results provide a deeper understanding of the statistical results. In some cases, the interpretation could suggest possible new quantitative analyses based on the qualitative-informed explanations. Interpretations in exploratory sequential designs hinge on an analysis of how the new quantitative feature (e.g., a new instrument) was enriched through the insights provided in the initial qualitative strand.

In arriving at meta-inferences in an MM study, researchers must actively engage in meaning making. Interpretation can be enhanced by allowing the two strands of a study to "talk to each other" in a meaningful, reflexive, and thought-provoking way. Tashakkori et al. (2020) offered several guidelines for making appropriate inferences at the interpretive stage of an MM study. Their "golden rule" is especially noteworthy: "*Know thy participants*" (p. 289). Mixed methods research offers great potential for getting a rounded picture of the complex lives of human beings.

QUALITY CRITERIA IN MIXED METHODS RESEARCH

The issue of quality criteria for mixed methods research has received considerable recent attention, in part because several controversies have emerged. One issue is similar to the one discussed in Chapter 26—what to *call* the quality goal. Terms like *quality, rigor,* and *validity* have been recommended by some, but rejected by others. Some experts have proposed terms that are deliberately different from those used in QUAN or QUAL studies. One prominent team of scholars, for example, have proposed *inference quality* as the MM substitute for validity (Tashakkori et al., 2020), while another team suggested the term *legitimation* (Onwuegbuzie & Johnson, 2006). Creswell and Plano Clark (2018) and other experts are urging greater consistency in quality terminology, but it is too early in the development of MM methodology to know what terms will be adopted.

> **TIP** In Teddlie and Tashakkori's (2009) classic framework, *inference quality* incorporates notions of both internal validity and statistical conclusion validity within a quantitative framework, and credibility within a qualitative framework. Inference quality essentially refers to the believability and accuracy of the inductively and deductively derived conclusions from an MM study. They also proposed *inference transferability* as a criterion that encompasses external validity (QUAN) and transferability (QUAL). Inference transferability is the degree to which the mixed methods conclusions can be applied to other similar people, contexts, settings, and time periods.

In terms of criteria to guide efforts to attain high quality, dozens of quality criteria frameworks for MM studies have been proposed. Fàbregues and Molina-Azorin (2017) undertook a systematic review of the MM literature and offered a metasummary of the most prevalent quality criteria that have been proposed. Some criteria concern excellence in reporting MM research and are helpful to those wishing to critically appraise a mixed methods study. Several criteria for *doing* high-quality mixed methods research, as proposed in many frameworks in Fàbregues and Molina-Azorin's (2017) review, are as follows:

1. A strong rationale exists for collecting and analyzing both QUAN and QUAL data.
2. The QUAN and QUAL strands are well implemented and adhere to the quality criteria of each tradition.
3. The QUAN and QUAL components of the study are well integrated.
4. The sampling, data collection, and data analysis procedures for both strands are linked to the study intent and the research questions.
5. Inferences are consistent with the study findings and with the study intent.

In a subsequent study, Fàbregues and colleagues (2018) compared how researchers in different disciplines conceptualized and operationalized quality in MM research. An international sample of 44 MM researchers, including 11 in nursing, were interviewed about their perspectives on quality. All five quality criteria noted earlier were highly rated by these experts, and the most frequently mentioned quality criteria were equally prevalent in the four disciplinary groups. However, nurses were especially likely to believe that the MM research community should reach a consensus on a set of quality criteria for conducting and appraising MM studies.

CRITICAL APPRAISAL OF MIXED METHODS RESEARCH

Individual components of mixed methods studies can be critically appraised using guidelines we have offered throughout this book. Key appraisal questions for quantitative studies (Box 5.2) and qualitative studies (Box 5.3) were presented in Chapter 5.

Box 27.1 offers supplementary questions that are specific to the mixed methods aspects of a study. Many of these questions were derived from the systematic review of Fàbregues and Molina-Azorin (2017) and therefore reflect a synthesis of widely promoted criteria for critical appraisals of mixed methods study. Formal tools for appraising mixed methods studies, such as the Mixed Methods Appraisal Tool have also been developed (Hong et al., 2018).

The overarching consideration in MM studies is whether true integration of the strands occurred and contributed to strong meta-inferences about the phenomenon under scrutiny. Integration is the cornerstone for the added value of MM research—it is a foundational principle. Researchers who report their QUAL and QUAN findings in separate papers should, ideally, write a third integrative paper. The separate single-method (QUAL or QUAN) papers should communicate, in the Discussion section, the kinds of integrative work that has been or will be undertaken.

TIP In critically appraising single-method qualitative or quantitative studies, it is worth considering whether a mixed methods approach would have enhanced the insights and value of the research.

RESEARCH EXAMPLE OF A MIXED METHODS STUDY

Study: Vicarious posttraumatic growth in NICU nurses (Beck & Casavant, 2020).

Statement of purpose: The purposes of this study were to assess (1) the level of vicarious posttraumatic growth in NICU nurses, (2) the degree that NICU nurses examine their core beliefs, (3) the description of their experiences of this type of growth, and (4) the integration of the qualitative and quantitative results to provide a more complete picture.

Methods: A convergent design (QUAL and QUANT) was used. The two strands were of equal priority and were collected in a single phase. Pragmatism was the paradigm guiding this research. Researchers recruited a sample of neonatal nurses from the National Association of Neonatal Nurses through their message board. A total of 109 nurses participated in the quantitative strand where they completed the Posttraumatic Growth Inventory and the Core Beliefs Inventory. Sixty-one nurses (55%) completed the qualitative strand where they described their experiences of any positive changes in their beliefs or life as a result of caring for critically ill infants.

BOX 27.1 Guidelines for Critically Appraising Mixed Methods Studies

1. Did the researcher provide an explicit and persuasive rationale for conducting a mixed methods (MM) study?
2. Did the researcher state an overarching MM intent and an explicit MM question?
3. Did the researcher identify the research design? Was the design clearly described in terms of purpose, sequencing, and priority? Is the design appropriate for the research questions and study intent? Was the design concurrent or sequential? Which strand (if either) was given priority? Was mixed methods design notation (or a visual diagram) used to communicate key aspects of the design?
4. What sampling strategy was used (identical, parallel, nested, multilevel), and was this strategy appropriate for the study intent? Was the sampling strategy described in sufficient detail?
5. How were study data gathered? Were the methods appropriate for the study intent? In sequential designs, did the second-phase data collection (and sampling) flow from the analysis of data gathered in the initial phase?
6. Were the qualitative and quantitative components carefully implemented? Were procedures used to enhance rigor/trustworthiness of the components?
7. Were data analysis procedures sufficiently described? What specific analytic techniques were used to promote analytic integration (e.g., was data transformation or a meta-matrix used)? Do the findings answer the mixed methods question? Were joint displays effectively used to communicate mixed methods findings?
8. Was the process of integrating the strands described? How did integration occur? Were the components integrated in an effective manner?
9. Do the integrated findings yield richly textured information and added-value insights? If there were inconsistencies between the strands, were they sufficiently described? If the findings from each strand are conflicting or qualifying, are well-conceived explanations for the discrepancies offered?
10. Are the researcher's meta-inferences consistent with the individual findings? Are the inferences consistent with the study intent? Do the meta-inferences adequately encompass and integrate inferences from each strand?

Data analysis and integration: Descriptive statistics were used to analyze the prevalence and degree of posttraumatic growth and examination of core beliefs of neonatal nurses. Correlation procedures were used to assess the relationship between the Posttraumatic Growth Inventory and the Core Beliefs Inventory scores and correlations of the demographic variables with both instruments' scores. Multiple regression analyses were also done. The qualitative data were analyzed using Krippendorff's content analysis using the five dimensions of posttraumatic growth to categorize NICU nurses' descriptions of their posttraumatic growth. The data from both the quantitative and qualitative strands were integrated by creating joint displays (Figure 27.4).

Key findings: NICU nurses reported a moderate degree of vicarious posttraumatic growth and close to a moderate degree of disruption of their core beliefs. The total Posttraumatic Growth Inventory scores and the Core Belief Inventory scores were significantly ($r = 0.77$, $p < .001$) correlated; this indicated that the greater the challenge to a nurse's core beliefs, the higher the level of posttraumatic growth. In the content analysis of the neonatal nurses' experiences of posttraumatic growth, Appreciation of Life was the Posttraumatic Growth Inventory dimension that reflected the highest growth in the nurses, while Spiritual Change reflected the lowest growth. The integration of the qualitative and quantitative findings provided a richer and more complete picture of both the degree of vicarious posttraumatic growth and core belief disruption in NICU nurses and their complex experiences.

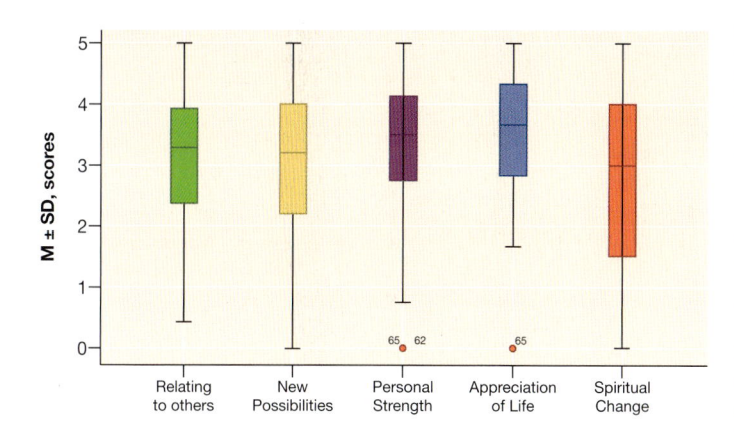

Relating to Others
"I believe the greatest change in my beliefs as a result of caring for babies in the NICU has been my passion and awareness of the struggles of others and appreciating that most people carry around silent trauma and pain."

New Possibilities
"Because of my experiences caring for critically ill infants and supporting the families through the unknown, I pursued what had been on my heart and making a difference for our families. I am in the process of preparing for certification in perinatal mental health."

Personal Strength
"I find that I can use the experience of taking care of critically ill infants as a strength for coping in other areas of my life. I tell myself, 'if I can hold a 23-weeker in the palm of my hand, I can do this'."

Appreciation of Life
As this nurse reflected, "staring at a mother while in kangaroo-care with her 2 lb baby really helps me reflect on the little things that make up the big picture. It helps to remind me to take a deep breath and cherish the little things with my own family even when the days are long and hard. I might be having a hard day but I always know someone else is having a harder one."

Spiritual Change
"There are so many experiences in the NICU that led me to where I am now. The fact that they have deepened my faith as a born again Christian is probably the most important to me. My NICU experience only makes sense to me with the faith context knowing that I have a GREAT GOD who uses everything for good!"

FIGURE 27.4 Joint display from Beck and Casavant's (2020) study of posttraumatic growth in NICU nurses. The vertical axis shows values of scale item responses, from 0 (not at all) to 5 (to a very great degree). Each boxplot represents the middle 50% of cases, between the 25th and 75th percentiles. To the right of the boxplots are illustrative quotes from the NICU nurses' qualitative data. (Printed with permission from Beck, C. T., & Casavant, S. (2020). Vicarious posttraumatic growth in NICU nurses. *Advances in Neonatal Care, 20*(4), 324–332.)

SUMMARY POINTS

- **Mixed methods** (MM) research involves the collection, analysis, and integration of both qualitative and quantitative data within a study or coordinated set of studies, often with an overarching goal of achieving enhanced insights.
- Mixed methods research has numerous advantages, including the complementarity of qualitative and quantitative data and the practicality of using methods that best address a question. MM research has many applications, including the development and testing of instruments, interventions, and programs.
- The paradigm often associated with MM research is **pragmatism**, which is considered to offer an umbrella worldview and has as a major tenet "the dictatorship of the research question."
- Mixed methods studies involve asking at least two questions that require different types of data, but high-quality MM research also asks integrative questions that focus on linking the two strands.
- **Integration** is a central feature of MM research—a centerpiece that distinguishes it from other methodologies. Integration ideally occurs throughout a project.
- Key decisions in designing an MM study involve how to sequence the components, which **strand** (if either) will be given priority, and how to integrate the two strands. Researchers also decide whether to use a "fixed" MM design or an emergent one that is devised as the study unfolds.
- In terms of **sequencing**, MM designs are either **concurrent designs** (both strands occurring in one simultaneous phase) or **sequential designs** (one strand occurring prior to and informing the second strand).
- Notation for MM research often designates both **priority**—all capital letters for the *dominant strand* and all lower-case letters for the *nondominant strand*—and sequence. An arrow is used for

sequential designs, and a "+" is used for concurrent designs. QUAL → quan, for example, is a sequential, qualitative-dominant design.
- *Core designs* for MM research in the Creswell and Plano Clark taxonomy include the **convergent design** (QUAL + QUAN); **explanatory sequential design** (QUAN → qual or quan → QUAL); and **exploratory sequential design** (e.g., QUAL → quan + qual → QUAN). More complex MM designs are sometimes adopted, involving intersecting core designs with other components or approaches.
- Sampling strategies can be described as **identical** (the same participants are in both strands); **nested** (some participants from one strand are in the other strand); **parallel** (participants are either in one strand or the other, drawn from the same population); or **multilevel** (participants are not the same and are drawn from different populations at different levels in a hierarchy).
- Data collection in MM research can involve all methods of structured and unstructured data. In sequential designs, decisions about data collection for the second phase often are based on findings from the first phase.
- Data analysis in MM research should involve integration of the strands, to arrive at META-**inferences** about the phenomenon under study. The integrative focus in many concurrent designs is to assess congruence and to explore complementarity.
- Methods of integration of qualitative and quantitative data during analysis include **data transformations**, such as qualitizing quantitative data or quantitizing qualitative data, and the use of a **meta-matrix** in which both qualitative and quantitative data are arrayed in a spreadsheet-type matrix.
- **Joint displays** are visual displays, either in tables or figures, that present integrated findings from both the qualitative and quantitative strands.
- Goals and criteria for the integrity of MM studies are still evolving. One framework proposes the goals of *inference quality* (the believability and accuracy of inductively and deductively derived conclusions) and *inference transferability* (the degree to which conclusions can be applied to other similar people or contexts).
- A key criterion for the conduct of an MM study is the rigorous implementation of both strands, each according to the quality criteria of each. Another criterion is thoughtful and thorough integration of the two strands.

REFERENCES CITED IN CHAPTER 27

Bazely, P. (2009a). Analysing mixed methods data. In Andrew, S., & Halcomb, E. (Eds.), *Mixed methods research for nursing and the health sciences* (pp. 84–117). Blackwell-Wiley.

Bazely, P. (2009b). Integrating data analyses in mixed methods research. *Journal of Mixed Methods Research, 3*, 203–207.

Bazely, P. (2012). Integrative strategies for mixed data sources. *American Behavioral Scientist, 56*, 814–828.

Beck, C. T., & Casavant, S. (2020). Vicarious posttraumatic growth in NICU nurses. *Advances in Neonatal Care, 20*(4), 324–332. https://doi.org/10.1097/anc.0000000000000689

Beck, C. T., & Harrison, L. (2016). Mixed methods research in the discipline of nursing. *Advances in Nursing Science, 39*(3), 224–234.

Bocquier, A., Branchereau, M., Gauchet, A., Bonnay, S., Simon, M., Ecollan, M., Chevreul, K., Mueller, J. E., Gagneux-Brunon, A., Thilly, N., & PrevHPV Study Group. (2023). Promoting HPV vaccination at school: A mixed methods study exploring knowledge, beliefs and attitudes of French school staff. *BMC Public Health, 23*(1), 486. https://doi.org/10.1186/s12889-023-15342-2

Bults, M., van Leersum, C. M., Olthuis, T. J. J., Bekhuis, R. E. M., & den Ouden, M. E. M. (2022). Barriers and drivers regarding the use of mobile health apps among patients with Type 2 diabetes mellitus in the Netherlands: Explanatory sequential design study. *JMIR Diabetes, 7*(1), e31451. https://doi.org/10.2196/31451

Creamer, E. (2018). *An introduction to fully integrated mixed methods research*. Sage Publications.

Creswell, J., Klassen, A., Plano Clark, V., & Smith, K. (2011). *Best practices for mixed methods research in the health sciences*. NIH.

Creswell, J. W., & Plano Clark, V. L. (2018). *Designing and conducting mixed methods research* (3rd ed.). Sage Publications.

Cullinen, K., Hill, M., Anderson, T., Jones, V., Nelson, J., Halawani, M., & Zha, P. (2021). Improving sexually transmitted infection screening, testing, and treatment among people with HIV: A mixed method needs assessment to inform a multi-site, multi-level intervention and evaluation plan. *PloS One, 16*(12), e0261824. https://doi.org/10.1371/journal.pone.0261824

Dickson, V. V., Jun, J., & Melkus, G. D. (2021). A mixed methods study describing the self-care practices in an older working population with cardiovascular disease (CVD): Balancing work, life and health. *Heart & Lung: The Journal of Critical Care, 50*(3), 447–454. https://doi.org/10.1016/j.hrtlng.2021.02.001

Dickson, V. V., & Page, S. D. (2021). Using mixed methods in cardiovascular nursing research: Answering the why, the how, and the what's next. *European Journal of Cardiovascular Nursing, 20*(1), 82–89. https://doi.org/10.1093/eurjcn/zvaa024

Durante, A., Ahtisham, Y., Cuoco, A., Boyne, J., Brawner, B., Juarez-Vela, R., & Vellone, E. (2022). Informal caregivers of people with heart failure and resilience: A convergent mixed methods study. *Journal of Advanced Nursing, 78*(1), 264–275. https://doi.org/10.1111/jan.15078

Fàbregues, S., & Molina-Azorin, J. (2017). Addressing quality in mixed methods research: A review and recommendations for a future agenda. *Quality & Quantity, 51*, 2847–2863.

Fàbregues, S., Pare, M., & Meneses, J. (2018). Operationalizing and conceptualizing quality in mixed methods research: A multiple case study of the disciplines of education, nursing, psychology, and sociology. *Journal of Mixed Methods Research, 13*(4), 424–445. doi:10.1177/1558689817751774

Fetters, M., Curry, L., & Creswell, J. (2013). Achieving integration in mixed methods designs: Principles and practices. *Health Services Research, 48*(6 pt 2), 2134–2156.

Fetters, M., & Freshwater, D. (2015). The 1 + 1 = 3 integration challenge. *Journal of Mixed Methods Research, 9*, 115–117.

Fetters, M., & Molina-Azorin, J. (2017a). Principles for bringing new and divesting of old language of the field. *Journal of Mixed Methods Research, 11*, 3–10.

Fetters, M., & Molina-Azorin, J. (2017b). The mixed methods research integration trilogy and its dimensions. *Journal of Mixed Methods Research, 11*, 291–307.

Fetters, M., & Molina-Azorin, J. (2017c). Perspectives of past editors on the current state of the field and future directions. *Journal of Mixed Methods Research, 11*, 423–432.

Forde, M. F., Coffey, A., & Hegarty, J. (2020). Bedside handover at the change of nursing shift: A mixed-methods study. *Journal of Clinical Nursing, 29*(19–20), 3731–3742. https://doi.org/10.1111/jocn.15403

Frels, R., Newman, I., & Newman, C. (2015). Mentoring the next generation in mixed methods research. In Hesse-Biber, S., & Johnson, R. (Eds.), *The Oxford handbook of multimethod and mixed methods research inquiry* (pp. 333–353). Oxford University Press.

Gale, N., Heath, G., Cameron, E., Rashid, S., & Redwood, S. (2013). Using the Framework Method for the analysis of qualitative data in multi-disciplinary health research. *BMC Medical Research Methodology, 13*, 117.

Gore, J., Toliver, J., Moore, M. A., Aycock, D., & Epps, F. (2022). A mixed-methods formative evaluation of a dementia-friendly congregation program for Black churches. *International Journal of Environmental Research and Public Health, 19*(8), 4498. https://doi.org/10.3390/ijerph19084498

Guetterman, T., Babchuk, W., Smith, M., & Stevens, J. (2019). Contemporary approaches to mixed methods-grounded theory research. *Journal of Mixed Methods Research, 93*, S154–S163.

Guetterman, T., Fetters, M., & Creswell, J. (2015). Integrating quantitative and qualitative results in health science mixed methods research through joint displays. *Annals of Family Medicine, 13*(6), 554–561.

Happ, M., Dabbs, A., Tate, J., Hricik, A., & Erlen, J. (2006). Exemplars of mixed methods data combination and analysis. *Nursing Research, 55*(2 suppl), S43–S49.

Hesse-Biber, S. (2016). Doing interdisciplinary mixed methods health care research: Working the boundaries, tensions, and synergistic potential of team-based research. *Qualitative Health Research, 26*(5), 649–658.

Hong, Q., Gonzalez-Reyes, A., & Pluye, P. (2018). Improving the usefulness of a tool for appraising the quality of qualitative, quantitative and mixed methods studies, the Mixed Methods Appraisal Tool (MMAT). *Journal of Evaluation in Clinical Practice, 24*(3), 459–467.

Johnson, R., Grove, A., & Clarke, A. (2019). Pillar integration process: A joint display technique to integrate data in mixed methods research. *Journal of Mixed Methods Research, 13*, 301–320.

Lippe, M. P., & Davis, A. (2023). Development of a primary palliative nursing care competence model and assessment tool: A mixed-methods study. *Nursing Education Perspectives, 44*(2), 76–81. https://doi.org/10.1097/01.NEP.0000000000001056

Logsdon, M. C., Lauf, A., Stikes, R., Revels, A., & Vickers-Smith, R. (2020). Partnering with new mothers to develop a smart phone app to prevent maternal mortality after hospital discharge: A pilot study. *Journal of Advanced Nursing, 76*(1), 324–327. https://doi.org/10.1111/jan.14219

Luo, S., & Creswell, J. (2016). Designing and developing an app for a mixed methods research design approach. *International Journal of Designs for Learning, 7*, 62–71.

Macedo, J. C. L., Soares, D. A., de Carvalho, V. C. H. D. S., Cortes, T. B. A., Mistro, S., Kochergin, C. N., Rumel, D., & Oliveira, M. G. (2022). Self-care in patients with non-optimal diabetes management in Brazilian rural areas: A mixed-methods study. *Patient preference and adherence, 16*, 1831–1842. https://doi.org/10.2147/PPA.S373302

Mayoh, J., & Onwuegbuzie, A. (2015). Toward a conceptualization of mixed methods phenomenological research. *Journal of Mixed Methods Research, 9*, 91–107.

Mendlinger, S., & Cwikel, J. (2008). Spiraling between qualitative and quantitative data on women's health behaviors: A double helix model for mixed methods. *Quantitative Health Research, 18*(2), 280–293.

Miles, M., Huberman, M., & Saldaña, J. (2020). *Qualitative data analysis: A methods source book* (4th ed.). Sage Publications.

Moffatt, S., White, M., Mackintosh, J. & Howel, D. (2006). Using quantitative and qualitative data in health services research—what happens when mixed method findings conflict? *BMC Health Services Research, 6*, 28.

Morse, J. M. (1991). Approaches to qualitative-quantitative methodological triangulation. *Nursing Research, 40*(2), 120–123.

Morse, J. M. (2012). Simultaneous and sequential qualitative mixed method designs. In Munhall, P. L. (Ed.), *Nursing research: A qualitative perspective* (pp. 553–569). Jones & Bartlett Learning.

Morse, J. M. (2017). *Essentials of qualitatively-driven mixed-method designs*. Routledge.

Ocak, G., Günhan, R., Uzun, A. M. & Karakuyu, A. (2023). Development and validation of a screen fatigue scale.

Participatory Educational Research, *10*(3), 226–246. https://doi.org/10.17275/per.23.53.10.3

O'Cathain, A. (2009). Mixed methods research in the health sciences: A quiet revolution. *Journal of Mixed Methods Research*, *3*, 3–6.

Odberg, K. R., Hansen, B. S., & Wangensteen, S. (2019). Medication administration in nursing homes: A qualitative study of the nurse role. *Nursing Open*, *6*(2), 384–392. https://doi.org/10.1002/nop2.216

Onwuegbuzie, A., & Collins, K. (2007). A typology of mixed methods sampling designs in social science research. *The Qualitative Report*, *12*, 281–316.

Onwuegbuzie, A., & Johnson, R. (2006) The validity issue in mixed methods research. *Research in the Schools*, *13*, 48–63.

Othman, S., Steen, M., & Fleet, J. A. (2021). A sequential explanatory mixed methods study design: An example of how to integrate data in a midwifery research project. *Journal of Nursing Education and Practice*, *11*(2), 75. https://doi.org/10.5430/jnep.v11n2p75

Patton, M. Q. (2015). *Qualitative research & evaluation methods* (4th ed.). Sage Publications.

Piil, K., Christensen, I. J., Grunnet, K., & Poulsen, H. S. (2022). Health-related quality of life and caregiver perspectives in glioblastoma survivors: A mixed-methods study. *BMJ Supportive & Palliative Care*, *12*(e6), e846–e854. https://doi.org/10.1136/bmjspcare-2019-001777

Plano Clark, V. L., Anderson, N., Wertz, J., Zhou, Y., Schumacher, K., & Miaskowski, C. (2015). Conceptualizing longitudinal mixed methods designs: A methodological review of health sciences research. *Journal of Mixed Methods Research*, *9*, 297–319.

Plano Clark, V., & Ivankova, N. (2016). *Mixed methods research: A guide to the field*. Sage Publications.

Polit, D. F., London, A., & Martinez, J. (2000). *Food security and hunger in poor, mother-headed families in four U.S. cities*. MDRC.

Powell, K. R., Deroche, C. B., & Alexander, G. L. (2021). Health data sharing in US nursing homes: A mixed methods study. *Journal of the American Medical Directors Association*, *22*(5), 1052–1059. https://doi.org/10.1016/j.jamda.2020.02.009

Prompahakul, C., Keim-Malpass, J., LeBaron, V., Yan, G., & Epstein, E. G. (2021). Moral distress among nurses: A mixed-methods study. *Nursing Ethics*, *28*(7–8), 1165–1182. https://doi.org/10.1177/0969733021996028

Saint Arnault, D., Hatashita, H., & Suzuki, H. (2016). Semantic examination of a Japanese Center for epidemiologic studies depression: A cautionary analysis using mixed methods. *Canadian Journal of Nursing Research*, *48*(3–4), 80–92.

Sandelowski, M. (2001). Real qualitative researchers do not count: The use of numbers in qualitative research. *Research in Nursing & Health*, *24*(3), 230–240.

Sandelowski, M. (2003). Tables or tableaux? The challenges of writing and reading mixed methods studies. In Tashakkori, A., & Teddlie, C. (Eds.), *Handbook of mixed methods in social and behavioral research* (pp. 321–350). Sage Publications.

Sandelowski, M., Voils, C., & Knafl, G. (2009). On quantitizing. *Journal of Mixed Methods Research*, *3*, 208–222.

Tashakkori, A., & Creswell, J. (2007). The new era of mixed methods. *Journal of Mixed Methods Research*, *1*, 3–7.

Tashakkori, A., Johnson, R. B., & Teddlie, C. (2020). *Foundations of mixed methods research: Integrating quantitative and qualitative approaches in the social and behavioral sciences* (2nd ed.). Sage Publications.

Teddlie, C., & Tashakkori, A. (2009). *Foundations of mixed methods research*. Sage Publications.

Tonkin-Crine, S., Anthierens, S., Hood, K., Yardley, L., Cals, J., Francis, N., Coenen, S., van der Velden, A. W., Godycki-Cwirko, M., Llor, C., Butler, C. C., Verheij, T. J. M., Goossens, H., Little, P., Little, P.; GRACE INTRO/CHAMP consortium. (2016). Discrepancies between qualitative and quantitative evaluation of randomised controlled trial results: Achieving clarity through mixed methods triangulation. *Implementation Science*, *11*, 66.

Uprichard, E., & Dawney, L. (2019). Data diffraction: Challenging data integration in mixed methods research. *Journal of Mixed Methods Research*, *13*(1), 19–32.

Valenta, S., Miaskowski, C., Spirig, R., Zaugg, K., Rettke, H., & Spichiger, E. (2021). Exploring learning processes associated with a cancer pain self-management intervention in patients and family caregivers: A mixed methods study. *Applied Nursing Research*, *62*, 151480. https://doi.org/10.1016/j.apnr.2021.151480

Watkins, D. C. (2023). *Secondary data in mixed methods research*. Sage.

Younas, A., & Durante, A. (2023). Decision tree for identifying pertinent integration procedures and joint displays in mixed methods research. *Journal of Advanced Nursing*, *79*(7), 2754–2769. https://doi.org/10.1111/jan.15536

28 Developing Complex Nursing Interventions Using Mixed Methods Research

Learning Objectives

1. Understand the process for developing, implementing, and testing nursing interventions.
2. Describe the factors that contribute to complex interventions.
3. Recognize several frameworks for developing and testing complex interventions.
4. Appreciate the importance of the development stage, including literature reviews, developing a diverse team, and gaining an in-depth understanding of the problem and the target population.
5. Articulate the importance of intervention theory in the development, timing, dose, intensity, modification, and individualization of the intervention to achieve desired outcomes.
6. Realize the importance of pilot studies and mixed method research in the process of intervention development and testing.

INTRODUCTION

This chapter discusses research-based efforts to develop innovative nursing interventions. Historically, there has been much more guidance on how to test interventions than on how to develop them, but that situation is changing. There is a growing recognition that new interventions should be designed based on research evidence and strong conceptualizations of the problem. Such endeavors benefit from mixed methods designs.

NURSING INTERVENTION RESEARCH

The term *intervention research* is used by nurse researchers to describe a research approach characterized not only by its research methods but by a distinctive *process* of developing, implementing, testing, and disseminating interventions (e.g., Richards & Rahm Hallberg, 2015; Sidani, 2015; Sidani & Braden, 2011). Naylor (2003) defined **nursing intervention research** as "studies either questioning existing care practices or testing innovations in care that are shaped by nursing's values and goals, guided by a strong theoretical basis, informed by recent advances in science, and designed to improve the quality of care and health of individuals, families, communities, and society" (p. 382).

Some nursing interventions are simple and do not require extensive development. For example, Lee and colleagues (2018) undertook a randomized controlled trial (RCT) to test the effect of music on anxiety, heart rate, and blood pressure in patients undergoing mechanical ventilation in the intensive care unit. The intervention was relatively simple—one 30-minute session of music therapy—and the researchers did not "develop" the intervention; rather, they developed a protocol for its implementation. Many nursing interventions that are currently being tested, however, are complex and created by nurses by themselves or in interprofessional teams, usually within a focused program of research involving an integrated series of studies.

Complex Interventions

The term **complex intervention** has become a buzzword in research circles and has been the topic of dozens of discussion articles, including several in the nursing literature (e.g., Corry et al., 2013). We begin by discussing what the term means.

The Medical Research Council (MRC) in the United Kingdom updated their framework for developing and testing complex interventions. Figure 28.1 shows the four phases of the MRC framework. They include (1) "the development or identification of an intervention, (2) assessment of feasibility of the intervention and evaluation design, (3) evaluation of the intervention, and (4) impactful implementation" (Skivington et al., 2021, p. 1). According to the MRC reports, complexity in an intervention can arise along several dimensions, including the following:

- The number of different components within the intervention ("bundling") and interactions between the components;
- The number of different behaviors required by those delivering or receiving the intervention, and the difficulty level of those behaviors;
- The number of different groups or organizational levels targeted by the intervention;
- The number and diversity of intervention outcomes targeted; and
- The degree to which the intervention can be tailored to individual patients.

Intervention complexity exists along a continuum, not as a dichotomy. There is no single point at which a simple intervention becomes complex. Lewin and colleagues (2017) have developed a complexity assessment tool in which interventions can be evaluated for complexity along 10 dimensions. Nursing interventions often are complex along multiple dimensions.

Complex interventions are likely to be needed when complex problems are being treated, when a conceptual framework suggests multiple mediating forces, or when prior research suggests that simple interventions are ineffective. The more complex the intervention, the stronger the need for an intervention framework.

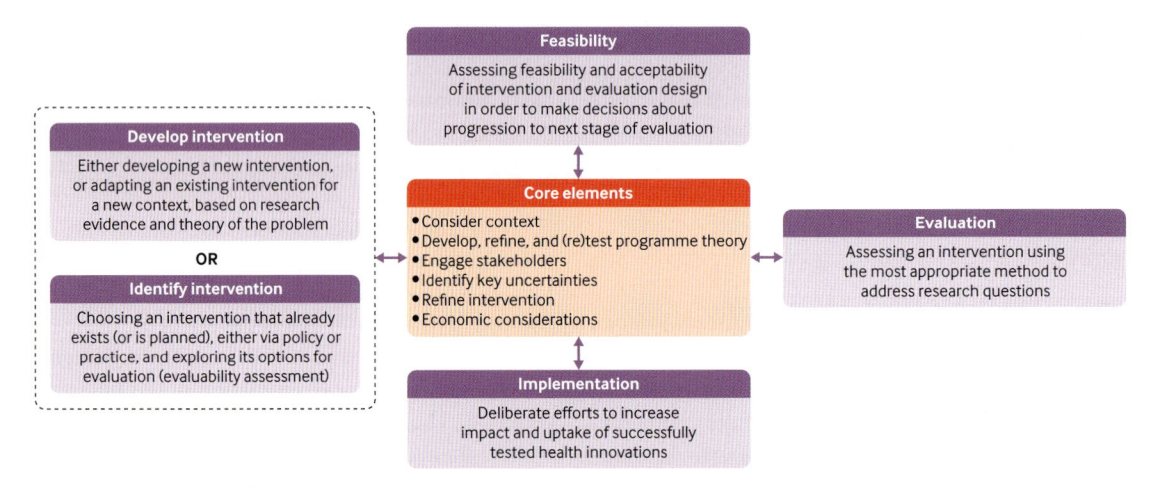

FIGURE 28.1 Medical Research Council's new framework for developing and evaluating complex interventions. (Skivington, K., Matthews, L., Simpson, S. A., Craig, P., Baird, J., Blazeby, J. M., Boyd, K. A., Craig, N., French, D. P., McIntosh, E., Petticrew, M., Rycroft-Malone, J., White, M., & Moore, L. (2021). A new framework for developing and evaluating complex interventions: update of Medical Research Council guidance. *BMJ (Clinical research ed.), 374*, n2061.)

TIP The issue of complexity has received considerable recent attention. Some writers have, for example, criticized the MRC framework for its absence of engagement with complexity theories (e.g., De Silva et al., 2014). One concern is that the interaction between interventions and *context* has not been conceptualized as a key complexity issue (Fletcher et al., 2016).

Frameworks for Developing and Testing Complex Interventions

Proponents of using a framework to guide the intervention development and testing process have rejected the simplistic and atheoretical approach that has often been used with healthcare interventions. The widely recommended process for intervention research involves an in-depth understanding of the problem and the target population, careful integration of diverse evidence, and the use of a guiding intervention theory. The recommendations call for a systematic, progressive sequence that places evidence-based developmental work at a premium.

Several frameworks for health interventions have been proposed. Table 28.1 lists a few of these frameworks, including two that have long served in the development of health promotion interventions (the Intervention Mapping and PRECEDE–PROCEED models) and one for nursing interventions.

The most prominent framework to date for complex health interventions is the **Medical Research Council framework**, which was first described in the literature in 2000 (Campbell et al., 2000). The original MRC framework was conceptualized as a five-phase process and is similar in some regards to the four-phase sequence delineated by the National Institutes of Health for clinical trials, as described in Chapter 11.

The MRC framework considers the "design and conduct research with a diversity of perspectives and appropriate choice of methods" (Skivington et al., 2021, p. 1). The phases of the MRC are not meant to be linear, but rather iterative. We have organized much of this chapter in terms of four broad "phases" of the MRC. The central focus of this chapter is on the first phase of the MRC framework, the development phase.

TABLE 28.1 • Frameworks for Health-Related Intervention Development

FRAMEWORK	COMMENTS
Intervention Mapping framework (Bartholomew Eldredge et al., 2016)[a]	Six-phase model geared to the development of health promotion interventions
PRECEDE–PROCEED model (Green & Kreuter, 2005)[a]	A model with two major components: PRECEDE (a series of planned assessments in five phases) and PROCEED (strategic implementation in four phases); used in health promotion programs
6SQuID (Wight et al., 2016)[a]	Framework with six "essential" steps for quality intervention Development (6SQuID), aimed primarily at public health interventions
Behavior Change Wheel (Michie et al., 2011)	A model that identifies intervention functions and policy categories for interventions in which behavioral change is sought
Evidence-based Nursing Interventions (van Meijel et al., 2004)	A model to guide the development of nursing interventions, involving strong development of interventions with a theoretical rationale
Medical Research Council Framework (Skivington et al., 2021)	An iterative framework with four broad stages for developing and testing complex health interventions

Key Features of Complex Intervention Research

Considerable effort has been put into fleshing out—and using—the MRC guidance. It has become clear that certain features of intervention research are critical to success. Here we identify a few key features.

First, there is strong support for *mixed methods approaches*. In moving from a problem to be solved to the rigorous testing of a new intervention, a wide variety of questions that require diverse methods need to be answered. Borglin (2015) has described the value of mixed methods in complex intervention research.

Second, intervention research is undertaken in the context of coordinated *teamwork*, and efforts to develop high-quality complex interventions are often multidisciplinary. Nurses are increasingly collaborating with other health professionals (e.g., physicians, physical therapists, psychologists, nutritionists) on thorny problems requiring a multi-faceted solution.

Another feature of intervention research is that it requires many years of work. The MRC framework calls for a sequence of activities that involve a long investment of time to "get it right." Commentators have begun to note that there is a lot of *research waste*—research that gets little or no *return on investment* because some researchers do not ask the right questions, do not take into account what is already known, use weak research methods, or fail to disseminate their work promptly and effectively (e.g., Chalmers et al., 2014; Ioannidis, 2016). Research on complex interventions benefits from being embedded in an ongoing, dedicated program of research (Rahm Hallberg, 2015). Coordinated efforts to understand a problem, integrate relevant evidence, develop and test an intervention, and promote its wider adoption are strategies for reducing research waste.

Finally, there is growing realization that *patient and public involvement* is imperative throughout the process of developing and testing complex interventions (Richards, 2015a). The literature on complex interventions is filled with cautions about potential challenges and pitfalls. Many pitfalls concern resistance on the part of patients, family members/caretakers, and healthcare staff in the settings where interventions get tested. In embarking on the pathway of complex intervention research, it is important to understand that a lot of things *can* go wrong, and so strategies should be designed to prevent them from happening to the extent possible. That is why skillful foundational work during the development phase is so crucial, including attempts to understand the perspectives of patients and other stakeholders.

> **TIP** One common pitfall is that intervention developers tend to be overly optimistic and fail to develop or identify evidence to support the links in the chain between the problem, the intervention components, and the outcomes of interest (Wight et al., 2016).

Desirable Features of Nursing Interventions

Nursing interventions are developed to improve health outcomes. Before embarking on an intervention development project, nurse researchers should carefully consider the relative importance of achieving certain goals.

Box 28.1 identifies features that may be considered "ideal" for nursing interventions—although in any situation, some features would be more vital than others. In some cases, the desirable features compete with one another—for example, cost and efficacy often involve trade-offs. Indeed, most of the ideals could plausibly be achieved if cost were not an issue.

Yet, practical issues *are* important considerations. Especially in this time of heightened consciousness about healthcare costs, an intervention should be one that has potential to be cost-effective. In designing new ways to address health needs, nurse researchers should give upfront thought to whether the intervention is feasible from a resource perspective in real-world settings. As noted by Richards (2015b), "We should consider the 'implementability' of our complex interventions from the moment we begin the process of design, testing, and evaluation" (p. 333). Some of the ideals in Box 28.1 may need to be relaxed in the face of cost

> **BOX 28.1** Features of an "Ideal" Nursing Intervention
>
> **An ideal clinical intervention would be:**
> - **Salient**—addresses a pressing problem
> - **Efficacious**—leads to improved client outcomes
> - **Safe**—avoids any adverse outcomes, burdens, or stress
> - **Conceptually sound**—has a theoretical underpinning
> - **Cost-effective**—is affordable and has economic benefits to clients or society
> - **Feasible**—can be implemented in real-world settings and integrated into current models of care
> - **Developmentally appropriate**—is suitable for the age group for whom it is intended
> - **Culturally sensitive**—demonstrates sensitivity to various groups
> - **Accessible**—can be easily accessed by the people for whom it is intended
> - **Acceptable**—is viewed positively by clients and other stakeholders, including family members, nurses, physicians, administrators, policy makers
> - **Adaptable**—can be tailored to local contexts
> - **Readily disseminated**—can be sufficiently described and packaged for adoption in other locales

constraints, but this should be a conscious decision and not left to serendipity. One ideal feature that should never be relaxed is the first one on the list—having an intervention that addresses a pressing problem.

PHASE 1: INTERVENTION DEVELOPMENT

The best current practice is to develop interventions in a systematic fashion, drawing on good evidence and an appropriate theory of how the intervention would achieve desired effects. In other words, interventions should be evidence based from the start, and this can require extensive and diverse types of foundational work.

Each phase in the intervention development and testing process can be thought of as having three aspects: (1) key *issues* that must be addressed during this stage, (2) *actions* and strategies that can be brought to bear on those issues, and (3) *products* that pave the way for moving on to the next phase. Table 28.2 summarizes issues, actions, and products during Phase I development.

Key Issues in Intervention Development

Conceptualization and in-depth understanding of the problem are key issues during Phase 1. The starting point of an intervention project is the problem itself, which must be thoroughly understood.

In Chapter 5, we discussed how those doing a literature review must "own" the literature. When it comes to intervention development, researchers must "own" the problem.

A thorough understanding of the target group—their needs, fears, preferences, and circumstances—is part of that ownership. It is only through such understanding that researchers can know whether key intervention pitfalls might be relevant in their situation. Ownership of the problem also requires a thorough grasp of existing evidence on similar interventions—and an understanding of current practices and why they are deficient.

Another development issue involves identifying key *stakeholders*—people who have a stake in fixing the problem—and getting them "on board." Interventions sometimes fail because researchers have not developed the relationships needed to ensure that the intervention will be given a fair test. In addition to the target group, stakeholders might include family members, advocates, community leaders, service providers in multiple disciplines, intervention agents, healthcare administrators, support staff in intervention settings, and content experts. The intervention team should think broadly about whose support could affect their ability to undertake the project.

Relationship building can contribute to the content of the intervention itself, because stakeholders can offer insight into the scope and depth of the problem. Relationships with stakeholders are also

TABLE 28.2 • Key Issues, Activities, and Products of Phase I Developmental Work for Nursing Interventions

KEY ISSUES	MAJOR ACTIVITIES	PRODUCTS AND OUTCOMES
• Conceptualization of the problem • Understanding of current practices and why they are deficient • Articulation of an evidence base for the intervention • Conceptualization of the context • Conceptualization of solutions, strategies, and outcomes • Construct validation of the intervention • Identification of potential pitfalls within the implementation context • Cultivation of relationships	• Critical synthesis of relevant literature • Concept and theory development • Exploratory and descriptive research • Consultation with experts; content validation • Brainstorming with colleagues, team building, partnerships with stakeholders • Modeling and designing the intervention	• An intervention theory • Preliminary specification of the content, intensity, dose, timing, setting, and delivery method of the intervention • Preliminary identification of key outcomes • Strategies to overcome pitfalls in implementing and testing the intervention • An implementation plan • A design for a pilot study • A plan for sponsorship of the pilot study

important because researchers must figure out not only *what* to deliver but also *how* to deliver it. The intervention must be delivered in a manner that will gain the support of administrators and healthcare staff, appeal to the target group, enhance recruitment and retention of participants, and strengthen intervention fidelity in later phases.

Relatedly, the project team should develop a firm understanding of the context in which the intervention will be implemented. As noted by Hawe and colleagues (2009), contextual factors will almost surely shape how an intervention is delivered, how it will work, and who is likely to benefit. Fletcher and colleagues (2016) have emphasized the value of conceptualizing the contextual conditions necessary for the intervention mechanisms to function as planned.

Activities and Strategies in Intervention Development

Developmental issues can be addressed through a variety of activities. The importance of adequate development cannot be overemphasized.

Synthesizing Existing Evidence

As shown in the MDC framework in Figure 28.1, development work includes identifying the evidence base, and thus development work often begins with close scrutiny of the literature. The research team needs to thoroughly understand the nature and scope of the problem, and how it is manifested in different groups or settings. The literature also needs to be searched for guidance about the content and mechanisms of possible interventions—the active ingredients. Systematic reviews may be available for evidence about specific strategies but preparing a new or updated one might be necessary (Chapter 30).

Researchers' efforts to understand the problem and possible solutions are an important, but not exhaustive, part of a literature review effort. Table 28.3 provides examples of other questions that should be addressed through a scrutiny of existing evidence during the development phase. When relevant literature is thin or nonexistent, other sources to address remaining uncertainties need to be pursued.

> **Example of Using the Literature in Intervention Research**
> In an effort to increase the transparency of the process and the ability to replicate their study, Jordens and colleagues (2022) described the implementation of a complex nursing intervention to reduce the decline of older postcardiac surgical patients in 12 cardiac surgical centers in the Netherlands. They noted that they used the literature to adapt existing interventions based on the situational local context.

TABLE 28.3 • Examples of Literature Review Questions for Designing an Evidence-Based Intervention

ISSUE	QUESTIONS FOR WHICH EVIDENCE CAN BE SOUGHT IN A LITERATURE REVIEW
Conceptualizing the problem	What is known about the nature and causes of this problem and possible solutions? What theories help to explain the problem? What are key mediators in the pathway between the causes or contributing factors and the outcomes?
Focusing the target group	Who or what have been the targets of efforts to address the problem—individuals? families? healthcare providers? healthcare systems? What populations appear to be most amenable to the intervention?
Developing intervention content and components	What is the content of other similar interventions? Is the presence of certain types of components linked to better outcomes? Are interventions generic or individualized?
Selecting outcomes and assessment strategies	What behaviors or outcomes have been targeted by similar interventions? Have the interventions had significant effects on these outcomes? Have they had an effect on key mediators? What assessment approaches and measures have been used with other similar interventions?
Making decisions about dose	How intense have other similar interventions been? Has dose been found to be related to outcomes?
Making decisions about timing of intervention	When are interventions of this type typically delivered? Is timing related to outcomes?
Making decision about mode of delivery	How have similar interventions been delivered? In face-to-face situations (group or individual delivery)? by telephone? Internet? video? Is there evidence that some delivery modes are especially effective?
Making decisions about timing of outcome measurement	When have data for this type of intervention typically been collected? Does the literature suggest that effects deteriorate?
Making decisions about settings and agents	Where (in what types of settings) have interventions of this type been delivered? Do impacts vary by type of setting? Who usually delivers them? Do outcomes vary by type of agent?
Assessing acceptability of the intervention	Is there evidence of strong (or weak) rates of participation in interventions of this type? Have recruitment or retention problems been reported?
Assessing cultural appropriateness	Is there evidence that cultural issues affect implementation of similar interventions? Is there cultural variation in outcomes?

Exploratory and Descriptive Research

Most researchers find that evidence from the literature is insufficient to satisfactorily address the questions suggested in Table 28.3. Almost inevitably, the developmental phase involves undertaking mixed methods exploratory and descriptive research. Insights from qualitative inquiries are virtually essential to the success of intervention development efforts. Morden and colleagues (2015) offer a compelling argument about the importance of qualitative research in developing and implementing complex interventions.

As previously noted, efforts to design acceptable and efficacious interventions require understanding clients' perspectives. Examples of questions that could be pursued in exploratory research with clients include the following: What is it like to have this problem? What strategies to address it have been tried and why have they not worked? What are clients' goals—what do *they* want as an intervention outcome? Answers to questions such as these could help to shape the intervention and make it more effective, tolerable, and appropriate for the group for whom the intervention is designed.

Exploratory research with other stakeholders can also be valuable. Many of the pitfalls of intervention research involve lack of cooperation, support, or trust among key stakeholders, including those who deliver the intervention. Stakeholders should be engaged in the development process to the extent possible.

Exploratory work can also be undertaken to understand the context within which an intervention would unfold (McGuire et al., 2000). It may also be important to understand institutional issues such as staff turnover, staff morale, nurse workload, and nurse autonomy. Van Meijel and colleagues (2004) recommended undertaking a "current practice analysis" to understand the status quo of how the problem under scrutiny is being addressed.

The nursing literature has hundreds of examples of descriptive or exploratory studies done as part of intervention development. Research strategies can include a wide range of approaches, such as focus group interviews, needs assessment surveys, in-depth or critical-incident interviews, records reviews, and observations in clinical settings. It is not unusual for researchers to conduct three or four small descriptive studies during the development phase of an intervention project.

Example of Qualitative Research for Developing a Nursing Intervention
Duggleby and colleagues (2020) described how they used qualitative research findings to adapt a web-based intervention for family caregivers of persons with dementia who were residing in long-term care (LTC). The process resulted in a feasible and acceptable web-based intervention to support the family caregivers.

Consultation With Experts

Experts in the content area of the problem can play a crucial role during the development of an intervention. Expert consultants are especially useful if the evidence base is thin and resources for exploratory research are limited. Many of the questions in Table 28.3 that are not answered by evidence in the research literature or from new descriptive studies are good candidates for discussion with experts.

TIP In selecting expert consultants, think in an interdisciplinary fashion. For example, the use of a cultural consultant may be valuable to assess the cultural sensitivity and appropriateness of some interventions. A developmental psychologist could help assess developmental suitability.

Often, experts are asked to review preliminary intervention protocols, to corroborate their utility, and to make suggestions for strengthening them. Curiously, this process is less often formalized than the process for reviewing new measurement scales. Procedures used to assess the *content validity* of new instruments using an expert panel (Chapter 16) can also be used to review draft intervention protocols. If the intervention is intended for use in diverse settings or contexts, content validation is likely to be a valuable approach.

Example of Content Validation of a Nursing Intervention
Cardoso and colleagues (2023) used a panel of 74 nurses with expertise in gerontological nursing and nursing diagnosis to assess the content validity of the nursing diagnosis "Readiness for enhanced healthy aging." Using the content validity index, they noted the score was acceptable at 0.81.

Brainstorming and Team Building

Development work is usually interpersonal and involves cultivating relationships. At the team level, this entails putting together an enthusiastic and committed project team with diverse clinical and research skills. (If development work is undertaken for a dissertation, the "team" includes the dissertation committee, so members of this committee should be chosen carefully.)

Ideally, brainstorming sessions occur frequently during the development period to discuss evidence summaries, descriptive findings, expert feedback, and preliminary protocols. Technological advances such as videoconferencing make it possible to include team members from different locations. The team may include key stakeholders as participating partners.

TIP It is wise to develop mechanisms for ongoing communication and collaboration with stakeholders. For example, it can be useful to form an advisory group of stakeholders and to have a project-specific website or Facebook page.

for extending the findings of a qualitative study by identifying intervention strategies related to the phenomenon of concern.

Example of a Qualitatively Derived Intervention Theory

Harvey Chochinov and other researchers (including nurse researchers) developed a theory of dignity based on in-depth interviews with hospice patients. The theory formed the basis for an intervention (Dignity Therapy) to promote dignity and reduce stress at the end of life. Nunziante and colleagues (2021) developed and tested a nurse-led Dignity Therapy intervention that was delivered to patients with advanced cancer who were receiving palliative care in the hospital setting.

Intervention Theory Development

A critical activity in the development phase is to delineate the conceptual basis for the intervention (Skivington et al., 2021). An **intervention theory** offers an explanation for the problem and guides what must be done to achieve desired outcomes. The theory provides a theoretical rationale for why an intervention should "work." In conceptualizing what is causing a problem, the research team needs to identify which factors are modifiable and which would have the greatest impact on improving outcomes of interest.

The intervention theory can be an existing one that has been well validated. Examples of theories that have been used in nursing intervention studies include the Health Promotion Model, the Transtheoretical Model, Social Cognitive Theory, the Health Belief Model, and the Theory of Planned Behavior (see Chapter 6). These theories provide guidance on how to fashion an intervention because they propose mechanisms to explain human behavior and behavior change. Abraham and colleagues (2015) offer perspectives on the theoretical basis of behavior change interventions.

Intervention theories can also be developed from qualitatively derived theory, a point made most eloquently by Morse (2006). Morse and colleagues (2000) developed a strategy called *qualitative outcome analysis* (QOA), which is a process

Modeling and Designing the Intervention

The MRC framework (Figure 28.1) includes "modeling processes and outcomes" as a component of intervention development. Modeling involves synthesizing the information gleaned during the development phase (Figure 28.2), constructing components of the intervention and visualizing the pathways that patients will take in going through the intervention. As described by Sermeus (2015), the aim of modeling is to unravel the "black box" between intervention components and desired outcomes.

An evidence-based intervention theory lays the groundwork for proceeding with the modeling task and developing intervention content. A visual *logic model* for the intervention should identify the active components and show how they are expected to work on the outcomes of interest. It should also describe how the active components relate to each other.

Example of a Logic Model in a Complex Intervention Study

Yip and colleagues (2021) described the evolution of a complex intervention to create an integrated care model in newly developed information and advice centers for home-dwelling older adults in Canton Basel-Landschaft, Switzerland. They created a logic model to describe "how" and the "what" including the resources needed, activities, anticipated outcomes, and anticipated impact of the overall program.

Intervention content can sometimes be adapted from other similar interventions. In addition to content, however, the research team needs to make many decisions about the intervention's ingredients, including decisions about the following:

1. **Dose and intensity.** The treatment must be sufficiently powerful to achieve a desired, measurable effect on outcomes of interest, but cannot be so powerful that it is cost prohibitive or burdensome to clients. Among the dose-related issues that need to be decided are the *potency* or *intensity* of the treatment (how much content is appropriate, and will it be given individually or in groups?); the *amount* of dose per session; the *frequency* of administering doses (number of sessions); and the *duration* of the intervention over time.

2. **Timing.** In some cases, it is important to decide when, relative to other events, the intervention will be delivered. The question is, When is the optimal point (in terms of an illness or recovery trajectory, individual development, or severity of a problem) to administer the intervention? Ideally, the intervention theory would suggest the most advantageous timing.

3. **Outcomes.** Two major decisions concern which outcomes will be targeted and when they will be measured. Thought should be given to selecting outcomes that are nursing sensitive and important to clients. One issue is whether the focus will be on proximal outcomes or more distal ones. *Proximal outcomes* are immediate and directly connected to the intervention—and thus usually most sensitive to intervention effects. For example, knowledge gains from a teaching component of an intervention are proximal. *Distal outcomes* are potentially more important, but more difficult to affect (e.g., eating behavior). Consideration should also be given to the information needs of people making decisions about using the intervention—what outcomes would affect uptake by administrators or policy makers? Another crucial outcome is cost: interventions are hard to "sell" without information about monetary costs and benefits.

4. **Setting.** Another design decision involves the setting for the intervention. Settings can vary in terms of ease of implementation, costs, and access. In deciding about settings (and sites), researchers need to think about the type of setting that will be acceptable and accessible to clients, offer good potential for impacts, provide needed resources or supports, and serve clients whose needs and characteristics are compatible with the intervention.

5. **Agents.** Researchers must decide who will deliver the intervention, and how intervention agents will be trained. In many cases, the agents will be nurses, but nurses are not necessarily the best choice. For example, some clients might feel more comfortable if the interventionists were community members or patients who have experienced a similar illness or problem (i.e., peers).

6. **Delivery mode.** With technological innovations occurring regularly, options for delivering interventions—or components of interventions—have broadened tremendously. Among the possibilities are face-to-face delivery, video or audio recordings, print materials, telephone communication, texts, emails, Internet discussion boards, and social networking sites. Care should be taken to match any technological delivery methods to the needs of the clients and to the requirements of the content. The latest technology is not always optimal.

7. **Individualization.** Another decision concerns the extent to which the intervention will be tailored to the needs and circumstances of a particular group (e.g., older adults) or individualized to particular clients. When individual information is used to guide content, the intervention is inherently more complex than a one-size-fits-all treatment but may be more effective and attractive to participants (Lauver et al., 2002).

These various decisions should be evidence based to the extent possible, using synthesized evidence from various sources. The development work should provide the basis for the intervention to be piloted in the next phase. As noted by the authors of the MRC framework, the intervention should be developed in a way that can reasonably be expected to be impactful (Skivington et al., 2021). The four phases of the MRC framework are the development or identification of the intervention, feasibility, evaluation, and implementation.

Products of Phase 1 Development

Phase I typically results in several products (Table 28.2). These include an intervention theory and a conceptual map or logic model, preliminary intervention components and protocols, and an implementation plan that includes strategies for addressing potential implementation pitfalls. Hopefully, the research team will have documented the development work and major decisions in an ongoing fashion. Detailed written information about the theory, the intervention components and strategies, and expected outcomes will be valuable for writing reports about the intervention and for making funding requests.

> **TIP** A matrix can often be useful in summarizing *key decisions* in one column and *supporting evidence* for those decisions in another. Such a matrix is a good communication tool for discussing decisions with others.

If the development work provides support for moving forward with a pilot test of the intervention, another product of Phase 1 work will be a design for a pilot study, usually in the form of a research proposal (Chapter 33).

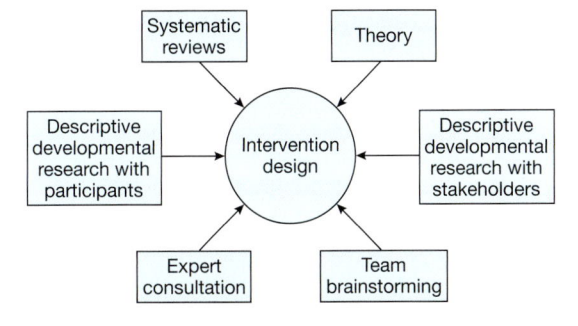

FIGURE 28.2 Synthesis of evidence sources for intervention development.

OTHER PHASES OF INTERVENTION RESEARCH

Other phases of intervention research include feasibility and implementation/pilot testing; a rigorous evaluation to assess efficacy; and implementation of the intervention (should it prove to be effective) into real-world settings with ongoing monitoring and longer-term follow-up. These other phases are briefly described next.

Phases 2: Pilot Testing and the Feasibility of the Intervention

The second phase of intervention research is to pilot test of the newly developed intervention. Key issues are *feasibility* (Can the intervention be implemented as conceptualized?), *acceptability* (Do recipients and other key stakeholders find the intervention relevant and appropriate?), and *promise* (Is it plausible that the intervention will result in desired effects on key outcomes?). The central *activities* of Phase 2 are undertaking a **pilot study** and analyzing pilot data. An important *product* of a pilot study is documentation of the results and the "lessons learned."

Although each pilot test yields its own context-specific and intervention-specific lessons, some "lessons" are recurrent. In particular, you should expect the reality of piloting the intervention to be different from the intervention that was developed on paper, and these differences—and reasons for them—should be documented. If the intervention proves feasible and promising, Phase 2 products include a formal intervention protocol for testing in a full Phase 3 trial. Another product is a formal plan for a Phase 3 evaluation, often in the form of a grant application. Chapter 29 discusses pilot tests of interventions in greater detail.

> **Example of a Mixed Methods Pilot Intervention Study**
> In the study by Yip and colleagues (2021) previously described, the research team used a mixed method approach to pilot test the intervention. The quantitative approach used descriptive statistics to analyze the secondary data of a subset of the population. The team then conducted qualitative interviews to help explain the survey results.

Phase 3: Evaluation of the Intervention

The third phase of a complex intervention project is a full test of the intervention, almost always using a randomized design. Many important issues of a Phase 3 evaluation were discussed in Chapter 10, which outlined various threats to the validity of quantitative studies and presented some strategies to address those threats. Whereas construct validity is particularly salient in the development phase of an intervention project, internal validity and statistical conclusion validity are key issues during the evaluation.

Although a major goal of Phase 3 is to assess the *efficacy* of the intervention, it is better to think of the trial as ongoing development rather than as simply "confirmatory." Even with a strong pilot study, problems and issues almost always emerge in the full test. As part of a process analysis (Chapter 11), problems should be identified, and researchers should make recommendations for how the intervention could be improved, how its implementation could be made smoother, or how context helped to shape the delivery or efficacy of the intervention.

The MRC has provided useful guidance about planning and implementing a process evaluation of complex evaluations (Moore et al., 2015), and a mixed methods approach is strongly advocated. Some of the goals of collecting qualitative data during Phase 3 might include the following:

1. **Assessing Intervention Fidelity.** Mixed methods research is needed to inform judgments about whether the intervention was faithfully implemented, and how it was delivered in real-world settings. If intervention effects are modest, one possibility is that it was not implemented according to the plan. The protocols or training materials, for example, might need revamping.
2. **Clarifying the Intervention.** A qualitative component in a randomized trial can help to clarify the nature and course of the intervention in its natural context. It is useful to understand how intervention recipients and other stakeholders experience the intervention in real life—and to identify possible barriers to widespread implementation.
3. **Understanding the Context.** Factors external to the intervention can facilitate or impede its implementation. Some of these factors can be measured (e.g., population characteristics, staff–patient ratios), but a full understanding of context usually requires deeper exploration. Pfadenhauer and colleagues (2017) have developed a framework to facilitate the conceptualization of context and implementation of complex interventions.
4. **Probing for Clinical Significance.** Quantitative results from a randomized trial indicate whether the results are statistically significant, and methods have been developed to quantitatively assess clinical significance (Chapter 21). Qualitative information could shed additional light—clinically relevant effects sometimes can be discerned qualitatively even when treatment effects are not statistically significant.
5. **Interpreting Results.** Quantitative results indicate *whether* an intervention had beneficial effects—but do not explain *why* effects occurred. A strong conceptual framework offers a theoretical rationale for explaining the results but may not tell the whole story if the effects were weaker than expected or if they were observed for some outcomes but not for others. Moreover, even if there are specific theory-driven intervention effects, it is inevitable that people will pose "black box" questions about what is *driving* the results. Such questions often stem from practical concerns, reflecting a desire to streamline successful interventions when resources are tight.

> **Example of Using Qualitative Data to Interpret Evaluation Results**
>
> Guided by the MRC framework, McGrattan and colleagues (2021) developed educational resources related to the Mediterranean diet and lifestyle. In the pilot test, 20 participants were enrolled, but 50% withdrew. Qualitative findings indicate those who remained in the study reviewed the intervention favorably. However, the authors note that recruitment and retention issues, as well as missing data, highlight the complexity of the study. They also indicate that feasibility could not be established.

> **TIP** Quantitative results do not have much "sex appeal." As astutely pointed out by Sandelowski (1996), qualitative research embedded in intervention studies can enhance the power of the study findings: "Storied accounts of scientific work are often the more compelling and culturally resonant way to communicate research results to diverse audiences, including patient groups and policy-makers" (p. 361).

A Phase 3 evaluation, then, includes both an analysis of intervention effectiveness and an in-depth process evaluation that provides rich information about the roll-out of the intervention and the processes of change that occurred. One final evaluation component is crucial to the intervention's potential for widespread adoption: a cost–benefit analysis. Interventions are unlikely to be integrated into healthcare systems if their cost outweighs any benefits, and so the evaluation team should strive to understand economic implications. Payne and Thompson (2015) provide an overview of economic evaluations of complex interventions.

The primary product of Phase 3 is a report summarizing the evaluation results. Often, single papers are insufficient for providing the full range of information about the project, particularly if a mixed methods approach was used. Ideally, one report would integrate findings from the qualitative and quantitative components and offer recommendations for further adoption of (or revisions to) the intervention.

> **TIP** Several groups have called for researchers to undertake *realist evaluations* (Chapter 11) in coming to conclusions about complex interventions (e.g., Fletcher et al., 2016; Hansen & Jones, 2017). Their position is that realist evaluations do a better job than traditional evaluations of answering questions about what works, for whom, and under what circumstances. The realist approach involves developing and testing theories about **context-mechanism-outcome (CMO)** configurations. Realist evaluations almost inevitably used mixed methods designs.

Phase 4: Implementation

In the MRC framework, the final phase of intervention research is the *implementation* of a complex intervention that has been found to have beneficial effects and favorable economic results. Implementation involves embedding a new and promising intervention into routine health and nursing services. The process of implementation is sometimes called *normalization*.

Increasingly, researchers have come to recognize that their work does not end with the publication of a research report on the findings from a Phase 3 trial. A whole new field of *implementation science* has burgeoned in efforts to help researchers plan for implementation challenges.

Several conceptual models and frameworks have been devised to guide the implementation process. One widely used framework is called **normalization process theory (NPT)** (May 2013; May et al., 2016). NPT is an action theory that focuses on how new interventions or programs become embedded within social contexts. NPT involves four core constructs that represent the kinds of work and activity that people do when implementing a new practice: Coherence, Cognitive Participation, Collective Action, and Reflexive Monitoring. A measure called NoMAD (Normalization MeAsure Development) is available to assess these four constructs in practice settings (Finch et al., 2013). Several chapters in Richards and Rahm Hallberg (2015) are devoted to issues of relevance during the implementation of complex interventions.

> **Example of Using Normalization Process Theory**
> Al-Shammari et al. (2022) describe a study protocol for a multisite parallel pragmatic trail in which they plan to use Normalization Process Theory to evaluate the effect of a complex intervention of a web-based training course. They hypothesized that post the training, nurses across five healthcare settings in Babylon, Iraq would be able to provide palliative care to the pediatric population as needed.

MIXED METHODS DESIGNS FOR INTERVENTION RESEARCH

The full cycle of research activity for developing and testing complex interventions addresses myriad questions that can only be answered using a rich blend of methods. Creswell and Plano Clark (2018) identified as a possible advanced mixed methods design what they called the *mixed methods intervention design,* which involves incorporating qualitative data into a trial before, during, and (or) after the experimental treatment has been implemented. They also identified another complex design, the *mixed methods program evaluation design,* which is consistent with the MRC's intervention framework.

Visual diagrams for two possible two-stage mixed methods intervention designs are presented in Figure 28.3. Models such as these can work reasonably well for interventions that are closer to the "simple" end of the simple → complex continuum. They might also be appropriate for a small-scale study (such as a dissertation project) in which the main QUAN component is essentially a pilot study.

For complex interventions such as those described in the MRC framework, it is better to think of a separate design structure for each phase, because each has its own purpose, research questions, design, sampling plan, and data collection strategy. For the project overall, QUAN typically has priority. Yet, foundational work in the development phase often involves QUAL-dominant research.

Figure 28.4 shows some design possibilities for a three-phase intervention project, and many others are possible. The overall project design is inherently sequential, but within each phase, the design could be either sequential or concurrent. Both qualitative and quantitative approaches are often used in each phase.

It is difficult to offer guidance on which of design to adopt because many factors influence which is most appropriate. Fewer design components may be required for simpler interventions, for "mainstream" target populations, for studies in a familiar site, and for studies of adaptations of well-tested interventions. Also, resources may force researchers to forgo components they would have liked to include. The design for the Phase 3 trial is also likely to be affected by which of the five goals for qualitative inquiry (as described in the previous section) is most salient. For example, if the desire to monitor intervention fidelity is the primary objective of including a qualitative component, a QUAN + qual design would be needed.

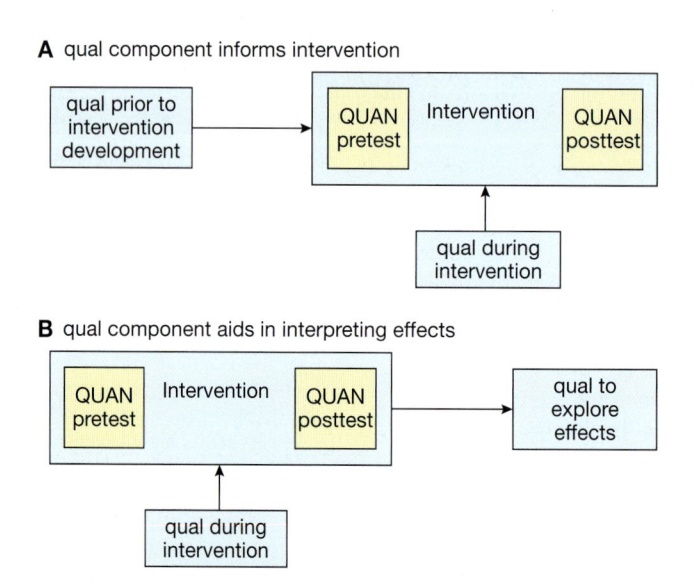

FIGURE 28.3 Mixed methods designs for a two-phase intervention project. (Adapted from Creswell, J. W., & Plano Clark, V. L. (2018). *Designing and conducting mixed methods research* (3rd ed.). Thousand Oaks, CA: Sage.)

Nursing Intervention Diagram

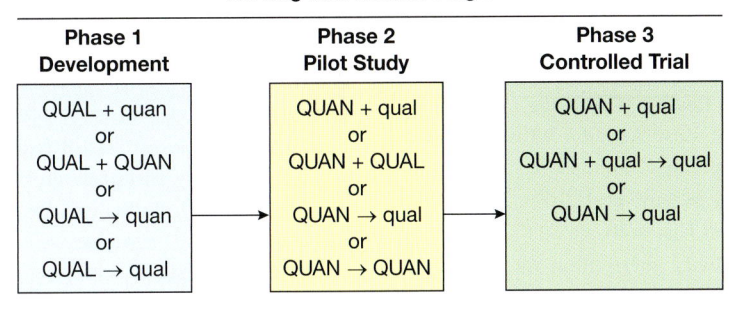

Phase 1 Development	Phase 2 Pilot Study	Phase 3 Controlled Trial
QUAL + quan or QUAL + QUAN or QUAL → quan or QUAL → qual	QUAN + qual or QUAN + QUAL or QUAN → qual or QUAN → QUAN	QUAN + qual or QUAN + qual → qual or QUAN → qual

FIGURE 28.4 Possible mixed methods designs for a three-phase nursing intervention project.

Sampling designs, as discussed in Chapter 27, also differ in the three phases. During Phase 1, a multilevel sampling approach is often used to gather in-depth QUAL data from different populations—for example, from patients, family members, and healthcare staff. In Phases 2 and 3, by contrast, sampling is likely to be either identical or nested—although multilevel sampling may also be useful for understanding intervention fidelity. Samples for qualitative questions are typically purposively selected along dimensions likely to influence the implementation and effectiveness of the intervention.

In summary, researchers can be creative in developing an overall design that matches their needs, circumstances, and budgets. Inevitably, however, strong research for developing and testing complex interventions will rely on a mixed methods design.

CRITICAL APPRAISAL OF INTERVENTION RESEARCH

Many chapters of this book offer guidelines for evaluating methodologic aspects of studies that would be included in an intervention project. For example, guidelines in Chapters 9 and 10 would be useful for critically appraising the Phase 3 design. Qualitative components can be evaluated using guidelines in Chapters 22 through 26, and the previous chapter included suggestions for appraising mixed methods research.

BOX 28.2 Guidelines for Critically Appraising Aspects of Intervention Projects

1. On a simple-to-complex continuum, where would you locate the intervention? If the intervention is complex, along which dimensions is complexity found (e.g., number of components, complexity of behaviors required, number of intervention sessions, time required, and so on)?
2. Is there an intervention theory, and is it adequate? Is there an explanation of how the theory was selected, adapted, or developed? Was a logic model presented?
3. What strategies were used to identify and create evidence in support of intervention development? Was a systematic review performed? Were expert consultants involved? Were descriptive or exploratory studies undertaken? Overall, was developmental work adequate?
4. What *was* the intervention? Was it described in sufficient detail in terms of content, target population, dose, outcomes, timing, individualization, intervention agents, and so on?
5. Was there a pilot study? Was pilot work sufficient for a decision to move forward with a full clinical trial?
6. For the overall project and for individual phases, was a mixed methods approach used? Which design was adopted, and is the design appropriate for the goals of different phases of the project?
7. Does the final report integrate key findings from the various strands of research?
   Does the report offer recommendations for replication, extension, or adaptation of the intervention or for use in different settings or with different populations?

EXAMPLE OF MIXED METHODS INTERVENTION RESEARCH

Study: A Virtual Reality Exergame to Engage Adolescents in Physical Activity: Mixed Methods Study Describing the Formative Intervention Development Process (Farič et al., 2021).

Statement of purpose: This study aimed to develop and test a physical activity intervention for adolescents using virtual gaming to promote exercise.

Phase 1: The team for this study included both academics and industry partners. The academic team had experts in the following areas: a behavioral scientist with a focus on physical activity (PA) for the prevention and treatment of health conditions, a sports scientist, an epidemiologist, and other members with expertise in health informatics, statistics, and psychology. The industry partners were commercial game designers with expertise in developing exercise-based apps. In phase one, the team conducted a literature review to determine the factors that may influence adolescents' PA. They found that the core constructs of competence, autonomy, and relatedness most closely aligned with the Self-Determination Theory of motivation.

Phase 2: Phase 2 involved pilot testing in which they recruited participants 13 to 24 years of age from two London-based schools for a user group. Using a cross-sectional sample of adolescents, they pilot tested a quantitative survey in 511 adolescents. They then conducted qualitative interviews with a subset of the adolescents ($N = 31$) and parents ($N = 18$). The next phase involved doing a thematic analysis of 498 public available reviews of the virtual reality exercise app to determine which features of the app were favorable or not.

Lastly, the team recruited a cross-sectional sample of users of the app to qualitatively explore their experiences of using the app. Future steps for phase 2 include refinement of the virtual reality app and linking it to smartphones and others who are using the app. Phase 2 also includes empirically testing the app and its potential to enhance motivation and change behavior.

SUMMARY POINTS

- **Nursing intervention research** involves a distinctive *process* of developing, implementing, testing, and disseminating nursing interventions—particularly complex interventions.
- *Complexity* in **complex interventions** can arise along several dimensions, including number of components, number of outcomes targeted, number and complexity of behaviors required, and the time needed for the full intervention to be delivered.
- Several frameworks for developing and testing complex interventions have been proposed. The most widely cited one is the **Medical Research Council (MRC) framework** (United Kingdom), which was first published in 2000 and then revised in 2008 and 2021.
- Most frameworks emphasize the critical importance of strong development efforts at the outset, followed by pilot tests of the intervention, and then a rigorous controlled trial to assess efficacy and evaluate the implementation process. The frameworks are idealized models; the process is rarely linear. Virtually all frameworks for intervention development and testing call for mixed methods (MM) research.
- Conceptualization and in-depth understanding of the problem and the target population are key issues during Phase 1 development work. An important product during Phase 1 is a carefully conceived **intervention theory** from which the design of the intervention flows. The theory indicates what inputs are needed to effect improvements on specific outcomes and is often incorporated into a *logic model*.
- In addition to theory, resources for creating an evidence-based intervention and intervention strategies during Phase 1 development include systematic reviews, descriptive research with the target population or key stakeholders, consultation with experts, and brainstorming with a dedicated and diverse team.

- In developing an intervention, researchers must make decisions about not only the *content* of the intervention but also about dose and intensity, timing of the intervention, outcomes to target and when to measure them, intervention setting, intervention agents, mode of delivery, and individualization.
- In a Phase 2 **pilot study**, the preliminary intervention is tested for feasibility and preliminary effectiveness. Pilots often include supplementary qualitative components to understand the experience of being in the intervention and any problems with recruitment, retention, and acceptability.
- A mixed methods approach can strengthen the test of the intervention during the Phase 3 controlled trial. The inclusion of qualitative components can shed light on intervention fidelity, clinical significance, and interpretive ambiguities.
- Mixed methods designs are appropriate in all phases of an intervention project. Broadly speaking, the design is sequential, but each phase can involve the use of various mixed methods designs. In Phase 1, QUAL often has priority, while in Phases 2 and 3, QUAN is usually dominant.

REFERENCES CITED IN CHAPTER 28

Abraham, C., Denford, S., Smith, J., Dean, S., Greaves, C., Lloyd, J., Tarrant, M., White, M. P., & Wyatt, K. (2015). Designing interventions to change health-related behaviour. In Richards, D., & Rahm Hallberg, I., (Eds.), *Complex interventions in health: An overview of research methods* (pp. 103–110). Routledge.

Al-Shammari, M. A., Yasir, A., Aldoori, N., & Mohammad, H. (2022). Using normalization process theory to evaluate an end-of-life pediatric palliative care web-based training program for nurses: Protocol for a randomized controlled trial. *JMIR Research Protocols*, *11*(11), e23783. https://doi.org/10.2196/23783

Bartholomew Eldredge, L., Markham, C., Ruiter, R., Fernandez, M., Kox, G., & Parcel, G. (2016). *Planning health promotion programs: An intervention mapping approach* (4th ed.). Jossey-Bass.

Borglin, G. (2015). The value of mixed methods for researching complex interventions. In Richards, D., & Rahm Hallberg, I., (Eds.), *Complex interventions in health: An overview of research methods* (pp. 29–45). Routledge.

Campbell, M., Fitzpatrick, R., Haines, A., Kinmonth, A. L., Sandercock, P., Spiegelhalter, D., & Tyrer, P. (2000). Framework for design and evaluation of complex interventions to improve health. *BMJ*, *321*(7262), 694–696.

Cardoso, R. B., Caldas, C. P., Brandão, M. A. G., de Souza, P. A., & Santana, R. F. (2023). "Readiness for enhanced healthy aging" nursing diagnosis: Content validation by experts. *International Journal of Nursing Knowledge*, *34*(1), 65–71.

Chalmers, I., Bracken, M., Djulbegovic, B., Garattini, S., Grant, J., Gulmezoglu, A, Howells, D. W., Ioannidis, J. P. A., Oliver, S., & Oliver, S. (2014). How to increase value and reduce waste when research priorities are set. *The Lancet*, *383*(9912), 156–165.

Corry, M., Clarke, M., While, A., & Lalor, J. (2013). Developing complex interventions for nursing: A critical review of key guidelines. *Journal of Clinical Nursing*, *22*(17–18), 2366–2386.

Creswell, J. W., & Plano Clark, V. L. (2018). *Designing and conducting mixed methods research* (3rd ed.). Sage.

De Silva, M., Breuer, E., Lee, L., Asher, L., Chowdhary, N., Lund, C., & Patel, V. (2014). Theory of change: A theory-driven approach to enhance the Medical Research Council's framework for complex interventions. *Trials*, *15*, 267.

Duggleby, W., Peacock, S., Ploeg, J., Swindle, J., Kaewwilai, L., & Lee, H. (2020). Qualitative research and its importance in adapting interventions. *Qualitative Health Research*, *30*(10), 1605–1613.

Farič, N., Smith, L., Hon, A., Potts, H. W. W., Newby, K., Steptoe, A., & Fisher, A. (2021). A virtual reality exergame to engage adolescents in physical activity: Mixed methods study describing the formative intervention development process. *Journal of Medical Internet Research*, *23*(2), e18161. https://doi.org/10.2196/18161

Finch, T., Rapley, T., Girling, M., Mair, F., Murray, E., Treweek, S., McColl, E., Steen, I. N., & May, C. R. (2013). Improving the normalization of complex interventions: Measure development based on normalization process theory (NoMAD)— Study protocol. *Implementation Science*, *8*, 43.

Fletcher, A., Jamal, F., Moore, G., Evans, R., Murphy, S., & Bonell, C. (2016). Realist complex intervention science: Applying realist principles across all phases of the Medical Research Council framework for developing and evaluating complex interventions. *Evaluation*, *22*(3), 286–303.

Green, L., & Kreuter, M. (2005). *Health program planning: An educational and ecological approach* (4th ed.). McGraw Hill.

Hansen, A., & Jones, A. (2017). Advancing "real world" trials that take account of social context and human volition. *Trials*, *18*(1), 531.

Hawe, P., Shiell, A., & Riley, T. (2009). Theorising interventions as events in systems. *American Journal of Community Psychology*, *43*(3–4), 267–276.

Ioannidis, J. (2016). Why most clinical research is not useful. *PLoS Medicine*, *13*(6), e1002049.

Jordens, Y. J., Ettema, R. E., Bleijenberg, N., Schuurmans, M. J., & Schoonhoven, L. (2022). Implementation design of a complex nursing intervention in Dutch hospitals: A methods paper. *Global Implementation Research and Applications*, *2*(1), 42–52.

Lauver, D. R., Ward, S. E., Heidrich, S. M., Keller, M. L., Bowers, B. J., Brennan, P. F., Kirchhoff, K. T., & Wells, T. J. (2002). Patient-centered interventions. *Research in Nursing & Health*, *25*(4), 246–255.

Lee, C., Lee, C., Hsu, M., Lai, C., Sung, Y., Lin, C., & Lin, L. (2017). Effects of music intervention on state anxiety and physiological indices in patients undergoing mechanical ventilation in the intensive care unit. *Biological Research for Nursing*, *19*(2), 137–144.

Lewin, S., Hendry, M., Chandler, J., Oxman, A., Michie, S., Shepperd, S., Reeves, B. C., Tugwell, P., Hannes, K., Rehfuess, E. A., Welch, V., Mckenzie, J. E., Burford, B., Petkovic, J., Anderson, L. M., Harris, J., & Noyes, J. (2017). Assessing the complexity of interventions within systematic reviews: Development, content and use of a new tool (iCAT_SR). *BMC Medical Research Methodology*, *17*(1), 76.

May, C. (2013). Towards a general theory of implementation. *Implementation Science*, *8*, 18.

May, C., Johnson, M., & Finch, T. (2016). Implementation, context and complexity. *Implementation Science*, *11*(1), 141.

McGrattan, A. M., McEvoy, C. T., Vijayakumar, A., Moore, S. E., Neville, C. E., McGuinness, B., McKinley, M. C., & Woodside, J. V. (2021). A mixed methods pilot randomised controlled trial to develop and evaluate the feasibility of a Mediterranean diet and lifestyle education intervention 'THINK-MED' among people with cognitive impairment. *Pilot and Feasibility Studies*, *7*(1), 3. https://doi.org/10.1186/s40814-020-00738-3

McGuire, D., DeLoney, V., Yeager, K., Owen, D., Peterson, D., Lin, L., & Webster, J. (2000). Maintaining study validity in a changing clinical environment. *Nursing Research*, *49*(4), 231–235.

Michie, S., van Stralen, M., & West, R. (2011). The behaviour change wheel: A new method for characterising and designing behaviour change interventions. *Implementation Science*, *6*, 42.

Moore, G., Audrey, S., Barker, M., Bond, L., Bonell, C., Hardeman, W., Moore, L., O'Cathain, A., Tinati, T., Wight, D., & Baird, J. (2015). Process evaluation of complex interventions: *Medical research guidance*. *BMJ*, *350*, h1258.

Morden, A., Ong, B., Brooks, L., Jinks, C., Porcheret, M., Edwards, J., & Dziedzic, K. (2015). Introducing evidence through research "push": Using theory and qualitative methods. *Qualitative Health Research*, *25*(11), 1560–1575.

Morse, J. M. (2006). The scope of qualitatively derived clinical interventions. *Qualitative Health Research*, *16*(5), 591–593.

Morse, J., Penrod, J., & Hupcey, J. (2000). Qualitative outcome analysis: Evaluating nursing interventions for complex clinical phenomena. *Journal of Nursing Scholarship*, *32*(2), 125–130.

Naylor, M. D. (2003). Nursing intervention research and quality of care: Influencing the future of healthcare. *Nursing Research*, *52*(6), 380–385.

Nunziante, F., Tanzi, S., Alquati, S., Autelitano, C., Bedeschi, E., Bertocchi, E., Dragani, M., Simonazzi, D., Turola, E., Braglia, L., Masini, L., & Di Leo, S. (2021). Providing dignity therapy to patients with advanced cancer: A feasibility study within the setting of a hospital palliative care unit. *BMC Palliative Care*, *20*, 1–12.

Payne, K., & Thompson, A. J. (2015). Economic evaluations of complex interventions. In Richards, D., & Rahm Hallberg, I., (Eds.), *Complex interventions in health: An overview of research methods* (pp. 326–333). Routledge.

Pfadenhauer, L., Gerhardus, A., Mozygemba, K., Lysdahl, K. B., Booth, A., Hofmann, B., Wahlster, P., Polus, S., Burns, J., Brereton, L., Rehfuess, E., & Rehfuess, E. (2017). Making sense of complexity in context and implementation: The Context and Implementation of Complex Interventions (CICI) framework. *Implementation Science*, *12*(1), 21.

Rahm Hallberg, I. (2015). Knowledge for health care practice. In Richards, D., & Rahm Hallberg, I. (Eds.), *Complex interventions in health: An overview of research methods* (pp. 16–28). Routledge.

Richards, D. A. (2015a). The critical importance of patient and public involvement for research into complex interventions. In Richards, D., & Rahm Hallberg, I. (Eds.), *Complex interventions in health: An overview of research methods* (pp. 46–50). Routledge.

Richards, D. A. (2015b). A few final thoughts. In Richards, D., & Rahm Hallberg, I. (Eds.), *Complex interventions in health: An overview of research methods* (pp. 326–333). Routledge.

Richards, D. A., & Rahm Hallberg, I. (Eds.). (2015). *Complex interventions in health: An overview of research methods*. Routledge.

Sandelowski, M. (1996). Using qualitative methods in intervention studies. *Research in Nursing & Health*, *19*, 359–365.

Sermeus, W. (2015). Modelling process and outcomes in complex interventions. In Richards, D., & Rahm Hallberg, I. (Eds.), *Complex interventions in health: An overview of research methods* (pp. 111–126). Routledge.

Sidani, S. (2015). *Health intervention research: Understanding research design & methods*. Sage.

Sidani, S., & Braden, C. J. (2011). *Design, evaluation, and translation of nursing interventions*. Wiley-Blackwell.

Skivington, K., Matthews, L., Simpson, S. A., Craig, P., Baird, J., Blazeby, J. M., Boyd, K. A., Craig, N., French, D. P., McIntosh, E., Petticrew, M., Rycroft-Malone, J., White, M., & Moore, L. (2021). A new framework for developing and evaluating complex interventions: Update of Medical Research Council guidance. *BMJ*, *374*, n2061. https://doi.org/10.1136/bmj.n2061

Van Meijel, B., Gamel, C., van Swieten-Duijfjes, B., & Grypdonck, M. (2004). The development of evidence-based nursing interventions: Methodological considerations. *Journal of Advanced Nursing, 48*(1), 84–92.

Wight, D., Wimbush, E., Jepson, R., & Doi, L. (2016). Six steps in quality intervention development (6SQuID). *Journal of Epidemiology and Community Health, 70*(5), 520–525.

Yip, O., Huber, E., Stenz, S., Zullig, L. L., Zeller, A., De Geest, S. M., Deschodt, M., & INSPIRE consortium. (2021). A contextual analysis and logic model for integrated care for frail older adults living at home: The INSPIRE Project. *International Journal of Integrated Care, 21*(2), 9. https://doi.org/10.5334/ijic.5607

29 Feasibility and Pilot Studies of Interventions Using Mixed Methods

Learning Objectives

1. Distinguish the difference between a feasibility study and pilot study.
2. Articulate the purpose of pilot studies.
3. Understand the various objectives of pilot studies.
4. Appreciate the potential for "lessons learned" and how they can inform future work.
5. Elucidate the various methods used in pilot studies.
6. Realize the importance of publishing pilot work.

INTRODUCTION

In the Medical Research Council's (MRC) framework for complex interventions, as described in Chapter 28, mixed methods are used to develop a preliminary intervention (Craig et al., 2008). In the next phase, researchers assess whether the intervention, and ideas about rigorously testing it, make sense—that is, whether it is feasible, acceptable, and shows promise of positive effects.

There is considerable agreement in the healthcare literature that pilot studies are often poorly designed and reported. Until recently, there was little guidance on planning and conducting pilot work. Indeed, in their often cited "tutorial" on pilot studies, Thabane and colleagues (2010) stated with regard to coverage of pilot work in research methods textbooks, "We are not aware of any textbook that dedicates a chapter on this issue" (p. 2). We have remedied this situation by devoting this chapter to a discussion of feasibility assessments and pilot tests of interventions. Many other resources that offer excellent and cutting-edge advice for conducting pilot work have become available (e.g., Arain et al., 2010; Moore et al., 2011; Richards & Rahm Hallberg, 2015), and an open-access journal devoted to this topic (*Pilot and Feasibility Studies*) was inaugurated in 2015.

TIP Wisdom regarding the value of advance planning can be seen in many cultures. For example, a 10th century bowl with a Kufic inscription on display in the Metropolitan Museum of Art in New York bears a relevant Iranian proverb: "Planning before work protects you from regret." Another proverb comes from Africa: "Only a fool tests the depth of a river with both feet."

BASIC ISSUES IN PILOTING INTERVENTIONS

This section lays the groundwork for conducting successful pilot work, the focus of which is to address *uncertainties* about the intervention or the planned evaluation.

Definition of Pilot and Feasibility Studies

The term *pilot study* has been defined in dozens of ways in the research literature and the terms "pilot study" and "feasibility study" are often used interchangeably. An international panel of experts recently came to a consensus about definitions and interrelationships, as delineated in a recent conceptual framework (Eldridge et al., 2016).

According to the expert panel, pilot studies are a subset of feasibility studies. *Feasibility* is an overarching concept—all pilot studies are feasibility studies, but not all feasibility studies are pilots. A **feasibility study** addresses whether something can be done: Should the team proceed with a project and, if so, how? The broad category of feasibility study includes three types of studies: randomized pilot studies, nonrandomized pilot studies, and other feasibility studies that are not pilots.

A **pilot study** is designed to assess the feasibility of mounting an intervention, but also has a specific goal of testing, on a smaller scale, features of a larger, more definitive future study. Pilot studies are designed to support refinements of the protocols, methods, and procedures to be used in a larger scale trial of an intervention. The emphasis in pilot studies is on assessing the feasibility of an entire set of procedures for a full-scale evaluation, including recruitment, protocol implementation, data collection procedures, outcome measurement, blinding, and the capacity to avoid contamination across treatment groups. Some pilot studies involve a randomized design—for example, to test whether people are willing to be randomized to treatment groups. Other pilot studies adopt quasiexperimental designs. Taylor and colleagues (2015) offer suggestions for when a pilot study requires randomization.

The third type of feasibility study is what the expert panel called "other" feasibility studies—which in this chapter we will call *feasibility assessments*. Such studies are often undertaken to test specific and discrete aspects of a new intervention or potential trial. For example, a feasibility assessment might evaluate whether a 10-week intervention is feasible and acceptable. Or, a feasibility assessment might explore whether a sufficient number of sites can be enlisted to participate in a multisite trial. Feasibility studies do not focus on intervention outcomes, but rather examine parameters that are integral to the conduct of a full intervention trial. Feasibility assessments typically do not use a randomized design.

For some interventions, it might be necessary for researchers to undertake both a feasibility assessment and a pilot trial. Lessons learned in an early feasibility assessment might, for example, lead to further development work, as suggested in the MRC framework (Figure 28.1). In other cases, especially if there is a strong evidence base and a well-conceived intervention theory, a single pilot study might suffice.

The distinction between a feasibility assessment and a pilot study is important for researchers doing them—for example, a study should be properly labeled in seeking funding or in publishing findings. However, to streamline our presentation in this chapter, we will for the most part describe activities under a general rubric of *pilot work*. Pilot work is sometimes undertaken for nonintervention studies (e.g., for a large-scale survey), but in this chapter we focus on intervention research.

TIP Some writers distinguish between an internal and external pilot. An *external pilot* is a stand-alone study, the findings from which inform the design and implementation of a full RCT. An *internal pilot* is an early phase of a large trial and the findings are typically used to adjust sample size projections. In this chapter, we primarily discuss stand-alone (external) pilot work.

Overall Purpose of Pilot Work

The overall purpose of pilot work is to avoid a costly fiasco. Fully powered RCTs are extremely expensive. Without piloting, a full-scale trial can result in wasted resources and erroneous conclusions. A strong pilot can enhance the likelihood that a full test will be methodologically and conceptually sound, ethical, and informative. As mentioned in Chapter 28, there is growing concern about waste and inefficiency in healthcare research (e.g., Ioannidis, 2016), and pilots represent an important tool in combatting these problems in a responsible manner (Treweek & Born, 2014). Large-scale trials often cannot get funded without adequate pilot work.

> **TIP** Thousands of studies in the healthcare literature are described as "pilots," but many are inappropriately labeled—they are often simply small studies. The term should not be used unless there is an explicit goal of learning how best to design and implement a larger and more definitive study.

Recent guidance on pilot work has emphasized an important point that is often not appreciated by those conducting pilots: *the purpose of a pilot is not to test hypotheses about the efficacy of the intervention*. That is, a goal should *not* be to test the effectiveness of an intervention on key outcomes—and if statistical hypothesis tests are used in pilot work, they should be interpreted cautiously (Arain et al., 2010; Thabane et al., 2010). Given the small sample size of pilots, hypothesis tests are typically underpowered and result in effect size estimates that are unreliable. We discuss this issue again later in the chapter.

> **TIP** Moore and colleagues (2011) bemoaned the cycle of nonproductive work than can ensue when young researchers undertake a pilot, find nonsignificant results, abandon their ideas, and then pursue another topic. When hypothesis testing is a major objective of a pilot, disappointment is typically high, and results are often unreported.

Lessons From Pilot Work

An important product of pilot work is a description of the "lessons learned." Almost inevitably, the pilot will reveal that the intervention did not play out in "real life" the way it was designed "on paper." A review of published reports on lessons learned in pilot studies reveals some recurrent themes. The following are among the most frequently mentioned lessons from pilot intervention studies:

- Fewer people meet the eligibility criteria than anticipated
- Recruitment of participants is more difficult and takes longer than expected
- Materials intended for direct use by participants (e.g., pamphlets, educational materials) need to be simplified
- Participant burden, especially regarding data collection, needs to be reduced
- Effect sizes tend to be larger in the pilot than in the main trial
- Key ingredients of the intervention should be front-loaded—that is, delivered early—because greater attention and higher attendance occurs early
- When there is a control condition, diffusion and contamination are recurrent problems
- Even expert interventionists need to be trained (including researchers themselves)
- Relationships with others need to be continuously nurtured

Researchers who undertake pilot work should keep these lessons in mind and try to design their study in such a way that frequently occurring problems are avoided or minimized.

> **Example of an Important Lesson Learned in Pilot Work**
> Chidebe and Pratt-Chapman (2022) conducted a pilot study on online patient navigation training among Nigerian nurses, patient advocates, and cancer survivors, with the goal of improving the confidence and performance of core patient navigation tasks. Although the findings provided data to support the efficacy of the training, the authors also reported several lessons learned including the need for improved staff resources, better technology, and expert support for larger scale implementation.

OBJECTIVES AND CRITERIA IN PILOT WORK

Writers who offer advice about the conduct of feasibility and pilot studies almost invariably encourage researchers to carefully articulate explicit objectives. For any given pilot study, the specific objectives can be wide ranging. Thabane and colleagues (2010) organized pilot objectives into four broad categories: process, resources, management, and scientific. We use this organization to describe some objectives that are good targets for pilot work. Our examples are not exhaustive, but hopefully they will suggest ideas for how pilot work can inform decisions about a full trial of an intervention.

Process-Related Objectives

Process-related objectives focus on the feasibility of planned procedures for launching and maintaining the study. These include such issues as eligibility criteria, recruitment, retention, comprehension, adherence, acceptability, and ethics. Each objective can be addressed by gathering data to answer various questions, examples of which are shown in Table 29.1. As the table indicates, process-related objectives are often best addressed by collecting both quantitative and quantitative data. Pilot studies and feasibility assessments are a good way of investigating potential problems in mounting an intervention—and exploring ways to remedy those problems.

Although preliminary answers to some of the questions in Table 29.1 are sometimes obtained during intervention development, those answers often need to be confirmed. For example, there may be a big difference between patients saying they *would be* interested in an intervention and actually *agreeing* to participate. Moreover, a person might be willing to participate in an intervention but may *not* be willing to be randomized to a control group. Or, even if a person is willing and interested, motivation may wane over the course of a multisession intervention. Thus, development work alone cannot answer important questions about feasibility of an intervention implemented in real-world settings.

Pilot work can reveal the adequacy of the initial eligibility criteria and suggest how eligibility criteria affect recruitment, retention, and protocol adherence. Decisions about eligibility criteria must address numerous concerns, including substantive ones (Should some people be excluded because they might not benefit?), ethical ones (Might certain people be harmed?), methodologic ones (How will eligibility criteria be measured? Will the criteria yield an adequate pool for the full-scale trial?), and scientific ones (Will eligibility criteria constrain the generalizability of the findings?). Pilot data can be used to fine-tune decisions about eligibility and about the time needed to recruit a sufficiently large sample.

TIP Unrealistic optimism about the size of the pool of eligibles is common—indeed, it is so common that it has been given a name: *Lasagna law* (van der Wouden et al., 2007). Carlisle and colleagues (2015) found, in analyzing nearly 500 trials that had either terminated because of failed sample accrual or completed with a much smaller sample than intended, that unsuccessful accrual was strongly associated with having a high number of eligibility criteria.

A particularly important process issue concerns recruitment—not only of study participants, but also of sites and research staff. If a multisite trial is envisioned for the full RCT, the feasibility of enlisting cooperative sites should be explored early. It is not just an issue of getting enough sites to achieve an adequate sample size, but also of making sure that there are sites that represent the diversity of the target population of participants. Also, if exploration of sites suggests a high rate of refusals, researchers might want to explore what factors led to refusals by administrators—especially if those factors are relevant for the eventual uptake of the intervention, should the RCT reveal promising results. For example, if concerns about staff time are a key consideration, the intervention may have little hope of being translated on a large scale.

Recruitment of participants is a perennial problem in clinical trials and is becoming more challenging. For example, a study found that in publicly funded trials in the United Kingdom, 45% failed to reach the targeted sample size (Sully et al., 2013), and similar findings were reported by Walters et al. (2017). Quantitative data from pilot work can answer questions about the feasibility of recruiting a sufficient number for a full trial, but qualitative data may suggest how key barriers could be eliminated or how additional recruitment techniques could be pursued. Treweek (2015) offers useful advice about participant recruitment.

Poor retention of participants in the study and low protocol adherence (on the part of participants or intervention agents) are two other problems that are strong candidates for scrutiny in pilot work. Attrition can reduce the final sample size for

TABLE 29.1 • Examples of Process-Related Objectives and Questions for Pilot Work

OBJECTIVE	QUESTIONS (QUANTITATIVE)	QUESTIONS (QUALITATIVE)
Recruitment: To assess the feasibility of recruiting an adequate number of study participants	• How many people were screened for eligibility each week/month? • What percentage of eligible people agreed to participate (and what percentage actually did participate)? • How many eligibles are enrolled each week/month? • What are the characteristics of those who do vs. those who did not agree to participate? • How long did it take to recruit the needed sample?	• Why did eligibles decline to participate? What would make the intervention (or study participation) more appealing? Was randomization a factor in their decision? • What barriers exist in the research sites regarding successful recruitment? • Did certain recruitment strategies work well? Work poorly?
Eligibility Criteria: To assess the adequacy of the eligibility criteria	• How many eligible people are there in each site? What proportion of all clients/patients are eligible? • Which eligibility criterion was associated with the biggest loss of potential participants? • Was attrition from the pilot associated with a particular eligibility criterion?	• Were procedures for identifying eligibles clear and manageable? • Would loosening or tightening the eligibility criteria be acceptable to some stakeholders (e.g., family members)? Would it affect ease of recruitment?
Retention: To assess the ability to retain an adequate proportion of participants	• What percentage of initial study participants remained in the study as they moved through the trial? • Were there differences in attrition by study group (intervention vs. control)? • What were the characteristics of those who remained and those who did not? • At what point did attrition occur?	• Why did participants decide to withdraw from the study? • What factors in the research sites contributed to poor retention?
Protocol Adherence: To assess the degree to which participants adhere to protocols	• What percentage of participants got the full "dose" of the intervention? What "dose" of the intervention did the typical participant get? • What are the characteristics of those who adhered and those who did not? • Were there particular components for which adherence was especially poor?	• Why did participants not adhere to the intervention protocol (or not adhere to particular components)? • What factors in the research sites contributed to successful adherence?

(continued)

TABLE 29.1 • Examples of Process-Related Objectives and Questions for Pilot Work (Continued)

OBJECTIVE	QUESTIONS (QUANTITATIVE)	QUESTIONS (QUALITATIVE)
Acceptability: To assess the extent to which the intervention/research is acceptable to recipients and key stakeholders	• How satisfied were recipients (or other stakeholders) with the intervention, or with specific components of the intervention? • What percentage of recipients were allocated to their preferred treatment condition? • To what extent did recipients feel overburdened by the data collection demands?	• What did recipients/stakeholders like and dislike about the intervention? What changes to the intervention protocol would make it more acceptable? • What did recipients most dislike about research aspects (e.g., the amount of time needed, the frequency of data collection?)
Ethics: To assess the adequacy of human protections	Were there any breeches of human protections (e.g., privacy, confidentiality)?	Did participants feel that they their rights and privacy were adequately protected?

analyses and can also lead to biases in estimating the intervention's potential benefits. High attrition, low adherence to protocols, and low levels of satisfaction suggest that an intervention is not yet ready for a full RCT.

Ethical issues also can be explored during the pilot phase. In particular, researchers need to be vigilant during a pilot regarding any unanticipated ethical transgressions that would need to be remedied before a main trial could be undertaken. Pilots are also a good place to get feedback about the consent process. Several commentators have pointed out the absence of any special guidelines for the ethical conduct of pilot studies. There is some agreement, however, that researchers have an obligation to disclose the feasibility nature of pilot studies during informed consent procedures (Arain et al., 2010; Thabane et al., 2010).

Example of Pilot Work Addressing Process Objectives

Hoyt and colleagues (2023) developed and pilot tested a goal-focused Emotion-regulation Therapy (GET) and compared it to an active control intervention in young testicular cancer survivors. In comparing the two interventions, the acceptability, treatment fidelity, engagement, and tolerability of each intervention were considered. Primary efficacy outcomes were focused on the emotional symptoms of anxiety and depression from baseline to 3 months postintervention. Findings indicated that those in the GET arm vs. the control had similar intervention completion rates. Fidelity to the GET intervention was 87% and those in the GET arm experienced greater reductions in depressive and anxiety symptoms. This pilot work suggests the GET is an acceptable and feasible intervention for survivors of testicular cancer that can be tested further in larger trials.

Resource-Related Objectives

Pilot work is often a useful way to get a handle on the resources that would be needed in a full-scale trial. Resource objectives typically concern the following aspects of a study:

- Monetary costs
- Time demands
- Institutional capacity
- Personnel requirements and availability
- Other resource needs such as equipment, technology, and lab facilities

Tickle-Degnen (2013) provided some good examples of resource-related questions asked in a pilot study of a self-management intervention for patients with Parkinson disease. Here are a few of them: (1) Do we have the capacity to handle the desired number of participants? (2) Do we have phone and communication technology capacity to stay in touch with and coordinate participants? and (3) Do we have institutional willingness and capacity to carry through with project-related tasks and to support investigator time and effort?

A full-scale RCT of a complex intervention costs many thousands of dollars. A pilot study can help researchers develop a realistic budget for such a trial. It can also shed light on whether the costs of the intervention are likely to be commensurate with the benefits. Even at an early stage, researchers should consider whether it is realistic to pursue a costly trial for an intervention that is unlikely to be translated into real-world applications because of prohibitive costs or modest benefits.

> **Example of Pilot Work and Resource Objectives**
> Danesh and colleagues (2021) described lessons learned from pilot work that was focused on self-management strategies across several chronic conditions. One of the findings was related to maximizing the resources around time. The researchers suggest that delivering the intervention asynchronously or through teleconference would allow patients the flexibility to do the intervention on their schedule, which in turn would minimize the need for scheduling in-person visits, decrease time spent to attend, and increase access.

Management-Related Objectives

Another category of objectives for pilot work concerns the ability for the research team to manage the effort and work productively as a team. Pilot work can help to identify management "glitches" that should be addressed before moving on to a full-scale trial. The management-related objectives in pilot work include assessing feasibility in terms of the following:

- Viability of the site or sites
- Motivation and competence of project staff
- Adequacy of reporting, monitoring, technological, and other systems
- Ability to manage or nurture interpersonal relationships

In articles that have described "lessons learned" from pilot work, a recurrent theme is that interpersonal relationships can create problems. These can be the result of tensions among staff, between staff and management, and between staff and study participants or their family members. Researchers have found that it is often useful to give various stakeholders a sense of ownership, and an opportunity to make suggestions or air complaints.

In the previously mentioned paper on pilot work for a self-management intervention for patients with Parkinson disease, Tickle-Degnen (2013) addressed various feasibility questions relating to management objectives. For example, what are the challenges and strengths of the investigators' administrative capacity to: (1) Manage the planned RCT? (2) Design systems to document participant progress through the trial? (3) Enter data and perform quality checks? and (4) Manage the ethical aspects of the trial?

Scientific-Related Objectives: Substantive Issues

Scientific objectives are the fourth category in Thabane and colleagues' (2010) classification system. For this crucial class of objectives, we discuss two subcategories. The first set of scientific objectives is substantive, concerning the intervention itself. The second set of scientific objectives is methodologic, concerning the feasibility of rigorously testing the intervention. In this section, we discuss substantive scientific objectives for pilot work.

Intervention Attributes

A pilot test provides an opportunity to evaluate whether the decisions made during the development phase regarding intervention content, dose, timing, setting, sequencing, and so on were sensible ones (Feeley & Cossette, 2015). A pilot study is an ideal time to revise the intervention protocols, based on feedback from participants and intervention staff and on such indicators as attendance and attrition.

Safety and Tolerability

Assessing the safety of patients in trials of a new intervention and the tolerability of the intervention are crucial objectives of many pilot studies. Unfortunately, it is widely acknowledged that pilots do a poor job of providing reliable safety and tolerability data because of small sample sizes. For example, in a pilot with 30 patients, observing no adverse events does not necessarily mean that there are no safety risks.

Leon and colleagues (2011) advised that group-specific adverse events rates in pilots should be reported, with 95% confidence intervals. They further recommended that when no adverse event is observed, the *rule of three* should be used to estimate the upper bound of the 95% CI. This "rule" uses as the upper bound the value of $3/n$. Thus, if there are 30 participants per group, and zero adverse events are observed in the intervention group, the 95% CI for the adverse event rate for that group would be estimated as 0% to 10% (3/30 = 10). Such a calculation, which suggests the possibility that one out of 10 participants could experience an adverse event, illustrates the tenuous nature of pilot data relating to safety and tolerability.

It is nevertheless important to monitor safety and tolerability if the intervention has potential for even minor adverse events such as fatigue or dizziness. Moreover, as noted by Leon et al. (2011), pilots are useful for testing the adequacy of safety monitoring systems. Pilots may also suggest the desirability of requiring permission to participate in the trial from participants' physicians. Feedback from participants about perceptions of safety and tolerability is also very useful for evaluating potential safety problems.

Example of Pilot Work and Safety Assessment
Saleem et al. (2021) aimed to assess the role of mindful organizing on the impact of workforce agility and Malaysian nurses' safety behavior. Findings indicate that workforce agility is a possible predictor of mindful organizing. Mindful organizing had a significant impact on safety compliance, a positive impact on safety participation, and was positively associated with safety performance.

Intervention Efficacy

Most pilot studies are undertaken with the objective of gaining preliminary evidence of the intervention's potential to be beneficial. As previously noted, hypothesis testing is not considered appropriate in pilot tests because of the high risk of making a Type II error (i.e., falsely concluding that the intervention is not effective, even when it was).

Effect size (ES) estimates provide information about the potential of an intervention to achieve beneficial effects on key outcomes, but extreme caution is needed in interpreting pilot ES results. We illustrate the problem by presenting 95% confidence intervals around effect size estimates (d) of different magnitude for various sample sizes that are common in pilot studies (Table 29.2). As a reminder, the effect size d is computed by dividing the difference between two group means (i.e., intervention and control group postintervention means on an outcome) by the pooled standard deviation. For example, suppose that in a pilot study with 40 participants (20 per group) we calculated d for the primary outcome to be 0.50, which is a moderately strong ES. As Table 29.2 indicates, in this scenario there is a 95% probability that the *true* effect size lies somewhere between −0.13 (i.e., the intervention is mildly detrimental) and +1.13 (i.e., the intervention is extremely beneficial). Increasing the sample size decreases the width of the estimated range and thus offers stronger evidence of the intervention's potential effectiveness. For example, with a sample size of 100 pilot participants (50 per group), the 95% CI for a d of 0.50 ranges from 0.10 (mildly favorable) to 0.90 (strongly favorable). (As we discuss later, a 95% CI is considered by some experts to be too stringent for pilot work, although it is the conventional standard.) The pilot effect size should at least be encouraging. For example, an obtained d of 0.02 is unlikely to instill confidence about the intervention's benefits.

Because the objective in a pilot is to obtain preliminary (and not definitive) evidence of the intervention's potential benefits, researchers should use additional methods to draw conclusions about an intervention's effects. In-depth interviews with program participants and intervention agents concerning their perceptions of benefits or disappointments are an especially important means of augmenting statistical results. For example, the plausibility of weak beneficial effects (based on the lower limit of the confidence limit) can sometimes be challenged through participants' feedback about the intervention's value to them. If there is a consistent pattern of positive ES estimates for several key outcomes, and if there is corroborating qualitative data, researchers may be well poised to conclude that intervention efficacy is promising.

> **Example of Pilot Work and Effect Size Estimates**
> Brislane and colleagues (2021) conducted a pilot study testing the impact of structured exercise on 18 healthy pregnant women. The women were assigned to either a control group or a moderate intensity exercise group. Their findings provided data on the effect size estimates for change in maternal and offspring vascular structures as well as estimates for sample size for future trials.

> **TIP** Major changes to the intervention based on pilot work (e.g., to the intervention content or dose) may put into question the accuracy of the pilot effect size as an estimate of what would be obtained in a full trial.

Clinical Significance

Another possible objective for pilot work is an early assessment of the intervention's clinical significance. At the group level, effect size estimates are often used to draw conclusions about clinical significance, as discussed in Chapter 21. This means that the researchers should establish in advance the size of the effect that would be regarded as clinically significant. The criterion could be based on a consensus reached by an advisory panel. Arnold and colleagues (2009) advised that an intervention can be declared to have potential efficacy if the 95% CI around the estimated effect size includes a predesignated minimal for clinical significance. However, given the width of 95% CIs when the sample is small, this may be too liberal a standard. For example, with a sample of 50 pilot participants (25 per group), and a criterion of 0.50 for a clinically significant d, even an obtained d of 0.00 would meet this criterion (95% CI = −0.57 to + 0.57). Thus, it might be more prudent for the advisory group to establish not only the criterion for clinical significance, but also the acceptable range. For example, if the criterion were 0.50, experts might set the lower bound for clinical significance at an ES of 0.20.

As described in Chapter 21, there is another approach to evaluating clinical significance. If the primary outcome is one with an established MIC (minimal important change) benchmark, the percentage of participants who achieved a clinically significant change can be computed. Even in the absence of statistical significance, if a sizable percentage of intervention recipients had clinically meaningful improvement, this could support the conclusion that the intervention showed promise.

Scientific-Related Objectives: Methodologic Issues

Scientific objectives encompass not only substantive concerns about the intervention, but also methodologic concerns about the feasibility of undertaking a rigorous controlled trial. This section focuses on pilot objectives relating to the methods of testing a new intervention.

Research Design

Preliminary evidence about feasibility can be obtained in feasibility assessments using fairly simple designs, such as a one-group pretest–posttest design. However, for a pilot study, the design ideally should be a trial run of the full-scale test. Many experts recommend that a pilot study use a randomized design rather than a quasiexperimental one to gain confidence that an RCT of the full trial is feasible (e.g., Conn et al., 2010; Thabane et al., 2010). As noted by Leon and colleagues (2011), the inclusion of a randomized control group in a pilot study "allows for a more realistic examination of recruitment, randomization, implementation of intervention, blinded assessment procedures, and retention" (p. 627).

A crucial issue in randomized trials is whether there is any contamination between the treatment groups. Pilot trials provide a good opportunity to assess whether any cointerventions could inflate intervention benefits (if those in the intervention receive them) or dilute benefits (if control group members receive them).

Intervention Fidelity

Pilot studies offer researchers the opportunity to examine whether intervention agents can successfully implement the intervention as planned.

Researchers also can assess the adequacy of intervention fidelity procedures for the full trial. Both quantitative and qualitative data play an important role in helping researchers understand how successful the implementation of the intervention was, and identify barriers to full enactment of the intervention protocols. Quantitative data can be used to calculate actual rates of achieving fidelity, and qualitative data can help researchers understand factors that made fidelity difficult to accomplish.

Example of Pilot Work and Intervention Fidelity
Pedersen et al. (2022) conducted a pilot study to test the feasibility and implementation fidelity of a walking program (WALK-Copenhagen) for hospitalized older adult medical patients during hospitalization. Fidelity of the intervention was measured through observing the delivery of the six components of the intervention. Findings suggested three of the six intervention components were only partially implemented as planned and three were not implemented.

Data Collection Protocols and Instruments

Researchers make many decisions about data collection instruments and procedures for intervention studies, and a pilot trial offers researchers an opportunity to assess those decisions. Data quality and participant burden are two key areas of inquiry. A pilot provides an opportunity to examine patterns of missing data, to evaluate internal consistency of any scales, to assess participant comprehension, to explore variability in responses, and to estimate how much time is required to administer the research instruments. Given the evidence that people often drop out of studies because of a burdensome schedule of data collection, it is important to understand the practicality of proposed methods. Lengthy data collection instruments are not only risky in terms of attrition, but also have cost implications for data collection staff, data entry, and analysis. The pilot study might lead researchers to eliminate one or more outcomes, to select shorter instruments, or to alter the schedule for measuring outcomes. Van Teijlingen and Hundley (2001) offer explicit advice about pilot testing instruments for use in a full-scale study.

Sample Size

Many pilot studies are conducted to inform sample size decisions for the main trial, but using a pilot effect size in a power analysis is risky. A large pilot effect size (e.g., $d = 0.80$) could reflect an inflated positive result. If this d were used as the estimated effect size in a power analysis, it likely would result in an underpowered full-scale trial, and the sample size projection would be too small. On the other hand, small pilot ES estimates could reflect a Type II error and could lead to a decision to abandon a potentially promising intervention.

> **TIP** Vickers (2003) found that many trials published in four major medical journals were considerably underpowered when sample size needs were estimated based on a pilot trial. He found, for example, that about one out of four of the full-scale trials needed five times as many participants as had been estimated.

Several approaches to this problem have been proposed. One is to calculate confidence intervals around the pilot ES and then use the lower limit of the CI in the power calculations. However, because the 95% CI results in a range that is unreasonably large with small pilot samples (Table 29.2), less conservative CIs have been suggested, such as an 80% CI (Cocks & Torgerson, 2013; Lancaster et al., 2004), a 75% CI (Lee et al., 2014), or a 68% CI (Hertzog, 2008).

As an example, suppose that in a pilot study with 30 participants (15 per group), we estimated the pilot ES as $d = 0.50$. As shown in Table 29.2, the 95% CI around 0.50 for this sample size ranges from −0.23 to +1.23. However, the 80% CI around a d of 0.50 ranges from −0.03 to 0.97, and the 68% CI ranges from 0.12 to +0.88. Using the lower limit for d of 0.12, the needed sample size for the final trial would still be prohibitive—over 1,000 subjects per group for power = 0.80 and alpha = 0.05 for a two-tailed test.

In many cases, researchers can draw on additional evidence to support their sample size projections. For example, if there were consistent evidence from trials of similar interventions that group differences on the primary outcome would

TABLE 29.2 • 95% Confidence Intervals[a] Around d, for Various Ns and ds

D	N = 20 10 PER GROUP	N = 30 15 PER GROUP	N = 40 20 PER GROUP	N = 50 25 PER GROUP	N = 60 30 PER GROUP	N = 100 50 PER GROUP
0.20	−0.69 to 1.09	−0.53 to 0.93	−0.43 to 0.83	−0.37 to 0.77	−0.32 to 0.72	−0.20 to 0.60
0.30	−0.59 to 1.19	−0.43 to 1.03	−0.33 to 0.93	−0.27 to 0.87	−0.22 to 0.82	−0.10 to 0.70
0.40	−0.49 to 1.29	−0.33 to 1.13	−0.23 to 1.03	−0.17 to 0.97	−0.12 to 0.92	0.00 to 0.80
0.50	−0.39 to 1.39	−0.23 to 1.23	−0.13 to 1.13	−0.07 to 1.07	−0.02 to 1.02	0.10 to 0.90
0.60	−0.29 to 1.49	−0.13 to 1.33	−0.03 to 1.23	0.03 to 1.17	0.08 to 1.12	0.20 to 1.00
0.70	−0.19 to 1.59	−0.03 to 1.43	0.07 to 1.33	0.13 to 1.27	0.18 to 1.22	0.30 to 1.10

[a]Approximation of 95% CI using formula provided in (Leon et al., 2011): $d + (4 \div \sqrt{N})$; assumes two groups of equal size.

favor the intervention group, we might be willing to use a one-tailed test. This would result in a needed sample size of about 850 per group for the main trial for an estimated d of +0.12.

Additional avenues for deriving sample size estimates can be pursued when there is evidence from trials of similar interventions. To continue with our example of an observed $d = 0.50$ from our pilot, suppose there were three prior RCTs of a similar intervention. In these trials, the values of d were 0.26, 0.34, and 0.42 for the same primary outcome (e.g., pain)—values that all fall within the 95% CI of our pilot d of 0.50. We could argue that triangulating the evidence provides the best basis for estimating sample size requirements for a full-scale RCT. We might choose to use $d = 0.26$ (because it is the most conservative of the four estimates); or we might elect to use $d = 0.34$ (if the study with that ES was the most rigorous); or we might use $d = 0.38$ (the average of the four trials, including our own pilot). (Essentially, this is analogous to conducting a crude mini meta-analysis.) For a two-tailed test, these decisions would result in projected sample size needs of 233, 136, and 109, respectively, per group. If we had simply used our $d = 0.50$ in a power analysis, our projected sample size needs would have been 63 per group, which very well could have resulted in an underpowered full trial and a Type II error with nonsignificant results. On the other hand, if we had used $d = 0.12$ (the lower bound of the 68% CI around 0.50), we likely would not have pursued a full trial because it would have required a total sample size of over 2,000 participants.

A supplementary strategy is to factor in clinical significance in the power calculations (Kraemer et al., 2006). The rationale is that if the intervention cannot achieve benefits that are significant clinically, it may not matter that the trial is underpowered. Thus, in our example, suppose the judgment of the research team or an advisory group is that the effect size would need to be at least 0.40 to be clinically significant. In other words, there is a consensus that an ES of 0.40 is the threshold below which clinicians are unlikely to be interested in the intervention. If we used $d = 0.40$, the estimated sample size for the full trial would be about 100 per group for a two-group design. Based on our pilot results, an ES of 0.40 is plausibly attainable because it falls well within a 95% CI for a d of 0.50. And its attainability is supported by the results from another trial of a similar intervention in which $d = 0.42$ was obtained.

In short, the most defensible strategy for sample size calculation is to consider a totality of evidence to estimate the size of the effect that is plausibly attainable and clinically meaningful in a main test. More detailed and sophisticated guidance is provided by Ukoumunne et al. (2015) and Bell et al. (2018).

Criteria and Pilot Objectives

We have presented a wide range of objectives as potentially relevant in pilot work for interventions. Clearly, no pilot or feasibility study can address all the objectives we described. It is crucial to identify the objectives of the pilot work in advance, however, because important design and data collection decisions for the pilot depend on what the objectives are.

We recommend that researchers select pilot objectives based on several considerations. First, choose objectives for which information is genuinely lacking—that is, objectives that address key *uncertainties*. You may already have a good estimate of how much attrition to expect, for example, based on your own previous work with the target population or based on attrition rates in other similar trials. Second, select objectives that impinge most significantly on the feasibility of a full-scale trial. For example, if you cannot recruit a sufficient number of participants for the pilot, a large trial may be impossible. Thus, assessing and enhancing recruitment would be important objectives. And third, focus on objectives about which funders will be particularly vigilant. These might include recruitment and efficacy, for example, and might also include resource requirements.

The importance of articulating key pilot objectives stems from the fact that pilot work should lead to a decision about "next steps." Essentially, there are three options. One decision would be to proceed to a full clinical trial. A second decision would be to revise the intervention protocols, methodologic protocols, or procedural processes. The decision to make changes might lead to further Phase I (developmental) work, and perhaps to a second pilot if the revisions are major. A third decision would be to abandon the entire effort because of poor prospects of feasibility or lack of adequate evidence that the intervention could be effective.

How do researchers make the critical decision about what course to take next? One widely advocated approach is to articulate not only objectives but also the criteria for making decisions (e.g., Arain et al., 2010; Arnold et al., 2009; Thabane et al., 2010). Prior to launching the pilot, the research team should formulate threshold criteria for claiming the feasibility of a full-scale RCT.

TIP An alternative (or supplementary) approach to decision-making after a pilot study has been suggested by Bugge and colleagues (2013). Their framework involves a systematic analysis of pilot problems and assessments of possible solutions.

Table 29.3 provides examples of pilot objectives and criteria for drawing conclusions about the feasibility of a full trial. As these examples suggest, the quantitative criteria can be expressed either as raw numbers or as rates. For example, the second and third entries in this table focus on the objective of assessing recruitment in the pilot. In objective #2, the benchmark for success involves having a certain percentage of all eligible people agreeing to participate in the pilot (in this example, 60%). In objective #3, by contrast, recruitment success is defined as getting a specific number of eligible people each week to agree to participate in the pilot.

The criteria would be based on judgments of the research team, but the judgments ideally would be informed by evidence gathered during the development phase (e.g., based on recruitment rates from other similar trials). The criteria should achieve a balance between what is ideal (e.g., 100% recruitment success) and what is realistic. Proposed criteria often can best be developed with the aid of an advisory group of experts and stakeholders. We emphasize that the criteria included in Table 29.3 are only *examples*—they should not be adopted literally without considering the actual context of pilot work, including the nature of the intervention, the site, and the target population.

Articulating criteria for the pilot's success makes decision-making about "next steps" easier. In the recruitment example, if only 30% of eligible patients in the pilot agreed to participate, the next step probably should not be to move forward to a full trial. Exploratory (qualitative) inquiry might help to reveal why the recruitment effort went awry. Perhaps different recruitment techniques are needed, perhaps the intervention or the research is too burdensome, or perhaps the eligibility criteria need to be adjusted. Without criteria for a pilot's success, researchers may be tempted to overinterpret their pilot data in the desired direction and move forward to a full trial before it is wise to do so.

The decision about "next steps" is likely to depend on how many criteria are not met, and the degree of deficiency in meeting them. For example, a 30% recruitment rate when 60% or higher was the benchmark might lead to major rethinking of the project, but a 50% recruitment rate might lead to adjustments to enhance recruitment. If identified problems cannot readily be rectified, then researchers might be forced to "go back to the drawing board" in efforts to address a clinical problem.

The decision to move forward to a full trial should be a carefully considered one. In preparing a proposal to fund a rigorous RCT, the research team should be persuaded that: (1) the intervention and the research methods are feasible; (2) any pitfalls for a rigorous test have been identified and solutions to potential problems have been identified; (3) there is preliminary evidence that the intervention will be effective; and (4) important stakeholders are "on board."

Example of Stakeholder Issues
Motl et al. (2022) reviewed findings from clinical trials on exercise and physical activity interventions for people with multiple sclerosis and provided expert opinion on lessons learned. They report that much of the work area is done in tightly controlled settings, but the further implementation does not translate well to other settings (e.g., long-term care, home settings make larger trials challenging). This presents as a stakeholder issue.

THE DESIGN AND METHODS OF PILOT STUDIES

In this section, we offer recommendations relating to the design and conduct of pilot work.

Research Design in Pilot Work

We encourage using a randomized design for a pilot trial, especially if the plan is to use the pilot as the basis for requesting funding for a full-scale trial. To the extent possible, all design features for the full trial should be tested, including the control group strategy, procedures for blinding, outcome measures, and the schedule of data collection. Arnold and colleagues (2009) have suggested that it might be constructive to conduct a pilot trial in multiple sites. A multisite pilot gives project managers experience in multisite supervision.

In a feasibility assessment, simpler designs are usually adequate. Simple descriptive designs may suffice—for example, if a major goal is to assess the number of eligible people or to estimate how many sites could be recruited. One-group designs are often used to assess aspects of the intervention itself, such as whether participants find the intervention acceptable.

It is advantageous to use mixed methods (MM) designs in pilot work, because feasibility questions concern not only whether key objectives can be met, but also why they might have fallen short. Thus, in many cases, the appropriate design for a pilot trial will be either concurrent MM designs (e.g., QUAN + qual or QUAN + QUAL) or sequential ones (e.g., QUAN → qual or QUAN → QUAL).

Example of a Research Design for a Pilot Study
Akinci and colleagues (2022) conducted a pilot study using a single-blind randomized controlled trial design. The aim of the study was to test the feasibility and safety of a Qigong intervention in physically inactive adults. Thirty-four participants were randomly assigned to either an asynchronous online format or a video-conference-based approach. The primary outcomes related to the feasibility were the retention rate and attendance rate. Safety was determined by self-report of injury during the intervention period. Other measures include satisfaction, sleep, stress anxiety, physical activity, and a 1-minute sit-to-stand test. No safety concerns were reported in either group. Each group met the threshold for attendance of 15 out of 18 sessions, but the asynchronous online video attended all 18 sessions. Retention rates indicate that the online rate was 100% and the video conference rate was 88.2%.

Sampling in Pilot Work

The sample used in pilot work should be drawn from the same population as that for the main trial. This means that the eligibility criteria should be the same—although these criteria might be adjusted during the pilot if researchers run into unanticipated problems.

The sample size for pilot studies is typically small. Hertzog (2008) examined pilot studies that had been funded by the National Institute of Nursing Research between 2002 and 2004 and found that for studies with two-group designs, the median number of participants per group was about 25. Billingham and colleagues (2013) did an audit of 79 pilot clinical studies in the United Kingdom and found that the median sample size per group in publicly funded trials was 33.

Several experts have suggested using confidence intervals around feasibility outcomes to estimate the sample size needed in the pilot (Arnold et al., 2009; Hertzog, 2008; Thabane et al., 2010). For example, suppose we decided that a full-scale trial would be feasible if the rate of attrition from the study was no more than 20% at a 3-month follow-up. Based on evidence from other similar trials or Phase I development work, we predict that the *actual* rate of attrition will be 12%. If we used a confidence interval of 95% around the expected rate of 12%, we would need a total sample size of 64 for the upper bound of the confidence interval not to exceed the criterion of 20% attrition (95% CI around 12% = 4% to 20% for $N = 64$). If we relaxed our standard to a less stringent 90% CI for the same scenario, the needed total sample size for the pilot would be 46 (90% CI around 12% = 4% to 20% for $N = 46$).

The ideal sample size for a pilot will vary from study to study because of differences in objectives and populations. Bell and colleagues (2018) provide "rules of thumb" for pilot size as a function of the targeted effect size. For example, if the target effect size is a *d* between 0.10 and 0.30 for an 80% powered main trial, they recommend a sample of 20 per arm in the pilot, but if the target *d* is greater than 0.70, a sample of 10 per arm would suffice. Hertzog (2008), however, has recommended a pilot size of at least 30 to 40 per group if funding for the pilot is being sought.

Data Collection in Pilot Work

The data collection plan for pilots is typically complex, because the pilot data serve two purposes: to test the viability of the instruments that would be used in the main trial and to address the various objectives of the pilot itself.

In terms of the second purpose, the type of data to be collected depends on the objectives. For example, if a key objective is to assess the acceptability of the intervention (Table 29.3), then a quantitative measure of participant satisfaction would be needed.

Detailed documentation about the trial and its progress should be maintained to help illuminate what went right and what went wrong. It is useful to keep a diary or journal to record impressions and observations about the pilot experience. Diary entries are probably best organized thematically rather than chronologically. For example, journal sections could be devoted to each pilot objective. Entries for each objective should be made at least weekly.

Thought needs to be given to how best to "get inside" the workings of the pilot through the collection of in-depth data. This is likely to include unstructured observations of various intervention activities (e.g., recruitment, consent procedures, intervention sessions). Participants in both the intervention and control groups could be asked to complete **exit interviews.** Focus group interviews could also be conducted with various stakeholders, including participants, family members, and pilot study staff.

Example of Data Collection in a Pilot Trial
Flanagan, one of the authors of this textbook, and colleagues (2022) conducted a pilot study to test the feasibility of a nurse-coached walking intervention for informal caregivers of people with dementia. They collected quantitative data to gather data on recruitment, attrition, user ease of the technology, fidelity, adherence, and effect size. They collected qualitative data to understand participants' experience related to the pedometer use and nurse coaching.

Data Analysis in Pilot Work

The analysis of quantitative data from a pilot study focuses mainly on the pilot objectives and, therefore, tends to involve mainly descriptive statistics. For example, the analysis might indicate what percentage of eligible people agreed to participate or consented to be randomized. Means and *SD*s are likely to be calculated (e.g., mean number of

TABLE 29.3 • Examples of Pilot Objectives and Criteria for Success

OBJECTIVE	CRITERION	MEASUREMENT
1. To assess the willingness of the site to screen prospective participants for eligibility	At least 50 patients per month will be screened for eligibility	Number of patients screened per month (and, possibly, number of patients not screened)
2. To assess the feasibility of recruiting study participants	60% of eligible people will agree to participate	Number agreeing to participate, divided by all eligibles
3. To assess the feasibility of recruiting study participants	At least three participants per week will be successfully recruited at each study site	Number of people agreeing to participate, per site
4. To assess the willingness of people to sign consent forms and be randomized	95% of people who agree to participate will be randomized to a treatment group	Number randomized, divided by number originally agreeing to participate
5. To assess the initiation of the intervention in a timely manner	90% of the people randomized to the intervention group will begin within 7 d of randomization	Number beginning the intervention within 7 d of randomization, divided by total number randomized
6. To assess adherence to the intervention	80% of those in the intervention group will complete at least 8 of the 10 intervention sessions	Number completing 8+ sessions, divided by the number randomized to the intervention
7. To assess the efficiency of the data collection protocols	90% of participants will complete the data collection package in <30 min	Number completing package within 30 min, divided by all completing the package
8. To assess trial retention rates	80% of participants in both study groups will complete 3-mo follow-up instruments	Number of people in each group completing 3-mo follow-ups, divided by number randomized to each group
9. To assess the intervention's acceptability	75% of participants will say they are "satisfied" or "completely satisfied" with the intervention	Number of patients who are satisfied, divided by number of intervention participants
10. To assess the preliminary efficacy of the intervention	Lower limit of the 68% confidence interval (CI) around the value of d will be at least 0.20	Lower limit of d for 68% CI around obtained d
11. To assess the clinical significance of the intervention	40% of those in the intervention group will have a reduction of 8+ cm on a visual analog scale (VAS) for pain (the minimal important change [MIC]) at 3 mo postbaseline	Number in the intervention group whose follow-up VAS pain score is > 8 cm lower than that at baseline, divided by the number randomized to the intervention group

sessions completed, mean length of time to complete the data collection forms). Effect size estimates may also be computed. In most of these cases, it is a good idea to compute confidence intervals around estimates. An upfront decision should be made about the desired level of precision (e.g., 68%, 80%, etc.).

It has been argued that researchers should pay more attention to individual results in pilot studies than to group averages. Shih and colleagues (2004), for example, suggest that the emphasis should be on testing whether *any* person experienced a beneficial effect, and provided statistical guidance for such an approach. One method is to assess whether, for each person, a reliable improvement has occurred (Chapter 15), or whether clinically significant change has occurred in a *responder analysis* (Chapter 21). If the main outcomes are ones for which MIC benchmarks have not been established, the research team can decide how large an improvement is needed to be deemed meaningful.

The results of the quantitative data analysis from pilots can be used to guide decisions about how to proceed, based on a comparison of the results to the pre-established criteria. Analysis of the qualitative can confirm the wisdom of that decision and can also help researchers make modifications to improve the likelihood that a full trial will be successful in giving the intervention a fair test.

PRODUCTS OF PILOT WORK

Pilot work should result in several products. As previously noted, one product should be a description of "lessons learned," which ideally would be drafted and reviewed by the research team, advisory panel, and key stakeholders for accuracy and completeness. Other products may include the following:

- Revised protocols for the intervention, its implementation, and the research plan (or, if major revisions are needed, a plan for further descriptive and exploratory research)
- A finalized list of outcomes
- A formal proposal for a full Phase III trial (or for another pilot) and a plan for seeking funding
- A written manuscript for publication in a professional journal

There has been considerable discussion about the desirability—and the obligation—of publishing results from pilots (e.g., Conn et al., 2010; Thabane et al., 2010). Moore and colleagues (2011) lamented that some researchers fail to publish pilot results because they "didn't find anything" (p. 3). This may well be the conclusion of researchers who focus on hypothesis tests of the intervention's efficacy, which are often nonsignificant. However, as we have discussed in this chapter, the main purpose of pilot work is *not* to test the statistical significance of intervention effects, but to assess the feasibility of a full-scale rigorous trial.

Even if a pilot trial suggests that the intervention has little hope of being effective, that knowledge should be shared. Others working on the same or a similar problem can benefit from learning about failures as well as successes. A related issue is the importance of including findings from pilots in meta-analyses and systematic reviews, especially if the pilot does not translate into a full trial. As we discuss in Chapter 30, meta-analysts struggle with the issue of *publication bias*—that is, the tendency of researchers to publish studies only when there are statistically significant results. Such a tendency does a disservice to evidence-based practitioners who are then using a biased subset of the evidence.

Several commentators have also noted that there is an ethical obligation to communicate the results from a pilot (e.g., Thabane et al., 2010; van Teijlingen et al., 2001). The argument is that participants have agreed to volunteer their time for an endeavor they believed would be helpful scientifically, and researchers fail to fulfill their end of the bargain if the findings are not shared. Moreover, precious research funds spent on pilots are wasted if the results are not published so that others can learn from what was done.

The quality of reporting of pilot studies has been criticized by many recent writers. Reports should clearly state the objectives of the pilot, as well the criteria used to make decisions about next steps. Given that the emerging advice on pilot testing is relatively new, researchers may have to "educate" reviewers and journal editors about the focus on feasibility objectives and not on hypothesis testing, citing the leading experts' advice about the risks of interpreting p values in pilots.

> **TIP** Researchers sometimes wonder if the data from an external pilot can be pooled with the data from a main study—in other words, treating the pilot participants as the early participants in the larger trial. This practice is considered acceptable only if there have been no changes in the intervention or study protocols, and if the population is the same. This is not likely to be the case in most circumstances. Lancaster et al. (2004) discuss the biases that can result from the practice of pooling data from the pilot into a main trial.

CRITICAL APPRAISAL OF FEASIBILITY AND PILOT STUDIES

Reports of pilot studies should provide descriptions of the study methods (e.g., the design, sampling and data collection plans, and so on). The intervention theory and development of the intervention should be explained, or a reference should be provided to any previously published papers on intervention development work. Readers should be able to draw their own conclusions about the potential feasibility and efficacy of the intervention, and so information about the key features of the intervention itself needs to be included.

A critical appraisal of pilot work should focus on the researchers' description of the pilot objectives, the criteria used to make decisions about feasibility, and the methods associated with the assessments. Readers should question the omission of explicitly stated objectives. If objectives and criteria were reported, readers can assess their reasonableness and judge whether the methods used to test them were adequate.

We have stressed that the small sample sizes of pilot trials make hypothesis testing for intervention efficacy a risky business. However, we do not recommend that pilot studies be criticized for including such information. Many journals expect such analyses, and editors may reject manuscripts that do not report them. Confidence intervals around the point estimates for outcomes or around effect size estimates would ideally be provided. However, if a pilot study does report the results of hypothesis testing, the researchers should be cautious in their interpretation of the results. Whether the results are statistically significant or not, the researchers should warn readers that the results are preliminary and that the sample size precludes definitive conclusions.

Box 29.1 offers some questions that can be used to appraise a report of a pilot study. The overarching question is whether the researchers were successful in securing the data needed to make a decision about what the next steps should be.

EXAMPLE OF A PILOT TRIAL

Study: A Group Videogame-Based Physical Activity Program Improves Walking Speed in Older Adults Living with a Serious Mental Illness (Leutwyler et al., 2022).

Statement of Purpose: The purpose of this study was to describe the impact of a pilot videogame-based physical activity program on walking speed in older adults with serious mental illness (SMI).

Research Design and Methods: A one group pre- and posttest design was used. Participants were recruited from mental health programs in the community. All participants had to be able to provide capacity to consent. The protocol called for the participants to play a video game for 50 minutes 3 times a week for 10 weeks.

Measures: In addition to clinical and sociodemographic data, measures included overall mobility as measured by the Short Physical Performance Battery (SPPB), and walking speed, which was assessed by a timed 3-minute walk test. Measures were taken at baseline and at 5 and 10 weeks.

Results: The group's mean score for the walking speed over the 10-week period was 0.10 m/s (BC CI LL = 0.04, UL = 0.15). This finding was clinically and statistically significant ($p \leq 0.05$). The SPPB score increased on average 0.06 points (BC CI LL = −0.01, UL = 0.12) over the entire 10-week study period, but this was not clinically or statistically significant.

Discussion and Implications: Walking speed is an important measure of cardiometabolic fitness. People

BOX 29.1 Guidelines for Critically Appraising Aspects of Pilot Work

1. Did the title and abstract of the paper describe the study as a pilot or feasibility study? Which term was used? Was the term "pilot" used appropriately—or was the study simply a small-scale or exploratory study with no mention of its role as part of a larger-scale effort?
2. Did the report state the explicit objectives of the study? Were specific feasibility outcomes identified, and was a description of how they were measured provided?
3. If objectives were stated, were they ones that would provide important knowledge about the design and conduct of a full-scale trial? Were potentially important objectives overlooked? Were too many objectives tested?
4. Did the researchers state the criteria that would be used as a basis for decision-making about "next steps"? If no, was there any discussion of how decisions might be made?
5. If there were explicit criteria for the pilot objectives, were the criteria reasonable ones? Were they too liberal or too strict?
6. To what extent did the design mirror the likely design for a full-scale trial? If randomization was not used, was that decision adequately justified?
7. How large was the pilot sample? Was the sample size adequate for addressing the study objectives?
8. Was the data collection plan adequate for measuring feasibility outcomes and for testing data collection protocols for a larger trial? Were both quantitative and qualitative data judiciously collected and integrated to provide a strong portrayal of feasibility?
9. Were confidence intervals around key variables reported? Was intervention effectiveness tested for key outcomes using statistical hypothesis testing procedures? If so, was sufficient caution used in interpreting the results?
10. Did the report describe important lessons learned? Did the discussion section describe how the intervention or the trial methods might be altered on the basis of the pilot?
11. Overall, was pilot work sufficient for a decision to move forward with a full clinical trial?

with serious mental illness have higher morbidity and mortality than the general public. They would benefit from physical activity. These findings suggest that engagement in a group videogame-based physical activity program was low-cost and engaging and improved walking speed in older adults with SMI.

SUMMARY POINTS

- Although the terms *feasibility study* and *pilot study* are sometimes used interchangeably in intervention research, an emerging trend is for greater definitional precision. A **feasibility study** is undertaken to assess whether something can be done (is feasible). *Feasibility* is an umbrella term.
- A **pilot study** is a small-scale version of a full trial, designed to assess feasibility and an entire set of procedures for implementing and evaluating an intervention, often using a randomized design. Pilot studies are feasibility studies but not all feasibility studies are pilots. Nonpilot *feasibility assessments* can be undertaken to test specific, discrete aspects of an emerging intervention, often using a simple design.
- Full-scale evaluations of new interventions are costly. The overall purpose of pilot work is to avoid a costly failure.
- There is a growing consensus among experts in pilot study methods that the purpose of pilot work should *not* be to test hypotheses about the effectiveness of the intervention, because sample sizes in pilots are too small to yield reliable results.
- Pilot work can address a variety of objectives, and researchers should articulate their objectives at the outset. The objectives can focus on processes (e.g., recruitment, retention, acceptability); resources (e.g., monetary costs, time

demands); management issues (e.g., system adequacy, interpersonal relationships); and scientific issues.
- Scientific objectives can concern the substantive aspects of the intervention, such as intervention content and dose, safety, preliminary evidence of efficacy, and clinical significance.
- Preliminary effect size estimates for key outcomes are often computed from pilot data, together with confidence intervals (CIs). Because only preliminary evidence of efficacy is sought in pilots, CIs that are not stringent (e.g., 68% CI) may be sufficient.
- Scientific objectives also concern questions about methodologic aspects of a trial, such as whether randomization is feasible. A major issue in many pilots is the estimation of the sample size that would be needed to adequately power a full trial. Using the effect size estimate from a pilot to estimate sample size needs directly is unwise, because such an estimate often leads to Type II errors (i.e., underpowered full-scale trials).
- Pilot studies are meant to inform the decision about whether to (1) move forward with a full trial, (2) make revisions that require an additional pilot, or (3) abandon the project altogether. To make this decision, researchers should articulate criteria for each objective in advance and then assess the degree to which the criteria were met.
- Mixed methods designs are especially well suited for pilot work. Quantitative data can be used to assess whether feasibility criteria were met, and qualitative data can elucidate *why* they were not met, or how the intervention or study protocols could be improved.
- Sample sizes for pilots are typically small. Some experts recommend at least 30 to 40 subjects per group, especially if funding for the pilot is sought.
- A major product from pilot work is a description of "lessons learned." Another product, if the intervention has been found to be feasible, acceptable, and promising, is a proposal for a full-scale trial.
- Ideally, regardless of the outcome, the findings from pilot work will be published so that others can benefit from learning about both successes and failures.

REFERENCES CITED IN CHAPTER 29

Akinci, B., Dayican, D. K., Deveci, F., Inan, C., Kaya, S., Sahin, O., & Onursan, Z. (2022). Feasibility and safety of Qigong training delivered from two different digital platforms in physically inactive adults: A pilot randomized controlled study. *European Journal of Integrative Medicine*, 54, 102171. https://doi.org/10.1016/j.eujim.2022.102171

Arain, M., Campbell, M., Cooper, C., & Lancaster, G. (2010). What is a pilot or feasibility study? A review of current practice and editorial policy. *BMC: Medical Research Methodology*, 10, 67.

Arnold, D., Burns, K., Adhikari, N., Kho, M., Meade, M., & Cook, D. (2009). The design and interpretation of pilot trials in clinical research in critical care. *Critical Care Medicine*, 37(1 Suppl. l), S69–S74.

Bell, M., Whitehead, A., & Julious, S. (2018). Guidance for using pilot studies to inform the design of intervention trials with continuous outcomes. *Clinical Epidemiology*, 10, 153–157.

Billingham, S., Whitehead, A., & Julious, S. (2013). An audit of sample sizes for pilot and feasibility trials being undertaken in the United Kingdom registered in the United Kingdom Clinical Research Network database. *BMC Medical Research Methodology*, 13, 104.

Brislane, Á., Jones, H., Holder, S. M., Low, D. A., & Hopkins, N. D. (2021). The effect of exercise during pregnancy on maternal and offspring vascular outcomes: A pilot study. *Reproductive Sciences*), 28(2), 510–523. https://doi.org/10.1007/s43032-020-00302-7

Bugge, C., Williams, B., Hagen, S., Logan, J., Glazener, C., Pringle, S., & Sinclair, L. (2013). A process for Decision-making after Pilot and feasibility Trials (ADePT): Development following a feasibility study of a complex intervention for pelvic organ prolapse. *Trials*, 14, 353.

Carlisle, B., Kimmelman, J., Ramsay, T., & MacKinnon, N. (2015). Unsuccessful trial accrual and human subjects protections: An empirical analysis of recently closed trials. *Clinical Trials*, 12(1), 77–83.

Chidebe, R. C. W., & Pratt-Chapman, M. L. (2022). Oncology patient navigation training: Results of a pilot study in Nigeria. *Journal of Cancer Education*, 37(4), 1172–1178. https://doi.org/10.1007/s13187-020-01935-7

Cocks, K., & Torgerson, D. (2013). Sample size calculations for pilot randomized trials: A confidence interval approach. *Journal of Clinical Epidemiology*, 66(2), 197–201.

Conn, V. S., Algase, D., Rawl, S., Zerwic, J., & Wyman, J. (2010). Publishing pilot intervention work. *Western Journal of Nursing Research*, 32(8), 994–1010.

Craig, P., Dieppe, P., Macintyre, S., Michie, S., Nazareth, I., & Petticrew, M. (2008). *Developing and evaluating complex interventions: New guidance*. MRC.

Danesh, V., Zuñiga, J. A., Timmerman, G. M., Radhakrishnan, K., Cuevas, H. E., Young, C. C., Henneghan, A. M., Morrison, J., & Kim, M. T. (2021). Lessons learned from eight teams: The value of pilot and feasibility studies in self-management science. *Applied Nursing Research, 57*, 151345. https://doi.org/10.1016/j.apnr.2020.151345

Eldridge, S., Lancaster, G., Campbell, M., Thabane, L., Hopewell, S., Coleman, C., & Bond, C. (2016). Defining feasibility and pilot studies in preparation for randomised controlled trials: Development of a conceptual framework. *PLoS One, 11*(3), e0150205.

Feeley, N., & Cossette, S. (2015). Testing the waters: Piloting a complex intervention. In Richards, D. & Rahm Hallberg, I. (Eds.), *Complex interventions in health: An overview of research methods* (pp. 166–174). Routledge.

Flanagan, J., Post, K., Hill, R., & DiPalazzo, J. (2022). Feasibility of a nurse coached walking intervention for informal dementia caregivers. *Western Journal of Nursing Research, 44*(5), 466–476. https://doi.org/10.1177/01939459211001395

Hertzog, M. A. (2008). Considerations in determining sample size for pilot studies. *Research in Nursing & Health, 31*(2), 180–191.

Hoyt, M. A., Wang, A. W., Ceja, R. C., Cheavens, J. S., Daneshvar, M. A., Feldman, D. R., Funt, S. A., & Nelson, C. J. (2023). Goal-focused emotion-regulation therapy (GET) in young adult testicular cancer survivors: A randomized pilot study. *Annals of Behavioral Medicine, 57*(9), 777–786. Advance online publication. https://doi.org/10.1093/abm/kaad010

Ioannidis, J. P. (2016). Why most clinical research is not useful. *PLoS Medicine, 13*(6), e1002049.

Kraemer, H. C., Mintz, J., Noda, A., Tinklenberg, J., & Yesavage, J. (2006). Caution regarding the use of pilot studies to guide power calculations for study proposals. *Archives of General Psychiatry, 63*(5), 484–489.

Lancaster, G., Dodd, S., & Williamson, P. (2004). Design and analysis of pilot studies: Recommendations for good practice. *Journal of Evaluation in Clinical Practice, 10*, 307–312.

Lee, E., Whitehead, A., Jacques, R., & Julious, S. (2014). The statistical interpretation of pilot trials: Should significance thresholds be reconsidered? *BMC Medical Research Methodology, 14*, 41.

Leon, A., Davis, L., & Kraemer, H. (2011). The role and interpretation of pilot studies in clinical research. *Journal of Psychiatric Research, 45*(5), 626–629.

Leutwyler, H., Hubbard, E., & Cooper, B. (2022). A group video-game-based physical activity program improves walking speed in older adults living with a serious mental illness. *Innovation in Aging, 6*(6), igac049. https://doi.org/10.1093/geroni/igac049

Moore, C., Carter, R., Nietert, P., & Stewart, P. (2011). Recommendations for planning pilot studies in clinical and translational research. *Clinical & Translational Science, 4*(5), 332–337.

Motl, R. W., Fernhall, B., McCully, K. K., Ng, A., Plow, M., Pilutti, L. A., Sandroff, B. M., & Zackowski, K. M. (2022). Lessons learned from clinical trials of exercise and physical activity in people with MS—guidance for improving the quality of future research. *Multiple Sclerosis and Related Disorders, 68*, 104088. https://doi.org/10.1016/j.msard.2022.104088

Pedersen, B. S., Kirk, J. W., Olesen, M. K., Grønfeldt, B. M., Stefánsdóttir, N. T., Brødsgaard, R., Tjørnhøj-Thomsen, T., Nilsen, P., Andersen, O., Bandholm, T., & Pedersen, M. M. (2022). Feasibility and implementation fidelity of a co-designed intervention to promote in-hospital mobility among older medical patients-the WALK-Copenhagen project (WALK-Cph). *Pilot and Feasibility Studies, 8*(1), 80. https://doi.org/10.1186/s40814-022-01033-z

Richards, D. A., & Rahm Hallberg, I., (Eds.). (2015). *Complex interventions in health: An overview of research methods*. Routledge.

Saleem, M. S., Isha, A. S. N., Mohd Yusop, Y., Awan, M. I., & Naji, G. M. A. (2021). Agility and safety performance among nurses: The mediating role of mindful organizing. *Nursing Reports (Pavia, Italy), 11*(3), 666–679. https://doi.org/10.3390/nursrep11030063

Shih, W. J., Ohman-Strickland, P., & Lin, Y. (2004). Analysis of pilot and early phase studies with small sample sizes. *Statistics in Medicine, 23*(12), 1827–1842.

Sully, B., Julious, S., & Nicholl, J. (2013). A reinvestigation of recruitment to randomised controlled, multicenter trials: A review of trials funded by two UK funding agencies. *Trials, 14*, 166.

Taylor, R., Ukoumunne, O., & Warren, F. (2015). How to use feasibility and pilot trials to test alternative methodologies and methodological procedures prior to a full-scale trial. In Richards, D. & Rahm Hallberg, I. (Eds.), *Complex interventions in health: An overview of research methods* (pp. 136–144). Routledge.

Thabane, L., Ma, J., Chu, R., Cheng, J., Ismaila, A., Rios, L., Robson, R., Thabane, M, Giangregorio, L, & Goldsmith, CH (2010). A tutorial on pilot studies: The what, why and how. *BMC Medical Research Methodology, 10*, 1.

Tickle-Degnen, L. (2013). Nuts and bolts of conducting feasibility studies. *American Journal of Occupational Therapy, 67*(2), 171–176.

Treweek, S. (2015). Addressing issues in recruitment and retention using feasibility and pilot trials. In Richards, D. & Rahm Hallberg, I. (Eds.), *Complex interventions in health: An overview of research methods* (pp. 155–165). Routledge.

Treweek, S., & Born, A. (2014). Clinical trial design: Increasing efficiency in evaluating new healthcare interventions. *Journal of Comparative Effectiveness Research, 3*, 233–236.

Ukoumunne, O., Warren, F., Taylor, R., & Ewings, P. (2015). How to use feasibility studies to derive parameter estimated in order to power a full trial. In Richards, D. & Rahm Hallberg, I. (Eds.), *Complex interventions in health: An overview of research methods* (pp. 145–154). Routledge.

Van der Wouden, J., Blankenstein, A., Huibers, M., van der Windt, D., Stalman, W., & Verhagen, A. (2007). Survey among 78 studies showed that Lasagna's law holds in Dutch primary care research. *Journal of Clinical Epidemiology, 60*(8), 819–824.

Van Teijlingen, E. R., & Hundley, V. (2001). The importance of pilot studies. *Social Research Update, 35*.

Van Teijlingen, E. R., Rennie, A., Hundley, V., & Graham, W. (2001). The importance of conducting and reporting pilot studies: The example of the Scottish Births Survey. *Journal of Advanced Nursing, 34*(3), 289–295.

Vickers, A. J. (2003). Underpowering in randomized trials reporting a sample size calculation. *Journal of Clinical Epidemiology, 56*(8), 717–720.

Walters, S., Bonacho Dos Anjos Henriques-Cadby, I., Bortolami, O., Flight, L., Hind, D., Jacques, R., Knox, C, Nadin, B, Rothwell, J, Surtees, M, Julious, SA, & Julious, S. (2017). Recruitment and retention of participants in randomised controlled trials: A review of trials funded and published by the United Kingdom Health Technology Assessment Programme, *BMJ Open, 7*(3), e015276.

Part 6

BUILDING AN EVIDENCE BASE FOR NURSING PRACTICE

Chapter 30 Systematic Reviews of Research Evidence
Chapter 31 Applicability, Generalizability, and Relevance: Toward Practice-Based Evidence
Chapter 32 Disseminating Evidence: Reporting Research Findings
Chapter 33 Writing Proposals to Generate Evidence

30 Systematic Reviews of Research Evidence

Learning Objectives

1. Understand the purpose and various approaches to systematic reviews.
2. Articulate when it is appropriate to consider a meta-analysis.
3. Recognize the major steps in the systematic review process.
4. Provide examples of searchable databases for the purpose of data extraction.
5. Discern the various approaches to apprising the evidence.
6. Consider various ways to display the data findings.

INTRODUCTION

This chapter discusses systematic reviews, which are considered a cornerstone of evidence-based practice (EBP). As noted in Chapter 2, systematic reviews are at the pinnacle of most evidence hierarchies and level-of-evidence scales.

RESEARCH INTEGRATION AND SYNTHESIS

A **systematic review (SR)** carefully and transparently integrates research evidence about a specific research question using methodical procedures that are spelled out in advance. Systematic reviewers use methods that are disciplined, reproducible, and verifiable. Compared to a simple literature review, systematic reviews involve the rigorous development of, and adherence to, a protocol with explicit rules for gathering data from **primary studies** (i.e., original research inquiries that addressed a specific question).

The field of research integration is expanding rapidly, in terms of both the number of reviews being conducted and techniques used to perform them. Methods for conducting systematic reviews are also evolving, making it challenging to offer guidance. We provide only a brief introduction to this complex topic. Our advice for those embarking on a review project is to keep abreast of developments in this field and to seek more detailed information in websites devoted to the topic—or to participate in training that has become available through organizations focused on evidence integration, such as PRISMA, the Cochrane Collaboration and the Joanna Briggs Institute (JBI).

> **TIP** The Cochrane Collaboration's reviewer's manual is a major resource for the conduct of systematic reviews. The 6.3 version of the manual, published in 2022 (Higgins et al., 2022), is referenced extensively in this chapter and is available online (https://training.cochrane.org/handbook/current).

TYPES OF SYSTEMATIC REVIEWS

Systematic reviews can take various forms and result in different products. No simple taxonomy for classifying systematic reviews has emerged; we look at review types along several dimensions.

Systematic Reviews of Quantitative, Qualitative, and Mixed Methods Research

Systematic reviews in healthcare fields have largely been syntheses of quantitative evidence from randomized controlled trials (RCTs)—syntheses that focus on the question: Does *this* work? In other words, systematic reviews have most often integrated evidence from primary studies that addressed Therapy/intervention questions. Researchers have also conducted systematic reviews of other types of quantitative research, such as reviews of studies addressing etiology, prognosis, or diagnosis questions (Munn et al., 2018).

Qualitative researchers have also created techniques to integrate evidence from multiple studies, and nurse researchers have played an important role in this area. Their products are often called **metasyntheses**. Metasyntheses typically involve integrations of studies focused on abstract phenomena and experiences (e.g., grief following the death of a child). However, there is an emerging interest among healthcare researchers in synthesizing information on qualitative aspects of interventions, such as patient acceptance, implementation processes, and barriers to implementation). Such reviews are often called **qualitative evidence syntheses (QES)**.

Mixed studies reviews (MSRs) (or mixed research syntheses) are another type of systematic review that integrates findings from qualitative *and* quantitative studies and from mixed methods studies.

Narrative vs. Statistical Integration (Meta-Analysis)

In systematic reviews, the "data" are findings from studies that addressed a question of interest. Data from the included studies can be integrated in a narrative fashion or statistically. Qualitative systematic reviews, and some quantitative reviews, involve a narrative synthesis.

Many systematic reviews of quantitative studies—especially those that focus on intervention effects—use statistical integration, in what are called **meta-analyses**. The essence of a meta-analysis is that information from each study in the review is used to develop a common metric, an *effect size*. Effect sizes are averaged across studies, yielding aggregated information about not only the *existence* of a relationship between variables, but also an estimate of its *magnitude*. Most systematic reviews in the Cochrane Collaboration involve a meta-analysis.

For integrating quantitative evidence, meta-analysis offers these advantages:

- *Objectivity.* In narrative reviews, reviewers use unidentified or subconscious criteria to integrate disparate results. In a meta-analysis, decisions are explicit, and the integration itself is objective. Two meta-analysts using the same dataset would reach the same conclusions.
- *Power.* Power is the probability of detecting a true relationship between variables. By combining results from multiple studies, power is increased. In a meta-analysis, it is possible to conclude, with a given probability, that a relationship is real (e.g., that an intervention is effective), even when several small studies yielded nonsignificant findings. In a narrative review, multiple nonsignificant findings would likely be interpreted as lack of evidence of a relationship, which could be erroneous.
- *Precision.* Meta-analysts draw conclusions about the size of an intervention's effect, with a specified probability that the results are accurate. Estimates of effect size across multiple studies yield smaller confidence intervals than individual studies, and thus precision is enhanced.

Special Types of Review

Most of this chapter is devoted to "basic" systematic reviews. However, in the evolving field of evidence synthesis, special types of review have emerged, and references to them are appearing regularly in the literature. In this section, we briefly describe a few special review types.

Integrative Reviews

The **integrative review** (IR) is a type of systematic review, but unlike the systematic review the question is directed at a gap in the existing literature and the question is generally broader. Like the systematic approach, the IR process includes several steps such as the literature search, data extraction, analysis, evidence appraisal, and the synthesis of the literature. The IR differs from a classic systematic review in that the synthesis does not include a statistical analysis of the findings (Oermann & Knafl, 2021; Toronto & Remington, 2020; Whittemore & Knafl, 2005). Because the question in an IR is generally broader and based on what is known or absent in the literature, it is important to note that the first critical step to the IR is knowing the literature in an area of concern and identifying the gap in knowledge. Due to the broad question being asked, the evidence included in an IR is not limited and can include theoretical or conceptual papers as well as papers that utilize varying research approaches. The goal of the IR is a more holistic understanding of the problem rather than a specific question about the available evidence to address a problem (Oermann & Knafl, 2021; Toronto & Remington, 2020; Whittemore & Knafl, 2005). Published IR follow the PRISMA guidelines and appraise or grade the evidence. Nurses often favor using the IR for several reasons. There is often not adequate nursing research on a topic of concern. Nurses may define the concept differently than others in the health field, and the approach allows for the exploration and integration of theories into the question being asked.

> **Example of a Question in an Integrative Review**
> Michel-Schuldt et al. (2020) conducted an integrative review to examine midwifery care delivery in low- and middle-income countries. The specific question was to understand how, where, and by whom has midwife-led care been provided in these countries. The authors stated they chose this approach so that they could include a wide range of studies and methods.

Scoping Reviews

A **scoping review** is a preliminary investigation that clarifies the range and nature of the evidence base. Unlike a systematic review, a scoping review addresses broad questions, uses flexible procedures, draws on both research and nonresearch work (e.g., policy papers), and typically does not formally evaluate evidence quality. Scoping reviews can suggest strategies for a full systematic review and can indicate whether statistical integration (meta-analysis) is feasible. Scoping reviews are also used to identify areas in need of further research (Aromataris & Munn, 2020; Peters et al., 2020).

> **Example of a Scoping Review**
> Vaartio-Rajalin et al. (2020) did a scoping review to describe the existing knowledge on nurses' use of art-based art therapy across adult healthcare settings, including home care. They reported on 42 studies that examined art-based therapies and found that group-based art therapies were most often used with adults 65 and older; there was an absence of art-based therapies in home settings, and individual narrative/story telling was a common art-based therapy used by nurses in other settings.

Rapid Reviews

Systematic reviews are considered the "gold standard" in knowledge synthesis, but they typically require up to 2 years to complete. **Rapid reviews** of research evidence are a type of evidence synthesis that has emerged. Rapid reviews are often used to inform emergent decisions facing clinicians in healthcare settings (Munn et al., 2015). This type of review was particularly prevalent during the COVID pandemic so that information about treatment effectiveness could be swiftly shared. Rapid reviews are typically done within a period of weeks; they do not involve statistical integration and involve a less rigorous search for available evidence so as to produce findings in a timely manner. Klerings and colleagues (2023) have a paper on rapid reviews and provide guidance on search strategies. The Cochrane Collaboration has a special methods group devoted to rapid reviews.

> **Example of a Rapid Review**
> Gordon and colleagues (2022) did a rapid review to explore the use of telehealth as a way to deliver palliative care to remote areas. They reported on 18 studies. Due to the diversity of methods used on the studies, they analyzed and reported on them narratively. They found that palliative care delivered by telehealth was effective for consultation, medication monitoring, and specialists' appointments.

Overview of Reviews (Umbrella Reviews)

With the dramatic rise in the number of systematic reviews being undertaken, reviews that integrate findings from multiple reviews now appear in the literature with some regularity. These are often referred to as **overviews of reviews** (Pollock et al., 2022; Higgins et al., 2022). JBI also offers a chapter on umbrella reviews (Aromataris & Munn, 2020). Umbrella reviews provide a broad overview of a topic. The goal of this type of review is to determine if the questions being asked around a topic or the evidence being reported is consistent. Hunt et al. (2018) noted that "overviews have evolved to address a growing need to filter the information overload" (p. 1).

> **Example of an Umbrella Review**
> Treacy et al. (2022) undertook an umbrella review to examine the evidence of mobility training, safety, and overall benefit to overall functioning and mobility in community dwelling frail older people. The review included 12 randomized control trials with a total of 1,317 participants across 9 countries.

Living Systematic Reviews

Systematic reviews can quickly get out-of-date. The time between starting and publishing a review is typically over a year, and (for one study) the median time from primary study publication to inclusion in a published systematic review ranged from 3 to 7 years. Elliott and his group have proposed the conduct of timely **living systematic reviews** that are updated as new research becomes available and are published as online-only evidence summaries. Their approach relies, in part, on new methods of automating the retrieval and extraction of relevant information. Guidelines for living systematic reviews were presented in a series of papers in the *Journal of Clinical Epidemiology* (e.g., Elliott et al., 2017; Thomas et al., 2017).

"Next-Generation" Systematic Reviews

Ioannidis (2017), in a medical journal editorial, mentioned several "next-generation" types of quantitative systematic reviews, including the following two:

- **Individual patient-level meta-analysis.** Reviewers sometimes obtain the raw data from multiple trialists and then use the individual-level data in the analysis. A primary benefit of this approach is the ability to make statistical adjustments for confounding variables and to perform analyses for distinct subgroups (Tierney et al., 2022).
- **Network meta-analysis (NMA).** Systematic reviews of interventions typically make direct pairwise comparisons, such as differences in outcomes between an intervention group vs. a control group—often a placebo or "usual care." Network reviews involve incorporating direct and indirect evidence to draw conclusions about the effects of alternative interventions for a health problem—even if they have not been directly compared in trials (Tonin et al., 2017). This approach is popular in comparative effectiveness research. The new Cochrane reviewer's manual devotes a chapter to NMA (Chaimani et al., 2022).

> **Example of a Network Meta-Analysis**
> Zhang and colleagues (2021a) conducted a network meta-analysis to assess the effect of all exercise-based interventions to improve social participations in patients post a cerebral vascular event. Sixteen randomized control trials were included in the analysis. They found that among 12 interventions, the motor relearning program was ranked as the most effective of all of the exercise interventions.

PLANNING A SYSTEMATIC REVIEW

Systematic reviews follow many of the same steps as for primary studies. Like other research endeavors, the conduct of a systematic review requires advance preparation and planning. We briefly discuss a few things to consider when planning a review.

Broad Steps in a Systematic Review

Despite the evolution of methods for conducting systematic reviews, some steps are fairly standard in rigorous efforts to synthesize research evidence. In sections that follow, we describe aspects of systematic review procedures in greater detail, but here is a brief summary of steps that are typical, especially for quantitative reviews:

1. Formulate the question(s) for the review
2. Define eligibility criteria for the primary studies
3. Prepare a protocol for the review
4. Search for and retrieve primary studies
5. Select studies for inclusion in the review
6. Assess the quality of the selected primary studies
7. Extract data from the studies
8. Analyze and synthesize the data
9. Evaluate the degree of confidence in the results
10. Present the findings in a systematic review report

Progress in conducting the review is less linear than this list suggests—there are typically feedback loops in the process.

Preparing to Conduct a Systematic Review

Some activities need to be addressed even before the actual review process gets underway.

Preliminary Groundwork

Before initiating a systematic review project, reviewers need to make sure that a review is necessary. One of the Institute of Medicine's standards for the conduct of high-quality systematic reviews is this: Confirm the need for a new review (IOM, 2011, Standard 2.5.1). An early search of important databases (including ones dedicated to systematic reviews) is warranted. Such a search might not reveal reviews that are underway, so it is important to also search for reviews in **PROSPERO**, an international prospective registry of systematic reviews.

The Review Team

Unlike literature reviews, systematic reviews require a team. Assembling the right team is an important planning activity. Several tasks in a systematic review (e.g., appraising study quality) require two reviewers and often a third who can serve as a tie-breaker. With multiple reviewers, the work load is shared and subjectivity is reduced. The team should involve content experts and a methodologic or statistical expert who is familiar with systematic review methods. The team should include a librarian or information specialist who has training in systematic reviews.

Review teams for systematic reviews increasingly include other stakeholders, such as patients and other members of the public. The Cochrane Collaboration explicitly encourages that the author team includes consumers of healthcare, clinicians, and people from various regions, and the region impacted by the issue of concern in particular (Cumpston & Chandler, 2022). The advisory group should be established to solicit input from people with a range of experiences.

The Review Auspices

Review teams may decide to undertake a systematic review independently—for example, in response to a locally identified problem. Some teams prepare a systematic review under the auspices of a national or international organization, such as the Cochrane Collaboration, the JBI, the Agency for Healthcare Research and Quality, or the Centre for Reviews and Dissemination. The process differs depending on the organization, but typically a review idea is submitted for approval prior to its conduct. Major review organizations also offer guidance to review teams working independently, through training opportunities and handbooks such as those by the Cochrane Collaboration (Higgins et al., 2022) and JBI (Aromataris & Munn, 2020). These handbooks focus primarily on quantitative reviews but have chapters on qualitative synthesis.

Computer Software

Systematic reviews involve massive amounts of data that need to be managed and analyzed. Computer software is usually used to facilitate the process. Dozens of software packages have been created, including text mining software (e.g., SWIFT-Review, TERMINE), citation management software (e.g., EndNote, Mendeley, RefWorks), deduplication software (e.g., DistillerSR), software to assist in screening (e.g., Covidence, DistillerSR, Rayyan), data extraction software (DistillerSR, Covidence), and software for meta-analysis (e.g., DistillerSR, Meta-Easy). Macros are also available for doing meta-analyses within major software packages such as SPSS and SAS. For qualitative systematic reviews, researchers often use NVivo or other software described in Chapter 25. The Cochrane Collaboration's popular software, called *RevMan*, includes tools that perform many of the functions for systematic reviews. Similarly, the JBI offers a comprehensive package of review software called *SUMARI*. The SRToolbox is a resource for identifying relevant software (http://systematicreviewtools.com/index.php).

Schedule for a Systematic Review

Systematic reviews typically take 9 to 18 months to complete. Before embarking on the project, a timeline should be constructed to help the project stay on track. Typically, the most time-consuming activities in the systematic review process are searching for and retrieving relevant studies, following up to obtain information that is missing in the study reports, and undertaking quality assessments.

In developing a project schedule, the team should plan for pilot tests of important decisions. For example, early in the search process, it is a good idea to pilot test the eligibility criteria to ensure that relevant primary studies are not filtered out. Quality assessment strategies and data extraction methods should also be pilot tested to ensure optimal results.

SYSTEMATIC REVIEWS OF QUANTITATIVE RESEARCH

In this section, we describe major steps in the conduct of a systematic review of quantitative research. The guidance applies to systematic reviews of quantitative research in general, but most advice has been developed for studies that address Therapy questions. Supplementary advice is available in both the JBI and Cochrane reviewers' manuals for integrating findings from observational studies, public health initiatives, economic evaluations, and diagnostic test accuracy research. The Agency for Healthcare Research and Quality (AHRQ, 2014) has also issued guidelines for reviews of comparative effectiveness studies.

Formulating the Review Question

A focused systematic review begins with a carefully framed question. Good review questions often follow the PICO format described in Chapter 2, with specification of the Population, the Intervention or Influence, the Comparison against which the intervention/influence is contrasted, and Outcomes. Question templates such as those provided in Chapters 2 or 4 serve as a good starting place.

> **TIP** Munn and colleagues (2018) suggest question formats for several types of systematic review. For example, for prevalence and incidence reviews, they use the acronym CoCoPop (Condition, Context, Population).

Systematic review questions vary in scope. For example, a review might address a broad question regarding whether exercise interventions (in general) are effective as a weight-loss therapy for obese adolescents. Alternatively, a review might address whether a particular intervention (e.g., high-intensity interval training) is an effective weight-loss strategy. Table 2.3.a in the Cochrane manual (Higgins et al., 2022) summarizes advantages and disadvantages of broad vs. narrow review questions. Broad reviews tend to be demanding of time and resources.

Finalizing the review question is likely to involve multiple iterations of refinement. Team members should all be "on board" with the question, and the process is likely to benefit from the opinions of a diverse group of stakeholders. Scoping reviews sometimes play a vital role in formulating the question for a systematic review.

The reviewers need to be careful about specifying outcomes for the review. The handbook for

Cochrane reviews recommends developing a list of possible outcomes and then prioritizing them. The "main outcomes" are those that are essential for decision-making and usually include two to three primary outcomes and a small number of secondary outcomes. For intervention studies, outcomes should include possible adverse effects.

> **Example of a Question from a Quantitative Systematic Review**
> Hughes and colleagues (2023) conducted a systematic review to explore if e-health interventions delivered to parents impacted infant procedural pain. The questions focused on the parental outcomes (e.g., stress, anxiety), use and acceptability of the e-intervention, parents' involvement in infant pain management, and infant outcomes such as pain, morbidity, and length of stay.

Defining Eligibility Criteria

In systematic reviews, inclusion and exclusion criteria must be specified before a search for primary studies gets underway. Sampling criteria for a systematic review typically cover substantive, methodologic, and practical elements, such as the following:

- **Study participants.** Inclusion criteria normally indicate the disease or condition of interest (e.g., patients with cancer, low-birth-weight babies) and any relevant demographic characteristics, such as age.
- **Intervention/influence.** Reviewers need to stipulate the essential characteristics of the intervention or influence of interest, including features such as mode or timing of delivery.
- **Study design.** Some reviews stipulate a study design for eligible primary studies—most often, a randomized design when the review focuses on a Therapy question.
- **Other criteria.** From a practical standpoint, the criteria might exclude reports written in a language other than English, or reports published before a certain date. The criteria might also stipulate whether both published and unpublished reports will be included in the review, a topic we discuss in a later section.

For some reviews, the inclusion criteria specify the outcomes of interest. However, for reviews focused on Therapy questions, the handbook for Cochrane reviews cautions against including or excluding studies with specific outcomes and would seek all rigorous studies to compare interventions in a population regardless of the outcomes measured (Higgins et al., 2022).

Criteria for eligibility are not always straightforward.

> **Example of Eligibility Criteria for a Quantitative Review**
> Neo and Tho (2022) have developed a protocol for a systematic review to determine the accuracy of images of wound care as compared to in-person assessment. Inclusion criteria include studies that are peer reviewed including those in the gray literature that compare in-person assessment to images of chronic wounds. Exclusion criteria are acute wounds and studies not comparing images to in-person assessment.

Preparing a Review Protocol

Review teams are increasingly expected to prepare—and often to publish—a **protocol** of the proposed systematic review. The protocol, which promotes transparency, serves as the road map for the review. Review protocols, which are typically 10 to 15 single-spaced pages, usually include the following information:

- The title of the review
- Members of the review team
- Proposed schedule, with beginning and end dates
- The research questions
- Background/argument for the review
- Eligibility criteria for studies in the review
- Search strategy (anticipated databases, keywords, supplementary search strategies)
- Review methods (assessment of methodologic quality, method of data extraction, analysis methods, assessment of bias)
- Assessment of confidence in the findings

> **TIP** Some software for systematic reviews, such as the software for Cochrane and JBI reviews, provide fill-in-the-blank forms for creating protocols.

Once a protocol has been developed, it is advisable to register the protocol with PROSPERO and, if relevant, with the Cochrane Collaboration, JBI, or other review group.

Example of a Systematic Review Protocol
Arantes et al. (2020) registered a protocol in PROSPERO. The team seeks to search the following databases MEDLINE SciELO, CINAHL, EMBASE, and LILACS to explore if the Timed Up and Go test is an accurate tool to identify older adults at risk of falling in community-based settings.

Searching for and Screening Primary Studies

Systematic reviewers should aim for an exhaustive search of primary studies that meet the eligibility criteria. Exhaustive searching requires a greater emphasis on sensitivity (ensuring retrieval of all relevant studies) than on specificity (minimizing retrieval of nonrelevant results). Preliminary search plans are spelled out in the protocol, but reviewers need to continuously assess and refine their strategies.

Traditionally, the keywords are the main research variables; many researchers use the PICO elements as keywords for a literature search. There is some evidence, however, that the use of a full PICO query may fail to retrieve all relevant articles. Ho et al. (2016), for example, found that using two or three of the PICO terms retrieved more articles than using all four, findings similar to those of Agoritsas et al. (2012). Chapter 4 on searching in the Cochrane Handbook explicitly recommends against including Outcome or Comparison as search terms for systematic reviews of interventions (Higgins et al., 2022). Pilot testing alternative search strategies is recommended.

Aromataris and Riitano (2014) provide advice on searching. They suggest creating a *logic grid* that begins as a matrix with PICO elements in four columns. An early step in a search is to identify alternative terms or synonyms for the concepts in the grid, and to then add them into the grid.

Searching for primary studies should be undertaken in multiple bibliographic databases and should include repositories of existing systematic reviews such as the Cochrane and JBI databases. Searching in MEDLINE, EMBASE, and CINAHL is essential. The Cochrane handbook (Higgins et al., 2022) includes lists of numerous national and regional databases, subject-specific databases, and citation indexes to consider. Bramer and colleagues (2017) estimated that 60% of published reviews fail to retrieve 95% of all relevant references as a result of not searching important databases. Their analysis suggested that Google Scholar should be included in the search strategy.

TIP It seems likely that technologic advances soon will result in new algorithms for automating several activities in producing systematic reviews, including search and screening activities (e.g., Beller et al., 2018; Tsafnat et al., 2018).

There is some disagreement about whether reviewers should limit their sample to published studies or should cast as wide a net as possible and include **gray literature**—that is, studies with a more limited distribution, such as dissertations, conference presentations, and so on. Some people restrict their sample to published reports in peer-reviewed journals, arguing that the peer review system is an important, tried-and-true screen for findings worthy of consideration as evidence.

The limitations of excluding nonpublished findings, however, have been widely noted. A primary issue is **publication bias**—the tendency for published studies to overrepresent statistically significant findings. (This bias is increasingly being referred to as one type of **dissemination bias**.) Publication bias is widespread: authors tend to refrain from submitting manuscripts with negative findings, reviewers and editors tend to reject such papers when they are submitted, and users of evidence tend to ignore the findings when they are published. The exclusion of gray literature in a systematic review can lead to the overestimation of effects (Conn et al., 2003; Dwan et al., 2013).

TIP In addition to the bias favoring publication of reports with statistically significant results, there is good evidence of another type of dissemination bias—selective reporting of only those outcomes with positive results, sometimes called *outcome reporting bias*.

We recommend retrieving as many relevant studies as possible, because methodologic weaknesses in unpublished reports can be dealt with later. Aggressive search strategies are essential and may include the following:

- **Handsearching** journals known to publish relevant content—that is, doing a manual search of the tables of contents of a few key journals
- *Snowballing* (the ancestry approach or footnote chasing, such as tracking down references in bibliographies of relevant studies) and *digital snowballing* (using "related citations" features in electronic databases)
- Identifying and contacting key researchers in the field to see if they have done studies that have not (yet) been published, and networking with researchers at conferences
- Doing an "author search" of key researchers in the field in databases and on the Internet
- Reviewing abstracts from trial registries and conference proceedings
- Searching for unpublished reports, such as dissertations and theses, government reports, and registries of studies in progress (e.g., in the United States, through the NIH RePORTER http://projectreporter.nih.gov/reporter.cfm)
- Contacting foundations, government agencies, or corporate sponsors of the type of research under study to get leads on work in progress or recently completed

Once potentially relevant studies are identified, the search results should be merged (often, using reference management software), and duplicates should be removed. The next step is to perform an initial screening of abstracts to remove obviously irrelevant articles. Next, full-texts of the articles that passed the screening need to be retrieved and reviewed to determine if they do, in fact, meet the eligibility criteria. All decisions relating to exclusions should be made by at least two reviewers, with conflicts resolved either by consensus or by a third reviewer.

Example of a Search Strategy from a Systematic Review
In a systematic review of universal newborn hearing screening programs, Yoshinaga-Itano et al. (2021) had two of the members of the review team search the electronic databases of PubMed, Cochrane library, Google Scholar, Web of Science, and One Search. They also searched the citations from papers they identified from the literature search. To conduct the word searches, they used text-word searches and MeSH terms. After removing duplicates and reviewing titles and abstracts, they assessed 220 papers for eligibility. From that, they removed 190 studies due to inclusion/exclusion criteria. No studies were eligible for quantitative synthesis/meta-analysis, but they were able to proceed with a qualitative synthesis of 30 studies.

TIP The reports of studies that meet the sampling criteria do not always contain complete information needed for a meta-analysis. Be prepared to devote time and resources to communicating with researchers to obtain supplementary information.

Evaluating Study Quality and Risk of Bias

In systematic reviews, the evidence from primary studies needs to be evaluated to determine how much confidence to place in the findings. Assessments of study quality sometimes involve quantitative ratings of study features. Dozens of quality assessment scales that yield summary scores of overall study quality have been developed (Zeng et al., 2015). A frequently used scale to appraise RCTs is the Jadad scale (Jadad et al., 1996). The Newcastle-Ottawa Scale (Stang, 2010) can be used to appraise nonrandomized studies. A carefully developed scale, called ROBINS-I, was developed to assess bias in nonrandomized studies but is also used for RCTs (Sterne et al., 2016). Scales, however, are sometimes criticized because of concerns about their validity and reliability. Quality criteria vary from instrument to instrument, and the result is that study quality can be rated differently with different assessment tools and by different assessors.

Another strategy is to use a quality assessment checklist with several discrete items that are not summed. An important example is the Critical Appraisal Tools developed by the JBI for evaluating different types of primary studies (e.g., RCTs, prevalence studies, case–control studies). The JBI Critical Appraisal tool for RCTs includes 13 items, each of which is rated as yes, no, unclear, or not applicable. For example, one item is, "Were outcomes measured in a reliable way?" After completing the checklist, the appraiser makes an assessment about whether to include the study in the review, exclude it, or seek more information.

The Cochrane Collaboration takes an approach that emphasizes risk of bias (RoB) rather than study quality, using a "component" approach (Higgins et al., 2022, Chapter 8). **Risk of bias** in intervention studies refers to the likelihood of an inaccuracy in the estimate of a causal effect—that is, a threat to internal validity. In Cochrane reviews, reviewers rate each study for seven bias risks (Table 30.1). Each component is rated low risk, high risk, or unclear RoB. Cochrane's risk-of-bias tool is primarily relevant for studies addressing Therapy questions; a comparable domain-based tool for nonrandomized studies, called ACROBAT-NRSI, has been developed (Bilandzic et al., 2016).

Regardless of approach, quality appraisals should be undertaken by at least two qualified individuals. If there are disagreements between the reviewers, there should be a discussion until a consensus has been reached or, if necessary, a third person should resolve the difference. Interrater reliability can be calculated to demonstrate adequate agreement on study quality.

TIP In the revised Cochrane Collaboration's reviewer's manual (Higgins et al., 2022), the RoB tool has been modified and is referred to as RoB2.

There is some disagreement about what to do with quality appraisal information. JBI recommends using their checklists as the basis for excluding studies of low quality (Porritt et al., 2014). Jüni and colleagues (2001), however, who advocated Cochrane's component approach, noted that

TABLE 30.1 • The Cochrane Collaboration's Tool for Assessing Risk of Bias

COMPONENT	SPECIFIC RISK
Selection bias	**Random sequence generation:** Was random sequence generation likely to produce comparable groups?
	Allocation concealment: Was the allocation sequence adequately concealed?
Performance bias	**Blinding of participants and personnel:** Were steps taken to blind participants and study personnel regarding receipt of the intervention?
	Blinding of outcome assessment: Were outcome assessors blinded to which intervention a participant received?
Attrition bias	**Incomplete outcome data:** How complete are the data for each outcome, including attrition and exclusions from the analysis?
Reporting bias	**Selective reporting:** Were all outcomes reported or was there selective reporting of outcomes?
Other bias	**Other sources of bias:** Are there important concerns about other types of bias not previously covered?

Adapted with permission from in Higgins, and Thomas. (Eds.). (2022). *Cochrane handbook for systematic reviews of interventions (version 6.3)*. The Cochrane Collaboration. Each primary study is rated as "low risk of bias," "high risk of bias," or "unclear risk of bias" for each risk factor. A new Risk of Bias tool has been developed, as outlined in the Toolkit.

excluding low-quality studies might sometimes be justified "but could exclude studies that might contribute valid information" (p. 45). They recommended excluding only studies with "gross deficiencies," and then handling quality at the analysis phase. Further information about quality assessments in systematic reviews is provided by Cooper (2017) and Viswanathan et al. (2018).

> **Example of Quality Assessments in a Systematic Review**
> Zhang and colleagues (2021b) conducted a systematic review to evaluate the effectiveness of using standardized terminologies in nursing. After searching the databases of PubMed, Web of Science, CINAHL, and OVID, the team used the Effective Public Health Practice Project's Quality Assessment Tool for Quantitative Studies to assess the quality of the studies. Of the 14 studies that were included in the final analysis, five were of high quality, one was of moderate quality, and eight were of weak quality.

Extracting and Encoding Data for Analysis

The next step in a systematic review is to extract information about study characteristics and findings from each report. A data extraction form must be developed, along with a coding manual to guide those who will be extracting information. Reviewers often begin with paper-and-pencil forms, but then input the data into an electronic system. Options include spreadsheets (e.g., Excel), database software (e.g., Access), web-based surveys repurposed for data extraction (e.g., SurveyMonkey), and review software such as Cochrane's RevMan (Elamin et al., 2009).

Basic data source information should be recorded for all studies. This includes such features as year of publication, country of participants, and language in which the report was published. Supplementary information might include whether the study was funded (and by whom) and the year in which data were collected.

In terms of methodologic information, a critical element is sample size. Design information also needs to be coded (e.g., RCT, quasiexperiment, case–control). Measurement issues may be important. For example, codes can be used to designate specific instruments used to measure outcomes. For scales, information is needed about whether a high or low score is desirable. In longitudinal studies, rates of attrition and length of time between waves of data collection are essential. Quality appraisal information needs to be included in the record for each study.

In intervention studies, features of the intervention should be recorded, such as type of setting, dose or length of intervention, and modality of delivering the intervention. Attributes of the comparison condition also needed to be extracted and recorded.

Characteristics of the study participants must be encoded as well, including both clinical and demographic traits. Categorical characteristics that could be represented as percentages include sex, race/ethnicity, educational level, and illness/treatment information (e.g., percentages of participants with comorbidities). Age usually should be recorded as mean age of sample members.

Finally, the findings must be encoded. Either effect sizes (discussed in the next section) or statistical information for computing effect sizes is essential for a meta-analysis. Effect size information is often recorded for multiple outcomes and may also be recorded for different subgroups of study participants (e.g., effects for males vs. females).

Extraction and coding of information should be completed by two or more people, for at least a portion of the studies, to allow for an assessment of interrater agreement. Reviewer training in data extraction and monitoring is essential: studies have found high rates of extraction errors in systematic reviews (Mathes et al., 2017). Further guidance on data extraction and the creation of data extraction forms is offered by Higgins et al. (2022), Chapter 5, and Pedder et al. (2016).

> **Example of Data Extraction in a Systematic Review**
> Dukuzumuremyi et al. (2020) conducted a systematic review to examine mothers' knowledge, attitude, and practice of exclusive breastfeeding in east Africa. The team used a data-extraction form they designed to extract data from each study. This included study characteristics (e.g., author, location of study, sample size and study aims) and whether the study assessed mothers' knowledge, attitude, and practice about exclusive breast feeding.

Analyzing and Synthesizing the Data

Once data extraction for the eligible studies has been completed, reviewers can proceed to analyze their data. In quantitative studies, a major analytic goal is to gain insight into *effects*—that is, the effect of an intervention or other causative factor on outcomes. Whether the analysis is narrative or statistical, reviewers are typically interested in integrating the data to answer the following questions: (1) What is the direction of the effect? (e.g., are there positive effects for the intervention group?); (2) How big is the effect? and (3) How consistent is the effect across studies? Supplementary questions may include the following: (4) Are effects similar for different subgroups of participants? and (5) Are effects similar for studies that vary in quality?

Narrative syntheses involve the creation of evidence summary tables and then the use of judgment to answer these questions, but reviewers often prefer to answer them by performing a meta-analysis. Statistical integration is not always possible, however, so reviewers often begin by considering the feasibility of a meta-analysis.

> **TIP** We focus mainly on meta-analytic procedures, but the Institute of Medicine (2011) recommends beginning with a narrative integration to gain insights, even if meta-analysis is ultimately performed. An older approach to quantitatively integrating results, called *vote counting*, involves adding up significant and nonsignificant findings to assess the preponderance of evidence. Yet another alternative is to construct graphic displays known as *harvest plots* to synthesize evidence when meta-analysis is not possible (Higgins et al., 2022; Ogilvie et al., 2008, Chapter 12).

Criteria for Using Meta-Analysis in a Systematic Review

A basic criterion for a meta-analysis is that the research question across studies is the same. This means that the independent variable, outcomes, and study populations must be sufficiently similar to merit integration. Variables may be operationalized differently, to be sure. Interventions to promote physical activity among diabetics could take the form of a 4-week clinic-based program in one study and a five-session web-based intervention in another, for example. The outcome (physical activity levels) could be measured differently across studies. Yet, a study of the effects of a 1-hour lecture to improve *attitudes* toward physical activity among obese adults would be a poor candidate to include in such a meta-analysis. This is frequently called the "apples and oranges" or "fruit" problem. A meta-analysis should not be about *fruit*—that is, a broad, encompassing category—but about a specific question addressed in multiple studies—such as "apples."

A second criterion concerns whether there is a sufficient knowledge base for statistical integration. If there are only a few studies, or if all studies are weakly designed and harbor extensive bias, it usually is not sensible to compute an "average" effect.

A final issue concerns consistency of the evidence. When the same hypothesis has been tested in multiple studies and results are highly conflicting, meta-analysis usually is not appropriate. As an extreme example, if half the studies testing an intervention found benefits for those in the intervention group, but the other half found benefits for the controls, it would be misleading to compute an average effect. A more appropriate strategy would be to do an in-depth narrative analysis of why the findings are at odds. The issue of *heterogeneity* of results is important even when a decision is made to move forward with a meta-analysis.

Calculating Effects in a Meta-Analysis

Meta-analyses involve the calculation of an index that encapsulates the relationship between the independent variable (the intervention or influence) and the outcome in each study. Because effects are captured differently depending on the variables' level of measurement, there is no single formula for calculating an effect size. In nursing, the most common situations for meta-analysis involve comparisons of two groups on a continuous outcome (e.g., the body mass index or BMI), comparisons of two groups on a dichotomous outcome (e.g., obese vs. not obese), or correlations between two continuous variables (e.g., the correlation between BMI and depression scores).

For simplicity, much of our discussion focuses on the first situation, comparison of group means. When the outcomes across studies are on identical scales (e.g., weight in pounds), the effect can be captured by simply subtracting the mean for one group from the mean for the other in each study. For example, if the mean weight in an intervention group were 182.0 lb and that for a control group were 190.0 lb, the effect would be −8.0. Outcomes often are measured on different scales, however. For example, postpartum depression might be measured by Beck's Postpartum Depression Screening Scale in one study and by the Edinburgh Postnatal Depression Scale in another. In such situations, mean differences across studies cannot be averaged—we need an index that is neutral to the metric used in the primary study. Cohen's d, described in Chapter 18, is the effect size (ES) index often used. It may be recalled that the formula for d is the group difference in means, divided by the pooled standard deviation, or:

$$d = \frac{\overline{X}_1 - \overline{X}_2}{SD_P}$$

where $\overline{X}_1$ is the mean of group 1, $\overline{X}_2$ is the mean of group 2, and SD_P is the pooled standard deviation. This effect size index transforms all effects to standard deviation units. That is, if d were 0.50, it means that the mean for one group was one-half a standard deviation higher than that for the other group—regardless of the original measurement scale.

> **TIP** The term for the effect size d in Cochrane reviews is **standardized mean difference** or SMD. Cooper (2017) describes another similar index, called the *g index*, which adjusts d for possible bias in the *SD* estimate when study samples are small.

If meta-analysis software is used in the meta-analysis, effect size statistics do not need to be calculated manually—the program can calculate them based on means and *SD*s. But what if this information is absent from the report? Fortunately, there are alternative formulas for calculating d from information in primary study reports. For example, it is possible to derive the value of d when the report gives the value of t or F, an exact probability value, or a 95% confidence interval around the mean group difference. If the necessary statistical information is not available in a report, authors must be contacted for additional information.

When the outcomes in the primary studies are dichotomies, meta-analysts have a choice of effect size index, but the most usual are ones we discussed in earlier chapters—the relative risk (RR) index, the odds ratio (OR), and absolute risk reduction (also called the risk difference). Guidance on computing these indexes was provided in Table 16.6. The selection of a summary effect index depends on several criteria, such as mathematical properties, ease of interpretation, and consistency. The odds ratio is difficult for many users of systematic reviews to interpret but is often used as the effect size index for dichotomous outcomes in the nursing literature.

For nonexperimental studies, a common statistic used to express the relationship between an influence and an outcome is Pearson's r. If the primary studies in a meta-analysis provide statistical information in the form of a correlation coefficient, the r itself serves as the indicator of the magnitude and direction of effect.

Sometimes findings are not all reported using the same level of measurement. For example, if the variable *weight* (a continuous variable) was our key outcome, some studies might present findings for weight as a dichotomous outcome (e.g., *obese* vs. *not obese*). One approach is to re-express some of the effect indicators so that all effects can be pooled. For example, an odds ratio can be converted to d, as can a value of r—and vice versa. Formulas for converting effect size information are available online (http://cebcp.org/practical-meta-analysis-effect-size-calculator/).

> **TIP** Our discussion of calculating effects sizes glosses over several complexities. Alternative methods sometimes may be needed (e.g., when the unit of analysis was not individual people, if a crossover design was used, if data were severely skewed). Those embarking on a complex meta-analysis project should seek guidance from statisticians.

Analyzing Data in a Meta-Analysis

Meta-analysis is a two-step analytic process. In the first step, a summary statistic that captures an effect is computed for each study, as just described. In the second step, a pooled effect estimate is computed as a **weighted average** of the effects for individual studies. A weighted average is defined as follows, with ES representing effect size estimates from each study:

$$\text{weighted average} = \frac{\text{sum of} (ES \times \text{weight for that ES})}{\text{sum of the weights}}$$

Weights reflect the amount of information that each study provides. The bigger the weight given to a study, the more that study will contribute to the weighted average. One widely used approach is the **inverse variance method**, which uses the inverse of the variance of the effect size estimate (that is, one divided by the square of its standard error) as the weight. Larger studies, which have smaller standard errors, are given greater weight than smaller ones. The data needed for this type of analysis are the estimate of the effect size and its standard error, for each study.

Meta-analysts make many decisions during the analysis. In this brief overview, we present basic information about the following topics: identifying and testing heterogeneity; deciding whether to use a fixed effects or random effects model; incorporating clinical and methodologic diversity into the analysis; and handling study quality.

Testing for Heterogeneity. An important analytic issue concerns the consistency of results across primary studies, which is referred to as **statistical heterogeneity**. Just as there is variation within studies (participants do not have identical scores on outcomes), there is inevitably variation in effects across studies. If results are highly variable (e.g., conflicting results), a meta-analysis may be inappropriate. But heterogeneity is a concern for analysts even when statistical pooling is justified.

Visual inspection of heterogeneity can most readily be accomplished by constructing a forest plot, which can be generated using meta-analysis software. **Forest plots** graph the estimated effect size for each study and the 95% CI around each estimate. Figure 30.1 depicts two forest plots for situations in which there is low (A) and high (B) heterogeneity for five studies that used the odds ratio as the effect size index. In Panel A, all ES estimates favor the intervention group and are statistically significant for three of them (studies 2, 4, and 5). In Panel B, results are "all over the map": two studies favor controls at significant levels (studies 1 and 5) and two favor the treatment group (studies

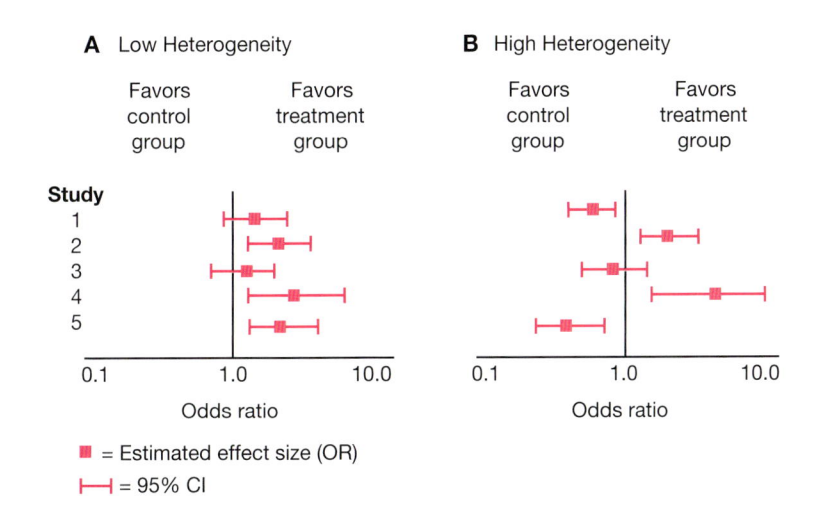

FIGURE 30.1 Two forest plots for five studies with low (A) and high (B) heterogeneity of effect size estimates.

2 and 4). A meta-analysis is not appropriate for the studies in B.

A procedure should be used to test the null hypothesis that heterogeneity across studies reflects random fluctuations. The test—traditionally the *Q test*—yields a *p* value indicating the probability of obtaining ES differences as large as those observed if the null hypothesis were true. An alpha of 0.05 is usually used as the significance criterion but, because the test is underpowered when the meta-analysis involves a small number of studies, an α of 0.10 is sometimes considered an acceptable criterion. Reviewers now often use the *I^2 test*, which adjusts for the number of studies in the analysis. This index yields values on a scale from 0% to 100%; a value greater than 50% usually is considered as moderate to high heterogeneity.

Deciding on a Statistical Model. Two basic statistical models can be used in a meta-analysis, and the choice relates to heterogeneity. In a **fixed effects model**, it is assumed that a single true effect size underlies all study results and that observed estimates vary only as a function of chance. The error term in a fixed effects model represents only within-study variation; between-study variation is ignored. A **random effects model**, by contrast, assumes that each study estimates different, yet related, true effects, and that the estimates are normally distributed around a mean effect size. A random effects model takes both within- and between-study variation into account.

When there is little heterogeneity, both models yield nearly identical results. With extensive heterogeneity, however, the analyses yield different estimates of the average effect size. Moreover, when there is heterogeneity, the random effects model yields wider confidence intervals than the fixed effects model and so is more conservative. But it is precisely when there *is* extensive heterogeneity that a random effects model should be used.

Some argue that a random effects model is needed only when the test for heterogeneity is statistically significant (or when $I^2 > 50\%$). Others argue that a random effects model is almost always more tenable. A recommended approach is to perform a **sensitivity analysis**—a test of how sensitive the results of an analysis are to changes in the way the analysis was done. This would involve using both models to assess how the results are affected. If the results differ substantially, it is prudent to report estimates from the random effects model.

Examining Factors Affecting Heterogeneity. Many meta-analysts seek to understand determinants of effect size variation through formal analyses. Such analyses should always be considered exploratory because they are inherently nonexperimental (observational)—any causal interpretations are necessarily speculative. To be considered scientifically appropriate, explorations of heterogeneity should be specified before doing the review (i.e., in the protocol), to minimize the risk of finding spurious associations.

Heterogeneity across studies could reflect systematic differences regarding clinical or methodologic characteristics, and both can be explored. *Clinical heterogeneity* can result from participant differences (e.g., males vs. females) or in the way that the independent variable was operationalized. For example, in intervention studies, variation in effects could reflect who the agents were (e.g., nurses vs. others) or what the setting or delivery mode was.

Methodologic heterogeneity could reflect design features, such when the outcomes were measured (e.g., 3 vs. 4 months after an intervention) or whether a randomized design was used. Explorations of methodologic diversity focus mainly on the possibility that results are affected by bias. Explorations of clinical diversity, on the other hand, are more substantively relevant: they examine the possibility that effects differ in relation to clinically relevant factors (e.g., are effects larger for certain types of people?).

Two strategies can be used to explore *moderating effects* on effect size: subgroup analysis and metaregression. **Subgroup analysis** involves splitting effect size information from studies into distinct subgroups—for example, gender groups. Effects for studies with all-male (or predominantly male) samples could be compared to those for studies with all or predominantly female samples, using some threshold for predominance (e.g., 80%

or more of participants). Of course, if it is possible to derive separate effect size estimates for males and females directly from study data, it is advantageous to do so, but this is seldom possible without contacting the researchers. Caution is important in undertaking subgroup analyses, as subgroup effects are often found to be spurious. (Subgroup analyses in primary studies are discussed at length in Chapter 31.)

When variables thought to influence study heterogeneity are continuous (e.g., "dose" of the intervention), or when there is a mix of continuous and categorical factors, then meta-regression might be appropriate. **Meta-regression** involves predicting the effect size based on possible explanatory factors. As in ordinary regression, the statistical significance of regression coefficients indicates a nonrandom linear relationship between effect sizes and the explanatory variable.

Example of Investigating Heterogeneity
Salari and colleagues (2020) conducted a systematic review and meta-analysis to examine the prevalence of the symptoms of stress, anxiety, and depression in the general population during the COVID-19 pandemic. Because there was heterogeneity in the studies, they were able to examine publication bias of three clinical symptoms by using a random effects model in the analysis of findings. They found that there was not significant publication bias.

Addressing Study Quality. There are four basic strategies for dealing with study quality in a meta-analysis. One is to set a quality threshold for study inclusion. Exclusions could reflect requirements for certain features (e.g., only randomized studies) or for a sufficiently high score on a quality assessment scale. We prefer other alternatives that allow reviewers to summarize the full range of evidence in an area, but quality-based exclusions might in some cases be justified.

A second strategy is to perform sensitivity analyses to see whether the exclusion of lower-quality studies changes the results. Conn and colleagues (2003) described as one option beginning the meta-analysis with high-quality studies and then sequentially adding studies of progressively lower quality to evaluate how robust the effect size estimates are to variation in quality.

Example of a Sensitivity Analysis for Study Quality
Qian et al. (2021) conducted a systematic review and to examine the effect of m-health interventions on breast feeding. M-health interventions improved breast feeding rates. The sensitivity analysis showed the results were stable at the timepoints of 1, 2, 3 and 6 months.

A third approach is to test indicators of bias as factors influencing heterogeneity of effects. For example, do effects vary as a function of the study's score on a quality assessment scale? Individual study components ratings (as in Table 30.1) and overall study quality can be used in subgroup analyses and metaregressions.

A fourth strategy is to weight studies according to quality criteria. Meta-analyses routinely give more weight to larger studies, but effect sizes can also be weighted by quality scores, thereby placing more weight on the estimates from rigorous studies. Jüni and colleagues (2001), however, warned that this approach is problematic for several reasons, such as the unknown validity of quality assessment scales and the unreliability of ratings.

A mix of strategies, with appropriate sensitivity analyses, is probably the most prudent approach to dealing with variation in study quality.

TIP Quality information, using a scale or component approach, is important descriptively and should be reported. For example, with a 25-point quality scale, reviewers should report the mean scale score across primary studies, or the percentage scoring above a threshold (e.g., 20 or higher).

Graphic Output From a Meta-Analysis. Dedicated meta-analysis software generates graphics to summarize aspects of the review. The most important graphic is the previously mentioned *forest plot*. A forest plot (Figure 30.2) visually communicates the effect in each primary study in the review (the point estimate for which is shown as a square with lines extending to show the 95% CI) and the overall meta-analysis results (shown as a diamond). The size of the squares corresponds to the weight assigned to each study, based on sample size. In this example, the overall effect for the risk ratio effect size, using a random effects model, was 1.49, a

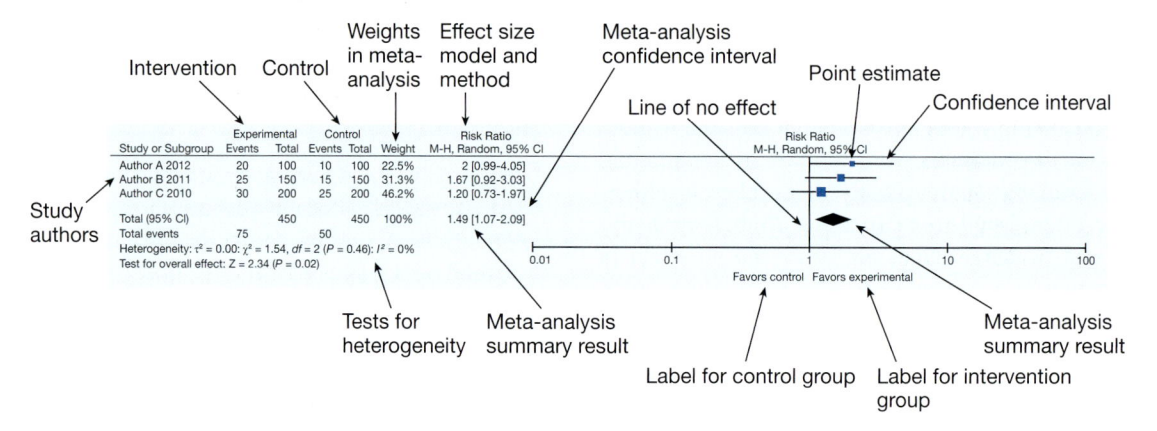

FIGURE 30.2 Annotated illustration of a forest plot from meta-analysis software. (Reprinted with permission from Munn, Z., Tufanaru, C., & Aromataris, E. (2014). JBI's systematic reviews: Data extraction and synthesis. *American Journal of Nursing, 114*(7), 49–54.)

statistically significant effect favoring those in the experimental group (p = .02). Heterogeneity for the three studies in the analysis was not significant ($\chi^2 = 1.54$, p = .46, $I^2 = 0\%$).

Meta-analysis software often provides other graphics to facilitate interpretation. For example, Cochrane's RevMan software creates a figure that summarizes RoB ratings for the components in Table 30.1 for every study in the review, as illustrated in Figure 30.3. Another useful risk-of-bias graph illustrates the proportion of studies with each of the three risk appraisal ratings (low, high, unclear) for the six bias components.

Example of Graphic Output

Lee and colleagues (2020) conducted a systematic review and meta-analysis to explore the debriefing methods and learning outcomes in simulation in nurse education. Eighteen studies were included in the systematic review and seven were included in the meta-analysis. They examined symmetry to estimate publication bias and presented the results in a funnel plot. The symmetric shape of the plot suggested there was no evidence of selective reporting.

Interpreting Results and Assessing Degree of Confidence: GRADE

Until a few years ago, reviewers typically moved from analyzing their data to writing a report of the findings. Increasingly, reviewers are taking one further step. Many systematic reviews now include a systematic effort to appraise the entire body of evidence—that is, to draw conclusions about how much *confidence* can be placed in the results of the review. Numerous organizations internationally, including the Cochrane Collaboration and JBI,

Study	A	B	C	D	E	F
Allen et al., 2017	+	−	+	+	+	−
Chisolm & Evans, 2016	+	+	+	+	+	?
Denny et al., 2018	+	?	−	−	?	−
Friesen et al., 2015	+	?	+	+	+	+
Koretzky & Forman, 2017	+	+	+	+	+	+
Strohl & O'Connor, 2018	+	+	−	−	?	−

KEY: A = Random sequence generation
B = Allocation concealment
C = Blinding participants/ personnel
D = Blinding of outcome assessment
E = Incomplete outcome data
F = Reporting bias

Green (+) = Low risk of bias
Red (−) = High risk of bias
Yellow (?) = Unclear risk of bias

FIGURE 30.3 Example of a risk of bias summary figure for studies in a review. (Adapted with permission from Figure 8.6a in Higgins and Thomas (Eds.). (2022). *Cochrane handbook for systematic reviews of interventions (version 6.3)*. The Cochrane Collaboration. Retrieved from http://training.cochrane.org/handbook)

have adopted the Grading of Recommendations, Assessment, Development and Evaluation (**GRADE**) approach to grading quality of evidence (Guyatt et al., 2008, 2011).

GRADE involves a two-part process designed to facilitate the development of clinical guidelines. In the first part of the process, the quality of the evidence about an intervention's effect is graded for each outcome. In the second part, a recommendation is made about using/not using the intervention, together with the strength of the recommendation (strong or weak). For those preparing a systematic review, only the first part is completed—that is, reviewers do not make clinical recommendations.

GRADE ratings are done on an outcome-by-outcome basis and usually are applied to only a subset of outcomes in a review—the patient-important outcomes judged to be critical to those making decisions about an intervention. Thus, an initial step is to decide which outcomes from the review will be graded.

> **TIP** GRADE was developed initially for evaluating the quality of a body of evidence for studies addressing Therapy questions, but guidelines have been developed for grading other types of studies, such as prognosis studies (Iorio et al., 2015), economic evaluations (Brunetti et al., 2013), and diagnostic test assessments (Schünemann et al., 2008).

Although evidence quality lies on a continuum, GRADE involves making a categorical determination of the *confidence* one can place in the systematic review results—that is, whether confidence in the evidence for a specified outcome (regardless of effect size) is High (++++), Moderate (+++), Low (++), or Very low (+). The second column of Table 30.2 shows GRADE's description of these classifications. A rating of High, for example, corresponds to high confidence that the *true* effect is close to the effect estimated in the review.

The review team begins by assigning an a priori "High" score (corresponding to 4 points) if the review integrated findings from randomized studies (column 1 of Table 30.2) or a "Low" score (2 points) if the primary studies were observational (nonexperimental). Evidence can be downgraded based on assessments of five criteria (column 3 of Table 30.2):

- **Risk of bias.** Important limitations in RCTs include lack of allocation concealment, lack of blinding, loss to follow up, and selective outcome reporting bias. Key limitations in observational studies include failure to control confounders, flawed measurement of exposure and outcome, and faulty eligibility criteria. Reviewers make a judgment about RoB (low, serious, very serious) *across all studies in the review* for the specified outcome.
- **Inconsistent results.** Results are inconsistent if point estimates vary widely across studies, the CIs for studies show minimal overlap, the test for heterogeneity has a low *p*-value, and/or the I^2 is large.
- **Indirectness of evidence.** Direct evidence comes from studies that directly compare interventions on outcomes of interest (e.g., not surrogate outcomes) in populations of direct interest (e.g., population of interest is people in long-term care but evidence is from hospital patients).
- **Imprecision.** Wide CIs for the specified outcome for studies in the review (usually because of small sample size) may result in downgrading the rating.
- **Publication bias.** Publication bias can result in substantial overestimates of effects, so a body of evidence can be downgraded if the risk of publication bias is likely.

The rating for a specific outcome in non-RCTs can be upgraded under three circumstances (column 4 of Table 30.2):

- **Large effect.** Confidence in evidence from observational studies can be upgraded when an effect is so large that the biases common to such studies could not account for the magnitude of the effect.
- **Dose–response gradient.** Confidence is enhanced when the effect is proportional to the degree of exposure.

TABLE 30.2 • GRADE Scoring for the Quality of Evidence for the Effect of an Intervention on a Specific Outcome[a]

STUDY DESIGN	QUALITY OF EVIDENCE	SUBTRACT POINTS IF:	ADD POINTS IF:
Randomized controlled trials (RCTs) (Start at 4 points, High)	High (++++): We are very confident that the true effect lies close to that of the estimate of the effect.	**Risk of bias** −1 Serious risk −2 Very serious risk **Inconsistent results:** −1 Serious concern −2 Very serious concern	**Large magnitude of effect:** +1 Large +2 Very large **Dose–response gradient:** +1 Evidence of a gradient
Downgraded RCTs or Upgraded observational studies	Moderate (+++): We are moderately confident in the effect estimate: The true effect is likely to be close to the estimate of the effect, but there is a possibility that it is substantially different.	**Indirectness of evidence:** −1 Serious concern −2 Very serious concern	**All plausible confounding:** would reduce a demonstrated effect or would suggest a spurious effect when results show no effect +1
Observational studies or double-downgraded RCTs	Low (++): Our confidence in the effect estimate is limited: The true effect may be substantially different from the estimate of the effect.	**Imprecision (Wide CIs):** −1 Serious concern −2 Very serious concern	
Downgraded studies of all types of design	Very low (+): We have very little confidence in the effect estimate: The true effect is likely to be substantially different from the estimate of effect	**Publication bias:** −1 Likely −2 Very likely	

[a]This table is a composite/adaptation of several tables created by the GRADE group.

- **Implausible confounders.** The score can be upgraded when possible confounders would probably *diminish* the observed effect, and so the actual effect likely is larger than the calculated effect size suggests.

The use of GRADE inevitably involves subjective judgments. For example, would a review of 10 RCTs be downgraded from High to Moderate if only two studies did not use blinding? The developers of GRADE acknowledge the need to "take an overall or gestalt view of the body of evidence" in scoring (Guyatt et al., 2011, p. 154). Evaluating confidence in the evidence using GRADE is not completely objective, but what it offers is transparency, requiring reviewers to explicitly provide a rationale for grading decisions.

Systematic reviewers who apply the GRADE approach often use software called GRADEpro, which generates two types of tables. The first is an **evidence profile** that provides detailed information about the grading judgments for each outcome. The rows of evidence profiles indicate each outcome that has been graded. Columns correspond to features of the scoring—such as RoB, inconsistency, and so on. The entries in the cells explain why any downgrading occurred.

GRADEpro can also produce **Summary of Findings** (SoF) tables. These tables show, for each outcome (shown in the rows), the results of the meta-analysis, number of participants and studies on which the effect size was based, and then the quality of evidence score (Table 30.3).

TABLE 30.3 • **Summary of Findings Table**

Educational or behavioral interventions compared to standard care for adherence to phosphate control in adults receiving hemodialysis

Patient or population: Adults receiving hemodialysis
Intervention: Educational or behavioral interventions
Comparison: Standard care

OUTCOME	NUMBER OF PARTICIPANTS			MEAN DIFFERENCE[a]	TEST FOR OVERALL EFFECT	QUALITY OF THE EVIDENCE (GRADE)
	EDUCATION OR BEHAVIORAL INTERVENTION				STANDARD CARE	TOTAL
Serum phosphate level	$n = 408$	$n = 382$	$n = 790$ (8 RCTs)	$d = -0.23$ mmol/L 95% CI ($-0.37, -0.08$)	$Z = 3.01$, $p = .003$	⊕⊕⊕○ MODERATE[b]

[a]Mean difference in serum phosphate level is expressed as intervention group minus standard care group.
[b]No explanation was given on blinding of data collectors and allocation concealment in four studies.

CI, Confidence interval; d, Mean difference; Z, Z-score.

Reprinted with permission from Milazi, M., Bonner, A., & Douglas, C. (2017). Effectiveness of educational or behavioral interventions on adherence to phosphate control in adults receiving hemodialysis: A systematic review. *JBI Database of Systematic Reviews and Implementation Reports, 15*(4), 971–1010.

Example of Using GRADE
Dias et al. (2021) conducted a systematic review to determine if exercise-based rehabilitation delivered through telehealth improved pain, physical function and quality of life in adults with physical disabilities. Two members of the team used the GRADE system to determine the strength of the recommendations and a third reviewer resolved discrepancies.

Writing a Quantitative Systematic Review

The final step in a systematic review project is to prepare a report to disseminate the results. Such reports typically follow much the same format as reports for primary studies, with an introduction, method section, results section, and discussion (see Chapter 32).

Particular care should be taken in preparing the method section. Readers of the review need to be able to assess the rigor of the review, and so methodologic decisions and their rationales should be described. Often, reports of systematic reviews include several appendixes that show details (e.g., the search strategy or quality appraisals of individual studies). If the reviewers decided that a meta-analysis was not justified, the reason for this decision must be made clear. The Cochrane *Handbook* (Higgins et al., 2022) offers excellent suggestions for preparing reports for a systematic review. There is also an explicit reporting guideline for meta-analyses of RCTs called **PRISMA** or Preferred Reporting Items for Systematic reviews and Meta-Analyses (Liberati et al., 2009) and another for meta-analyses of observational studies called **MOOSE** (Meta-analysis of Observational Studies in Epidemiology (Stroup et al., 2000)). Our critical appraisal guidelines later in this chapter also suggest types of information to include.

A thorough discussion section is also important. The discussion should present an assessment of the overall quality of the body of evidence and the consistency of findings across studies—as well as an interpretation of why there might be inconsistencies. If GRADE was used to evaluate confidence in the results, that information is usually included in the discussion section. Implications of the review should also be described, including a discussion of further research needed to improve the evidence base and the clinical implications of the review.

Tables and figures typically play a key role in reports of systematic reviews. Forest plots are almost always presented, as well as SoF tables. A table usually summarizes characteristics of studies in the review. Also, the PRISMA guidelines call for the inclusion of a flow chart that documents the identification, screening, and inclusion of studies in a systematic review.

Finally, full citations for the entire sample of studies included in the review should be provided in the bibliography. Often these are identified separately from other references—for example, by noting them with asterisks.

QUALITATIVE SYSTEMATIC REVIEWS

The systematic integration of qualitative findings is a rapidly evolving and sometimes perplexing field. Dozens of approaches have been proposed and hundreds of articles describing, explaining, or critiquing them have been published in the last 10 years alone. The field is also filled with controversies and debates. Some prominent qualitative scholars have challenged the prominence of *systematic* reviews as an approach to synthesizing healthcare knowledge (e.g., Greenhalgh et al., 2018). Others have embraced the expansion of systematic reviews to include qualitative evidence.

Terminology in this field can also be confusing. Indeed, there is not even a consensus on what to call the entire enterprise. The most frequently used "umbrella" terms are *qualitative metasynthesis, qualitative systematic review, qualitative evidence synthesis,* and *qualitative research synthesis* (Booth et al., 2016).

It is beyond the scope of this book to provide detailed descriptions of the various approaches to synthesizing qualitative evidence. Even summarizing the state of this field adequately is challenging. Several groups have put effort into developing comparison tables for various approaches along multiple dimensions as aids to helping reviewers select the "right" approach. Our goal in this chapter is to present a broad overview of a few approaches.

Aggregative and Interpretive Qualitative Reviews

Several scholars have characterized systematic reviews as being either *aggregative* or *interpretive/configurative* (e.g., Booth et al., 2018; Gough et al., 2012). We will use the aggregative/interpretive distinction to highlight several features of qualitative reviews, but we emphasize that most qualitative reviews have elements of both aggregation and interpretation and that the boundaries between these two broad categories are permeable.

The decision on which broad (and specific) qualitative synthesis approach to use depends on several factors, including the nature of the question and the philosophical leanings of the reviewers. Other important factors may include time and resource constraints, the expertise of the review team, and the intended audience for the review (Booth et al., 2018; Paterson, 2013). For students, the decision may also be affected by the preferences of their advisers.

Aggregative Qualitative Reviews

Qualitative reviews that are predominantly aggregative are similar in many respects to quantitative systematic reviews. Aggregative reviews involve the *pooling* of findings (that is, themes, categories, or processes) across the qualitative studies in the review. Other features that make aggregative qualitative reviews similar to quantitative systematic reviews include the following:

- The review process tends to be fairly structured, following a well-defined series of steps;
- The questions these reviews address are predetermined and, often, fairly focused;
- Exhaustive searching for primary studies is expected;
- Assessment of the quality of the primary studies is considered essential;
- Efforts are made to minimize subjectivity or bias; and
- A goal of the review is to provide direct and useable guidance for action.

Certain research questions are especially well-suited to an aggregative qualitative approach. Often these questions concern how best to address a healthcare problem—questions typically addressed in descriptive qualitative inquiries. Examples of such questions include the following: Why do people who know the risks of smoking continue to smoke? What strategies do people use in efforts to quit smoking? What are patients' barriers to participating in a smoking cessation intervention? What features of a smoking intervention lead to lapses in implementation fidelity?

Both the JBI and the Cochrane Collaboration, who typically use the umbrella term **qualitative evidence synthesis (QES)**, provide guidance for reviews that would best be characterized as aggregative. At JBI, qualitative reviews use an approach to evidence synthesis called **meta-aggregation** (Aromataris & Munn, 2020; Hannes & Lockwood, 2011). The JBI approach is described in a later section.

Interpretive Qualitative Reviews

Qualitative reviews that are predominantly interpretive in nature emphasize the creation of integrated conceptualizations and theories by interpreting and reconfiguring findings from qualitative studies. Interpretive syntheses tend to have the following features:

- The approach tends not to be highly structured;
- The questions addressed by interpretive reviews often evolve during a process of discovery;
- Purposive sampling of studies is sometimes preferred to comprehensive searching;
- Assessment of the quality of the primary studies is not always considered essential;
- Interpreters' insights are valued; and
- The goal of the review is to provide enlightenment through new ways of understanding phenomena.

Interpretive syntheses most often focus on questions about meanings, feelings, experiences, and processes—questions typically addressed through phenomenologic, ethnographic, or grounded theory research. Examples of such questions include the following: What is it like for smokers to lose a loved one to lung cancer? Is smoking an important part of the culture among those in the military? What is the process by which previous smokers succeed in quitting?

In nursing, the term **metasynthesis** has predominated as the umbrella term for qualitative synthesis, usually referring to syntheses that are interpretive. In fact, nurse researchers have contributed more to the field of qualitative research synthesis than scholars in other health-related disciplines (Tricco et al., 2016). In the next section, we discuss metasynthesis but note that nurse researchers have used other interpretive synthesis approaches, including critical interpretive synthesis or CIS (Dixon-Woods et al., 2006), and thematic synthesis (Thomas & Harden, 2008).

TIP The book by Hannes and Lockwood (2012) has completely worked out examples of a meta-ethnography, a critical interpretive synthesis, and a meta-aggregation.

Metasynthesis

Over a decade ago, five leading thinkers on qualitative integration used the term "metasynthesis" as an umbrella term, with metasynthesis broadly representing "a family of methodologic approaches to developing new knowledge based on rigorous analysis of existing qualitative research findings" (Thorne et al., 2004), p. 1343). There are diverse approaches to doing a metasynthesis.

There is more agreement on what a metasynthesis is not than on what it is. Metasynthesis is not a literature review—nor a collation of research findings—nor is it a concept analysis. Many writers have followed the definition of metasynthesis offered by Schreiber and colleagues (1997): "…the bringing together and breaking down of findings, examining them, discovering the essential features and, in some way, combining phenomena into a transformed whole" (p. 314). Most metasyntheses involve a transformational process.

Two important approaches to interpretive metasynthesis are **metaethnography** (Noblit & Hare, 1988) and **metastudy** (Paterson et al., 2001). An approach called **metasummary** (Sandelowski & Barroso, 2007) is more of an aggregative than interpretive approach; it is described in this section because of its link to metasynthesis. For the most part, differences in these approaches concern how the data from qualitative studies are analyzed and synthesized.

Preliminary Steps in a Metasynthesis

Many of the steps in qualitative syntheses are similar to ones we described for quantitative systematic reviews, and so details will not be repeated here. However, we point out a few distinctive issues relating to qualitative integration.

Formulating the Question. In metasynthesis, researchers begin with a broad research question or an investigative focus. Booth et al. (2018) have described the research question in an aggregative review as an "anchor," but more like a "compass" in interpretive reviews. One issue concerns the scope of the inquiry. Finfgeld (2003) recommended that the scope be broad enough to fully capture the phenomenon of interest, but sufficiently focused to yield findings that are meaningful to clinicians or other researchers.

In metasyntheses, the research question may evolve over the course of the review. It may not be evident at first whether the initial question can be answered, or whether the scope of the review should be expanded or contracted. In their reports, metasynthesists sometimes state an overall study purpose rather than a research question.

> **Example of a Statement of Purpose in a Meta-Ethnography**
> Reeder (2022) stated that her aim was to synthesize the findings from qualitative studies on the experiences of people who are incarcerated in accessing mental healthcare with the goal of better understanding the scope of these experiences and identifying gaps in custodial mental healthcare.

Designing a Metasynthesis. Metasyntheses require advance planning. Having a team of at least two researchers to design and implement the study is often advantageous. Investigator triangulation is one strategy for enhancing the integrity of the metasynthesis.

> **TIP** Meta-analyses often are undertaken by researchers who did not do one of the primary studies in the review. Metasyntheses, by contrast, are often completed by researchers whose area of interest has led them to do both original studies and metasyntheses on the same topic. Prior work in an area offers advantages in terms of researchers' ability to grasp subtle nuances and to think abstractly about a topic, but a disadvantage may be a certain degree of partiality about one's own work.

Metasynthesists make several decisions about sampling. One issue is whether their sample of studies will be exhaustive (i.e., including all relevant studies) or purposive. Some approaches to metasynthesis, notably metaethnography, may involve purposive strategies in which studies are selected for conceptual purposes. For those opting for a purposive strategy, one guideline for sampling adequacy is whether categories in the metasynthesis are theoretically saturated (Finfgeld, 2003; Toye et al., 2014). Thus, the number of studies included in a metasynthesis is likely to be affected by the conceptual richness of the studies themselves. When purposive sampling is adopted, it is often difficult to articulate an up-front sampling strategy.

Another issue is whether to include findings only from peer-reviewed journals in the synthesis. One advantage of including nonpublished sources is that journal articles are constrained in what can be reported because of space limitations. Finfgeld (2003), in her metasynthesis on *courage,* used dissertations even when a peer-reviewed journal article was available from the same study because the dissertation offered richer data.

An aspect of sampling that has been controversial in metasynthesis concerns whether to integrate studies from different research traditions. Some researchers have argued against combining studies from different traditions. Others, however, advocate combining findings across traditions and methods. Which path to follow is likely to depend on the focus of the inquiry, its intent vis-à-vis theory development, and the nature of the available evidence.

Example of Sampling Decisions
Bayuo and colleagues (2023) conducted a metaethnography on the qualitative findings of the experiences of people living with postburn scars. Inclusion criteria included (1) primary qualitative or mixed methods studies with a qualitative strand exploring scarring experiences after moderate to severe burns, (2) reported in English, and (3) published between 2010 and 2020. Preprints and gray literature were excluded.

Regardless of whether sampling for the review will be exhaustive or purposive, metasynthesists must develop inclusion and exclusion criteria. These are likely to include language restrictions, and perhaps restrictions on settings (e.g., rural; long-term care settings), demographic characteristics (e.g., people older than 60 years), or research tradition.

Searching the Literature for Data. It is sometimes difficult to find relevant qualitative studies for a synthesis. Booth (2016) identified numerous challenges in searching for qualitative studies, including nonstandardized terminology, inadequate database indexing, interdatabase differences in indexing terminology, and the variety of qualitative methodologies. It is likely to be helpful to search using not only broad search terms (qualitative) but also specific names of traditions (e.g., grounded theory, phenomenolog*, ethnograph*). Booth's suggested search terms include *interview* and *experience*. Further search guidance is offered by DeJean et al. (2016).

TIP Mnemonics other than PICO have been proposed for qualitative evidence searches (Booth, 2016). These include 3WH (What [topic], Who [population], When [temporal], and How [methodologic]); SPIDER (Sample, Phenomenon of Interest, Design, Evaluation, Research type), and PICo (Population, phenomenon of Interest, Context).

Appraising Study Quality. In general, there is less of an emphasis on assessing the methodologic quality of primary studies in interpretive syntheses than in aggregative ones. Nevertheless, critical appraisal is often used in metasyntheses, sometimes simply to describe the sample of studies in the review but in other cases to make sampling decisions.

There is no consensus about whether quality should be a criterion for eliminating studies for a metasynthesis. Sandelowski and Barroso (2003a) advocated inclusiveness: "Excluding reports of qualitative studies because of inadequacies in reporting…, or because of what some reviewers might perceive as methodologic mistakes, will result in the exclusion of reports with findings valuable to practice that are not necessarily invalidated by these errors" (p. 155). Finfgeld (2003) suggested that, at a minimum, studies included in the review must have used accepted qualitative methods and must have findings that are supported by raw data (i.e., quotes from participants).

Noblit and Hare (1988) advocated including all relevant studies, but also suggested giving more weight to higher-quality studies. A more systematic application of assessments in a metasynthesis is to use quality information in a sensitivity analysis that explores whether interpretations are altered when low-quality studies are removed (Thomas & Harden, 2008).

Several instruments have been created to appraise qualitative studies for a metasynthesis. Many nurse researchers use the 10-question assessment tool from the Critical Appraisal Skills Programme (CASP) of the Centre for Evidence-Based Medicine in the United Kingdom (CASP, 2016). Others use the tool created for JBI qualitative evidence summaries, which we describe later in this chapter. Majid and Vanstone (2018) undertook a detailed analysis of appraisal instruments and recommended that those who are novices or looking for an easy-to-follow tool should use CASP.

Example of a Quality Appraisal in a Metasynthesis
Wang and Tocchi (2023) conducted a meta-ethnography of partners' experiences of informal caregiving for people with heart failure. The ten included studies were appraised using the CASP instrument. Two researchers compared study scores and any scoring disagreements were resolved through discussion. Nine out of the ten studies received a high rating and one study received a moderate rating.

Extracting Data for Analysis. Information about various features of the study needs to be abstracted and coded as part of the project. Metasynthesists usually record data source information (e.g., year of publication, country), characteristics of the sample (e.g., number of participants, mean age, gender distribution), and methodologic features (e.g., research tradition).

Most important, information about study findings must be extracted and recorded. Sandelowski and Barroso (2003b) have defined *findings* as the "data-based and integrated discoveries, conclusions, judgments, or pronouncements researchers offered regarding the events, experiences, or cases under investigation (i.e., their interpretations, no matter the extent of the data transformation involved)" (p. 228). Others characterize findings as the key themes, metaphors, categories, concepts, or phrases from each study.

As Sandelowski and Barroso (2002) have noted, however, *finding* the findings is not always easy. Qualitative researchers intermingle data with interpretation and findings from other studies with their own. Noblit and Hare (1988) advised that, just as primary study researchers must read and reread their data before they can proceed with a meaningful analysis, metasynthesists must read the primary studies multiple times to fully grasp the categories or metaphors being explicated. A metasynthesis becomes "another 'reading' of data, an opportunity to reflect on the data in new ways" (McCormick et al., 2003, p. 936).

Synthesizing and Interpreting the Data

Strategies for metasynthesis diverge most at the analysis stage. We briefly describe three approaches and advise you to consult other resources for more guidance. Regardless of approach, metasynthesis is a complex task that involves "carefully peeling away the surface layers of studies to find their hearts and souls in a way that does the least damage to them" (Sandelowski et al., 1997, p. 370).

Meta-Ethnography. Noblit and Hare's (1988) meta-ethnographic approach has been influential among nurse researchers. Noblit and Hare argued that the synthesis should focus on constructing interpretations rather than analyses (i.e., interpretation in lieu of aggregation). Their approach includes seven phases that overlap and repeat as the synthesis progresses, the first three of which are preanalytic: (1) deciding on the phenomenon, (2) deciding which studies are relevant for the synthesis, and (3) reading and rereading each study. Phase 7 involves writing up the synthesis. Phases 4 through 6 concern the analysis:

Phase 4: Deciding how the studies are related to each other. In this phase the researcher makes a list of the key metaphors in each study and their relation to each other. Noblit and Hare used the term "metaphor" to refer to themes, perspectives, and/or concepts that emerged from the primary studies. Studies can be related in three ways: *reciprocal* (directly comparable), *refutational* (in opposition to each other), and in *lines of argument* rather than either reciprocal or refutational.

Phase 5: Translating the qualitative studies into one another. Noblit and Hare noted that "translations are especially unique syntheses because they protect the particular, respect holism, and enable comparison. An adequate translation maintains the central metaphors and/or concepts of each account in their relation to other key metaphors or concepts in that account" (p. 28). *Reciprocal translation analysis* (RTA) involves exploring and explaining similarities and contradictions between studies and is similar to constant comparison.

Phase 6: Synthesizing translations. In this phase, the challenge is to make a whole into more than the individual parts imply. Syntheses involve building up a new picture of the whole (e.g., a whole culture or phenomenon) from a scrutiny of its parts.

Atkins and colleagues (2008), noting that some aspects of metaethnography were not well-defined by Noblit and Hare, offered further guidance. Campbell and colleagues (2011) prepared a useful open-access document that presents an evaluation of metaethnographic methods. More recently, Toye and colleagues (2014) identified challenges and offered suggestions for building on the metaethnographic approach.

> **Example of a Meta-Ethnography**
> Zipf and colleagues (2022) used metaethnography to synthesize findings on the experiences of nurses during the COVID-19 pandemic from 13 studies. Using Noblit and Hare's method, four themes were identified: (1) Fear and moral conflict: Unprepared and scared for safety; (2) Duty: A sense of calling and obligation; (3) Mental and physical side effects: Exhaustion; and (4) Growth: A renewed sense of professional identify and calling.

Metastudy. Paterson and colleagues' (2001) metastudy method of metasynthesis involves three components: metadata analysis, metamethod, and metatheory. These components often are conducted concurrently, and the metasynthesis results from the integration of findings from these three components. Paterson and colleagues define **metadata analysis** as the study of results of reported research in a specific substantive area of investigation by means of analyzing the "processed data." **Metamethod** is the study of the methodologic approaches and rigor of the studies included in the metasynthesis. Lastly, **metatheory** refers to the analysis of the theoretical underpinnings on which the studies are grounded. Metastudy uses metatheory to describe and deconstruct theories that shape a body of inquiry. The end product is a metasynthesis that results from bringing back together the findings of these three components.

Example of a Metastudy
Kersey and colleagues (2022) conducted a metastudy to explore midlife women's understanding and perception of their alcohol consumption, what factors influence drinking, and the theoretical underpinnings of the qualitative studies exploring midlife women's drinking. The findings suggest midlife women's use of alcohol is influenced by social influences including material circumstances, a perception that drinking is acceptable and encouraged, and how they feel and look rather than health or other consequence.

Sandelowski and Barroso's Metasummary and Metasynthesis. The strategies developed by Sandelowski and Barroso (2007) are the results of a multiyear methodologic project. They proposed a continuum relating to how much data transformation occurs in a primary study. Further, they dichotomized studies based on level of synthesis and interpretation. Reports are described as *summaries* if the findings are descriptive synopses of the qualitative data, usually with lists and frequencies of topics and themes, without conceptual reframing. *Syntheses* are findings that are more interpretive and explanatory and that involve conceptual or metaphorical reframing. Sandelowski and Barroso argued that only syntheses should be used in a metasynthesis.

Both summaries and syntheses can, however, be used in a **metasummary**, which can lay a foundation for a metasynthesis. Sandelowski and Barroso (2003a) provided an example of a metasummary in which they used both summaries and syntheses of mothering within the context of HIV infection. The first step, extracting findings, resulted in almost 800 complete sentences from the 45 reports. The 800 sentences were then reduced to 93 thematic statements, or abstracted findings.

The next step in the metasummary was to calculate **manifest effect sizes** (i.e., effect sizes calculated from the manifest content pertaining to motherhood within the context of HIV as represented in the 93 abstracted findings). Qualitative effect sizes should not be confused with treatment effects: the "…calculation of effect sizes constitutes a quantitative transformation of qualitative data in the service of extracting more meaning from those data and verifying the presence of a pattern or theme" (Sandelowski & Barroso, 2003a, p. 231). They argued that by calculating effect sizes, integration can avoid the possibility of over- or underweighting findings.

Two types of manifest effect size can be calculated. A **frequency effect size**, which indicates the magnitude of a finding, is the number of reports with unduplicated information that contain a given finding, divided by all unduplicated reports. For example, Sandelowski and Barroso (2003a) calculated an overall frequency effect size of 60% for the finding of mothers struggling with whether or not to disclose their HIV status to their children. In other words, 60% of the 45 reports had a finding of this nature. Such effect size information can be calculated for subgroups of reports (e.g., for published vs. unpublished reports, for reports from different research traditions, and so on).

An **intensity effect size** indicates the concentration of findings *within* each report. It is calculated by dividing the number of different findings in a report, divided by the total number of findings in all reports. As an example, one primary study had 29 out of the 93 findings, for an intensity effect size of 31% for that study (Sandelowski & Barroso, 2003a).

Metasyntheses can build on metasummaries, but require findings that are interpretive (i.e., from reports characterized as syntheses). Metasyntheses require reviewers to piece the individual syntheses together and craft a new coherent explanation of a target event or experience. Several analytic methods can be used to achieve this goal, including, "…for example, constant comparison, taxonomic analysis, the reciprocal translation of in vivo concepts, and the use of imported concepts to frame data" (Sandelowski in Thorne et al., 2004, p. 1358).

> **Example of Sandelowski and Barroso's Approach**
> Shorey and Pereuram (2022) undertook a meta summary of fathers' experiences caring for children with neuro-developmental disorders. The researchers provided step-by-step description using Sandelowski and Barroso's approach to synthesize 38 studies. Four themes emerged: (1) The illness is all the time: An overwhelming experience; (2) Navigating healthcare and educational systems; (3) Strong alone, stronger together; and (4) My child is different not less: A different perspective. For each extracted theme, the effect size ranged from 76.3% to 92.1%.

Writing a Metasynthesis Report

Metasynthesis reports are similar to quantitative systematic review reports, except that the results section contains the new interpretations rather than quantitative findings. When a metasummary has been done, metafindings would typically be presented in a table.

The method section of a metasynthesis report should describe the sampling criteria, search procedures, study appraisal methods, and efforts to enhance the integrity of the integration. Key features of the sample of studies are usually summarized in a table. A PRISMA-type flowchart highlighting sampling decisions and outcomes is often included. Reporting guidelines for qualitative systematic reviews are called **ENTREQ** (Enhancing Transparency in Reporting the synthesis of Qualitative research) (Tong et al., 2012). France et al. (2019) offer reporting guidelines for metaethnographies called eMERGe.

Meta-Aggregation

The JBI uses an aggregative, structured approach to synthesizing qualitative evidence. JBI maintains that regardless of whether the evidence is quantitative or qualitative, the same review process should be used, with certain steps tailored to accommodate the special nature of the findings. Hannes and Lockwood (2011) have described the JBI approach as aligned with pragmatism, wherein the synthesis is connected to the idea of "practical usefulness." The JBI **meta-aggregation** method is aimed at delivering synthesized findings to inform clinical decision-making.

The JBI reviewer's manual (Aromataris & Munn, 2020) offers prescriptive guidance on preparing a *qualitative evidence synthesis* using meta-aggregation. Researchers at JBI have also published a series of articles describing their approach to systematic reviews in *The American Journal of Nursing* in 2014 (e.g., Munn et al., 2014; Porritt et al., 2014). Additionally, the qualitative working group at the Cochrane Collaboration has published guidance on QES in six papers published in the *Journal of Clinical Epidemiology* (e.g., Noyes et al., 2018; Tugwell et al., 2018). Although less prescriptive than JBI, the Cochrane guidelines also favor aggregative approaches. In this section, we briefly touch on a few issues relating to the JBI approach.

Preliminary Steps in a JBI Qualitative Evidence Synthesis

In a meta-aggregation synthesis, an explicit review question is formulated upfront. JBI recommends using the PICo format (**P**opulation, phenomenon of **I**nterest, **Co**ntext) for articulating the question (Stern et al., 2014). Reviewers are expected to do comprehensive and exhaustive searching for relevant evidence, including a search of the gray literature. For JBI reviews, a protocol describing plans for the QES—including the review question, search strategies, and inclusion criteria—must be prepared. Data are extracted by two independent reviewers using a JBI extraction form, and the information is input into the JBI software, SUMARI. In the extraction form, findings are listed, together with a supporting illustrative quote from the study's raw data.

Quality appraisals of the studies are undertaken using the 10-item JBI Critical Appraisal Checklist for Qualitative Research. In addition to appraising each study for its overall methodologic quality, the JBI approach calls for ratings of the *credibility* of each finding in a study. Reviewers assign a rating of *unequivocal* (a finding is beyond a reasonable doubt), *credible* (finding is open to challenge), and *unsupported* (findings not supported by the data).

Analysis Through Meta-Aggregation

Data synthesis using meta-aggregation is a three-step process that begins with the extraction of findings and illustrations from all included studies. In the second step, findings that are sufficiently similar or related conceptually are collapsed into categories. Each category must have two or more findings. In the final step, the reviewers develop one or more synthesized findings that encompass at least two categories. Reviewers are expected to explain what data they considered as a "finding," the process by which findings were identified, and how findings were grouped to create categories.

Munn et al. (2014a) presented a figure illustrating the analysis for a meta-aggregation of qualitative evidence on how patients experience high-technology medical imaging like MRIs. For example, three findings were: "An alien experience," "Being in another world," and "Swallowed and sinking," and these were grouped into the category "Out of this world, alien experience." One of the synthesized findings derived from this and other categories was this: "Scanning is a unique, out-of-this world experience that must be experienced by the person to be truly understood" (p. 53).

Assessment of Confidence

Inspired by the GRADE rating system for quantitative reviews, a working group at JBI developed a system to rate confidence in the synthesized findings of a QES (Munn et al., 2014b). The **ConQual** approach, as it is called, requires a score—on a scale from four (high) to one (very low)—summarizing the reviewers' confidence in each finding. Essentially, a synthesized qualitative finding is given an initial score of "high" that can be downgraded because of low credibility (e.g., a mix of unequivocal and credible findings results in the loss of a point) or low dependability. The dependability score is based on answers to five specific questions from the critical appraisal tool.

The end product is a SoF table, similar to the one produced using GRADE. The table presents a synthesized finding for the meta-aggregation analysis in each row, together with the following information: type of research, dependability score, credibility score, the ConQual score, and comments explaining the scoring.

TIP A separate effort was undertaken by a group working with GRADE to develop a means of rating confidence in the findings from a qualitative synthesis. A seven-paper series was published in the journal *Systematic Reviews* in 2018 to explain the **GRADE-CERQual** (Confidence in the Evidence from Reviews of Qualitative Research) (see Lewin et al., 2018). The GRADE-CERQual approach considers four aspects for each finding: methodologic limitations, coherence, data adequacy, and relevance. Dissemination bias also plays a role. The system yields a Summary of Qualitative Findings table and an evidence profile. Like GRADE, there are four levels of confidence: High, Moderate, Low, and Very Low confidence. Although ConQual and CERQual develop similar rankings, the criteria for scoring in the two systems differ.

Writing a Meta-Aggregation Report

JBI's reviewer's manual provides explicit direction on preparing a qualitative evidence report. Many JBI reviews include a table that lists the studies included in the review in the rows and then answers to the 10 critical appraisal questions in the columns (yes, no, unclear, or not applicable). A diagram showing the progression from findings to categories and then to synthesized findings is encouraged. A SoF table, with ConQual ratings, is essential. Discussing the relevance of the findings to key stakeholders (e.g., patients, clinicians) is recommended.

Example of the JBI Meta-Aggregation Approach
Easton and colleagues (2022) undertook a JBI qualitative review of 24 studies on the experience of food insecurity during and following homelessness in high-income countries. Using JBI approach, their meta-aggregation yielded four themes: (1) Imposed food options as a determinant of health: out of my control; (2) Obtaining food for survival despite stigma or other consequences; (3) Situated within a system that maintains food insecurity; and (4) Surviving hardship.

SYSTEMATIC MIXED STUDIES REVIEWS

The growing recognition of the complexity of healthcare problems has given rise to interest in systematic reviews that integrate findings from a methodologic array of studies. Reviews that integrate qualitative and quantitative evidence have been called *mixed methods systematic reviews* (Pearson et al., 2014); *mixed methods reviews* (Harden & Thomas, 2005); *mixed research syntheses* (Sandelowski et al., 2013); *mixed method syntheses* (Noyes et al., 2018); and *mixed method research synthesis* (Heyvaert et al., 2017).

We use the term systematic **mixed studies review** (Pluye et al., 2016; Pluye & Hong, 2014) to refer to a systematic review that uses disciplined procedures to integrate and synthesize findings from qualitative, quantitative, and mixed methods studies. We prefer a term that does not include the phrase "mixed method," to clarify that such reviews are not syntheses of mixed methods studies alone, but rather efforts to synthesize findings from diverse primary studies.

Rationale for Mixed Studies Reviews

MSRs reflect the growing awareness that single-method reviews can seldom provide full information for making healthcare decisions in real-world settings. MSRs combine information about the human experience of illness and health with information on the prevalence of health problems, the effectiveness of interventions, or the prognosis of disease conditions. Syntheses of qualitative studies give voice to the concerns and experiences of clients and providers, and syntheses of quantitative studies provide information about outcomes and effects. Single-method reviews often present an incomplete picture that constrains their utility in evidence-based decisions. MSRs "have the capacity to present a very high level of evidence" (Pearson et al., 2014, p. 16).

In a review of MSRs, Hong and colleagues (2017) identified 459 published MSRs and found that the number had increased by 1,000% (from 10 to 101) between 2007 and 2014. The reasons for performing an MSR fell into several categories, including: (1) to acknowledge the complexity of the problem itself; (2) to address related but different questions (what, how, and why); (3) to attain a thorough understanding or provide a complete picture; (4) to strengthen confidence in results through corroboration; and (5) to provide more meaningful evidence for practice.

TIP The advantages of MSRs need to be considered within the context of potential obstacles. MSRs are more time consuming and expensive than single-method reviews and require a team with diverse skills. Moreover, the evidence may be insufficient in one of the strands to provide meaningful integration.

Another impetus for MSRs is the growing interest in complex interventions. As noted by Petticrew and colleagues (2015), complex interventions present "unique challenges" for those conducting systematic reviews. A growing body of papers to guide MSRs for complex interventions has emerged, including a series of seven papers published in the *Journal of Clinical Epidemiology* in 2017 (e.g., Pigott et al., 2017). The revised Cochrane Manual includes a chapter on reviews relating to intervention complexities (Higgins et al., 2022, Chapter 17).

Conducting Mixed Studies Reviews

In this section, we briefly review some issues relating to the conduct of MSRs but acknowledge that this is a field with new ideas and methods emerging weekly. We do not describe steps in the conduct of MSRs that are covered in earlier sections of this paper, such as searching for reports or extracting findings, but focus instead on issues unique to MSRs.

TIP An issue that has led to debate and controversy in all systematic reviews concerns quality appraisal of included studies; MSRs are no exception. Criteria for appraising the quality of quantitative, qualitative, and mixed methods study for MSRs have been proposed and tested (e.g., Pace et al., 2012; Pluye et al., 2009).

Research Questions for MSRs

As in mixed methods research, the "dictatorship of the research question" is a driving force behind MSRs. Harden and Thomas (2005), whose work focused on health promotion interventions, noted that their reviews "were beginning to answer multiple questions" and that their reviews increasingly involved "more than one section in which the results of studies are brought together" (p. 261).

In an MSR, there must be at least two questions, one requiring quantitative data and the other needing qualitative data. In many cases, the quantitative question in an MSR concerns the effects of an intervention, which is the case for all MSRs undertaken within the Cochrane Collaboration (Harden et al., 2018). In such reviews, there is a Therapy question and sometimes a question about intervention costs (economic evaluations). Qualitative questions can address diverse intervention-related issues, such as: What are patients' experiences with an intervention or with the health problem the intervention was designed to address? What are the experiences of patients unable to access the intervention? In what contexts was the intervention implemented and how did context shape the implementation and the outcomes? Which components or aspects of the intervention are perceived as most or least beneficial? MSRs can also address non-Therapy questions, including Prognosis, Etiology, and prevalence questions.

Although not always explicitly stated, MSR reviewers also address integrative questions. That is, the diverse evidence needs to be integrated to discern whether the qualitative findings corroborate, qualify, refute, or expand the quantitative ones.

Example of Questions in a Mixed Studies Review

Beck, one of the authors of this textbook, and Vo (2020) conducted a mixed research synthesis on fathers' stress related to their infants' NICU hospitalization. Using findings from 10 quantitative studies and 11 qualitative studies, the review addressed four research questions:
1. What are the stress levels of fathers whose infants are in the NICU?
2. What interventions have been tested to decrease stress in fathers while their infants are in the NICU?
3. What are the NICU experiences of fathers during their infants' stay in the NICU?
4. How do the quantitative and qualitative sets of findings develop a more comprehensive picture of stress in fathers whose infants are hospitalized in the NICU?

Designs for Mixed Studies Reviews

MSRs are a relatively new endeavor; both terminology and approaches are evolving at a rapid pace. Several typologies have been developed, some of which rely on category schemes associated with mixed methods designs (e.g., Heyvaert et al., 2013; Pluye & Hong, 2014).

A basic design issue concerns the timing of the reviews—that is, whether the review of quantitative results and the review of qualitative results are conducted concurrently (*convergent* designs) or *sequentially* (Hong et al., 2017). MSRs for the Cochrane Collaboration are all sequential; often a "posthoc" qualitative review is undertaken following a standard Cochrane review on intervention effectiveness, to offer enriched guidance to clinicians (Harden et al., 2018).

Sandelowski et al., 2006 described three MSR designs that vary in approach and goals. In a *segregated design,* two separate syntheses are undertaken, one of qualitative and the other of quantitative findings, and then the mixed synthesis integrates the two. This approach is appropriate when qualitative and quantitative findings are seen as complementing each other, as opposed to confirming or refuting each other. Complementarity occurs when the qualitative and quantitative research has addressed different but connected questions. The segregated design model characterizes many MSRs and has been found to be useful in integrating information about both effectiveness and context/processes in intervention research. The JBI has adopted segregated designs as its approach to MSR (Pearson et al., 2014).

The second model is an *integrated design* (Sandelowski et al., 2006), which can be used when qualitative and quantitative findings in an area of inquiry are perceived as able to confirm, extend, or refute each other. In an integrated design, studies are grouped not by method but by findings viewed as answering the same research question. The analytic approach may involve transforming the findings (quantitizing qualitative findings or qualitizing quantitative findings) to enable them to be combined.

A third model is a *contingent design* (Sandelowski et al., 2006) that involves a coordinated and sequential series of syntheses. In such a design, the findings from the systematic synthesis to answer one research question are used to address a second research question—which may lead to yet another synthesis addressing a different question. For example, a qualitative synthesis can precede a quantitative review and may help to define key outcomes or key variables for an analysis of heterogeneity for the meta-analysis.

In Hong et al.'s (2017) review of 459 MSRs, fewer than 5% were contingent/sequential. Most

MSRs used what they called "data-based convergent" designs, which they described as being most akin to Sandelowski et al.'s (2006) integrated design.

> **TIP** The chapter on mixed studies reviews in the JBI reviewer's manual (Chapter 8) has tables that outline Sandelowski's three MSR designs (Pearson et al., 2014).

Approaches to Analysis and Integration

Many approaches to analysis and integration in MSRs have been described. Techniques such as textual narrative, content analysis, narrative summary, thematic synthesis, and critical interpretive synthesis (an adaptation of meta-ethnography) were identified in Hong et al.'s (2017) review of MSRs; the most common method was thematic synthesis.

Another approach is *Bayesian synthesis*, which is used in MSRs at the JBI. Bayesian synthesis involves transforming data into a compatible format—that is, either converting qualitative findings to quantitative ones or vice versa (e.g., Voils et al., 2009). The JBI method involves transforming quantitative data into qualitative themes that are then synthesized through meta-aggregation (Pearson et al., 2014).

> **TIP** Lucas and colleagues (2007) provide a worked-out example of two alternative approaches to MSRs (thematic synthesis and textual narrative) and Flemming (2010) offers a step-by-step guide to using critical interpretive synthesis in an MSR. A chapter in the book by Hannes and Lockwood (2012) includes a worked example of a Bayesian approach to MSRs.

The Cochrane working group identified five "tools" or methods for integrating qualitative evidence with intervention effectiveness reviews: (1) juxtaposing findings in a matrix; (2) using logic models or conceptual frameworks; (3) analyzing intervention theory; (4) testing hypotheses derived from qualitative evidence statistically via subgroup analysis; and (5) qualitative comparison analysis (Harden et al., 2018). All five tools can be used with MSRs whose design is sequential/contingent, but only the first three can be used with convergent designs.

The third tool, analyzing intervention or program theory, is a strategy often associated with realist reviews. The aim of **realist reviews** (or *realist syntheses*) is to understand theory-driven *Context-Mechanism-Outcome* *(CMO)* configurations in studies of interventions—especially complex interventions. The overall goal of a realist review is to gain insights into what works, for whom, and under what circumstances (Emmel et al., 2019; Pawson, 2013).

According to a realist perspective, interventions work by altering the context for the people acting within it. Contexts are defined as the institutional or spatial locations in which interventions are situated. Context includes the norms, values, and interrelationships within the intervention setting, all of which establish boundaries on intervention mechanisms. The mechanisms, in turn, include the beliefs, feelings, choices, and motivations of people and groups of people, which affect behaviors that are considered outcomes. Realist reviews combine qualitative and quantitative findings to "unpack" how an intervention works in different contexts, through the development of theoretical explanations. Evidence from RCTs usually contributes to the outcome and mechanism components of a realist CMO analysis, and evidence from qualitative and implementation studies contributes to the context and mechanism components.

In Hong et al.'s (2017) review of 459 MSRs, only six were realist reviews, but interest in realist reviews is growing and several nurse researchers have been on teams that completed such reviews.

> **Example of a Realist Review**
> Caswell and colleagues (2022) undertook a systematic realist review related to providing a supportive environment for disclosure of sexual violence and based in a sexual and reproductive healthcare setting. The reviewers sought to develop and refine theories that explain how, for whom, and in what context sexual and reproductive healthcare services facilitate disclosure. A total of 28 papers were included in this review.

It is almost certain that guidance (and debate) on how best to conduct MSRs will continue in the years ahead.

BOX 30.1 Guidelines for Critically Appraising Systematic Reviews

The Problem
- Did the report clearly state the research problem and/or research questions? Is the scope of the project appropriate?
- Is the topic of the review important for nursing?
- Were concepts, variables, or phenomena adequately defined?

Search Strategy
- Did the report clearly describe criteria for selecting primary studies, and are those criteria reasonable?
- Were the databases used by the reviewers identified, and are they appropriate and comprehensive? Were search terms identified, and are they exhaustive?
- Did the reviewers use adequate supplementary efforts to identify relevant studies?
- Was a PRISMA-type flow chart included to summarize the search results?

The Sample
- Were inclusion and exclusion criteria clearly articulated, and were they defensible?
- Did the search strategy yield a strong and comprehensive sample of studies? Were strengths and limitations of the sample identified?
- If an original report was lacking key information, did reviewers attempt to contact the original researchers for additional information—or did the study have to be excluded?
- If studies were excluded for reasons other than insufficient information, did the reviewers provide a rationale for the decision?

Quality Appraisal
- Did the reviewers appraise the quality of the primary studies? Did they use a defensible and well-defined set of criteria or a respected quality appraisal scale?
- Did two or more people do the appraisals and was interrater agreement reported?
- Was the appraisal information used in a well-defined and defensible manner in the selection of studies or in the analysis of results?

Data Extraction
- Was adequate information extracted about methodologic and administrative aspects of the study, sample characteristics, and study findings?
- Were steps taken to enhance the integrity of the dataset (e.g., were two or more people used to extract and record information for analysis)?

Data Analysis—General
- Did the reviewers explain their method of pooling, integrating, and synthesizing the data?
- Was the analysis of data thorough and credible?
- Were tables, figures, and text used effectively to summarize findings?
- Did the reviewers use GRADE or another approach to evaluate confidence in the review findings?

Data Analysis—Quantitative
- If a meta-analysis was not performed, was there adequate justification for using a narrative integration method? If a meta-analysis was performed, was this justifiable?
- For meta-analyses, were appropriate procedures followed for computing effect size estimates for relevant outcomes?
- Was heterogeneity of effects adequately dealt with? Was the decision to use a random effects model or a fixed effects model sound?
- Were appropriate subgroup analyses undertaken—or was the absence of subgroup analyses justified?
- Was the issue of publication bias adequately addressed?

> **BOX 30.1** Guidelines for Critically Appraising Systematic Reviews *(Continued)*
>
> **Data Analysis—Qualitative**
> - Was the analytic approach mainly aggregative or interpretive?
> - In a metasynthesis, did the reviewers describe the techniques they used to compare the findings of each study, and did they explain their method of interpreting their data?
> - If a metasummary was undertaken, did the abstracted findings seem appropriate and convincing? Were appropriate methods used to compute effect sizes? Was information presented effectively?
> - In a metasynthesis, did the synthesis achieve a fuller understanding of the phenomenon to advance knowledge? Do the interpretations seem well-grounded? Was there a sufficient amount of data included to support the interpretations?
> - In a meta-aggregation, does the integration of findings into categories and categories into synthesized findings appear insightful and justifiable?
>
> **Conclusions**
> - Did the reviewers draw reasonable conclusions about the quality, quantity, and consistency of evidence relating to the research question?
> - Were limitations of the review/synthesis noted?
> - Were implications for nursing practice and further research clearly stated?

All systematic reviews/research syntheses.
Systematic reviews of quantitative studies.
Metasyntheses/qualitative evidence syntheses.

CRITICAL APPRAISAL OF SYSTEMATIC REVIEWS

Systematic reviews should be appraised before the findings are deemed trustworthy and relevant. Supplementary questions are likely to be needed for some reviews—for example, for MSRs.

Several tools have been developed to assess systematic reviews. One rigorously developed tool is called Assessment of Multiple Systematic Reviews (AMSTAR) (Shea et al., 2007). Although AMSTAR has been revised (AMSTAR 2), there continue to be debates about some limitations, and further study into its reliability and usability is underway (Gates et al., 2018). The PRISMA guidelines are an additional resource for assessing whether a review included sufficient information (Box 30.1).

In drawing conclusions about a research synthesis, a major issue concerns the nature of the decisions the reviewers made. Sampling decisions, approaches to handling quality of the primary studies, and analytic methods should be carefully evaluated. Another aspect, however, is envisioning how you might use the evidence in clinical practice.

RESEARCH EXAMPLE

We conclude this chapter with a description of an integrative review conducted by a team that included one of the authors of this book.

Study: Physical and Behavioral Health Characteristics of Aging Homeless Women in the United States: An Integrative Review (Dickins et al., 2021).

Purpose: This study aimed to understand the physical and behavioral health characteristics of older homeless women in the United States.

Eligibility Criteria: Studies published in English between 2002 and 2019 focused on the physical and behavioral characteristics of women who were older than age 50 and currently homeless were eligible. Exclusion criteria included women who were not actively homeless. Literature that was not peer reviewed or empirical (e.g., a study protocol) was also excluded.

Search Strategy: The databases searched included Medline, Embase, Ovid Nursing Database, Cochrane Library, the Cumulative Index to Nursing and Allied Health Literature, and Web of Science.

Sample and Data Extraction: A total of 6,185 records were initially retrieved, but once duplicates were removed 3,177 records remained. The papers were then loaded into Covidence, a software system for the management of systematic reviews. After two members of the team screened the records, 3,089 records did not meet eligibility criteria, leaving 88 papers for full text screening and, of those, 78 did not meet eligibility criteria.

Quality Appraisal: Ten studies were reviewed using the Johns Hopkins Nursing Evidence-Based Practice (JHNEBP) Research Evidence Appraisal Tool for the level and quality of evidence.

Data Analysis: The team used an inductive thematic synthesis approach to analyze the data and develop categories. They were physical health, behavioral health, social health, and spiritual health.

Sample Characteristics: Collectively the studies were representative of all regions of the United States. The sample sizes within studies ranged from 5 to 223. The women were mostly either Black or White. Four of the 10 studies were qualitative and the 6 were mixed methods. The studies designs were descriptive and nonexperimental, with 90% being of good quality.

Key Findings: The findings from this review suggest that aging homeless women had physical health concerns related to poor nutrition and preventative health. Additionally, they had elevated rates of mental health issues that were compounded by substance use disorders and interpersonal trauma. While economic challenges, family, and social concerns contributed to social woes, spiritual health was found to be a protective factor.

SUMMARY POINTS

- EBP relies on rigorous integration of research evidence on a topic through systematic reviews.
- A **systematic review** methodically and transparently integrates findings from multiple **primary studies** about a specific research question using careful procedures that are spelled out in advance in a **protocol.**
- Systematic reviews are undertaken to synthesize quantitative findings, qualitative findings, or mixed findings. Reviews of quantitative studies often involve statistical integration of findings through **meta-analysis**, a procedure whose advantages include objectivity, enhanced power, and precision; meta-analysis is not appropriate, however, for broad questions or when there is substantial inconsistency of findings.
- In the rapidly evolving field of evidence synthesis, special types of reviews have emerged. **Integrative reviews** are based on what is known or absent in the research literature, allow for a broad approach to the literature searched, and include studies using all methods as well as theoretical and conceptual papers. **Scoping reviews** are preliminary efforts to map the literature on a topic and assess the possibility of a systematic review. **Rapid reviews** are less rigorous than systematic reviews but are intended to yield timely information. **Umbrella reviews** are systematic reviews of multiple systematic reviews. **Network meta-analyses** are reviews in which multiple interventions are compared using both direct and indirect comparisons.
- Major steps in a systematic review typically involve the following: formulating the question, defining eligibility criteria, preparing a protocol, searching for and selecting primary studies, evaluating study quality, extracting data, analyzing the data, interpreting the findings and evaluating confidence in them, and reporting the findings. To minimize the risk of duplication, a systematic review protocol can be registered in a database called **PROSPERO.**
- In most cases, reviewers undertake a comprehensive search, using a wide range of methods, including a search in multiple bibliographic databases, **handsearching** in key journals, *snowballing,* and searching in trial registries.
- Reviewers are increasingly likely to search for **gray literature**—such as unpublished

- reports—out of concern for **publication bias** (a form of **dissemination bias**) that results in the underrepresentation of nonsignificant findings in published literature.
- There are many approaches to appraising the quality of evidence of primary studies, including the use of various scales and checklists. In the Cochrane approach, each study is rated on separate **risk-of-bias** domains.
- In a meta-analysis, findings from primary studies are represented by an **effect size** index that quantifies the magnitude and direction of relationship between variables (e.g., an intervention and its outcomes). Common effect size indexes include d (the **standardized mean difference** or SMD), the OR, RR index, and Pearson's r.
- Effects from individual studies are pooled to yield an estimate of the population effect size by calculating a **weighted average** of effects, often using the **inverse variance** as the weight—which gives greater weight to larger studies.
- **Statistical heterogeneity** (diversity in effects across studies) affects decisions about using a **fixed effects model** (which assumes a single true effect size) or a **random effects model** (which assumes a distribution of effects). Heterogeneity can be examined using a **forest plot** and tested statistically—most often using a chi square test or the I^2 **test.**
- Nonrandom heterogeneity (moderating effects) can be explored through **subgroup analyses** or **meta-regression**, in which the purpose is to identify clinical or methodologic features systematically related to variation in effects.
- Quality assessments are sometimes used to exclude weak studies from reviews, but they can also be used to differentially weight studies or in **sensitivity analyses** to test whether including or excluding weaker studies changes conclusions.
- Systematic reviewers are increasingly likely to use the **GRADE** (Grading of Recommendations, Assessment, Development, and Evaluation) approach to rate the degree of *confidence* that the review team has in the estimated effect, for outcomes in a review.
- Qualitative systematic reviews have been described as either **aggregative** (in which findings from multiple studies are pooled) or **interpretive** (in which the goal is to discover new ways of understanding phenomena). Aggregative reviews are often called **qualitative evidence syntheses**; the umbrella term most often used in nursing for interpretive reviews is **metasynthesis.** Most qualitative reviews in nursing have elements of both aggregation and interpretation.
- Metasynthesis methods often used by nurse researchers include meta-ethnography, metastudy, and metasummary.
- Metasynthesists do not necessarily start with a predetermined question—questions often emerge during the process of discovery. Metasynthesists may not undertake an exhaustive review—the sampling of studies may be purposive.
- One approach to qualitative integration, **meta-ethnography** as proposed by Noblit and Hare, involves listing key themes or metaphors across studies and then reciprocally translating them into each other. Key metaphors can be translated in one of three ways: *reciprocal, refutational,* or *lines-of-argument.*
- Paterson and colleagues' **metastudy** method integrates three components: (1) **metadata analysis,** the study of results in a specific substantive area through analysis of the "processed data"; (2) **metamethod,** the study of the studies' methodologic rigor; and (3) **metatheory,** the analysis of the theoretical underpinnings on which the studies are grounded.
- Sandelowski and Barroso distinguish qualitative findings in terms of whether they are *summaries* (descriptive synopses) or *syntheses* (interpretive explanations of the data). Both summaries and syntheses can be used in a **metasummary**, which can lay the foundation for a metasynthesis.
- A metasummary involves developing a list of abstracted findings from the primary studies and calculating **manifest effect sizes. A frequency effect size** is the percentage of studies in a sample of studies that contain a given finding. An **intensity effect size** indicates the percentage of all findings that are contained within any given report.

- In the Sandelowski and Barroso approach, only studies described as *syntheses* can be used in a metasynthesis, which can use a variety of approaches to analysis and interpretation (e.g., constant comparison).
- The approach to QES used at the JBI is **meta-aggregation**, which is more structured than a metasynthesis and relies on comprehensive searching and systematic quality appraisals. In a meta-aggregation, similar findings across studies are grouped into *categories,* which in turn are grouped into *synthesized findings.* In JBI qualitative reviews, confidence in the findings is assessed using a rating system called **ConQual.** Another similar system, inspired by GRADE, is called **GRADE-CerQual.**
- **Systematic mixed studies reviews (MSRs)** are systematic reviews that use disciplined procedures to integrate and synthesize findings from qualitative, quantitative, and mixed methods studies.
- Designs for MSRs are either concurrent/convergent (qualitative and quantitative syntheses undertaken concurrently) or sequential. Sandelowski proposed three designs: *segregated* (two separate syntheses followed by integration); *integrated* (when qualitative and quantitative findings are viewed as answering the same question); or *contingent* (a coordinated, sequential series of syntheses). JBI MSRs use a segregated design, while Cochrane MSRs use a sequential design.
- Many approaches have been suggested for analyzing and synthesizing data in an MSR, including content analysis, narrative summary, critical interpretive synthesis, and *Bayesian synthesis.*
- A special type of MSR is called a **realist synthesis,** the goal of which is to understand theory-driven *Context-Mechanism-Outcome* (CMO) configurations. Realist syntheses are often used in reviews of complex interventions.
- **PRISMA** (Preferred Reporting Items for Systematic reviews and Meta-Analyses) is a useful reporting guideline for writing up a systematic review of RCTs; another called **MOOSE** (Meta-analysis of Observational Studies in Epidemiology) is for meta-analyses of observational studies. **ENTREQ** is a reporting guideline for qualitative systematic reviews.
- Most systematic reviews include a flow chart (showing search efforts and results), forest plots (for meta-analyses), and a **summary of findings** (SoF) table.

REFERENCES CITED IN CHAPTER 30

Agency for Healthcare Research and Quality. (2014). *Methods guide for effectiveness and comparative effectiveness reviews.* AHRQ.

Agoritsas, T., Merglen, A., Courvoisier, D., Combescure, C., Garin, N., Perrier, A., & Perneger, T. (2012). Sensitivity and predictive value of 15 PubMed search strategies to answer clinical questions rated against full systematic reviews. *Journal of Medical Internet Research, 14*(3), e85.

Arantes, P., Sirineu, D., Castro, J., & Cunha, J. (2020). *Accuracy of timed up and Go test to predict fall risk in community-dwelling older: Protocol for a systematic review.* PROSPERO CRD42020161189. Available from https://www.crd.york.ac.uk/prospero/display_record.php?ID=CRD42020161189

Aromataris, E., Fernandez, R., Godfrey, C., Holly, C., Khalil, H., & Tungpunkom, P. (2020). Chapter 10: Umbrella reviews. In: Aromataris, E., Munn, Z. (Eds.). *JBI manual for evidence synthesis.* JBI. https://doi.org/10.46658/JBIMES-20-11

Aromataris, E., & Munn, Z., (Eds). (2020). *JBI manual for evidence synthesis.* JBI. https://doi.org/10.46658/JBIMES-20-01

Aromataris, E., & Riitano, D. (2014). Constructing a search strategy and searching for evidence: A guide to the literature search for a systematic review. *American Journal of Nursing, 114*(5), 49–56.

Atkins, S., Lewin, S., Smith, H., Engel, M., Fretheim, A., & Volmink, J. (2008). Conducting a meta-ethnography of qualitative literature: Lessons learnt. *BMC Medical Research Methodology, 8,* 21.

Bayuo, J., Wong, F. K. Y., Lin, R., Su, J. J., & Abu-Odah, H. (2023). A meta-ethnography of developing and living with post-burn scars. *Journal of Nursing Scholarship, 55*(1), 319–328. https://doi.org/10.1111/jnu.12811

Beck, C. T., & Vo, T. (2020). Fathers' stress related to their infants' NICU hospitalization: A mixed research synthesis. *Archives of Psychiatric Nursing, 34*(2), 75–84. https://doi.org/10.1016/j.apnu.2020.02.001

Beller, E., Clark, J., Tsafnat, G., Adams, C., Diehl, H., Lund, H., Ouzzani, M., Thayer, K., Thomas, J., Turner, T., Xia, J., Robinson, K., Glasziou, P., Glasziou, P., founding members of the ICASR group. (2018). Making progress with the automation of systematic reviews: Principles of the International

Collaboration for the Automation of Systematic Reviews (ICASR). *Systematic Reviews*, 7(1), 77.

Bilandzic, A., Fitzpatrick, T., Rosella, L., & Henry, D. (2016). Risk of bias in systematic reviews of non-randomized studies of adverse cardiovascular effects of thiazolidinediones and Cyclooxygenase-2 inhibitors: Application of a new Cochrane risk of bias tool. *PLoS Medicine*, 13(4), e1001987.

Booth, A. (2016). Searching for qualitative research for inclusion in systematic reviews: A structured methodological review. *Systematic Reviews*, 5, 74.

Booth, A., Noyes, J., Flemming, K., Gerhardus, A., Wahlster, P., van der Wilt, G., Mozygemba, K., Refolo, P., Sacchini, D., Tummers, M., Rehfuess, E., & Rehfuss, E. (2018). Structured methodology review identified seven (RETREAT) criteria for selecting qualitative evidence synthesis approaches. *Journal of Clinical Epidemiology*, 99, 41–52.

Booth, A., Noyes, J., Flemming, K., Gerhardus, A., Wahlster, P., van der Wilt, G., & Rehfuss, E. (2016). *Guidance on choosing qualitative evidence synthesis methods for use in health technology assessments of complex interventions.* Retrieved from http://www.integrate-hta.eu/downloads/

Bramer, W., Rethlefsen, M., Kleijnen, J., & Franco, O. (2017). Optimal database combinations for literature searches in systematic reviews: A prospective exploratory study. *Systematic Reviews*, 6(1), 245.

Brunetti, M., Shemilt, I., Pregno, S., Vale, L., Oxman, A., Lord, J., Sisk, J., Ruiz, F., Hill, S., Guyatt, G. H., Jaeschke, R., Helfand, M., Harbour, R., Davoli, M., Amato, L., Liberati, A., Schünemann, H. J., & Schünemann, H. (2013). GRADE guidelines: 10. Considering resource use and rating the quality of economic evidence. *Journal of Clinical Epidemiology*, 66(2), 140–150.

Campbell, R., Pound, P., Morgan, M., Daker-White, G., Britten, N., Pill, R., Yardley, L., Pope, C., Donovan, J., & Donovan, J. (2011). Evaluating meta-ethnography: Systematic analysis and synthesis of qualitative research. *Health Technology Assessment*, 15(43), 1–164.

Caswell, R. J., Ross, J. D. C., Maidment, I., & Bradbury-Jones, C. (2023). Providing a supportive environment for disclosure of sexual violence and abuse in a sexual and reproductive healthcare setting: A realist review. *Trauma, Violence, & Abuse*, 24(4), 2661–2679. https://doi.org/10.1177/15248380221111466

Chaimani, A, Caldwell, D. M., Li, T, Higgins, J. P. T., & Salanti, G. (2022). Chapter 11: Undertaking network meta-analyses. In: Higgins, J. P. T., Thomas, J., Chandler, J., Cumpston, M., Li, T., Page, M. J., & Welch, V. A. (Eds.). *Cochrane handbook for systematic reviews of interventions.* version 6.3 (updated February 2022). Cochrane. Available from www.training.cochrane.org/handbook

Conn, V., Valentine, J., Cooper, H., & Rantz, M. (2003). Grey literature in meta-analyses. *Nursing Research*, 52(4), 256–261.

Cooper, H. (2017). *Research synthesis and meta-analysis: A step-by-step approach* (5th ed.). Sage Publications.

Critical Appraisal Skills Programme. (2016). *CASP qualitative research checklist.* Retrieved from http://www.cask-uk.net/casp-tools-checklists

Cumpston, M., & Chandler, J. (2022). Chapter II: Planning a Cochrane review. In: Higgins, J. P. T., Thomas, J., Chandler, J., Cumpston, M., Li, T., Page, M. J., & Welch, V. A. (Eds.). *Cochrane handbook for systematic reviews of interventions* version 6.3. Cochrane.

DeJean, D., Giacomini, M., Simeonov, D., & Smith, A. (2016). Finding qualitative research evidence for health technology assessment. *Quality Health Research*, 26(10), 1307–1317.

Dias, J. F., Oliveira, V. C., Borges, P. R. T., Dutra, F. C. M. S., Mancini, M. C., Kirkwood, R. N., Resende, R. A., & Sampaio, R. F. (2021). Effectiveness of exercises by telerehabilitation on pain, physical function and quality of life in people with physical disabilities: A systematic review of randomised controlled trials with GRADE recommendations. *British Journal of Sports Medicine*, 55(3), 155–162. https://doi.org/10.1136/bjsports-2019-101375

Dickins, K. A., Philpotts, L. L., Flanagan, J., Bartels, S. J., Baggett, T. P., & Looby, S. E. (2021). Physical and behavioral health characteristics of aging homeless women in the United States: An integrative review. *Journal of Womens Health*, 30(10), 1493–1507. https://doi.org/10.1089/jwh.2020.8557

Dixon-Woods, M., Cavers, D., Agarwal, S., Annandale, E., Arthur, A., Harvey, J., Hsu, R., Katbamna, S., Olsen, R., Smith, L., Riley, R., Sutton, A. J., & Sutton, A. (2006). Conducting a critical interpretive synthesis of the literature on access to healthcare by vulnerable groups. *BMC Medical Research Methodology*, 6, 35.

Dukuzumuremyi, J. P. C., Acheampong, K., Abesig, J., & Luo, J. (2020). Knowledge, attitude, and practice of exclusive breastfeeding among mothers in east Africa: A systematic review. *International Breastfeed Journal*, 15(1), 70. https://doi.org/10.1186/s13006-020-00313-9

Dwan, K., Gamble, C., Williamson, P., & Kirkham, J., Reporting Bias Group. (2013). Systematic review of the empirical evidence of study publication bias and outcome reporting bias: An updated review. *PLoS One*, 8(7), e66844.

Easton, C., Oudshoorn, A., Smith-Carrier, T., Forchuk, C., & Marshall, C. A. (2022). The experience of food insecurity during and following homelessness in high-income countries: A systematic review and meta-aggregation. *Health & Social Care in the Community*, 30(6), e3384–e3405. https://doi.org/10.1111/hsc.13939

Elamin, M., Flynn, D., Bassler, D., Briel, M., Alonso-Coello, P., Karanicolas, P., Guyatt, G. H., Malaga, G., Furukawa, T. A., Kunz, R., Schünemann, H., Murad, M. H., Barbui, C., Cipriani, A., Montori, V. M., & Montori, V. (2009). Choice of data extraction tools for systematic reviews depends on resources and review complexity. *Journal of Clinical Epidemiology*, 62(5), 506–510.

Elliott, J., Synnot, A., Turner, T., Simmonds, M., Akl, E., McDonald, S., Salanti, G., Meerpohl, J., MacLehose, H., Hilton, J., Tovey, D., Shemilt, I., & Thomas, J., Living Systematic Review Network, (2017). Living systematic review: 1. Introduction—the why, what, when, and how. *Journal of Clinical Epidemiology*, 91, 23–30.

Emmel, N., Greenhalgh, J., Manzano, A., Monaghan, M., & Dalkin, S. (Eds.). (2019). *Doing realist research.* Sage Publications.

Finfgeld, D. (2003). Metasynthesis: The state of the art—so far. *Qualittive Health Research*, 13(7), 893–904.

Flemming, K. (2010). Synthesis of quantitative and qualitative research: An example using Critical Interpretive Synthesis. *Journal of Advanced Nursing*, 66(1), 201–217.

France, E., Cunningham, M., Ring, N., Uny, I., Duncan, E., Jepson, R., Maxwell, M., Roberts, R. J., Turley, R. L., Booth, A., Britten, N., Flemming, K., Gallagher, I., Garside, R., Hannes, K., Lewin, S., Noblit, G. W., Pope, C., Thomas, J., … Noyes, J. (2019). Improving reporting of meta-ethnography: The eMERGe reporting guidance. *Journal of Advanced Nursing*, 75(5), 1126–1139.

Gates, A., Gates, M., Duarte, G., Cary, M., Becker, M., Prediger, B., Vandermeer, B., Fernandes, R. M., Pieper, D., Hartling, L., & Hartling, L. (2018). Evaluation of the reliability, usability, and applicability of AMSTAR, AMSTAR 2, and ROBIS: Protocol for a descriptive analytic study. *Systematic Review*, 7(1), 85.

Gordon, B., Mason, B., & Smith, S. L. H. (2022). Leveraging telehealth for delivery of palliative care to remote communities: A rapid review. *Journal of Palliative Care*, 37(2), 213–225. https://doi.org/10.1177/08258597211001184

Gough, D., Thomas, J., & Oliver, S. (2012). Clarifying differences between review designs and methods. *Systematic Review*, 1, 28.

Greenhalgh, T., Thorne, S., & Malterud, K. (2018). Time to challenge the spurious hierarchy of systematic over narrative reviews? *European Journal of Clinical Investigaion*, 48(6), e12931.

Guyatt, G. H., Oxman, A., Akl, E., Kunz, R., Vist, G., Brozek, J., Norris, S., Falck-Ytter, Y., Glasziou, P., DeBeer, H., Jaeschke, R., Rind, D., Meerpohl, J., Dahm, P., Schünemann, H. J., & Schunemann, H. (2011). GRADE guidelines: 1. Introduction—GRADE evidence profiles and summary of findings tables. *Journal of Clinical Epidemiology*, 64(4), 383–394.

Guyatt, G., Oxman, A., Vist, G., Kunz, R., Falck-Ytter, Y., Alonso-Coello, P., & Schünemann, H., GRADE Working Group. (2008). GRADE: An emerging consensus on rating quality of evidence and strength of recommendations. *BMJ*, 336(7650), 924–926.

Hannes, K., & Lockwood, C. (2011). Pragmatism as the philosophical foundation for the Joanna Briggs meta-aggregative approach to qualitative evidence synthesis. *Journal of Advanced Nursing*, 67(7), 1632–1642.

Hannes, K., & Lockwood, C. (2012). *Synthesizing qualitative research: Choosing the right approach*. Wiley-Blackwell.

Harden, A., & Thomas, J. (2005). Methodologic issues in combining diverse study types in systematic reviews. *International Journal of Social Research Methodology*, 8, 257–271.

Harden, A., Thomas, J., Cargo, M., Harris, J., Pantoja, T., Flemming, K., Booth, A., Garside, R., Hannes, K., Noyes, J., & Noyes, J. (2018). Cochrane Qualitative and Implementation Methods Group guidance series—paper 5: Methods for integrating qualitative and implementation evidence within intervention effectiveness reviews. *Journal of Clinical Epidemiology*, 97, 70–78.

Heyvaert, M., Hannes, K., & Onghena, P. (2017). *Using mixed methods research synthesis for literature reviews*. Sage Publications.

Heyvaert, M., Maes, B., & Onghena, P. (2013). Mixed methods research synthesis: Definition, framework, and potential. *Quality and Quantity*, 47, 659–676.

Higgins, J. P. T, Thomas, J., Chandler, J., Cumpston, M., Li, T., Page, M. J., & Welch, V. A. (Eds.). (2022). *Cochrane handbook for systematic reviews of interventions* version 6.3. Cochrane, 2022. Available from www.training.cochrane.org/handbook

Ho, G., Liew, S., Ng, C., Hisham Shunmugam, R., Glasziou, P. (2016). Development of a search strategy for an evidence-based retrieval service. *PLoS One*, 11(12), e0167170.

Hong, Q., Pluye, P., Bujold, M., & Wassef, M. (2017). Convergent and sequential synthesis designs: Implications for conducting and reporting systematic reviews of qualitative and quantitative evidence. *Systematic Review*, 6(1), 61.

Hughes Née Richardson, B., Benoit, B., Rutledge, K., Dol, J., Martin-Misener, R., Latimer, M., Smit, M., McGrath, P., & Campbell-Yeo, M. (2023). Impact of parent-targeted eHealth educational interventions on infant procedural pain management: A systematic review. *JBI Evidence Synthesis*, 21(4), 669–712. https://doi.org/10.11124/JBIES-21-00435

Hunt, H., Pollock, A., Campbell, P., Estcourt, L., & Brunton, G. (2018). An introduction to overviews of reviews: Planning a relevant research question and objective for an overview. *Systematic Review*, 7(1), 39.

Institute of Medicine. (2011). *Finding what works in health care: Standards for systematic reviews*. The National Academies Press.

Ioannidis, J. (2017). Next-generation systematic reviews: Prospective meta-analysis, individual-level data, networks and umbrella reviews. *British Journal of Sports Medicine*, 51(20), 1456–1458.

Iorio, A., Spencer, F., Falavigna, M., Alba, C., Lang, E., Burnand, B., McGinn, T., Hayden, J., Williams, K., Shea, B., Wolff, R., Kujpers, T., Perel, P., Vandvik, P. O., Glasziou, P., Schunemann, H., Guyatt, G., & Guyatt, G. (2015). Use of GRADE for assessment of evidence about prognosis: Rating confidence in estimates of event rates in broad categories of patients. *BMJ*, 350, h870.

Jadad, A. R., Moore, R., Carroll, D., Jenkinson, C., Reynolds, D., Gavaghan, D., & McQuay, H. (1996). Assessing the quality of reports of randomized controlled trials. *Control Clinical Trials*, 17, 1–12.

Jüni, P., Altman, D., & Egger, M. (2001). Systematic reviews in health care: Assessing the quality of controlled clinical trials. *BMJ*, 323(7303), 42–46.

Kersey, K., Lyons, A. C., & Hutton, F. (2022). Alcohol and drinking within the lives of midlife women: A meta-study systematic review. *International Journal of Drug Policy*, 99, 103453. https://doi.org/10.1016/j.drugpo.2021.103453

Klerings, I., Robalino, S., Booth, A., Escobar-Liquitay, C. M., Sommer, I., Gartlehner, G., Devane, D., Waffenschmidt, S.; Cochrane Rapid Reviews Methods Group. (2023). Rapid reviews methods series: Guidance on literature search. *BMJ*

Evidence Based Medicine, 28(6), 412–417. Advance online publication. https://doi.org/10.1136/bmjebm-2022-112079

Lee, J., Lee, H., Kim, S., Choi, M., Ko, I. S., Bae, J., & Kim, S. H. (2020). Debriefing methods and learning outcomes in simulation nursing education: A systematic review and meta-analysis. *Nurse Education Today*, 87, 104345. https://doi.org/10.1016/j.nedt.2020.104345

Lewin, S., Booth, A., Glenton, C., Munthe-Kaas, H., Rashidian, A., Wainwright, M., Bohren, M. A., Tunçalp, Ö., Colvin, C. J., Garside, R., Carlsen, B., Langlois, E. V., Noyes, J., & Noyes, J. (2018). Applying GRADE-CERQual to qualitative evidence synthesis findings: Introduction to the series. *Implementation Science*, 13(Suppl. 1), 2.

Liberati, A., Altman, D., Tetzlaff, J., Mulrow, C., Gøtzsche, P. C., Ioannidis, J., Clarke, M., Devereaux, P. J., Kleijnen, J., Moher, D. (2009). The PRISMA statement for reporting systematic reviews and meta-analyses of studies that evaluate health care interventions: Explanation and elaboration. *Journal of Clinical Epidemiology*, 62(10), e1–e34.

Lucas, P., Baird, J., Arai, L., Law, C., & Roberts, H. (2007). Worked examples of alternative methods for the synthesis of qualitative and quantitative research in systematic reviews. *BMC Medical Research Methodology*, 7, 4.

Majid, U., & Vanstone, M. (2018). Appraising qualitative research for evidence syntheses: A compendium of quality appraisal tools. *Qualitative Health Research*, 28(13), 2115–2131.

Mathes, T., Klassen, P., & Pieper, D. (2017). Frequency of data extraction errors and methods to increase data extraction quality: A methodological review. *BMC Medical Research Methodology*, 17(1), 152.

McCormick, J., Rodney, P., & Varcoe, C. (2003). Reinterpretations across studies: An approach to meta-analysis. *Qualitative Health Research*, 13(7), 933–944.

Michel-Schuldt, M., McFadden, A., Renfrew, M., & Homer, C. (2020). The provision of midwife-led care in low- and middle-income countries: An integrative review. *Midwifery*, 84, 102659. https://doi.org/10.1016/j.midw.2020.102659

Munn, Z., Lockwood, C., & Moola, S. (2015). The development and use of evidence summaries for point of care information systems: A streamlined rapid review approach. *Worldviews Evidence Based Nursing*, 12(3), 131–138.

Munn, Z., Porritt, K., Lockwood, C., Aromataris, E., & Pearson, A. (2014b). Establishing confidence in the output of qualitative research synthesis: The ConQual approach. *BMC Medical Research Methodology*, 14, 108.

Munn, Z., Stern, C., Aromataris, E., Lockwood, C., & Jordan, Z. (2018). What kind of systematic review should I conduct? A proposed typology and guidance for systematic reviewers in the medical and health sciences. *BMC Medical Research Methodology*, 18(1), 5.

Munn, Z., Tufanaru, C., & Aromataris, E. (2014a). JBI's systematic reviews: Data extraction and synthesis. *American Journal of Nursing*, 114(7), 49–54.

Neo, N. W. S., & Tho, P. C. (2022). Diagnostic accuracy and validity of image-assisted versus face-to-face wound assessments for the management of chronic wounds: A systematic review protocol. *JBI Evidence Synthesis*, 20(10), 2572–2578. https://doi.org/10.11124/JBIES-21-00293

Noblit, G., & Hare, R. D. (1988). *Meta-ethnography: Synthesizing qualitative studies.* Sage Publications.

Noyes, J., Booth, A., Cargo, M., Flemming, K., Garside, R., Hannes, K., Harden, A., Harris, J., Lewin, S., Pantoja, T., & Thomas, J. (2018). Cochrane qualitative and implementation methods group guidance series—paper 1: Introduction. *Journal of Clinical Epidemiology*, 97, 35–38.

Oermann, M. H., Knafl, K. A. (2021). Strategies for completing a successful integrative review. *Nurse Author & Editor*, 31(3–4), 65–68. https://doi.org/10.1111/nae2.30

Ogilvie, D., Fayter, D., Petticrew, M., Sowden, A., Thomas, S., Whitehead, M., & Worthy, G. (2008). The harvest plot: A method for synthesising evidence about the differential effects of interventions. *BMC Medical Reserach Methodology*, 8, 8.

Pace, R., Pluye, P., Bartlett, G., Macaulay, A. C., Salsberg, J., Jagosh, J., & Seller, R. (2012). Testing the reliability and efficiency of the pilot Mixed Methods Appraisal Tool (MMAT) for systematic mixed studies review. *International Journal of Nursing Studies*, 49(1), 47–53.

Paterson, B. (2013). Metasynthesis. In Beck, C. T., (Ed.). *Routledge international handbook of qualitative nursing research* (pp. 331–346). Routledge.

Paterson, B. L., Thorne, S. E., Canam, C., & Jillings, C. (2001). *Meta-study of qualitative health research.* Sage Publications.

Pawson, R. (2013). *The science of evaluation: A realist manifesto.* Sage Publications.

Pearson, A., White, H., Bath-Hextall, F., Apostolo, J., Salmond, S., & Kirkpatrick, P. (2014). *Methodology for JBI mixed methods systematic reviews. The Joanna Briggs Institute Reviewers' Manual 2014, chapter 8.* JBI.

Pedder, H., Sarri, G., Keeney, E., Nunes, V., & Dias, S. (2016). Data extraction for complex meta-analysis (DECiMAL) guide. *Systematic Review*, 5(1), 212.

Peters, M. D. J., Marnie, C., Tricco, A. C., Pollock, D., Munn, Z., Alexander, L., McInerney, P., Godfrey, C. M., & Khalil, H. (2020). Updated methodological guidance for the conduct of scoping reviews. *JBI Evidence Synthesis*, 18(10), 2119–2126. https://doi.org/10.11124/JBIES-20-00167

Petticrew, M., Anderson, L., Elder, R., Grimshaw, J., Hopkins, D., Hahn, R., Krause, L., Kristjansson, E., Mercer, S., Sipe, T., Tugwell, P., Ueffing, E., Waters, E., & Welch, V. (2015). Complex interventions and their implications for systematic reviews: A pragmatic approach. *International Journal of Nursing Studies*, 52(7), 1211–1216.

Pigott, T., Noyes, J., Umscheid, C., Myers, E., Morton, S., Fu, R., Sanders-Schmidler, G. D., Devine, B., Murad, M. H., Kelly, M. P., Fonnesbeck, C., Kahwati, L., & Beretvas, S. N. (2017). AHRQ series on complex intervention systematic reviews-Paper 5: Advanced analytic methods. *Journal of Clinical Epidemiology*, 90, 37–42.

Pluye, P., Gagnon, M., Griffiths, F., & Johnson-Lafleur, J. (2009). A scoring system for appraising mixed methods research, and concomitantly appraising qualitative, quantitative, and mixed methods primary studies in Mixed Studies

Reviews. *International Journal of Nursing Studies*, 46(4), 529–546.

Pluye, P., & Hong, Q. N. (2014). Combining the power of stories and the power of numbers: Mixed methods research and mixed studies reviews. *Annual Review of Public Health*, 35, 29–45.

Pluye, P., Hong, Q.N., Bush, P., & Vedel, I. (2016). Opening-up the definition of systematic literature review: The plurality of worldviews, methodologies and methods for reviews and syntheses. *Journal of Clinical Epidemiology*, 73, 2–5.

Pollock, M., Fernandes, R. M., Becker, L. A., Pieper, D., Hartling, L. (2022). Chapter V: Overviews of reviews. In: Higgins, J. P. T., Thomas, J., Chandler, J., Cumpston, M., Li, T., Page, M. J., & Welch, V. A. (Eds.). *Cochrane handbook for systematic reviews of interventions* version 6.3. Cochrane. Available from www.training.cochrane.org/handbook

Porritt, K., Gomersall, J., & Lockwood, C. (2014). JBI's systematic reviews: Study selection and critical appraisal. *American Journal of Nursing*, 114(6), 47–52.

Qian, J., Wu, T., Lv, M., Fang, Z., Chen, M., Zeng, Z., Jiang, S., Chen, W., & Zhang, J. (2021). The value of mobile health in improving breastfeeding outcomes among perinatal or postpartum women: Systematic review and meta-analysis of randomized controlled trials. *JMIR Mhealth Uhealth*, 9(7), e26098. https://doi.org/10.2196/26098

Reeder, A. L. (2023, April-June 01). The experiences of people who are incarcerated in accessing mental health care: A qualitative meta-ethnography. *Journal of Forensic Nursing*, 19(2), 131–139, https://doi.org/10.1097/jfn.0000000000000405

Salari, N., Hosseinian-Far, A., Jalali, R., Vaisi-Raygani, A., Rasoulpoor, S., Mohammadi, M., Rasoulpoor, S., & Khaledi-Paveh, B. (2020). Prevalence of stress, anxiety, depression among the general population during the COVID-19 pandemic: A systematic review and meta-analysis. *Global Health*, 16(1), 57. https://doi.org/10.1186/s12992-020-00589-w

Sandelowski, M., & Barroso, J. (2002). Finding the findings in qualitative studies. *Journal of Nursing Scholarship*, 34(3), 213–219.

Sandelowski, M., & Barroso, J. (2003a). Toward a metasynthesis of qualitative findings on motherhood in HIV-positive women. *Research in Nursing and Health*, 26(2), 153–170.

Sandelowski, M., & Barroso, J. (2003b). Creating metasummaries of qualitative findings. *Nursing Research*, 52(4), 226–233.

Sandelowski, M., & Barroso, J. (2007). *Handbook for synthesizing qualitative research*. Springer Publishing Company.

Sandelowski, M., Docherty, S., & Emden, C. (1997). Qualitative metasynthesis: Issues and techniques. *Research in Nursing & Health*, 20, 365–377.

Sandelowski, M., Voils, C., & Barroso, J. (2006). Defining and designing mixed research synthesis studies. *Reseach in the Schools*, 13(1), 29.

Sandelowski, M., Voils, C. I., Crandell, J. L., & Leeman, J. (2013). Synthesizing qualitative and quantitative research findings. In Beck, C. T. (Ed.), *Routledge international handbook of qualitative nursing research* (pp. 347–356). Routledge.

Schreiber, R., Crooks, D., & Stern, P. N. (1997). Qualitative meta-analysis. In Morse, J. M. (Ed.), *Completing a qualitative project* (pp. 311–326). Sage Publications.

Schünemann, H., Oxman, A., Brozek, J., Glasziou, P., Jaeschke, R., Vist, G., Williams, J. W. Jr, Kunz, R., Craig, J., Montori, V. M., Bossuyt, P., Guyatt, G. H., GRADE Working Group. (2008). Grading quality of evidence and strength of recommendations for diagnostic tests and strategies. *BMJ*, 336(7653), 1106–1110.

Shea, B., Grimshaw, J., Wells, G. Boers, M., Andersson, N., Hamel, C., Porter, A. C., Tugwell, P., Moher, D., Bouter, L. M., & Bouter, L. (2007). Development of AMSTAR: A measurement tool to assess the methodological quality of systematic reviews. *BMC Medical Research Methodology*, 7, 10.

Shorey, S., & Pereuram, T. L. B. (2022). Experiences of fathers caring for children with neurodevelopmental disorders: A meta-synthesis. *Family Process*, 62(2), 754–774. https://doi.org/10.1111/famp.12817

Stang, A. (2010). Critical evaluation of the Newcastle-Ottawa scale for the assessment of the quality of nonrandomized studies in meta-analyses. *European Journal of Epidemiology*, 25(9), 603–605.

Stern, C., Jordan, Z., & McArthur, A. (2014). JBI's systematic reviews: Developing the review question and inclusion criteria. *American Journal of Nursing*, 114(4), 53–56.

Sterne, J., Hernán, M. A., Reeves, B., Savovic, J., Berkman, N., Viswanathan, M., Henry, D., Altman, D. G., Ansari, M. T., Boutron, I., Carpenter, J. R., Chan, A. W., Churchill, R., Deeks, J. J., Hróbjartsson, A., Kirkham, J., Jüni, P., Loke, Y. K., Pigott, T. D., ... Higgins, J. (2016). ROBINS-I: A tool for assessing risk of bias in non-randomised studies of interventions. *BMJ*, 355, i4919.

Stroup, D., Berlin, J., Morton, S., Olkin, I., Williamson, G., Rennie, D., Moher, D., Becker, B. J., Sipe, T. A., & Thacker, S. (2000). Meta-analysis of observational studies in epidemiology: A proposal for reporting. Meta-Analysis of Observational Studies in Epidemiology (MOOSE). *Journal of the American Medical Association*, 283, 208–212.

Thomas, J., & Harden, A. (2008). Methods for the thematic synthesis of qualitative research in systematic reviews. *BMC Medical Research Methodology*, 8, 45.

Thomas, J., Noel-Storr, A., Marshall, I., Wallace, B. McDonald, S., Mavergames, C., Glasziou, P., Shemilt, I., Synnot, A., Turner, T., & Elliott, J., Living Systematic Review Network. (2017). Living systematic reviews: 2. Combining human and machine effort. *Journal of Clinical Epidemiology*, 91, 31–37.

Thorne, S., Jensen, L., Kearney, M., Noblit, G., & Sandelowski, M. (2004). Qualitative metasynthesis: Reflections on methodological orientation and ideological agenda. *Qualitative Health Research*, 14(10), 1342–1365.

Tierney, J. F., Stewart, L. A., & Clarke, M. (2022). Chapter 26: Individual participant data. In: Higgins, J. P. T., Thomas, J., Chandler, J., Cumpston, M., Li, T., Page, M. J., & Welch,

V. A. (Eds.). *Cochrane handbook for systematic reviews of interventions* version 6.3 (updated February 2022). Cochrane. Available from www.training.cochrane.org/handbook

Tong, A., Flemming, K., McInnes, E., Oliver, S., & Craig, J. (2012). Enhancing transparency in reporting the synthesis of qualitative research: ENTREQ. *BMC Medical Research Methodology, 12*, 181.

Tonin, F., Rotta, I., Mendes, A., & Pontarolo, R. (2017). Network meta-analysis: A technique to gather evidence from direct and indirect comparisons. *Journal of Pharmacy Practice, 15*(1), 943.

Toronto, C. E., & Remington, R. (Eds.). (2020). *A step-by-step guide to conducting an integrative review*. Springer.

Toye, F., Seers, K., Allcock, N., Briggs, M., Carr, E., & Barker, K. (2014). Meta-ethnography 25 years on: Challenges and insights for synthesising a large number of qualitative studies. *BMC Medical Research Methodology, 14*, 80.

Treacy, D., Hassett, L., Schurr, K., Fairhall, N. J., Cameron, I. D., & Sherrington, C. (2022). Mobility training for increasing mobility and functioning in older people with frailty. *Cochrane Database Systematic Review, 6*(6), CD010494. https://doi.org/10.1002/14651858.CD010494.pub2

Tricco, A., Soobiah, C., Antony, J., Cogo, E., MacDonald, H., Lillie, E., Tran, J., D'Souza, J., Hui, W., Perrier, L., Welch, V., Horsley, T., Straus, S. E., & Kastner, M. (2016). A scoping review identifies multiple emerging knowledge synthesis methods, but few studies operationalize the method. *Journal of Clinical Epidemiology, 73*, 19–28.

Tsafnat, G., Glasziou, P., Karystianis, G., & Coiera, E. (2018). Automated screening of research studies for systematic reviews using study characteristics. *Systematic Review, 7*(1), 64.

Tugwell, P., Knottnerus, J., McGowan, J., & Tricco, A. (2018). Systematic Review Qualitative Methods Series reflect the increasing maturity in qualitative methods. *Journal of Clinical Epidemiology, 97*, vii-viii.

Vaartio-Rajalin, H., Santamäki-Fischer, R., Jokisalo, P., & Fagerström, L. (2021). Art making and expressive art therapy in adult health and nursing care: A scoping review. *International Journal of Nursing Science, 8*(1), 102–119. https://doi.org/10.1016/j.ijnss.2020.09.011

Viswanathan, M., Patnode, C., Berkman, N., Bass, E., Chang, S., Hartling, L., Murad, M. H., Treadwell, J. R., & Kane, R. L. (2018). Recommendations for assessing the risk of bias in systematic reviews of health-care interventions. *Journal of Clinical Epidemiology, 97*, 26–34.

Voils, C., Hassselblad, V., Crandell, J., Chang, Y., Lee, E., & Sandelowski, M. (2009). A Bayesian method for the synthesis of evidence from qualitative and quantitative reports: The example of antiretroviral medication adherence. *Journal of Health Services Research & Policy, 14*(4), 226–233.

Wang, Z., & Tocchi, C. (2023). Partners' experience of informal caregiving for patients with heart failure: A meta-ethnography. *Journal of Cardiovascular Nursing, 38*(2), E40–E54. https://doi.org/10.1097/jcn.0000000000000903

Whittemore, R., & Knafl, K. (2005). The integrative review: Updated methodology. *Journal of Advanced Nursing, 52*(5), 546–553. https://doi.org/10.1111/j.1365-2648.2005.03621.x

Yoshinaga-Itano, C., Manchaiah, V., & Hunnicutt, C. (2021). Outcomes of universal newborn screening programs: Systematic review. *Journal of Clinical Medicine, 10*(13), 2784. https://doi.org/10.3390/jcm10132784

Zeng, X., Zhang, Y., Kwong, J., Zhang, C., Li, S., Sun, F., Niu, Y., & Du, L. (2015). The methodological quality assessment tools for preclinical and clinical studies, systematic review and meta-analysis, and clinical practice guideline: A systematic review. *Journal of Evidence Based Medicine, 8*(1), 2–10.

Zhang, Q., Schwade, M., Smith, Y., Wood, R., & Young, L. (2021a). Exercise-based interventions for post-stroke social participation: A systematic review and network meta-analysis. *International Journal of Nursing Studies, 111*, 103738. https://doi.org/10.1016/j.ijnurstu.2020.103738

Zhang, T., Wu, X., Peng, G., Zhang, Q., Chen, L., Cai, Z., & Ou, H. (2021b). Effectiveness of standardized nursing terminologies for nursing practice and healthcare outcomes: A systematic review. *International Journal of Nursing Knowledge, 32*(4), 220–228. https://doi.org/10.1111/2047-3095.12315

Zipf, A. L., Polifroni, E. C., & Beck, C. T. (2022). The experience of the nurse during the COVID-19 pandemic: A global meta-synthesis in the year of the nurse. *Journal of Nursing Scholarship, 54*(1), 92–103. https://doi.org/10.1111/jnu.12706

31

Applicability, Generalizability, and Relevance: Toward Practice-Based Evidence

Learning Objectives

1. Articulate the goal of practice-based evidence.
2. Recognize the difference between the applicability, generalizability, and relevance of evidence.
3. Understand the relevance of comparative effectiveness research and pragmatic clinical trials.
4. Distinguish the differences in multiphase optimization strategy (MOST) trials in developing targeted adaptive interventions.

INTRODUCTION

This chapter covers new ground in this edition. It differs from some of the other chapters in that it is not prescriptive—that is, it does not outline the steps that researchers should take to enhance the integrity of their inquiries. Rather, it presents a rationale for why greater attention should be paid to the *applicability* and *relevance* of research evidence in real-world settings and offers several suggestions for accomplishing these goals. This chapter reflects emerging trends in developing and testing targeted, personalized, and precision healthcare initiatives.

Because this chapter covers a lot of new ideas, we have included an extensive reference list with many open-access articles.

EVIDENCE-BASED PRACTICE AND PRACTICE-BASED EVIDENCE

The evidence-based practice (EBP) movement has made significant and enduring contributions to the well-being of human beings. Clinicians no longer rely exclusively on a repository of knowledge acquired during their training—they are expected to be lifelong learners who seek and utilize evidence from rigorous studies about how best to address pressing health problems.

Yet, EBP has limitations that are not always acknowledged. In particular, concerns are increasingly expressed that EBP fails to provide "evidence to guide decisions in clinical care for individual patients" (Horwitz & Singer, 2017). Several commentators have noted that high-quality patient care requires **practice-based evidence**—evidence that is developed in real-world settings and is responsive to the needs and circumstances of specific patients and contexts (Concato, 2012; Horwitz et al., 2017; Sacristán & Dilla, 2018).

In this section, we briefly point out some limitations of EBP with respect to the applicability of research findings for clinical decision-making. Many concerns stem from EBP's reliance on randomized controlled trials (RCTs), which are considered the "gold standard" design for understanding intervention effects on health outcomes. An entire issue of the journal *Social Science & Medicine* was devoted to discussions about RCTs (e.g., Deaton & Cartwright, 2018; Horwitz & Singer, 2018), and although commentators acknowledged that RCTs are "clearly indispensable," they noted ways in which they are "often flawed" or "mostly useless" (Ioannidis, 2018, p. 53).

Evidence-Based Practice and Population Models

EBP is based on evidence about *populations* of people, such as a population of preterm infants or a population of adolescents with obesity. Systematic reviews of RCTs, at the pinnacle of evidence hierarchies, are the cornerstone of EBP. Yet, systematic reviews of RCTs cannot affirm that *all* patients receiving an effective intervention will benefit from it—only that the "average" patient in a specified population probably would. Clinicians, however, do not treat "average" patients—they care for people with varying and distinctive traits, preferences, and health risks.

Subramanian and colleagues (2018) were especially eloquent about this issue, noting that inferences about **average treatment effects** can be misleading or even harmful when responses to an intervention diverge—a situation that is called **heterogeneity of treatment effects (HTEs)**. They noted that the "average patient" is a construct, not a reality, and provided some evidence for their claim that "most people taking RCT-validated, effective treatments derive no benefit from them" (p. 78). For a few interventions, it is possible that beneficial effects from an intervention are nearly universal—but this is unlikely to be the case for nursing interventions aimed at affecting complex behaviors or emotions. Universal effects should seldom be assumed. Subramanian et al. provided one example regarding evidence that the widely used drug Nexium, although found to be effective based on RCT results, "works for only 1 in 25 people who take it for heartburn" (p. 78)—that is, the number needed to treat (NNT) is 25. Yet, not unreasonably, clinicians recommend Nexium to treat heartburn because, *on average*, patients who used it in trials had a lower incidence of heartburn than those who did not. It is not that trial information about average effects is unimportant, but it is often insufficient. For an individual patient, the average effect is of little interest—an intervention either is or is not beneficial.

TIP Randomized trials were initially used in agriculture: different strategies were experimentally tested with the goal of improving crop yield. However, those experimental strategies were never about the welfare of individual plants (Rolfe, 2009).

Average treatment effects, such as the ones estimated in systematic reviews, are problematic from another perspective: averages strip away *context*. Context shapes how interventions are implemented and influences their effectiveness. However, population models of EBP provide context-free conclusions about the delivery of effective care.

Evidence-Based Practice and External Validity

In Chapter 10, we pointed out the tensions between efforts to enhance a study's internal validity (inferences that an intervention *caused* an effect) and external validity (inferences that causal claims generalize across people, settings, and time). Strategies to reduce threats to internal validity tend to negatively impact external validity and vice versa.

Researchers who seek to generate evidence for practice have traditionally resolved the tension between internal and external validity in favor of internal validity. Evidence hierarchies, for example, rank study designs based on their ability to eliminate threats to internal validity; external validity is ignored. In systematic reviews, evaluations of study quality almost invariably focus on internal rather than external validity. The GRADE system for evaluating reviewers' *confidence* in evidence from systematic reviews (Chapter 30), which emphasizes internal validity, gives a nod to external validity by including a criterion of consistency of results (Table 30.2), but the underlying concern is the *replicability* of a causal inference and not its generalizability (i.e., not whether the results are maintained across different settings or populations).

Traditional RCTs undermine the generalizability of the results in diverse ways. Table 31.1 lists

TABLE 31.1 • **Constraints on Generalizability in Traditional (Explanatory) Randomized Controlled Trials (RCTs)[a]**

TYPE OF ISSUE	NATURE OF THE PROBLEM
Research Design	Confounding influences on the outcomes are tightly controlled, unlike what typically occurs.
	Follow-up period in the trial is often shorter than what a usual course of treatment might be; long-term outcomes are seldom studied to see if benefits are sustained or if harms emerge.
	Participants are prohibited from receiving other treatments, unlike what happens in the normal course of life.
	Comparing the intervention to no treatment or to a placebo leaves questions about clinical decision-making unanswered.
Intervention	The trial is often undertaken in high-skill, resource-rich settings, not in "typical" settings.
	Intervention typically is administered by highly skilled and well-trained staff, unlike what occurs in normal settings.
	The intervention is adequately funded and carefully managed.
	Participants often undergo stringent tests/screenings to be eligible to participate, unlike what occurs in normal settings.
	The intervention in trials may be limited to a specified time interval rather than having treatment determined by need.
	Adherence and intervention fidelity are higher in trials than in normal practice settings.
Sampling	Exclusion criteria often eliminate people who might most benefit from (or who might most be harmed by) the intervention (e.g., older patients, ones with comorbidities).
	Low rates of participation in trials result in biases; RCT samples include only those willing to be randomized and might exclude people (or clinicians) who have strong treatment preferences.
Outcomes/ Measurement	Studies are not always focused on outcomes of greatest interest to patients (e.g., quality of life).
	Studies seldom focus on outcomes of greatest interest to administrators (costs, resource requirements).
	Insufficient information on adverse events is gathered.
	Heavy response burden can contribute to attrition from the study.
Analysis	Focus is on "average" effects, not on the distribution of effects.
	Subgroup analyses, when undertaken, are not well conceived.

[a]Identified in such papers as those by Gross and Fogg (2001) and Rothwell (2005b; 2006).

features often used to enhance the internal validity of RCTs. These features indicate that RCTs have typically been conducted under ideal conditions rather than in normal, real-world situations. All aspects of the study are tightly controlled, including what the exact intervention is, who the interventionists are, where the study takes place, and who participates in the study.

Sampling issues are particularly troublesome for generalizing the results of RCTs. To reduce confounding, trialists often impose exclusion criteria that eliminate key groups of people—often, older people and those with comorbidities, who might especially benefit from, or be harmed by, the intervention under study. Other groups are often left out simply because they are not served in large healthcare centers where the trials are conducted (e.g., low income groups, rural residents). These limits on generalizability are compounded by low rates of participation in RCTs, with refusal rates sometimes approaching 90%. The bottom line is that, in general, patients are usually very different from those included in RCTs.

Example of an RCT With a High Rate of Refusal
Zolotarova et al. (2023) undertook a RCT to explore the impact of an educational intervention on COVID-19 vaccine uptake. The intervention was individually delivered to people imprisoned across prisons in Canada. Of the 303 that met eligibility criteria, 202 were invited to participate in the study, but 32% declined to participate.

The combined effect of relying on a population model of average effects and using data from highly select study participants is that EBP is often based on evidence of whether an intervention works for a hypothetical "average" patient under ideal, context-neutral conditions. Although the RCT results may be unbiased from an internal validity standpoint, they may be less useful than one would hope in making decisions about individual patients who are neither "ideal" nor "average."

Applicability, Generalizability, and Relevance

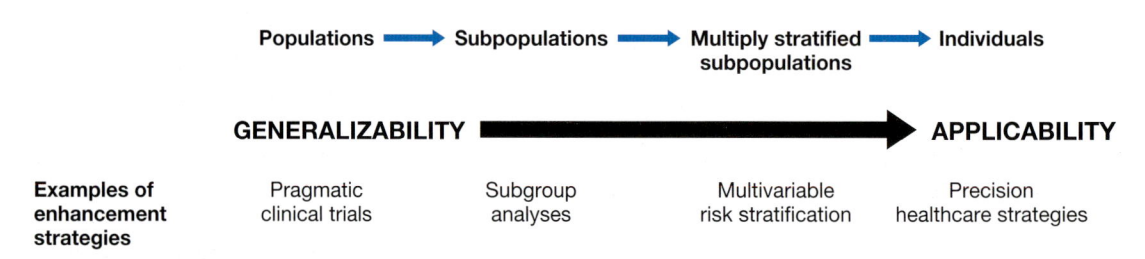

The terms *generalizability* and *applicability* have often been used interchangeably, but there is a growing view that they are quite distinct (Sacristán & Dilla, 2018; Treweek & Zwarenstein, 2009). Generalizability is a term associated with populations—researchers identify characteristics of a population to which their findings might reasonably be generalized. As astutely noted by Lincoln and Guba (1985), however, "The trouble with generalizations is that they don't apply to particulars" (p. 110).

We define **applicability** as the degree to which research evidence can be applied to individuals, small groups of individuals, or local contexts. Applicability is relevant to clinical decision-making because of human heterogeneity—averages are not of much value as decision guides if there is wide diversity in whether an intervention works or how it is viewed, experienced, adhered to, or incorporated into normal life. Sacristán and Dilla (2018) noted that "As healthcare decisions are becoming more patient centric, the term 'applicability' should evoke 'individual patient' rather than 'average patient'" (p. 165).

Figure 31.1 shows a hypothetical continuum along which evidence can move from generalizable to applicable. The bottom of the figure shows examples of strategies that researchers can use along the continuum. We discuss several ideas for enhancing applicability and generalizability—as well as relevance—in this chapter. In the context of practice-based evidence, we define **relevance** as

Populations ⟶ Subpopulations ⟶ Multiply stratified subpopulations ⟶ Individuals

GENERALIZABILITY ⟶ APPLICABILITY

Examples of enhancement strategies: Pragmatic clinical trials | Subgroup analyses | Multivariable risk stratification | Precision healthcare strategies

FIGURE 31.1 Generalizability and applicability.

evidence that is important to key stakeholders and has the potential to be actionable. **Patient-centered research**, which focuses on developing evidence that is meaningful and valuable to patients, involves efforts to attain relevance.

Producing evidence that is applicable, relevant, and generalizable requires researchers to be vigilant, creative, and insightful in an ongoing way. The task of applying research evidence to solve healthcare problems is a responsibility of practitioners, but researchers need to take steps to enrich the readiness of their evidence for "reasonable extrapolation" (Patton, 2015).

New Directions in Healthcare Research

Concern about the limitations of EBP for guiding decisions about individuals in real-world contexts has led to the emergence of new ideas and innovative methods for *optimizing* evidence. Efforts at optimization have taken various forms, such as *precision healthcare, individualized healthcare, stratified healthcare, personalized healthcare,* and *patient-centered healthcare*. Research in these domains has gone in broadly similar directions, but sometimes with different emphases. Such research typically strives for evidence that is practice based.

Comparative effectiveness research (CER) is an important manifestation of emerging directions in healthcare research. CER emphasizes patient-centeredness and involves direct comparisons of clinical interventions to facilitate decision-making (Chapter 11). As noted by Greenfield and Kaplan (2012), "CER calls for substantial changes in the way clinical research is conducted, interpreted, and practically applied …the evolving CER paradigm requires … innovations that address three basic questions: what works? for whom? and in whose hands?" (p. 263).

The Institute of Medicine's (2009) report on priorities for CER offered six defining characteristics of CER:

1. *CER's objective is to directly inform clinical decisions.* CER places a high value on the ability to generalize results to real-world decision-making. Because the goal is to contribute to important decisions, a broad range of relevant stakeholders and decision-makers (including patients) should be included in setting priorities, designing studies, and implementing results.
2. *CER involves comparisons of two or more alternative treatments, each of which has potential to be* "best practice." CER avoids the use of placebos, attention controls, or no intervention as comparators in testing an intervention. For this reason, CER trials are sometimes referred to as "head-to-head" trials.
3. *CER seeks evidence at both the population and the subgroup level.* A goal of CER is to help providers and patients in individualizing decisions—going beyond "average effects" to effects for people with similar characteristics.
4. *CER uses outcomes that are important to patients.* CER strives to include and give weight to patient-reported outcomes and to attend to benefits, harms, and unintended consequences of healthcare interventions. In turn, this means that CER is often focused on long-term outcomes. Costs are also considered important in CER because they can influence decisions.
5. *CER uses diverse research designs and methods.* Some comparative effectiveness studies involve experimental designs, but CER also uses other designs, including nonexperimental (observational) approaches. CER also draws on diverse data sources, such as data from electronic health records (EHRs), administrative claims, and clinical registries.
6. *CER is conducted in real-world settings.* CER studies the effectiveness of interventions in settings similar to those where an intervention would actually be used.

These characteristics of CER diverge in many important respects from the research model that has come to be established under EBP, which focuses on internal validity and adheres rather rigidly to evidence from RCTs. Note that these characteristics of CER embody concerns about generalizability (defining characteristic 1), applicability (defining characteristic 3), and relevance (defining characteristic 4). In the remainder of this chapter, we offer some suggestions for optimizing evidence and generating practice-based evidence. Many of these suggestions rely on ideas emerging in the context of CER, methods for which are still evolving.

STRATEGIES TO ENHANCE APPLICABILITY, GENERALIZABILITY, AND RELEVANCE

We organize this section on strategies to develop practice-based evidence according to major steps of a research project. We consider our suggestions merely a starting place and hope that we will inspire insights on how to make evidence more useful to practitioners in real-world settings.

Planning a Study for Practice-Based Evidence

A good place to begin with efforts to enhance applicability is to ask the right questions—questions that patients and clinicians want answered. There is a growing awareness of the importance of "co-designing" studies with a range of stakeholders and *end-users* of research evidence (Rycroft-Malone, 2012). Collaboration with patients, practitioners in varied disciplines, and administrators throughout the research process can result in better interprofessional "buy-in" and greater relevance of research results. Stakeholder involvement can also offer practical advantages, including greater ease of recruiting study participants and study sites. The Patient-Centered Outcomes Research Institute (PCORI) has played a lead role in spurring stakeholder involvement in health research and is a key funder of CER projects (Forsythe et al., 2018; Newhouse et al., 2015).

TIP Several models of stakeholder and patient engagement have been proposed (e.g., Concannon et al., 2014; Sofolahan-Oladeinde et al., 2017). Research thus far suggests that stakeholder involvement can be challenging but results in research deemed to be highly relevant.

Site selection is important. A local focus, as in quality improvement projects or action research, greatly enhances applicability but may constrain generalizability. In planning a project, consideration needs to be given to which of these goals is more salient. Implementing the project in multiple sites is often a useful strategy, but then a decision must be made about whether the sites are essentially *replicates* (in a manner that might enhance applicability to certain contexts) or are deliberately selected to allow conclusions to be generalized to different types of contexts or people. In the latter case, care must be taken to identify key dimensions of difference for the selected sites (e.g., rural/urban; public/private institutions, etc.).

As Figure 31.1 suggests, one approach to moving from generalizability to greater applicability is to study whether intervention effects differ for different subpopulations. We encourage researchers to give thought early in the planning process to studying *subgroup effects*, so that appropriate design and sampling strategies, described later, can be put in place. It is especially important to develop hypotheses about subgroup effects in advance and to develop a cogent rationale for such hypotheses.

During the planning stage, researchers should also consider using a framework to guide the design and implementation of a study aimed at enhancing relevance. One such framework is called **R**each, **E**ffectiveness, **A**doption, **I**mplementation, and **M**aintenance or **RE-AIM** (Battaglia & Glasgow, 2018). RE-AIM was explicitly developed with the goal of elevating awareness about external validity.

TIP Numerous frameworks have been devised to facilitate translation and implementation projects. This chapter is not designed to assist researchers who are focused on translating evidence from efficacy trials into real-world settings. Rather, our goal is to illustrate how researchers can take steps to enhance relevance and applicability from the get-go. Although RE-AIM is most often used in implementation science, some of its strategies are useful to any researcher interested in developing practice-based evidence.

Designing a Study for Practice-Based Evidence

Table 31.1 identifies several features of a traditional RCT—all of which suggest opportunities for design modifications that could increase the relevance of intervention research. Here we mention a few design considerations, most of which are consistent with CER, but we acknowledge that this is an area in which innovations occur daily and which is ripe for further methodologic creativity.

Pragmatic Clinical Trials

As we have noted, features of the traditional RCT designs are so tightly controlled that the relevance of the findings to real-life situations can be questioned. Concern about this problem has led to interest in **pragmatic clinical trials (PCTs)**, which are designed to maximize external validity with minimal negative effect on internal validity (Ford & Norrie, 2016; Glasgow et al., 2005; Treweek & Zwarenstein, 2009). Tunis and colleagues (2003), in a seminal paper, defined pragmatic (practical) clinical trials as "trials for which the hypotheses and study design are formulated based on information needed to make a decision" (p. 1626). Thus, pragmatic trials are consistent with the goals of CER.

> **TIP** Pragmatic trials are more squarely focused on *effectiveness* rather than *efficacy* (Chapter 10). Pragmatic trials sometimes are part of a translational project—that is, they involve tests in usual care settings of an intervention previously found to be efficacious in a traditional RCT. But *pragmatism* as a construct can be applied in most studies. As noted by Sacristán and Dilla (2018), pragmatism is not so much a design type but a "mindset"—pragmatic attitudes can be used in all types of research. Indeed, pragmatism is the paradigm underlying mixed methods research.

Compared to more traditional **explanatory trials** conducted under optimal conditions with carefully selected participants, PCTs address practical questions about the benefits and risks of an intervention—as well as its costs—as they would unfold in routine clinical practice. Tunis and co-authors (2003) made these recommendations for PCTs: enrollment of diverse populations with fewer exclusions of high-risk patients; recruitment of participants from a variety of practice settings; follow-up over a longer period; inclusion of economic outcomes; and comparisons of clinically viable alternatives.

Trials cannot readily be categorized as *pragmatic* or *explanatory*, because they do not represent a dichotomy. As noted by Treweek and Zwarenstein (2009), "there is a continuum rather than a dichotomy… with the pragmatic attitude explicitly favoring design choices that maximise applicability of the trial results to usual care settings" (p. 2).

A tool called **PRECIS-2** (**P**referred **E**xplanatory **C**ontinuum **I**ndicator **S**ummary) has been developed to help researchers evaluate how pragmatic their trial is and to help ensure that their designs are congruent with their intended aims (Loudon et al., 2015). The tool covers nine domains (e.g., patient eligibility, patient recruitment), each of which is rated from 1 (very explanatory) to 5 (very pragmatic). For example, the question for the eligibility domain is this: To what extent are the participants in the trial similar to those who would receive this intervention if it was part of usual care?

> **TIP** Nurse researchers have demonstrated growing interest in PCTs. A methods conference at the 2017 meeting of the Council for the Advancement of Nursing Science was devoted to pragmatic trials, and a special issue of *Nursing Outlook* included several papers based on presentations at the conference. In that issue, Battaglia and Glasgow (2018) asserted that pragmatic research "is an area of tremendous opportunity for the nursing science community" (p. 430). Littleton-Kearney (2018) described funding of PCTs at the National Institute of Nursing Research. Zenk (2022), the Director of the NINR, provided a keynote presentation on PCTs to the NIH Pragmatic Trials Collaboratory.

Glasgow and colleagues (2005) proposed several research designs for pragmatic trials. The most promising (and widely used) include cluster randomization (randomization of groups rather than individuals) and delayed treatment designs (everyone gets the intervention eventually). When a delay-of-treatment strategy is combined with cluster randomization, the result is a **stepped wedge design**, which involves having clusters randomized to receive the intervention at different points (Battaglia & Glasgow, 2018).

> **Example of a PCT With Cluster Randomization**
> Kua et al. (2021) conducted a multidisciplinary, pragmatic, multicenter, stepped-wedge cluster randomized control trial. Led by pharmacists, the trial examined the effectiveness of a deprescribing intervention aimed at reducing falls in long-term care facilities. The team used cluster randomization to assign patients to either receive the deprescribing intervention or usual care. Although the intervention group did have a reduction in medication prescribing, the findings did not indicate that they experienced a decrease in falls.

PCTs protect internal validity by using familiar bias-reducing strategies such as randomization, allocation concealment, and blinding. Moreover, cluster randomized pragmatic trials can promote internal validity by guarding against contamination of treatments. However, Eckardt and Erlanger (2018) have noted possible threats to validity in pragmatic trials. One issue is that the interventions are often less standardized in different real-world settings, perhaps resulting in differential "dosing" of the intervention and different degrees of intervention fidelity.

Another issue with PCTs is that *precision* can be affected: PCTs allow (and encourage) greater diversity in settings and participants, and so confidence intervals around treatment effects tend to be wider. This implies that larger sample sizes might be needed for pragmatic than explanatory trials.

Adaptive Interventions and Adaptive Trial Designs

Researchers are using a variety of strategies to individualize interventions and to target them more effectively. Recently, researchers have begun to use a framework called the **multiphase optimization strategy (MOST)**, which has been used for optimization in both fixed interventions and in dynamic multicomponent interventions that evolve over time (Collins et al., 2014).

Adaptive, dynamic treatments are common in clinical practice—clinicians begin with an intervention, assess whether it is working, and then make another decision (e.g., continuing with the treatment, strengthening it, trying something else). **Adaptive interventions** are ones in which there are multiple decision points over time, and decisions are based on individual responses. Adaptive interventions sometimes take the form of *stepped care interventions* in which care begins with a low-intensity strategy that is increased if goals are not reached, or with a high-intensity strategy that is stepped down if they are reached. Adaptive interventions involve four main components:

1. *Decision points.* Points in time when a treatment decision is made.
2. *Tailoring variables.* Information about individuals that is used to make treatment decisions.
3. *Intervention options.* Options regarding type, dose, intensity, duration, or delivery mechanism of the intervention.
4. *Decision rules.* Links between the tailoring variables and the treatment options at the decision points.

The MOST framework for optimizing adaptive interventions often involves using a **sequential, multiple assignment, randomized trial (SMART)** design to answer questions about individualized sequences of interventions (Almirall et al., 2014; Lei et al., 2012; Wilbur et al., 2016). SMART typically uses a factorial design to obtain information for optimization. SMART studies always involve at least two stages (decision points), with randomization occurring at each stage. SMART designs can be used to identify the best decision points, tailoring variables, intervention options, or decision rules.

There are two types of tailoring variables. *Baseline tailoring variables* are ones for which information obtained prior to the intervention is used to make tailored treatment decisions at the first or at a subsequent decision stage. For example, in a weight loss intervention, participants might be given longer or more intensive treatment in the first phase if they are classified as "obese" rather than "overweight." *Intermediate tailoring variables,* obtained after baseline, are often preliminary "outcomes," that is, indicators of whether the initial intervention has promise of effectiveness. Using a pre-established threshold, these tailoring variables are used to distinguish *responders* and *nonresponders* to the initial treatment, and this in turn is used to tailor the intervention in the second stage.

Figure 31.2 presents a hypothetical example in which an intermediate tailoring variable was used. At the outset, all study participants are randomized to Intervention A or Intervention B (in our example, individual [A] vs. group [B] counseling for weight loss). Six weeks later, all study participants are evaluated for their response to the intervention—that is, whether they have reached the responder threshold based on a pre-established criterion (e.g., weight loss >3.0% of baseline weight). Benchmarks might be established by a panel of stakeholders or by referencing established thresholds for clinical significance on the primary outcome (Chapter 21). In both arms of the trial, responders and non-responders are further randomized. Responders in both arms are randomized to either "maintenance" (e.g., continuation of the intervention) or discontinuation. Nonresponders are randomized to either an intensified version of the original treatment (e.g., longer or more frequent sessions) or to an augmented treatment (Intervention C) in which they receive a supplementary component (e.g., meal replacements).

In this example, the first *decision point* is at the outset (identifying people who are overweight and want to lose weight) and the second is 6 weeks later. The *tailoring variable* is whether the person showed adequate weight loss progress after getting an intervention. The *intervention options* included: (1) individualized weight loss counseling; (2) group weight loss counseling; (3) intensified counseling of both types; and (4) a supplementary intervention. The *decision rules* were to offer an initial intervention and to then tailor it depending on the response.

The goal of a SMART study is to construct and optimize a tailored intervention before it is brought to a full traditional (or pragmatic) randomized trial. At each stage of a SMART, researchers use randomization to address a

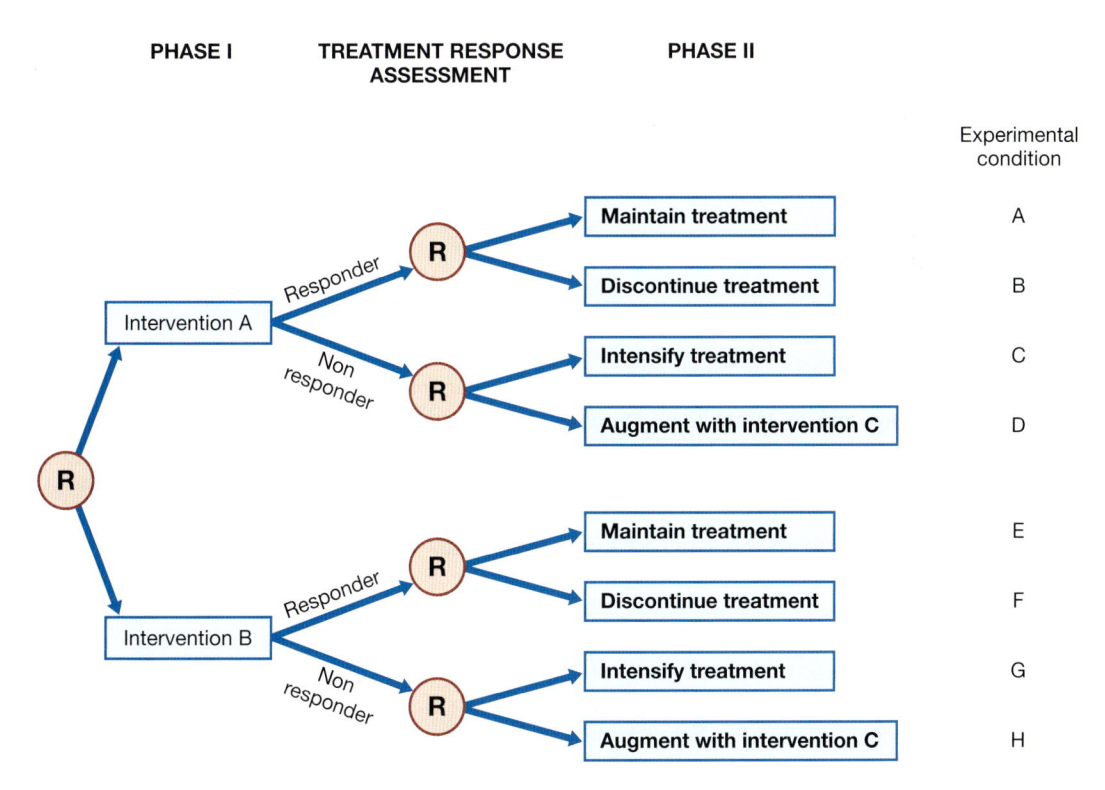

FIGURE 31.2 Example of a Sequential Multiple Assignment Randomized Trial (SMART). Note: R = randomization to treatment condition.

question about treatment options, and those options are tailored to individual circumstances or responses. Randomization in a SMART design permits unbiased comparisons between treatment components at each stage in the development of an adaptive intervention.

Several variants of SMART designs have been proposed. For example, Dai and Shete (2016) suggested a time-varying SMART design in which participants are rerandomized to the second stage interventions as soon as the predesignated intermediate response is observed—in our example, as soon as a participant achieves a weight loss greater than 3% of weight at baseline.

Example of SMART Design
Yan et al. (2021) conducted a study to compare a SMART design trial to a conventional RCT to identify the best sequence for two telemedicine modalities for titration of insulin dosing in patients initiating insulin therapy for type 2 diabetes mellitus. One intervention was delivered through a smartphone app and the other was a telephone-delivered nurse consultation. The primary outcome of the study was the HbA1c. The study findings support the use of the SMART design over a conventional RCT for evaluating sequences of therapies.

SMART studies are used to develop adaptive interventions, but they do not typically involve an **adaptive trial design** in which the trial design itself is altered during the course of the trial (Bhatt & Mehta, 2016). Adaptive designs are used to learn if a treatment is safe and effective and who will derive the most benefit (Heckman-Stoddard & Smith, 2014). In an adaptive trial design, the results of interim analyses are used to make adjustments to features of the study design. For example, the interim analyses may lead to stopping the trial early, adaptively assigning doses, dropping or adding study arms, focusing more attention on responder groups, or changing the proportion of participants randomized to each arm of the trial. Adaptive trial designs (and other innovative types of designs such as *basket* trials) are often used in tests of gene therapies in connection with precision healthcare (Biankin et al., 2015; Pallmann et al., 2018).

TIP The emergence of "just-in-time" adaptive interventions using mHealth (mobile health) technologies has given rise to other innovations in experimental design, including *microrandomization*, which involves randomly assigning intervention options at multiple decision points—that is, at the points at which a particular component might be efficacious (Klasnja et al., 2015).

N-of-1 Trials

The ultimate approach to individualization is to test an intervention with individual study participants. **N-of-1 trials** (also called **single-subject experiments**) are studies in which different treatments are tested in an individual patient over time. N-of-1 trials typically are randomized crossover trials conducted on a single patient. These trials are characterized by alternating an active treatment phase and a placebo phase (or alternating two active treatments). The simplest N-of-1 trial design is exposure to one treatment condition (A) and then exposure to another condition (B). When the sequence is randomly determined, this results in an AB or BA allocations. However, preferred designs involve the repetition of treatment sequences to protect against various sources of biases—for example, designs such as ABAB or ABBAABBA. N-of-1 trials have been strongly advocated by proponents of patient-centered research: such designs are uniquely capable of leading to evidence-informed clinical decisions for individual patients. In some cases, N-of-1 studies can be profitably aggregated (Schork, 2018).

Example of a Single-Subject ABA Design
Shams and colleagues (2021) used an ABA single-subject design to assess the feasibility and efficacy of basic movements of Azeri dance on the balance and static posture in a person with Parkinson disease. At baseline (A), measures were taken four times over a 2-week period. In the third week, the Azeri dance intervention (B) was implemented for 45 minutes, three times per week over 4 weeks, and measures were assessed after each session. Lastly, the measures were assessed post the intervention (A2) at 2, 4, and 6 weeks to establish the withdrawal phase.

The *Journal of Clinical Epidemiology* published a series of papers on N-of-1 trials in 2016, consistent with the growing research interest in the personalization of healthcare (e.g., Knottnerus et al., 2016; Vohra, 2016). Punja and colleagues (2016) identified numerous potential advantages of single-subject trials, including the following: (1) intervention approaches are individualized; (2) results are applicable and directly relevant to participants; (3) participants quickly learn the results; and (4) the cost is low compared to traditional RCTs. Methodologic safeguards are traditionally implemented in N-of-1 trials (e.g., randomization and blinding). Indeed, the Oxford Centre for Evidence-Based Medicine considers evidence from such trials as Level 1 evidence. Kravitz and Duan (2014) offer excellent guidance on single-subject trials.

TIP Some studies that are called "N-of-1" trials do not involve alternating treatments but rather are tests of interventions that are personalized for each participant.

Example of a Personalized (N-of-1) Study Platform
Konigorski et al. (2022) describe a StudyU platform that is available for free and can be used by researchers to design and conduct digital N-of-1 trials to assess the effects of different interventions on individual's health. The authors' goal is to create personalized treatments and evidence to optimize health.

Alternatives to Randomized Trials: Quasi-Experiments

Randomized designs are the gold standard for enhancing internal validity and coming to conclusions about causal relationships, but they are often removed from clinical realities. As pointed out by Gross and Fogg (2001), nurse researchers should consider "reasonable alternatives" to random assignment. Participation in an intervention study can be far more acceptable to prospective participants (and to research site administrators) if randomization of patients is not involved—which is precisely what makes cluster randomization attractive in pragmatic trials. Higher rates of participation, in turn, enhance generalizability.

Quasiexperimental designs are sometimes a useful alternative to an RCT, but researchers need to be strategic in designing quasiexperiments to minimize threats to internal validity. Also, in 2017, the *Journal of Clinical Epidemiology* published a useful series of 13 papers on the utility of quasiexperimental designs (e.g., Bärnighausen et al., 2017; Rockers et al., 2017). Partially randomized patient preference designs (Chapter 9) can also be useful for enhancing applicability—such designs include both randomized and nonrandomized components and can provide valuable information about what patients prefer.

Alternatives to Randomized Trials: Nonexperimental Research

Observational (nonexperimental) studies are even lower than quasiexperiments on traditional evidence hierarchies. Yet, there is growing awareness that carefully conducted observational studies can yield evidence with high internal validity—and with far greater external validity than explanatory RCTs because they tend to involve broader and more representative samples (e.g., Booth & Tannock, 2013; Concato & Horwitz, 2018). CER embraces the contribution of observational studies in assessing the benefits and harms of alternative interventions (Marko & Weil, 2010).

Observational studies can be used to evaluate the effects of alternative interventions in situations in which patients have not been randomized to the treatment. Although there have been concerns about "overestimation bias" in observational studies of treatment effects when there is self-selection into treatments, new approaches to designing studies that mimic RCT protocols are emerging. Such methodologic strategies as aligning eligibility criteria to an RCT, establishing a "zero time" for treatment, and using sophisticated methods such as propensity score analysis and *instrumental variables* to address confounding variables are being pursued (Armstrong, 2012; Frieden, 2017).

Observational studies with large administrative or epidemiological databases can contribute to practice-based evidence in other ways. For example, large observational studies can help researchers to understand the representativeness of samples from traditional or pragmatic RCTs (Greenhouse et al., 2008). In that vein, some have suggested "nesting" RCTs within large population databases or electronic health record (EHR) databases to get a better handle on the generalizability of the RCT results (Angus, 2015; Dahabreh, 2018).

Other important uses of observational data from large databases include the following: learning the uptake and outcomes of new interventions in routine practice; identifying potential harms or adverse effects associated with new interventions; expanding tailored clinical decision support mechanisms (Angus, 2015); and developing prediction models about the types of people most likely to have a favorable response to an intervention (Iwashyna & Liu, 2014).

Booth and Tannock (2013) argued that RCTs and population-based observational research should be considered partners in the evolution of healthcare evidence. They recommend a two-prong approach in which rigorous RCTs powered to detect clinically meaningful improvements are followed by observational studies that "evaluate patterns of care, toxicity, and the effectiveness of treatment in routine practice" (p. 553).

Mixed Methods Designs

Developing practice-based evidence requires the thoughtful integration of qualitative and quantitative data, especially in studies of intervention effectiveness (Battaglia & Glasgow, 2018). Qualitative data offer insights into why, how, and with whom effects are observed.

There are several ways in which mixed methods designs are especially valuable with regard to the applicability of evidence. Qualitative information can provide a rich understanding of the *context* in which interventions are delivered. Contextualized understandings can lead to insights into the kinds of environments in which an intervention does or does not "work."

Qualitative data can also play a crucial role in untangling the enigma of "average treatment effects." For individual participants, the effects might be much greater than the average, while for others, the intervention might have no benefit. Sometimes quantitative subgroup analyses can be undertaken, but these are productive only if the dimension along which variation occurs is a measurable attribute about which hypotheses have been developed in advance. A qualitative study of participants who experienced the intervention differently could illuminate how to target the intervention more effectively in the future or how to improve it to reach a more diverse audience. A qualitative component also can lay the foundation for more formal subgroup analysis or for developing interventions tailored to individual needs and circumstances. Qualitative methods are well suited to exploring the HTEs (Holtrop et al., 2018). Realist evaluations, described earlier in this book, usually use mixed methods to address a range of questions about an intervention, including applicability.

Sampling for Practice-Based Evidence

A major problem with the evidence from traditional RCTs—evidence that forms the basis for most clinical practice guidelines—is that the samples exclude many types of people to whom the evidence is supposed to be applied. Pragmatic trials, which typically have fewer exclusion criteria, tend to yield samples that are closer to real-world populations. Thus, one obvious suggestion for generating practice-based evidence is to make efforts to ensure that research samples reflect the full range of people who could benefit from an intervention.

Other advice concerning strategies to enhance applicability and generalizability includes the following:

- *Clearly identify the target population.* The starting point for selecting a heterogeneous "real-world" sample to which study results can be generalized is to clearly define the characteristics of the people (and settings) of interest. All too often, researchers seem to begin with a nonrepresentative sample from an ill-defined and restrictive population and then hope for the best. Stakeholder involvement in identifying the target population is likely to be productive.

- *Use purposive sampling strategies.* Convenience samples of "ideal" (e.g., no comorbidities) and cooperative people are all too common in quantitative research. Quota sampling is a step in the right direction—it is used to ensure a sufficient number of sample members within key population strata. In general, researchers would do far better at achieving representative samples if they had a more purposive approach to sampling (Polit & Beck, 2010). When researchers know in advance the characteristics of their target population, they can monitor sample characteristics in an ongoing fashion and then recruit types of participants who are not yet adequately represented. Sampling totally by convenience is seldom justified if the goal is to produce practice-based evidence.
- *Sample from multiple sites.* It is often useful to recruit sample members from multiple sites, being strategic about site selection. For example, if people in a single site are homogeneous with regard to a characteristic that might affect intervention outcomes, then an important way to broaden understanding about intervention effects is to select sites that vary on important dimensions (e.g., low-income vs. affluent communities).
- *Aim for a sample size that permits subgroup analyses.* The sample size should be large enough to support relevant subgroup analyses that are sufficiently powered. Sample size projections should also take into consideration requirements for studying clinical significance, which is more patient-centric than statistical significance.
- *Sample participants carefully for in-depth inquiry in mixed methods studies.* A nested sample (Chapter 27) of participants from the full sample may be especially useful for in-depth explorations of heterogeneity of effects, as well as other issues such as variation in adherence. Multilevel samples may provide rich insights into the research context.

Collecting Data for Practice-Based Evidence

Several steps can be taken to improve the data collection efforts of researchers striving for practice-based evidence. First and foremost, there is growing awareness that researchers do not always focus on the needs and interests of key stakeholders, including both patients and clinicians. Studies ideally would be cocreated with people who can provide input regarding patient-important outcomes. For example, patients are much less likely to care about whether an intervention can bring about a 5-point improvement on a composite scale—or even a 5% decrease in blood pressure—than about functional outcomes (e.g., regaining the ability to walk up a flight of stairs). People are more likely to cooperate in research if they perceive the research to be relevant to them, and selecting relevant outcomes is a path to patient-centered evidence.

In Chapter 15, we describe psychometric criteria for selecting high-quality measures for research purposes—notably reliability, validity, and responsiveness. Additional criteria should be considered for creating practice-based evidence. Glasgow and Riley (2013) offered four primary criteria for "*pragmatic measures*":

- Important to stakeholders (outcomes are deemed important by diverse stakeholder groups);
- Low response burden (requires minimal time and effort to complete);
- Actionable (enhances application in busy, real-world settings; easy to interpret and useful in decision-making); and
- Sensitive to change (capable of tracking progress).

For certain outcomes, the use of measures from the Patient-Reported Outcome Measurement Information System (PROMIS®) offers many advantages (Kroenke et al., 2015). PROMIS® covers dozens of outcomes with high relevance to patients (e.g., pain, physical function, sleep disturbance), and, because of computer adaptive testing, the measures are extremely efficient yet precise. Another important feature of PROMIS® is that scoring is instantaneous and yields feedback about performance relative to normed samples (for many measures, separate norms by sex and age). Scoring is on a common metric (a T-score), where a score of 50 equals the mean of the U.S. general population—this, in turn, makes scores interpretable and actionable by patients and clinicians. Finally, PROMIS® includes measures that are sensitive to change and minimizes floor and ceiling effects. PROMIS® measures are available for use with the general population, as well as with adult and pediatric populations with chronic conditions. PROMIS® measures are available for free online, and most have been translated into several languages.

Patients and clinicians are likely to find the *clinical significance* of outcomes of greater relevance to them than statistical significance. This suggests the desirability of including outcome measures for which a minimal important change (MIC) benchmark has been estimated. (Alternatively, researchers can take steps to estimating it themselves, as we discuss in Chapter 21.) The best approach to estimating an MIC value involves getting input about meaningfulness directly from patients.

Qualitative data are also important for building practice-based evidence. Qualitative data can potentially shed light on *why* or *with whom* an intervention was effective—or why it was not. Qualitative data can also illuminate implementation processes and contextual features that are important to those interested in translating an intervention into other settings.

> **TIP** Information about study contexts are most often qualitative descriptions. However, in some cases, it might make sense to formally measure contextual elements—especially in multisite studies. Carole Estabrooks and her colleagues (2011), for example, have developed the Alberta Context Tool to measure organizational contextual factors.

In addition to traditional methods of measurement and data collection, thought should also be given to the use of Big Data in nursing studies, which can be used to address questions about broad groups and populations (with potential enhancements to generalizability) and about variations in treatment effects (with potential enhancements to applicability). **Big Data** refers to large, complex datasets that are often difficult to process using customary analytic methods. Big Data has been described as having three features: high volume of data, high velocity of data flow, and high variety of data types (Wang & Krishnan, 2014). Big Data can come from aggregated clinical datasets, administrative datasets (e.g., Medicare), EHR datasets, and from large dedicated surveys, such as data from the diverse 1 million-person research cohort "All of Us" in the United States (Lyles et al., 2018). As noted previously, observational data from large datasets can be exploited to improve both generalizability of results about treatment effects and to improve applicability with the development of predictive models to guide individualized decisions. Big Data has another important advantage over traditional clinical research methods—they are better suited than data from RCTs for tracking people's health and symptoms trajectories over years or decades (Concato & Horwitz, 2018).

Finally, with the rapidly emerging interest in precision healthcare, researchers should consider gathering data on relevant biomarkers that might facilitate understanding of individual health. Corwin and Ferranti (2016) urge that nurse researchers integrate biomarkers into their studies to be "better able to precisely tailor and test nursing interventions to improve the health and well-being of patients and families across the lifespan" (p. 293). They argued that studying biomarkers and their contribution to disease and symptoms in observational studies can pave the way for precision nursing interventions.

Analyzing Data for Practice-Based Evidence

The analysis of research data is a major avenue for enhancing applicability. In particular, analytic strategies can be used to better understand HTEs. Strategies to enhance practice-based evidence range from simple approaches to complex, sophisticated ones.

Know Your Data

With the focus on *average effects* in many RCTs and systematic reviews, quantitative researchers may seldom feel the need to get close to their data. The sheer ease with which complex statistical analyses can be undertaken can result in a "disconnect" between researchers and their data—and this is especially true if statisticians are called in to do the analysis.

With respect to statistical analyses, it is always a good idea to begin with a thorough exploration of the dataset. Researchers should learn how the data on key outcomes are distributed—for example, whether heterogeneity is extensive, whether there are extreme outliers, whether the data are skewed, and so on. Focusing on heterogeneity is crucial—if there was no variation, the "average" would apply to everyone in the sample.

Qualitative researchers are expected to be immersed in their data; quantitative researchers could benefit from greater immersion as well. One strategy is for researchers to look at their data horizontally (within cases) and not simply vertically (across cases). By careful scrutiny of the complete records of selected cases—for example, people who improved greatly, deteriorated, remained unchanged, and so on—researchers often can illuminate "what is going on" in a dataset in a way that computing an average cannot (Polit & Beck, 2010). Integrating quantitative information about extreme cases or typical cases with in-depth qualitative information about such cases can potentially lead to powerful insights into constraints on generalizability and approaches to enhancing applicability.

Exploring and Representing the Outcomes

It is inevitable that researchers will continue to calculate and report average treatment effects, but they should consider other ways to look at their data. For example, if the distribution for key outcomes is skewed, it would be wise to report both median and mean values (Green & Glasgow, 2006).

In analyzing data from clinical trials, researchers often test for group differences on mean postintervention outcomes for the intervention and control groups. Assuming that outcomes were measured at baseline, it is prudent to also examine the *change scores:* How diverse were the changes in the intervention group and what was typical? Both patients and clinicians are likely to find it more relevant to know what percentage of people receiving an intervention improved than what a mean value on an outcome is.

For insights into potential intervention effects on individuals, several experts have noted the importance of calculating the absolute risk reduction (ARR)—rather than relative risk—for key outcomes. Rothwell and colleagues (2005) noted that the "absolute risk reductions in large pragmatic RCTs are…the best guide to the probable effects of treatment of individuals in routine practice" (p. 257). The ARR, which indicates the probability that an individual will benefit from an intervention on a specified outcome, is the mathematic equivalent of the NNT. For example, an ARR of 25% equals an NNT of 4: 1 patient out of 4 patients treated would benefit. As noted in Chapter 21, the NNT is considered an index of clinical significance at the group level.

ARRs and NNTs are calculated with dichotomous outcomes (e.g., did/did not fall), but continuous outcomes can be dichotomized. As described in Chapter 21, there are various approaches to estimating a benchmark for meaningful change (e.g., the minimal important change or MIC). Such benchmarks create an opportunity for dichotomizing outcomes (did/did not have meaningful change) and calculating the NNT. Even in the absence of an MIC benchmark, many measures have "cutpoints" for interpreting scores that can be used to dichotomize people—for example, a threshold for clinical depression on depression scales. Finally, some researchers use the median value of the outcome to divide a sample into responder and nonresponder groups.

It is particularly useful, from the point of view of patient-centeredness, to estimate the percentage of people who experienced clinically meaningful change. Researchers who are interested in developing relevant evidence should make efforts to analyze meaningful improvement (or deterioration), which is calculated at the level of individual participants. *Responder analyses* of those in intervention and control groups who have and have not had meaningful change are a vital tool in the analytic arsenal for improving applicability.

TIP Sometimes insights into differential effectiveness of an intervention can be gained by undertaking a *dose–response analysis*—that is, whether getting different "doses" of an intervention or exposure results in different outcomes. Some researchers create treatment groups with different amounts of an intervention, but more often, in dose–response analyses, "dose" is not under the researchers' control. If the "dose" is not experimentally manipulated, then caution would be needed in coming to conclusions about whether different doses yielded different outcomes—or whether different people self-selected into different doses.

Heterogeneity of Treatment Effects and Subgroup Analyses

Many researchers try to develop evidence that is applicable to well-defined groups of people (rather than to entire populations) by conducting subgroup analyses. A **subgroup analysis** involves efforts to disentangle HTEs for subpopulations of people. For example, a subgroup analysis might suggest that an intervention is effective for males but not for females, or more effective for people with comorbidities than for those without them.

Subgroup analyses, which are intuitively appealing to those interested in individualizing care, are often undertaken in the context of RCTs. Reviews of RCTs in medicine have consistently suggested that subgroup analyses of primary outcomes are undertaken and reported in 50% to 60% of published trials (Gabler et al., 2009, 2016; Sun et al., 2012). Evidence suggests that the rate of subgroup analysis is increasing, perhaps because of its prominence in CER. Subgroup analyses are also performed in many cohort studies that examine treatment effects (Dahan et al., 2018).

Subgroup analyses are, however, controversial, in part because they are frequently not undertaken properly (e.g., Burke et al., 2015; Sun et al., 2014). The struggle between wanting to go beyond population averages on the one hand and the statistical challenges of subgroup analysis on the other was described by renowned clinical epidemiologist Alvan Feinstein as a "clinicostatistical tragedy" (Feinstein, 1998, p. 297).

The statistical challenge in subgroup analyses involves addressing the strong risk of both Type I and Type II errors. False positives (Type I errors) are common because researchers often test multiple subgroups without making adjustments to probabilities. The probability of a false positive might be 5% for one test, but for three independent tests, the risk is 14% (Chapter 18). This problem has resulted in many reported subgroup effects that could not be replicated. Potential subgroup effects are also at high risk of being missed because of a Type II error. If a study is adequately powered for the entire sample, it will likely be underpowered when the sample is divided into subgroups.

Because of increased interest in personalized healthcare, the number of scholarly papers devoted to subgroup analyses and HTE tripled between 2005 and 2014 (Tanniou et al., 2016). We describe a few of the recommended subgroup analyses strategies here, with particular emphasis on analyses within randomized trials, and urge readers to seek additional guidance in referenced papers.

- *Specify hypotheses in advance.* Subgroup analysis should be a hypothesis-testing effort, not a fishing expedition. Tables showing 5 to 10 subgroup test results, without a priori hypotheses, are common in reports of RCTs. Multiple subgroup tests are especially suspect when there is no overall significant effect—the researchers appear to be searching for a subgroup "rescue" for disappointing results. Hypotheses about differential effects should be based on sound theoretical reasoning, biologic plausibility, or previous empirical evidence. This, in turn, means that hypotheses should be directional, specifying which group is expected to experience greater benefit. Plans for subgroup analyses should be specified in the trial protocol, and preferably the trial would be registered. When there is a strong basis for a subgroup hypothesis, researchers might consider using stratified randomization—although Kaiser (2016) found that stratification is not always needed for prespecified subgroup analyses.

TIP Burke et al. (2015) distinguished *primary* subgroup analyses (based on a priori hypotheses) and *secondary* subgroup analyses that are not stipulated in advance but can sometimes *generate* hypotheses. They reasoned that positive hypothesis-testing analyses can influence decisions about patient care, but that positive hypothesis-generating analyses require confirmatory research.

- *Restrict the number of subgroup analyses.* Burke and colleagues (2015) argued that only rarely should more than one or two primary subgroup analyses be performed. The problem with large numbers of tests is twofold. First, the risk of a Type I error increases as the number of tests goes up. Another problem is that the same people are in multiple subgroups. If we hypothesized, for example, that women would benefit more from an intervention than men (gender subgroup) and that younger people would benefit more than older people (age subgroup), what would be the expectation for older women or younger men? (This is an issue we discuss in the next section.) It is probably safest to specify a single primary subgroup analysis and to consider subgroup tests beyond that one as exploratory and to adjust the probabilities using a Bonferroni-type procedure. For exploratory (hypothesis-generating) analyses, some have suggested relaxing the criterion for significance, for example, to $p < .10$ (Gabler et al., 2009).
- *Restrict subgroup tests to the primary outcome.* Several experts have recommended that subgroup analyses should be undertaken only for the primary outcome in a trial, not for secondary ones (e.g., Assmann et al., 2000; Rothwell, 2005a).
- *Avoid severely underpowered subgroup analyses.* Many trials are powered to find an overall true treatment effect 80% of the time, but subgroup tests inevitably have lower statistical power. Power is probably closer to 20% to 30% for subgroup effect sizes that are similar in magnitude to the expected main treatment effect (Burke et al., 2015). This suggests the desirability of using a more stringent power standard for the overall sample (e.g., 90% to 95% power) when a subgroup analysis is planned. Also, power is modestly enhanced if there are an equal proportion of participants in the subgroups (e.g., 50% male and female). Although the term "subgroup" suggests categorical groupings, the variable for which HTE is hypothesized can be continuous (e.g., age, body mass index [BMI]), and continuous variables can yield substantial improvements in statistical power (Hayward et al., 2006).
- *Base the analyses on variables defined at baseline.* As noted by Sun and colleagues (2014), subgroup analyses should be based on baseline characteristics, not on ones that emerge during the study (e.g., length of stay in the ICU). The most frequently used variables for HTE analyses in medical RCTs include risk factors for the outcome (e.g., smoking status, disease severity, comorbidity), sex, and age (Gabler et al., 2009, 2016). In multisite studies, subgroup analyses are often undertaken to assess whether similar effects are observed across sites.
- *Analyze for subgroup differences using tests for interactions.* Most analyses for subgroup effects are done incorrectly (e.g., Gabler et al., 2009, 2016). The typical approach is to test for intervention effects *within* each subgroup—for example, testing intervention–control group differences separately for males and females—and then comparing the results. If, for example, there is a significant intervention effect for males but not for females, this is often considered evidence of a subgroup effect. However, such analyses could lead to totally erroneous conclusions—for example, the differences might simply be the result of differential subgroup sample sizes. The question that should be addressed in tests of HTE is this: *Are subgroup treatment effects significantly different from each other?* The null hypothesis is that the treatment effect is the same in the subgroups. To test this hypothesis, the analysis should test for an **interaction**—that is, an interaction between the treatment variable and the subgroup variable. Such analyses of HTE are sometimes referred to as **moderator analyses** (Kraemer et al., 2006; Wang & Ware, 2013). When formal tests for interaction are undertaken, they should be reported as the estimated difference in the effect of the intervention in the subgroups, with a confidence interval.
- *Calculate ARRs/NNTs for subgroups if possible.* Rothwell and colleagues (2005) advise that both overall results and subgroup results should be expressed as absolute risk reductions.

Because the risk of statistical errors is high, it is wise to be cautious in interpreting subgroup results.

The most convincing evidence for a subgroup effect comes from replicated results—especially if the effect is supported by a persuasive biologic or theoretic rationale. Corroboration can occur in the context of a systematic review (Chapter 30). As noted by Sun et al. (2014), it is appropriate to consider the likelihood of a true subgroup effect "on a continuum ranging from 'certainly true' to 'certainly false'" (p. 406).

> **TIP** Consistent *lack* of support for subgroup effects is also illuminating: it suggests that using the overall average may be appropriate in applying the evidence.

> **Example of a Subgroup Analysis**
> Wallström et al. (2020) conducted a study to evaluate the effects of a person-centered telephone intervention to address the issue of fatigue in patients with heart failure. Patients received either usual care or a telephone intervention. Measures of fatigue were taken at baseline and at 6 months. A subgroup analysis indicated that in the intervention group, motivation improved significantly from baseline to the 6-month follow-up compared with the control group.

Multivariable Risk-Stratified Analyses

A growing number of experts have noted the limitations of subgroup analysis for understanding HTEs, even when analyses are rigorously conducted. The basic problem is that subgroup analysis is a "one-variable-at-a-time" approach—despite the fact that people may have many traits that could moderate the effects of an intervention and they belong to dozens of potential subgroups. Sometimes analysts create multifactorial subgroups by combining traits—for example, older men, older women, younger men, and younger women. However, this approach involves only two variables at a time and increases the risk of a Type II error.

An approach that is gaining momentum is **multivariable risk stratification** (MRS) in analyses of intervention effects (e.g., Dahabreh et al., 2016; Hayward et al., 2006; Kent et al., 2010). To perform an MRS analysis, researchers use a tool that has been developed to predict the risk of the primary outcome. For example, if the intervention of interest was designed to reduce the risk of pressure ulcers (PUs), then a prediction tool such as the Braden Scale (Bergstrom et al., 1987) or other PU prediction tools (e.g., Deng et al., 2017) could be used. Scores on the risk index are then included in the MRS analysis instead of a subgroup variable in tests for interaction. The tool should be one that has been rigorously evaluated for discriminant validity—usually using receiver operating curves—and found to be adequate (e.g., area under the curve >0.60). The components of risk prediction tools often are easily obtainable clinical variables that are available in EHRs (e.g., age, sex, smoking status, BMI, etc.). Risk prediction tools have been developed for many outcomes of interest to nurse researchers. Some measures of disease severity (APACHE) have broad predictive scope and could be useful.

> **TIP** Experts typically recommend using an externally developed risk prediction tool in risk-stratified analyses. However, such tools are not always available. Kent and colleagues (2010) have discussed developing "internal" risk models using baseline data from the trial itself to predict the outcome, using blinded logistic regression analysis.

Table 31.2 presents an example of results from a risk-stratified analysis, using fictitious data from an RCT testing an intervention to prevent falls in hospitals. The table shows the absolute risk for those in the intervention and control groups, the relative risk reduction, and the NNT for study participants who were predicted to have low, moderate, or high risk of falling, based on their scores on a fall risk prediction scale. This table shows that those in the low-risk group did not benefit from the intervention, whereas those in the moderate- and (especially) high-risk groups did benefit. Typically, the actual risk-stratified analysis uses the full risk score rather than creating risk subgroups—unless there are reasons to suspect that the effect of the risk variable is nonlinear; however, results may be easier to communicate in a subgroup format.

When a risk-stratified analysis is possible, it offers many advantages over subgroup analysis for understanding HTEs. First, MRS analyses are consistent

TABLE 31.2 • Risk-Stratified Analysis: Fictitious Example of Fall Outcomes in a Fall Prevention Intervention Trial, Stratified on Predicted Risk of Falling

PREDICTED RISK OF A FALL[a]	EXPERIENCED A FALL AT END OF TRIAL		RELATIVE RISK REDUCTION (RRR) (95% CI)	P	NUMBER NEEDED TO TREAT (NNT)
	INTERVENTION GROUP	CONTROL GROUP			
<3%	8/500 (1.6%)	6/500 (1.2%)	−33% (−28%, 50%)	.79	−250[b]
3%–10%	10/400 (2.5%)	24/400 (6.0%)	58% (14%, 80%)	.02	29
>10%	8/100 (8%)	20/100 (20%)	60% (14%, 82%)	.025	8
Overall	26/1,000 (2.6%)	50/1,000 (5.0%)	48% (17%, 67%)	.007	42

[a]The predicted risk of a fall is based on a score of a fall risk prediction tool. The results are shown in three risk categories to facilitate interpretation, but the risk-stratified analysis to test for heterogeneity of effects should be based on the full continuous scores on the risk prediction tool.
[b]The negative sign indicates the number needed to **harm**; this was not statistically significant.

with the fact that outcomes are affected by multiple independent contributing factors. Second, this analytic approach uses the full sample size because it does not divide the sample into discrete subgroups. This means that MRS analyses almost invariably have superior statistical power to subgroup analyses (Hayward et al., 2006). The results of a risk-stratified MRS analysis provide insights into who best can benefit from an intervention—or who might not be helped very much. In turn, this can help to target interventions to the people for whom they are most likely to be effective.

Heterogeneity in treatment effects can arise for different reasons (Hayward et al., 2006). One is that people differ in their risk for a bad outcome (e.g., a fall) even before any intervention. Risk-stratified analysis is especially useful to help with targeting decisions in such situations. If, however, HTE reflects differential benefits from the treatment itself, then a subgroup analysis based on a strong theoretical rationale may be advantageous. Thus, Hayward et al. suggest that a risk-stratified analysis should sometimes supplement rather than replace subgroup analyses.

Risk-stratified analyses of trial data are less common than subgroup analyses, but this approach is growing in popularity in medical RCTs. Gabler and colleagues, in their reviews of studies exploring HTE, found only three studies that used MRS in their 2009 review of 319 trials (0.9%), compared to 33 studies in their 2016 review of 416 trials (7.9%). Kent and colleagues (2016) illustrate how such analyses are done, using data from 32 large clinical trials.

TIP MRS analyses offer avenues of opportunity for innovative nursing research. For example, risk-stratified analyses of HTE sometimes can be undertaken as a reanalysis of trial data by researchers not involved in the trial. Another opportunity lies in developing and validating risk prediction tools for outcomes of importance to nursing.

Precision/Personalized Healthcare

A fundamental tenet of **precision healthcare** (a term sometimes used interchangeably with *personalized healthcare* or *stratified healthcare*) is that interventions can be individually tailored to people based on their unique genetic, physiologic, behavioral, lifestyle, and environmental profile. The goal is not necessarily to develop a unique treatment for every individual, but rather to tailor interventions for those with tightly grouped biologic and other features—moving beyond what is possible with risk-stratified analyses. Personalized healthcare is being driven by advances in molecular genomics and is heavily dependent on data linkages and integration, data analytics, and machine learning for the identification of patterns in large datasets (Big Data).

The term *precision healthcare* has been strongly connected with advances in genomics. However, genomics and other "omic" data (e.g., metabolomics, proteomics) are not the only sources of data in personalized healthcare. A wide range of biomarkers, data from EHRs, and data from wearable sensors are examples of data with relevance to precision healthcare, suggesting the inevitability of complex multivariate models that will be needed for mapping dynamic factors that affect individual health (Mutch et al., 2018). Multivariate stratification algorithms using machine learning systems are likely to play an important role.

Precision science is advancing rapidly, which bodes well for improving targeted and efficient healthcare with high levels of applicability. Hickey and colleagues (2019) provide a description of the Nursing Science Precision Health Model.

Example of Nursing Involvement in the Precision Health Initiative

Nowak and colleagues (2022) conducted a study that contributes to nursing knowledge and understanding of epigenomic research, a type of precision health. This team's work is focused on preventing negative birth outcomes such as preterm birth in underrepresented populations. This team suggests that by using genomics, women at risk can be identified early so that appropriate interventions can be put in place to reduce risk and ultimately improve birth outcomes.

TIP Ralph Horwitz and his colleagues, proponents of practice-based evidence, have proposed the development of a large library of patient profiles that could be searched for tailored healthcare decisions for individual patients. The profiles would be derived from EHRs, clinical trials, and longitudinal observational studies. Their view is that the profiles would comprise an "*n* of many" comparison group of patients who have and have not been exposed to many different interventions (e.g., Horwitz & Singer, 2017, 2018).

Reporting Results for Practice-Based Evidence

Enhancing the applicability and relevance of research evidence requires that great care be taken in reporting study results and discussing their implications. We encourage researchers to provide sufficient information in their reports so that readers can make judgments about the utility of the information for individual patients or groups of patients. Here are a few specific suggestions:

- *Begin with an "applicability" attitude.* Committing to applicability as an important goal will likely sharpen efforts to have a strong dissemination plan. Researchers should ask themselves: What would I need to know if I were making a decision about using this evidence? Treweek and Zwarenstein (2009) noted that "trialists can and should report their trials in ways that make it easier for others to make judgements about their applicability" (p. 2).
- *Seek stakeholder input.* An important way to gain perspective on the applicability of the evidence is to involve key stakeholders in planning analyses, interpreting results, and reviewing drafts of reports. An explicit request for feedback on applicability should be made to diverse stakeholders.
- *Disseminate widely.* One way to enhance applicability is to share the evidence broadly. This means making deliberate efforts to disseminate results to various stakeholders (e.g., clinicians, patients, and their families, advocacy groups)—preferably in face-to-face meetings or at conferences. Especially when presenting results to lay audiences, be thoughtful about how results are presented—for example, talking about the percentage of people who improved rather than mean improvement.
- *Seek opportunities to provide supplementary information.* Page constraints in journals may make it difficult to provide as much information to inform relevance/applicability judgments as desired. Open-access journals (Chapter 32) are often less restrictive in terms of article length than traditional journals, but many traditional

journals offer the possibility of online supplements in which more extensive information can be included. Alternatively, researchers can publish a separate paper focused explicitly on study methods, with a focus on methods that enhance both rigor and applicability.
- *Clearly describe the sample.* Research reports almost always describe the research samples on key characteristics, but they may neglect to report important information, such as baseline risk on the primary outcome. If a risk prediction tool is available, it is useful to describe the distribution of risk, which can provide a richer understanding of the sample than one-variable-at-a-time descriptions (e.g., mean age, mean BMI).
- *Clearly describe the target population.* Research reports are not always clear about who the target population was. Users cannot envision the use of evidence in their own settings without understanding the intended population—which needs to be described beyond just stipulating the eligibility criteria. Readers should be able to discern whether the population is similar to the patients in their care.
- *Provide details about the research context.* Potential users of evidence judge the relevance of research evidence not only in terms of the target population but also in terms of the context in which the research was conducted. Rich qualitative descriptions about the study sites should be provided—together with information about how and why the research sites were selected. Make explicit efforts to evaluate whether contextual descriptions are sufficiently "thick," and involve others in this evaluation, if possible. Readers of the report should be able to draw conclusions about whether it would make sense to implement the findings of a study in their own practice setting.
- *Call readers' attention to aspects of the results that relate to applicability.* If possible, include information about the components identified in the PRECIS tool, whether the study is "pragmatic" or not. Also, an effort should be made to call readers' attention to the heterogeneity of the results, not just to "average" results.
- *Provide guidance in the discussion.* The discussion section of the report should emphasize constraints on applicability and generalizability. A discussion about what heterogeneity of effects might mean in terms of clinical decision-making—and future research—can help to shine a spotlight on applicability issues. If subgroup analyses were performed, readers should be cautioned about not overinterpreting their significance, but evidence supporting the consistency of subgroup results should be noted.

MOVING TOWARD PRACTICE-BASED EVIDENCE

The push for EBP has led to impressive improvements in healthcare in all health disciplines, and ongoing commitment to EBP is warranted. However, for maximum benefit, efforts to generate evidence based on population models will have to be integrated with evidence for individualized care.

Several forces in health research are converging to encourage greater demand for and interest in evidence that is patient-centered, practice-based, and personalized. These include frustration about the limitations of EBP on the part of many clinicians, the growth of interest in and funding for CER, and the emerging excitement over opportunities that will become available through precision healthcare research and Big Data initiatives. The messages in this chapter are consistent with the priorities of the PCORI in the United States—an institute in which nurse researchers have played a big role. For example, two of its research priorities are as follows: Identifying patient differences in response to therapy and Understanding differences in effectiveness across groups (Barksdale et al., 2014).

Conducting rigorous research has never been an easy process, but there have been well-accepted "blueprints" for minimizing bias and coming to conclusions about the quality of the resulting evidence. We are moving into an era that will be even more demanding because person-centered and practice-based evidence require greater creativity and scrupulous vigilance: researchers cannot make findings relevant to real-world settings and applicable to individuals by mechanically following standard "steps" of research. We have provided a few ideas about strategies for moving toward practice-based evidence, but we are confident that many nurse researchers will be inventive in their efforts to make their research relevant and applicable.

TIP We note that interprofessional collaboration is likely to prove vital to the advancement of person-centered research and practice-based evidence. Disciplinary "silos" are likely to be unproductive in efforts to personalize healthcare.

New challenges and new rewards are in store for those who wish to facilitate patient-centered care based on patient-centered evidence. Thus, the overall message of this chapter to those conducting research is this: Strive to consider in an ongoing way the needs of the users of evidence in planning and designing your studies, analyzing your data, interpreting your results, and reporting your findings.

CRITICAL APPRAISAL OF APPLICABILITY, GENERALIZABILITY, AND RELEVANCE

Box 31.1 provides a few suggestions for those who wish to consider whether researchers have provided sufficient information for coming to conclusions about a study's applicability, generalizability, and relevance. In many cases, the researchers' lack of attention to the issues discussed in this chapter may be disappointing. The absence of information on applicability may reflect page constraints in the journal. It may also reflect the fact that most

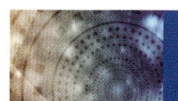

BOX 31.1 Guidelines for Critically Appraising a Study's Applicability, Generalizability, and Relevance[a]

1. Were patients or other stakeholders involved in codesigning the study? In what way were they involved (e.g., identifying the research question, designing the study, disseminating or using the results?) If there was no such involvement, what steps (if any) did the researcher take to enhance the relevance of the research?
2. Did the researchers mention that the study was comparative effectiveness research? If yes, did the study match the six characteristics of CER described in the text? If the study was a clinical trial, what was the comparator?
3. If the study was a clinical trial, where on the pragmatic-to-explanatory continuum did the trial lie? To what extent was the study conducted in "real-world" circumstances with a broad range of study participants? Did the researchers claim that the trial was pragmatic? Was the PRECIS-2 tool used?
4. To what extent could the measures used in the study be considered *pragmatic*?
5. If the study involved an intervention, did the researchers make any efforts to *tailor* the intervention to individual participants? Was there any effort to *target* the intervention to particular types of people—for example, was an adaptive intervention tested or was an adaptive trial design used?
6. What are some of the constraints on the generalizability of the results? For example, could the study context limit generalizability? Do the eligibility criteria for the sample constrain generalizability? Did a high percentage of people invited to participate in the study decline?
7. Were subgroup effects examined? If yes, were the subgroup analyses done properly (e.g., a priori hypotheses of a small number of subgroup effects; appropriate test for interaction)? Was a multivariable risk-stratified analysis undertaken?
8. Did the Discussion section of the report adequately address the issues of applicability, generalizability, and relevance?

[a]These questions are primarily relevant for quantitative or mixed methods studies, especially for trials of an intervention.

researchers use conventional standards in preparing their articles—standards that have not taken applicability into account. Moreover, the peer review of most articles is undertaken by researchers who may not yet be attuned to changes taking place in healthcare research. We hope that in the future researchers will do more to help clinicians answer questions about applicability, generalizability, and relevance.

> **TIP** A carefully developed checklist for the appraisal of moderators and predictors is available to appraise studies with subgroup analyses (van Hoorn et al., 2017). Another useful resource for appraisal is a guideline for reporting pragmatic clinical trials (Zwarenstein et al., 2008).

RESEARCH EXAMPLE

In this section, we present a description of a protocol for a project that incorporated several strategies described in this chapter.

Study: The ACHRU-CPP vs. usual care for older adults with type 2 diabetes and multiple chronic conditions and their family caregivers: study protocol for a randomized controlled trial (McAiney et al., 2022).

Background: An interdisciplinary team in Canada has developed a program of research called the Aging, Community and Health Research Unit (ACHRU). The research program, which is devoted to research on the promotion of optimal aging at home for older adults with multimorbidities, is described by the team as patient-oriented and is devoted to interagency and intersectoral partnerships with community-based agencies, policy makers, and health and social service agencies (Markle-Reid et al., 2018). The team describes a protocol for a two-armed, multisite, pragmatic, mixed-methods RCT to examine the effectiveness and implementation of the ACHRU-Community Partnership Program, a nurse-led interprofessional program. The program promotes T2DM self-management in adults age 65 and older with multiple comorbidities and provides support for their caregiving network.

Program Outcomes: The primary proposed outcome of this protocol is an improvement in physical functioning and secondary goals are improvements in measures of depression, anxiety, and self-efficacy. Caregiver outcomes include health-related quality of life and depressive symptoms.

Methods: This study protocol describes a two-armed, multisite, pragmatic, mixed-methods RCT examining the effectiveness and implementation of the ACHRU-CPP program. Registered nurses and dieticians will deliver the intervention over 6 months. They plan to enroll and randomly assign 160 Canadian participants in two arms: usual care and intervention. The study will also compare healthcare service costs between the two groups. A subgroup analysis is planned to determine which individuals benefit the most from the program. They will also collect descriptive characteristics and qualitative data to examine program implementation and the impact of the program on interprofessional/team collaboration.

SUMMARY POINTS

- The EBP movement has made significant contributions to healthcare worldwide. However, a variety of forces are combining to demand greater attention to **practice-based evidence**—*patient-centered evidence* from real-world settings that is responsive to the needs and circumstances of specific patients and local contexts.
- EBP is based on evidence about populations of people; it relies heavily on results from randomized controlled trials (RCTs)—which (especially when integrated in systematic reviews) yield **average treatment effects** within the population of interest.
- **Applicability** is the degree to which research evidence can be applied to individuals, small groups of individuals, or local contexts.
- **Generalizability** concerns the ability to extrapolate evidence from samples to a specified population.
- **Relevance**, in the context of this chapter, is the degree to which research evidence is important to key stakeholders and has the potential to be actionable. A key strategy for developing practice-based evidence is to involve stakeholders as cocreators of the research process.

- RCTs are seldom designed with the goals of generalizability or applicability in mind. In traditional **explanatory trials**, researchers value internal validity at the expense of external validity and focus on average effects at the expense of understanding **heterogeneity of treatment effects (HTEs)**—individual variation in response to interventions.
- Researchers have begun to address these issues with innovative methodologic strategies, some of which are described in this chapter. In particular, there is growing interest in **comparative effectiveness research**, whose defining characteristics are in line with person-centered research and practice-based evidence.
- Concerns about explanatory RCTs (e.g., restrictive eligibility criteria, tight controls) have led to the development of **pragmatic clinical trials** that enroll diverse people from real-world settings and are designed to enhance external validity. The degree to which a trial is "pragmatic" can be evaluated using a tool called **PRECIS-2**.
- A strategy called the **multiphase optimization strategy (MOST)** is being used to develop targeted adaptive interventions. **Adaptive interventions** are ones that have multiple decision points, and decisions are based on individual responses. The MOST framework for adaptive interventions often uses a tool called **sequential, multiple assignment, randomized trial (SMART)**, which uses *targeting variables* (e.g., response to an initial intervention) to tailor an intervention in a second round of randomization.
- The ultimate design for individualization is an **N-of-1 trial (single-subject experiment)** in which different treatments are tested in an individual or a small number of patients over time. These trials usually are characterized by alternating an active treatment phase and a placebo phase (or alternating two active treatments), such as in an AB or ABAB arrangement.
- Randomized trials are considered the gold standard design for yielding rigorous evidence for EBP, but alternatives (e.g., quasiexperiments, observational designs) have attractive features in the movement toward personalized and precision healthcare. Mixed methods designs also are important for practice-based evidence because they can incorporate rich contextual information and in-depth insights into why "average effects" are misleading and provide clues into sources of variation of effects.
- Sampling strategies for practice-based evidence include clarifying the target population, using purposive sampling strategies, and recruiting a large enough sample for subgroup analyses.
- In terms of data collection, researchers should consider *pragmatic measures*—ones that are important to stakeholders, actionable, and sensitive to change and that minimize response burden (e.g., measures from the Patient-Reported Outcome Measurement Information System or PROMIS®).
- **Big Data** (large complex datasets) potentially can be exploited to improve generalizability of evidence about populations and to improve applicability through the development of predictive models to guide individualized decisions.
- **Subgroup analyses** are efforts to disentangle heterogeneity of treatment effects for subpopulations. Subgroup analyses have been controversial because of risks of both Type I and Type II errors, but guidance for rigorously conducting them has emerged (e.g., prespecification of hypotheses, limiting analyses to a small number of subgroups, testing for interactions).
- In lieu of "one-variable-at-a-time" subgroup analyses, it is sometimes possible to undertake **multivariable risk stratification** that uses a person's score on a multicomponent index of risk rather than a subgroup variable. The results of a risk-stratified analysis can provide insights into who can best benefit from an intervention.
- Advances in technology and research methods, coupled with increased interest in personalized and precision healthcare, will likely advance the promise of practice-based and patient-centered evidence and contribute to its applicability.

REFERENCES CITED IN CHAPTER 31

Almirall, D., Nahum-Shani, I., Sherwood, N., & Murphy, S. (2014). Introduction to SMART designs for the development of adaptive interventions: With application to weight loss research. *Translational Behavioral Medicine, 4*(3), 260–274.

Angus, D. C. (2015). Fusing randomized trials with big data. *Journal of the American Medical Association*, *314*(8), 767–768.

Armstrong, K. (2012). Methods in comparative effectiveness research. *Journal of Clinical Oncology*, *30*, 4208–4214.

Assmann, S., Pocock, S., Enos, L., & Kasten, L. (2000). Subgroup analysis and other (mis)uses of baseline data in clinical trials. *The Lancet*, *355*(9209), 1064–1069.

Barksdale, D., Newhouse, R., & Miller, J. (2014). The patient-centered outcomes Research Institute (PCORI): Information for academic nursing. *Nursing Outlook*, *62*(3), 192–200.

Bärnighausen, T., Tugwell, P., Røttingen, J., Shemilt, I., Rockers, P., Geldsetzer, P., Lavis, J., Grimshaw, J., Daniels, K., Brown, A., Bor, J., Tanner, J., Rashidian, A., Barreto, M., Vollmer, S., Atun, R., & Atun, R. (2017). Quasi-experimental study designs series—paper 4: Uses and value. *Journal of Clinical Epidemiology*, *89*, 21–29.

Battaglia, C., & Glasgow, R. (2018). Pragmatic dissemination and implementation research models, methods and measures and their relevance for nursing research. *Nursing Outlook*, *66*(5), 430–445.

Bergstrom, N., Braden, B., Laguzza, A., & Holman, V. (1987). The Braden Scale for predicting pressure sore risk. *Nursing Research*, *36*(4), 205–210.

Bhatt, D., & Mehta, C. (2016). Adaptive designs for clinical trials. *New England Journal of Medicine*, *375*(1), 65–74.

Biankin, A., Piantadosi, S., & Hollingsworth, S. (2015). Patient-centric trials for therapeutic development in precision oncology. *Nature*, *526*(7573), 361–370.

Booth, C., & Tannock, F. (2014). Randomised controlled trials and population-based observational research: Partners in the evolution of medical evidence. *British Journal of Cancer*, *110*(3), 551–555.

Burke, J., Sussman, J., Kent, D., & Hayward, R. (2015). Three simple rules to ensure reasonably credible subgroup analyses. *British Medical Journal*, *351*, h5651.

Collins, L., Nahum-Shani, I., & Almirall, D. (2014). Optimization of behavioral dynamic treatment regimens based on the sequential, multiple assignment, randomized trial (SMART). *Clinical Trials*, *11*(4), 426–434.

Concannon, T., Fuster, M., Saunders, T., Patel, K., Wong, J., Leslie, L., & Lau, J. (2014). A systematic review of stakeholder engagement in comparative effectiveness and patient-centered outcomes research. *Journal of General Internal Medicine*, *29*(12), 1692–1701.

Concato, J. (2012). Is it time for medicine-based evidence? *Journal of the American Medical Association*, *307*(15), 1641–1643.

Concato, J., & Horwitz, R. (2018). Randomized trials and evidence in medicine: A commentary on deaton and cartwright. *Social Science & Medicine*, *210*, 32–36.

Corwin, E., & Ferranti, E. (2016). Integration of biomarkers to advance precision nursing interventions for family research across the lifespan. *Nursing Outlook*, *64*(4), 292–298.

Dahabreh, I. (2018). Randomization, randomized trials, and analyses using observational data: A commentary on deaton and cartwright. *Social Science & Medicine*, *210*, 41–44.

Dahabreh, A., Hayward, R., & Kent, D. (2016). Using group data to treat individuals: Understanding heterogeneous treatment effects in the age of precision medicine and patient-centred evidence. *International Journal of Epidemiology*, *45*, 2184–2193.

Dahan, M., Scemama, C., Porcher, R., & Biau, D. (2018). Reporting of heterogeneity of treatment effect in cohort studies: A review of the literature. *BMC Medical Research Methodology*, *18*(1), 10.

Dai, T., & Shete, S. (2016). Time-varying SMART design and data analysis methods for evaluating adaptive intervention effects. *BMC Medical Research Methodology*, *16*(1), 112.

Deaton, A., & Cartwright, N. (2018). Understanding and misunderstanding randomized controlled trials. *Social Science & Medicine*, *210*, 2–21.

Deng, X., Yu, T., & Hu, A. (2017). Predicting the risk for hospital-acquired pressure ulcers in critical care patients. *Critical Care Nursing*, *37*(4), e1–e11.

Eckardt, P., & Erlanger, A. (2018). Pragmatic study lessons learned: Methods and analyses. *Nursing Outlook*, *66*(5), 446–454.

Estabrooks, C., Squires, J., Hutchinson, A., Scott, S., Cummings, G. G., Kang, S., Midodzi, W. K., Stevens, B., & Stevens, B. (2011). Assessment of variation in the Alberta Context Tool: The contribution of unit level contextual factors and specialty in Canadian pediatric acute care settings. *BMC Health Services Research*, *11*, 251.

Feinstein, A. R. (1998). The problem of cogent subgroups: A clinicostatistical tragedy. *Journal of Clinical Epidemiology*, *51*(4), 297–299.

Ford, I., & Norrie, J. (2016). The changing face of clinical trials: Pragmatic trials. *New England Journal of Medicine*, *375*(5), 454–463.

Forsythe, L., Heckert, A., Margolis, M., Schrandt, S., & Frank, L. (2018). Methods and impact of engagement in research, from theory to practice and back again: Early findings from the patient-centered outcomes research institute. *Quality of Life Research*, *27*(1), 17–31.

Frieden, T. R. (2017). Evidence for health decision-making: Beyond randomized, controlled trials. *New England Journal of Medicine*, *377*(5), 465–475.

Gabler, N., Duan, N., Liao, D., Elmore, J., Ganiats, T., & Kravitz, R. (2009). Dealing with heterogeneity of treatment effects: Is the literature up to the challenge? *Trials*, *10*, 43.

Gabler, N., Duan, N., Raneses, E., Suttner, L., Ciarametaro, M. Cooney, E., Dubois, R. W., Halpern, S. D., Kravitz, R. L., & Kravitz, R. (2016). No improvement in the reporting of clinical trial subgroup effects in high-impact general medical journals. *Trials*, *17*(1), 320.

Glasgow, R. E., Magid, D., Beck, A., Ritzwoller, D., & Estabrooks, P. (2005). Practical clinical trials for translating research to practice: Design and measurement recommendations. *Medical Care*, *43*(6) 551–557.

Glasgow, R., & Riley, W. (2013). Pragmatic measures: What they are and why we need them. *American Journal of Preventive Medicine*, *45*(2), 237–243.

Green, L., & Glasgow, R. (2006). Evaluating the relevance, generalization, and applicability of research: Issues in external validation and translation methodology. *Evaluation & the Health Professions*, *29*(1), 126–153.

Greenfield, S., & Kaplan, S. (2012). Building useful evidence: Changing the clinical research paradigm to account for comparative effectiveness research. *Journal of Comparative Effectiveness Research*, *1*(3), 263–270.

Greenhouse, J., Kaizar, E., Kelleher, K., Seltman, H., & Gardner, W. (2008). Generalizing from clinical trial data: A case study. The risk of suicidality among pediatric antidepressant users. *Statistics in Medicine*, *27*(11), 1801–1813.

Gross, D., & Fogg, L. (2001). Clinical trials in the 21st century: The case for participant-centered research. *Research in Nursing and Health*, *24*(6), 530–539.

Hayward, R., Kent, D., Vijan, S., & Hofer, T. (2006). Multivariable risk prediction can greatly enhance the statistical power of clinical trial subgroup analysis. *BMC Medical Research Methodology*, *6*, 18.

Heckman-Stoddard, B., & Smith, J. (2014). Precision medicine clinical trials: Defining new treatment strategies. *Seminars in Oncology Nursing*, *30*(2), 109–116.

Hickey, K., Bakken, S., Byrne, M., Bailey, D., Demiris, G., Docherty, S., & Dorsey, S. G., Guthrie, B. J., Heitkemper, M. M., Jacelon, C. S., Kelechi, T. J., Moore, S. M., Redeker, N. S., Renn, C. L., Resnick, B., Starkweather, A., Thompson, H., Ward, T. M., McCloskey, D. J., Austin, J. K., & Grady, P. A. (2019). Precision health: Advancing symptom and self-management science. *Nursing Outlook*, *67*(4), 462–475.

Holtrop, J., Rabin, B., & Glasgow, R. (2018). Qualitative approaches to use of the RE-AIM framework: Rationale and methods. *BMC Health Services Research*, *18*(1), 177.

Horwitz, R., Hayes-Conroy, A., Caricchio, R., & Singer, B. (2017). From evidence based medicine to medicine based evidence. *American Journal of Medicine*, *130*(11), 1246–1250.

Horwitz, R., & Singer, B. (2017). Why evidence-based medicine failed in patient care and medicine-based evidence will succeed. *Journal of Clinical Epidemiology*, *84*, 14–17.

Horwitz, R., & Singer, B. (2018). Introduction: What works? And for whom? *Social Science and Medicine*, *210*, 22–25.

Institute of Medicine of the National Academies. (2009). *Initial priorities for comparative effectiveness research*. IOM.

Ioannidis, J. (2018). Randomized controlled trials: Often flawed, mostly useless, clearly indispensable—A commentary on deaton and cartwright. *Social Science and Medicine*, *210*, 53–56.

Iwashyna, T., & Liu, V. (2014). What's so different about Big Data? *Annals of the American Thoracic Society*, *11*(7), 1130–1135.

Kaiser, L. D. (2016). Stratification of randomization is not required for a pre-specified subgroup analysis. *Pharmaceutical Statistics*, *12*, 43–47.

Kent, D., Nelson, J., Dahabreh, I., Rothwell, P., Altman, D., & Hayward, R. (2016). Risk and treatment effect heterogeneity: Re-Analysis of individual participant data from 32 large clinical trials. *International Journal of Epidemiology*, *45*(6), 2075–2088.

Kent, D., Rothwell, P., Ioannidis, J., Altman, D., & Hayward, R. (2010). Assessing and reporting heterogeneity in treatment effects in clinical trials: A proposal. *Trials*, *11*, 85.

Klasnja, P., Hekler, E., Shiffman, S., Boruvka, A., Almirall, D., Tewari, A., & Murphy, S. (2015). Micro-randomized trials: An experimental design for developing just-in-time adaptive interventions. *Health Psychology*, *34S*(0), 1220–1228.

Knottnerus, J., Tugwell, P., & Tricco, A. (2016). Individual patients are the primary source and the target of clinical research. *Journal of Clinical Epidemiology*, *76*, 1–3.

Konigorski, S, Wernicke, S, Slosarek, T, Zenner, A. M., Strelow, N., Ruether, D. F., Henschel, F., Manaswini, M., Pottbäcker, F., Edelman, J. A., Owoyele, B., Danieletto, M., Golden, E., Zweig, M., Nadkarni, G. N., & Böttinger, E. (2022). StudyU: A platform for designing and conducting innovative digital N-of-1 trials. *Journal of Medical Internet Research*, *24*(7), e35884. https://doi.org/10.2196/35884

Kraemer, H., Frank, E., & Kupfer, D. (2006). Moderators of treatment outcomes: Clinical, research, and policy importance. *Journal of the American Medical Association*, *296*(10), 1286–1289.

Kravitz, R. L., & Duan, N. (2014). *Design and implementation of N-of-1 trials: A user's guide*. Agency for Healthcare Research and Quality.

Kroenke, K., Monahan, P., & Kean, J. (2015). Pragmatic characteristics of patient-reported outcome measures are important for use in clinical practice. *Journal of Clinical Epidemiology*, *68*(9), 1085–1092.

Kua, C. H., Yeo, C. Y. Y., Tan, P. C., Char, C. W. T., Tan, C. W. Y., Mak, V., Leong, I. Y., & Lee, S. W. H. (2021). Association of deprescribing with reduction in mortality and hospitalization: A pragmatic stepped-wedge cluster-randomized controlled trial. *Journal of the American Medical Directors Association*, *22*(1), 82–89.e3. https://doi.org/10.1016/j.jamda.2020.03.012

Lei, H., Nahum-Shani, I., Lynch, K., Oslin, D., & Murphy, S. (2012). A "SMART" design for building individualized treatment sequences. *Annual Review of Clinical Psychology*, *8*, 21–48.

Lincoln, Y., & Guba, E. (1985). *Naturalistic inquiry*. Sage.

Littleton-Kearney, M. (2018). Pragmatic clinical trials at the National Institute of Nursing Research. *Nursing Outlook*, *66*(5), 470–472.

Loudon, K., Treweek, S., Sullivan, F., Donnan, P., Thorpe, K., & Zwarenstein, M. (2015). The PRECIS-2 tool: Designing trials that are fit for purpose. *British Medical Journal*, *350*, h2147.

Lyles, C., Lunn, M., Obedin-Maliver, J., & Bibbins-Domingo, K. (2018). The new era of precision population health: Insights for the all of us research program and beyond. *Journal of Translational Medicine*, *16*(1), 211.

Markle-Reid, M., Ploeg, J., Valaitis, R., Duggleby, W., Fisher, K., Fraser, K., Ganann, R., Griffith, L. E., Gruneir, A., McAiney, C., … Williams, A. (2018). Protocol for a program of research from the Aging, Community and Health Research Unit: Promoting optimal aging at home for older adults with comorbidities. *Journal of Comorbidity*, *8*, 1–16.

Marko, N., & Weil, R. (2010). The role of observational investigations in comparative effectiveness research. *Value Health*, *13*(8), 989–997.

McAiney, C., Markle-Reid, M., Ganann, R., Whitmore, C., Valaitis, R., Urajnik, D. J., Fisher, K., Ploeg, J., Petrie, P., McMillan, F., & McElhaney, J. E. (2022). Implementation of the Community Assets Supporting Transitions (CAST) transitional care intervention for older adults with multimorbidity and depressive symptoms: A qualitative descriptive study. *PloS One*, *17*(8), e0271500. https://doi.org/10.1371/journal.pone.0271500

Mutch, D., Zulyniak, M., Rudkowska, I., & Tejero, M. (2018). Lifestyle genomics: Addressing the multifactorial nature of personalized health. *Lifestyle Genomics*, *11*, 1–8.

Newhouse, R., Barksdale, D. J., & Miller, J. (2015). The patient-centered outcomes research institute: Research done differently. *Nursing Research*, *64*(1), 72–77.

Nguyen, H., Moy, M., Fan, V., Gould, M., Xiang, A., Bailey, A., Desai, S., Coleman, K. J., & Coleman, K. (2018). Applying the pragmatic-explanatory continuum indicator summary to the implementation of a physical activity coaching trial in chronic obstructive pulmonary disease. *Nursing Outlook*, *66*(5), 455–463.

Nowak, A. L., Giurgescu, C., Ford, J. L., Mackos, A., Ohm, J., Tan, A., Pietrzak, M., & Anderson, C. M. (2022). Methodologic considerations for epigenomic investigation of preterm birth in African American women. *Western Journal of Nursing Research*, *44*(1), 81–93. https://doi.org/10.1177/01939459211030339

Pallmann, P., Bedding, A., Choodari-Oskooei, B., Dimairo, M., Flight, L., Hampson, L., Holmes, J., Mander, A. P., Odondi, L., Sydes, M. R., Villar, S. S., Wason, J. M. S., Weir, C. J., Wheeler, G. M., Yap, C., Jaki, T., & Jaki, T. (2018). Adaptive designs in clinical trials: Why use them, and how to run and report them. *BMC Medicine*, *16*(1), 29.

Patton, M. Q. (2015). *Qualitative research & evaluation methods* (4th ed.). Sage.

Polit, D. F., & Beck, C. T. (2010). Generalization in quantitative and qualitative research: Myths and strategies. *International Journal of Nursing Studies*, *47*(11), 1451–1458.

Punja, S., Bukutu, C., Shamseer, L., Sampson, M., Hartling, L., Urichuk, L., & Vohra, S. (2016). N-of-1 trials are a tapestry of heterogeneity. *Journal of Clinical Epidemiology*, *76*, 47–56.

Rockers, P., Tugwell, P., Røttingen, J., & Bärnighausen, T. (2017). Quasi-experimental study designs series—paper 13: Realizing the full potential of quasi-experiments for health research. *Journal of Clinical Epidemiology*, *89*, 106–110.

Rolfe, G. (2009). Complexity and uniqueness in nursing practice. *International Journal of Nursing Studies*, *46*, 1156–1158.

Rothwell, P. M. (2005a). Treating individuals 2. Subgroup analysis in randomised controlled trials: Importance, indications, and interpretation. *The Lancet*, *365*(9454), 176–186.

Rothwell, P. M. (2005b). External validity of randomised controlled trials: "To whom do the results of this trial apply?" *The Lancet*, *365*(9453), 82–93.

Rothwell, P. M. (2006). Factors that can affect the external validity of randomised controlled trials. *PLoS Clinical Trials*, *1*, e9.

Rothwell, P. M., Mehta, Z., Howard, S., Gutnikov, S., & Warlow, C. (2005). Treating individuals 3: From subgroups to individuals—General principles and the example of carotid endarterectomy. *The Lancet*, *365*(9455), 256–265.

Rycroft-Malone, J. (2012). Implementing evidence-based practice in the reality of clinical practice. *Worldviews Evidence Based Nursing*, *9*, 1.

Sacristán, J., & Dilla, T. (2018). Pragmatic trials revisited: Applicability is about individualization. *Journal of Clinical Epidemiology*, *99*, 164–166.

Schork, N. J. (2018). Randomized clinical trials and personalized medicine: A commentary on deaton and cartwright. *Social Science and Medicine*, *210*, 71–73.

Shams, A. S., Rezaei, M., Havaei, N., & Mohammadi, A. (2021). Feasibility of the basic movements of Azeri dance in the balance and posture of a person with Parkinson's disease: ABA single subject design. *International Journal of Therapy Rehabilitation*, *28*(12), 1–8. https://doi.org/10.12968/ijtr.2020.0119

Sofolahan-Oladeinde, Y., Newhouse, R., Lavallee, D. C., Huang, J. C., & Mullins, C. D. (2017). Early assessment of the 10-step patient engagement framework for patient-centred outcomes research studies: The first three steps. *Family Practice*, *34*(3), 272–277.

Subramanian, S., Kim, R., & Christakis, N. (2018). The "average" treatment effect: A construct ripe for retirement. A commentary on deaton and cartwright. *Social Science & Medicine*, *210*, 77–82.

Sun, X., Briel, M., Busse, J., You, J. J., Akl, E. A., Mejza, F., Bala, M. M., Bassler, D., Mertz, D., Diaz-Granados, N., Vandvik, P. O., Malaga, G., Srinathan, S. K., Dahm, P., Johnston, B. C., Alonso-Coello, P., Hassouneh, B., Walter, S. D., Heels-Ansdell, D., … Guyatt, G. (2012). Credibility of claims of subgroup effects in randomised controlled trials: Systematic review. *British Medical Journal*, *344*, e1553.

Sun, X., Ioannidis, J., Agoritsas, T., Alba, A., & Guyatt, G. (2014). How to use a subgroup analysis: Users' guide to the medical literature. *Journal of the American Medical Association*, *311*(4), 405–411.

Tanniou, J., van der Tweel, I., Teerenstra, S., & Roes, K. (2016). Subgroup analyses in confirmatory clinical trials: Time to be specific about their purposes. *BMC Medical Research Methodology*, *16*, 20.

Treweek, S., & Zwarenstein, M. (2009). Making trials matter: Pragmatic and explanatory trials and the problem of applicability. *Trials*, *10*, 37.

Tunis, S. R., Stryer, D., & Clancy, C. (2003) Practical clinical trials: Increasing the value of clinical research for decision making in clinical and health policy. *Journal of the American Medical Association*, *290*(12), 1624–1632.

Van Hoorn, R., Tummers, M., Booth, A., Gerhardus, A., Rehfuess, E., Hind, D., Bossuyt, P. M., Welch, V., Debray, T. P. A., Underwood, M., Cuijpers, P., Kraemer, H., van der Wilt, G. J., Kievit, W., & Kievet, W. (2017). The development of CHAMP: A checklist for the appraisal of moderators and predictors. *BMC Medical Research Methodology*, *17*(1), 173.

Vohra, S. (2016). N-of-1 trials to enhance patient outcomes: Identifying effective therapies and reducing harms, one patient at a time. *Journal of Clinical Epidemiology*, *76*, 6–8.

Wallström, S., Ali, L., Ekman, I., Swedberg, K., & Fors, A. (2020). Effects of a person-centred telephone support on fatigue in people with chronic heart failure: Subgroup analysis of a randomised controlled trial. *European Journal of Cardiovascular Nursing*, *19*(5), 393–400. https://doi.org/10.1177/1474515119891599

Wang, W., & Krishnan, E. (2014). Big data and clinicians: A review of the state of the science. *Journal of Medical Informatics*, *1*, e1.

Wang, R., & Ware, J. (2013). Detecting moderator effects using subgroup analyses. *Prevention Science*, *14*(2), 111–120.

Wilbur, J., Kolanowski, A., & Collins, L. (2016). Utilizing MOST frameworks and SMART designs for intervention research. *Nursing Outlook*, *64*(4), 287–289.

Yan, X., Matchar, D. B., Sivapragasam, N., Ansah, J. P., Goel, A., & Chakraborty, B. (2021). Sequential multiple assignment randomized trial (SMART) to identify optimal sequences of telemedicine interventions for improving initiation of insulin therapy: A simulation study. *BMC Medical Research Methodology*, *21*(1), 200. https://doi.org/10.1186/s12874-021-01395-7

Zenk, S. N. (2022, June 15–16). Pragmatic clinical trials: The role of nursing science [keynote address]. Critical questions for pragmatic clinical trialists—Insights from the NIH pragmatic trials Collaboratory's first decade, virtual workshop. https://dcricollab.dcri.duke.edu/sites/NIHKR/KR/2022%20NIH%20Workshop_Keynote.pdf

Zolotarova, T., Dussault, C., Park, H., Varsaneux, O., Basta, N. E., Watson, L., Robert, P., Davis, S., Mercer, M., Timmerman, S., Bransfield, M., Minhas, M., Kempis, R., & Kronfli, N. (2023). Education increases COVID-19 vaccine uptake among people in Canadian federal prisons in a prospective randomized controlled trial: The EDUCATE study. *Vaccine*, *41*(8), 1419–1425. https://doi.org/10.1016/j.vaccine.2023.01.040

Zwarenstein, M., Treweek, S., Gagnier, J., Altman, D., Tunis, S., Haynes, B., Oxman, AD, Moher, D; CONSORT group, Pragmatic Trials in Healthcare Practihc group. (2008). Improving the reporting of pragmatic trials: An extension of the CONSORT statement. *British Medical Journal*, *337*, a2390.

32 | Disseminating Evidence: Reporting Research Findings

Learning Objectives

1. Understand the importance of identifying the intended audience, journal aims, and scope in selecting the appropriate journal for potential publication.
2. Recognize the aspects of ethical publication including establishing who is an author, the order of authors, duplicative publication, and the importance of indexed journals.
3. In organizing the paper, implement the appropriate format and existing guidelines for reporting study findings.
4. Appreciate the importance of figures and tables in highlighting major findings or processes.
5. Articulate the elements of the discussion section that are necessary for successful publication.
6. Realize the value of peer review and how to appropriately respond for successful publication.

INTRODUCTION

No study is complete until the findings have been shared with others. This chapter offers guidance on disseminating research results. Several books on publishing research findings offer further assistance (e.g., Long & Beck, 2017; Oermann, 2023; Saver, 2021). Also, the *American Journal of Nursing* published four articles that take nurses through the publication process (Roush, 2017a; 2017b; 2017c; 2017d).

GETTING STARTED ON DISSEMINATION

Researchers consider various issues in developing a dissemination plan, as we discuss in this section.

Selecting a Communication Medium and Outlet

Researchers can communicate their findings orally or in writing. Oral presentations (typically at professional conferences) can be a formal talk in front of an audience or integrated with written material in a *poster session*. Major advantages of conference presentations are that they can be done soon after study completion (or while it is in progress) and they offer opportunities for dialogue with people interested in the topic. Written reports can take the form of theses/dissertations or journal articles published in traditional or open-access journals. A major advantage of journal articles, especially ones that are open-access, is worldwide accessibility. Our advice is relevant for most types of dissemination, but publication in journals is featured.

Knowing the Audience

Good research communication requires researchers to think about the audience they hope to reach. Here are some questions to consider:

1. Will the audience be nurses only, or will it likely include professionals from other disciplines

(e.g., physicians, psychologists, physical therapists)?
2. Will the audience be researchers, or will it include clinicians or other professionals (e.g., healthcare policy makers)?
3. Are patients or other lay people a potential audience?
4. Will the audience include people whose native language is not English?
5. Will reviewers, editors, and readers be experts in the field?

Researchers often write with multiple audiences in mind, which means writing clearly and avoiding technical jargon to the extent possible. It also means that researchers sometimes must develop a multi-prong strategy—for example, publishing a report for researchers in a journal such *Nursing Research*, and then publishing a summary for clinicians in a specialty publication or an institutional newsletter.

Although writing for a broad audience may be a goal, it is also important to keep in mind the needs of the *main* intended audience. If the readers are mostly clinical nurses, it is essential to explain what the findings mean for practice. If the audience is administrators or policy makers, information should be included about implications for such outcomes as *cost* and *accessibility*. If researchers are the primary audience, information about methodologic strategies, study limitations, and implications for future research should be provided.

Developing a Plan

Before writing a report, researchers should have a plan, part of which involves how best to coordinate the actual tasks of preparing a **manuscript** (i.e., an unpublished paper).

Deciding on Authorship

When a study is undertaken by a team, division of labor and authorship must be addressed. The International Committee of Medical Journal Editors (ICMJE, 2023) advises that authorship credit should be based on (1) making a substantial contribution to the study's conception and design, or to data acquisition, data analysis, and interpretation; (2) drafting or revising the manuscript for intellectual content; (3) approving the final version of the manuscript to be published; and (4) agreeing to be accountable for all aspects of the work. The **lead author**, usually the first-named author, has overall responsibility for the report. The lead author and coauthors should reach an agreement in advance about responsibilities for producing the manuscript. To avoid possible conflicts, they should also decide beforehand the order of authors' names. Ethically, it is most appropriate to list names in the order of authors' contribution to the work, not according to status. When contributions of coauthors are comparable, an alphabetical listing is appropriate. The editorial board of the *Western Journal of Nursing Research* has prepared guidelines for coauthorship (Conn et al., 2015), as has the past editor of *Research in Nursing & Health* (Kearney, 2014).

TIP A taxonomy called Contributor Roles Taxonomy (CRediT) has been created to help people identify specific author contributions to scholarly written work. More guidance on authorship credit, roles, and responsibilities is offered by Alfonso, and Editors' Network European Society of Cardiology ESC Task Force (2019).

Deciding on Content

In many studies, more data are collected than can be presented in one report, and multiple publications are thus possible. And, if there are multiple research questions, more than one paper may be required to communicate results adequately. In such situations, an early decision involves which findings to present in a given paper. In mixed methods research, separate reports are sometimes needed to summarize qualitative and quantitative findings—although there should also be a report integrating findings from both strands.

It is, however, inappropriate and even unethical to write several papers when one would suffice—a practice known as "salami slicing" (Gennaro, 2021; Sullivan-Bolyai et al., 2022). Each paper from a study should make an independent contribution. Editors, reviewers, and readers expect original work, so unnecessary overlap should be avoided. It is also unethical to submit essentially the same or similar paper to two journals simultaneously. Oermann (2023) offers guidelines regarding duplicate and redundant publications, and Happell (2016) provides practical tips for dealing with multiple papers from one dataset.

Assembling Materials

Planning also involves assembling the materials needed to begin a draft, including information about manuscript requirements. Traditional and online journals issue guidelines for authors, and these guidelines should be retrieved and understood.

Other materials also need to be gathered, including relevant literature; details about instruments used in the study; descriptions of the study sample; output of computer analyses; relevant analytic memos or reflexive notes; figures or photographs that illustrate some aspect of the study; and permissions to use copyrighted materials. Style manuals that provide information about both grammar and language use (e.g., Strunk & Campbell, 2018) are important tools, as are specific guides for writing professional and scientific papers (e.g., American Psychological Association, 2020; ICMJE, 2023).

> **TIP** For authors whose native language is not English but who plan to submit their work to an English-language journal, a review of the manuscript by someone proficient in English is advisable. For authors from developing countries, assistance may be available through AuthorAID (https://www.authoraid.info/en/).

Finally, a written outline and a timeline should be developed, especially if there are multiple coauthors who have responsibility for different sections of the paper. The overall outline and individual assignments, together with due dates, should be developed collaboratively.

Writing Effectively

Many people have a hard time putting their ideas down on paper. It is beyond the scope of this book to teach good writing skills, but we can offer a few suggestions. One suggestion, quite simply, is: *do it*. Get in the habit of writing, even if it is only 15 minutes a day. *Writer's block* is probably responsible for thousands of unfinished (or never-started) manuscripts each year. So, just begin somewhere, and keep at it regularly—writing gets easier with practice.

Writing *well* is, of course, important, and several resources offer suggestions on how to write compelling sentences, select good words, and organize your ideas effectively (e.g., Silvia, 2018). It is usually better to write a draft in its entirety, and then go back later to rewrite awkward sentences, correct errors, reorganize, and generally polish it up.

In a survey of 61 nursing journal editors, Northam and colleagues (2014) found that the two most common reasons for rejecting a manuscript were that (1) the article provided no new information and (2) it was poorly written. A frequently mentioned suggestion by these editors was to have others review the manuscript before submitting it. In another survey of 53 editors, Kennedy and colleagues (2017) reported common problems that editors found in student papers submitted to journals, such as failure to follow author guidelines, poor writing, and insufficient detail. Griffiths and Norman (2016) also noted that poor writing is a common concern of peer reviewers of papers submitted to the *International Journal of Nursing Studies* (IJNS).

> **TIP** It should go without saying that plagiarism should be avoided. In some cases, this means avoiding "plagiarizing" yourself. Most journals now have powerful plagiarism detection software that will trigger an editorial response, and you may be asked to rewrite sentences that you "lifted" from your own prior publications.

CONTENT OF RESEARCH REPORTS

Research reports vary in terms of audience, purpose, and length. Theses or dissertations document students' ability to perform scholarly work and therefore tend to be long. Journal articles, by contrast, are short because they compete for limited journal space and are read by busy professionals. Nevertheless, the form and content of research reports are often similar. Chapter 3 summarized the major sections of research reports, and here we offer a few additional tips. Distinctions among various kinds of reports are described later in the chapter.

Quantitative Research Reports

Quantitative reports typically follow the **IMRAD format**, which involves organizing content into four sections—the **I**ntroduction, **M**ethod, **R**esults, and **D**iscussion. These sections, respectively, address the following questions:

- Why was the study done? (I)
- How was the study done? (M)
- What was learned? (I)
- What does it mean? (D)

The Introduction

The introduction acquaints readers with the research problem, its significance, and its context. The introduction sets the stage by describing existing literature, the study's conceptual framework, the problem, research questions, or hypotheses, and the study rationale. Although the introduction includes multiple components, it should be concise. A common critique of research manuscripts by reviewers is that the introduction is too long.

Introductions are often written in a funnel-shaped structure, beginning broadly to establish a framework for understanding the study and then narrowing to the specifics of what researchers sought to learn. The end point of the introduction should be a succinct delineation of the research questions or hypotheses, which provides a good transition to the method section.

> **TIP** An up-front, clearly stated problem statement is of immense value. The first paragraph should be written with special care, because the goal is to grab readers' attention.

The introduction typically includes a summary of related research to provide a pertinent context. Except for dissertations, the literature review should be a brief summary, not an exhaustive review. The summary should make clear what is known and what the deficiencies are, thus helping to clarify the contribution of the new study.

The introduction also should describe the study's theoretical or conceptual framework. The framework should be sufficiently explained so that readers who are unfamiliar with it can understand its main thrust.

The various background strands need to be convincingly and cogently interwoven to persuade readers that, in fact, the new study holds promise for adding evidence important to nursing. The introduction, in other words, lays out the *argument* for new research.

> **TIP** Many journals articles begin without an explicit heading labeled *Introduction*. In general, all the material before the method section is considered the introduction. Some introductions include subheadings such as *Literature Review* or *Hypotheses*.

The Method Section

To critically appraise the quality of a study's evidence, readers need to know exactly what methods were used to answer research questions. In traditional dissertations, the method section should provide sufficient detail that another researcher could replicate the study. In journal articles and conference presentations, the method section is condensed, but the degree of detail should permit readers to draw conclusions about the integrity of the findings. Faulty method sections are a leading cause of manuscript rejection by journals. Your job in writing the method section of a quantitative report is to persuade readers that evidence from your study is sufficiently robust to merit consideration.

> **TIP** The method section is often subdivided into several parts, which helps readers to locate vital information. As an example, the method section might contain the following subsections: Research Design; Sample; Data Collection Instruments; Procedures; and Data Analysis.

The method section usually begins with the description of the research design. The design is often given detailed coverage in clinical trials, with information about what specific design was adopted, how participants were assigned to groups, and whether and with whom blinding was used. Reports for studies with multiple points of data collection should indicate the number of times data were collected and the amount of time elapsed between those points. In all types of quantitative studies, it is important to identify the methods used to control confounding variables. The method section also addresses steps taken to safeguard participants' rights.

Readers also need to know about study participants. This subsection (which may be labeled *Research Sample*, *Subjects*, or *Study Participants*) normally specifies the eligibility criteria, to clarify the population to whom results can be generalized. The method of sample selection and its rationale, recruitment techniques, and sample size should be indicated. If a power analysis was undertaken to estimate sample size needs, this should be described. There should also be information about response rates and, if possible, about response bias (or attrition bias, if this is relevant). Basic characteristics of study participants (e.g., age, gender, health status) should also be described—although this is sometimes presented in the results section.

TIP Readers who are interested in using study evidence in practice need to learn not only about characteristics of the sample, but also about key contextual features so they can judge whether study findings are relevant in their setting.

Data collection methods, another critical component of the method section, may be presented in a subsection called *Instruments*, *Measures*, or *Data Collection*. A description of study instruments, and a rationale for their use, should be provided. If instruments were constructed specifically for the project, the report should describe their development. Any special equipment that was used (e.g., to gather biomarker data) should be described, including information about the manufacturer. The report should also indicate who collected the data (e.g., the authors, research assistants, staff nurses) and how they were trained. The report must convince readers that data collection methods were sound. Information relating to data quality, and procedures used to evaluate reliability and validity, should be described.

In intervention research, there is usually a procedures subsection with information about the intervention. What exactly did the intervention entail? How and by whom was the treatment administered? What was the control group condition? How much time elapsed between the intervention and measurement of the outcome? How was intervention fidelity monitored?

Analytic procedures are also described in the method section. It is usually sufficient to identify the statistical tests used; formulas or references for commonly used statistics such as a multiple regression are not necessary. For unusual procedures, a technical reference justifying the approach should be noted. If confounding variables were controlled statistically, the variables controlled should be identified. The level of significance is typically set at 0.05 for two-tailed tests, which may not be stated; however, if a different significance level or one-tailed tests were used, this must be specified.

Explicit guidelines for reporting key information for various types of studies are now available (Table 32.1). The most well known is the Consolidated Standards of Reporting Trials or **CONSORT guideline**. These and other guidelines for various types of studies are regularly being updated or expanded on the EQUATOR Network site (https://www.equator-network.org/reporting-guidelines/consort/). The EQUATOR site offers resources in Spanish and other languages.

The CONSORT guideline focuses on reporting information about randomized controlled trials (RCTs); extensions have been developed for specific designs, such as cluster randomized trials and pilot trials. The CONSORT guideline has been adopted by most major medical and nursing journals; it includes a checklist of information to include in reports of RCTs (Butcher et al., 2022; Moher et al., 2010). The CONSORT website offers an interactive checklist with detailed information about checklist components. A special reporting

TABLE 32.1 • Reporting Guidelines for Various Types of Papers

TYPE OF STUDY	GUIDELINE
Parallel group randomized controlled trials (RCTs)	CONSORT[a]: CONsolidated Standards Of Reporting Trials (Butcher et al., 2022; Moher et al., 2010)
Development and evaluation of complex interventions in healthcare	CReDECI 2: Criteria for Reporting the Development and Evaluation of Complex Interventions (Möhler et al., 2015)
Description of features of an intervention	TIDieR: Template for Intervention Description and Replication (Hoffman et al., 2014)
Protocols for clinical trials	SPIRIT: Standard Protocol Items: Recommendations for Interventional Trials (Chan et al., 2013)
Evaluations of interventions using quasiexperimental designs	TREND: Transparent Reporting of Evaluations with Nonrandomized Designs (Des Jarlais et al., 2004)
Nonexperimental (observational) studies	STROBE: Strengthening the Reporting of Observational Studies in Epidemiology (von Elm et al., 2014)
Implementation studies of complex interventions	StaRI: Standards for Reporting Implementation studies (Pinnock et al., 2017)
Observational studies using routinely collected health data	RECORD: Reporting of studies Conducted using Observational Routine-collected health Data (Benchimol et al., 2015)
Qualitative studies	SRQR: Standards for Reporting Qualitative Research (O'Brien et al., 2014)
Qualitative studies (focus groups and interview studies)	COREQ: COnsolidated criteria for REporting Qualitative research (Tong et al., 2007)
Studies of measurement reliability and agreement	GRRAS: Guidelines for Reporting Reliability and Agreement Studies (Kottner et al., 2011)
Diagnostic accuracy studies	STARD: Standards for Reporting of Diagnostic accuracy (Cohen et al., 2016)
Health care quality improvement studies	SQUIRE 2: Standards for QUality Improvement Reporting Excellence (Ogrinc et al., 2015)
Health economic evaluations	CHEERS: Consolidated Health Economic Evaluation Reporting Standards (Husereau et al., 2013)
Meta-analyses of RCTs	PRISMA[b]: Preferred Reporting Items for Systematic Reviews and Meta-Analyses (Moher et al., 2009)
Meta-analysis of observational studies	MOOSE: Meta-analysis Of Observational Studies in Epidemiology (Stroup et al., 2000)
Synthesis of qualitative research	ENTREQ: ENhancing Transparency in REporting the synthesis of Qualitative research (Tong et al., 2012)

[a]CONSORT extensions are available for several types of design-specific trials, such as the following: Pilot and feasibility trials (Eldridge et al., 2016); N-of-1 trials (Vohra et al., 2016); within-person (crossover) trials (Pandis et al., 2017); pragmatic trials (Zwarenstein et al., 2008); noninferiority and equivalence trials (Piaggio et al., 2012); cluster randomized trials (Campbell et al., 2012); trials of nonpharmacological interventions (Boutron et al., 2008); trials with patient reported outcomes (Calvert et al., 2013); and trials for psychological interventions (Montgomery et al., 2013).

[b]Numerous extensions of PRISMA have been developed. See http://www.equator-network.org/reporting-guidelines/prisma/.

CHAPTER 32 Disseminating Evidence: Reporting Research Findings • 711

guideline has been prepared for pragmatic trials (Zwarenstein et al., 2008), which should be scrutinized by those interested in enhancing the applicability of their findings.

> **TIP** Reporting guidelines are also available for manuscripts using the style of the American Psychological Association (APA), a style used by many nursing journals.

Several guidelines recommend inclusion of a flow chart to track participants through a study, from eligibility screening through analysis of outcomes. Flow charts should be as detailed as possible, within space constraints, about reasons for losing participants during the study. Figure 32.1 provides an example of such a flow chart for a RCT. This chart summarizes withdrawals from the intervention, as well as participant losses during follow-up. It also shows that data for all participants were analyzed in an intention-to-treat analysis, which is recommended in CONSORT (Polit & Gillespie, 2010).

In response to critiques about inadequate reporting of intervention features several relevant guidelines have emerged. The **CReDECI** guidelines (Möhler et al., 2015) offer criteria for reporting the phases researchers have undertaken in developing, piloting, and evaluating complex interventions. CReDECI is useful for providing information about the *processes* of intervention research. The **TIDieR** guidelines (Hoffmann et

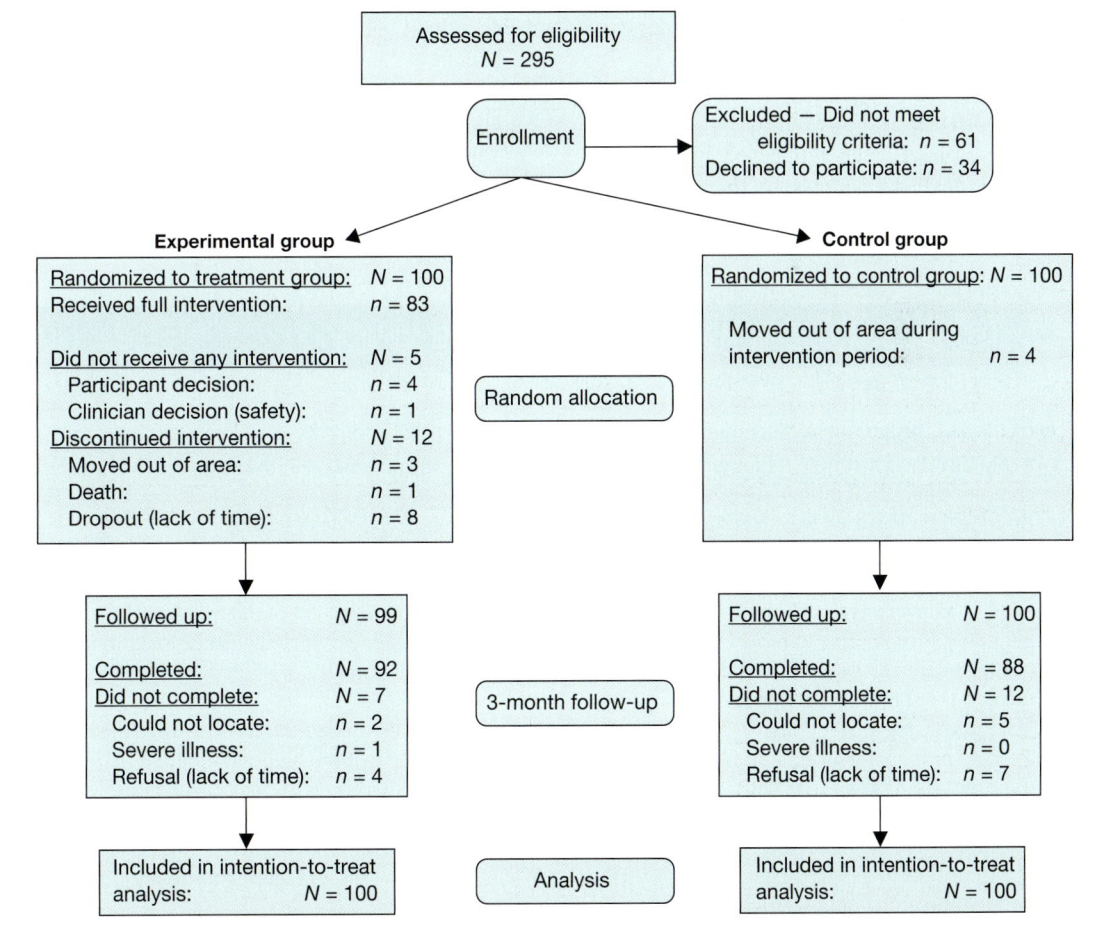

FIGURE 32.1 Example of CONSORT guidelines flowchart: progression of participants in an intervention study.

al., 2014) offer a template for a thorough description of interventions. Key intervention features should always be summarized in a report of a trial, but a separate article describing the intervention in greater detail might be needed.

The Results Section

Readers scrutinize the method section to learn if the study was done with rigor, but the results section is the heart of the report. In a quantitative study, the results of the statistical analyses are summarized in a factual manner. Descriptive statistics are ordinarily presented first, to provide an overview of study variables. If key research questions involve comparing groups with regard to dependent variables (e.g., in an experimental or case–control study), the results section often begins with information about the groups' comparability on baseline variables, so readers can evaluate the risk of selection bias.

Research results are usually ordered in terms of overall importance. If, however, research questions or hypotheses have been numbered in the introduction, the analyses addressing them should be ordered in the same sequence.

When reporting results of hypothesis-testing statistical tests, three pieces of information are typically stated: the value of the calculated statistic, degrees of freedom, and the exact probability level. For instance, a report might state, "Patients who received the intervention were significantly less likely to develop decubitus ulcers than patients in the control group (χ^2 = 8.23, df = 1, p = .008)." However, the current publication manual of the American Psychological Association (2020) urges authors to report confidence intervals: "Because confidence intervals combine information on location and precision and can often be directly used to infer significance levels, they are, in general, the best reporting strategy" (p. 34). The manual also strongly encourages reporting effect sizes, which can facilitate meta-analyses.

When results from several statistical analyses are reported, they should be summarized in a **table**. Good tables, with precise titles, headings, and footnotes, are an important way to avoid dull, repetitious statements. When tables are used, the text should refer to the table by number (e.g., "As shown in Table 2, patients in the intervention group…"). Box 32.1 presents some suggestions regarding the construction of effective statistical tables.

BOX 32.1 Guidelines for Preparing Statistical Tables

1. Number tables so they can be referenced in the text.
2. Give tables a brief but clear explanatory title.
3. Avoid both overly simple tables with information more efficiently presented in the text, and overly complex tables that intimidate or confuse readers.
4. Arrange data in such a way that patterns are obvious at a glance.
5. Give each column and row of data a heading that is succinct but clear. Table headings should establish the logic of the table structure.
6. Express data values to the number of decimal places justified by the precision of the measurement. In general, it is preferable to report numbers to one decimal place (or to two decimal places for correlation coefficients) because rounded values are easier to absorb than more precise ones. Report all values in a table to the same level of precision.
7. Make each table a "stand-alone" presentation, capable of being understood without referring to the text.
8. Indicate probability levels, either as actual p values or with confidence intervals. In correlation matrixes, use the system of asterisks with a probability level footnote. The usual convention is one asterisk when $p < .05$, two when $p < .01$, and three when $p < .001$.
9. Indicate units of measurement for numbers in the table whenever appropriate (e.g., pounds, milligrams).
10. Use footnotes to explain abbreviations or special symbols used in the table, except commonly understood abbreviations such as N.

> **TIP** Do not simply repeat statistical information in text and tables. Tables should display information that would be monotonous to present in the text—and to display it in such a way that patterns are evident. The text can be used to highlight major findings.

Figures may also be used to communicate results. Figures that display the results in graphic form are used less as an economy than as a means of dramatizing important findings and relationships. Figures are especially helpful for displaying information on phenomenon over time or for portraying conceptual or empirical models.

> **TIP** Research evidence does not constitute *proof* of anything, and so the report should never claim that the data proved, verified, confirmed, or demonstrated that hypotheses were correct or incorrect. Hypotheses are supported or not supported, accepted or rejected.

The Discussion Section

The discussion section is devoted to a thoughtful (and, hopefully, insightful) analysis of the findings and their clinical and theoretical utility. A typical discussion section addresses the following questions: What were the main findings? What do the findings mean? What evidence is there that the results and the interpretations are valid? What limitations might threaten validity? How do the results compare with prior knowledge on the topic? What are the implications of the findings for future research? What are the implications for nursing practice?

> **TIP** The discussion is often the most challenging section to write. It deserves your most intense intellectual effort—and careful review by peers. Peers should be asked to comment on how reasonable your inferences are, how well organized the section is, and whether it is too long—a common flaw. Griffiths and Norman (2016) noted that faulty conclusions are a common reason for rejecting manuscripts submitted to the *International Journal of Nursing Studies*.

Typically, the discussion section begins with a summary of key findings. The summary should be brief, however, because the focus of the discussion is on making sense of (and not merely repeating) the results.

Interpretation of results is a global process, encompassing the findings, methodologic strengths and limitations, sample characteristics, related research findings, clinical and contextual aspects, and theoretical issues. Researchers should justify their interpretations, stating why alternative explanations have been ruled out. If the findings conflict with those of earlier studies, tentative explanations should be offered. The generalizability of study findings should also be discussed.

Implications of study findings are speculative and so should be couched in tentative terms, as in the following example: "The results *suggest* that nurses' communication about advanced directives is inconsistent, and that nurses' years of experience affect the nature and amount of communication." The interpretation is, in essence, a hypothesis that can be tested in another study. The discussion should include recommendations for testing such hypotheses.

Finally, implications of the findings for nursing practice, policy, education, and/or research need to be discussed. There are several questions that can guide the implication section. Are aspects of the evidence clinically significant—and, if so, how might the evidence be used by nurses? What research is needed to support the findings and to advance the knowledge gained from this study? Are there policy implications and, if so, how can they be addressed? Are there implications for nursing education and how can these be addressed? The importance of addressing implications for nursing is critical for successful publication.

Other Aspects of the Report

The materials covered in the four IMRAD sections are found in some form in most quantitative research reports. Other aspects of the report deserve mention.

Title. Every research report needs a title articulating the nature of the study. Insofar as possible, the independent variables and outcomes (or central constructs under study) should be named in the title. It is also desirable to indicate the study population. Yet, the title should be brief (no more than about 15 words), so writers must balance clarity with brevity. The length of titles can often be reduced by omitting unnecessary terms such as "A Study of…" or "An Investigation to Examine the Effects of…" The title should communicate concisely what was studied and stimulate interest in the research. A few journals, however, such as the IJNS, request that the basic method or design be stated in the title, often after a colon. For example, Markopoulos and colleagues (2019) published a paper in IJNS titled "Bladder training prior to urinary catheter removal in total joint arthroplasty: A randomized controlled trial."

Abstract. Research reports usually include abstracts—brief descriptions of the problem, methods, and findings of the study, written so that readers can decide whether to read the entire report. As noted in Chapter 3, journal abstracts are sometimes written as an unstructured paragraph of 100 to 200 words, or in a structured form with subheadings. Pearce and Ferguson (2017) offer tips on writing strong abstracts.

> **TIP** Take the time to write a compelling abstract, which is your first main point of contact with reviewers and readers. It should convey that your study is important clinically and that it was done with conceptual and methodologic rigor. The abstract should contain words that will help people find your paper if they search for articles on your topic.

Keywords. It is often necessary to include keywords that will be used in databases to help others locate your study. Sometimes authors are given a list of keywords from which to choose (often Medical Subject Headings or MeSH terms), but additional keywords sometimes can be added. Substantive, methodologic, and theoretical terms can be used as keywords.

References. Each report concludes with a list of references cited in the text, using a reference style specified by the journal or institution. References can be cumbersome to prepare, but software can facilitate the preparation of reference lists (e.g., EndNote, ProCite, Reference Manager, Format Ease). Penders (2018) offers some guidance on responsible referencing.

Acknowledgments. People who helped with the research but whose contribution does not qualify them for authorship can be acknowledged in the report. This might include statistical consultants, data collectors, or people who reviewed the manuscript. Acknowledgments should also give credit to organizations that made the project possible, such as funding agencies or organizations that helped with participant recruitment.

Checklist. Some journals, such as the IJNS, require the completion of an author checklist that obliges authors to state their compliance with various conditions, such as total word count, declaration of keywords, and so on.

Qualitative Research Reports

There is no single style for reporting qualitative findings, but qualitative research reports often follow the IMRAD format or something akin to it. The most used guideline for reporting qualitative research is the Consolidated Criteria for Reporting Qualitative Research (**COREQ**) (Tong et al., 2007).

The Introduction

Qualitative reports usually begin with a problem statement, in a similar fashion to quantitative reports. The types of questions the researchers sought to answer are usually tied to the research tradition underlying the study (e.g., grounded theory, ethnography), which is usually stated in the introduction. Prior research on the phenomenon under study may be summarized in the introduction but is sometimes described in the discussion section.

In qualitative studies, it is essential to explain the study's cultural or social context. For studies with an ideologic orientation (e.g., critical theory), it is also important to describe the sociopolitical context. For studies using phenomenologic or grounded theory designs, the philosophy of phenomenology or symbolic interaction, respectively, may be described.

As another aspect of explaining the study's background, qualitative researchers sometimes provide information about relevant personal experiences or qualifications. If a researcher is studying decisions about long-term care placements is caring for two older parents and participates in a caregiver support group, this is relevant for readers' understanding of the study. In descriptive phenomenologic studies, researchers may discuss their personal experiences in relation to the phenomenon being studied to communicate what they bracketed.

The concluding paragraph of the introduction usually offers a summary of the purpose of the study or the research questions.

The Method Section

Although the research tradition of the study usually is noted in the introduction, the method section elaborates on specific methods used in conjunction with that tradition. Design features such as whether the study was longitudinal should also be stated. Beck (2022) identified how to avoid the most common pitfalls in qualitative research methods when trying to publish your study.

The method section should provide a good description of the research setting, so that readers can assess transferability of findings. Study participants and methods by which they were selected should also be described. Even when samples are small, it is often useful to provide a table summarizing participants' key characteristics. If researchers have a personal connection to participants, this connection should be noted. To disguise a group or institution, it may be necessary to omit or modify potentially identifying information.

Qualitative reports usually do not provide much specific information about data collection, but some researchers provide a sample of questions, especially if a topic guide was used. The description of data collection methods should include how data were collected (e.g., interview or observation), who collected the data, and how the data were recorded.

Information about quality and integrity is particularly important in qualitative studies. The more information included in the report about steps researchers took to describe reflexivity and to ensure the trustworthiness of the data, the more confident readers can be that the findings are credible.

Quantitative reports typically have only brief descriptions of data analysis techniques because standard statistical procedures are widely understood. By contrast, analytic procedures are often described in some detail in qualitative reports because readers need to understand how researchers organized, synthesized, and made sense of their data.

The Results Section

In their results sections, qualitative researchers summarize their themes, categories, taxonomic structure, or theory. The results section can be organized in a number of ways. For example, if a process is being described, results may be presented chronologically, corresponding to the unfolding of the process. Key themes, metaphors, or domains are often used as subheadings, organized in order of salience to participants or to a theory.

> **Example of Organization of Qualitative Results**
> Mattson et al. (2024) in their grounded theory study of self-management of opioid recovery through pregnancy and early parenting interviewed 16 women who had given birth during the past 12 months and used medication for opioid use disorder for recovery. The researchers identified the central process of Growing as a Healthy Dyad which consisted of maintaining vigilance, performing self-care, putting in the work of recovery, advocating, navigating social support, and acquiring skills and knowledge.

Because of the richness of qualitative data, researchers must decide which story, or how much of it, they want to tell. They must also decide how best to balance description and interpretation. The results section in a qualitative paper, unlike that in a quantitative one, intertwines data and interpretations of those data. It is important, however, to give sufficient emphasis to the voices and experiences of participants themselves so that readers can appreciate their lives and worlds. Most often, this occurs through the inclusion of direct quotes to illustrate key points. Because of space constraints in journals, quotes cannot be extensive; great care must be exercised in selecting the best possible exemplars.

Thorne (2021) offers guidance on integrating quotes appropriately in writing the findings section of qualitative research reports.

> **TIP** Using quotes is a complex process. When inserting quotes in the results section, pay attention to how the quote is introduced and how it is put in context. Quotes should not be used haphazardly or listed one after the other in a string.

Figures, diagrams, and word tables that organize concepts are often useful in summarizing an overall conceptualization of the phenomena under study. Grounded theory studies are especially likely to benefit from a schematic presentation of the basic social process.

Discussion

In qualitative studies, findings and interpretation are typically interwoven in the results section because the task of integrating qualitative materials is essentially interpretive. The discussion section of a qualitative report, therefore, is not so much designed to give meaning to the results, but to summarize them, link them to other research, and suggest possible implications for theory, research, or nursing practice.

Other Aspects of a Qualitative Report

Qualitative reports, like quantitative ones, include abstracts, keywords, references, and acknowledgments. Abstracts for journals that feature qualitative reports (e.g., *Qualitative Health Research*) tend to be the traditional (single-paragraph) type, rather than structured abstracts.

The titles of qualitative reports usually state the central phenomenon under scrutiny. Phenomenologic studies often have titles that include such words as "the lived experience of..." or "the meaning of...". Grounded theory studies often indicate something about the *findings* in the title—for example, mentioning the core category or basic social process. Ethnographic titles usually indicate the culture being studied. Two-part titles are not uncommon, with substance and method, research tradition and findings, or theme and meaning separated by a colon. For example, Ghafourifard and colleagues (2022) published a paper with this title: "Compassionate nursing care model: Results from a grounded theory study."

> **TIP** Preparing a report for a mixed methods (MM) study has challenges of its own—particularly regarding the integration of the qualitative and quantitative strands. Creswell and Plano Clark (2018) offer useful guidance for writing up integrated MM reports.

THE STYLE OF RESEARCH REPORTS

Research reports, especially for quantitative studies, are written in a distinctive style. Some style issues were discussed previously, but additional points are elaborated here.

A research report is not an essay. It is an account of how and why a problem was studied, and what was discovered as a result. The report should not include overtly subjective assertions or emotionally laden statements. This is not to say that the research story should be told in a dreary manner. Indeed, in qualitative reports there are ample opportunities to enliven the narration with rich description, direct quotes, and insightful interpretation. Authors of quantitative reports, although somewhat constrained by structure and the need to include numeric information, should strive to keep the presentation lively.

Quantitative researchers often avoid personal pronouns such as "I," "my," and "we" because impersonal pronouns, and use of the passive voice, may suggest greater impartiality. Qualitative reports, by contrast, are sometimes written in the first person and in an active voice. Even among quantitative researchers, however, there is a trend toward striking a greater balance between active and passive voice. If a direct presentation can be made without suggesting bias, a more readable product usually results.

It is not easy to write simply and clearly, but these are important goals of scientific writing. The use of technical jargon does little to enhance the communicative value of the report and should be avoided in conveying findings to practicing nurses. The style should be concise and straightforward. If writers can add elegance to their reports without interfering with clarity and accuracy, so much the better, but the product is not expected to be a literary achievement.

A common flaw in reports of novice researchers is inadequate organization. The overall structure is fairly standard, but organization within sections and subsections also needs attention. Sequences should be in an orderly progression with appropriate transitions. Continuity and logical thematic development are critical to good communication.

It may seem a trivial point, but methods and results should be described in the past tense. For example, it is inappropriate to say, "Nurses who receive special training perform triage functions significantly better than those without training." In this sentence, "receive" and "perform" should be changed to "received" and "performed" to reflect the fact that the statement pertains only to a particular sample whose behavior occurred in the past.

TYPES OF RESEARCH REPORTS

This section describes features of several major kinds of research reports: theses and dissertations, traditional or online journal articles, and presentations at professional meetings. Reports for class projects are excluded—not because they are unimportant but rather because they so closely resemble theses on a smaller scale.

Theses and Dissertations

Most doctoral degrees, and some master's degrees, are granted on the successful completion of a study. Most universities have a preferred format for their dissertations. Until recently, most schools used a traditional format with the following organization:

- Front Matter: Title Page; Abstract; Copyright Page; Approval Page; Acknowledgment Page; Table of Contents; List of Tables; List of Figures; List of Appendices
- Main Body: Chapter I. Introduction; Chapter II. Review of the Literature; Chapter III. Methods; Chapter IV. Results; Chapter V. Discussion and Summary
- Supplementary Pages: Bibliography; Appendices; Curriculum vita

The **front matter** (preliminary pages) for dissertations is similar to those for a scholarly book. The title page indicates such information as the title of the study, the author's name, the degree requirement being fulfilled, and the name of the university awarding the degree. The acknowledgment page gives writers the opportunity to thank those who contributed to the project. The table of contents outlines major sections and subsections of the report, indicating on which page readers will find material of interest. The lists of tables and figures identify by number, title, and page the tabular and graphic material in the text.

The main body of a traditionally formatted dissertation incorporates the IMRAD sections described earlier. The literature review often is so extensive that a separate chapter may be devoted to it. When a short review is sufficient, the first two chapters may be combined. In some cases, a separate chapter may also be required to elaborate the study's conceptual framework.

> **TIP** In some traditional dissertations, the early chapters describe students' intellectual journey, including a description of the paths they took and decisions they made in selecting their final research question and methodology.

The supplementary pages include a bibliography or list of references and one or more appendixes. An appendix contains materials that are either too lengthy or too tangential to be incorporated into the body of the report. Data collection instruments, scoring instructions, codebooks, cover letters, permission letters, IRB approval, category schemes, and peripheral statistical tables are examples of appendix materials. Sometimes a *curriculum vita* of the author is required.

Many nursing programs offer the **paper format thesis** or **publication option** (Graves et al., 2018). In a typical paper format thesis, there is an introduction, two or more publishable papers, and a conclusion that includes a synthesis or the findings and implications for nursing policy, research, education, and practice. Formats for the paper format thesis vary and are typically decided by the program. Universities generally require that a certain number of the publishable papers (e.g., two out of three) be data-based—that is, reports of original research. Other papers within the dissertation, however, might be publishable concept analyses or methodologic papers (e.g., describing the development of an instrument).

While some students opt for the traditional dissertation option, the manuscript style of dissertation is advantageous in that it assures that students will have published some aspect of their dissertation in a professional journal. The manuscript option requires clear expectations around faculty–student mentorship and roles, the manuscript dissertation formatting, and authorship. Universities must also provide clear guidelines on the expectations around the requirements for the status of publication of papers for successful program completion (e.g., under review, accepted, or *in press*).

If an academic institution does not accept paper format theses, students need to adapt their dissertations before submission to a journal. Ahern (2012) provides some guidance on converting a traditional dissertation into a manuscript. Roush (2016) has written a useful guide on writing theses and dissertations.

> **TIP** Another innovation involves publishing theses and dissertations electronically. In some fields, online repositories of dissertations are widely used, but this has not been the case in nursing (Macduff et al., 2016). Electronic Theses and Dissertations (ETDs) have the advantage of making scholarly work widely accessible—and ETDs can incorporate such features as film and audio clips. A new initiative is underway to promote nursing's engagement with ETDs (www.inetdin.net).

Journal Articles

Traditional dissertations, which are too lengthy for widespread use and often difficult to access, are read only by a handful of people. Publication in a professional journal ensures broader circulation of research findings, and it is professionally advantageous to publish. This section discusses the publication of research reports in journals.

> **TIP** The Nurse Author & Editor website at https://onlinelibrary.wiley.com/journal/17504910 is a valuable resource for nurse authors.

Traditional and Open-Access Journals

An important issue facing authors concerns whether to publish in a traditional journal or an open-access journal. Traditional journals are typically available both in print and online, but access to the online version is restricted to individuals and institutions paying a subscription fee. **Open-access journals** are available online free of charge to those with access to the Internet.

A major benefit is that open-access formats offer a worldwide audience of readers and hence can increase the visibility and impact of the authors' research. Also, unlike traditional journals in which the journal publishers maintain the copyright for all publications, open-access journals usually allow authors to retain copyright. The legal basis for open access is the consent of the copyright holder, i.e., the authors. In many cases, copyright holders demonstrate their consent to use open access by using something called the *Creative Commons licenses*. When authors consent to open access, they are usually consenting upfront to unrestricted access, reading, downloading, copying, printing, and sharing of the work.

An article accepted by an open-access journal typically gets published more quickly than is true for traditional print journals. Another advantage is that online journals are much less strict about page limits. Qualitative researchers may benefit from this feature because it allows them to include more extensive verbatim quotes. Quantitative researchers can include more figures and tables than is true in traditional journal articles (although some traditional journals publish online supplements that can be used to share additional material).

> **TIP** In selecting examples of nursing studies in this edition, we deliberately sought studies published as open-access articles, so that readers around the world would be able to obtain them. We identify open-access articles in the chapter reference lists.

One drawback is that open-access journals usually charge a fee to cover the cost of producing the journal. For example, in 2019, the open-access journal *BMC Nursing* charged authors $2290 (EUR), 2690 (USD), 2090 (GBP) for an accepted article. However, many nurse authors are affiliated with institutions that are members of BioMed Central, in which case there is no fee. In other cases, institutions pay publication fees for faculty members. (The fee for open-access journal publication is often waived for authors from low-income countries and is sometimes reduced for students.) Publishing in nonnursing journals became a popular option for some nurse authors due to a lack of open-access nursing journals. However, with the ever-increasing number of open-access nursing journals, nurses can now choose this option for timely publication in nursing journals in order to reach their audience as opposed to publishing in nonnursing journals.

TIP The Directory of Open Access Journals indexes and provides information for about 13,234 open-access journals, 297 of which were classified as having *Nursing* as a subject code in 2023 (https://doaj.org/). Examples include *Nursing Plus Open*, *SAGE Open Nursing*, *Global Qualitative Nursing Research*, and *BMC Nursing*. Many open-access nursing journals are subsidized by national governments (e.g., in Brazil). The Cochrane Collaboration publishes their systematic reviews as open access: https://www.cochranelibrary.com/cdsr/reviews.

Many traditional journals have moved to a hybrid model, in which authors can elect to have individual articles published as open access, usually for an article-processing fee. However, many government agencies that fund health research (such as the National Institutes of Health in the United States and Research Councils [United Kingdom]) now require that articles reporting government-funded studies be published as open access.

Some journals allow articles to be uploaded into *open-access repositories* in academic networks such as Research Gate or Academia.edu, or in institutional repositories. If open access is important but unaffordable, researchers should check a journal's policy about uploading to open-access repositories—including whether there is a period of *embargo*. When there is an embargo, an article cannot be uploaded to the repository for a period after it first appears in print (e.g., 12 months). As noted by Griffiths (2014), publishers and journals vary in their policies regarding costs and embargos (or permission to upload at all), so authors "need to be wary to avoid breaking copyright laws" (p. 690).

When the open-access movement got underway, many expressed concerns that low-quality articles would increasingly find their way into publication. And, in fact, there has been an alarming surge in **predatory journals** that charge fees, fail to provide adequate review and editorial services, and publish articles of poor quality (Oermann et al., 2018). In their study of predatory nursing journals, Oermann et al., 2016 identified 140 such journals, most of which solicit manuscripts through spam emails. Several nursing editors offer advice on how to avoid predatory nursing journals (Hulsey et al., 2023; Oermann et al., 2019).

Nevertheless, many high-quality open-access journals are fully peer reviewed, and many have attained high prestige. All major open-access initiatives insist on the importance of high-quality scientific review of submitted articles.

Selecting a Journal

Hundreds of nursing journals exist and are indexed in CINAHL and PubMed. Journals differ in focus, prestige, acceptance rates, word limits, and reference styles. Journals also vary in their goals, types of manuscript sought, review methods, and readership. These various factors need to be matched against personal ambitions and realistic assessments of the study. Writers should develop a clear idea of the journal to which a manuscript will be submitted before writing begins.

TIP Several "journal selection" websites have been created and are designed to help researchers identify appropriate journals (Cuschieri, 2018). Some services are free but others charge a fee.

All journals release goal statements, as well as guidelines for preparing and submitting a manuscript. This information is published on journal websites.

> **Example of a of Journal Goal Statement From the Website**
> Consistently ranked as one of the most-read and most assigned journals by faculties of graduate programs in nursing, *Advances in Nursing Science* (ANS) is intellectually challenging, innovative and progressive, and features articles from a wide range of scholarly traditions. The primary purposes of ANS are to advance the development of nursing knowledge and to promote the integration of nursing philosophies, theories, and research with practice. The journal particularly encourages works that speak to the need for global sustainability and that take an intersectional approach, recognizing class, color, sexual and gender identity, and other dimensions of human experience related to health. Articles in ANS are peer reviewed and chosen for their pioneering perspectives and for their significance in contributing the evolution of the discipline of nursing (https://journals.lww.com/advancesinnursingscience/pages/default.aspx).

Many authors would like to know a journal's acceptance rate, but this information is seldom available. Northam and colleagues (2014) conducted a survey of journal editors and reported on the acceptance rate for 61 nursing journals. Some journals were more competitive than others. For example, *Nursing Research* accepted only 20% of submitted manuscripts, whereas the acceptance rates for some specialty journals was greater than 50%. Competition for journal publication likely became keener in the years since the survey was conducted.

> **TIP** Some nursing journals provide acceptance information on their websites. For example, the website for *Oncology Nursing Forum* stated in 2018 that the journal accepted 36% of manuscripts on first submission and 52% after revision. The website also noted that the peer review process took, on average, 6 to 8 weeks, and that the time to publication was 7 to 10 months. In a paper by editors of the prestigious *International Journal of Nursing Studies* (IJNS), Griffiths and Norman (2016) explained that about 70% of manuscripts submitted to IJNS are rejected even before being sent out for peer review.

Authors are often guided in their selection of a journal by the journal's *prestige*. Several metrics have been developed to capture a journal's impact, including indexes called *impact factor*, *Cite Score*, and *Source Normalized Impact per Paper (SNIP)*.

A journal's **impact factor (IF)** is the most widely used status index. The IF is a measure of citation frequency for an average article in a journal. Specifically, a journal's IF for, say, 2019 is the number of times in 2019 that articles published in the journal in the two prior years (2017 and 2018) were cited, divided by the number of the journal's articles in those 2 years that *could* have been cited (i.e., number of actual citations divided by the number of potentially citable articles) (Polit & Northam, 2011). IF information can be found in *Journal Citation Reports* and on the websites of journals that have an IF. Although some nursing journals are not evaluated for IF, increasingly they are and this is true of open-access nursing journals as well. However, many open-access medical journals have high IFs that make them appealing options for some nurses, especially those working in interdisciplinary teams. Open-access journals have been found to have more citations overall than traditional journals (Cuschieri, 2018). Because a journal's IF can be influenced by a single article that is cited numerous times, another potentially useful metric is the *percentage* of articles in a journal that are cited. This metric is available in InCites by Clarivate Analytics.

> **TIP** Citation impact metrics are available not only for journals, but also for specific articles and for authors. The best-known measure of author-level citations is the *h-index*, which attempts to capture both the productivity and citation impact of a scholar's publications. An alternative approach (often referred to as *altmetrics*) is to measure impact based on usage data, such as the number of article downloads.

Query Letters

It is sometimes useful to send a **query letter** to a journal to ask the editor whether there is interest in a manuscript. The query letter should briefly describe the topic and methods, title, and a tentative submission date. Query letters are not essential if you have done a lot of homework about the journal's goals, but they might help to avoid impediments in some circumstances (e.g., if editors have recently accepted several papers on a similar topic and do not wish to consider another). Query letters can be submitted by e-mail using contact information provided on the journal's website.

Query letters can be sent to multiple journals simultaneously, but ultimately the manuscript can be submitted only to one—or rather, to one at a time. If several editors express interest in reviewing a manuscript, journals can be prioritized according to criteria previously described. The priority list should be preserved because the manuscript can be resubmitted to the next journal on the list if the journal of first choice rejects it.

TIP A useful strategy in selecting a journal is to inspect your citation list. Journals that appear in your list have shown an interest in your topic and likely are good candidates for publishing new studies on that topic.

Preparing the Manuscript

Once a journal has been selected, the information in the journal's **Instructions to Authors** should be carefully reviewed to avoid what is known as a "desk reject," an issue addressed by several nursing editors in guiding potential authors toward successful publication (Flanagan, 2021; Lake, 2020). These instructions typically give authors such information as the maximum page length; permissible fonts and margins; the type of abstract desired; the reference style that should be used; and how to submit the manuscript online. It is important to adhere to the journal's guidelines to avoid rejection for nonsubstantive reasons.

TIP Before you begin to write, it can be helpful to examine a research article that can serve as a model. Select a journal article on a topic similar to your own in the journal you have selected as first choice. When you have written a draft, a review by colleagues or advisers can be invaluable in getting feedback about possible improvements.

Typically, a manuscript for journals should be no more than 15 to 20 pages, double-spaced, not counting references and tables. The greatest amount of space usually should be allocated to methods and results. A frequent complaint of journal editors is that submitted manuscripts are too long.

Care should be taken in using and preparing citations. Some nursing journals suggest that there be no more than 15 references in total or no more than three citations supporting a single point. In general, only published work can be cited (e.g., not papers presented at a conference). The reference style of the American Psychological Association (APA, 2020) is the style used by many nursing journals. Another popular style is that of the American Medical Association.

TIP There is a wealth of resources to assist you with the APA style, including tutorials from university libraries such as https://owl.purdue.edu/.

Submission of a Manuscript

When the manuscript is ready for journal submission, a *cover letter* should be drafted. The cover letter should state the title of the paper and the name and contact information of the **corresponding author** (the author who communicates with the journal, usually the lead author). The letter may include assurances that (1) the paper is original and has not been published or submitted elsewhere; (2) all authors have read and approved the manuscript; and (3) there are no conflicts of interest. Most traditional journals also require a signed *copyright transfer* form, which transfers all copyright ownership of the manuscript to the journal and warrants that all authors signing the form participated sufficiently in the research to justify authorship.

In submitting an article online, it is usually necessary to upload several files containing different parts of your manuscript. The title page, which has author-identifying information, should be in the first file. The next file usually contains the abstract, main text, and reference list. Tables and figures are submitted separately, one file at a time. In other words, if there are two tables and one figure, these would be submitted in three files. At the end of the process, a pdf file that contains all the elements is created for your review prior to submission. The entire process often requires a fair amount of time, but fortunately it is usually possible to begin the process and return later if you need to track down information, such as the addresses of coauthors.

TIP Nurses publish articles in many health-related journals, not just in nursing journals. Nurse researchers, who increasingly work in interprofessional teams, are coauthors on papers published in diverse journals.

Manuscript Review

Most nursing journals with research content have a policy of independent **peer review** of manuscripts by two or more experts in the field. Reviewers are typically independent—they do not collaborate to achieve consensus. The ultimate decision rests in the hands of journal editors. Peer review usually is a *blind review*, the idea being that greater candor is possible if there is anonymity. In a double-blind review, reviewers do not know the identity of the authors, and authors do not learn the identity of reviewers. Journals with peer reviewers are **refereed journals** and are held in higher esteem than nonrefereed journals. When submitting a manuscript to a refereed journal, authors' names should not appear anywhere except on the title page.

TIP It takes skill to be a good reviewer. In an ideal scenario, experienced reviewers would mentor their students in this important professional role. The website Nurse Author & Editor provides several resources for peer reviewers that can be found online at https://onlinelibrary.wiley.com/page/journal/17504910/homepage/for-reviewers.

Peer reviewers make recommendations to the editors about whether to accept the manuscript for publication, accept it contingent on revisions, or reject it. It is rare that a manuscript is accepted on first submission—substantive and editorial revisions are the norm.

Example of Reviewer Recommendation Categories
The journal *Research in Nursing & Health* asks reviewers to make one of five recommendations: (1) Accept; (2) Minor revision; (3) Major revision; (4) Reject and resubmit; and (5) Reject.

Authors are sent information about the editors' decision, together with reviewers' comments. In many cases, the initial review results in an invitation to resubmit the manuscript. As noted by Algase (2016), the revise-and-resubmit decision reflects the editor's view that the paper has appeal but has some flaws that make it unacceptable in its initial form. The editor typically gives a deadline for the revised submission. Authors can accept the invitation, but if the authors decline to resubmit, the paper should be withdrawn from consideration.

When resubmitting a revised manuscript to the same journal, each reviewer recommendation should be addressed, either by making the requested change, or by explaining in a cover letter the rationale for not revising. Defending some aspect of a paper against a reviewer's recommendation often requires a strong supporting argument and citations (https://onlinelibrary.wiley.com/page/journal/17504910/homepage/for-reviewers). Southgate (2022) has offered advice about responding to reviewers. Typically, many months go by between submission of the original manuscript and the publication of a journal article, especially if there are revisions, as there usually are.

Example of Journal Timeline
Beck and Twomey (2023) published a paper in *MCN: The American Journal of Maternal Child Nursing* titled, Posttraumatic growth after postpartum psychosis. The timeline for acceptance and publication of this manuscript, which was fast, was as follows:

March 29, 2023	Manuscript submitted to *MCN: The American Journal of Maternal Child Nursing* for review
April 28, 2023	Letter from editor informing of a revise-and-resubmit decision
May 9, 2023	Revised manuscript resubmitted
June 6, 2023	Revised manuscript accepted for publication
August 17, 2023	Published ahead of print
November/December 2023	Publication in *MCN: The American Journal of Maternal Child Nursing*

Many manuscripts are rejected because of keen competition. If a manuscript is rejected, the reviewers' comments should be taken into consideration before submitting it to another journal.

TIP Author reviews of their experiences with journals are available in SciRev. The reviews for a specific discipline can be found at www.SciRev.sc by entering the discipline name in the search field; specific journals can also be searched.

Presentations at Professional Conferences

Many international, national, and regional organizations sponsor meetings at which nursing studies are presented, either in an oral report or as a visual display in a poster session. Professional conferences are good forums for presenting results to clinical audiences. Researchers can take advantage of meeting and talking with other conference attendees who are working on similar problems in different geographic regions. Becker's (2014) book on conference presentations is a useful resource, and Joshua (2017) has written about the learning opportunities of presenting at a conference.

TIP **Predatory conferences** are set up to look like legitimate professional conferences but, in reality, they are an exploitative method to make money from registration fees. Guidelines called "Think. Check. Attend." can be used to judge the legitimacy of a conference.

The mechanism for submitting a presentation to a conference is simpler than for journal submission. The association sponsoring the conference ordinarily publishes an announcement or **Call for Abstracts** on its website or sends an email to its members, 6 to 9 months before the meeting date. The notice indicates topics of interest, submission requirements, and deadlines for submitting a proposed paper or poster. Most universities and major healthcare agencies receive and post Call for Abstracts notices. In addition, Sigma Theta Tau posts a schedule of nursing conferences on its website (https://www.sigmanursing.org).

Oral Reports

Most conferences require prospective presenters to submit online abstracts of 250 to 1,000 words. Each conference has its own guidelines for abstract content and form. Abstracts are sometimes submitted to the organizer of a particular session; in other cases, conference sessions are organized after-the-fact, with related papers grouped together. Abstracts are evaluated based on the quality and originality of the research and the paper's appropriateness for the conference audience. If abstracts are accepted, researchers are committed to appear at the conference to make a presentation.

Oral reports at meetings usually follow the IMRAD format. The time allotted for presentation usually is about 10 to 15 minutes, with 5 minutes or so for audience questions. Thus, only the most important aspects of the study, with emphasis on the results, can be shared. It is especially challenging to condense qualitative findings to a brief oral summary without losing the rich, in-depth character of the data.

A handy rule of thumb is that a page of double-spaced text requires 2½ to 3 minutes to read aloud. Although presenters often prepare a written paper or a script, presentations are most effective if they are delivered informally or conversationally, rather than if they are read verbatim. The presentation should be rehearsed to gain comfort with the script and to ensure that time limits are not exceeded.

TIP Most conferences presentations include visual materials—notably PowerPoint slides. Visual materials should be kept simple for biggest impact. Tables are difficult to read on a slide but sometimes can be distributed to the audience in hard copy form.

The question-and-answer period can be a good opportunity to expand on aspects of the research and to get early feedback. Audience comments can be helpful in turning the conference presentation into a manuscript for journal submission. It is important to note that the same abstract for an oral or paper presentation should not be submitted multiple times. The guidelines for this sort of potential "duplicative" publication are not as clear as they are for written papers. However, the generally accepted premise is that a poster presentation is the first presentation of findings. Ideally, feedback will guide the presenter in refining the work and, ultimately, the abstract for a paper or podium presentation. The oral presentation will again provide an opportunity for feedback that will shape the development of the abstract and full paper to be submitted for publication. For this reason, the abstracts for each should vary. This is particularly the case if the abstract for a poster or podium presentation at a conference is to be published. Recycling the same abstract in these cases can result in self-plagiarism unless the abstract is cited. However, given it is rare to not modify an abstract based on feedback, the journal editor should be queried prior to submission. An exception to this is for a presentation that is given to varied audiences with little to no overlap, such as work that is presented at a conference and then later delivered to colleagues in a university school or hospital setting. Although it is primarily intended for biomedical and industry sponsored presentations and publications, Foster et al., 2019; DeTora et al., 2022 offer some guidance on this topic.

Poster Presentation

Researchers sometimes present their findings or study protocols in **poster sessions**. Abstracts, often similar to those required for oral presentations, must be submitted to conference organizers according to specific guidelines. In poster sessions, several researchers simultaneously present visual displays summarizing study features, and conference attendees circulate around the exhibit area perusing displays. Those interested in a poster topic can discuss the study with the researcher and bypass posters dealing with topics of less interest. Poster sessions are efficient and encourage one-on-one discussions. Poster sessions are typically 1 to 2 hours in length. Researchers are expected to stand near their posters throughout the session to allow discussion.

It is challenging to design an effective poster. The poster must convey essential information about the background, design, and results of a study, in a format that can be perused in minutes. Bullet points, graphs, and photos are useful for communicating information quickly. Large, bold fonts are essential, because posters are often read from a short distance. It is important to follow conference guidelines regarding such matters as poster size, format, and display materials. For those traveling long distances, lightweight fabric posters can be created.

Several authors have offered advice on preparing for poster sessions (e.g., Berg & Hicks, 2017; Kohtz et al., 2017; Siedlecki, 2017, 2022). Software for producing posters is also available (e.g., www.postersw.com).

Electronic Dissemination

Computers and the Internet have changed forever how information is disseminated. Earlier we discussed publishing in open-access online-only journals, but there are other ways to disseminate research findings on the Internet. For example, some researchers or research teams develop their own web page with information about their studies. When there are hyperlinks embedded in the websites, consumers can navigate between files and websites to retrieve relevant information on a topic of interest. Links to unpublished papers can also be uploaded on to the websites of individual researchers, their institutions, special interest organizations, and online repositories.

Such online dissemination avenues ensure timely distribution of information. One drawback of such dissemination opportunities, however, is that the papers are not peer reviewed. Researchers who want their evidence to have an impact on nursing practice should seek publication in outlets that subject manuscripts to expert external review.

TIP McGrath and Brandon (2016) offer advice on how to "market" your research on social media, such as Facebook or Twitter.

CRITICAL APPRAISAL OF RESEARCH REPORTS

Although various aspects of study methodology can be evaluated using guidelines presented throughout this book, the manner in which study information is communicated in the research report can also be scrutinized in a comprehensive appraisal. Box 32.2 summarizes major points to consider in evaluating the presentation of a research report.

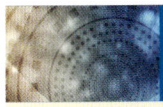

BOX 32.2 Guidelines for Critically Appraising the Presentation of a Research Report

1. Does the report include a sufficient amount of detail to permit a thorough appraisal of the study's purpose, conceptual framework, design and methods, handling of ethical issues, analysis of data, and interpretation?
2. Is the report well written and grammatical? Are pretentious words or jargon used when simpler wording would have been possible?
3. Is the report well organized? Is there an orderly, logical presentation of ideas?
4. Does the report effectively combine text with tables or figures?
5. Are overt biases, exaggerations, and distortions avoided? Are conclusions logical?
6. Is the report written using appropriately tentative language?
7. Is sexist or insensitive language avoided?
8. Does the title of the report adequately capture the key concepts and the population under investigation? Does the abstract adequately summarize the research problem, study methods, and important findings?

An important issue is whether the report provided sufficient information for a thoughtful appraisal of other dimensions. When vital pieces of information are missing, researchers leave readers little choice but to assume the worst because this would lead to the most cautious interpretation of the results. For example, if there is no mention of blinding, then the safest conclusion is that blinding did not occur.

Styles of writing differ for qualitative and quantitative reports, and it is unreasonable to apply the standards considered appropriate for one paradigm to the other. Regardless of style, however, you should be alert to indications of overt biases or exaggerations.

In summary, a research report is meant to be an account of how and why a problem was studied and what results were obtained. The report should be clearly written, cogent, and concise, and written in a manner that piques readers' interest.

SUMMARY POINTS

- In developing a dissemination plan, researchers select a communication outlet (e.g., journal article, conference presentation), identify the audience whom they wish to reach, and decide on the content that can be effectively communicated.
- In the planning stage, researchers need to decide authorship credits (if there are multiple authors), who the **lead author** and **corresponding author** will be, and in what order authors' names will be listed.
- Quantitative reports (and many qualitative reports) follow the **IMRAD format**, with the following sections: Introduction, Method, Results, and Discussion.
- The *introduction* acquaints readers with the research problem. It includes the problem statement and study purpose, the research hypotheses or questions, a brief literature review, and description of a framework. In qualitative reports, the introduction indicates the research tradition and, if relevant, the researchers' connection to the problem.
- The *method section* explains what researchers did to address the research problem. It includes a description of the study design (or an elaboration of the research tradition); the sampling approach and a description of study participants; instruments and procedures used to collect and evaluate the data; and methods used to analyze the data.
- In the *results section*, findings from the analyses are summarized. Results sections in qualitative reports necessarily intertwine description and interpretation. Quotes from transcripts are essential for giving voice to study participants.

- Both qualitative and quantitative researchers include **figures** and **tables** that dramatize or succinctly summarize major findings or conceptual schema.
- The *discussion section* presents the interpretation of results, how the findings relate to earlier research, study limitations, and implications of the findings for nursing practice and future research.
- Standards for reporting methodologic elements now abound. Researchers reporting an RCT follow the **CONSORT guideline** (Consolidated Standards of Reporting Trials), which includes use of a flow chart to shows the flow of study participants. Guidelines for reporting aspects of an intervention include **CReDECI** and **TIDieR**. The most used guideline for reporting qualitative research is the Consolidated Criteria for Reporting Qualitative Research (**COREQ**)
- The major types of research reports are theses and dissertations, journal articles, and presentations at professional meetings.
- Theses and dissertations normally follow a standard IMRAD format, but some schools now accept **paper format theses**, which include an introduction, two or more publishable papers, and a conclusion.
- In selecting a journal for publication, researchers consider the journal's goals and audience, its prestige, and how often it publishes. Another major consideration is whether to publish in a traditional journal or in an online **open-access journal.** An advantage of open-access journals is speedy, worldwide dissemination.
- Researchers need to be wary of the many **predatory journals** that solicit manuscripts and collect article processing charges for a profit, but then fail to provide adequate editorial services and tend to publish articles of poor quality.
- One proxy for a journal's prestige is its **impact factor,** the ratio between citations to a journal and recent citable items published.
- Before beginning to prepare a **manuscript** for submission to a journal, researchers need to carefully to review the journal's **Instructions to Authors.**
- Most nursing journals that publish research reports are **refereed journals** with a policy of basing publication decisions on **peer reviews** that are usually **double-blind reviews** (identities of authors and reviewers are not divulged).
- Nurse researchers can also present their research at professional conferences, either through a 10- to 15-minute oral report to a seated audience, or in a **poster session** in which the "audience" moves around a room perusing research summaries attached to posters. Sponsoring organizations usually issue a **Call for Abstracts** for the conference 6 to 9 months before it is held.

REFERENCES CITED IN CHAPTER 32

Ahern, K. (2012). How to create a journal article from a thesis. *Nursing Research*, 19(4), 21–25.

Alfonso, F., & Editors' Network European Society of Cardiology ESC Task Force. (2019). Authorship: From credit to accountability—Reflections from the editors' network. *Netherlands Heart Journal*, 27(6), 289–296. https://doi.org/10.1007/s12471-019-1273-y

Algase, D. L. (2016). Revise and resbumit: Now what? *Research and Theory for Nursing Practice*, 28, 195–198.

American Psychological Association. (2020). *Publication manual of the American Psychological Association* (7th ed.). Author.

Beck, C. T. (2022). Avoiding potential pitfalls in qualitative research methods. *Journal of Obstetric, Gynecologic, & Neonatal Nursing*, 51(5), 473–476. https://doi.org/10.1016/j.jogn.2022.08.002

Beck, C. T., & Twomey, T. (2023). Posttraumatic growth after postpartum psychosis. *MCN The American Journal of Maternal Child Nursing*, 48(6), 303–311. https://doi.org/10.1097/nmc.0000000000000954

Becker, L. (2014). *Presenting your research: Conferences, symposiums, poster presentations and beyond*. Sage.

Benchimol, E., Smeeth, L., Guttman, A., Harron, K., Moher, D., Petersen, I., Sørensen, H. T., von Elm, E., Langan, S. M., RECORD Working Committee, Langan, S. (2015). The reporting of studies conducted using observational routinely-collected health data (RECORD) statement. *PLoS Med*, 12(10), e1001885.

Berg, J., & Hicks, R. (2017). Successful design and delivery of a professional poster. *Journal of American Association of Nurse Practitioners*, 29(8), 461–469.

Boutron, I., Moher, D., Altman, D., Schulz, K., Ravaud, P., & CONSORT Group. (2008). Extending the CONSORT statement to randomized trials of nonpharmacologic treatment:

Explanation and elaboration. *Annals of Internal Medicine*, *148*(4), 295–309.

Butcher, N. J., Monsour, A., Mew, E. J., Chan, A. W., Moher, D., Mayo-Wilson, E., Terwee, C. B., Chee-A-Tow, A., Baba, A., Gavin, F., Grimshaw, J. M., Kelly, L. E., Saeed, L., Thabane, L., Askie, L., Smith, M., Farid-Kapadia, M., Williamson, P. R., Szatmari, P., ... Offringa, M. (2022). Guidelines for reporting outcomes in trial reports: The CONSORT-outcomes 2022 extension. *JAMA*, *328*(22), 2252–2264. https://doi.org/10.1001/jama.2022.21022

Calvert, M., Blazeby, J., Altman, D., Revicki, D., Moher, D., Brundage, M., & CONSORT PRO Group. (2013). Reporting of patient-reported outcomes in randomized trials: The CONSORT PRO extension. *Journal of the American Medical Association*, *309*(8), 814–822.

Campbell, M., Piaggio, G., & Elbourne, D. R., Altman, D. G., & CONSORT Group. (2012). CONSORT 2010 statement: Extension to cluster randomised trials. *British Medical Journal*, *345*, e5661.

Chan, A. W., Tetzlaff, J., Gøtzsche, P. C., Altman, D., Mann, H., Berlin, J., Dickersin, K., Hróbjartsson, A., Schulz, K. F., Parulekar, W. R., Krleza-Jeric, K., Laupacis, A., Moher, D., & Moher, D. (2013). SPIRIT 2013 explanation and elaboration: Guidance for protocols of clinical trials. *British Medical Journal*, *346*, e7586.

Cohen, J., Korevaar, D., Altman, D., Bruns, D., Gatsonis, C., Hooft, L., Irwig, L., Levine, D., Reitsma, J. B., de Vet, H. C. W., Bossuyt, P. M. M., & Bossuyt, P. (2016). STARD 2015 guidelines for reporting diagnostic accuracy studies: Explanation and elaboration. *BMJ Open*, *6*(11), e012799.

Conn, V. S., Ward, S., Herrick, L., Topp, R., Alexander, G., Anderson, C., Smith, C. E., Benefield, L. E., Given, B., Titler, M., Larson, J. L., Fahrenwald, N. L., Cohen, M. Z., & Georgesen, S. (2015). Managing opportunities and challenges of co-authorship. *Western Journal of Nursing Research*, *37*(2), 134–163.

Creswell, J. W., & Plano Clark, V. L. (2018). *Designing and conducting mixed methods research* (3rd ed.). Sage.

Cuschieri, S. (2018). Is open access publishing the way forward? A review of the different ways in which research papers can be published. *Early Human Development*, *121*, 54–57.

Des Jarlais, D., Lyles, C., Crepaz, N., & TREND Group. (2004). Improving the reporting quality of nonrandomized evaluations of behavioral and public health interventions: The TREND statement. *American Journal of Public Health*, *94*(3), 361–366.

DeTora, L. M., Toroser, D., Sykes, A., Vanderlinden, C., Plunkett, F. J., Lane, T., Hanekamp, E., Dormer, L., DiBiasi, F., Bridges, D., Baltzer, L., & Citrome, L. (2022). Good publication practice (GPP) guidelines for company-sponsored biomedical research: 2022 update. *Annals of Internal Medicine*, *175*(9), 1298–1304. https://doi.org/10.7326/M22-1460

Eldridge, S., Chan, C., Campbell, M., Bond, C., Hopewell, S., Thabane, L., Lancaster, G., & PAFS Consensus Group. (2016). CONSORT 2010 statement: Extension to randomised pilot and feasibility trials. *British Medical Journal*, *355*, i5239.

Flanagan, J. (2021). Avoiding the desk reject. *International Journal of Nursing Knowledge*, *32*(2), 87. https://doi.org/10.1111/2047-3095.12325

Foster, C., Wager, E., Marchington, J., Patel, M., Banner, S., Kennard, N. C., Panayi, A., Stacey, R., & GPCAP Working Group. (2019). Good practice for conference abstracts and presentations: GPCAP. *Research Integrity and Peer Review*, *4*, 11. https://doi.org/10.1186/s41073-019-0070-x

Gennaro, S. (2021). Text recycling and salami slicing. *Journal of Nursing Scholarship*, *53*(5), 531–532. https://doi.org/10.1111/jnu.12700

Ghafourifard, M., Zamanzadeh, V., Valizadeh, L., & Rahmani, A. (2022). Compassionate nursing care model: Results from a grounded theory study. *Nursing Ethics*, *29*(3), 621–635. https://doi.org/10.1177/09697330211051005

Graves, J. M., Postma, J., Katz, J. R., Kehoe, L., Swalling, E., & Barbosa-Leiker, C. (2018). A national survey examining manuscript dissertation formats among nursing PhD programs in the United States. *Journal of Nursing Scholarship*, *50*(3), 314–323. https://doi.org/10.1111/jnu.12374

Griffiths, P. (2014). Open access publication & the International Journal of Nursing Studies: All that glitters is not gold. *International Journal of Nursing Studies*, *51*(5), 689–690.

Griffiths, P., & Norman, I. (2016). Why was my paper rejected? Editors' reflections on common issues which influence decisions to reject papers submitted for publication in academic nursing journals. *International Journal of Nursing Studies*, *57*, A1–A4.

Happell, B. (2016). Salami: By the slice or swallowed whole? *Applied Nursing Research*, *30*, 29–31.

Hoffmann, T. C., Glasziou, P. P., Boutron, I., Milne, R., Perera, R., Moher, D., Altman, D. G., Barbour, V., Macdonald, H., Johnston, M., Lamb, S. E., Dixon-Woods, M., McCulloch, P., Wyatt, J. C., Chan, A. W., Michie, S., & Michie, S. (2014). Better reporting of interventions: Template for intervention description and replication (TIDieR) checklist and guide. *British Medical Journal*, *348*, g1687.

Hulsey, T., Carpenter, R., Carter-Templeton, H., Oermann, M. H., Keener, T. A., & Maramba, P. (2023). Best practices in scholarly publishing for promotion or tenure: Avoiding predatory journals. *Journal of Professional Nursing*, *45*, 60–63. https://doi.org/10.1016/j.profnurs.2023.01.002

Husereau, D., Drummond, M., Petrou, S., Carswell, C., Moher, D., Greenberg, D., Augustovski, F., &Briggs, A. H., Mauskopf, J., Loder, E., & CHEERS Task Force, (2013). Consolidated Health Economic Evaluation Reporting Standards (CHEERS) statement. *BMC Medicine*, *11*, 80.

International Committee of Medical Journal Editors. (2023). *Recommendations for the conduct, reporting, editing, and publication of scholarly work in medical journals—updated 2023*. Retrieved from www.icmje.org

Joshua, B. (2017). Reflecting on the learning opportunities of presenting at a conference. *Nurse Researcher*, *24*(4), 27–30.

Kearney, M. H. (2014). Be a responsible co-author. *Research in Nursing and Health*, *37*, 1–2.

Kennedy, M., Newland, J., & Owens, J. (2017). Findings from the INANE survey on student papers submitted to nursing journals. *Journal of Professional Nursing*, *33*(3), 175–183.

Kohtz, C., Hymer, C., Humbles-Pegues, P. C., Hymer, C., & Humbles-Pegues, P. (2017). Poster creation: Guidelines and tips for success. *Nursing*, *47*(3), 43–46.

Kottner, J., Audigé, L., Brorson, S., Donner, A., Gajewski, B. J., Hróbjartsson, A., Roberts, C., Shoukri, M., Streiner, D. L., & Streiner, D. (2011). Guidelines for Reporting Reliability and Agreement Studies (GRRAS) were proposed. *International Journal of Nursing Studies*, *48*(6), 661–671.

Lake, E. T. (2020). Why and how to avoid a desk-rejection. *Research in Nursing & Health*, *43*(2), 141–142. https://doi.org/10.1002/nur.22016

Long, T. L., & Beck, C. T. (2017). *Writing in nursing: A brief guide*. Oxford University Press.

Macduff, C., Goodfellow, L., Leslie, G., Copeland, S., Nolfi, D., & Blackwood, D. (2016). Harnessing our rivers of knowledge: Time to improve nursing's engagement with Electronic Theses and Dissertations. *Journal of Advanced Nursing*, *72*(10), 2255–2258.

Markopoulos, G., Kitridis, D., Tsikopoulos, K., Georgiannos, D., & Bisbinas, I. (2019). Bladder training prior to urinary catheter removal in total joint arthroplasty: A randomized controlled trial. *International Journal of Nursing Studies*, *89*, 14–17.

Mattson, N. M., Ohlendorf, J. M., & Haglund, K. (2024). Grounded theory approach to understand self-management of opioid recovery through pregnancy and early parenting. *Journal of Obstetric, Gynecologic, & Neonatal Nursing*, *53*(1), 34–45. https://doi.org/10.1016/j.jogn.2023.09.001

McGrath, J., & Brandon, D. (2016). Scholarly publication and social media: Do they have something in common? *Advances in Neonatal Care*, *16*, 245–248.

Moher, D., Hopewell, S., Schulz, K. F., Montori, V., Gøtzsche, P. C., Devereaux, P., Elbourne, D., Egger, M., & Altman, D. G. (2010). CONSORT 2010 explanation and elaboration: Updated guidelines for reporting parallel-group randomised trials. *British Medical Journal*, *340*, c869.

Moher, D., Liberati, A., Tetzlaff, J., Altman, D., & PRISMA Group. (2009). Preferred reporting items for systematic reviews and meta-analyses: The PRISMA statement. *British Medical Journal*, *339*, b2535.

Möhler, R., Köpke, S., & Meyer, G. (2015). Criteria for reporting the development and evaluation of complex interventions in healthcare: Revised guideline (CReDECI 2). *Trials*, *16*, 204.

Montgomery, P., Grant, S., Hopewell, S., Macdonald, G., Moher, D., Michie, S., & Mayo-Wilson, E. (2013). Protocol for CONSORT-SPI: An extension for social and psychological interventions. *Implementation Science*, *8*, 99.

Northam, S., Greer, D., Rath, L., & Toone, A. (2014). Nursing journal editor survey results to help nurses publish. *Nurse Educator*, *39*(6), 290–297.

O'Brien, B., Harris, I., Beckman, T., Reed, D., & Cook, D. (2014). Standards for reporting qualitative research: A synthesis of recommendations. *Academic Medicine*, *89*(9), 1245–1251.

Oermann, M.. (2023). *Writing for publication in nursing* (5th ed.). Springer Publication.

Oermann, M., Conklin, J., Nicoll, L., Chinn, P., Ashton, K., Edie, A., Amarasekara, S., & Budinger, S. C. (2016). Study of predatory open access nursing journals. *Journal of Nursing Scholarship*, *48*(6), 624–632.

Oermann, M. H., Nicoll, L. H., Carter-Templeton, H., Woodward, A., Kidayi, P. L., Neal, L. B., Edie, A. H., Ashton, K. S., Chinn, P. L., & Amarasekara, S. (2019). Citations of articles in predatory nursing journals. *Nursing Outlook*, *67*(6), 664–670. https://doi.org/10.1016/j.outlook.2019.05.001

Oermann, M., Nicoll, L., Chinn, P., Ashton, K., Conklin, J., Edie, A., Amarasekara, S., & Williams, B. L. (2018). Quality of articles published in predatory nursing journals. *Nursing Outlook*, *66*(1), 4–10.

Ogrinc, G., Davies, L., Goodman, D., Batalden, P., Davidoff, F., & Stevens, D. (2015). SQUIRE 2.0 (Standards for QUality Improvement Reporting Excellence): Revised publication guidelines from a detailed consensus process. *Journal of Nursing Care Quality*, *31*, 1–8.

Pandis, N., Chung, B., Scherer, R., Elbourne, D., & Altman, D. (2017). CONSORT 2010 statement: Extension checklist for reporting within person randomised trials. *British Medical Journal*, *357*, j2835.

Pearce, P., & Ferguson, L. (2017). How to write abstracts for manuscripts, presentations, and grants: Maximizing information in a 30-s sound bite world. *Journal of the American Association of Nurse Practitioners*, *29*(8), 452–460.

Penders, B. (2018). Ten simple rules for responsible referencing. *PLoS Computational Biology*, *14*(4), e1006036.

Piaggio, G., Elbourne, D., Pocock, S., Evans, S., Altman, D., & CONSORT Group. (2012). Reporting of noninferiority and equivalence randomized trials: Extension of the CONSORT 2010 statement. *Journal of the American Medical Association*, *308*(24), 2594–2604.

Pinnock, H., Barwick, M., Carpenter, C., Eldridge, S., Grandes, G., Griffiths, C., Rycroft-Malone, J., Meissner, P., Murray, E., Patel, A., Sheikh, A., Taylor, S. J. C., StaRI Group, & Taylor, S. (2017). Standards for reporting Implementation studies (StaRI): Explanation and elaboration document. *BMJ Open*, *7*(4), e013318.

Polit, D. F., & Gillespie, B. (2010). Intention-to-treat in randomized controlled trials: Recommendations for a total trial strategy. *Research in Nursing & Health*, *58*, 391–399.

Polit, D. F., & Northam, S. (2011). Impact factors in nursing journals. *Nursing Outlook*, *59*(1), 18–28.

Roush, K. (2016). *A nurse's step-by-step guide to writing your dissertation or capstone*. Sigma Theta Tau.

Roush, K. (2017a). Becoming a published writer. *American Journal of Nursing*, *117*(3), 63–66.

Roush, K. (2017b). Writing your manuscript: Structure and style. *American Journal of Nursing*, *117*(4), 56–61.

Roush, K. (2017c). What types of articles to write. *American Journal of Nursing*, *117*(5), 68–71.

Roush, K. (2017d). Navigating the publishing process. *American Journal of Nursing*, *117*(6), 62–67.

Saver, C. (2021). *Anatomy of writing for publication in nursing* (4th ed.). Sigma Theta Tau International.

Siedlecki, S. L. (2017). Original research: How to create a poster that attracts an audience. *American Journal of Nursing, 117*(3), 48–54.

Siedlecki, S. L. (2022). Presenting your research findings: Tips from a conference chair. *Clinical Nurse Specialist, 36*(5), 233–240. https://doi.org/10.1097/NUR.0000000000000692

Silvia, P. (2018). *How to write a lot: A practical guide to productive academic writing.* American Psychological Association.

Southgate, A. (2022). Writing for publication: Responding to peer review feedback. *British Journal of Nursing, 31*(3), 180. https://doi.org/10.12968/bjon.2022.31.3.180

Stroup, D., Berlin, J., Morton, S., Olkin, I., Williamson, G., Rennie, D., Moher, D., Becker, B. J., Sipe, T. A., & Thacker, S. (2000). Meta-analysis of observational studies in epidemiology: A proposal for reporting. *Journal of the American Medical Association, 283*, 208–2012.

Strunk, W., & Campbell, V. (2018). *The elements of style: Simplified & illustrated for busy people.* Campbell & Co. Literary.

Sullivan-Bolyai, S., Ratta, C. D., Flanagan, J., Pudasainee-Kapri, S., & Sefcik, J. S. (2022). Salami slicing and other fatal flaws to avoid in publishing qualitative findings. *Journal of Pediatric Nursing, 66*, A9–A10. https://doi.org/10.1016/j.pedn.2022.08.003

Thorne, S. (2021). On the use and abuse of verbatim quotations in qualitative research reports. *Nurse Author & Editor, 30*(3), 4–6. https://doi.org/10.1111/nae2.2

Tong, A., Flemming, K., McInnes, E., Oliver, S., & Craig, J. (2012). Enhancing transparency in reporting the synthesis of qualitative research: ENTREQ. *BMC Medical Research Methodology, 12*, 181.

Tong, A., Sainsbury, P., & Craig, J. (2007). Consolidated criteria for reporting qualitative research (COREQ): A 32-item checklist for interviews and focus groups research (COREQ)—A 32-item checklist for interviews and focus groups. *International of Journal of Quality in Health Care, 19*(6), 349–357.

Vohra, S., Shamseer, L., Sampson, M. Bukutu, C., Schmid, C., Tate, R., Nikles, J., Zucker, D. R., Kravitz, R., Guyatt, G., Altman, D. G., Moher, D., & CENT Group. (2016). CONSORT extension for reporting N-of-1 trials (CENT) 2015 statement. *Journal of Clinical Epidemiology, 76*, 9–17.

Von Elm, E., Altman, D., Egger, M., Pocock, S., Gøtzsche, P. C., Vandenbroucke, J., & STROBE Initiative. (2014). The Strengthening the Reporting of Observational studies in Epidemiology (STROBE) statement: Guidelines for reporting observational studies. *International Journal of Surgery, 12*, 1495–1499.

Zwarenstein, M., Treweek, S., Gagnier, J., Altman, D., Tunis, S., Haynes, B., Oxman, A. D., Moher, D., CONSORT Group, Pragmatic Trials in Healthcare Practihc group, & Moher, D. (2008). Improving the reporting of pragmatic trials: An extension of the CONSORT statement. *British Medical Journal, 337*, a2390–a2398.

33 Writing Proposals to Generate Evidence

Learning Objectives

1. Understand the skills required to achieve successful grant funding.
2. Recognize the various sources and types of funding available both through the government and private entities.
3. Be familiar with the NIH as a resource for funding, including the various calls for proposals, application requirements, and deadlines.
4. Appreciate the necessary steps in the process of developing a strong research plan.
5. Realize the importance of peer critique in the development and refinement of the proposal.

INTRODUCTION

Research proposals communicate a research problem and proposed methods of solving it to an interested party. Research proposals are written both by students seeking faculty approval for studies and by researchers seeking financial support. In this chapter, we offer tips on how to improve the quality of research proposals and how to develop proficiency in **grantsmanship**—the set of skills needed to secure research funding.

OVERVIEW OF RESEARCH PROPOSALS

This section provides some general information about research proposals, most of which applies equally to dissertation proposals and grant applications.

Functions of a Proposal

Proposals are a means of opening communication between researchers and other parties. Those parties typically are either funding agencies or faculty advisers, whose job it is to accept or reject the proposed plan or to request modifications. An accepted proposal is a two-way contract: those accepting the proposal are effectively saying, "We are willing to offer our (professional or financial) support for a study that proceeds as proposed," and those writing the proposal are saying, "If you offer support, then the study will be conducted as proposed."

Proposals often serve as the basis for negotiating with other parties as well. For example, a proposal may be shared with administrators when seeking institutional approval to conduct a study (e.g., for gaining access to participants). Proposals may also be incorporated into submissions to research ethics committees or Institutional Review Boards.

Proposals help researchers to clarify their own thinking. By committing ideas to writing, ambiguities are eliminated at an early stage. When proposals are undertaken collaboratively, they help ensure that all parties are "on the same page" about how the study is to proceed. Reviewers also play an important role by suggesting conceptual and methodologic improvements.

Proposal Content

Proposal reviewers want a clear idea of what the researcher plans to study, why the study is needed, what methods will be used to achieve study goals, how and when tasks will be accomplished, and whether the researcher has the skills to complete the project successfully. Proposals are evaluated on a number of criteria, including the importance of the question, the adequacy of the methods, and, if money is requested, the reasonableness of the budget.

Proposal writers are usually given instructions about how to structure proposals. Funding agencies often supply an application kit that includes forms to be completed and specifies the format for organizing proposal content. Universities issue guidelines for dissertation proposals. The content and organization of most proposals are broadly similar to that for a research report, but proposals are written in the future tense (i.e., indicating what the researcher *will* do) and obviously do not include results and conclusions.

Proposals for Qualitative Studies

Preparing a proposal for qualitative research entails special challenges. Methodologic decisions typically evolve in the field, and therefore it is seldom possible to provide thorough information about such matters as sample size or data collection strategies. Sufficient detail needs to be provided, however, so that reviewers gain confidence that the researcher will assemble rich data from a good sample and will do justice to the data collected.

Qualitative researchers must persuade reviewers that the topic is important and worth studying, that they are sufficiently knowledgeable about the challenges of field work and adequately skillful in eliciting rich data, and, in short, that the project would be a good risk.

Resources are available to help qualitative researchers with proposal development. For example, in Terrell's (2022) book *Writing a Proposal for Your Dissertation*, there is a chapter devoted to qualitative research proposals. Another book by Amanfi (2019) focuses on writing a qualitative proposal. A third book by Schneider and Fuller (2018) on writing research proposals in the health sciences incorporates a creative way to describe the step-by-step process of proposal development using the journey of Liang and Natasha, two fictional researchers, who are developing their research proposals. Liang develops a quantitative proposal while Natasha, a midwife, develops a qualitative proposal to study pregnant women's strategies of coping and their impact on fear and anxiety in the first trimester of pregnancy.

TIP DeCuir-Gunby and Schutz (2017) provide guidance on developing proposals for mixed methods studies.

Proposals for Theses and Dissertations

Dissertation proposals are sometimes a bigger hurdle than dissertations themselves. Many doctoral candidates founder at the proposal development stage rather than when writing or defending the dissertation. Much of our advice—especially in our "Tips" section later in the chapter—applies equally to proposals for theses and dissertations as for grant applications, but some additional advice might prove helpful.

The Dissertation Committee

Choosing the right dissertation adviser or chair (if a chair is chosen rather than appointed) is almost as important as choosing the right research topic. The ideal chair is a mentor, an expert with a strong reputation in the field, a good teacher, a patient and supportive coach and critic, and an advocate. Ideally, the chair also has sufficient time and interest to devote to your research and will stick with your project until its completion. This means that it might matter whether the prospective chair has plans for a sabbatical leave or is nearing retirement.

Dissertation committees often involve three or more members. If the chair lacks certain "ideal" characteristics, those characteristics can be balanced across committee members by seeking people with complementary talents. Putting together a group who will work well together can, however, be tricky. Advisers can usually offer suggestions about other committee members.

Once a committee has been formed, it is important to develop a good working relationship with members and to learn about their viewpoints before and during the proposal development stage. This means, at a minimum, becoming familiar with their research and the methodologic strategies they have favored. It also means meeting with them and sounding them out with ideas about topics and methods. If the suggestions from two or more members are at odds, it is prudent to seek your chair's counsel on how to resolve this.

> **TIP** When meeting with your chair and committee members, take notes about their suggestions and write them out in more detail after the meeting while they are still fresh in your mind. The notes should be reviewed while developing the proposal.

Practices vary from one institution to another and from adviser to adviser, but some faculty require a *prospectus* before giving approval to prepare a full proposal. The prospectus is usually a three- to four-page paper outlining the research questions and proposed methods.

Content of Dissertation Proposals

Specific requirements regarding the length and format of dissertation proposals vary in different settings, and it is important to know at the outset what is expected. Typically, dissertation proposals are 20 to 40 pages in length. In some cases, however, committees prefer "mini-dissertations," that is, a document with fully developed sections that can be inserted with minor adaptation into the dissertation itself. For example, the review of the literature, theoretical framework, hypotheses, and the bibliography may be sufficiently refined at the proposal stage that they can be incorporated into the final product.

Literature reviews are often the most important section of a dissertation proposal, at least for quantitative studies. Committees may not desire lengthy literature reviews, but they want to be assured that students are in full command of knowledge in their field of inquiry.

Dissertation proposals sometimes include elements not normally found in proposals to funding agencies. One such element may be table shells (see Chapter 20), which can demonstrate that the student knows how to analyze data and present results effectively. Another element in proposals is the table of contents for the dissertation. The table of contents serves as an outline for the final product and demonstrates that the student knows how to organize material.

Several books provide additional advice on writing a dissertation proposal, including Hyatt (2023) and Terrell (2022). Bloomberg (2022) has written specifically about qualitative dissertations.

FUNDING FOR RESEARCH PROPOSALS

Funding for research projects is becoming increasingly difficult to obtain because of keen competition. Successful proposal writers need to have good research and proposal-writing skills, and they must also know from whom funding is available. Ahn and Reifsnider (2021) offered specific recommendations on how to develop successful grant proposals for nursing research. Wisdom et al. (2015), in their synthesis of grant-writing advice in 53 papers, emphasized the importance of doing appropriate background investigation to identify the goals and missions of potential funders.

> **TIP** Because competition for research funding is fierce, Conn and colleagues (2015) suggested creative approaches to undertaking "science on a shoestring"—that is, research that is less costly to carry out. Examples include secondary analyses, research using data from electronic health records or social media, and collaborative efforts involving *practice-based research networks* (PRBNs).

Government Funding

Government Funding in the United States

The largest funder of research activities in the United States is the federal government. For healthcare researchers, the National Institutes of Health (NIH), the Agency for Healthcare Research and Quality (AHRQ), and the Patient-Centered Outcomes Research Institute (PCORI) are leading agencies. Two major types of federal disbursements are grants and contracts. **Grants** are awarded for studies conceived by researchers themselves, whereas **contracts** are for studies desired by the government.

There are several mechanisms for NIH grants, which can be awarded to researchers in both domestic and foreign institutions. Most grant applications are unsolicited and reflect the research interests of individual researchers. Unsolicited applications should be consistent with the broad objectives of an NIH institute, such as the National Institute of Nursing Research (NINR). Investigator-initiated applications are submitted in response to **Parent Announcements**, which are covered under omnibus *Funding Opportunity Announcements* (FOAs).

NIH also issues periodic **Program Announcements** (PAs) that describe new, continuing, or expanded program interests. For example, in January 2023, NINR issued a PA titled "Addressing the Impact of Structural Racism and Discrimination on Minority Health and Health Disparities" (PAR-23-112). The purpose of this PA, which expires in 2026, is to encourage applications for projects that "support intervention research that addresses structural racism and discrimination (SRD) in order to improve minority health or reduce health disparities."

Another grant mechanism allows federal agencies to identify a *specific* topic area in which they are interested in receiving proposals. **Requests for Applications** (RFAs) are one-time opportunities with a single submission date. As an example, NIH issued an RFA titled "The Intersection of Sex and Gender Influences on Health and Disease" (RFA-OD-22-028) in October 2022, with grant applications due November 2024. The purpose of the RFA is "to invite R01 applications on the influence and intersection of sex and gender in health and disease." The *NIH Guide for Grants and Contracts* (available online at https://grants.nih.gov/funding/index.htm) contains announcements about RFAs, PAs, and Parent Announcements.

Some federal agencies—notably PCORI—award contracts to do specific studies. Contract offers are announced in a **Request for Proposals** (RFPs), which details the study that the government wants. Contracts, which are often awarded to only one competitor, constrain researchers' activities. Federal RFPs are announced in Federal Business Opportunities (https://www.fbo.gov/) or on the agencies' websites.

> **TIP** Kulage et al. (2015) have pointed out the very high costs associated with applying for NIH grants. An analysis in one school of nursing indicated that costs per grant application ranged from about $5,000 to $13,500.

Government Funding in Countries Other Than the United States

Government funding for nursing research is also available in many other countries. In Canada, for example, various types of health research are sponsored by the Canadian Institutes of Health Research. In Australia, major government funding for health research comes from the National Health and Medical Research Council. In the United Kingdom, the major funder of health research is the Medical Research Council.

Private Funds

Healthcare research is supported by numerous philanthropic foundations, professional organizations, and corporations. Many researchers prefer private funding rather than government support because there is less "red tape."

Information about philanthropic foundations that support research in the United States is available through the Foundation Center (http://foundationcenter.org). A comprehensive resource for identifying funding opportunities is the Center's *Foundation Directory*, available online for a fee. The directory lists the purposes and activities of foundations and information for contacting them. The Foundation Center also offers seminars and training on grant-writing and funding opportunities in many locations in the United States. Another resource for information on funding is the Community of Science's database on funding opportunities. Hassmiller (2017) noted that it may be easier to get initial funding from smaller regional foundations; the United Philanthropy Forum is a resource for such foundations.

> **TIP** The Robert Wood Johnson Foundation has been an especially strong supporter of nursing projects. It funds research to support a collaborative framework called a Culture of Health, which has as its goal that each person is able to live the healthiest life possible (Hassmiller, 2017).

Professional associations (e.g., the American Nurses' Foundation, Sigma Theta Tau, the American Association of Critical-Care Nurses) offer funds for conducting research. Health organizations, such as the American Heart Association and the American Cancer Society, also support research activities.

Finally, research funding is sometimes donated by private corporations, particularly those dealing with healthcare products. The Foundation Center publishes a directory of corporate grantmakers and provides links through its website to corporate philanthropic programs. Additional information about corporate requirements and interests should be obtained from the organization directly or from staff in the research administration offices of the institution with which you are affiliated. Conn and colleagues (2015) also noted that the local business community, which prefers supporting local causes, may be another resource worth exploring.

GRANT APPLICATIONS TO NIH

NIH funds many nursing studies through NINR and other institutes. Because of the importance of NINR as a funding source for nurse researchers, this section describes the process of proposal submission and review at NIH. AHRQ, which also funds nurse-initiated studies, uses the same application kit and similar procedures. Although the specifics of applying for funding vary across funders, many of the points made in this section are relevant for other funding sources.

> **TIP** NIH has 27 institutes and centers that make grant awards, each of which has a website that explains its mission and priorities (e.g., for NINR: https://www.ninr.nih.gov/aboutninr/what-we-do). If you have an idea for a study and are not sure which type of grant program is suitable—or are unsure whether NINR or another NIH institute might be interested—you should contact NINR directly (Telephone number: 301-496-0207, email: info@ninr.nih.gov). NINR Program Officers can provide feedback about whether your proposed study matches NINR's program interests.

Types of NIH Grants and Awards

NIH awards different types of grants, and each has its own objectives and review criteria. The basic grant program—and the primary funding mechanism for independent research—is the traditional **Research Project Grant (R01)**. The objective of R01 grants is to support specific projects in areas reflecting the interests and competencies of a Principal Investigator (PI) and their team. It is NIH's most commonly used grant program. Note that there are two separate Parent Announcements for R01 grants—one for clinical trials and one for other types of projects.

Three other grant programs available through NIH are worth noting. A special program (R15) has been established for researchers working in institutions that have not been major participants in NIH programs. These **Academic Research Enhancement Awards (AREAs)** are designed to stimulate research in institutions that provide baccalaureate training for many individuals who go on to do health-related research. There is also a **Small Grant Program** (R03) that provides support for pilot or feasibility studies, methodology development, and secondary analyses. R03 grants provide a maximum of $50,000 of direct support for up to 2 years and are not renewable. Finally, the R21 grant mechanism—the **Exploratory/Developmental Research Grant Award**—is intended to encourage new, exploratory, and developmental projects by providing support for early stages of research.

NIH and other agencies also offer individual and institutional predoctoral and postdoctoral fellowships, as well as career development awards. Individual fellowship mechanisms available through the National Research Service Award (NRSA) program within NINR include the following:

- F31, Ruth Kirschstein Individual Predoctoral NRSA Fellowships, support nurses in a supervised training leading to a doctoral degree in areas related to the NINR mission.
- F32, Ruth Kirschstein Individual Postdoctoral NRSA Fellowships, support postdoctoral training to nurses to broaden their scientific background.

> **TIP** Advice on developing a proposal for an NRSA (F31) fellowship has been offered in a paper by Rawl (2014).

Three important Career Development Awards offered through NINR are as follows:

- K01, Mentored Research Scientist Development Award, available to doctorally prepared scientists who would benefit from a mentored experience with an expert sponsor
- K23, Mentored Patient-Oriented Research Career Development Award, supports the career development of investigators who are committed to focusing on patient-oriented research
- K99, Pathway to Independence Awards, provides for postdoctoral research activity leading to the submission of an independent research project application

> **TIP** Botham et al. (2017) have described "10 simple rules" for preparing a career development award proposal. Also, Lor et al. (2019) have prepared a resource guide for postdoctoral opportunities for nurses.

NIH Forms and Processing Schedule

The SF424 application form, accessed through the online portal Grants.gov, is used for the types of grants and awards described in the previous section, although supplemental components are needed for some of them. Researchers use Adobe Reader to "fill in" and complete this application. There is abundant information online about the application process, and NIH offers training sessions on how to submit applications electronically. Several options can be used to submit an application, one of which is the use the NIH ASSIST system to prepare and submit the application and another is to use an institutional system-to-system process.

New grant applications are usually processed in three cycles annually. Different types of grants have different deadlines, as shown in Table 33.1. For most new applications, except fellowships in the F series and AIDS-related research, the deadline for receipt is in February, June, and October. The scientific merit review dates are about 4 to 5 months after each submission date. For example, applications submitted for the February cycle are reviewed in June or July; the earliest project start date for applications funded in that cycle would be in September or December (depending on when the applications are reviewed by the NIH Advisory Council). Individual applicants should begin a registration process through the Electronic Research Administration (eRA) Commons at least 6 weeks prior to the submission date. Once submitted, applications can be tracked through eRA Commons (https://www.era.nih.gov/).

Preparing a Grant Application for NIH

Although many substantive aspects of the NIH grant application have remained stable, the forms and procedures for NIH grant applications have been changing. It is crucial to carefully review up-to-date instructions for grant application submission rather than relying on information in this chapter.

Forms: Screens and Uploaded Attachments

The SF424 form set has numerous components. The "front matter" of SF424 consists of various forms that appear on a series of fillable screens. These forms help in processing the application. Some of the major forms include the following:

- *SF424 Form.* This form, used in all grant applications, collects information about the type of submission, type of applicant, proposed project dates, and other administrative data. Applicants must also state a brief descriptive title of the project.

TABLE 33.1 • Schedule for Selected New Research Applications, National Institutes of Health

APPLICATION DUE DATE[a]	MECHANISM OF SUPPORT (TYPE OF AWARD)				
	R01 (NEW)	R03, R21	R15	K SERIES	F SERIES
Cycle I[b]	February 5	February 16	February 25	February 12	April 8
Cycle II[c]	June 5	June 16	June 25	June 12	August 8
Cycle III[d]	October 5	October 16	October 25	October 12	December 8

[a]Note: AIDS-related applications are on a different schedule: May 7, September 7, January 7 for new applications.
[b]Cycle I: Scientific Merit Review: June–July; Earliest start date: September or December.
[c]Cycle II: Scientific Merit Review: October–November; Earliest start date: April.
[d]Cycle III: Scientific Merit Review: February–March; Earliest start date: July.

TIP The project title should be given careful thought. It is the first thing that reviewers see and should be crafted to create a good impression. The title, which is limited to 200 characters, should be concise, informative, and should also be compelling.

- *R&R Other Project Information Form.* This form is the mechanism for submitting key information for all grant applications. The form begins with questions about human subjects and vertebrate animals. The last few items require attachments to be uploaded, including a project summary, a project narrative, bibliography, and facilities and equipment information. Attachments, which must be in PDF format, have strict size limitations. The **Project Summary** serves as a succinct description of aims and methods of the proposed study and must be no longer than 30 lines. The **Project Narrative** is a brief (two to three sentences) description of the relevance of the research to public health. The *Bibliography* is a list of references cited in the research plan; any reference style is acceptable. The *Facilities* attachment is used to describe needed and available resources (e.g., laboratories). The *Equipment* attachment is used to list major items of equipment already available for the project.
- *Senior/Key Person Profile Form.* For each key person, the form requests basic identifying information and calls for an attachment, a Biographical Sketch. The sketch should list education and training, as well as the following: (1) a Personal Statement describing the qualifications that make the person well suited for their role; (2) Positions and Honors; (3) Contributions to Science in which up to five contributions are described, each of which can provide citations for up to four publications or interim research products relevant to that contribution; and (4) Research Support (ongoing and completed projects) and/or Scholastic Performance. A maximum of five pages is permitted for each person.
- *Budget Form.* For NIH applications, researchers must choose between two budget options—the R&R Budget Component or the PHS 398 Modular Budget Component. Detailed R&R budgets showing specific projected expenses are required if annual direct project costs exceed $250,000.

TIP Cover letters are no longer recommended except under special circumstances (e.g., an application is late and a cover letter explains extraordinary circumstances that caused a delay). Requests to be assigned (or to *not* be assigned) to a particular review group should be submitted on a special form called the PHS Assignment Request Form. This form also allows applicants to identify individuals who should *not* review the application and the reason for such a request.

For grant applications to NIH and other public health service agencies, additional forms referred to as PHS 398 components are required and include the following:

- *PHS 398 Modular Budget Form.* **Modular budgets**, paid in modules of $25,000, are appropriate for R-series applications (e.g., R01s) from domestic organizations requesting $250,000 or less per year of direct costs. (**Direct costs** include specific project-related costs such as staff and supplies; **indirect costs** are institutional **overhead** costs.) This form provides budget fields for annual summaries of projected costs for up to 5 years of support. A *budget justification* attachment, detailing primarily personnel costs, must be uploaded.

> **TIP** Even though modular budget forms ask only for summaries of the funds needed to complete a study, you should prepare a more detailed budget to arrive at a reasonable projection of needed funds. Beginning researchers are likely to require the assistance of a research administrator or an experienced, funded researcher in developing their first budget.

- *PHS 398 Research Plan Form.* The PHS 398 Research Plan form requires information, in the form of attachments, about the proposed study and the research plan. Research plan requirements, the heart of the proposal, are described in the next section.
- *PHS Human Subjects and Clinical Trials Information.* Researchers who plan to collect data from human beings must submit a form relating to the protection of participants. Applicants must either address the involvement of humans and describe protections from research risks or provide a justification for exemption. The application must also include various types of information regarding the inclusion of women, minorities, and children. For example, applicants must complete an Inclusion Enrollment Report and Cumulative Inclusion Enrollment Report, which ask for expectations for enrollment of participants from various racial and ethnic categories, separately by gender. Additional attachments include a recruitment and retention plan and a study timeline. An attachment describing the data safety monitoring plan is required if the proposed study is a clinical trial.

The Research Plan Component

The Research Plan component consists of 12 items, not all of which are relevant to every application—for example, item 1 is an Introduction but is required only for a resubmission or revision. Each item involves uploading a separate PDF attachment. In this section, we briefly describe guidelines for several items, with emphasis on items 2 and 3. We also present some advice based on a study (Inouye & Fiellin, 2005) in which the researchers content analyzed the criticisms in the review sheets of 66 applications (R01s) submitted to a clinical research review group (not NINR). Thus, the advice relating to specific pitfalls is "evidence-based," i.e., based on identified problems in actual applications. To our knowledge, this helpful analysis has not been updated.

Based on their study, Inouye and Fiellin (2005) created a grant-writing checklist designed as a self-assessment tool for proposal developers.

Specific Aims. On this attachment, which is restricted to a single page, researchers must provide a succinct summary of the research problem and the specific objectives of the study, including any hypotheses to be tested. The aims statement should indicate the scope and importance of the problem. Care should be taken to be precise and to identify a problem of manageable proportions. Santen et al. (2017) describe the Specific Aims section as the "jewel in the crown" of a grant proposal—the most important component because reviewers read it first and form an immediate opinion.

Inouye and Fiellin (2005) found that the most frequent critique of the Specific Aims section was that the goals were overstated, overly ambitious, or unrealistic (18% of the reviews). Other complaints were that the project was poorly conceptualized (15%) or that hypotheses were not clearly articulated (12%).

Research Strategy. Unless otherwise specified in an FOA, the Research Strategy section is restricted to 12 pages for R01 and R15 applications and to 6 pages for R03, R21, and F-series applications.

For other funding mechanisms, page restrictions are specified in the FOA.

> **TIP** Career Development Awards (K-series) involve completion of a special form, requiring attachments that include a description of the applicant's background, a statement of career goals and objectives, career development or training activities during the award period, and training in the responsible conduct of research. The applicant's institution and mentor must also submit a letter describing their commitment to the candidate and to their development.

The Research Strategy section is organized into three subsections: Significance, Innovation, and Approach. In the Significance section, researchers must convince reviewers that the proposed study idea has clinical or theoretical relevance and that the study will contribute to scientific knowledge or clinical practice. Applicants should describe how the concepts, treatments, services, or interventions that drive the field will be changed if the project aims are achieved. Researchers describe the study context in this section through a brief analysis of existing knowledge and gaps on the topic. Researchers should demonstrate command of current knowledge in a field, but this section must be very tightly written. Inouye and Fiellin (2005) found that a frequent critique expressed by reviewers about this section was that the need for the study was not adequately justified (29%).

In the Innovation section, researchers should describe how the proposed study challenges, refines, or improves current research or clinical practice paradigms. The application should describe novel theoretical concepts, instrumentation, or interventions to be developed or implemented, and explain their advantage over existing ones. An innovative grant application often proposes approaches to solve a persistent problem in new ways.

The proposed design and methods for the study are described in the third subsection, Approach. This section, which is the heart of the application, should be written with extreme care and reviewed with a self-critical eye. The Approach section needs to be concise but with sufficient detail to persuade reviewers that methodologic decisions are sound and that the study will yield important and reliable evidence.

> **TIP** In 2018, NIH launched initiatives to enhance the accountability and transparency of clinical research—especially for clinical trials. A special website—Research Methods Resources—has been developed that offers help to investigators in satisfying new requirements (https://researchmethodsresources.nih.gov/).

The Approach section typically describes the following: (1) the research design, including comparison group strategies and methods of controlling confounding variables (for qualitative studies, the research tradition should be described); (2) the experimental intervention, if applicable, including a description of the treatment and control group conditions; (3) procedures, such as how participants will be assigned to groups and what type of blinding, if any, will be achieved; (4) the sampling plan, including eligibility criteria and sample size; (5) data collection methods and the measurement properties of measures that will be used; and (6) data analysis strategies. The Approach should identify potential methodologic problems and intended strategies for handling such problems. In proposals for qualitative studies, steps that will be taken to enhance the integrity and trustworthiness of the study should be described.

Inouye and Fiellin (2005) found that *all* of the reviews they analyzed had one or more criticism of this section, the most general of which was that the description of methods was underdeveloped (15%). A few of the most persistent criticisms were as follows:

- Inadequate blinding for outcome assessment (36%)
- Sample was flawed—biased or unrepresentative (36%)
- Important confounding variables inadequately controlled (32%)
- Inadequate sample size or inadequate power calculations (26%)
- Insufficient description of the approach to data analysis (24%)

- Outcome measures inadequately specified or described (23%)

Although some of these concerns relate to clinical trials (e.g., blinding), many have broad relevance. Small sample size, sample biases, and poorly described data collection and analysis plans can be problematic in any type of study.

The Approach section must also include information on Preliminary Studies. In new applications, researchers must describe the PI's preliminary or developmental studies and any experience pertinent to the application. This section must persuade reviewers that you have the skills and background needed to do the research. Any pilot work that has served as a foundation for the proposed project should be described. Inouye and Fiellin's (2005) analysis is especially illuminating with regard to Preliminary Studies. They found that the single biggest criticism across the 66 reviews was that more pilot work was needed, mentioned in 41% of the reviews.

Other Research Plan Sections. Most remaining items of the research plan (items 5-11) are not universally relevant. These include such items as a description and justification of the use of vertebrate animals (item 5) and a leadership plan if there are multiple PIs (item 7). One item (item 9), however, has relevance to many applications: Letters of support. This item requires you to attach letters from individuals agreeing to provide services to the project, such as consultants and collaborators. A letter of support should also be provided from proposed host organizations (preferably on their letterhead), indicating that the project is embraced by the organization and would be supported in moving forward as proposed.

Appendix Materials. In 2017, NIH initiated restrictions on appendix materials. Allowable materials include clinical trial protocols (for clinical trials), blank informed consent forms, and blank questionnaires or data collection instruments. Other items may be included only if the FOA requires it. The consequence of including disallowed items is nonreview of the application.

TIP In terms of content, the research plan for NIH applications is similar to what is required in most research proposals—although emphases and page restrictions may vary and supplementary information may be required.

The Review Process

Grant applications submitted to NIH are reviewed for completeness, relevance, and adherence to instructions by the NIH Center for Scientific Review. Acceptable applications are assigned to an appropriate Institute or Center, and to a peer review group.

NIH uses a sequential, dual review system for informing decisions about its grant applications. The first level involves a panel of peer reviewers (not NIH employees), who evaluate applications for their scientific merit. These review panels are called **scientific review groups** (SRGs) or, more commonly, **study sections**. Each panel consists of about 10 to 20 researchers with backgrounds appropriate to the study section for which they have been selected and usually with a track record of NIH funding. Appointments to the review panels are for 4-year terms and are staggered so that about one-fourth of each panel is new each year.

TIP Applications by nurse researchers usually are assigned to the Nursing and Related Clinical Sciences Study Section (acronym NRCS). However, applications by nurse researchers can be reviewed in other study sections, such as Health Disparities and Equity Promotion (HDEP) or Health Services Organization and Delivery (HSOD).

The second level of review is by a National Advisory Council, which includes scientific and lay representatives. The Advisory Council considers not only the scientific merit of an application but the relevance of the proposed study to the programs and priorities of the Center or Institute to which the application has been submitted, as well as budgetary considerations.

During the first round of review in a study section, applications are assigned to primary and secondary (and sometimes a tertiary) reviewers for detailed analysis. Each assigned reviewer prepares comments and assigns scores according to five core review criteria.

1. *Significance.* Does this study address an important problem? If the aims of the application are achieved, how will scientific knowledge or clinical practice be advanced? What will be the effect of the study on the concepts or methods that drive this field?
2. *Investigator.* Is the PI appropriately trained and well suited to carry out this work? Is the proposed work appropriate to the experience level of the PI and other researchers? Do Early-Stage Investigators have appropriate training and experience?
3. *Innovation.* Does the project employ novel concepts, approaches, or methods? Are the aims original and innovative? Does the project challenge existing paradigms or develop new methods or technologies?
4. *Approach.* Are the overall strategy, design, methods, and analyses adequately developed, and appropriate to the aims of the project? Does the applicant acknowledge potential problem areas and consider alternative tactics?
5. *Environment.* Does the scientific environment in which the work will be done contribute to the probability of success? Do the proposed experiments take advantage of unique features of the scientific environment or employ useful collaborative arrangements?

In addition to these five criteria, other factors are relevant in evaluating proposals, including the adequacy of protections for human or animal subjects and the appropriateness of the sampling plan in terms of including women, minorities, and children as participants. These factors are not, however, formally scored.

Scoring of applications changed in 2010. In the current system, each of the five core criteria is scored on a scale from 1 (exceptional) to 9 (poor). Assigned reviewers score applications and submit their scores before attending a study section meeting and submit a preliminary overall **impact score** (also called a **priority score**) on the same 1 to 9 scale. An impact score reflects a reviewer's assessment of the extent to which the study will exert a powerful influence in an area of research. Based on preliminary impact scores, applications with unfavorable scores (usually those in the lower half) are not discussed or scored by the entire study section in its meeting. This streamlined process was instituted so that study section members could focus their discussion on the most meritorious applications.

For applications that *are* discussed in the meeting, each study section member (not just those who were assigned as reviewers) designates an impact score, based on their own critique of the application and the committee's discussion. Individual impact scores from all committee members are averaged, and the mean is then multiplied by 10 to arrive at a final score. Thus, final impact scores for applications that are discussed can range from 10 (the best possible score) to 90 (the worst possible score). Final scores tend to cluster in the 10 to 50 range, however, because the least meritorious applications were previously screened out and not scored by the full study section. Among the scored applications, only those with the best priority scores actually obtain funding. Cutoff scores for funding vary from institute to institute and year to year, but a score of 20 or lower is usually needed to secure funding.

TIP Some NIH institutes (but not NINR) calculate and publish a *payline*—a percentile-based funding cutoff point for impact scores, up to which nearly all R01 applications are funded.

Within a few days after a study section meeting, applicants can learn their priority score and percentile ranking online via the NIH eRA Commons, and within about 30 days they can access a summary of the evaluation. These **summary statements** include critiques written by the assigned reviewers, a summary of the study section's discussion, study section recommendations, and administrative notes of special consideration (e.g., human subjects issues). All applicants receive a summary sheet, even if their applications were unscored. Applicants of unscored applications also learn how the assigned reviewers scored the five core criteria.

Revisions and Resubmissions

Unless an unfunded proposal is criticized in some fundamental way (e.g., the problem area was not judged to be significant), applications often should be resubmitted, with revisions that reflect the concerns of the peer reviewers. Noble (2017) has offered "10 simple rules" for preparing a response to reviewers. Although his guidance was in relation to reviews of manuscripts submitted to a journal, the advice is also useful for addressing concerns of proposal reviewers. Examples of his tips include respond to every point raised by the reviewer; be polite and respectful of reviewers; and do what the reviewer asks, when possible.

When a proposal is resubmitted, the next review panel members are given a copy of the original application and the summary sheet so that they can evaluate the degree to which concerns have been addressed. Revised applications to NIH can be submitted only once.

TIPS ON PROPOSAL DEVELOPMENT

Although it is impossible to tell you exactly what steps to follow to produce a successful proposal, we conclude this chapter with some advice that might help to improve the process and the product. Many of these tips are especially relevant for those preparing proposals for funding. We draw heavily in this section on the many papers that have appeared in the healthcare literature on writing successful grant proposals and on a synthesis of advice by Wisdom et al. (2015). Further suggestions for writing effective grant applications may be found in Funk and Tornquist (2016), Gerin et al. (2018), and Karsh and Fox (2014).

Things to Do Before Writing Begins

Advance planning is essential to the development of a successful proposal. This section offers suggestions for things you can do to prepare for the actual writing.

Start Early

Writing a proposal and attending to the details of a formal submission process are time consuming and almost always take longer than envisioned. Be sure to budget enough time that the product can be reviewed and rereviewed by members of the team (including any faculty mentors) and by willing colleagues. Build in adequate time for administrative issues such as securing permissions and getting budgets approved.

Having a proposal timeline is a good way to impose discipline on the proposal development process. Figure 33.1 presents one example, but the list of tasks is merely suggestive. Of course, it is advantageous to build pilot or preliminary work into your proposal development schedule, which may add many months to your timeline. As noted earlier, NIH reviewers frequently criticize the absence of adequate pilot work. Incremental knowledge building is attractive to reviewers. When you apply for funding, you are asking funders to make an *investment* in you; they will have the sense of being offered a better investment opportunity if some groundwork for a study has already been completed.

Select an Important Problem

A factor that is critical to the success of a proposal is selecting a problem that has clinical or theoretical significance. The proposal must articulate a persuasive argument that the research could make a contribution to evidence on a topic that is important and appealing to reviewers.

Researchers can sometimes profit by taking advantage of certain "hot topics" that have the special attention of the public and government officials. For example, *patient safety* emerged as a key topic in the early part of this century. Other "buzz words" in healthcare have included *integrated care, patient-centered care,* and *precision medicine* and the more recent focus is on health equity and social determinants of health.

Researchers should be sensitive to social, cultural and political realities. Sometimes there is an emerging hot topic that allows researchers to "catch and ride the wave" (Wiseman et al., 2013, p. 229). In the United States, one way of keeping abreast of emerging health topics is to visit the website for the "Healthy People" initiative that focuses on key health topics for the coming decade. Healthy People 2030 reduced the number of objectives from over

Task	Timeline (Months Before Submission)
	12+ | 12 | 11 | 10 | 9 | 8 | 7 | 6 | 5 | 4 | 3 | 2 | 1
Identify/conceptualize the problem	X
Undertake a literature review	X
Identify and approach possible data collection sites	X
Initiate descriptive or pilot work	X
Analyze pilot data, assess feasibility	XXXXX
Develop a "brief," outlining significance & preliminary thoughts about overall study design	XX
Identify methodologic and content experts; solicit input and possible collaboration	XXX
Begin building a team of co-investigators and consultants	XXXX
Identify and contact funder/program officer (as needed)	XX
Obtain/download all application forms and instructions	XX
Review funding agencies' priorities; review recently funded grants	XXX
Develop research plan, identify instruments, etc.; consult with statisticians, psychometricians, etc., as needed	XXXXXXX
Collect site data for describing site, staff, clients	XXX
Obtain written letters of agreement and/or support from data collection sites	XXX
Prepare an outline of the proposal; develop writing assignments	XX
Write draft of proposal	XXXXXXX
Draft a budget	XX
Draft other ancillary components (bio sketches, etc.)	XX
Review application package internally (team members)	XXX
Make revisions based on review	XXX
Review application package externally by colleagues or mentors; convene mock review	XXX
Review all comments; make final revisions	XXX
Write abstract/summary	XX
Finalize budget and other ancillary components	X
Prepare all final documents, get needed signatures	X

FIGURE 33.1 Example of a grant-writing timeline.

1,000 in Healthy People 2020 to 359 core objectives. More about these can be found here: https://health.gov/healthypeople/objectives-and-data/browse-objectives. Data will now be tracked three times over the decade to monitor the progress of achieving core objectives ranging from "baseline" (progress unknown because only initial data exists) to "getting worse" meaning the target is further away than it was at the beginning of the decade. More about this tracking can be found at https://health.gov/healthypeople/objectives-and-data/about-objectives.

Know Your Audience

Learn as much as possible about the audience for your proposal. For dissertations, this means getting to know your committee members and learning about their expectations, interests, and schedules. If you are writing a proposal for funding, you should obtain information about the funding organization's priorities. It is also a good idea to learn about recently funded projects. For NIH applications, you may be able to learn about the interests and preferred methods of reviewers by finding a roster of study section members for the likely review group.

Another aspect to "knowing your audience" concerns appreciating reviewers' perspective. Reviewers for funding agencies are busy professionals who are taking time away from their own work to consider the merits of proposed new studies. They are likely to be methodologically sophisticated and experts in *their* field—but they may have limited knowledge of your area of research. It is therefore imperative to help time-pressured reviewers to grasp the merits of your proposed study, without relying on jargon or specialized terminology.

Identify and Consult With a Mentor

An experienced grant-writer who is willing to provide guidance and support can play an invaluable role for novice researchers. A mentor may be willing to share their own experience in writing or reviewing proposals. Ideally, you would find a mentor who is willing to discuss early ideas, help you navigate the budgeting process, and review preliminary products. You should also ask your mentor to review your proposal timeline (and then commit to adhering to it). Mentors can often help young researchers through the "what-was-I-thinking" stage of proposal writing (Conn, 2013).

Review a Successful Proposal

Although there is no substitute for actually writing a proposal as a learning experience, novice proposal writers can profit by examining a successful proposal. It is likely that some of your colleagues or fellow students have written a proposal that has been accepted (either by a funding sponsor or by a dissertation committee), and some people are willing to share their successful efforts with others. Also, proposals funded by the government are usually in the public domain—that is, you can ask for a copy of funded proposals. To obtain a funded NIH project, for example, you can contact the NIH Freedom of Information Coordinator for the appropriate institute. An important alternative is to communicate directly with the PI of previously funded projects to inquire if they might be willing to share their proposal with you.

A chapter in the book by DeCuir-Gunby and Schutz (2017) includes a full mixed methods research proposal. Although the proposal is not in a health field and it is longer than proposals to NIH, it offers a useful perspective on good grant writing. Finally, one NIH institute (the National Institute of Allergy and Infectious Diseases) offers sample applications and summary statements for several types of funding mechanisms, such as R01, R03, R15, K01, and F31.

Create a Strong Research Team

For funded research, it is important to think strategically in putting together a team because reviewers often give considerable weight to researchers' qualifications. Having a team of competent people is insufficient—it is necessary to have the right *mix* of competence. Gaps and weaknesses can often be compensated for by the judicious use of consultants.

Another shortcoming of some project teams is that there are too many researchers with small-time commitments. It is unwise to propose a staff with five or more top-level professionals who can contribute only 5% to 10% of their time to the project. Such projects often run into management problems because no one is in control of the work flow. Although collaborative work is commendable, you should be able to justify the inclusion of every person.

Things to Do as You Write

If you have planned well and drafted a realistic schedule, the next step is to move forward with the development of the proposal. Some suggestions for the writing stage follow.

Adhere to Instructions

Funding agencies (and universities) provide instructions on what is required in a research proposal. It is crucial to read these instructions carefully and to follow them precisely. Proposals are sometimes rejected without review if they do not adhere to such guidelines as minimum font size or page limitations.

Build a Clear and Persuasive Case

In a proposal, whether or not funding is sought, you need to persuade reviewers that you are asking the right questions, that you are the right person to ask those questions, and that you will use rigorous methods to obtain valid and credible answers. You must also convince them that the answers will make a difference to nursing and its clients.

Beginning proposal writers sometimes forget that they are *selling* a product: themselves and their ideas. It is appropriate, therefore, to think of the proposal as a marketing opportunity. It is not enough to have a good idea and sound methods—you must have a persuasive presentation. When funding is at stake, the challenge is greater because *other applicants are trying to persuade reviewers that their proposal is more worthy of funding than yours.*

Reviewers know that most applications they review will *not* get funded. For example, in fiscal year 2022, the *success rate* for new and competing grant applications to NINR for a R01 was 18.2%, for an R 15 it was 0%, and R 21 it was 9.9%. (For F-series training grants, the success rate tends to be higher, about 33%–45%.) The reviewers' job is to identify the most scientifically worthy applications. In writing the proposal, you must consciously include features that will put your application in a positive light. That is, you should think of ways to gain a competitive edge. Be sure to give thought to issues persistently identified as problematic by reviewers (Inouye & Fiellin, 2005) and use a well-conceived checklist to ensure that you have not missed an opportunity to strengthen your proposal.

The proposal should be written in a positive, self-assured tone. If you do not sound convinced that the proposed study is important and will be rigorously done, then reviewers will not be persuaded either. It is unwise to promise what cannot be achieved, but you should think about ways to create enthusiasm.

Justify Methodologic Decisions

Many proposals fail because they do not instill confidence that key decisions have a good rationale. Methodologic decisions should be made carefully, keeping in mind the benefits and drawbacks of alternatives, and a compelling—if brief—justification should be provided. To the extent possible, make your decisions evidence-based and *defend* the proposed methods with citations demonstrating their utility. Insufficient detail and scanty explanation of methodologic choices can be perilous, although page constraints often make full elaboration impossible.

Address the Review Criteria

As you write, be conscious of the review criteria and emphasize the parts of the proposal that are relevant to those criteria. Every paragraph should be scrutinized to evaluate whether it addresses at least one of the criteria by which the proposal will be judged. If you ask others to review the proposal, be sure that they understand the review criteria.

Begin and End With a Flourish

The abstract or summary to the proposal should be crafted with extreme care. Because it is one of the first things that reviewers read, you need to be sure that it will create a favorable impression. (For NIH applications, nonassigned reviewers may read *only* the summary and not the entire application.) The ideal abstract is one that generates excitement and inspires confidence in the proposed study's rigor. Although abstracts appear at the beginning of a proposal, they are often written last.

Proposals typically conclude with material that is somewhat unexciting, such as a data analysis plan. A brief, upbeat concluding paragraph that summarizes the significance and innovativeness of the proposed project can help to remind reviewers of its potential to contribute to nursing practice and nursing science.

Pay Attention to Presentation

Reviewers are put in a better frame of mind if the proposals they read are well organized, grammatical, and easy to read. Glitzy figures are not needed, but the presentation should be professional and show respect for weary reviewers. In Inouye and Fiellin's (2005) study, 20% of the grant applications were criticized for such presentation issues as typographical or grammatical errors, poor layout, inconsistencies, and omitted tables.

Have the Proposal Critiqued

Before formal submission of a proposal, a draft should be reviewed by others. Reviewers should be selected for both substantive and methodologic expertise. If the proposal is being submitted for funding, one reviewer ideally would have first-hand knowledge of the funding source. If a consultant has been proposed because of specialized expertise that you believe will strengthen the study, they should be asked to participate by reviewing the draft and making recommendations for its improvement.

In universities, mock review panels are often convened prior to submission to a funding agency. Faculty and students are invited to these mock reviews and provide valuable feedback for enhancing a proposal. Kulage and Larson (2018) found, in one school of nursing, that applications that had undergone a mock review had a significantly higher rate of funding than those that had not. They describe protocols for mock reviews.

RESEARCH EXAMPLES

NIH makes available the abstracts of all funded projects through its Research Portfolio Online Reporting Tools (RePORTER). Abstracts can be searched by subject, researcher, institute, type of funding mechanism, year of support, and so on. Abstracts for two projects funded through NINR are presented here.

Example of a Funded Clinical Trial (R01) Project

Dr. Hyochol Ahn, who is the associate dean for research and professor at Florida State University's College of Nursing, prepared the following abstract for the project entitled "Combination Therapy of Home-based Transcranial Direct Current Stimulation and Mindfulness-based Meditation for Self-management of Clinical Pain and Symptoms in Older Adults with Knee Osteoarthritis." The project was reviewed by the Clinical Management of Patients in Community-based Settings Study Section panel and received NINR funding in April 2020. The project is scheduled for completion in January 2024. The total funding for this project is $476,652.

Project Summary: The long-term goal of this project is to improve clinical pain and symptoms for older adults with knee osteoarthritis (OA) using home-based nonpharmacological approaches. Knee OA is one of the most common pain conditions among people over 45 years old, and the management of OA pain is challenging because existing pharmacological approaches often produce significant adverse events, and the treatment benefits may decrease over time. Also, knee OA pain is characterized by increased pain-related brain activation, possibly explaining the limited success of existing peripherally based treatments that target the pain locally in the area of the knee. Therefore, innovative nonpharmacological interventions targeting pain-related brain function are needed. Two nonpharmacological pain treatments, transcranial direct current stimulation (tDCS), and mindfulness-based meditation (MBM) have been shown to improve pain-related brain function in older adults with knee OA. The rationale for the proposed research is that because tDCS promotes neuroplasticity, it may potentiate the effect of MBM, which also stimulates adaptive changes in the brain. However, no investigations to date have examined whether remotely supervised tDCS paired with MBM at home can enhance pain-related brain function and reduce OA-related clinical pain and symptoms. Home-based interventions are critical because older adults with knee OA have limited mobility, and recent technological advances have created the potential for home interventions with real-time monitoring through a secure videoconferencing platform. The central hypothesis is that remotely supervised tDCS paired with MBM at home will decrease clinical pain and OA-related clinical symptoms, improve physiopsychological pain processing, and increase participant satisfaction with treatment. This hypothesis will be tested by pursuing the following specific aims: determine the effects of active tDCS paired with active MBM on clinical pain and OA-related clinical symptoms (specific aim 1); determine the effects of active tDCS paired with active MBM on physiopsychological pain processing (specific aim 2); and determine the effects of active tDCS paired with active MBM on participant satisfaction with treatment (specific aim 3). The proposed study will directly investigate the effects of remotely supervised tDCS paired with MBM at home in 200 older adults with symptomatic knee OA using a double-blind, randomized, sham-controlled, phase II parallel group (1:1:1:1 for four groups defined by 2×2 factorial design) design. The proposed research is significant because it is expected to provide valuable insight into an exciting new modality of nonpharmacological pain self-management that is extremely easy, safe, and noninvasive with minimal side effects.

Example of a Funded Mixed Methods Training (F31) Project

Amy Goh, a doctoral student at Boston College, submitted a successful application for an NRSA predoctoral (F31) fellowship. The project was funded by NINR in June 2023 and is scheduled to end in June 2024. She prepared the following abstract for a study entitled "Respectful Communication and Patient Portal Usage in Pregnant People of Color."

Project Summary: Pregnant people of color consistently report poor communication, being dismissed, ignored, discriminated against, and disrespected. Racially-based mistreatment contributes to worse experiences and increased labor interventions. Improvements in patient-provider communication (PPC) are urgently needed in prenatal care. With the increasing numbers of digital modalities, such as the patient portal, it is essential to examine the impact of these digital tools on PPC. Patient portals have emerged as an effective and valuable strategy to improve PPC providers in the general population. Research on patient portal usage in the general population, including in pregnant people, demonstrates lower portal usage in communities of color creating the digital divide. One aspect of this divide is digital health literacy (DHL). Few studies have examined DHL in pregnancy in the United States. No study has examined the relationship between PPC, patient portal usage and DHL in pregnant people of color. With the persistent perinatal health inequities and the rapid integration of digital health tools, the time is now to better understand PPC, patient portal usage, and DHL in pregnant people of color. The long-term goal of the proposed research is to improve respect and quality in perinatal care through the creation of an inclusive, culturally relevant digital health intervention to address PPC for pregnant people of color. The specific aims are Aim 1—quantify the relationships between PPC, patient portal usage, and DHL in pregnant people of color; and Aim 2—identify the facilitators and barriers to optimal digital communication in pregnant people of color. This multimethod study will recruit 130 self-identified pregnant people of color from an urban safety net hospital. Survey data will be collected on demographic and clinical information, as well as participant perceptions of PPC in pregnancy, patient portal usage, and DHL. Exploratory qualitative questions will be posed at the end of the survey to inquire about facilitators and barriers to optimal digital PPC. For Aim 1, regression analysis will examine the associations among respectful PPC, DHL, and patient portal usage in pregnant people of color, after controlling for covariates. In Aim 2, thematic analysis will be applied to understand how optimal communication develops through patient portal utilization by individual experiences of the participants. This research is significant because it proposes to examine a potentially modifiable influence on PPC, a public health priority. This study addresses the NINR's research lenses to advance health equity and social determinants of health research. Without data on how PPC within the patient portal and utilization barriers faced by pregnant people of color, the benefit of this digital modality will be inequitable and disparities exacerbated.

SUMMARY POINTS

- A **research proposal** is a written document specifying what a researcher intends to study; proposals are written by students seeking approval for dissertations and theses and by researchers seeking financial or institutional support. The set of skills associated with developing proposals for funding is called **grantsmanship**.
- Preparing proposals for qualitative studies is especially challenging because some methodologic decisions are made in the field; qualitative proposals need to persuade reviewers that the proposed study is important and a good risk.
- Students preparing a proposal for a dissertation or thesis need to work closely with a well-chosen committee and chair. Dissertation proposals are sometimes "mini-dissertations" that include sections that can be incorporated into the dissertation.
- The federal government is the largest source of research funds for health researchers in the United States. Regular grants programs are

- described through **Parent Announcements** (which are covered under *Funding Opportunity Announcements* or FOAs). Federal agencies such as the National Institutes of Health (NIH) also announce special opportunities in the form of **Program Announcements (PAs)** and **Requests for Applications (RFAs)** for **grants** and **Requests for Proposals (RFPs)** for **contracts**.
- Nurses can apply for a variety of grants from NIH, the most common being **Research Project Grants** (R01 grants), **AREA Grants** (R15), **Small Grants** (R03), or **Exploratory/Developmental Grants** (R21). NIH also awards training fellowships through the National Research Service Award (NRSA) program as F-series awards and Career Development Awards (K-series awards).
- Grant applications to NIH are submitted online using the SF424, which has a series of special forms (fillable screens) that require uploaded PDF attachments.
- The heart of an NIH grant application is the **research plan component**, which includes two major sections for new applications: *Specific Aims* and *Research Strategy*. The latter, which is restricted to 12 pages for R01 applications, includes subsections called Significance, Innovation, and Approach.
- NIH grant applications also require budgets, which can be abbreviated **modular budgets** if requested funds for R01 grants do not exceed $250,000 in direct costs per year.
- Grant applications to NIH are reviewed three times a year in a dual-review process. The first phase involves peer review by a **scientific review group** (SRG, usually called a **study section**) that evaluates each proposal's scientific merit; the second phase is a review by an Advisory Council.
- In NIH's review procedure, the study section assigns **priority (impact) scores** only to applications judged to be in the top half of proposals based on a preliminary appraisal by assigned reviewers. A final priority score of 10 by the study section is the best possible score and 90 is the poorest score.
- All applicants for NIH grants are sent a **summary statement**, which offers a critique of the proposal. Applicants of scored proposals also receive information on the impact/priority score and percentile ranking.
- Some suggestions for writing a strong proposal include several for the planning stage (e.g., starting early, selecting an important topic, learning about the audience, reviewing a successful proposal, creating a strong team) and several for the writing stage (adhering to proposal instructions, building a persuasive case, justifying methodologic decisions, ensuring that review criteria are addressed, beginning and ending with a flourish, and having the draft proposal critiqued by reviewers).

REFERENCES CITED IN CHAPTER 33

Ahn, H., & Reifsnider, E. (2021). A guide to writing grant proposals for nursing research. *Research. In Nursing & Health*, *44*(4), 596–597.

Amanfi, M. (2019). *Step-by-step guide on writing the proposal: Using the qualitative methodology.* Independent Publisher.

Bloomberg, L. (2022). *Completing your qualitative dissertation: A road map from beginning to end* (5th ed.). Sage.

Botham, C., Arribere, J., Brubaker, S., & Beier, K. (2017). Ten simple rules for writing a career development award proposal. *PLoS Computational Biology*, *13*(12), e1005863.

Conn, V. (2013). Welcome to the dark side of grant writing. *Western Journal of Nursing Research*, *35*(8), 967–969.

Conn, V., Topp, R., Dunn, S., Hopp, L., Jadack, R., Jansen, D., Jefferson, U Moch, S. D. (2015). Science on a shoestring: Building nursing knowledge with limited funding. *Western Journal of Nursing Research*, *37*(10), 1256–1268.

DeCuir-Gunby, J., & Schutz, P. (2017). *Developing a mixed methods proposal: A practical guide for beginning researchers.* Sage.

Funk, S. G., & Tornquist, E. M. (2016). *Writing winning proposals for nurses and health care professionals.* Springer Publishing Co.

Gerin, W., Kinkade, C., & Page, N. (2018). *Writing the NIH grant proposal: A step-by-step guide* (3rd ed.). Sage.

Hassmiller, S. B. (2017). How to engage funders and get money: The 10Rs you need to know. *American Journal of Nursing*, *117*(4), 63–65.

Hyatt, L. (2023). *The dissertation journey: A practical guide to planning, writing, and defending your dissertation* (4th ed.). Sage.

Inouye, S. K., & Fiellin, D. A. (2005). An evidence-based guide to writing grant proposals for clinical research. *Annals of Internal Medicine*, *142*(4), 274–282.

Karsh, E., & Fox, A. (2014). *The only grant-writing book you'll ever need* (4th ed.). Basic Books.

Kulage, K., & Larson, E. (2018). Intramural pilot funding and internal grant reviews increase research capacity at a school of nursing. *Nursing Outlook, 66*(1), 11–17.

Kulage, K., Schnall, R., Hickey, K., Travers, J., Zezulinski, K., Torres, F., Burgess, J, Larson, E. L., & Larson, E. (2015). Time and costs of preparing and submitting an NIH grant application at a school of nursing. *Nursing Outlook, 63*(6), 639–649.

Lor, M., Oyesanya, T., Chen, C., Cherwin, C., & Moon, C. (2019). Postdoctoral opportunities for nursing PhD graduates: A resource guide. *Western Journal of Nursing Research, 41*(3), 459–476. https://doi.org/10.1177/0193945918775691

Noble, W. S. (2017). Ten simple rules for writing a response to reviewers. *PLoS Computational Biology, 13*(10), e1005730.

Rawl, S. M. (2014). Writing a competitive individual National research service award (F31) application. *Western Journal of Nursing Research, 36*(1), 31–46.

Santen, R., Barrett, E., Siragy, H., Farhi, L., Fishbein, L., & Carey, R. (2017). The jewel in the crown: Specific aims section of investigator-initiated grant proposals. *Journal of the Endocrine Society, 1*(9), 1194–1202.

Schneider, Z., & Fuller, J. (2018). *Writing research proposals in the health sciences: A step-by-step guide*. Sage.

Terrell, S. R. (2022). *Writing a proposal for your dissertation: Guidelines and examples* (2nd ed.). Gilford Press.

Wisdom, J., Riley, H., & Myers, N. (2015). Recommendations for writing successful grant proposals: An information synthesis. *Academic Medicine, 90*(12), 1720–1725.

Wiseman, J., Alavi, K., & Milner, R. (2013). Grant writing 101. *Clinics in Colon and Rectal Surgery, 26*(4), 228–231.

Appendix:
Statistical Tables of Theoretical Probability Distributions

TABLE A.1 • Critical Values for the *t* Distribution

df	α, 2-Tailed Test:	.10	.05	.02	.01	.001
	α, 1-Tailed Test:	.05	.025	.01	.005	.0005
1		6.314	12.706	31.821	63.657	636.619
2		2.920	4.303	6.965	9.925	31.598
3		2.353	3.182	4.541	5.841	12.941
4		2.132	2.776	3.747	4.604	8.610
5		2.015	2.571	3.376	4.032	6.859
6		1.953	2.447	3.143	3.707	5.959
7		1.895	2.365	2.998	3.449	5.405
8		1.860	2.306	2.896	3.355	5.041
9		1.833	2.262	2.821	3.250	4.781
10		1.812	2.228	2.765	3.169	4.587
11		1.796	2.201	2.718	3.106	4.437
12		1.782	2.179	2.681	3.055	4.318
13		1.771	2.160	2.650	3.012	4.221
14		1.761	2.145	2.624	2.977	4.140
15		1.753	2.131	2.602	2.947	4.073
16		1.746	2.120	2.583	2.921	4.015
17		1.740	2.110	2.567	2.898	3.965
18		1.734	2.101	2.552	2.878	3.922
19		1.729	2.093	2.539	2.861	3.883
20		1.725	2.086	2.528	2.845	3.850
21		1.721	2.080	2.518	2.831	3.819
22		1.717	2.074	2.508	2.819	3.792
23		1.714	2.069	2.500	2.807	3.767
24		1.711	2.064	2.492	2.797	3.745
25		1.708	2.060	2.485	2.787	3.725
26		1.706	2.056	2.479	2.779	3.707
27		1.703	2.052	2.473	2.771	3.690
28		1.701	2.048	2.467	2.763	3.674
29		1.699	2.045	2.462	2.756	3.659
30		1.697	2.042	2.457	2.750	3.646
40		1.684	2.021	2.423	2.704	3.551
60		1.671	2.000	2.390	2.660	3.460
120		1.658	1.980	2.358	2.617	3.373
∞		1.645	1.960	2.326	2.576	3.291

TABLE A.2 • Critical Values for the F Distribution

	α = .05 (Two-Tailed)					α = .025 (One-Tailed)				
df_B / df_W	1	2	3	4	5	6	8	12	24	∞
1	161.4	199.5	215.7	224.6	230.2	234.0	238.9	243.9	249.0	254.3
2	18.51	19.00	19.16	19.25	19.30	19.33	19.37	19.41	19.45	19.50
3	10.13	9.55	9.28	9.12	9.01	8.94	8.84	8.74	8.64	8.53
4	7.71	6.94	6.59	6.39	6.26	6.16	6.04	5.91	5.77	5.63
5	6.61	5.79	5.41	5.19	5.05	4.95	4.82	4.68	4.53	4.36
6	5.99	5.14	4.76	4.53	4.39	4.28	4.15	4.00	3.84	3.67
7	5.59	4.74	4.35	4.12	3.97	3.87	3.73	3.57	3.41	3.23
8	5.32	4.46	4.07	3.84	3.69	3.58	3.44	3.28	3.12	2.93
9	5.12	4.26	3.86	3.63	3.48	3.37	3.23	3.07	2.90	2.71
10	4.96	4.10	3.71	3.48	3.33	3.22	3.07	2.91	2.74	2.54
11	4.84	3.98	3.59	3.36	3.20	3.09	2.95	2.79	2.61	2.40
12	4.75	3.88	3.49	3.26	3.11	3.00	2.85	2.69	2.50	2.30
13	4.67	3.80	3.41	3.18	3.02	2.92	2.77	2.60	2.42	2.21
14	4.60	3.74	3.34	3.11	2.96	2.85	2.70	2.53	2.35	2.13
15	4.54	3.68	3.29	3.06	2.90	2.79	2.64	2.48	2.29	2.07
16	4.49	3.63	3.24	3.01	2.85	2.74	2.59	2.42	2.24	2.01
17	4.45	3.59	3.20	2.96	2.81	2.70	2.55	2.38	2.19	1.96
18	4.41	3.55	3.16	2.93	2.77	2.66	2.51	2.34	2.15	1.92
19	4.38	3.52	3.13	2.90	2.74	2.63	2.48	2.31	2.11	1.88
20	4.35	3.49	3.10	2.87	2.71	2.60	2.45	2.28	2.08	1.84
21	4.32	3.47	3.07	2.84	2.68	2.57	2.42	2.25	2.05	1.81
22	4.30	3.44	3.05	2.82	2.66	2.55	2.40	2.23	2.03	1.78
23	4.28	3.42	3.03	2.80	2.64	2.53	2.38	2.20	2.00	1.76
24	4.26	3.40	3.01	2.78	2.62	2.51	2.36	2.18	1.98	1.73
25	4.24	3.38	2.99	2.76	2.60	2.49	2.34	2.16	1.96	1.71
26	4.22	3.37	2.98	2.74	2.59	2.47	2.32	2.15	1.95	1.69
27	4.21	3.35	2.96	2.73	2.57	2.46	2.30	2.13	1.93	1.67
28	4.20	3.34	2.95	2.71	2.56	2.44	2.29	2.12	1.91	1.65
29	4.18	3.33	2.93	2.70	2.54	2.43	2.28	2.10	1.90	1.64
30	4.17	3.32	2.92	2.69	2.53	2.42	2.27	2.09	1.89	1.62
40	4.08	3.23	2.84	2.61	2.45	2.34	2.18	2.00	1.79	1.51
60	4.00	3.15	2.76	2.52	2.37	2.25	2.10	1.92	1.70	1.39
120	3.92	3.07	2.68	2.45	2.29	2.17	2.02	1.83	1.61	1.25
∞	3.84	2.99	2.60	2.37	2.21	2.09	1.94	1.75	1.52	1.00

TABLE A.2 • Critical Values for the *F* Distribution (Continued)

	α = .01 (Two-Tailed)					α = .005 (One-Tailed)				
df_B / df_W	1	2	3	4	5	6	8	12	24	∞
1	4,052	4,999	5,403	5,625	5,764	5,859	5,981	6,106	6,234	6,366
2	98.49	99.00	99.17	99.25	99.30	99.33	99.36	99.42	99.46	99.50
3	34.12	30.81	29.46	28.71	28.24	27.91	27.49	27.05	26.60	26.12
4	21.20	18.00	16.69	15.98	15.52	15.21	14.80	14.37	13.93	13.46
5	16.26	13.27	12.06	11.39	10.97	10.67	10.29	9.89	9.47	9.02
6	13.74	10.92	9.78	9.15	8.75	8.47	8.10	7.72	7.31	6.88
7	12.25	9.55	8.45	7.85	7.46	7.19	6.84	6.47	6.07	5.65
8	11.26	8.65	7.59	7.01	6.63	6.37	6.03	5.67	5.28	4.86
9	10.56	8.02	6.99	6.42	6.06	5.80	5.47	5.11	4.73	4.31
10	10.04	7.56	6.55	5.99	5.64	5.39	5.06	4.71	4.33	3.91
11	9.65	7.20	6.22	5.67	5.32	5.07	4.74	4.40	4.02	3.60
12	9.33	6.93	5.95	5.41	5.06	4.82	4.50	4.16	3.78	3.36
13	9.07	6.70	5.74	5.20	4.86	4.62	4.30	3.96	3.59	3.16
14	8.86	6.51	5.56	5.03	4.69	4.46	4.14	3.80	3.43	3.00
15	8.68	6.36	5.42	4.89	4.56	4.32	4.00	3.67	3.29	2.87
16	8.53	6.23	5.29	4.77	4.44	4.20	3.89	3.55	3.18	2.75
17	8.40	6.11	5.18	4.67	4.34	4.10	3.78	3.45	3.08	2.65
18	8.28	6.01	5.09	4.58	4.29	4.01	3.71	3.37	3.00	2.57
19	8.18	5.93	5.01	4.50	4.17	3.94	3.63	3.30	2.92	2.49
20	8.10	5.85	4.94	4.43	4.10	3.87	3.56	3.23	2.86	2.42
21	8.02	5.78	4.87	4.37	4.04	3.81	3.51	3.17	2.80	2.36
22	7.94	5.72	4.82	4.31	3.99	3.76	3.45	3.12	2.75	2.31
23	7.88	5.66	4.76	4.26	3.94	3.71	3.41	3.07	2.70	2.26
24	7.82	5.61	4.72	4.22	3.90	3.67	3.36	3.03	2.66	2.21
25	7.77	5.57	4.68	4.18	3.86	3.63	3.32	2.99	2.62	2.17
26	7.72	5.53	4.64	4.14	3.82	3.59	3.29	2.96	2.58	2.13
27	7.68	5.49	4.60	4.11	3.78	3.56	3.26	2.93	2.55	2.10
28	7.64	5.45	4.57	4.07	3.75	3.53	3.23	2.90	2.52	2.06
29	7.60	5.42	4.54	4.04	3.73	3.50	3.20	2.87	2.49	2.03
30	7.56	5.39	4.51	4.02	3.70	3.47	3.17	2.84	2.47	2.01
40	7.31	5.18	4.31	3.83	3.51	3.29	2.99	2.66	2.29	1.80
60	7.08	4.98	4.13	3.65	3.34	3.12	2.82	2.50	2.12	1.60
120	6.85	4.79	3.95	3.48	3.17	2.96	2.66	2.34	1.95	1.38
∞	6.64	4.60	3.78	3.32	3.02	2.80	2.51	2.18	1.79	1.00

(*continued*)

TABLE A.2 • Critical Values for the F Distribution (Continued)

	α = .001 (Two-Tailed)						α = .0005 (One-Tailed)			
df_W \ df_B	1	2	3	4	5	6	8	12	24	∞
1	405,284	500,000	540,379	562,500	576,405	585,937	598,144	610,667	623,497	636,619
2	998.5	999.0	999.2	999.2	999.3	999.3	999.4	999.4	999.5	999.5
3	167.5	148.5	141.1	137.1	134.6	132.8	130.6	128.3	125.9	123.5
4	74.14	61.25	56.18	53.44	51.71	50.53	49.00	47.41	45.77	44.05
5	47.04	36.61	33.20	31.09	29.75	28.84	27.64	26.42	25.14	23.78
6	35.51	27.00	23.70	21.90	20.81	20.03	19.03	17.99	16.89	15.75
7	29.22	21.69	18.77	17.19	16.21	15.52	14.63	13.71	12.73	11.69
8	25.42	18.49	15.83	14.39	13.49	12.86	17.04	11.19	10.30	9.34
9	22.86	16.39	13.90	12.56	11.71	11.13	10.37	9.57	8.72	7.81
10	21.04	14.91	12.55	11.28	10.48	9.92	9.20	8.45	7.64	6.76
11	19.69	13.81	11.56	10.35	9.58	9.05	8.35	7.63	6.85	6.00
12	18.64	12.97	10.80	9.63	8.89	8.38	7.71	7.00	6.25	5.42
13	17.81	12.31	10.21	9.07	8.35	7.86	7.21	6.52	5.78	4.97
14	17.14	11.78	9.73	8.62	7.92	7.43	6.80	6.13	5.41	4.60
15	16.59	11.34	9.34	8.25	7.57	7.09	6.47	5.81	5.10	4.31
16	16.12	10.97	9.00	7.94	7.27	6.81	6.19	5.55	4.85	4.06
17	15.72	10.66	8.73	7.68	7.02	6.56	5.96	5.32	4.63	3.85
18	15.38	10.39	8.49	7.46	6.81	6.35	5.76	5.13	4.45	3.67
19	15.08	10.16	8.28	7.26	6.61	6.18	5.59	4.97	4.29	3.52
20	14.82	9.95	8.10	7.10	6.46	6.02	5.44	4.82	4.15	3.38
21	14.59	9.77	7.94	6.95	6.32	5.88	5.31	4.70	4.03	3.26
22	14.38	9.61	7.80	6.81	6.19	5.76	5.19	4.58	3.92	3.15
23	14.19	9.47	7.67	6.69	6.08	5.65	5.09	4.48	3.82	3.05
24	14.03	9.34	7.55	6.59	5.98	5.55	4.99	4.39	3.74	2.97
25	13.88	9.22	7.45	6.49	5.88	5.46	4.91	4.31	3.66	2.89
26	13.74	9.12	7.36	6.41	5.80	5.38	4.83	4.24	3.59	2.82
27	13.61	9.02	7.27	6.33	5.73	5.31	4.76	4.17	3.52	2.75
28	13.50	8.93	7.19	6.25	5.66	5.24	4.69	4.11	3.46	2.70
29	13.39	8.85	7.12	6.19	5.59	5.18	4.64	4.05	3.41	2.64
30	13.29	8.77	7.05	6.12	5.53	5.12	4.58	4.00	3.36	2.59
40	12.61	8.25	6.60	5.70	5.13	4.73	4.21	3.64	3.01	2.23
60	11.97	7.76	6.17	5.31	4.76	4.37	3.87	3.31	2.69	1.90
120	11.38	7.31	5.79	4.95	4.42	4.04	3.55	3.02	2.40	1.56
∞	10.83	6.91	5.42	4.62	4.10	3.74	3.27	2.74	2.13	1.00

TABLE A.3 • Critical Values for the χ^2 Distribution

df	\.10	\.05	\.02	\.01	\.001
1	2.71	3.84	5.41	6.63	10.83
2	4.61	5.99	7.82	9.21	13.82
3	6.25	7.82	9.84	11.34	16.27
4	7.78	9.49	11.67	13.28	18.46
5	9.24	11.07	13.39	15.09	20.52
6	10.64	12.59	15.03	16.81	22.46
7	12.02	14.07	16.62	18.48	24.32
8	13.36	15.51	18.17	20.09	26.12
9	14.68	16.92	19.68	21.67	27.88
10	15.99	18.31	21.16	23.21	29.59
11	17.28	19.68	22.62	24.72	31.26
12	18.55	21.03	24.05	26.22	32.91
13	19.81	22.36	25.47	27.69	34.53
14	21.06	23.68	26.87	29.14	36.12
15	22.31	25.00	28.26	30.58	37.70
16	23.54	26.30	29.63	32.00	39.25
17	24.77	27.59	31.00	33.41	40.79
18	25.99	28.87	32.35	34.81	42.31
19	27.20	30.14	33.69	36.19	43.82
20	28.41	31.41	35.02	37.57	45.32
21	29.62	32.67	36.34	38.93	46.80
22	30.81	33.92	37.66	40.29	48.27
23	32.01	35.17	38.97	41.64	49.73
24	33.20	36.42	40.27	42.98	51.18
25	34.38	37.65	41.57	44.31	52.62
26	35.56	38.89	42.86	45.64	54.05
27	36.74	40.11	44.14	46.96	55.48
28	37.92	41.34	45.42	48.28	56.89
29	39.09	42.56	46.69	49.59	58.30
30	40.26	43.77	47.96	50.89	59.70

TABLE A.4 • Critical Values of the r Distribution

	LEVEL OF SIGNIFICANCE FOR ONE-TAILED TEST				
	.05	.025	.01	.005	.0005
	LEVEL OF SIGNIFICANCE FOR TWO-TAILED TEST				
df	.10	.05	.02	.01	.001
1	.98769	.99692	.999507	.999877	.9999988
2	.90000	.95000	.98000	.990000	.99900
3	.8054	.8783	.93433	.95873	.99116
4	.7293	.8114	.8822	.91720	.97406
5	.6694	.7545	.8329	.8745	.95074
6	.6215	.7067	.7887	.8343	.92493
7	.5822	.6664	.7498	.7977	.8982
8	.5494	.6319	.7155	.7646	.8721
9	.5214	.6021	.6851	.7348	.8471
10	.4973	.5760	.6581	.7079	.8233
11	.4762	.5529	.6339	.6835	.8010
12	.4575	.5324	.6120	.6614	.7800
13	.4409	.5139	.5923	.5411	.7603
14	.4259	.4973	.5742	.6226	.7420
15	.4124	.4821	.5577	.6055	.7246
16	.4000	.4683	.5425	.5897	.7084
17	.3887	.4555	.5285	.5751	.6932
18	.3783	.4438	.5155	.5614	.5687
19	.3687	.4329	.5034	.5487	.6652
20	.3598	.4227	.4921	.5368	.6524
25	.3233	.3809	.4451	.5869	.5974
30	.2960	.3494	.4093	.4487	.5541
35	.2746	.3246	.3810	.4182	.5189
40	.2573	.3044	.3578	.3932	.4896
45	.2428	.2875	.3384	.3721	.4648
50	.2306	.2732	.3218	.3541	.4433
60	.2108	.2500	.2948	.3248	.4078
70	.1954	.2319	.2737	.3017	.3799
80	.1829	.2172	.2565	.2830	.3568
90	.1726	.2050	.2422	.2673	.3375
100	.1638	.1946	.2301	.2540	.3211

Glossary

5 Whys A process involving rounds of questioning that is used in some quality improvement projects to gain insight into the root cause of a problem.

6S hierarchy A 6-level hierarchy that ranks evidence sources (including preappraised evidence) in terms of ease of use in clinical settings.

absolute risk (AR) The proportion of people in a group who experienced an undesirable outcome.

absolute risk reduction (ARR) The difference between the absolute risk in one group (e.g., those exposed to an intervention) and the absolute risk in another group (e.g., those not exposed); sometimes called the *risk difference* or *RD*.

abstract A brief description of a completed or proposed study, usually located at the beginning of a report or proposal.

accessible population The population of people available for a particular study, often a nonrandom subset of the target population.

acquiescence response set A bias in self-report instruments, especially in psychosocial scales, created when participants characteristically agree with statements ("yea-say"), independent of content.

adaptive intervention An intervention in which there are multiple decision points over time and decisions are based on individual responses to the treatment.

adaptive trial design A strategy for testing an intervention that involves altering the design itself during the course of the trial (e.g., dropping or adding a study arm).

adherence to treatment The degree to which those in an intervention group adhere to protocols or continue getting the treatment.

after-only design An experimental design in which data are collected from participants only after an intervention has been introduced.

AGREE instrument A widely used instrument (Appraisal of Guidelines Research and Evaluation) for systematically assessing clinical practice guidelines.

allocation concealment The process used to ensure that the people enrolling participants into a clinical trial are unaware of upcoming assignments to treatment conditions.

alpha (α) (1) In tests of statistical significance, the significance criterion—the risk the researcher is willing to accept of making a Type I error; (2) in measurement, an index of internal consistency, i.e., Cronbach's alpha.

alternative hypothesis In hypothesis testing, a hypothesis different from the one actually being tested—usually, the alternative to the null hypothesis, sometimes called the *research hypothesis*.

analysis The organization and synthesis of data so as to answer research questions or test hypotheses.

analysis of covariance (ANCOVA) A statistical procedure used to test mean group differences on an outcome variable, while controlling for one or more covariates.

analysis of variance (ANOVA) A statistical procedure for testing mean differences among three or more groups by contrasting variability between groups to variability within groups, yielding an *F*-ratio statistic.

analytic generalization One of three models of generalization concerning researchers' efforts to generalize from particulars to broader conceptualizations and theories.

ancestry approach In literature searches, using citations from relevant studies to track down earlier research on the same topic (the "ancestors"), also called *snowballing*, *footnote chasing*, and *pearl growing*.

anchor-based approach An approach to estimating a measure's responsiveness and to developing a benchmark of importance for interpreting change scores that rely on a "gold standard" criterion as the anchor.

anonymity Protection of participants' confidentiality such that even the researcher cannot link individuals with the data they provided.

applicability The degree to which research evidence can be applied to individuals, small groups of individuals, or local contexts (as opposed to broad populations).

applied research Research aimed at finding a solution to a practical problem.

area under the curve (AUC) In ROC analysis, an index of the performance of a diagnostic or screening measure vis-à-vis diagnostic accuracy, summarized in a single value that typically ranges from .50 (no better than random classification) to 1.0 (perfect classification).

argument An explanation of what a researcher wants to study, with supportive evidence and background material linked in a manner that provides a rationale.

arm A particular treatment condition to which participants are allocated (e.g., the intervention *arm* or control *arm* of a controlled trial).

ascertainment bias Systematic differences between groups being compared in how outcome variables are measured, verified, or recorded when data collectors have not been blinded, also called *detection bias*.

assent The affirmative agreement of an individual (e.g., a child) to take part in a study, typically to supplement formal consent by a parent or guardian.

associative relationship An association between two variables that cannot be described as causal.

assumption A principle that is accepted as being true based on logic or reason, without proof.

asymmetric distribution A distribution of data values that is skewed, with two halves that are not mirror images of each other.

attention control group A control group that gets a similar amount of attention as those in the intervention group, without receiving the "active ingredients" of the treatment.

attrition The loss of participants over the course of a study, which can create bias by changing the composition of the sample initially drawn.

AUC See *area under the curve*.

audio-CASI (computer-assisted self-interview) An approach to collecting self-report data in which respondents listen through headphones to questions being read and respond by entering information onto a computer.

audit trail The systematic documentation of material that would allow an independent auditor of a qualitative study to draw conclusions about trustworthiness.

authenticity The extent to which qualitative researchers fairly and faithfully show a range of different realities in the collection, analysis, and interpretation of data.

autoethnography An ethnographic study in which researchers study their own culture or group.

axial coding The second level of coding in a grounded theory study using the Strauss and Corbin approach, involving the process of categorizing, recategorizing, and condensing first level codes by connecting a category and its subcategories.

back translation The translation of a translated text back into the original language, so that original and back-translated versions can be compared to assess semantic equivalence.

baseline data Data collected at an initial measurement (e.g., prior to an intervention), to enable an assessment of changes.

basic research Research designed to extend the base of knowledge in a discipline for the sake of knowledge production or theory construction rather than for solving a current problem.

basic social process (BSP) A central social process that is discovered through the analysis of grounded theory data; a type of *core variable*.

before–after design A design in which data are collected from participants both before and after the introduction of an intervention.

benchmark In measurement, a threshold value on a measure that signifies an important value, such as a threshold for interpreting whether a change in scores is meaningful or clinically significant.

beneficence An ethical principle that seeks to maximize benefits for study participants, and prevent harm.

beta (β) In statistical testing, the probability of a Type II error.

beta (β) weight In multiple regression, the standardized coefficients indicating the relative weights of the predictor variables in the equation.

between-subjects design A research design in which different groups of people are compared (e.g., smokers and nonsmokers; intervention and control group members).

bias Any influence that distorts the results of a study and undermines validity.

bibliographic database Data files containing bibliographic (reference) information that can be accessed electronically in conducting a literature search.

Big Data Large, complex datasets that have high velocity of data flow, high volume of data, and high variety in data types; analyses involve a search for patterns, trends, and associations.

bimodal distribution A distribution of data values with two peaks (high frequencies).

binomial distribution A statistical distribution with known properties describing the number of occurrences of an event in a series of observations; forms the basis for analyzing dichotomous data.

biomarker An objective, measurable characteristic of a biological process or condition.

bivariate statistics Statistical analysis of two variables to assess the empirical relationship between them.

Bland–Altman plot A graphic depiction of the degree of agreement between two sets of scores for people who have been measured twice on the same continuous measurement scale; the plot highlights random differences between the two measurements through the construction of a parameter called the *limits of agreement*.

Blind review The review of a manuscript or proposal such that neither the author nor the reviewer is identified to the other party.

blinding The prevention of those involved in a study (participants, intervention agents, data collectors, or healthcare providers) from having information that could lead to a bias, particularly information about which treatment group a participant is in; also called *masking*.

Bonferroni correction An adjustment made to establish a more conservative alpha level when multiple statistical tests are being run from the same data set; the correction is computed by dividing the desired α by the number of tests—e.g., .05/3 = .017.

bracketing In phenomenological inquiries, the process of identifying and holding in abeyance any preconceived beliefs and opinions about the phenomena under study, also called *epoché*.

bricolage The tendency in qualitative research to gather a complex array of data from a variety of sources using a variety of methods.

calendar question A question used to obtain retrospective information about the chronology of events and activities in people's lives.

carryover effect The influence that one treatment (or measurement) can have on subsequent treatments (or measurements), notably in a crossover design or in test-retest reliability assessments.

Case study A study involving a thorough in-depth analysis of an individual, group, or other social unit.

case–control design A nonexperimental design that compares "cases" (i.e., people with a specified condition, such as lung cancer) to matched controls (similar people without the condition), to examine differences that could have contributed to "caseness."

categorical variable A variable that involves discrete categories (e.g., blood type) rather than values along a continuum (e.g., weight).

category system In studies involving observation, the prespecified plan for recording the behaviors and events under observation; in qualitative studies, the system developed from the narrative data to organize the data.

causal modeling The development and statistical testing of an explanatory model of hypothesized causal relationships among phenomena.

causal (cause-and-effect) relationship A relationship between two variables wherein the presence or value of one variable (the "cause") affects the presence or value of the other (the "effect").

cause-probing research Research designed to illuminate the underlying causes of phenomena.

ceiling effect An effect resulting from restricted variation above a certain point on a measurement continuum, which limits discrimination at the upper end of the measure, constrains true variability, and reduces the amount of upward change that is detectable.

cell The intersection of a row and column in a table (matrix) with two or more dimensions; in a factorial design, the representation of an experimental condition in a schematic diagram.

census A survey covering an entire population.

central category The main category or pattern of behavior in grounded theory analysis, sometimes referred to as the *core category*.

central limit theorem A statistical principle stipulating that the larger the sample, the more closely the sampling distribution of the mean will approximate a normal distribution and that the mean of a sampling distribution will equal the population mean.

central tendency A statistical index of what is "typical" in a set of scores, derived from the center of the score distribution; indices of central tendency include the mode, median, and mean.

Certificate of Confidentiality A certificate issued by the National Institutes of Health in the United States to protect researchers against forced disclosure of confidential research information.

change score A person's score difference between two measurements on the same measure, calculated by subtracting the value at one point in time from the value at the other point.

chi-square test A statistical test used in various contexts, most often to assess differences in proportions, symbolized as χ^2.

classical test theory (CTT) A measurement theory that has traditionally been used in the development of multi-item scales; in CTT, any score on a measure is conceptualized as having a "true score" component and an error component, and the goal is to approximate the true score.

clinical practice guidelines Practice guidelines that typically combine a synthesis and appraisal of research evidence from systematic reviews with specific recommendations for clinical decisions.

clinical relevance The degree to which a study addresses a problem of significance to clinical practice.

clinical research Research designed to generate knowledge to guide practice in healthcare fields.

clinical significance The practical importance of research results in terms of whether they have genuine, palpable implications for patients' daily lives or for the healthcare decisions made on their behalf.

clinical trial A study designed to assess the safety, efficacy, and effectiveness of a new clinical intervention, sometimes involving several phases (e.g., Phase III typically is a *randomized controlled trial* using an experimental design).

clinimetrics An approach to the quantitative measurement of clinical phenomena such as symptoms and signs; an alternative approach to psychometrics for health measurement.

closed-ended question A question that offers respondents specific response options, also referred to as a *fixed alternative question*.

cluster randomization The random assignment of intact units or organizations (e.g., hospitals), rather than individuals, to treatment conditions.

cluster sampling A form of sampling in which large groupings ("clusters") are selected first (e.g., census tracts), typically with successive subsampling of smaller units (e.g., households) in a multistage approach.

Cochrane Collaboration An international organization that aims to facilitate well-informed healthcare decisions by sponsoring systematic reviews, primarily about the effects of healthcare interventions.

code of ethics The fundamental ethical principles established by a discipline or institution to guide researchers' conduct in research with human (or animal) participants.

codebook A record documenting categorization and coding decisions.

coding The process of transforming raw data into standardized form for data processing and analysis; in quantitative research, the process of attaching numbers to categories; in qualitative research, the process of identifying and indexing recurring salient words, themes, or concepts within the data.

coefficient alpha A widely used index of internal consistency, indicating the degree to which the items on a multi-item scale are measuring the same underlying construct, also referred to as *Cronbach's alpha*.

coercion In a research context, the explicit or implicit use of threats (or excessive rewards) to gain people's cooperation in a study.

cognitive questioning A method sometimes used in a pretest of an instrument in which respondents are asked to explain the process by which they answer questions; basic approaches include a *think-aloud* method and the use of targeted *probes,* also used in connection with content validity work.

cognitive test A performance test designed to assess cognitive skills or cognitive functioning (e.g., a test of cognitive impairment).

Cohen's *d* An effect size index for comparing two group means, computed by subtracting one mean from the other and dividing by the pooled standard deviation, also called *standardized mean difference* or *SMD*.

Cohen's kappa See *kappa*.

cohort design A nonexperimental design in which a defined group of people (a cohort) is followed over time to study outcomes for the cohorts or subgroups within it, also called a *prospective design*.

comparative effectiveness research (CER) A patient-centered research approach that focuses on comparisons of alternative approaches to bring about health improvements.

comparison group A group of study participants whose scores on an outcome are used to evaluate the outcome of the group of primary interest (e.g., nonsmokers as a comparison group for smokers); the term is often used in lieu of a control group when the study design is not a randomized experiment.

complex intervention An intervention in which complexity exists along one or more dimensions, including number of components, number of targeted outcomes, and the time needed for the full intervention to be delivered.

composite scale A measure of an attribute involving the aggregation of information from multiple items into a single numerical score that places people on a continuum with respect to the attribute.

computerized adaptive testing (CAT) An approach to measuring a latent trait in which computer algorithms are used to tailor a set of questions to individuals, usually using questions from an item bank created using item response theory; CAT offers precise measures of a trait with a small set of targeted items.

concealment A tactic involving the unobtrusive collection of research data without participants' knowledge or consent, used to obtain an accurate view of naturalistic behavior when the known presence of an observer would distort the behavior of interest.

concept An abstraction inferred from observation or self-reports of behaviors, situations, or characteristics (e.g., stress, pain).

concept analysis A systematic process of analyzing a concept or construct with the aim of identifying its boundaries, definitions, and dimensionality.

conceptual definition The abstract or theoretical meaning of a concept of interest.

conceptual equivalence The extent to which a construct of interest is comparable in another culture, which is of relevance in the translation or cultural adaptation of an instrument.

conceptual files A manual method of organizing qualitative data, by creating file folders for each category in the coding scheme and inserting relevant excerpts from the data.

conceptual map A schematic representation of a theory or conceptual model that graphically represents key concepts and linkages among them, also called a *schematic model*

conceptual model Interrelated concepts assembled in a rational and often explanatory scheme to illuminate relationships, but less formally than a theory, sometimes called a *conceptual framework*.

Concurrent design A mixed methods study design in which the qualitative and quantitative strands of data collection occur simultaneously, symbolically designated with a plus sign (e.g., QUAL + QUAN).

Concurrent validity A type of criterion validity that concerns the degree to which scores on an instrument are correlated with an external criterion, measured at the same time.

confidence interval (CI) The range of values within which a population parameter is estimated to lie at a specified probability (e.g., 95% CI).

confidence limit The upper (or lower) boundary of a confidence interval.

confidentiality Protection of study participants so that data provided are never publicly divulged.

confirmability A criterion for trustworthiness in a qualitative inquiry, referring to the objectivity or neutrality of the data and interpretations.

confirmatory factor analysis (CFA) A factor analysis designed to confirm a hypothesized measurement model, using maximum likelihood estimation; used in assessments of an instrument's structural validity.

confounding variable A variable that is extraneous to the research question and that confounds understanding of the relationship between the independent and dependent variables; confounding variables can be controlled in the research design or through statistical procedures.

consecutive sampling Involves sampling all the people from an accessible population who meet the eligibility criteria over a specific time interval or for a specified sample size.

consent form A written agreement signed by a study participant and a researcher concerning the terms and conditions of voluntary participation in a study.

CONSORT guidelines Widely adopted guidelines (Consolidated Standards of Reporting Trials) for reporting information for a randomized controlled trial, including a checklist and flow chart for tracking participants through the trial from recruitment through data analysis.

constant comparison A procedure used in qualitative analysis (especially in grounded theory) wherein new data are compared in an ongoing fashion with data obtained earlier to refine theoretically relevant categories.

constitutive pattern In hermeneutic analysis, a pattern that expresses the relationships among relational themes and is present in all the interviews or texts.

construct An abstraction or concept that is invented (constructed) by researchers based on inferences from human behavior or human traits (e.g., health locus of control), sometimes referred to as a *latent trait*.

construct validity The degree to which evidence about study particulars supports inferences about the higher order constructs they are intended to represent; in measurement, the degree to which a measure truly captures the focal construct.

constructivist grounded theory An approach to grounded theory, developed by Charmaz, in which the grounded theory is constructed from shared experiences and relationships between the researcher and study participants and interpretive aspects are emphasized.

constructivist paradigm An alternative to the positivist paradigm that holds that there are multiple interpretations of reality and that the goal of research is to understand how individuals construct reality within their context, associated with qualitative research, also called *naturalistic paradigm*.

contamination The inadvertent, unwanted influence of one treatment condition on another treatment condition when members of the control group receive the intervention, sometimes called *treatment diffusion*.

content analysis An approach to extracting, organizing, and synthesizing material from documents, often narrative data from a qualitative study, according to key concepts and themes.

content validity The degree to which a multi-item instrument has an appropriate set of relevant items reflecting the full content of the construct domain being measured.

content validity index (CVI) An index summarizing the degree to which a panel of experts agrees on an instrument's content validity; both item content validity (I-CVI) and the overall scale content validity (S-CVI) can be assessed.

continuous quality improvement An approach to healthcare that involves creating an environment in which management and staff strive to constantly improve quality.

continuous variable A variable that can take on an infinite range of values along a specified continuum (e.g., height); less strictly, a variable measured on an interval or ratio scale.

Control group Participants in an experimental study who do not receive the intervention being tested and whose performance provides a counterfactual against which the effects of the intervention can be compared (see also *comparison group*).

control, research The process of holding constant confounding influences on the outcome under study.

controlled trial A trial that has a control group with or without randomization.

convenience sampling Selection of the most readily available persons as participants in a study.

convergent design A concurrent mixed methods design in which complementary qualitative and quantitative (usually equal priority) data are gathered about a phenomenon, often symbolized as QUAL + QUAN.

convergent validity A type of construct validity concerning the degree to which scores on a focal measure are correlated with scores on measures of constructs with which there is a hypothesized correlation (i.e., the degree of conceptual convergence).

core category (variable) In a grounded theory study, the central phenomenon that is used to integrate all categories of the data and that is central in explaining what is going on.

correlation An association or bond between variables, with variation in one variable systematically related to variation in another.

correlation coefficient An index summarizing the strength of relationship between variables, typically ranging from +1.00 (for a perfect positive relationship) through .00 (for no relationship) to −1.00 (for a perfect negative relationship).

correlation matrix A two-dimensional display showing the correlation coefficients between all pairs of variables in a set of several variables.

correlational design An observational research design that explores interrelationships among variables of interest without researcher intervention.

COSMIN The **Co**nsensus-based **St**andards for the selection of health **M**easurement **In**struments, an initiative that developed an important measurement taxonomy and sought to standardize the definitions of measurement properties.

cost–benefit analysis An economic analysis in which both costs and outcomes of a program or intervention are expressed in monetary terms and compared.

cost-effectiveness analysis An economic analysis in which costs of an intervention are measured in monetary terms but outcomes are expressed in natural units (e.g., costs per added year of life).

cost–utility analysis An economic analysis that expresses the effects of an intervention as overall health improvement and describes costs for some additional utility gain—usually in relation to gains in quality-adjusted life years (QALY).

counterbalancing The process of systematically varying the order of presentation of stimuli or treatments to control for ordering effects, especially in a crossover design.

counterfactual The condition or group used as a basis of comparison in a trial, representing what would have happened *to the same people* exposed to a causal factor if they *simultaneously* were *not* exposed to the causal factor.

covariate A variable that is statistically controlled (held constant) in ANCOVA, typically a confounding influence on, or a preintervention measure of, the outcome variable.

covert data collection The collection of information in a study without participants' knowledge.

Cox regression A regression analysis in which independent variables are used to model the risk (or hazard) of experiencing an event at a given point in time, given that one has not experienced the event before that time.

Cramér's *V* An index describing the magnitude of relationship between nominal-level data, used when the contingency table to which it is applied is larger than 2 × 2.

credibility A criterion for evaluating trustworthiness in qualitative studies, referring to confidence in the truth of the data, analogous to internal validity in quantitative research.

Criterion sampling A purposive sampling approach used by qualitative researchers that involves selecting cases that meet a predetermined criterion of importance.

criterion validity The extent to which scores on a measure are an adequate reflection of (or predictor of) a criterion—i.e., a "gold standard" measure.

critical case sampling A qualitative sampling approach involving the purposeful selection of cases that are especially important or illustrative.

critical ethnography An ethnography that focuses on raising consciousness in the group or culture under study in the hope of effecting social change.

critical region The area in the sampling distribution representing values that are "improbable" if the null hypothesis is true.

critical theory An approach to studying phenomena that involves a critique of society, with the goal of envisioning new possibilities and effecting social change.

critique A critical appraisal that analyzes both weaknesses and strengths of a research report or proposal.

Cronbach's alpha A widely used index that estimates the internal consistency of a composite measure composed of several subparts (e.g., items), also called *coefficient alpha*.

cross-cultural validity The degree to which the items on a translated or culturally adapted scale perform adequately and equivalently, individually and in the aggregate, in relation to their performance on the original instrument, an aspect of construct validity.

crossover design An experimental design in which one group of participants is exposed to more than one condition or treatment in random order.

cross-sectional design A study design in which data are collected at one point in time in contrast to a longitudinal design; sometimes used to infer change over time when data are collected from different ages or developmental groups.

crosstabulation A calculation of frequencies for two variables considered simultaneously—e.g., gender (male/female) crosstabulated with smoking status (smoker/nonsmoker).

cutoff point (cut point) The point in a distribution of scores used to classify or divide people into different groups, such as cases and noncases for a disease or health problem (e.g., the cut point for classifying newborns as low birthweight is 5.5 pounds [2500 g]).

d An effect size index for comparing two group means, computed by subtracting one mean from the other and dividing by the pooled standard deviation, also called *Cohen's d* or *standardized mean difference*.

data The pieces of information obtained in a study; the singular is *datum*.

data analysis The systematic organization and synthesis of research data and, in most quantitative studies, the testing of hypotheses using those data.

data cleaning The preparation of data for analysis by performing checks to ensure that the data are correct.

data collection plan The plan for the gathering of information needed to address a research problem.

data collection protocols The formal procedures researchers develop to guide the collection of data in a standardized fashion.

data saturation The collection of qualitative data to the point where a sense of closure is attained because new data yield redundant information.

data set The total collection of data on all variables for all participants in a study.

data transformation A step undertaken before quantitative data analysis, to put the data in a form that can be meaningfully analyzed (e.g., recoding of values); in mixed method studies, qualitizing quantitative data or quantitizing qualitative data.

data triangulation The use of multiple data sources for the purpose of validating conclusions.

debriefing Communication with study participants after participation is complete regarding aspects of the study.

deception The deliberate withholding of information, or the provision of false information, to study participants usually to minimize potential biases.

deductive reasoning The process of developing specific predictions from general principles; see also *inductive reasoning*.

degrees of freedom (*df*) A statistical concept referring to the number of sample values free to vary (e.g., with a given sample mean, all but one value would be free to vary).

deidentified data Data or records from which identifying information is removed to protect the privacy of individuals.

delay of treatment design A design for an intervention study that involves putting control group members on a waiting list for the intervention until follow-up data are collected, also called a *wait-list design*.

Delphi survey A technique for obtaining judgments from an expert panel about an issue of concern; experts are questioned individually in several rounds, with a summary of the panel's views circulated between rounds, to achieve some consensus.

dendrogram A tree diagram sometimes used in qualitative studies to illustrate the arrangement of codes and categories in a hierarchically ordered system.

dependability A criterion for evaluating trustworthiness in qualitative studies, referring to the stability of data over time and over conditions; analogous to reliability in quantitative research.

dependent variable The variable hypothesized to depend on or be caused by the independent variable; the outcome variable of interest.

descendancy approach In literature searches, finding a pivotal early study and searching forward in citation indexes to find more recent studies ("descendants") that cited the key study.

Description question A question aimed at describing a health-related phenomenon.

descriptive research Research that has as a primary objective the accurate portrayal of people's characteristics or circumstances and/or the frequency with which certain phenomena occur.

descriptive statistics Statistics that describe and summarize data (e.g., means, percentages).

descriptive theory A broad characterization that thoroughly accounts for a phenomenon.

detection bias Systematic differences between groups being compared in how outcome variables are measured, verified, or recorded; a bias that can result when there is no blinding of data collectors.

determinism The belief that phenomena are not haphazard or random but rather have antecedent causes; an assumption in the positivist paradigm.

deviation score A score computed by subtracting an individual score from the mean of all scores.

diagnostic accuracy The degree to which a measure is accurate in diagnosing or predicting "caseness" and "noncaseness" for a condition, as established by a gold standard criterion.

Diagnosis/assessment question A question about the accuracy and validity of instruments to screen, diagnose, or assess patients.

dichotomous variable A variable having only two values or categories (e.g., alive/dead).

differential item functioning (DIF) The extent to which an item functions differently for one group than for another despite the groups' equivalence on the underlying latent trait.

direct costs Specific project-related costs incurred during a study (e.g., for salaries, supplies, etc.).

directional hypothesis A hypothesis that makes a specific prediction about the direction of the relationship between two variables.

disconfirming case In qualitative research, a case that challenges the researchers' conceptualizations; sometimes sought as part of a sampling strategy.

discourse analysis A qualitative tradition, from the discipline of sociolinguistics, that seeks to understand the rules, mechanisms, and structure of conversations.

discrete variable A variable with a finite number of values between two points, representing discrete quantities (e.g., number of children).

disproportionate sampling A sampling approach in which the researcher samples varying proportions of people from different population strata to ensure adequate representation from smaller strata.

dissemination bias A bias that occurs when the profile of a study's results depends on the direction or strength of its findings; one example is *publication bias*.

Distribution-based approach An approach to estimating a measure's responsiveness and to developing a benchmark of importance for interpreting change scores, that relies on distributional properties of the data—often the distribution of change scores.

divergent validity An approach to construct validation that involves gathering evidence that the focal measure is not a measure of a different construct, also called *discriminant validity*.

domain analysis One of Spradley's levels of ethnographic analysis, focusing on the identification of domains or units of cultural knowledge.

domain -sampling model The model underpinning scale development in the classical test theory framework, which conceptually involves the random sampling of a homogeneous set of items from a hypothetical universe of items relating to the construct.

dose–response analysis An analysis to assess whether larger doses of an intervention are associated with greater benefits.

double-blind study A study (usually a clinical trial) in which two sets of people are blinded with respect to the group that a study participant is in; often a situation in which neither the participants nor those who administer the treatment know who is in the experimental or control group.

dummy variable Dichotomous variables created for use in many multivariate statistical analyses, typically using codes of 0 and 1 (e.g., smoker = 1, non-smoker = 0).

ecological momentary assessment (EMA) Repeated assessments of people's feelings, experiences, or behaviors in real time, within their natural environment, using contemporary technologies such as smartphones.

ecological validity The extent to which study designs and findings have relevance and meaning in a variety of real-world contexts.

economic analysis An analysis of the costs and outcomes of alternative healthcare interventions.

effect A consequence of a causal factor (e.g., the effect of an intervention on an outcome).

effect size (ES) In quantitative research, an index summarizing the strength of relationship between variables, an example is *Cohen's d*; in metasynthesis, an index used to characterize the salience of a theme or category.

effectiveness study A clinical trial designed to test the effectiveness of an intervention under standard real-world conditions, often with an intervention already found to be efficacious in an efficacy study.

efficacy study A tightly controlled trial designed to establish the efficacy of an intervention under ideal conditions using a design that maximizes internal validity, sometimes called an *explanatory trial*.

eigenvalue The value equal to the sum of the squared weights for a linear composite, such as a factor in a factor analysis, indicating how much variance is accounted for in the solution.

element The most basic unit of a population for sampling purposes, typically a human being.

eligibility criteria The criteria designating the specific attributes of the target population by which people are selected for inclusion in a study or excluded from it.

emergent design A design that unfolds during the course of a qualitative study as the researcher makes ongoing design decisions reflecting what has already been learned.

emergent fit A concept in grounded theory that involves comparing new data and new categories with previous conceptualizations.

emic perspective An ethnographic term referring to the way members of a culture themselves view their world; the "insider's view."

empirical evidence Evidence rooted in objective reality and gathered using one's senses as the basis for generating knowledge.

endogenous variable In a causal model (path analysis), a variable whose variation is influenced by other variables within the model.

endpoint In a clinical trial, the target outcome of interest.

equivalence In the context of instrument translation, the degree to which the translated and original measures are comparable; types of equivalence include conceptual equivalence, content equivalence, semantic equivalence, technical equivalence, measurement equivalence, and factorial equivalence.

equivalence trial A trial designed to assess whether the outcomes of two treatments do *not* differ by no more than a prespecified amount judged to be clinically unimportant.

error of measurement The difference between the hypothetical true scores and the obtained scores of a measured characteristic.

error term The mathematic expression (e.g., in a regression analysis) that represents all unknown or unmeasurable attributes that affect the outcome variable.

estimation procedures Statistical procedures that estimate population parameters based on sample statistics.

eta squared In ANOVA, a statistic calculated to indicate the proportion of variance in the dependent variable explained by the independent variables, analogous to R^2 in multiple regression.

ethics In research, a system of moral values that is concerned with the degree to which research procedures adhere to professional, legal, and social obligations to study participants.

ethnography A branch of human inquiry, associated with anthropology, that focuses on the culture of a group of people with an effort to understand the world view and customs of those under study.

ethnonursing research The study of human cultures with a focus on a group's beliefs and practices relating to nursing care and related health behaviors.

etic perspective In ethnography, the "outsider's" view of the experiences of a cultural group.

Etiology question A question about the underlying cause of a health problem, such as an environmental cause or personal behavior (e.g., smoking).

evaluation research Research that assesses how well a program, practice, or policy works.

event history calendar A data collection matrix that plots time on one dimension and events or activities of interest on the other.

event sampling A type of observational sampling that involves the selection of integral behaviors or events to be observed.

evidence-based practice (EBP) A practice that involves making clinical decisions based on clinical judgment, patient preferences, and on the best available evidence, which often is evidence from disciplined research.

evidence hierarchy A ranked arrangement of the strength of research evidence based on the rigor of the method that produced it; the traditional evidence hierarchy is appropriate primarily for cause-probing research.

exclusion criteria Criteria specifying characteristics that a target population does *not* have, stipulated for the purpose of sampling.

exogenous variable In a causal model (path analysis), a variable whose determinants lie outside the model.

expectation bias The bias that can arise when study participants (or research staff) have expectations about treatment effectiveness in intervention research; the expectations can result in altered behavior.

expectation maximization (EM) A sophisticated imputation process that generates an estimated value for missing data in two steps (an expectation or E-step and a maximization or M-step), using maximum likelihood estimation.

experimental group The study participants who receive the experimental treatment or intervention.

experimental research A study using a design in which the researcher controls (manipulates) the independent variable by randomly assigning participants to different treatment conditions; randomized controlled trials use experimental designs.

explanatory design A sequential mixed methods design in which quantitative data are collected in the first phase and qualitative data are collected in the second phase to build on or explain quantitative findings.

explanatory trial A traditional clinical trial conducted under optimal conditions with carefully selected participants in an effort to enhance internal validity.

exploratory design A sequential mixed methods design in which qualitative data are collected in the first phase and quantitative data are collected in the second phase based on the initial in-depth exploration.

exploratory factor analysis (EFA) A factor analysis undertaken to explore the underlying dimensionality of a set of variables.

exploratory research A study that explores the dimensions of a phenomenon or that develops or refines hypotheses about relationships between phenomena.

external validity The degree to which study results can be generalized to settings or samples other than the one studied.

extraneous variable A variable that confounds the relationship between the independent and dependent variables and that needs to be controlled either in the research design or through statistical procedures, often called *confounding variable*.

extreme response set A bias resulting from a respondent's consistent selection of extreme alternatives (e.g., *strongly agree* or *strongly disagree*) to scale items regardless of item content.

***F*-ratio** The statistic obtained in several statistical tests (e.g., ANOVA) in which variation is attributable to different sources (e.g., between-group variation and within-group variation) is contrasted.

face validity The extent to which a measuring instrument looks as though it is measuring what it purports to measure.

factor analysis A statistical procedure for disentangling complex interrelationships among items and identifying the items that "go together" as a unified dimension.

factor extraction The first phase of a factor analysis, which involves the extraction of as much variance as possible through the successive creation of linear combinations of the variables in the analysis.

factor loading In factor analysis, the weight associated with a variable or item on a given factor.

factor matrix In a factor analysis of scale items, a matrix with items on one dimension and factors on the other, with matrix entries being factor loadings of the items on the factors; factor matrices can be either *rotated* or *unrotated*.

factor rotation The second phase of factor analysis during which the reference axes for the factors are pivoted to more clearly align items or variables with a single factor.

factorial design An experimental design in which two or more independent variables are simultaneously manipulated, permitting a separate analysis of the main effects of the independent variables and their interaction.

Failure Mode and Effect Analysis (FMEA) In quality improvement, a systematic approach to identifying and preventing problems before they occur.

feasibility study Research completed prior to a main intervention study to assess whether it is sensible to proceed with the project; as distinct from a *pilot study*, a *feasibility assessment* test's specific aspects of an intervention or the anticipated trial (e.g., the intervention's acceptability).

feminist research Research that seeks to understand how gender and a gendered social order shape women's lives and their consciousness.

field diary A daily record of events and conversations in the field, also called a log.

field notes The notes taken by researchers to record the unstructured observations made in the field, and the interpretation of those observations.

field research Research in which the data are collected "in the field" from people in their normal roles, with the aim of understanding the practices, behaviors, and beliefs of individuals or groups as they normally function in real life.

fieldwork The activities undertaken by qualitative researchers to collect data out in the field, i.e., in natural settings.

findings The results and interpretation of analyzed research data.

fishbone analysis A technique used in root cause analyses that is aimed at visualizing causal processes and identifying opportunities for quality improvement.

Fisher's exact test A statistical procedure used to test the significance of differences in proportions used when the sample size is small or cells in the crosstabs table have no observations.

fit An element in Glaserian grounded theory analysis in which the researcher develops categories of a substantive theory that fits the data.

fixed effects model In meta-analysis, a model in which studies are assumed to be estimating a single true effect; a pooled effect estimate is calculated under the assumption that observed variation between studies is attributable to chance.

floor effect An effect resulting from restricted variation below a certain point on a measurement continuum, which limits discrimination at the lower end of the measure, constrains true variability, and reduces the amount of downward change that is detectable.

focus group interview An interview with a small group of individuals assembled to discuss a specific topic, usually guided by a moderator using a semistructured topic guide.

focused interview A loosely structured interview in which an interviewer guides the respondent through a set of questions using a topic guide.

follow-up study A study undertaken to ascertain the outcomes of individuals who have a specified condition or who received a specific treatment.

forest plot A graphic representation of effects across studies in a meta-analysis, permitting a visual assessment of heterogeneity.

formal grounded theory A theory of a substantive grounded theory's core category that is extended by sampling other studies in a range of substantive areas.

formative index A multi-item measure whose items are viewed as "causing" or defining the construct of interest rather than being the effect of the construct, distinct from a *reflective scale*.

forward translation The translation of an item (or any text, such as scale instructions) from an original source language into a target language. See also *back translation*.

framework The conceptual underpinnings of a study—a *theoretical framework* in theory-based studies or a *conceptual framework* in studies based on a conceptual model.

framework analysis A method used to organize and manage qualitative analysis that yields a matrix that allows researchers, usually working in a team, to analyze data both by case and theme.

frequency distribution A systematic array of numeric values from the lowest to the highest, together with a count of the number of times each value was obtained.

frequency effect size In a qualitative metasummary, the percentage of reports that contain a given thematic finding.

frequency polygon A graphic display of frequency distribution information that shows the distribution's shape.

Friedman test A nonparametric analog of ANOVA used with paired groups or repeated measures situations.

full disclosure The communication of complete, accurate information to potential study participants.

functional relationship A relationship between two variables in which it cannot be assumed that one variable caused the other.

funnel plot A graphic display that plots a measure of study precision (e.g., sample size) against effect size to explore the possibility of publication bias.

gaining entrée The process of gaining access to study participants through the cooperation of key gatekeepers in a selected community or site.

general linear model (GLM) A large class of statistical techniques (including regression analysis and ANOVA) that describe the relationship between a dependent variable and one or more independent variables using straight-line solutions.

generalizability The degree to which the research methods justify the inference that the findings are true for a broader group than study participants, usually the inference that the findings can be generalized from the sample to the population.

global rating scale (GRS) A single item that provides a summary measurement of a person's status on a construct, or his/her perception of change on a construct over a specified interval, also referred to as a *health transition rating*.

"going native" A pitfall in ethnographic research wherein a researcher becomes emotionally involved with participants and loses the ability to observe objectively.

GRADE The Grades of Recommendation, Assessment, Development and Evaluation, an approach to grading the quality of an overall body of evidence.

grand theory A broad theory aimed at describing and explaining large segments of the physical, social, or behavioral world, also called a *macrotheory*.

grand tour question A broad question asked in an unstructured interview to gain a general overview of a phenomenon, on the basis of which more focused questions are subsequently asked.

grant A financial award made to a researcher to conduct a proposed study.

grantsmanship The set of skills and knowledge needed to secure financial support for a research idea.

graphic rating scale A scale in which respondents are asked to rate a concept along an ordered, numbered continuum, typically on a bipolar dimension (e.g., "very poor" to "excellent").

grey literature Unpublished, and thus less readily accessible, papers or research reports (e.g., a dissertation).

grounded theory An approach to collecting and analyzing qualitative data that aims to develop theories about social processes, grounded in data from real-world observations.

handsearching The searching of key journals on an article-by-article basis (i.e., by hand), to identify relevant reports that might be missed in electronic searches.

Hawthorne effect The effect on the outcome resulting from people's awareness that they are participants under study.

health transition rating scale A single item, often on a 7-point scale, that asks people to rate the extent to which they have improved/deteriorated (e.g., slightly, moderately, greatly), or stayed the same with regard to a focal attribute.

hermeneutic circle In hermeneutics, a methodologic and interpretive process in which, to reach understanding, there is continual movement between the parts and the whole of the text that are being analyzed.

hermeneutics A qualitative research tradition, drawing on interpretive phenomenology, that focuses on the lived experiences of humans and on how they interpret those experiences.

heterogeneity The degree to which objects are dissimilar (i.e., characterized by variability) on some attribute.

heterogeneity of treatment effects (HTE) Variation in the effectiveness of an intervention across a population—i.e., the intervention's benefits (or harms) are not universal.

hierarchical multiple regression A multiple regression analysis in which predictor variables are entered into the equation in a series of prespecified steps.

histogram A graphic display of frequency distribution information that shows the distribution's shape.

historical comparison group A comparison group chosen from a group observed at some time in the past or for whom existing data are available, often in records.

historical research Systematic studies designed to discover facts and relationships about past events.

history threat The occurrence of events external to an intervention, but concurrent with it, that can affect the outcome variable and threaten the study's internal validity.

homogeneity The degree to which objects are similar (i.e., characterized by low variability) on some attribute.

Hosmer–Lemeshow test A test used in logistic regression to evaluate the degree to which observed frequencies of predicted probabilities correspond to expected frequencies in an ideal model over the range of probability values; a good fit is indicated by lack of statistical significance.

hypothesis A statement of predicted outcomes, most often about predicted relationships between study variables.

hypothesis-testing validity The extent to which it is possible to corroborate hypotheses regarding how scores on a measure function in relation to scores on other variables; a key aspect of construct validity.

identical sampling An approach to sampling in mixed method studies in which all participants are included in both the qualitative and quantitative strands.

impact analysis An evaluation of the effects of a program or intervention on outcomes of interest, net of other factors influencing those outcomes.

impact factor An annual measure of citation frequency for an average article in a given journal over a 2-year period, i.e., the ratio between citations and citable items published in the journal in that period.

implementation analysis In evaluations, a descriptive analysis of the process by which a program or intervention was implemented in practice.

implementation potential The extent to which an innovation is amenable to implementation in a new setting, an assessment of which is sometimes made in an evidence-based practice project.

implementation research Research that focuses on solving problems in the implementation of healthcare improvements (e.g., a new program).

implied consent Consent to participate in a study that a researcher assumes has been given based on participants' actions, such as returning a completed questionnaire.

improvement science An emerging field that focuses on explorations of how to accelerate quality improvement and to do it rigorously.

imputation A class of methods used to address missing values problems by estimating (imputing) the missing values.

IMRAD format The standard organization of a research report into four sections: the **I**ntroduction, **M**ethod, **R**esults, and **D**iscussion sections.

incidence rate The rate of new cases with a specified condition, computed by dividing the number of new cases over a given period of time by the number at risk of becoming a new case (i.e., free of the condition at the outset of the time period).

independent variable The variable that is believed to cause or influence the dependent variable; in experimental research, the manipulated variable (the intervention).

index A multi-item measure, by convention differentiated from a *scale* in that the term *index* is used for a formative (rather than a reflective) measure.

indirect costs Administrative costs, over and above the specific (direct) costs of conducting the study, also called *overhead*.

inductive reasoning The process of reasoning from specific observations to more general rules (see also *deductive reasoning*).

inference In research, a conclusion drawn from study evidence, taking into account the methods used to generate that evidence.

inference quality An overarching criterion for the integrity of mixed methods studies, referring to the believability and accuracy of inductively and deductively derived conclusions.

inferential statistics Statistics that permit inferences about whether results observed in a sample are likely to be found in the population.

informant An individual who provides information to researchers about a phenomenon under study, term used mostly in qualitative studies.

informed consent An ethical principle that requires researchers to obtain people's voluntary participation after informing them of possible risks and benefits.

inquiry audit An independent scrutiny of qualitative data and supporting documents by an external reviewer to evaluate their dependability and confirmability.

insider research Research on a group or culture—usually in an ethnography—by a member of the group or culture; in ethnographic research, an *autoethnography*.

Institutional Review Board (IRB) A term used primarily in the United States to refer to the institutional group that convenes to review proposed and ongoing studies with respect to ethical considerations.

instrument The device used to collect data (e.g., a questionnaire or observation checklist).

instrumentation threat The threat to the internal validity of the study that can arise if the researcher changes the measuring instrument or measurement circumstances between two points of data collection.

intensity effect size In a qualitative metasummary, the percentage of all thematic findings that are contained in any given report.

intention-to-treat A strategy for analyzing data in a randomized controlled trial that includes all randomized participants in the group to which they were assigned, whether or not they received or completed the treatment associated with the group, and whether or not their outcome data were missing.

interaction effect The effect of two or more independent variables acting interactively on an outcome; subgroup analyses test for an interaction between a treatment variable and the subgroup variable.

intercoder reliability The degree to which two coders, working independently, agree on coding decisions.

internal consistency The degree to which the items on a composite scale are interrelated and are measuring the same attribute or dimension, usually as evaluated using coefficient alpha; a measurement property within the reliability domain.

internal validity The degree to which it can be inferred that an intervention (the independent variable), rather than confounding factors, caused the observed effect on the outcome.

Interpretability In measurement, the degree to which it is possible to assign qualitative meaning to an instrument's scores or change scores.

interpretation The process of making sense of the results of a study and examining their implications.

Interquartile range (*IQR*) A measure of variability indicating the difference between Q_3 (the third quartile or 75th percentile) and Q_1 (the first quartile or 25th percentile).

interrater (interobserver) reliability The degree to which two raters or observers, operating independently, assign the same ratings or score values for an attribute being measured.

interval estimation A statistical estimation approach in which the researcher establishes a range of values that is likely, within a given level of confidence, to contain the true population parameter.

interval measurement A measurement level in which an attribute or a variable is rank ordered on a scale that has equal distances between points on that scale (e.g., Fahrenheit degrees).

intervention In experimental research (clinical trials), the treatment is being tested.

intervention fidelity The extent to which the implementation of a treatment is faithful to its plan.

intervention protocol The specific details about what the intervention and alternative (or control) treatment conditions are and how they should be administered.

intervention research Research involving the development, implementation, and testing of an intervention.

intervention theory The conceptual underpinning of a healthcare intervention, which articulates the theoretical basis for the achievement of desired outcomes.

interview A data collection method in which an interviewer asks questions of a respondent, either face-to-face or by telephone.

interview schedule The formal instrument that specifies the wording of questions to be asked orally of respondents in studies collecting structured self-report data.

intraclass correlation coefficient (ICC) The statistical index used to assess the reliability (e.g., test-retest reliability) of a measure.

intrarater reliability The extent to which a rater or observer assigns the same score values for an attribute being observed on two separate occasions as an index of self-consistency.

intuiting The second step in descriptive phenomenology, which occurs when researchers remain open to the meaning attributed to the phenomenon by those who experienced it.

inverse relationship A relationship characterized by the tendency of high values on one variable to be associated with low values on the second variable, also called a *negative relationship*.

inverse variance method In meta-analysis, a method that uses the inverse of the variance of the effect estimate (one divided by the square of its standard error) as the weight in calculating a weighted average of effects.

investigator triangulation The use of two or more researchers to code, analyze, or interpret data, to enhance trustworthiness.

Iowa Model of Evidence-Based Practice A widely used framework that can be used to guide the development and implementation of a project to promote evidence-based practice.

item A single question on an instrument, such as on a scale.

item analysis A type of analysis used to assess whether items on a scale are tapping the same construct and are sufficiently discriminating.

item bank In item response theory, a large collection of previously tested items, usually with the aim of using the items in computerized adaptive testing (e.g., the PROMIS® item bank established by NIH).

item characteristic curve (ICC) In item response theory, a graphic representation of an item's performance that models the relationship between people's responses to the item and their level of the latent trait; typically an ICC is approximately S-shaped, and different parts of the curve yield information about different item parameters, such as difficulty and discrimination.

item discrimination A parameter in item response theory models that indicates the degree to which an item can differentiate between people with different levels of the latent trait.

item location A parameter in item response theory and Rasch models, indicating the amount of a latent trait a respondent must possess in order to "pass" (or endorse) an item, also referred to as *item difficulty*.

item pool A collection of items generated for possible inclusion in a multi-item scale.

item response theory (IRT) A "modern" measurement perspective, also called *latent trait theory*, that is gaining favor for developing precise multi-item measures of latent traits; in IRT, the focus is on understanding item characteristics, independent of the people who complete the items; an alternative to *classical test theory*.

joint display In mixed methods research, a visual display that presents integrated results from both the qualitative and quantitative strands.

jottings Short notes jotted down quickly while engaged in fieldwork so as to not distract researchers from their observations or their role as participating members of a group.

journal article A report (e.g., description of a study) appearing in a professional journal such as *Nursing Research* or *International Journal of Nursing Studies*.

journal club A group that meets in clinical settings (or online) to discuss and critically appraise research reports published in journals.

kappa A statistical index of chance-corrected agreement or consistency between two nominal or ordinal measurements, often used to assess interrater or intrarater reliability.

Kendall's tau A correlation coefficient used to indicate the magnitude of a relationship between ordinal-level variables.

key informant A person knowledgeable about a phenomenon or culture and who is willing to share information and insights with the researcher, most often in ethnographies.

keyword An important term used to search for references on a topic in a bibliographic database provided by authors or indexers to enhance the likelihood that the report will be found.

knowledge translation (KT) The exchange, synthesis, and application of knowledge by relevant stakeholders within complex systems to accelerate the beneficial effects of research aimed at improving healthcare.

known-groups validity A type of construct validity that concerns the degree to which a measure is capable of discriminating between groups known or expected to differ with regard to the construct of interest, also called *discriminative validity*.

Kruskal–Wallis test A nonparametric test used to test the difference between three or more independent groups, based on ranked scores.

last observation carried forward (LOCF) A method of imputing a missing outcome using the previous measurement of that same outcome.

latent trait An abstract human trait that is not directly observable or measurable, but that can be inferred from people's behavior or their responses to a set of questions; a term often used in the context of item response theory analyses, confirmatory factor analyses, and structural equations modeling. See also *construct*.

latent trait scale A scale developed within an *item response theory* framework, an alternative psychometric theory to *classical test theory*.

lean approach In quality improvement, a model whose aim is to improve quality and efficiency at lower costs, also called the Toyota Production System.

least-squares estimation A method of statistical estimation in which the solution minimizes the sums of squares of error terms, also called OLS (ordinary least squares).

level of evidence (LOE) scale A scale that rank orders evidence for cause-probing questions in terms of risk of bias, based on evidence hierarchies; level I evidence is typically a systematic review.

level of measurement A system of classifying measurements according to the nature of the measurement and the type of permissible mathematical operations; the levels are nominal, ordinal, interval, and ratio.

level of significance The risk of making a Type I error in a statistical analysis, with the criterion (alpha) established by the researcher beforehand (e.g., $\alpha = .05$).

life history A narrative self-report about a person's life experiences vis-à-vis a topic of interest.

likelihood ratio (LR) For a screening or diagnostic instrument, the relative likelihood that a given result is expected in a person with (as opposed to one without) the target attribute; LR indexes summarize the relationship between specificity and sensitivity in a single number.

likelihood ratio test A test for evaluating the overall model in logistic regression or to test improvement between models when predictors are added.

Likert scale A type of scale for measuring attitudes involving the summation of scores on a set of items that respondents rate for their degree of agreement or disagreement; more loosely, the name used for many summated rating scales.

limits of agreement (LOA) An estimate of the range of differences in two sets of scores that could be considered random measurement error, typically with 95% confidence; graphically portrayed on Bland–Altman plots.

linear regression An analysis for predicting the value of a dependent variable from one or more predictors by determining a straight-line fit to the data that minimizes deviations from the line.

listwise deletion A method of dealing with missing values in a data set that involves the elimination of cases with missing data.

literature review A summary of research on a topic of interest, often prepared to put a research problem in context; typically less rigorously conducted than a systematic review.

log In participant observation studies, the observer's daily record of events and conversations, also called a *field diary*.

logical positivism The philosophy underlying the traditional scientific approach; see also *positivist paradigm*.

logistic regression A multivariate regression procedure that analyzes relationships between two or more independent variables and a categorical outcome.

logit The natural log of the odds, used as the outcome variable in logistic regression, short for logistic probability unit.

longitudinal design A study design that involves the collection of data at more than one point in time over an extended period in contrast to a cross-sectional study.

macrotheory A broad theory aimed at describing and explaining large segments of the physical, social, or behavioral world, also called a *grand theory*.

main effect In a study with multiple independent variables, the effect of a single independent variable on the outcome.

manifest variable An observed, measured variable that serves as an indicator of an underlying construct/latent trait; a term used often in a confirmatory factor analysis or structural equations modeling.

manipulation The deliberate introduction of an intervention or treatment in experimental or quasi-experimental studies to assess its effect on outcomes of interest.

Mann–Whitney *U* test A nonparametric statistic used to test the difference between two independent groups, based on ranked scores.

MANOVA See *multivariate analysis of variance*.

masking See *blinding*.

matching The pairing of participants in one group with those in another group based on their similarity on one or more dimension to enhance the comparability of groups.

maturation threat A threat to the internal validity of a study that results when changes to the outcome variable result from the passage of time.

maximum likelihood estimation An estimation approach in which the estimators are ones that estimate the parameters most likely to have generated the observed measurements.

maximum variation sampling A sampling approach used by qualitative researchers involving the purposeful selection of cases with variation on dimensions of interest.

McNemar test A statistical test for comparing differences in proportions when values are derived from paired (nonindependent) groups.

mean A measure of central tendency computed by summing all scores and dividing by the total number of cases.

mean substitution A relatively weak approach for addressing missing data problems that involves substituting missing values on a variable with the sample mean for that variable.

Meaning/process question A question about what health-related phenomena mean to people or about how a process unfolds.

measure A device designed to quantify an attribute or a construct, i.e., to yield quantitative scores.

measurement The process of assigning numbers to represent the amount of a construct or attribute that is present in a person (or object) according to specified rules.

measurement error The systematic and random error of a person's score on a measure, reflecting factors other than the construct being measured and resulting in an observed score that is different from a hypothetical true score, a measurement property within the reliability domain.

measurement model In structural equations modeling, the model that stipulates the hypothesized relationships among manifest and latent variables.

measurement parameter A statistical index that estimates a measurement property of a measure (e.g., Cronbach's alpha is a measurement parameter for the property of internal consistency).

measurement property A characteristic reflecting a distinct aspect of a measure's quality; properties include reliability, validity, reliability of change, and responsiveness.

median A measure of central tendency; the point in a score distribution above and below which 50% of the cases fall.

mediating variable A variable that mediates or acts like a "go-between" in a causal chain linking two other variables, also called a *mediator*.

Medical Research Council framework A framework developed in the United Kingdom for developing and testing complex interventions.

member check A method of validating the credibility of qualitative data through debriefings and discussions with study participants.

MeSH Medical Subject Headings, used to index articles in MEDLINE; recommended by several nursing journals to help authors identify keywords for their articles.

meta-aggregation An approach to the synthesis of qualitative evidence in which findings are categorized and summarized rather than transformed.

meta-analysis A technique for quantitatively integrating the results of multiple studies addressing the same research question.

meta-ethnography An approach to the integration of findings from qualitative studies by translating and interpreting concepts and metaphors across studies, developed by Noblit and Hare.

meta-inference A higher-order conclusion that can be gleaned in a mixed methods study when findings from the two strands (qualitative and quantitative) are integrated and interpreted.

meta-matrix A two-dimensional data array, sometimes used in a mixed methods study, that permits researchers to recognize important patterns and themes across data sources.

metaphor A figurative comparison used by some qualitative analysts to evoke a visual or symbolic analogy.

meta-regression In meta-analyses, a method for statistically examining clinical, demographic, and methodologic factors contributing to the heterogeneity of effects.

metasummary A type of qualitative research synthesis that uses quantitatively oriented methods to aggregate qualitative findings; it involves the development of a list of abstracted findings from primary studies and calculating manifest effect sizes (frequency and intensity effect size).

metasynthesis An interpretive translation produced by integrating findings from multiple qualitative studies.

method triangulation The use of multiple methods of data collection about the same phenomenon to enhance coherence and validity.

methodologic study Research designed to develop or refine methods of obtaining, organizing, or analyzing data.

methods, research The steps, procedures, and strategies for designing a study and gathering and analyzing study data.

middle-range theory A theory that attempts to explain a piece of reality or human experience focusing on a limited number of concepts (e.g., a theory of stress).

minimal important change (MIC) A benchmark for interpreting change scores that represent the smallest change that is meaningful to patients or clinicians, and thus establish clinical significance.

minimal risk Anticipated risks from study participation that are no greater than those ordinarily encountered in daily life or during the performance of routine tests or procedures.

missing at random (MAR) Values that are missing from a data set in such a manner that missingness is unrelated to the value of the missing data after controlling for another variable; missingness is unrelated to the value of the missing data but *is* related to values of other variables.

missing completely at random (MCAR) Values that are missing from a data set in such a manner that missingness is unrelated to either the value of the missing data or the value of any other variable; the subsample with missing values is a totally random subset of the original sample.

missing not at random (MNAR) Values that are missing from a dataset in such a manner that missingness *is* related to the value of the missing data and usually to values of other variables as well.

missing values Values missing in a dataset for some participants due to such factors as refusals, withdrawals from the study, failure to complete forms, or researcher errors.

mixed design A design that lends itself to comparisons both within groups over time (within subjects) and between different groups of participants (between subjects).

mixed methods (MM) research Research in which both qualitative and quantitative data are collected and analyzed to address different but related questions.

mixed studies review A systematic review that integrates and synthesizes findings from qualitative, quantitative, and mixed methods studies on a topic.

modality A characteristic of a frequency distribution concerning the number of peaks, i.e., values with high frequencies.

mode A measure of central tendency; the value that occurs most frequently in a distribution of scores.

model A symbolic representation of concepts or variables, and interrelationships among them.

moderator variable A variable that affects (moderates) the strength or direction of a relationship between the independent and dependent variables.

mortality threat A threat to the internal validity of a study, referring to differential loss of participants from different groups.

multicollinearity A problem that can occur in multiple regression when predictor variables are too highly intercorrelated, which can lead to unstable estimates of the regression coefficients.

multilevel sampling An approach to sampling in mixed methods studies in which participants in the two strands are not the same and are drawn from different populations at different levels of a hierarchy (e.g., nurses, nurse administrators).

multimodal distribution A distribution of values with more than one peak (high frequency).

multiphase optimization strategy (MOST) A framework for optimizing behavioral and biobehavioral interventions and targeting them more effectively, often involving factorial designs.

multiple comparison procedures Statistical tests, normally applied after an ANOVA indicates statistically significant group differences that compare all pairs of groups, also called *post hoc tests*.

multiple correlation coefficient An index that summarizes the strength of a relationship between two or more independent (predictor) variables and a dependent variable symbolized as *R*.

multiple imputation (MI) The gold standard approach for addressing missing values involving the imputation of multiple (*m*) estimates of the missing value, which are later pooled and averaged.

multiple regression A statistical procedure for examining the effects of two or more independent (predictor) variables on a dependent variable.

multisite study A study in which data are collected in multiple sites, typically to enhance generalizability and to recruit a larger sample.

multistage sampling A sampling strategy that proceeds through stages from larger to smaller sampling units (e.g., from states, to census tracts, to households).

multitrait–multimethod matrix method A method of assessing an instrument's construct validity using multiple measures for a sample; the target instrument is valid to the extent that there is a strong relationship between it and other measures of the same attribute (convergent validity) and a weak relationship between it and measures presumed to measure a different attribute (divergent validity).

multivariable risk stratification An analytic approach designed to understand the link between patients' risks and their response to an intervention.

multivariate analysis of variance (MANOVA) A statistical procedure used to test the significance of differences between the means of two or more groups on two or more outcomes, considered simultaneously.

multivariate statistics Statistical procedures designed to analyze relationships among three or more variables (e.g., multiple regression, ANCOVA).

N The symbol designating the total number of participants (e.g., "the total *N* was 500").

n The symbol designating the number of participants in a subgroup or cell of a study (e.g., "each of the four groups had an *n* of 125, for a total *N* of 500").

***N*-of-one trial** A trial that tests the effectiveness of an intervention with a single person, typically using a time series design, which is sometimes called a *single-subject experiment*.

Nagelkerke R^2 A pseudo R^2 statistic used as an overall effect size index in logistic regression, analogous to R^2 in least-squares multiple regression but lacking the ability to capture the proportion of variance explained in the outcome variable.

narrative analysis A qualitative approach that focuses on the story as the object of the inquiry.

natural experiment A nonexperimental study that takes advantage of a naturally occurring event (e.g., an earthquake) that is explored for its effect on people's behavior or condition, typically by comparing people exposed to the event with those not exposed.

naturalistic setting A setting for the collection of research data that is natural to those being studied (e.g., homes, places of employment).

nay-sayers bias A bias in self-report scales created when respondents characteristically disagree with statements ("nay-say"), independent of content.

needs assessment A study designed to describe the needs of a group, community, or organization usually as a guide to policy planning and resource allocation.

negative case analysis The refinement of a theory or description in a qualitative study through the search for and inclusion of cases that appear to disconfirm earlier hypotheses.

negative predictive value (NPV) A measure of the usefulness of a screening/diagnostic test that can be interpreted as the probability that a negative test result is correct; calculated by dividing the number with a negative test that does not have the target condition by the number with a negative test.

negative relationship A relationship between two variables in which there is a tendency for high values on one variable to be associated with low values on the other (e.g., as stress increases, emotional well-being decreases), also called an *inverse relationship*.

negative results Results that fail to support the researcher's hypotheses.

negative skew An asymmetric distribution of data values with a disproportionately high number of cases at the upper end; when displayed graphically, the tail points to the left.

nested sampling An approach to sampling in mixed methods studies in which some, but not all, of the participants from the quantitative strand are included in the sample for the qualitative strand.

net impact The effect of an intervention or program on an outcome, over and above standard care, and sometimes after controlling for the effect of covariates statistically (e.g., through ANCOVA).

network sampling The sampling of participants based on referrals from others already in the sample, also called *snowball sampling*.

nominal measurement The lowest level of measurement involving the assignment of numbers to categories (e.g., married = 1; not married = 2).

nondirectional hypothesis A research hypothesis that does not stipulate the expected direction of the relationship between variables.

nonequivalent control group design A quasi-experimental design involving a comparison group that was not created through random assignment.

nonexperimental research Studies in which the researcher collects data without introducing an intervention, also called *observational research*.

noninferiority trial A trial designed to assess whether the effect of a new treatment is not worse than a standard treatment by no more than a prespecified amount judged to be clinically unimportant.

nonparametric statistical tests A class of statistical tests that do not involve stringent assumptions about the distribution of variables.

nonprobability sampling The selection of elements (e.g., participants) from a population using nonrandom procedures (e.g., convenience sampling).

nonrecursive model A causal model that predicts reciprocal effects (i.e., a variable can be both the cause of and an effect of another variable).

nonresponse bias A bias that can result when a nonrandom subset of people invited to be study participants decline to participate.

nonsignificant result The result of a statistical test indicating that group differences or observed relationships could have occurred by chance at a given probability level, sometimes abbreviated as NS.

normal distribution A theoretical distribution that is unimodal, bell-shaped, and symmetrical, also called a *Gaussian distribution*.

norms Measurement standards based on test or scale score information from a large, representative sample.

novelty effect A potential threat to design-related construct validity that can occur when participants or research agents alter their behavior because an intervention is new or different, not because of its inherent qualities.

null hypothesis A hypothesis stating no relationship between the variables under study, used primarily in statistical testing as the hypothesis to be rejected.

number needed to treat (NNT) An estimate of how many people would need to receive an intervention to prevent one undesirable outcome, computed by dividing 1 by the value of the absolute risk reduction.

nursing intervention research Studies either questioning existing care practices or testing innovations in care that are shaped by nursing's values and goals and are guided by an intervention theory.

nursing research Systematic inquiry designed to develop knowledge about issues of importance to the nursing profession.

nursing-sensitive outcome A patient outcome that improves if there is greater quantity or quality of nursing care.

objectivity The extent to which two independent researchers would arrive at similar judgments or conclusions (i.e., judgments not biased by personal values or beliefs).

oblique rotation In factor analysis, a rotation of factors such that the reference axes are allowed to move to acute or oblique angles and hence the factors are allowed to be correlated.

observation A method of collecting information and measuring constructs by directly watching and recording behaviors and characteristics.

observational notes An observer's in-depth descriptions of events and conversations observed in naturalistic settings.

observational research A study that does not involve an experimental intervention—i.e., nonexperimental research in which phenomena are merely observed.

observed (obtained) score The actual score or numerical value assigned to a person on a measure.

Odds A way of expressing the chance of an event; the probability of an event occurring relative to the probability that it will not occur, calculated by dividing the number of people who experienced an event by the number who did not.

odds ratio (OR) The ratio of one odds to another odds, e.g., the ratio of the odds of an event in one group to the odds of an event in another group; an odds ratio of 1.0 indicates no difference between groups.

one-tailed test A statistical test in which only values in one tail of a distribution are considered in determining significance; sometimes used when the researcher states a directional hypothesis.

open-access journal A journal that allows free online access to articles, without user subscription costs (authors or their institutions typically pay publication costs); traditional journals may include some articles that are open-access.

open coding The first level of coding in a grounded theory study, referring to the basic descriptive coding of the content of narrative materials.

open-ended question A question in an interview or questionnaire that does not restrict respondents' answers to preestablished response options.

operational definition The definition of a concept or variable in terms of the procedures by which it is to be measured.

operationalization The process of translating research concepts into measurable phenomena.

ordinal measurement A measurement level that involves sorting people (or objects) based on their relative ranking on an attribute.

ordinary least squares (OLS) regression Regression analysis that uses a least-squares criterion for estimating the parameters in the regression equation.

orthogonal rotation In factor analysis, a rotation of factors such that the reference axes are kept at right angles, and hence, the factors remain uncorrelated.

outcome analysis An evaluation of what happens to outcomes of interest after implementing a program or intervention, typically using a one group before–after design.

outcome variable A term often used, especially in intervention studies, to refer to the dependent variable, i.e., the outcome (endpoint) of an intervention.

outcomes research Research designed to document the effectiveness of healthcare services and the end results of patient care.

outlier A value that lies outside the normal range of values on a measure, especially in relation to other cases in a dataset.

***p* value** In statistical testing, the probability that the obtained results are due to chance; the probability of a Type I error.

pairwise deletion A method of dealing with missing values in a dataset that involves deleting cases with missing data selectively (i.e., on a variable by variable basis).

paradigm A way of looking at natural phenomena—a worldview—that encompasses a set of philosophical assumptions that guides one's approach to inquiry.

paradigm case In Benner's hermeneutic analysis, a strong exemplar of the phenomenon under study, often used early in the analysis to gain understanding of the phenomenon.

parallel sampling An approach to sampling in mixed methods studies in which the participants in one strand are completely different from those in the other strand, but sampling for both strands is from the same population.

parameter A characteristic of a population (e.g., the mean age of all practicing nurses).

parametric statistical tests A class of statistical tests that involves assumptions about the distribution of the variables and the estimation of a parameter.

pareto chart A chart used in quality improvement that graphically shows the distribution of factors contributing to a targeted problem and that can be useful in setting priorities.

partially randomized patient preference (PRPP) design A design that involves randomizing only patients without a strong preference for a treatment condition.

participant observation A method of collecting data through the participation in and in-depth observation of a group or culture, most often used in an ethnography.

participatory action research (PAR) A research approach with groups or communities that is based on the premise that the use and production of knowledge can be political and used to exert power.

path analysis A regression-based procedure for testing causal models, typically using correlational data.

path coefficient The weight representing the effect of one variable on another in a path analytic model.

path diagram A graphic representation of the hypothesized interrelationships and causal flow among variables.

patient-centered intervention (PCI) An intervention tailored to meet individual needs or characteristics.

patient-centered research Research that focuses on the development of evidence that is important and relevant to patients.

patient-reported outcome (PRO) A health outcome that is measured by directly asking the patient for information.

Pearson's *r* A correlation coefficient designating the magnitude of relationship between two variables measured on at least an interval scale, also called the *product-moment correlation coefficient.*

peer debriefing Sessions with peers to review and explore various aspects of a study, as an approach to enhancing trustworthiness in a qualitative study.

peer review A review and critique of a research report (or proposal) by one or more researchers that makes a recommendation about publishing (or funding) the research.

pentadic dramatism An approach for analyzing narratives, developed by Burke, that focuses on five key elements of a story—act (what was done), scene (when and where it was done), agent (who did it), agency (how it was done), and purpose (why it was done).

per protocol analysis Analysis of data from a randomized controlled trial that excludes participants who did not obtain the protocol to which they were assigned (or who received an incomplete dose of the intervention), sometimes called an *on-protocol analysis.*

percentile A value indicating the percentage of people who score below a particular score on a measure; the 50th percentile is the median for the distribution of scores.

perfect relationship A correlation between two variables such that the values of one variable permit perfect prediction of the values of the other, designated as 1.00 or −1.00.

performance bias In clinical trials, systematic differences in the care provided to members of different groups of participants, apart from the intervention that is the focus of the inquiry, which can occur when there is no blinding.

performance ethnography A scripted, staged reenactment of ethnographically derived findings that reflect an interpretation of the culture.

performance test A measure designed to assess a person's physical or cognitive abilities or achievements.

permuted block randomization Randomization that occurs for blocks of participants (e.g., 6 or 8 at a time), to ensure a balanced allocation to groups within cohorts of participants; the size of the blocks is varied (permuted).

persistent observation A qualitative researcher's intense focus on the aspects of a situation that are relevant to the phenomena being studied.

person triangulation The collection of data from different levels or types of persons, with the aim of validating data through multiple perspectives on the phenomenon.

person-item map A graphic display of information from a Rasch analysis that shows the distribution of respondents on one side of a latent trait continuum or "ruler," and the distribution of items on the other side.

personal interview A face-to-face interview between an interviewer and a respondent.

phenomenography A qualitative approach in which researchers strive to understand the qualitatively different ways in which people experience a phenomenon.

phenomenology A qualitative research tradition, with roots in philosophy and psychology, that focuses on the lived experience of humans.

phenomenon The abstract concept under study; a term often used by qualitative researchers in lieu of a *variable.*

phi coefficient A statistical index describing the magnitude of a relationship between two dichotomous variables.

photo elicitation An in-depth interview stimulated and guided by photographic images.

photovoice A method of collecting qualitative data that involves asking participants to take photographs of their culture or environment and then interpret the photos.

PICO framework A framework for asking well-worded questions and for searching for evidence, where P = population, I = intervention or influence, C = comparison, and O = outcome.

pilot study A small scale version, or trial run, of a study done in preparation for a major study; designed to assess the feasibility of, and support refinements to, the protocols, methods, and procedures to be used in a larger scale study, such as a clinical trial.

placebo A sham or pseudo intervention, sometimes used as a control group condition.

placebo effect Changes in the outcome attributable to the placebo condition because of expectations.

Plan-Do-Study-Act (PDSA) A quality improvement model that involves systematic, rapid cycles of activities, sometimes called *Plan-Do-Check-Act (PDCA)*.

plausibility analysis An analysis of the plausibility of alternative explanations (rival hypotheses) of study results; useful especially in designs without randomization.

point estimation A statistical procedure in which information from a sample (a statistic) is used to estimate the single value that best represents the population parameter.

point prevalence rate The number of people with a condition or disease divided by the total number at risk, multiplied by the total number for whom the rate is being established (e.g., per 1000 population).

population The entire set of individuals or objects having some common characteristics (e.g., all RNs in Canada), sometimes called *universe*.

positive predictive value (PPV) A measure of the usefulness of a screening/diagnostic test that can be interpreted as the probability that a positive test result is correct; calculated by dividing the number with a positive test that has the target condition by the number with a positive test.

positive relationship A relationship between two variables in which high values on one variable tend to be associated with high values on the other (e.g., as physical activity increases, heart rate increases).

positive results Research results that are consistent with the researcher's hypotheses.

positive skew An asymmetric distribution of values with a disproportionately high number of cases at the lower end; when displayed graphically, the tail points to the right.

positivist paradigm The paradigm underlying the traditional scientific approach, which assumes that there is an orderly reality that can be objectively studied, often associated with quantitative research.

post hoc test A test for comparing all possible pairs of groups following a significant test of overall group differences (e.g., in an ANOVA).

poster session A session at a professional conference in which several researchers simultaneously present visual displays summarizing their studies, while conference attendees circulate around the room perusing the displays.

posttest The collection of data after introducing an intervention.

posttest-only design An experimental design in which data are collected from participants only after the intervention has been introduced, also called an *after-only design*.

power The ability of a design or analysis to detect true relationships that exist among variables.

power analysis A procedure used to estimate sample size requirements prior to undertaking a study or to estimate the likelihood of committing a Type II error.

practice-based evidence Research evidence that is developed in real-world settings and is responsive to the needs and circumstances of specific patients and contexts.

pragmatic (practical) clinical trial A trial that addresses practical questions about the benefits, risks, and costs of an intervention as it would unfold in routine clinical practice to enhance clinical decision-making.

pragmatism The paradigm on which mixed methods research is often said to be based in that it acknowledges the practical imperative of the "dictatorship of the research question."

PRECIS-2 instrument A widely used instrument (**Pr**eferred **E**xplanatory **C**ontinuum **I**ndicator **S**ummary) for assessing where a trial design lies on a "pragmatic" to "explanatory" continuum.

precision The degree to which it can be inferred that repeated measurements (or parameter estimates) under unchanged conditions show the same results; usually expressed in terms of the width of the confidence interval.

precision healthcare A model that proposes the customization of healthcare, with decisions and treatments tailored to individual patients based on their unique genetic, physiologic, behavioral, lifestyle, and environmental profile.

prediction The use of empirical evidence to make forecasts about how variables will perform in a new setting and with a different sample.

predictive validity A type of criterion validity that concerns the degree to which a measure is correlated with a criterion measured at a future point in time.

predictor variable A variable (usually the independent variable) used to predict another variable (usually the outcome); term used primarily in the context of regression analysis.

pretest (1) The collection of data prior to an experimental intervention, sometimes called baseline data. (2) The trial administration of a newly developed measure to identify flaws or to gain better understanding of how the construct in question is conceptualized by respondents.

pretest–posttest design An experimental design in which data are collected from participants both before and after introducing an intervention, also called a *before–after design*.

prevalence The proportion of a population having a particular condition (e.g., ovarian cancer) at a given point in time.

primary source First-hand reports of facts or findings; in research, the original report prepared by the investigator who conducted the study.

primary study In a systematic review, an original study whose findings are the data in the review.

principal components analysis (PCA) An analysis that some consider a type of factor analysis; PCA analyzes all variance in the observed variables, not just common factor variance, with 1s on the diagonal of the correlation matrix.

principal investigator (PI) The person who is the lead researcher with primary responsibility of overseeing a study.

priority A feature of mixed methods designs, concerning which strand (qualitative or quantitative) will be given more emphasis; using symbols to represent a design, the dominant strand is in all capital letters, as QUAL or QUAN, and the nondominant strand is in lower case, as qual or quan.

PRISMA guidelines Guidelines for reporting meta-analyses of randomized controlled trials.

probability sampling The selection of elements (e.g., participants) from a population using random procedures (e.g., simple random sampling).

probe A method used in interviews to get detailed and reflective information from a respondent; in cognitive interviews, a method used to obtain information about how a question was processed and answered.

problem statement The articulation of a dilemma or disturbing situation that needs investigation.

process analysis In evaluations, a descriptive analysis of the process by which a program or intervention gets implemented and used in practice.

process consent In qualitative studies, an ongoing, transactional process of negotiating consent with study participants, allowing them to collaborate in decisions about their continued participation.

product moment correlation coefficient (r) A correlation coefficient designating the magnitude of relationship between two variables measured on at least an interval scale, also called *Pearson's r*.

Prognosis question A question about the consequences or long-term outcomes of a disease or health problem.

projective technique A data collection method designed to elicit information about a person's innermost feelings and emotions through the presentation of vague stimuli (e.g., the Rorschach inkblot test).

prolonged engagement In qualitative research, the investment of sufficient time during data collection to have an in-depth understanding of the group under study, thereby enhancing credibility.

propensity score A score that captures the conditional probability of exposure to a treatment, given various preintervention characteristics; can be used to match comparison groups or as a statistical control variable to enhance internal validity.

proportion of agreement In assessing agreement/consistency between two nominal or ordinal measurements, the proportion of cases for which there is total agreement.

proportional hazards model A model in which independent variables are used to predict the risk (hazard) of experiencing an event at a given point in time.

proportionate stratified sampling A sampling approach in which the researcher samples from different strata of the population in direct proportion to their representation in the population.

proposal A document for a proposed study that communicates a research problem, its significance, proposed methods for addressing the problem, and when funding is sought, how much the study will cost.

prospective design A study design that begins with an examination of presumed causes (e.g., cigarette smoking) and then goes forward in time to observe presumed effects (e.g., lung cancer); also called a *cohort design*.

proximal similarity model A conceptualization relating to generalization that concerns the contexts that are more or less like the one in a study in terms of a *gradient of similarity* for people, settings, times, and contexts.

pseudo R^2 A type of statistic used to evaluate overall effect size in logistic regression, analogous to R^2 in least-squares multiple regression; the statistic does not, strictly speaking, indicate the proportion of variance explained in the outcome variable.

psychometric assessment An evaluation of the quality of an instrument, in which its measurement properties (i.e., its reliability, validity, and responsiveness) are estimated.

psychometrics A field of inquiry concerned with the theory of measurement of abstract psychological constructs, and the application of the theory in the development and testing of measures.

publication bias A bias resulting from the fact that published studies overrepresent statistically significant findings, reflecting the tendency to not publish nonsignificant results; a form of *dissemination bias*, also called a *bias against the null hypothesis*.

purposive (purposeful) sampling A nonprobability sampling method in which the researcher selects participants based on a judgment about which ones will be most informative.

Q sort A data collection method in which participants sort statements into piles (usually 9 or 11) according to some bipolar dimension (e.g., most helpful/least helpful).

qualitative analysis The organization and interpretation of narrative data for the purpose of discovering important underlying themes, categories, and patterns of relationships.

qualitative data Information in narrative (nonnumeric) form, such as the information provided in a conversational (open-ended) interview.

qualitative descriptive research Qualitative studies that yield rich descriptions of phenomena, but that are not embedded in a qualitative tradition such as phenomenology.

qualitative evidence synthesis (QES) A systematic review of qualitative evidence, typically using an aggregative approach to evidence synthesis and often focused on qualitative aspects of an intervention or program (e.g., barriers to participation).

qualitative research The investigation of phenomena, typically in an in-depth fashion, through the collection of rich narrative materials using a flexible research design.

qualitizing The process of reading and interpreting quantitative data in a qualitative manner.

quality improvement (QI) Systematic efforts to improve practices and processes, typically within a specific organization or patient group.

quantitative analysis The exploration of numeric data through statistical procedures for the purpose of describing phenomena or assessing the magnitude and reliability of relationships among them.

quantitative data Information collected in a numeric (quantified) form.

quantitative research The investigation of phenomena that lend themselves to precise measurement and quantification, often involving a rigorous and controlled design and statistical analysis of data.

quantitizing The process of coding and analyzing qualitative data quantitatively.

quasi-experiment A type of design for an intervention study in which participants are not randomly assigned to treatment conditions, also called a *nonrandomized trial*.

quasi-statistics An "accounting" system sometimes used to assess the validity of conclusions derived from qualitative analysis.

query letter A letter to a journal editor to ask if there is interest in a proposed manuscript or to a funding source to ask if there is interest in a proposed study.

questionnaire A written or electronic instrument used to gather self-report data via self-administration of questions.

quota sampling A nonrandom sampling method in which "quotas" for certain subgroups (e.g., males, females) are established based on population proportions to increase the representativeness of the sample.

r The symbol for a bivariate correlation coefficient (*Pearson's r*), summarizing the magnitude and direction of a relationship between two variables measured on an interval or ratio scale.

R The symbol for the multiple correlation coefficient, indicating the magnitude (but not direction) of the relationship between an outcome variable and multiple independent (predictor) variables, taken together.

***R*^{2}** The squared multiple correlation coefficient, indicating the proportion of variance in the dependent variable explained by a group of independent (predictor) variables.

random assignment The assignment of participants to treatment conditions in a random manner (i.e., in a manner determined by chance alone), also called *randomization*.

random effects model In meta-analysis, a model in which studies are not assumed to be measuring the same overall effect, but rather different, yet related effects; often preferred to a fixed effect model when there is extensive statistical heterogeneity.

random number table A table displaying hundreds of digits (from 0 to 9) in random order; each number is equally likely to follow any other.

random sampling The selection of a sample such that each member of a population has an equal probability of being included.

randomization The assignment of participants to treatment conditions in a random manner (i.e., in a manner determined by chance alone), also called *random assignment*.

randomized controlled trial (RCT) A full experimental test of an intervention, involving random assignment of participants to different treatment groups.

randomness An important concept in quantitative research involving having certain features of the study established by chance rather than by design or personal preference.

range A measure of variability, computed by subtracting the lowest value from the highest value in a distribution of scores.

rapid review A streamlined and less rigorous approach to evidence synthesis than a systematic review, typically completed in a few weeks to meet information needs in a timely manner.

Rasch model A latent trait model, used to evaluate items for a scale or test, that estimates only item difficulty (location) parameters, which is mathematically similar to a one-parameter item response theory model.

rating scale A scale that requires ratings of an object or concept along a continuum.

ratio measurement A measurement level with equal distances between scores and a true meaningful zero point (e.g., body weight).

raw data Data in the form in which they were collected, without being transformed or analyzed.

reactivity A measurement distortion arising from the study participant's awareness of being observed, or more generally, from the effect of the measurement procedure itself.

readability The ease with which materials (e.g., a questionnaire) can be read by people with varying reading skills, often empirically evaluated through readability formulas.

realist evaluation A theory-driven approach to evaluating complex programs, designed to examine "What works for whom and under what circumstances?"

realist review An approach to synthesizing qualitative and quantitative evidence on complex interventions that seek to understand theory-driven Context-Mechanism-Outcome (CMO) configurations.

RE-AIM framework (*Reach, Efficacy, Adoption, Implementation,* and *Maintenance*) A model for designing and evaluating intervention research that addresses multiple forms of study validity, including external validity.

receiver operating characteristic curve (ROC curve) A statistical tool that involves plotting specificity against sensitivity for different scores on a measure to determine the best cutoff score for "caseness"; also used to generate an index (the *area under the curve*) that has relevance to assessing validity and responsiveness in some situations.

recursive model A path model in which the causal flow is unidirectional, without any feedback loops and distinct from a nonrecursive model.

reflective lifeworld research (RLR) Dahlberg's approach to phenomenologic research that enables researchers to reflect on taken-for-granted assumptions so that the phenomenon being studied can show itself more fully.

reflective notes Notes that document a qualitative researcher's personal experiences, reflections, and progress in the field.

reflective scale A multi-item scale whose items are conceptualized as having been "caused" by the underlying trait that is being measured; items are viewed as the "effects" of an underlying construct. See also *formative index*.

reflexivity In qualitative studies, critical self-reflection about one's own biases, preferences, and preconceptions.

regression analysis A statistical procedure for predicting values of a dependent variable based on one or more independent (predictor) variables.

relationship A bond or a connection between two or more variables.

relative risk (RR) An estimate of the risk of "caseness" in one group compared to another, computed by dividing the absolute risk for one group (e.g., a treated group) by the absolute risk for another (e.g., the untreated group); also called the *risk ratio*.

relative risk reduction (RRR) The estimated proportion of baseline (untreated) risk that is reduced through exposure to an intervention, computed by dividing the absolute risk reduction (ARR) by the absolute risk for the control group.

relevance In the context of patient-centered research, the degree to which evidence is meaningful and valuable to patients and other stakeholders and has the potential to be actionable.

reliability The accuracy and consistency of information in a study. In measurement, the extent to which a measurement is free from measurement error. In statistics, the degree to which the results support an inference about what is true in the population.

reliability coefficient A quantitative index, usually ranging in value from .00 to 1.00, that provides an estimate of how reliable an instrument is (e.g., the intraclass correlation coefficient).

reliable change index (RCI) An index used (used especially in psychotherapy) to estimate the threshold for a "real" change in scores—i.e., a change that, with 95% confidence, is beyond measurement error, which is similar in concept to the *smallest detectable change* but based on a different formula.

repeated-measures ANOVA An analysis of variance used when there are multiple measures of the outcome variable over time (e.g., in a crossover design).

repeated measures design A design that involves the collection of data multiple points in time, to track changes in an outcome.

replication The repetition of research procedures in a second investigation for the purpose of assessing whether earlier results can be confirmed.

representative sample A sample whose characteristics are comparable to those of the population from which it is drawn.

research Systematic inquiry that uses orderly, disciplined methods to answer questions or solve problems.

research control See *control, research*.

research design The overall plan for addressing a research question, including specifications for enhancing the study's integrity.

research hypothesis The actual hypothesis a researcher wishes to test (as opposed to the *null hypothesis*), stating the anticipated relationship between two or more variables.

research methods The techniques used to structure a study and to gather and analyze information relevant to a research question.

research misconduct Fabrication, falsification, plagiarism, or other practices that deviate from those that are commonly accepted within the scientific community for conducting or reporting research.

research problem An enigmatic or perplexing situation or condition that can be investigated through disciplined inquiry.

research proposal A document for a proposed study that communicates a research problem, its significance, proposed procedures for solving the problem, and when funding is sought, how much the study will cost.

research question The specific query the researcher wants to answer to address a research problem.

research report A document (often a journal article) summarizing the main features of a study, including the research question, the methods used to address it, the findings, and the interpretation of the findings.

research utilization The use of some aspect of a study in an application unrelated to the original research.

researcher credibility The faith that can be put in a researcher, based on his or her training, qualifications, and experiences.

residuals In regression analyses, the error term, i.e., unexplained variance.

respondent In a self-report study, the person responding to questions posed by the researcher.

responder analysis An analysis that compares the percentage of people who are *responders*, i.e., who reach a benchmark on a change score in different groups (e.g., a treatment group versus a control group).

response bias An influence that leads a person to select a response option that does not correspond to his or her hypothetical "true score" for an item.

response options The prespecified set of possible answers to a closed-ended question or item, also called *response alternatives*.

response rate The rate of participation in a study, calculated by dividing the number of people participating by the number of people invited to participate.

response set bias The systematic bias resulting from the tendency of some individuals to respond to items in characteristic ways (e.g., always agreeing), independently of item content.

responsiveness The ability of a measure to detect change over time in a construct that has changed, commensurate with the amount of change that has occurred.

results The answers to research questions, obtained through an analysis of collected data.

retrospective design A study design that begins with the manifestation of the outcome in the present (e.g., lung cancer), followed by a search for a presumed cause occurring in the past (e.g., cigarette smoking).

risk/benefit ratio The relative costs and benefits, to an individual person and to society at large, of participation in a study; also, the relative costs and benefits of implementing an innovation.

rival hypothesis An alternative explanation, competing with the researcher's hypothesis for interpreting the results of a study.

root cause analysis (RCA) In quality improvement, systematic efforts to identify the underlying causes of a problem that needs to be addressed (e.g., using the "5 whys" process).

sample A subset of a population comprising those selected to participate in a study.

sample size The number of people who participate in a study; an important factor in the *power* of the analysis and in statistical conclusion validity.

sampling The process of selecting a portion of the population to represent the entire population.

sampling bias Distortions that arise when a sample is not representative of the population from which it was drawn.

sampling distribution A theoretical distribution of a statistic, using the values of a statistic (e.g., means) computed from an infinite number of samples as the data points in the distribution.

sampling error The fluctuation of the value of a statistic from one sample to another drawn from the same population.

sampling frame A list of all the elements in the population from which the sample is selected.

sampling plan In quantitative research, a formal plan specifying a sampling method, desired sample size, and procedures for recruiting participants.

saturation The collection of qualitative data to the point where a sense of closure is attained because new data yield redundant information.

scale A composite measure of an attribute or trait, involving the aggregation of information from multiple items into a single numerical score that places people on a continuum with respect to the trait.

scatter plot A representation of the relationship between two continuous variables on a coordinate graph.

schematic model A representation of a theory or conceptual model that graphically represents key concepts and linkages among them, also called a *conceptual map*.

scientific merit The degree to which a study is methodologically and conceptually sound.

scientific method A set of orderly, systematic, controlled procedures for acquiring dependable, empirical—and typically quantitative—information; the methodologic approach associated with the positivist paradigm.

scoping review A preliminary review of research findings to clarify the range and nature of the evidence base, often to refine the questions and protocols for a systematic review.

score A numerical value derived from a measurement that communicates *how much* of an attribute is present in a person or whether the attribute is present or absent.

screening instrument An instrument used to ascertain whether potential participants for a study meet eligibility criteria or for determining whether a person tests positive for a specified condition.

secondary analysis A form of research in which the data collected in a study are reanalyzed (usually by another investigator) to answer new questions.

secondary source Secondhand accounts of events or facts; in research, a description of a study prepared by someone other than the original researcher.

selection threat (self-selection) A threat to the internal validity of the study resulting from preexisting differences between groups under study; the differences affect the outcome variable in ways extraneous to the effect of the independent variable (e.g., an intervention).

selective coding A level of coding in a grounded theory study that begins once the core category has been discovered; involves limiting coding to only those categories related to the core category.

self-determination A person's right to voluntarily decide whether to participate in a study.

self-report A method of collecting data that involves a direct verbal report of information by the person who is being studied (e.g., by interview or questionnaire).

semantic differential A method used to measure attitudes in which respondents rate concepts of interest on a series of bipolar rating scales.

semantic equivalence In a translation or adaptation of an instrument, the extent to which the meaning of an item is the same in the target culture after the item is translated as it was in the original.

semistructured interview An interview in which the researcher has a list of topics to cover rather than specific questions to ask.

sensitivity The ability of a measure to correctly identify a "case" or true positive, i.e., the correct diagnosis of a condition.

sensitivity analysis An effort to test how sensitive the results of a statistical analysis are to changes in assumptions or in the way the analysis was done (e.g., in a meta-analysis, assessing whether conclusions are sensitive to the quality of the studies included).

sequential clinical trial A trial in which data are continuously analyzed, and *stopping rules* are used to decide when the evidence about treatment efficacy is sufficiently strong that the trial can be stopped.

sequential design A mixed methods design in which one strand of data collection (qualitative or quantitative) occurs prior to the other, informing the second strand; symbolically shown with an arrow, as QUAL → QUAN.

sequential, multiple assignment, randomized trial (SMART) A trial design for optimizing adaptive interventions, involving multiple individualized sequences of interventions used to identify the best decision points, decision rules, intervention options, and tailoring variables for patients with varying response to intervention components.

setting The physical location in which data collection takes place in a study.

simple random sampling Basic probability sampling, involving the random selection of sample members from a sampling frame.

simultaneous multiple regression A multiple regression analysis in which all predictor variables are entered into the equation simultaneously.

single-blind study A study in which only one group (e.g., data collectors) does not know participants' status in terms of the group to which they have been assigned.

single-subject experiment An intervention study that tests the effectiveness of an intervention with a single person, typically using a time series design, which is often called an *N-of-1 experiment.*

site The overall location where a study is undertaken.

Six Sigma Model A quality improvement approach that focuses on improving outputs by minimizing variation in performance.

skewed distribution An asymmetric distribution of data values around a central point.

smallest detectable change (SDC) An index that estimates the threshold for a "real" change in scores—i.e., a change that, with 95% confidence, is beyond measurement error; the SDC is a change score that falls outside the limits of agreement on a Bland–Altman plot.

snowball sampling The selection of participants through referrals from earlier participants, also called *network sampling* and *chain sampling.*

social desirability response bias A bias in self-report instruments created when participants tend to misrepresent their opinions in the direction of views consistent with prevailing social norms.

space triangulation The collection of data on the same phenomenon in multiple sites to assess cross-site consistency and enhance the validity of the findings.

Spearman's rank-order correlation (Spearman's rho) A correlation coefficient indicating the magnitude of a relationship between variables measured on an ordinal scale.

specificity The ability of a screening or diagnostic instrument to correctly identify noncases (true negatives).

stakeholder In the context of healthcare, a person or group that has a direct interest in a healthcare decision or action.

standard deviation A statistic that describes the "average" amount of variability in a set of scores.

standard error The standard deviation of a sampling distribution, such as the sampling distribution of the mean.

standard error of measurement (SEM) An index that quantifies the amount of "typical" error on a measure and indicates the precision of individual scores.

standard score A score expressed in terms of standard deviations from the mean, with raw scores typically transformed to have a mean of zero and a standard deviation of one, sometimes called a *z* score.

standardized mean difference (SMD) In meta-analysis, the effect size index for comparing two group means, computed by subtracting one mean from the other and dividing by the pooled standard deviation, also called Cohen's *d.*

statement of purpose A broad declarative statement of the overall goals of a study.

statistic An estimate of a parameter, calculated from sample data.

statistical analysis The organization and analysis of quantitative data using statistical procedures, including both descriptive and inferential statistics.

statistical conclusion validity The degree to which inferences about relationships from a statistical analysis of the data are correct.

statistical control The use of statistical procedures to control confounding influences on the outcome variable.

statistical heterogeneity Diversity of effects across primary studies included in a meta-analysis.

statistical inference An inference about the population based on information from a sample using laws of probability.

statistical power The ability of a research design and analytic strategy to detect true relationships among variables.

statistical process control (SPC) A statistical method of monitoring a process unfolding over time, used originally to monitor quality in manufacturing processes, but SPC can be used to test hypotheses about changes over time (e.g., as the result of a quality improvement).

statistical significance A term indicating that the results from an analysis of sample data are unlikely to result from chance at a specified level of probability.

statistical test An analytic tool used to estimate the probability that results from a sample that reflects true population values.

stepped wedge design A design involving a delayed treatment strategy within a cluster randomized design (i.e., the clusters receive the intervention at different points in time).

stepwise multiple regression A multiple regression analysis in which predictor variables are entered into the equation in steps in the order in which the increment to *R* is greatest.

stimulated recall interview An approach that involves video recording study participants in social situations and then discussing participants' behavior in follow-up interviews.

stipend A monetary payment to individuals participating in a study as an incentive for participation and/or to compensate for time and expenses.

strata Subdivisions of the population based on a specified characteristic (e.g., gender); singular is *stratum*.

stratification The division of a sample of a population into smaller units (e.g., males and females), typically to enhance representativeness used in both sampling and in allocation to treatment groups.

stratified random sampling The random selection of study participants from two or more strata of the population independently.

structural equations modeling (SEM) A statistical modeling procedure that involves equations representing the magnitude of hypothesized relations among sets of variables; typically used to test a model or theory in a path analysis using maximum likelihood estimation.

structural validity The extent to which an instrument captures the hypothesized dimensionality of a broad construct, an aspect of construct validity.

structured data collection An approach to collecting data from participants, either through self-report or observation, in which categories of information (e.g., response options) are specified in advance.

study participant An individual who participates and provides information in a study.

study section Within the National Institutes of Health, a group of peer reviewers who evaluate grant applications in the first phase of a dual-review process.

subgroup analysis Analytic efforts to understand whether intervention effects vary for well-defined groups of people (e.g., men versus women); undertaken to disentangle heterogeneity of treatment effects (HTE).

subject An individual who participates and provides data in a study; term used primarily in quantitative research.

subscale A subset of items that measures one aspect or dimension of a multidimensional construct.

summated rating scale A composite scale consisting of multiple items that are added together to yield an overall continuous measure of an attribute (e.g., a Likert scale).

superiority trial A trial in which the researchers hypothesize that the focal intervention is "superior to" (more effective than) the control condition; most clinical trials are superiority trials.

surrogate outcome An outcome used as a substitute or proxy for an actual outcome of interest (e.g., continued smoking as a proxy for eventual lung cancer).

survey research Nonexperimental research that involves gathering information about people's activities, beliefs, preferences, and attitudes via direct questioning.

survival analysis A statistical procedure used when the outcome variable represents a time interval between an initial event (e.g., onset of a disease) and an end event (e.g., death).

symmetric distribution A distribution of values with two halves that are mirror images of each other.

systematic review A rigorous synthesis of research findings on a research question using systematic sampling, data collection, and data analysis procedures, and a formal protocol.

systematic sampling The selection of sample members such that every *kth* (e.g., every tenth) person or element in a sampling frame is chosen.

table shell A table without any numeric values, prepared in advance of data analysis to guide the analyses to be performed.

tacit knowledge Information about a culture that is so deeply embedded that members do not talk about it or may not even be consciously aware of it.

target population The entire population in which a researcher is interested and to which he or she would like to generalize study results.

taxonomy In an ethnographic analysis, a system of classifying and organizing terms and concepts developed to illuminate the domain's internal organization and the relationship among the categories of the domain.

test statistic A statistic used to assess the reliability of relationships between variables (e.g., chi-squared, *t*); sampling distributions of test statistics are known for circumstances in which the null hypothesis is true.

test-retest reliability The type of reliability that concerns the extent to which scores for people who have not changed are the same when a measure is administered twice; an assessment of a measure's stability.

testing threat A threat to a study's internal validity that occurs when the administration of a pretest or baseline measure of an outcome variable results in changes on the variable, apart from the effect of the independent variable.

theme A recurring regularity emerging from an analysis of qualitative data.

theoretical notes In field studies, notes detailing the researcher's interpretations of observed behavior and events.

theoretical sampling In qualitative studies, especially in grounded theory studies, the selection of sample members based on emerging findings to ensure adequate saturation of important theoretical categories.

theory An abstract generalization that presents a systematic explanation about relationships among phenomena or that thoroughly describes a phenomenon.

Therapy/intervention question A question focused on the effects of an intervention on patient outcomes.

thick description A rich and thorough description of the research context, study participants, and the phenomenon of interest in a qualitative study narrative.

think aloud method A qualitative method used to collect data about cognitive processes (e.g., decision-making) in which people's reflections on decisions or problem-solving are captured as they are being made, sometimes used in cognitive questioning during a pretest of a new instrument.

threats to validity In research design, reasons that an inference (e.g., about the effect of an independent variable, such as an intervention, on an outcome) could be wrong.

time sampling In structured observations, the sampling of time periods during which observations will take place.

time series design A quasi-experimental design involving the collection of data over an extended time period with multiple data collection points both before and after an intervention is introduced.

time triangulation The collection of data on the same phenomenon or about the same people at different points in time to assess congruence and enhance trustworthiness.

topic guide A list of broad question areas to be covered in a semistructured interview or focus group interview.

tracing Procedures used to relocate participants to reduce attrition in a longitudinal study.

transferability The extent to which qualitative findings can be extrapolated to other settings or groups, an aspect of trustworthiness.

translational research Research that focuses on how study findings can best be translated into practice.

treatment An intervention: in experimental research (a clinical trial), the condition being manipulated.

treatment group The group receiving the intervention being tested, the experimental group.

trend study A form of longitudinal study in which different samples from a population are studied over time with respect to some phenomenon (e.g., annual polls on attitudes toward abortion).

triangulation The use of multiple methods to collect and interpret data about a phenomenon so as to converge on an accurate representation of reality.

true score A hypothetical score that would be obtained if a measure were infallible.

trustworthiness The degree of confidence qualitative researchers have in their data and analyses, assessed using the criteria of credibility, transferability, dependability, confirmability, and authenticity.

***t*-test** A parametric statistical test for analyzing the difference between two group means.

two-tailed tests Statistical tests in which both ends of the sampling distribution are used to establish improbable values.

Type I error An error created by rejecting the null hypothesis when it is true (i.e., the researcher concludes that a relationship exists when in fact it does not—a false positive).

Type II error An error created by accepting the null hypothesis when it is false (i.e., the researcher concludes that *no* relationship exists when in fact it does—a false negative).

umbrella review A systematic review that integrates findings from multiple systematic reviews, also called an *overview of reviews*.

underpowered A characteristic of a study that lacks sufficient statistical power to minimize the risk of a Type II error (i.e., the risk of concluding that a relationship does not exist when, in fact, it does).

unidimensional scale A scale that measures only one construct or a unitary facet of a construct.

unimodal distribution A distribution of values with one peak (high frequency).

unit of analysis The basic unit or focus of a researcher's analysis—typically individual study participants.

univariate statistics Statistical analysis of a single variable for purposes of description (e.g., computing a mean).

unstructured interview An interview in which the researcher asks respondents questions without having a fixed plan regarding the content or flow of information to be gathered.

unstructured observation The collection of descriptive data through direct observation that is not guided by a formal, prespecified plan for observing, enumerating, or recording the information.

urn randomization A method of randomizing participants to groups, in which group balance is monitored and the allocation probability is adjusted when imbalances occur.

validity A quality criterion referring to the degree to which inferences made in a study are unbiased and well-founded; in measurement, the degree to which an instrument measures what it is intended to measure.

variability The degree to which values in a set of scores are dispersed.

variable An attribute that varies, that is, takes on different values (e.g., body temperature, heart rate).

variance A measure of variability or dispersion, equal to the standard deviation squared.

vignette A brief description of an event, person, or situation to which respondents are asked to express their reactions.

visual analog scale (VAS) A scaling procedure used to measure certain clinical symptoms (e.g., pain, fatigue) by having people indicate on a straight line the intensity of the symptom; usually measured on a 100-mm scale with values from 0 to 100.

vulnerable groups Special groups of people whose rights in studies need special protection because of their inability to provide meaningful informed consent or because their circumstances place them at higher-than-average risk of adverse effects (e.g., children, unconscious patients).

wait-list design A design for an intervention study that involves putting control group members on a waiting list for the intervention until follow-up data have been collected, also called a *delay of treatment design*.

Wald statistic A statistic used to evaluate the significance of individual predictors in a logistic regression equation.

web-based survey A questionnaire delivered over the Internet on a dedicated survey website for self-administration.

weighting A procedure used to adjust estimated population values when disproportionate sampling has been used.

Wilcoxon signed rank test A nonparametric statistical test for comparing two paired groups based on the relative ranking of values between the pairs.

wild code A coded value that is not legitimate within the coding scheme for that data set.

within-subjects design A research design in which a single group of participants is compared under different conditions or at different points in time (e.g., before and after surgery).

yea-sayers bias A bias in self-report scales created when respondents characteristically agree with statements ("yea-say"), independent of content.

***z* score** A standard score, expressed in terms of standard deviations from the mean; raw scores are transformed such that the mean equals zero and standard deviations are 1.

Quick Guide to an Evidence Hierarchy of Designs or Therapy/Intervention Questions

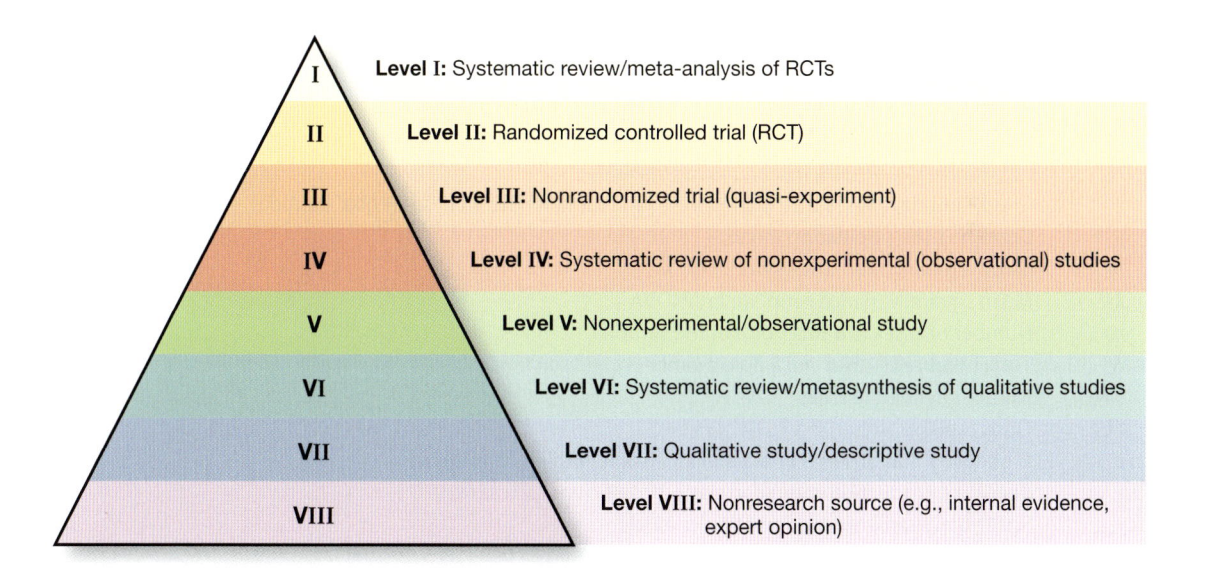

- **Level I:** Systematic review/meta-analysis of RCTs
- **Level II:** Randomized controlled trial (RCT)
- **Level III:** Nonrandomized trial (quasi-experiment)
- **Level IV:** Systematic review of nonexperimental (observational) studies
- **Level V:** Nonexperimental/observational study
- **Level VI:** Systematic review/metasynthesis of qualitative studies
- **Level VII:** Qualitative study/descriptive study
- **Level VIII:** Nonresearch source (e.g., internal evidence, expert opinion)

Glossary of Selected Statistical Symbols

This list contains some commonly used symbols in statistics. The list is in approximate alphabetical order, with English and Greek letters intermixed. Nonletter symbols have been placed at the end.

a	Regression constant, the intercept
α	Greek alpha; significance level in hypothesis testing, probability of Type I error; also, a reliability coefficient
b	Regression coefficient, slope of the line
β	Greek beta, probability of a Type II error; also, a standardized regression coefficient (beta weight)
χ^2	Greek chi squared, a test statistic for several statistical tests
CI	Confidence interval around estimate of a population parameter
d	An effect size index, a standardized mean difference
df	Degrees of freedom
η^2	Greek eta squared, index of variance accounted for in ANOVA context
f	Frequency (count) for a score value
F	Test statistic used in ANOVA, ANCOVA, and other tests
H_0	Null hypothesis
H_A	Alternative hypothesis; research hypothesis
λ	Greek lambda, a test statistic used in several multivariate analyses (Wilks' lambda)
μ	Greek mu, the population mean
M	Sample mean (alternative symbol for $\overline{X}$)
MS	Mean square, variance estimate in ANOVA
n	Number of cases in a subgroup of the sample
N	Total number of cases or sample members
NNT	Number needed to treat
OR	Odds ratio
p	Probability that observed data are consistent with null hypothesis
r	Pearson's product-moment correlation coefficient for a sample
r_s	Spearman's rank-order correlation coefficient
R	Multiple correlation coefficient
R^2	Coefficient of determination, proportion of variance in *dependent variable* attributable to *independent variables*
RR	Relative risk
ρ	Greek rho, population correlation coefficient
SD	Sample standard deviation
SEM	Standard error of the mean
σ	Greek sigma (lowercase), population standard deviation
Σ	Greek sigma (uppercase), sum of
SS	Sum of squares
t	Test statistics used in *t*-tests (sometimes called Student's *t*)
U	Test statistic for the Mann–Whitney *U*-test
$\overline{X}$	Sample mean
x	Deviation score
Y'	Predicted value of Y, dependent variable in regression analysis
z	Standard score in a normal distribution
$\|\ \|$	Absolute value
$\leq$	Less than or equal to
$\geq$	Greater than or equal to
$\neq$	Not equal to

Index

Note: Page numbers followed by f indicate figures, t indicate tables and b indicate boxes.
Page numbers in bold type indicate glossary entries.

3WH, evidence search, 659
5 Whys, 247–248, 247f, **755**
6S hierarchy, evidence search, 24–28, 25t, **755**
6SQuID framework, 597t

A

Absolute risk (AR), 375, **755**
Absolute risk reduction (ARR), 376, 648, 691, **755**
Abstract, 56–57, **755**
  call for, conferences and, 723
  in research reports, 714
Academic Research Enhancement Awards (AREAs), 734
Acceptability, pilot studies and, 605
Accessible population, 257–258, **755**
Acquiescence response set, 292, **755**
ACROBAT-NRSI, 645
Adaptation model, 117
Adaptive intervention, 684–686, 685f, **755**
Adaptive measure, 309
Adaptive trial design, 684–686, 685f, **755**
Adaptive trials, 187
Adequacy, 495
Adherence to treatment, **755**
Adjusted goodness-of-fit index (AGFI), 424
Adjusted means, 417
Adjusted odds ratio, 420
Adulatory Validity, 558
After-only design, **755**
Agency for Healthcare Research and Quality (AHRQ), 640, 732
Agents, intervention, 604
Aggregative qualitative review, 656–657
AGREE instrument, **755**
Allocation concealment, 182, **755**
Alpha (α), **755**
  significance level, 384
Alternative hypothesis, 384, **755**
Analysis, **755**
Analysis of covariance (ANCOVA), 415, **755**
  adjusted means and, 417
  covariate selection, 417
  procedures, 415–417, 416t
  uses of, 415
Analysis of variance (ANOVA), 391, **755**
  multifactor, 393–394

  multiple comparison procedures and, 393
  nonparametric, 395
  one-way, 392–393, 392t–393t
  repeated-measures ANOVA (RM-ANOVA), 394–395
  two-way, 393–394, 394t
Analysis triangulation, 559
Analytic generalization, 495, **755**
Analytic memos, qualitative research, 502, 524
Analytic notes, 515
Analytic phase, 53
Analyzing information, 106
Ancestry approach, **755**
Anchor-based approach, 330, 453, **755**
Anonymity, **755**
  absence confidentiality, 140–141
  definition, 140
  example of, 140
Applicability, 449, **755**
  generalizability and, 680f
  strategies to enhance, 682–697
Applied research, 13, **756**
Applying evidence, 37
Appraising evidence, 36–37
Appropriateness, 495
Area under the curve (AUC), 324, **756**
Argument, 73, **756**
Arm, **756**
Artificial Intelligence (AI), 528
Ascertainment, 184
  bias, **756**
Assembled information, 8
Assent, 142, **756**
Assimilatory biases, 296
Associative relationship, 48, **756**
Assumptions, 9, **756**
  testing for statistical tests, 436
Asymmetric distribution, **756**
ATLAS.ti software, 528
Attention control group, 179, **756**
Attrition, 163, 617, **756**
  bias, 436
Audience, 285
Audio-CASI (computer-assisted self-interview), **756**
Audio-computer-assisted self-interview (ACASI), 233

787

Audit trail, 556, **756**
Authenticity, **756**
 qualitative research and, 554
Authority, 7–8
Author, lead, 706
Authorship, research reports, 706
Autoethnography, 467–468, **756**
Available case analysis, 433
Average treatment effects, RCTs and, 678
Axial coding, 541, **756**

B

Back translation, **756**
Balanced design, 207
Bandura's social cognitive theory, 118–119
Baseline data, 183, **756**
Baseline tailoring variables, 684
Basic research, 13, **756**
Basic social process (BSP), 472, 537, **756**
Basic terminology, 65
Beck's Postpartum Depression Screening Scale, 648
Before–after design, **756**
Being-in-the-world, 468
Benchmarks for clinical significance, 451, **756**
Beneficence, 132, **756**
Benner's hermeneutic analysis, 536
Best evidence, 21–22
Beta (β), 398, **756**
 weight, **756**
 weights, in regression analysis, 413
Between-subjects designs, 159, **756**
Between-subjects effect, 418
Between-subjects tests, 387
Bias, 153–154, **756**
 ascertainment, **756**
 assessment of, 435–436
 attrition, 436
 credibility of quantitative results and, 444–445, 445*t*
 detection, 184, **762**
 dissemination, 643, **762**
 expectation, **763**
 Nay-sayers, **772**
 nonresponse, 271, 435
 publication, 629, 643
 risk of, 644–646, 645*t*
 selection, 436
Bibliographic databases, 88, 89–91, **756**
Bibliography, 736
Big Data, 690, **756**
Bimodal distribution, 366, **756**
Binomial distribution, 383, **756**
Biomarkers, 165, 297, **756**
 definition, 297
 evaluation of, 298–299
 selecting, 298
 types of, 297
Biophysiologic measures, 165
Bipolar scale, 281
Bivariate descriptive statistics, 370–373
Bivariate relationships, 397–398
Bivariate statistics, **756**
Bland–Altman plot, **757**
Blinding, 184–185, **757**

Blind review, **757**
Blog analysis, 507
Body of Evidence, 30
Bonferroni correction, 390, **757**
Boolean operators, 90
Bracketing, 469, **757**
Brainstorming, 602–603
Breach of confidentiality, 140
Bricolage, 462, **757**
Bridling, reflective lifeworld research, 471
British Nursing Index (BNI), 91
Budget justification, 737
Building blocks, 43–48

C

Calendar question, **757**
Carryover effect, 437, **757**
Case–control design, 193, **757**
Case mean substitution, 434
Case selection variant, 577
Case study, 474–475, **757**
Case-to-case translation, 495
Catalytic validity, 552
Categorical variable, **757**
Category system, 292–293, **757**
Causality
 counterfactual model, 175–176
 criteria for, 176
 qualitative research and, 464
 research design, 176
Causal modeling, 422–424, **757**
Causal relationship, 48
Causal (cause-and-effect) relationship, **757**
Cause-and-effect, 48
Cause-and-effect relationship, 176
Cause-probing, 13
 research, **757**
Ceiling effect, 435, **757**
Cells, 371, **757**
Censored data, 422
Census, 232, **757**
Central category, 541, **757**
Central limit theorem, 387, **757**
Central tendency, 366–368, **757**
Centre for Reviews and Dissemination, 640
Certificate of confidentiality, 141, **757**
Change scores, **757**
 reliability of, 328–330
Checklists, 281, 292–293
 for journal articles, 714
Chi-square (χ^2) test, 395–396, **757**
CI. *See* Confidence interval (CI)
CINAHL, 643
Citation management software, 641
Clarity, 285
Classical test theory (CTT), 308, **757**
Cleaning data, 430–432
Clinical heterogeneity, 650
Clinical nursing research, 2
Clinical practice guidelines, 27, **757**
Clinical question, 33–34
Clinical relevance, **757**
Clinical research, **757**

Clinical significance, 449–456, **758**
   benchmarks for, 451
   complex interventions and, 606
   conceptual definitions, 451–452
   group level, 450–451, 451*t*
   individual level, 451–456
   inquiries, 455–456
   Jacobson-Truax approach, 452
   minimal important change (MIC), 452–454
   operationalizing, 452–454, 453*f*
   pilot studies and, 622
   responder analysis and, 456
Clinical trials, 49, **758**
   definition, 224
   equivalence, 225–226
   explanatory, 683
   noninferiority, 225–226
   phases of, 224–225
   pilot studies for, 614–630
   pragmatic, 226
   pragmatic (practical), 683–684
   registry, 225
   sequential, 225–226
   superiority, 225–226
Clinimetrics, **758**
Closed-ended questions, 279, **758**
Cluster randomization, 184, 684, **758**
Cluster sampling, 265, **758**
Cmap Tools, 529
Cochrane Central Register of Controlled Trials (CENTRAL), 91
Cochrane Collaboration, 23, **758**
   risk of bias, 645*t*
   systematic review (SR), 636, 638. *See also* Systematic review (SR)
Codebook, 432, 527, **758**
Codes of ethics, 130, **758**
Coding, 524–529, **758**
   axial, 541
   categories and, 530*f*
   concept, 526
   descriptive, 526
   excerpt, 526*t*
   focused, 541
   holistic, 527
   initial, 541
   open, 536
   process, 526
   qualitative data, 527
   quantitative data, 428–430
   selective, 537
   theoretical, 538
   in vivo, 526
Coefficient alpha, 317, **758**
Coercion, 133, **758**
Cognitive questioning, 343, **758**
Cognitive tests, 283, **758**
Cohen's *d*, 399, **758**
Cohen's kappa, **758**
Cohort design, 194, **758**
Cohort studies, 163
Communicating, 70–74

Communication. *See also* Journal articles. *See also* Research report
   medium and outlet, 705
Comparative effectiveness research (CER), 7, 179, 229, **758**
   practice-based evidence, 681
Comparative value, 489–490
Comparison group, 188, **758**
Competing explanations, 559–560
Complete case analysis, 433
Complex intervention, 595–609, **758**
   critical appraisal of, 609
   definition of, 596
   desirable features of, 598–599, 599*b*
   development phase (phase 1), 599–605
   evaluation phase (phase 3), 606–607
   exploratory research and, 601–602
   frameworks for, 597, 597*t*
   key features of research on, 598
   Medical Research Council framework, 596–597, 596*f*
   mixed method research designs for, 608–609, 608*f*–609*f*
   pilot testing phase (phase 2), 605, 614–630
   synthesis of evidence sources, 605*f*
   theory, 603
Componential analysis, 532
Composite scale, **758**
Computer, analysis files for, 432
Computer-assisted personal interviewing (CAPI), 233
Computer-assisted qualitative data analysis software (CAQDAS), 528
Computer-assisted telephone interviewing (CATI), 233
Computerized adaptive testing (CAT), 309, **758**
Concealment, **758**
Concepts, 43, **758**
   analysis, **758**
   coding, 526
Conceptual definition, 45–46, **758**
Conceptual equivalence, **758**
Conceptual files, 528, **759**
Conceptual framework, 115
Conceptualization, 472
Conceptualizing, 54–55
Conceptual map, **759**
Conceptual models, 43–44, 115, 117, **759**
Conceptual phase, 50–51
Concurrent design, **759**
   mixed methods, 574
Concurrent validity, 321, **759**
Conducting, 55–56
Conference, professional, 723
Confidence interval (CI), **759**
   around a mean, 382–383
   around proportions, 383
   around risk indexes, 383
   for mean differences, 390–391
   precision of, 446
Confidence limits, 382, **759**
Confidentiality, **759**
   anonymity, 140–141
   certificates of, 141
Confirmability, 553, **759**
Confirmation, mixed methods (MM) research, 571
Confirmatory factor analysis (CFA), 352–353, **759**
Confirming cases, 491

Confirming evidence, 559
Confounding variable, **759**
ConQual approach, 663
Consecutive sampling, 262, **759**
Consensus-based Standards for the selection of health Measurement Instruments (COSMIN), 311
Consensus panel, 453
Consent form, 138, **759**
Consistency check, data cleaning, 432
CONSORT
    guidelines, **759**
    reporting guideline, 709, 710*t*, 711*f*
Constancy of conditions, 207
Constant comparison, 472, 536, **759**
Constitutive pattern, 535, **759**
Construct, **759**
Constructivist grounded theory, 474, 541–542, **759**
Constructivist paradigm, 9*t*, 10, **759**
Constructs, 43
Construct validity, 205–206, 324, **759**
    enhancing, 216–217
    evidence, 327
    threats to, 217
Consumer–producer continuum, 3–4
Contact information, 214
Contamination, **759**
Content, 56
    analysis, 477, 542–543, **759**
    interventions and, 602
    validity, 319–320, 343, **759**
Content validity index (CVI), 320, **759**
Context, complex interventions and, 602
Context-mechanism-outcome (CMO), 607
Contextualized description, 561–562
Continuous quality improvement (CQI), 241, **759**
Continuous variable, **759**
Contracts, government, 733
Control charts, 250
Control group, 178, **760**
Controlled trial, **760**
Controlling confounding participants
    control methods, evaluation of, 209–210
    crossover, 206
    homogeneity, 206–207
    matching, 207
    randomization, 206
    statistical control, 207–209
    stratification/blocking, 207
Control method, 10
Control, research, **760**
Convenience sampling, 260, 488, **760**
Convergent design, **760**
    mixed methods, 576–577
Convergent validity, 324–326, **760**
Corbin and Strauss approach, 540–541
Core category, 537, **760**
COREQ reporting guideline, 714
Correlation, 192, 371, **760**
Correlational, 192–193
Correlational designs, 192–193, **760**
Correlation coefficient, 312, 408, **760**
Correlation matrix, 373, 409*t*, **760**

COSMIN (Consensus-based Standards for the selection of health Measurement Instruments), **760**
Cost–benefit analysis, 227, **760**
Cost/economic analyses, 227–228
Cost-effectiveness analysis, 227, **760**
Cost–utility analyses, 227–228, **760**
Counterbalancing, 187, **760**
Counterfactual model, 175–176, **760**
Counts, variable creation, 436
Covariate, **760**
Cover letter, 285
Covert data collection, 133, **760**
Covidence, 641
Cox regression, 422, **760**
Cramér's *V*, 398, **760**
Creativity, 531
CReDECI reporting guideline, 711
Credibility, 153, **760**
    bias and, 444–445
    corroboration and, 445
    proxies and, 442–443, 442*f*, 443*t*, 444*f*
    qualitative research and, 553
    quantitative results, 442–445
    researcher, 552, 562
    validity and, 443–444
Criterion sampling, 491, **760**
Criterion validity, 320–324, **760**
Critical appraisal, 78–79, 79*t*
    of complex intervention, 609
    data collection, 300, 301*b*
    data quality, 332–333, 332*b*
    descriptive statistics, 376, 376*b*
    of dissemination, research results and, 724–725
    ethics, research, 147
    of evidence, 101–103, 104*b*–106*b*
    of inferential statistics, 402–403, 402*b*
    of interpretation of results, 456, 457*b*
    literature reviews, 101–103, 104*b*–106*b*
    of mixed methods (MM) research, 589
    of multivariate statistics, 424, 424*t*–425*t*
    of pilot study, 630
    planning, 169–170
    of practice-based evidence, 698–699, 698*b*
    of qualitative analysis, 545, 545*b*
    qualitative data, 517, 518*b*
    of qualitative sampling, 495, 496*b*
    of quality enhancements, qualitative studies, 563–564
    quality improvement (QI), 252–253, 252*b*
    quantitative sampling, 270–271, 271*b*
    quantitative studies, 234, 234*b*
    of research, 108–109
    of research design, qualitative studies, 480–481, 481*b*
    of research design, quantitative studies, 199, 200*b*
    research hypotheses, 78–79, 79*t*
    research questions, 78–79, 79*t*
    sampling, 270–271, 271*b*
    scale development, 356, 356*b*
    of systematic review (SR), 668
    theoretical frameworks, 125
    validity, 220, 220*b*
Critical Appraisal Skills Programme (CASP), 659
Critical case sampling, **760**
Critical ethnography, 478, **760**

Critical incidents technique, 507
Critical region, 385–386, 385*f*, **760**
Critical theory, 122, 478–479, 478*t*, **760**
Critique, **760**
Cronbach's alpha, 317, **761**
Cross-cultural validity, 328, **761**
Crossover design, 186–187, **761**
Cross-sectional designs, 161–162, **761**
Crosstabs tables, 370–371
Crosstabulation, **761**
Cultural consultants, 493
Cumulative Index to Nursing and Allied Health Literature (CINAHL), 91
Cutoff point, 323, **761**

D

d (Cohen's *d*), **761**
Data, 46–47, **761**
Data analysis, 53, **761**. *See also* Qualitative analysis
   mixed methods (MM) research and, 581–588
   pilot studies and, 627–629
   for practice-based evidence, 690–696
Data and safety monitoring board (DSMB), 144
Database of Promoting Health Effectiveness Reviews (DoPHER), 91
Data cleaning, 430–432, **761**
Data collection, 53, 529
   biomarkers, 297–299
   critical appraisal, 300, 301*b*
   data extracted from records, 299
   forms and procedures, 278
   identifying data needs, 275–276
   implementing, 299–300
   intensity of, 500–501
   measures, selecting types of, 276
   mixed methods (MM) research, 581
   physical performance tests, 299
   pilot studies and, 623, 627
   plan, 52, **761**
   planning, 275–278
   for practice-based evidence, 689–690
   pretesting, 277–278
   protocols, 278, **761**
   in qualitative research, 499–518
   quality-enhancement strategies, 554–558
   quantitative research, 275–301
   selecting/developing instruments, 276–277
   structured observation, 292–297
   structured self-report instruments, 278–292
Data conversion, 529
Data extraction software, 641
Data quality, 492
   assessment of, 435
   critical appraisal, 332–333, 332*b*
   critical appraisal of, 563–564
   measurement, 307–313
   qualitative research and, 551–564
   reliability, 319–330
   responsiveness. *See* Responsiveness
Data saturation, 56, 492, **761**
Dataset, 428, **761**
Data transformation, 436–437, **761**
   in mixed methods research, 576

Data triangulation, 556, **761**
Debriefing, 141, **761**
   peer, 560
Deception, 134, **761**
Dedoose, 528
Deductive hypotheses, 76
Deductive reasoning, 8, **761**
Deduplication software, 641
Default, statistical software, 433
Degrees of freedom, 388, **761**
Deidentified, 138
Deidentified data, **761**
Delay of treatment design, **761**
Deletion method, missing data, 433
Deliberative discussion, focus groups, 505
Delivery mode, intervention, 604
Delphi surveys, 234, **761**
Dendrogram, 530, **761**
Dependability, **761**
   qualitative research and, 553
Dependent variables, 44–45, **761**
Depth of questioning, 285
Descendancy approach, **761**
Description questions, 15–16, **761**
Descriptive coding, 526
Descriptive correlational research, 195
Descriptive notes, 515
Descriptive observation, 513
Descriptive phenomenology, 469, 533, 534*t*
Descriptive qualitative studies, 477
Descriptive research, **761**
   in intervention development, 601–602
Descriptive statistics, **761**
   bivariate descriptive statistics, 370–373
   central tendency, 366–368
   critical appraisal, 376, 376*b*
   frequency distributions, 364–366
   interval measurement, 363
   levels comparison, 364
   levels of measurement, 362–364
   nominal measurement, 362–363
   ordinal measurement, 363
   ratio measurement, 363
   risk indexes, 373–376
   variability, 368–370
Descriptive theory, 114, **761**
Design/planning phase, 51–53
Detailed approach, 533
Detection, 184
   bias, **762**
Determinism, 9, **762**
Development phase (phase 1), 599–605, 600*t*
   activities and strategies, 600–604
   key issues, 599–600
   products of, 605
Deviation score, 368, **762**
Diagnosis/assessment questions, 15, **762**
Diagnostic accuracy, 321, **762**
Diary, 282, 505–506
Dichotomous questions, 280
Dichotomous variable, **762**
Differential item functioning (DIF), **762**
Digital storytelling, 506

Diligence, 563
Direct costs, 737, **762**
Directional hypothesis, 77, **762**
Directional *vs.* nondirectional hypotheses, 77
Disciplined research, 8
Disconfirming cases, 491, **762**
Disconfirming evidence, 559–560
Discourse analysis, **762**
Discrete variable, **762**
Discriminant analysis, 419
Discussion section, 58
   in qualitative research reports, 716
   in quantitative research reports, 713
Disproportionate sampling, 265, **762**
Disseminating, 56
Dissemination, 705–725. *See also* Journal articles. *See also* Research report
   bias, 643, **762**
   critical appraisal of, 724–725
   electronic dissemination, 724
   getting started, 705–707
   journal articles, 718–723
   phase, 53–54
   professional conferences and, 723–724
   qualitative research reports, 714–716
   quantitative research reports, 708–714
   style of reports, 716–717
   theses and dissertations, 717–718
Dissertations, 717–718
   proposals for, 731–732
Distal outcomes, 604
DistillerSR, 641
Distribution-based approach, 331, 454, **762**
Divergent validity, 326–327, **762**
Documentation, 98
   of coding, 432
Domain analysis, 532, **762**
Domain sampling model, 340, **762**
Dose, intervention development, 604
Dose–response analysis, **762**
Dose–response design, 191
Dose–response effects, 179
Dose–response gradient, 653
Double-blind study, 185, **762**
Dummy variables, 410, 436, **762**

E

Ecological momentary assessment (EMA), 284, **762**
Ecological validity, **762**
Economic analysis, 227, **762**
Edinburgh Postnatal Depression Scale, 648
Effect(s), **762**
   average treatment, 678
   heterogeneity of, 678
   magnitude of, 446
   subgroup, 682
Effectiveness studies, 219, **762**
Effect size (ES), 268, 398–402, **762**
   calculations, 401–402
   Cohen's *d*, 399
   logistic regression, 421
   meta-analysis and, 648
   metasynthesis and, 661

   pilot studies and, 621–622
   systematic review (SR), 637
Efficacy, intervention, 606
   pilot studies and, 621–622
Efficacy studies, 219, **762**
Egocentric network analysis, 466
Eigenvalues, 348, **762**
Electroconvulsive therapy (ECT), 446
Electronic dissemination, 724
Electronic health records (EHRs), 252, 299
Elements, 259, **762**
Eligibility criteria, 258, **763**
   intervention/influence, 642
   qualitative sampling and, 488
   study design, 642
   study participants, 642
   systematic reviews and, 642
EMBASE, 643
Embedded design, 475
Embodiment, phenomenology and, 468
eMERGe, 662
Emergent design, 55, 462, **763**
Emergent fit, 540, **763**
Emergent sampling, 491
Emic perspective, 465, **763**
Emotional involvement, 501
Empathic neutrality, 500
Empirical evidence, 10–11, **763**
Empirical phase, 53
EndNote, 641
Endogenous variable, 422, **763**
Endpoint, 177, **763**
ENTREQ reporting guideline, 662
Environmental distractions, 501
EQUATOR Network, 709
Equivalence, **763**
   trials, 225–226, 448, **763**
Errors
   of leniency, 297
   of measurement, 308, **763**
   of prediction, 407
   of severity, 297
   term, **763**
Estimation procedures, **763**
Eta-squared, 400, **763**
Ethical dilemmas, 131–132
Ethics, research, **763**
   animals research, 145–146
   beneficence, 132–133
   codes of ethics, 130
   communications, 141–142
   confidentiality procedures, 140–141
   critical appraisal, 147
   debriefings, 141–142
   ethical dilemmas, 131–132
   external reviews, 143–144
   human rights protection, 143–144
   informed consent, 136–140
   justice, 134–135
   participant authorization, 136–140
   referrals, 141–142
   research misconduct, 146–147
   respect for human dignity, 133–134

Index • 793

risk/benefit assessments, 135–136, 135b
study design, 144–145
study participants protecting, government regulations for, 131
vulnerable groups, 142–143
Ethnography, 49–50, 464–468, **763**
   autoethnography, 467–468
   critical, 478, **760**
   data collection and, 499
   ethnonursing, 466–467
   focused, 465
   institutional, 467
   internet, 507
   interviewing, 503
   macroethnography, 464
   microethnography, 464
   participant observation and, 466
   performance, 466
   qualitative analysis and, 532–533
   sampling and, 493–494
   video-reflexive ethnography (VRE), 467
Ethnonursing research, 466–467, **763**
Etic perspective, 466, **763**
Etiology questions, 15, **763**
Evaluation research, **763**
   cost/economic analyses, 227–228
   definition, 226
   outcome/impact analyses, 227
   process/implementation analyses, 226
   realist evaluations, 228
Event history calendar, 281, **763**
Event sampling, 295, **763**
Evidence
   assembled information, 8
   authority, 7–8
   clinical experience, 8
   designs and, 198–199
   disciplined research, 8
   logical reasoning, 8
   sources of, 7–8
   tradition, 7–8
   trial and error, 8
Evidence-based practice (EBP), 2, 218, **763**
   apply the evidence, 37
   appraising evidence, 36–37
   best evidence, 21–22
   clinical expertise, 22
   clinical question, 33–34
   Cochrane Collaboration, 23
   components, 22f
   definition, 21–22
   evidence hierarchies, 28–30
   experiential evidence, 22
   external validity and, 678–680
   individual, 32–33
   knowledge translation (KT), 23
   models for, 30–31, 31b
   nursing research, study purposes, 16–17
   organizational, 32–33
   patient-centered care, 22
   practice-based evidence and, 677–681
   practice change outcomes, 37–38
   preprocessed/preappraised evidence, 24–28

quality improvement (QI), 24
research evidence, 34–36, 35t
research utilization (RU), 22–23
resources, 24–31
6S Hierarchy, 24–28
steps, 33–37
study purposes, 16–17
systematic review (SR), 636
translational research, 23–24
Evidence-based quality improvement (EBQI), 240
Evidence hierarchies, 28–30, **763**
Evidence profile, GRADE, 654
Excerpta Medica database (EMBASE), 91
Exclusion criteria, 258, **763**
Exemplars, 535
Exit interview, 627
Exogenous variable, 422, **763**
Expectation bias, 184, **763**
Expectation maximization (EM), 434, **763**
Expected frequencies, 396
Expedited review, 144
Experiential evidence, 22
Experiment, 176
Experimental group, **763**
Experimental research, 48–49, **763**
   basic experimental designs, 185–186
   crossover design, 186–187
   design features, 177–185
   factorial design, 186
   limitations, 187–188
   specific experimental designs, 185–187
   strengths, 187
Experts, intervention development and, 602
Explanatory design, **763**
   mixed methods, 577
Explanatory trial, 683, **764**
Explication, mixed methods (MM) research, 571
Exploratory design, **764**
Exploratory (sequential) design, mixed methods, 578
Exploratory/Developmental Research Grant Award, 734
Exploratory factor analysis (EFA), 347, **764**
Exploratory research, 601–602, **764**
External validity, 206, **764**
   enhancements, 218
   evidence-based practice (EBP) and, 678–680
   threats to, 218
Extracting information, 98–101
Extraneous variable, **764**
Extreme (deviant) case sampling, 490
Extreme outlier, 435
Extreme response set, 291, **764**

F

Facebook posts, 507
Face validity, 319–320, **764**
Factor analysis, 327, 347, **764**
Factor extraction, 348–349, **764**
Factorial design, 186, **764**
Factor loadings, 350, **764**
Factor matrix, **764**
Factor rotation, 349–351, **764**
Factors, 348
Failure Mode and Effect Analysis (FMEA), 246, **764**

794 • Index

Feasibility, 69, 605
   assessments, 615
   definition, 615
   pilot studies and, 614–615. *See also* Pilot study
   study, **764**
Feminist research, 479, **764**
Fidelity, intervention, 606, 622–623, **767**
Field diary, **764**
Field notes, 514, **764**
   content of, 514–515
   process of writing, 515–517
Field research, **764**
Fieldwork, 43, **764**
Figures, in reports, 713
Filter questions, 287
Findings, 57, **764**
Fishbone analysis, 248–249, 248*f*, **764**
Fisher's exact test, 397, **764**
Fit, 536, **764**
Fixed effects model, 650, **764**
Floor effect, 435, **764**
Focused coding, 541
Focused ethnography, 465
Focused interview, **765**
Focused observations, 513
Focus group data, 543–544
Focus group interviews, 504–505, **765**
Follow-up explanations variant, 577
Follow-up reminders, 290
Follow-up study, **765**
Food security, 588
Forced-choice questions, 281
Forest plot, 649, **765**
Form(s)
   for NIH grant application, 735–737
Formal grounded theory, 473, **765**
Formative indexes, 310, **765**
Formative measures, 310
Forward translation, **765**
Frameworks, 115–116, **765**
   analysis, **765**
F-ratio, **764**
   analysis of variance (ANOVA), 391
Frequency distributions, 364–366, **765**
Frequency effect size, 661, **765**
Frequency polygons, 365, **765**
Friedman test, 395, **765**
Front matter, dissertations and theses, 717
Full disclosure, 133, **765**
Functional relationship, 48, **765**
Funding for research, 732–734
   government, 732–733
   private, 733–734
Funding Opportunity Announcements (FOAs), 733
Funnel plot, **765**

G

Gaining entrée, 55, 512, **765**
Gatekeepers, 55
Generalizability, 11, 156, 679*t*, **765**
   applicability and, 680*f*
   discussion section of research reports, 713
   results, 449

   sampling, 270
   strategies to enhance, 682–697
Generalized estimating equation (GEE), 406
General linear model (GLM), 417, **765**
Generic qualitative inquiries, 477
Glaser and Strauss' grounded theory method, 473
Global rating scale (GRS), 330, 453, 453*f*, **765**
Going native, 501, **765**
Goodness-of-fit index (GFI), 424
Goodness-of-fit statistic, 421
Google Scholar (GS), 95–97, 643
Government funding
   other countries, 733
   United States, 732–733
GRADE, **765**
   dose–response gradient, 653
   implausible confounders, 654
   imprecision, 653
   inconsistent results, 653
   indirectness of evidence, 653
   large effect, 653
   meta-analyses and, 652–655
   publication bias, 653
   risk of bias, 653
GRADE-CERQual, 663
Grade-point averages (GPAs), 408
Grading of Recommendations Assessment, Development, and Evaluation (GRADE), 30
Grand theories, 114–115, **765**
Grand tour question, 502, **765**
Grant, **765**
Grant applications to NIH. *See also* Research proposal
   forms and processing schedule, 735
   preparing application, 735–738
   review process, 739–740
   revisions and resubmissions, 741
   types of grants and awards, 734–735
Grants, 732
Grantsmanship, 730, **765**
Grant-writing timeline, 742*f*
Graphic rating scale, 765
Gray literature, 643, **765**
Grounded theory, 49, 472–474, **765**
   alternative views of, 473
   basic social process (BSP), 472
   constructivist (Charmaz), 473–474
   core variable, 472
   data collection and, 502
   modification, 473
   qualitative analysis, 536–542, 537*t*
   sampling and, 494
Group-level clinical significance, 450–451

H

Halo effect, 296
Handsearching journals, 644, **765**
Hawthorne effect, 188, **765**
Health and Psychosocial Instruments database (HaPI), 91
Health Belief Model (HBM), 119–120, 603
Health Promotion Model (HPM), 118, 603
Health services research, 229–232
Health transition rating scale, 330, **765–766**
Heideggerian hermeneutics, 470

Hermeneutic circle, 470, 535, **766**
Hermeneutics, 470–472, 535–536, **766**
Heterogeneity, **766**
　meta-analysis and, 647, 649–651
Heterogeneity of treatment effects (HTE), 678, **766**
Heterogeneous variability, 44, 368
Hierarchical multiple regression, 411, **766**
Histograms, 365, **766**
Historical comparison group, 189, **766**
Historical research, **766**
History threat, 213, **766**
Holistic approach, 533
Holistic coding, 527
Holistic design, 475
Homogeneity, **766**
Homogeneous sampling, 490
Homogeneous variability, 44, 368
Hosmer–Lemeshow test, 421, **766**
Humanbecoming hermeneutic sciencing, 471
Humanbecoming Paradigm (Parse), 471
HyperRESEARCH software, 528
Hypotheses, 51, **766**
Hypothesis testing, 383
　between-subjects tests *vs.* within-subjects tests, 387
　critical regions, 385–386, 385*f*
　level of significance, 384–385
　nonparametric tests, 387
　null hypothesis, 383–384
　one-tailed and two-tailed tests, 386–387, 386*f*
　overview of procedures for, 387–389, 388*f*
　parametric tests, 387
　Type I and Type II errors, 384, 384*f*
Hypothesis-testing validity, 324, **766**
Hypothesized results, 446–447

I

Identical sampling, 580, **766**
Identification (ID) number, 140
Ideological perspectives in research, 477
　critical theory, 478–479, 478*t*
　feminist research, 479
　participatory action research (PAR), 479–480
Impact analysis, 227, **766**
Impact factor, journals and, 720, **766**
Impact score, 740
Implausible confounders, 654
Implementation analysis, **766**
Implementation phase, complex interventions, 607
Implementation potential, **766**
Implementation research, 234, **766**
Implications of results, 449
Implied consent, 138, **766**
Improvement science, 241–242, **766**
Improvement Science Research Network (ISRN), 242
Imputation, **766**
　missing data and, 433–435
IMRAD format, 56, 708, **766**
Inception cohort design, 194
Incidence rate (IR), 196, **766**
Incidence studies, 196
Inclusion criteria, 258
Incubation, 531

Independent variables, 44–45, **766**
In-depth interviews, 508–509
Index, 310, **766**
Indirect costs, 737, **766**
Individualization, intervention development and, 604
Individuals, 32–33
Inductive hypothesis, 76
Inductive reasoning, 8, **766**
Inference, 152, 205–210, **766**
　meta-inferences, mixed methods and, 587–588
　quality, mixed methods and, **767**
　statistical. *See* Inferential statistics
Inferential statistics, 362, 380–403, **767**
　chi-square test, 395–396
　confidence interval (CI), 396
　critical appraisal of, 402–403, 402*b*
　hypothesis testing, 383–389
　nonparametric tests, 395
　one-way ANOVA, 392–393
　parameter estimation, 382–383
　power analysis and effect size, 398–402
　repeated-measures ANOVA (RM-ANOVA), 394–395
　sampling distributions, 380–381, 381*f*
　testing correlations, 397–398
　two group means, 389–391
　two-way ANOVA, 393–394
Informants, 42, **767**
Informed consent, **767**
　comprehension of, 137–138
　documentation of, 138
　participant authorization, 136–140
Initial coding, 541
Initiative in long-term care settings (INTERACT), 241
Inquiry audit, 561, **767**
Insider research, 467, **767**
Insightful interpretation, 563
Institute of Medicine (IOM), 681
Institutional ethnography, 467
Institutional Review Board (IRB), 143, **767**
Instrument, **767**
Instrumental case study, 475
Instrumentation, 214
Instrumentation threat, **767**
Instruments, 276
Integration, mixed methods research, 572
Integrative review (IR), 638
Intensity effect size, 661, **767**
Intensity, intervention development, 604
Intensity sampling, 490
Intention-to-treat (ITT) analysis, 216, 435, **767**
Intent, mixed methods research and, 573, 582–583
Interaction effects, 393, 418, **767**
Intercoder reliability, **767**
Inter-item correlation, 347
Intermediate tailoring variables, 684
Intermethod mixing, 581
Internal consistency, 317–318, 351, **767**
Internal validity, 205, **767**
　data analysis, 215–216
　threats to, 212–215
International Committee of Medical Journal Editors (ICMJE), 706

Internet
  ethnography, 507
  interviews and, 506–508
  self-report narratives on, 506–507
Interpretability, 354, **767**
Interpretation, 53, **767**
Interpretation of results
  aspects of, 442
  clinical significance and, 449–456
  credibility of quantitative results and, 442–445
  critical appraisal of, 456, 457b
  discussion section of report and, 713
  quantitative research and, 441–449
Interpretive description, 477
Interpretive mindset, 441
Interpretive phenomenologic analysis (IPA), 470–471
Interpretive phenomenology, 470–472, 535–536
Interpretive qualitative reviews, 657
Interprofessional collaboration, 6
Interquartile range (IQR), 435, **767**
Interrater reliability, 313, 315, **767**
Interval estimation, 382, **767**
Interval measurement, 363, **767**
Intervention(s), **767**
  attributes, 620
  complex, 595–609
  efficacy of, 621–622
  logic model, 603
  protocol for, 602, **767**
  safety and tolerability, 620–621
  theory and, 603
Intervention fidelity, 606, **767**
  pilot studies and, 622–623
Intervention protocols, 52, 178
Intervention research, 14, **767**
Intervention theory, 603, **767**
Interviewer
  developing rapport and, 512
  focus group, 509
Interviews, **767**
  conducting, 509–510
  critical incidents technique, 507
  exit, 627
  focused, **765**
  focus group, 504–505, **765**
  in-depth, 508–509
  Internet, 508
  joint, 505
  life history, 507
  locations for, 507–508
  oral history, 507
  photo elicitation, 506
  postinterview procedures and, 510
  schedule, 278, **767**
  self-interview, reflexivity and, 555
  semistructured, 503–504
  think-aloud method, 507
  unstructured, 502–503
  videoconferencing, 508
  video-stimulated recall, 506
Intraclass correlation coefficient (ICC), **767**
Intramethod mixing, 581
Intrarater reliability, 313, 315, **767**
Intrinsic case study, 475

Intuiting, 469, **768**
Inverse/negative relationships, 312
Inverse relationship, **768**
Inverse variance method, **768**
  meta-analysis, 649
Investigation, 42
Investigator, 42
  triangulation, 558–559, **768**
In vitro measurement, 297
In vivo coding, 526
In vivo measurements, 297
Iowa Model of Evidence-Based Practice, **768**
Item, **768**
  analysis, 347, **768**
  bank, **768**
  discrimination, **768**
  intensity, 341
  location, **768**
  pool, 339, **768**
  reversals, 436
  time frames, 341
Item characteristic curve (ICC), **768**
Item content validity index (I-CVI), 320
Item-level content validity index (I-CVI), 345
Item response theory (IRT), 308, **768**
Item-scale correlations, 347
I^2 test, 650

J

Jacobson-Truax approach, 452
Joanna Briggs Institute (JBI), 640
  meta-aggregation, 662
  systematic review (SR), 636
Joint display, 585–587, 586f, **768**
Joint interviews, 505
Jottings, 516, **768**
Journal(s), 505–506
  impact factor (IF), 720
  open-access, 718–719
  peer review, 722
  predatory, 719, 723
  preparation of manuscripts for, 721
  refereed, 722
  reflexive, 555
  selecting, for publication, 719–720
  submission of manuscript to, 721–722
  traditional, 718–719
Journal articles, 56–59, 718–723, **768**
  abstract, 56–57
  content, 56
  discussion section, 58, 713
  introduction, 57
  method section, 57, 708–712, 715
  reading research reports tips, 58–59
  results section, 57–58, 712–713, 712b
  style of research, 58
  traditional and open-access, 718–719
Journal club, 4, **768**
Journals, handsearching, 644

K

Kappa, **768**
Kendall's tau, 397, **768**
Key informants, 466, 493, **768**

Keywords, 89, **768**
　research reports, 714
King's Brief Interstitial Lung Disease Questionnaire (K-BILD), 455
Knowledge translation (KT), 23, **768**
Known-groups validity, 326, **768**
Kruskal–Wallis test, 395, **768**

L

Last observation carried forward (LOCF), 435, **768**
Latent trait, 338, **768**
　scale, **768**
Laws of probability, 380
Lead author, 706
Lean approach, 244, **769**
Least-squares estimation, 407, **769**
Leininger's method, 533
Letting-go-of-validity, 552
Level I codes, 537
Level II codes, 537
Level III codes, 537
Level of evidence (LOE) scales, 28, **769**
Level of measurement, **769**
Level of significance, 57, **769**
　hypothesis testing and, 384–385
Levels of measurement, 362–364
Life history, 507, **769**
Likelihood index, 421
Likelihood ratios (LR), 322, 421, **769**
Likert scale, 282, **769**
Limits of agreement (LOA), 318, **769**
Lincoln and Guba qualitative integrity framework
　authenticity, 554
　confirmability, 553
　credibility, 553
　dependability, 553
　transferability, 554
Linear regression, **769**
　multiple, 408–414
　simple, 406–408, 407t
Listwise deletion, 433, **769**
Literature reviews, 50, **769**
　analyzing information, 106
　critical appraisal of evidence, 101–103, 104b–106b
　critical appraisal of research, 108–109
　definition, 83
　documentation, 98
　extracting and recording information, 98–101
　Google Scholar (GS), 95–97
　intervention development and, 600
　MEDLINE database, 94–95
　nurse researchers, electronic databases for, 91–94
　organization, 87–88
　primary questions, 85–86
　PubMed, 94–95
　purposes of, 83–84
　qualitative research, 83–85
　screening and gathering references, 97–98
　searching bibliographic databases, 89–91
　search strategy, 88–89
　secondary questions, 85–86
　sources for, 85
　steps and strategies, 86–87
　synthesizing information, 106

systematic review (SR), 636–668
writing, 106–108
Living systematic review, 639
Log, **769**
Logical positivism, **769**
Logical reasoning, 8
Logic model, interventions and, 603
Logistic regression, 419, **769**
　basic concepts, 419
　effect size (ES), 421
　odds ratio (OR), 420
　significance tests in, 420–421
　variables in, 420
Logit, 419, **769**
Longitudinal designs, 162–163, **769**
Longitudinal measurement properties, 354

M

Macroethnography, 464
Macrotheory, **769**
Magnitude of effects, 446
Main effects, 393, **769**
Management-related objectives, 620
Manifest effect sizes, 661
Manifest variable, **769**
Manipulation, **769**
　check, 212
　control condition, 178–180
　experimental intervention, 177–178
　intervention, 177
　treatment, 177
Mann–Whitney U test, 391, **769**
Manuscript, research report, 721
Masking, 184–185, **769**
Matching, 180, **769**
Matrix correlation, 409t
Maturation, 213
　threat, **769**
Maximum likelihood estimation (MLE), 419, **769**
Maximum variation sampling, 489–490, **769**
MAXQDA software, 528
McNemar test, 397, **769**
Mean, 367, **769**
　substitution, **770**
Meaning
　process questions, 16, **770**
　quantitative results and, 446–447
　units, 542
Mean square (MS), 393
Measure, **770**
Measurement, **770**
　advantages of, 308
　definition, 307
　errors of, 308–309
　major types of, 309–310
　parameters, 312
　properties, 310–313
　rules, 307
　statistics, 312–313
　taxonomy, 310–311, 311f
　theories of, 308
Measurement error, 318–319, **770**
Measurement model, 352, **770**
Measurement parameters, 312, **770**

798 • Index

Measurement property, **770**
Median, 367, **770**
Mediating variable, 72, **770**
Medical Literature On-Line (MEDLINE), 91
Medical Research Council (MRC) complex intervention framework, 596–597, 596f, 606. *See also* Complex intervention
Medical Research Council framework, **770**
Medical Subject Headings (MeSH), 94
MEDLINE database, 94–95, 643
Member check, 557–558, **770**
Mendeley, 641
MeSH, **770**
Meta-aggregation, 26, 657, **770**
    analysis, 662–663
    assessment of confidence, 663
    preliminary steps, 662
    writing report, 663
Meta-analysis, 25, 661, **770**
    analyzing data in, 649–652, 649f, 652f
    criteria for using, 647
    effects, calculation of, 647–648
    extracting and encoding data for, 646
    graphic output, 651–652
Meta-Easy, 641
Metaethnography, 657, **770**
Meta-inference, 570, **770**
Meta-matrices, 584–585, 584f, **770**
Metamethod, 661
Metaphor, **770**
Metaphorical emergings, 536
Metaphors, 531
Meta-regression, 651, **770**
Metastudy, 657
Metasummary, 658, **770**
Metasynthesis, 26, 657, **770**
    preliminary steps, 658–660
    Sandelowski and Barroso, 661–662
    synthesizing, 660–662
    systematic review (SR), 637
    writing report on, 662
Metatheory, 661
Methodologic heterogeneity, 650
Methodologic notes, 515
Methodologic studies, 234, **770**
Method section, 57
    in qualitative research reports, 715
    in quantitative research reports, 708–712
    research, **770**
Method triangulation, 556, **770**
Meticulousness, 563
Microethnography, 464
Middle-range theory, 115, 117–118, **770**
Minimal clinically important difference (MCID), 452
Minimal detectable change (MDC), 329
Minimal important change (MIC), 452, **770**
    anchor-based approach, 453
    benchmarks, 452–454
    consensus panel and, 453
    distribution-based approach, 454
    global rating scale (GRS), 453, 453f
    triangulation of methods, 454–455
Minimal important difference (MID), 452

Minimal risk, 135, **770**
Mishel's Uncertainty in Illness Theory, 118
Missing at random (MAR), 432, **770**
Missing completely at random (MCAR), 432, **771**
Missing information, 285
Missing not at random (MNAR), 432, **771**
Missing values, 429, **771**
    assessing and handling, 432–435
Missing Values Analysis (MVA) in SPSS, 433
Mixed design, 159, **771**
    RM-ANOVA and, 418
Mixed methods (MM) research, 13, 153, 569–589, **771**
    applications of, 570–572
    complementarity, 570
    complex interventions and, 598, 605, 608–609, 608f–609f. *See also* Complex intervention
    confirmation and explication, 571
    core design, 575–578, 576t
    critical appraisal of, 589
    data analysis and, 581–588
    data collection, 581
    definition of, 569–570
    designs for, 574–579
    enhanced validity, 570
    fixed *vs.* emergent designs, 574
    instrumentation, 571
    integration and, 572
    intervention and program evaluation, 571–572
    intervention development, 571
    joint displays, 585–587, 586f
    meta-inferences and, 587–588
    notation and diagramming, 575, 576f
    overview of, 569–573
    paradigm issues and, 570
    pilot studies and, 614–630
    practicality, 570
    prioritization, 575
    purpose/intent of, 573
    quality criteria for, 588–589
    research questions for, 573–574
    sampling in, 579–581
    sequencing, 574
    skills and resources for, 572–573
Mixed results, 448–449
Mixed studies reviews (MSRs), 637, 664, **771**
    approaches, 666
    conducting, 664–666
    designs, 665–666
    rationale for, 664
    research questions, 664–665
Mobile positioning, observations and, 513
Modality, 366, **771**
Mode, 367, **771**
Model, **771**
Modeling, intervention development, 603–605
Models of healthcare quality, 230
Models, qualitative research, 523
Moderators, 504
    analyses, 693
    effects, 650
    variable, 72, **771**
Modular budget, 737
MOOSE reporting guideline, 655

Mortality, 213
  threat, **771**
Multicollinearity, 409, **771**
Multifactor ANOVA, 393–394
Multilevel sampling, 580, **771**
Multimodal distribution, 366, **771**
Multiphase optimization strategy (MOST), 684, **771**
Multiphase timing, 574
Multiple case design, 475
Multiple-choice questions, 280
Multiple comparison procedures, 393, **771**
Multiple correlation, 406
  coefficient, **771**
Multiple correlation coefficient *(R)*, 409
Multiple imputation (MI), 434, **771**
Multiple paradigms, 12–13
Multiple positioning, observations and, 513
Multiple regression (analysis), 406, **771**
  adding predictors, 410
  basic concepts, 408–410, 409*t*
  handling predictors, 411–412
  hierarchical, 411
  overall equation and *R,* 410
  power analysis, 414, 415*t*
  relative contribution of predictors, 412–413
  results, 413–414
  simultaneous, 411
  stepwise, 411–412, 412*f*
  tests of significance and, 410–411
Multisite studies, 43, **771**
Multistage cluster sampling, 265
Multistage sampling, 259, **771**
Multitrait–multimethod matrix method, **771**
Multivariable risk stratification (MRS), 694–695, 695*t*, **771**
Multivariate analysis of covariance (MANCOVA), 419
Multivariate analysis of variance (MANOVA), 418–419, **769, 771**
Multivariate statistics, 406–425, **771**
  analysis of covariance (ANCOVA), 415–417
  causal modeling, 422–424
  critical appraisal of, 424, 424*t*–425*t*
  least-squares multivariate techniques, 417–418
  logistic regression, 419–421
  multiple linear regression, 408–414
  multivariate analysis of covariance (MANCOVA), 419
  multivariate analysis of variance (MANOVA), 418–419
  simple linear regression, 406–408, 407*t*
  survival analysis, 421–422
Mutual shaping, 464

N
N, **771**
n, **771**
Nagelkerke R^2, 421, **772**
Narrative analysis, 475–476, **772**
Narrative reviews, 6
National Institute of Nursing Research (NINR), 4, 733
National Institutes of Health (NIH), 732
National Quality Forum (NQF), 251–252
Natural experiment, 194–195, **772**
Naturalistic setting, **772**
Nay-sayers, 292
  bias, **772**

NCapture, 528
Needs assessments, 234, **772**
Negative case analysis, 560, **772**
Negatively skewed distribution, 366
Negative predictive value (NPV), 322, **772**
Negative relationship, **772**
Negative results, **772**
Negative skew, **772**
Negative stems, 341
Nested sampling, 580, **772**
Net impacts, 227, **772**
Network meta-analysis (NMA), 639
Network sampling, **772**
Next-generation systematic reviews
  individual patient-level meta-analysis, 639
  network meta-analysis (NMA), 639
N-of-one trial, **771**
N-of-1 trials, 187, 686–687
Nola Pender's Health Promotion Model (HPM), 118
NoMAD (Normalization MeAsure Development), 607
Nominal measurement, 362–363, **772**
Nondirectional hypothesis, 77, **772**
Nonequivalent control group design, **772**
Nonequivalent control group pretest–post-test design, 188
Nonexperimental/observational research, 48–49, **772**
  correlational designs, 192–193
  definition, 192
  descriptive research, 195–196
  limitations of, 196–197
  natural experiments, 194–195
  path analytic studies, 195
  prospective designs, 194
  retrospective designs, 193
  strengths, 197–198
Noninferiority trials, 225–226, 448, **772**
Nonparametric statistical tests, **772**
Nonparametric tests, 387
Nonparametric two-group tests, 391
Nonprobability sampling, **772**
  consecutive sampling, 262
  convenience sampling, 260
  evaluation of, 262–263
  purposive sampling, 262
  quota sampling, 260–261
Nonrecursive models, 423, **772**
Nonresponse bias, 271, 435, **772**
Nonsignificant results, 386, 447–449, **772**
Normal distribution, **772**
Normalization process theory (NPT), 607
Norms, 158, **772**
Novelty effect, **772**
Null hypotheses, 77, 383–384, **772**
Number needed to treat (NNT), 376, 450, 678, **772**
Nurse researchers, electronic databases for, 91–94
Nursing intervention research, 595, **772**. *See also* Complex intervention
Nursing processes and actions, 231
Nursing research, **773**
  Bandura's social cognitive theory, 118–119
  conceptual models, 117
  constructivist paradigm, 9*t*, 10
  consumer–producer continuum, 3–4
  current and future directions, 4–7, 5*t*–6*t*

Nursing research *(Continued)*
   definition, 2
   description questions, 15–16
   diagnosis/assessment questions, 15
   etiology questions, 15
   health belief model (HBM), 119–120
   historical perspective, 4
   importance of, 3
   meaning/process questions, 16
   middle-range theories, 117–118
   Mishel's uncertainty in illness theory, 118
   multiple paradigms, 12–13
   Nola Pender's Health Promotion Model (HPM), 118
   Orem's self-care deficit nursing theory, 117
   other models and theories, 118
   paradigms and methods, 8–9
   positivist paradigm, 9–10, 9*t*
   prognosis questions, 15
   purposes of, 13–17, 13*t*
   quantitative and qualitative research, 10–12
   Roy's adaptation model, 117
   study purposes and evidence-based practice, 16–17
   theories of nursing, 117
   theory/model selecting, 120
   therapy/intervention, 14, 14*t*
   Transtheoretical model, 119
   users assistance, 17
Nursing-sensitive outcomes, 231–232, **773**
Nursology, 120
NVivo software, 528, 641

O

Objectivity, 167, **773**
   systematic review (SR), 637
Oblique rotations, 349, **773**
Observation, 164–165, **773**
   persistent, 554–555
   recording methods, 514–517
Observational notes, 515, **773**
Observational research, **773**
Observational study, 49
Observed frequencies, 396
Observed/obtained score, 308, **773**
Observer biases, 165
Observer–participant role, 511
Odds, 419, **773**
Odds ratio (OR), 376, 383, 648, **773**
   adjusted, 420
   logistic regression and, 420
One-tailed tests, 386–387, 386*f*, **773**
One-way analysis of variance (ANOVA), 392–393, 392*t*–393*t*
Open-access journal movement, 97, 718–719, **773**
Open coding, 536, **773**
Open-ended questions, 279, **773**
Operational definition, 45–46, **773**
Operationalization, **773**
Opportunistic sampling, 491
Oral history, 507
Oral reports, 723–724
Ordering bias, 216
Ordinal measurement, 363, **773**
Ordinary least squares (OLS), 407, **773**
Orem's self-care deficit nursing theory, 117

Organization, 32–33, 87–88
Orthogonal rotation, 349, **773**
Outcome analysis, 227, **773**
Outcome/impact analyses, 227
Outcomes, 229–232, **773**
   challenges in, 232
   distal, 604
   in intervention development, 604
   proximal, 604
Outcome variable, 44, **773**
Outliers, 430, **773**
   sampling, 490
Overhead costs, 737
Overviews of reviews, 639

P

Paired *t*-tests, 391
Pair matching, 207
Pairwise deletion, 433, **773**
Paper format thesis, 717
Paradigm, 8, **773**
   pragmatism, 570
Paradigm cases, 535, **773**
Paradigms, 8–9, 65–66
Parallel databases variant, 576
Parallel sampling, 580, **773**
Parallel test reliability, 313, 316
Parameter, 362, **773**
   estimation, 382
Parametric statistical tests, **773**
Parametric tests, 387
Parent Announcement, NIH, 733
Pareto charts, 249, **773**
Parsesciencing, 471, 536
Parse's phenomenologic-hermeneutic research method, 471
Partially randomized patient preference (PRPP), 184, **774**
Partial randomization, 184
Participant-driven inquiry, 563
Participant observation, 466, 510–517, **774**
   establishing rapport, 512
   evaluation of, 517
   observer-participant role, 511
   recording observations and, 514–517
   unstructured observational data, 513–514
   windshield survey, 512
Participatory action research (PAR), 479–480, **774**
Path analysis, 195, 422, **774**
Path coefficients, 423, **774**
Path diagram, 422, 423*f*, **774**
Patient acceptable symptom state (PASS), 452
Patient and public involvement (PPI), 157
   complex interventions and, 598
Patient-centered care, 22
Patient-centered interventions (PCIs), 178, **774**
Patient centeredness, 7
Patient-Centered Outcomes Research Institute (PCORI), 229, 682, 732
Patient-centered research, **774**
Patient-reported outcomes (PROs), 164, 282, **774**
Patient-Reported Outcomes Measurement Information System (PROMIS®), 291
Patient risk adjustment, 231
Pearson's *r*, 312, 373, 397, **774**
   meta-analysis and, 648

Peer
  reviewers, 101
  reviews, **774**
Peer debriefing, 560, **774**
Peer review
  qualitative integrity and, 560–561
Pender's Health Promotion Model, 603
Pentadic dramatism, 476, **774**
Percentile, 354, **774**
Perfect relationship, 312, **774**
Performance bias, 184, **774**
Performance ethnography, 466, **774**
Performance tests, 299, **774**
Permuted block randomization, 184, **774**
Per-protocol analysis, 215, **774**
Persistent observation, 554–555, **774**
Personal interviews, 233, **774**
Personalized healthcare, 695–696
Personal notes, 515
Person-item map, **774**
Person triangulation, 556, **774**
Phenomena, 43
Phenomenography, 472, **774**
Phenomenology, 49, 468–472, **774**
  data collection and, 499
  descriptive, 469
  interpretive (hermeneutics), 470–472
  Parse's method, 471
  phenomenography, 472
  qualitative analysis and, 533–536
  reflective lifeworld research (RLR), 471
  sampling and, 494
Phenomenon, **774**
Phi coefficient, 398, **774**
Photo elicitation, 506, **774**
Photovoice, 506, **774**
Physical performance tests, 299
PICO framework, **774**
Pillar Integration Process, 587
Pilot study, 168, 605, 614–630, **775**
  basic issues, 614–616
  CONSORT guidelines and, 709
  criteria and pilot objectives, 625–626
  criteria for decision-making, 616–626
  critical appraisal of, 630
  data analysis, 627–629
  data collection, 627, 628t
  feasibility study and, 614–615
  lessons from, 616
  management-related objectives, 620
  overall purpose of, 615–616
  process-related objectives, 617–619, 618t–619t
  products of, 629–630
  research design, 626
  resource-related objectives, 619–620
  sampling, 626–627
  scientific/substantive issues in, 620–624
Placebo, 178, **775**
Placebo effects, 178, **775**
Plan-Do-Study-Act (PDSA), **775**
Planning a study, 54–55
  concepts, 152–157
  critical appraisal, 169–170

  data collection, 163–167
  project organization, 167–169
  research design features, 157–163
  tools, 152–157
Plausibility analysis, **775**
Point-biserial correlation coefficient, 397
Point estimation, 382, **775**
Point-of-care (PoC), 26
Point prevalence rate, **775**
Pooling, data, 437
Populations, 52, 257–258, **775**
Positively skewed distribution, 366
Positive predictive value (PPV), 322, **775**
Positive relationship, 312, **775**
Positive results, 446, **775**
Positive skew, **775**
Positive stems, 341
Positivism, 9
Positivist paradigm, 9–10, 9t, **775**
Poster session, 724, **775**
Post hoc test, **775**
Post positivist paradigm, 10
Posttest, **775**
Posttest-only design, 185, **775**
Power, **775**
  systematic review (SR), 637
Power analysis, 266, 398–402, **775**
  multiple regression situations, 414, 415t
Practical significance, 450
Practice-based evidence, 677–699, **775**
  critical appraisal of, 698–699, 698b
  data analysis for, 690–696
  data collection for, 689–690
  designing a study for, 682–688
  evidence-based practice and, 677–681
  planning a study to develop, 682
  reporting results for, 696–697
  sampling for, 688–689
Practice change outcomes, 37–38
Pragmatic clinical trials (PCTs), 226, **775**
  cluster randomization, 684
  practice-based evidence and, 683–684
Pragmatism, **775**
  paradigm, 570
Preanalysis phase, 428
  coding quantitative data, 428–430
Precise coding, 430
PRECIS-2 instrument, 683, **775**
Precision, **775**
  healthcare, 695–696, **775**
  of results, interpretation and, 445–446
  systematic review (SR), 637
Precoding, 524
Predatory
  conference, 723
  journals, 719
Prediction, **775**
Predictive validity, 321, **775**
Predictive values, 322
Predictor variables, 408, **775**
Preliminary groundwork, 640
Preprocessed/preappraised evidence, 24–28
Pretesting, 277, **776**

Pretest–posttest design, 185, **776**
Preunderstandings, 556
Prevalence, **776**
Prevalence rate (PR), 196
Prevalence studies, 195
Primary questions, 85–86
Primary source, 85, **776**
Primary studies, 24
Primary study, 636, **776**
Principal axis factor analysis, 348
Principal components analysis (PCA), 348, **776**
Principal investigator (PI), 42, **776**
Priority, 575, **776**
   score, 740
PRISMA guidelines, **776**
PRISMA reporting guideline, 636, 655
Privacy Boards, 144
Private funding, research proposals, 733–734
Probability sampling, **776**
   evaluation of, 266
   multistage cluster sampling, 265
   simple random sampling, 263–264
   stratified random sampling, 264–265
   systematic sampling, 265–266
Probes, 289, 343, **776**
Problem statements, 65, 73–74, **776**
Procedures manual, 212
Process analysis, **776**
Process coding, 526
Process consent, 137, **776**
Process/implementation analyses, 226
Process-related objectives, 617–619, 618*t*–619*t*
Product moment correlation coefficient (r), 372, **776**
Prognosis questions, 15, **776**
Program Announcement (PA), NIH, 733
Program of research, 78
Projective techniques, 164, **776**
Project Narrative, 736
Project Summary, 736
Prolonged engagement, 554–555, **776**
Propensity matching, 207
Propensity scores, 207, 417, **776**
Proportional hazards model, **776**
Proportionate stratified sampling, 265, **776**
Proportion of agreement, **776**
Proposal, 53, 730–745, **776**. *See also* Research proposal
Prospective design, 194, **776**
PROSPERO, 640
Protocol
   intervention, 602
   systematic reviews, 642–643
Proximal outcome, 604
Proximal similarity model, **776**
Pseudo R^2, 421, **776**
Psychology Information (PsycINFO), 91
Psychometric assessment, **776**
Psychometrics, 308, **777**
Publication bias, 629, 643, **777**
Publication option, dissertations, 717
PubMed, 94–95
Purposive sampling, 262
   representativeness/comparative value, 489–490
   sequentially, 491
   special/unique cases, 490–491

Purposive (purposeful) sampling, **777**
p value, **773**

Q

QDA Miner software, 528
Q sorts, 284, **777**
Qualitative analysis, 522–545, **777**
   analytic procedures, 529–532
   challenges, 522
   coding, 525–527
   content analysis, 542–543
   critical appraisal of, 545, 545*b*
   data management, 525–529
   decisions in, 522–524
   ethnography and, 532–533
   focus group data and, 543–544
   grounded theory, 536–542
   overview of, 524*f*
   phenomenology and, 533–536
   process of, 524–525
Qualitative data, 46, 47*b*, 499–518, **777**
   coding, 527–529
   computer software, 528–529
   critical appraisal of data collection, 517, 518*b*
   enhancing quality and integrity of, 554–562
   issues in collecting, 499–502, 500*t*
   management of, 525–529
   manual methods, 528
   quantitizing, 585
   self-reports and, 502–510
   transforming, 585
Qualitative descriptive research, 49, **777**
Qualitative evidence synthesis (QES), 637, **777**
Qualitative Health Research, 463
Qualitative outcome analysis (QOA), 603
Qualitative research, 10–12, 48–56, 83–85, **777**
   activities, 54–56
   conceptualizing, 54–55
   conducting, 55–56
   data collection and, 499–518
   disseminating, 56
   dissemination, research results and, 714–716
   ethnography, 49–50
   grounded theory, 49
   phenomenology, 49
   planning, 54–55
   qualitative descriptive research, 49
   research proposal and, 731
   rigor in, 551–564
Qualitative sampling, 487–496
   critical appraisal of, 495, 496*b*
   logic of, 487–488
   qualitative traditions and, 493–494
   sample size and, 492–493
   transferability and, 494–495
   types of, 488–492
Qualitative secondary data analysis, 544
Qualitative systematic review, 656–663
   aggregative *vs.* interpretive, 656–657
   meta-aggregation, 662–663
   metasynthesis, 657–662
Qualitizing, **777**
Qualitizing data, 585
Quality-adjusted life year (QALY), 228

Quality enhancement, qualitative research. *See also* Trustworthiness
  coding and analysis, 555–561
  critical appraisal of, 563–564
  debates about, 551–552
  presentation, 561–562
  quality-minded outlook and, 562–563
  strategies for, 554–558
  terminology and, 553
Quality improvement (QI), 24, **777**
  continuous quality improvement (CQI), 241
  critical appraisal, 252–253, 252*b*
  designs for projects, 249–251
  features of, 241
  impetus for improvement, health care, 240
  interventions, 242–244
  Lean approach, 244
  nursing and improvement science, 241–242
  Plan-Do-Study-Act (PDSA), 244–246, 245*f*
  research, 239–240
  Six Sigma approach, 244
  tools and methods, 247–252
  types of, 242–244
Quantitative analysis, **777**
  cleaning data, 430–432
  coding and, 428–430
  entering, 430–432
  preliminary assessments and actions, 432–437
  principal analyses, 437–438
  verifying, 430–432
Quantitative data, 46, **777**
  analysis of. *See* Quantitative analysis
  flow of tasks, 429*f*
  process-related objectives, 617
Quantitative information, 11
Quantitative portion of the entrance exam (EE-Q), 408
Quantitative research, 10–12, 48–56, 74–75, **777**
  analytic phase, 53
  clinical trial, 49
  conceptual phase, 50–51
  data collection, 275–301
  design and planning phase, 51–53
  dissemination phase, 53–54
  empirical phase, 53
  experimental research, 48–49
  nonexperimental research, 48–49
  observational study, 49
  research designs and. *See* Research design. *See* quantitative studies
  research report and, 708–714
  steps, 50–54, 51*f*
Quantitative sampling
  basic concepts, 257–260
  critical appraisal, 270–271, 271*b*
  implementing sampling plan, 268–270
  nonprobability sampling, 260–263
  probability sampling, 263–266
  sample size in, 266–268
Quantitative studies
  clinical trials, 224–226
  comparative effectiveness research (CER), 229
  critical appraisal, 234, 234*b*
  delphi surveys, 234
  evaluation research, 226–228

health services and outcomes research, 229–232
  implementation research., 234
  methodologic studies, 234
  needs assessments, 234
  replication studies, 234
  sample size in, 266–268
  secondary analysis, 234
  survey research, 232–233
  translational research, 234
Quantitative systematic review, 641–656
Quantitizing, **777**
  data, 585
Quasi-experimental designs
  comparison conditions, 191
  dose–response design, 191
  nonequivalent control group designs, 188–189
  other designs, 191
  strengths and limitations, 192
  time series designs, 189–191
Quasi-experiments, **777**
  comparison conditions, 191
  definition, 188
  designs, 188–191
  strengths and limitations, 192
Quasi-randomization, 184
Quasi-statistics, 561, **777**
Query letter, 720–721, **777**
Questioning route, focus group interviews, 504–505
Question, meta-ethnography, 658
Questionnaire, 278, **777**
  variant, 576
Questionnaires, 233
Quirkos software, 528
Quota sampling, 260–261, **777**

R
R, **777**
r, **777**
R^2, **777**
Random allocation, 180
Random assignment, 180, **777**
Random bias, 154
Random effects model, 650, **777**
Randomization, 180, **777**
  basic, 180–181
  definition, 180
  matching, 180
  principles, 180
  procedures, 182–184
  variants, 184
Randomized consent, 184
Randomized controlled trial (RCT), 176, 434, **778**. *See also* Experimental research
  CONSORT guidelines and, 709
  high rate of refusal, 680
  nonexperimental research, 687–688
  practice-based evidence and, 677
  quasi-experiments, 687
  subgroup analyses and, 692–694
  systematic review (SR), 637
Randomness, 155, **778**
Random number table, **777**
Random sampling, 263, **777**
Range, 368, **778**

Rank-order questions, 280
Rapid cycles, 245
Rapid response teams (RRTs), 189
Rapid reviews, 26, 638–639, **778**
Rapport, establishing, 512
Rasch model, **778**
Rating scales, 293–294, **778**
   questions, 281
Ratio measurement, 363, **778**
Raw data, 56, **778**
Rayyan, 641
Reactivity, 165, **778**
Readability, 342, **778**
   formula, 138
Reading research reports tips, 58–59
RE-AIM framework, 682, **778**
Realist evaluations, 228, **778**
Realist review, **778**
Receiver operating characteristic curve (ROC curve), 323, **778**
Recodes, data, 436
Recording equipment, types of, 514, 514*b*
Recording information, 98–101
Records, 165–166
Recursive model, 422, **778**
Reduction, phenomenologic, 469
Refereed journals, 722
Reference group, 420
References
   in research report, 714
Refining, 67–70
Reflective lifeworld research (RLR), 471, 536, **778**
Reflective notes, 515, **778**
Reflective scales, 310, **778**
Reflexive journal, 469
Reflexivity, 155–156, 555–556, 563, **778**
   data collection and, 501
RefWorks, 641
Regression analysis, 406, **778**
Regression coefficient *(b)*, 410–411
Relationships, 47–48, **778**
   complex interventions and, 599
Relative risk (RR), 196, 376, 648, **778**
Relative risk reduction (RRR), 376, **778**
Relevance, **778**
   patient-centered research and, 681
   strategies to enhance, 682–697
Reliability, 152–154, **778**
   coefficients interpretation, 316
   factors affecting, 316–317
   internal consistency, 317–318
   interrater reliability, 315
   intrarater reliability, 315
   measurement error, 318–319
   measuring change, 328–329
   parallel test reliability, 316
   test–retest reliability, 313–315
Reliability coefficients, 313, **778**
   interpretation of, 316
Reliable change index (RCI), 329–330, **778**
Repeated-measures ANOVA (RM-ANOVA), 394–395, 418, **779**
Repeated measures designs, 163, **779**

Replication, 552, **779**
   corroboration of results, 445
   studies, 234
Representativeness, 52, 489–490
Representative sample, 259, **779**
Reputational case sampling, 490
Request for Proposals (RFPs), 733
Requests for Applications (RFAs), 733
Research, 2, **779**
   building blocks, 43–48
   concepts, 43
   conceptual and operational definitions, 45–46
   constructs, 43
   data, 46–47
   Ethics Board, 143
   ethnonursing, **763**
   exploratory, 601–602, **764**
   faces, 42–43
   general questions, 59
   implementation, **766**
   journal articles, 56–59
   null hypotheses *vs.,* 77–78
   nursing intervention, 595
   phenomena, 43
   places of, 42–43
   quantitative/qualitative, 48–56
   relationships, 47–48
   terminology, 176
   theories/conceptual models, 43–44
   variables, 44–45
Researchability, 69
Research control, 154–155, **779**
Research critique, 103
Research design, 52, 462–481, **779**
   case studies, 474–475
   causality and, 464
   characteristics of, 462
   comparisons, 463
   critical appraisal of, 480–481, 481*b*
   descriptive studies, 477
   emergent design, 462
   ethnography, 464–468. *See also* Ethnography
   features of, 463
   grounded theory, 472–474. *See also* Grounded theory
   ideological perspectives and, 477–480
   narrative analysis, 475–476
   overview of, 464, 465*t*
   phenomenology, 468–472. *See also* Phenomenology
   pilot studies and, 622, 626
   planning and, 463
Research design, quantitative studies
   causality, 175–176
   construct validity, 216–217
   critical appraisal, 199, 200*b*
   designs, 198–199
   design terminology, 176
   experimental design, 176–185
   experiments, strengths and limitations of, 187–188
   external validity, 218
   internal validity, 212–216
   nonexperimental research, 192–198

observational research, 192–198
quasi-experiments. *See* Quasi-experiments
research evidence, 198–199
specific experimental designs, 185–187
statistical conclusion validity, 210–212
validity, 205–210, 219–220
Researcher, 42
  credibility, 552, 562, **779**
  expectancies, 217
  interest, 69–70
  obtrusiveness, 166–167
Research evidence, 34–36, 35*t*. *See also* Evidence
Research hypotheses, 77, **779**
  critical appraisal, 78–79, 79*t*
  derivation of, 76
  directional *vs*. nondirectional hypotheses, 77
  quantitative research, 74–75
  research *vs*. null hypotheses, 77–78
  testable hypotheses, 75–76
  testing and proof, 78
  wording of, 76–77
Research location, 159
Research methods, 10, **779**
Research misconduct, 146, **779**
Research Plan component, 737
Research problems, 65, **779**
  basic terminology, 65
  communicating, 70–74
  developing, 67–70
  evaluating, 68–70
  feasibility, 69
  paradigms, 65–66
  problem statements, 73–74
  refining, 67–70
  researchability, 69
  researcher interest, 69–70
  research questions, 71–73
  significance of, 68
  sources of, 66–67
  statements of purpose, 70–71
  terms relating examples, 66*t*
  topic narrowing, 67–68
  topic selecting, 67
Research Project Grant (R01), NIH, 734
Research proposal, 730–745, **779**
  functions of, 730
  funding for, 732–734
  grants from NIH and, 734–741
  proposal content, 730–731
  qualitative research and, 731
  theses and dissertations, 731–732
  tips for preparing, 741–745
Research questions, 65, 71–73, **779**
  communicating, 70–74
  critical appraisal, 78–79, 79*t*
  problem statements, 73–74
  qualitative studies, 72–73
  quantitative studies, 50, 71–72
  statements of purpose, 70–71
Research report, 53, **779**
  abstracts in, 714
  acknowledgments, 714
  assembling materials, 707

audiences for, 705–706
authorship and, 706
checklist, 714
communication outlets for, 705
deciding on content, 706–707
discussion section in, 713
introduction in, 705
keywords and, 714
method section in, 708–712
quantitative research and, 708–714
references in, 714
results section in, 712–713, 712*b*
titles of, 713–714
writing effectively, 707
Research utilization (RU), 22–23, **779**
Research waste, 598
Residuals, 407, **779**
Residual variables, 423
Resource-related objectives, 619–620
Respondent, **779**
Respondent-driven sampling (RDS), 260
Responder analysis, 456, 629, **779**
Response bias, 291, **779**
Response options, 279, 340–341, **779**
Response rates, 271, 285, **779**
Response sets, 291
  bias, **779**
Responsiveness, **779**
  construct approach, 331
  criterion approach to, 330–331
Results, **779**
  implications of, 449
  interpretation of, 441–458. *See also* Interpretation of results
  interpreting, 606–607
  magnitude of effects and, 446
  meaning of, 446–447
  mixed, 448–449
  nonsignificant, 447–449
  positive, 446
  precision of, 445–446
  regression, 413–414, 414*t*
Results section, 57–58
  in qualitative research reports, 715–716
  in quantitative reports, 712–713, 712*b*
Retrospective design, 193, **779**
Return on investment (ROI), 228, 598
Revelatory case sampling, 491
Review
  auspices, 640
  integrative, 638
  narrative, 637
  question, 641–642
  rapid, 638–639
  scoping, 638
  special types of, 637–639
  systematic, 636–668
  team, 640
  umbrella, 639
Review Manager (RevMan) software, 641
Rigor, qualitative research and, 551–564. *See also* Trustworthiness

Risk
  benefit assessment, 135
  benefit ratio, **779**
  of bias, 644–646, 645*t*, 652*f*
  difference, 648
  indexes, 373–376, 383
Rival hypothesis, 192, **779**
ROBINS-I, 644
Root cause analysis (RCA), 247, **779**
Rotated factor matrix, 350
Roy's adaptation model, 117
Rules, 307

S
Safety/tolerability of interventions, pilot studies and, 620–621
Samples, 258–259, **779**
Sample size, **779**
  bivariate tests, 400–401
  pilot studies and, 623–624
  qualitative studies and, 492–493
  two means, 399–400, 399*t*
Sample survey, 232
Sampling, 258–259, 579, **779**
  attrition, 268
  basics, 266–267
  bias, 259–260, **779**
  characteristics of, 381
  cluster, **758**
  confirming, 491
  consecutive, **759**
  convenience, 488
  cooperation, 268
  critical appraisal, 270–271, 271*b*
  decisions, 659
  disproportionate, **762**
  distribution, **779**
  distributions, 380–381, 381*f*
  effect size, 268
  error, 266, 380, **780**
  ethnography and, 493–494
  event, **763**
  frame, 263, 264*t*, **780**
  generalizing, 270
  grounded theory and, 494
  identical, **766**
  identical relationship, 580
  interval, 266
  maximum variation, **769**
  multilevel relationship, 580
  nested relationship, 580
  nonprobability. *See* Nonprobability sampling
  parallel relationship, 580
  phenomenology and, 494
  pilot studies and, 626–627
  plan, 257
  politically important cases, 491
  population, homogeneity of, 268
  practice-based evidence and, 688–689
  probability. *See* Probability sampling
  purposive, 489–491
  in qualitative research. *See* Qualitative sampling
  quantitative research, 257–271
  snowball, 488–489
  standard error of the mean (SEM), 381
  subgroup analyses, 268
  theoretical, 491–492
  transferability and, 494–495
Sampling plan, 52, **780**
Sandelowski and Barroso approach, metasynthesis and, 661–662
Saturation, **780**
Scale, 282, **780**
Scale content validity index (S-CVI), 320
Scale development
  conceptualization and item generation, 338–342
  critical appraisal of, 356, 356*b*
  data analysis, 346–351
  instrument field testing, 345–346
  preliminary evaluation of items, 342–345
  scale refinement and validation, 351–354
  scale scores, interpretability of, 354–355
Scatter plot, 371, **780**
Schematic models, 115, **780**
Scientific merit, 152, **780**
Scientific method, 10–11, **780**
Scientific-related objectives, 620–624
  clinical significance, 622
  data collection protocols and instruments, 623
  intervention attributes, 620
  intervention efficacy, 621–622
  intervention fidelity, 622–623
  methodologic issues, 622–624
  research design, 622
  safety and tolerability, 620–621
  sample size, 623–624, 624*t*
  substantive issues, 620–622
Scientific review groups (SRGs), 739
Scoping review, 638, **780**
Scores, **780**
  change, 328–330
Screening
  gathering references, 97–98
  instrument, 269, **780**
Searching bibliographic databases, 89–91
Search strategy, 88–89
Secondary analysis, 234, **780**
Secondary qualitative data analysis, 544
Secondary questions, 85–86
Secondary sources, 85, **780**
Selection bias, 436
Selection threat, **780**
Selective approach, 533
Selective coding, 537, 541, **780**
Selective observations, 513
Self-care deficit nursing theory, 117
Self-determination, 133, **780**
Self-efficacy theory, 118
Self-interview, reflexivity and, 555
Self-report(s), 164, 232, **780**
  diaries, 505–506
  focus group, 504–505
  joint, 505
  journals, 505–506
  narratives on internet, 506–507
  photo elicitation, 506

photovoice, 506
semistructured, 503–504
unstructured, 502–503
video-stimulated recall, 506
Self-selection, 196
SEM. *See* Standard error of the mean (SEM)
Semantic differential (SD) scales, 284, **780**
Semantic equivalence, **780**
Semistructured interviews, 503–504, **780**
Sensitivity, 321, **780**
  analysis, 438, 650, **780**
Sensitizing frameworks, 44
Sequential clinical trials, 225–226, **780**
Sequential design, 574, **780**
Sequential, multiple assignment, randomized trial (SMART), 684, **780**
Setting, 604, **780**
SF424 form, 735
Shadowed data, 492
Short form, 138
Show card, 288
Simple linear regression, 406–408, 407*t*, 408*f*
Simple random sampling, 263–264, **780**
Simultaneous multiple regression, 411, **780**
Single-blind study, 185, **781**
Single case study, 475
Single positioning, observations and, 513
Single-subject experiments, 686–687, **781**
Site, **781**
  selection, 159
  visits, 159
Six Sigma model, 244, **781**
Skewed distribution, 366, **781**
Skip patterns, 287
Smallest detectable change (SDC), 329, **781**
Small Grant Program, NIH (R03), 734
Snowballing, literature search, 644
Snowball sampling, 260, 488–489, **781**
Social cognitive theory, 118–119, 603
Social desirability response bias, 291, **781**
Source materials, 85
Source Normalized Impact per Paper (SNIP), 720
Space triangulation, 556, **781**
Spearman's rank-order correlation, **781**
Spearman's rho, 373, 397
Specificity, 321, **781**
Spradley's method, 532
SPSS (IBM SPSS Statistics)
  defaults and, 433
  Missing Values Analysis (MVA), 433
Squared semipartial correlation coefficients (sr^2), 413
SRToolbox, 641
Staged sampling, 259
Stakeholder(s), **781**
  complex interventions and, 599
  engagement, 156–157
  pilot work and, 626
Standard deviation, 368–369, **781**
Standard error, **781**
Standard error of measurement (SEM), 318, **781**
Standard error of the mean (SEM), 381
Standardized mean difference (SMD), 648, **781**
Standard scores, 355, **781**

Statements of purpose, 65, 70–71, **781**
Static measure, 309
Statistic(s), **781**
  bivariate, **756**
  descriptive, **761**
  inferential. *See* Inferential statistics
  multivariate. *See* Multivariate statistics
Statistical analysis, 53, **781**
Statistical Analysis System, 428
Statistical conclusion validity, 205, **781**
  low statistical power, 210–211
  restriction of range, 211
  treatment, unreliable implementation of, 211–212
Statistical control, **781**
Statistical heterogeneity, 649, **781**
Statistical inference, **781**
Statistically significant, 57
Statistical Package for the Social Sciences (SPSS), 428, 678
Statistical power, **781**
Statistical process control (SPC), 190, 250, **781**
Statistical significance, **781**
Statistical tests, 57, 384, **781**
  between-subjects *vs.* within-subjects, 387
  one-tailed and two-tailed tests, 386–387, 386*f*
  parametric and nonparametric tests, 387
  power of, 398
Statistics, 362
STEEEP, 240
Stepped wedge design, 683, **781**
Stepwise multiple regression, 411–412, 412*f*, **781**
Stimulated recall interview, **781**
Stipend, 133, **781**
Strand, mixed methods research, 574
Strata, 259, **782**
Stratification, **782**
Stratified purposive sampling, 490
Stratified randomization, 184
Stratified random sampling, 264–265, **782**
Structural equation modeling (SEM), 352, 423, **782**
Structural validity, 327–328, **782**
Structured data collection, 166, **782**
Structured methods, 166
Structured observation
  evaluation of, 296–297
  nonresearch observers, 296
  recording methods, 292–295
  sampling, 295
  technical aids, 295–296
Structured self-report instruments
  administering, 288–291
  composite scales and other structured self-reports, 282–285
  designing, 285–288
  evaluation of, 291–292
  interview data collecting, 288–289
  questionnaire data collecting, in-person distribution, 289
  questionnaire data collecting, internet, 290–291
  questionnaire data collecting, mail, 290
  structured questions, types of, 279–282
Structure of care, 230–231
Study participants, 42, 206–210, **782**
Study quality, 651
Study sections, 739, **782**

808 • Index

Study validity, tradeoffs and priorities in
   critical appraisal, 220
   external validity, 219
   internal validity, 219
   prioritization and design decisions, 219–220
Style of research, 58
Subgroup analysis, 650, 692–694, **782**
Subgroup effects, 268, 682
Subgroup mean substitution, 434
Subjects, 42, **782**
Subscale, **782**
Substantive analyses, 438
Substantive codes, 536
Substantive data analysis, 437–438
Substantive theory, 120, 473
SUMARI, 641
Summary of Findings (SoF) table, 654, 655*t*
Summary statements, 740
Summated rating scales, 282, **782**
Sum of squares
   error, 395
   between groups, 392
   within groups, 392
   subjects, 395
   treatments, 395
Superiority trials, 225–226, **782**
Supplementary data, 285
Surrogate outcomes, 163, 275, **782**
Survey, 232
   Delphi, **761**
   research, 232–233, **782**
Survival analysis, 421–422, **782**
Symbolic interaction, 121
Symmetric distribution, 366, **782**
Synthesized Member Checking (SMC), 557
Synthesizing information, 106
Systematic bias, 154
Systematic method, 10
Systematic mixed studies review, 26
Systematic review (SR), **6,** 636–668, **782**
   broad steps in, 640
   computer software, 640–641
   critical appraisal of, 668
   evidence-based practice and, 636
   mixed studies reviews, 663–666
   planning of, 639–641
   preliminary groundwork, 640
   qualitative studies and, 656–663
   quantitative studies and, 641–656
   review auspices, 640
   review team, 640
   schedule, 641
   types of, 637–639
Systematic sampling, 265–266, **782**

T
Table(s)
   in journal article submissions, 712
   random numbers, 181
   shell, 438, **782**
Tacit knowledge, 466, **782**
Tailored interventions, 178
Tailoring variable, 685

Target population, 257–258, **782**
Taxonomic analysis, 532
Taxonomy, 523, **782**
Team building, 602–603
Teamwork, complex interventions and, 598
Telephone interviews, 233
Terminology, research, 553
Terms relating examples, 66*t*
Testable hypotheses, 75–76
Testing, 214
   proof, 78
   threat, **782**
Test–retest reliability, 313–315, **782**
   analysis, 351
Test statistic, **782**
Thematic analysis, 477
Themes, 55, **782**
   analysis, 532
   qualitative research, 523
Theoretical coding, 536, 538, 539*t*
Theoretical frameworks, 115
   developing, 120–125
   research reports, critical appraisal in, 125
   testing, 120–125
   theories and models, 113–120
Theoretical notes, **782**
Theoretical sampling, 491–492, **782**
Theory, 43–44, 114, **782**
   Bandura's social cognitive theory, 118–119
   conceptual models, 117
   descriptive theory, 114
   developing, 120–125
   grand, 114–115
   health belief model (HBM), 119–120
   intervention, 603
   levels of, 114–115
   middle-range, 115, 117–118
   Mishel's uncertainty in illness theory, 118
   model selecting, 120
   Nola Pender's Health Promotion Model (HPM), 118
   nursing, 117
   Orem's self-care deficit nursing theory, 117
   organizing structure, 123
   origin of, 116
   other models and theories, 118
   problem fitting, 123
   qualitative research, 120–122
   quantitative research, 122–123
   quantitative study, 123–125
   research, 116–117
   role of, 116
   Roy's adaptation model, 117
   tentative nature of, 116
   testing, 120–125
   therapy/intervention, 14, 14*t*
   traditional theory, components of, 114
   Transtheoretical model, 119
Theory of Planned Behavior (Ajzen), 114, 603
Theory of Planned Behavior (TPB), 114
Theory triangulation, 558–559
Therapy/intervention questions, 14, 14*t*, **783**
Theses, 717–718
   proposals for, 731–732

Thick description, 495, 561–562, **783**
Think aloud method, 343, 507, **783**
Thoroughness, qualitative research and, 563
Threats to validity, 205, **783**
TIDieR reporting guideline, 711
Time sampling, 295, **783**
Time series design, 189, **783**
Time triangulation, 556, **783**
Timing, intervention development, 604
Title of research report, 713–714
Topic guide, 503, **783**
Topic narrowing, 67–68
Topic selecting, 67
Tracing, 214, **783**
Tradition, 7–8
Traditional journals, 718–719
Traditional theory, components of, 114
Training manual, 300
Transana, 528
Transferability, 156, **783**
    qualitative research, 554
    sampling and, 494–495
Transformative paradigm, 478
Translational research, 6, 23–24, 234, **783**
Transmogrifying, 536
Transparency, in researchers, 562–563
Transsubstantiating, 536
Transtheoretical model, 119
Transtheoretical Model (Prochaska), 603
Treatment, **783**
    adherence, 212
    group, **783**
Trend study, **783**
Trial/error, 8
Triangulation, 153, **783**
    data, 556
    investigator, **768**
    method, 556
    mixed methods (MM) research, 572
True score, 308, **783**
Trust, gaining participants, 500
Trustworthiness, 152–154, 551–564, **783**
    authenticity, 554
    confirmability, 553
    credibility, 553
    dependability, 553
    transferability, 554
T scores, 355
t-test, **783**
    Bonferroni correction, 390
    independent groups, 389–390, 389*t*
    one-sample, 389
    paired, 391
Two-dimensional matrices, 530
Two-tailed tests, 386–387, **783**
Two-way analysis of variance (ANOVA), 393–394, 394*t*
Type I error, 384, 384*f*, **783**
    Bonferroni correction, 390
Type II error, 384, 384*f*, **783**
    pilot studies and, 621
    power analysis and, 398
Typical case sampling, 490

U

Umbrella review, 639, **783**
Uncertainty in illness theory, 118
Underpowered, **783**
Unhypothesized results, 448
Unidimensional scale, **783**
Unimodal distribution, 366, **783**
Unit of analysis, 26, **783**
Univariate descriptive studies, 195–196
Univariate statistics, **783**
Unstructured data collection, 499–518
    field issues in, 499–501
    observations and, 510–517. *See also* Participant observation
    recording and storing data, 501–502
Unstructured interviews, 502–503, **783**
Unstructured methods, 166
Unstructured observation, **783**
Unstructured self-reports, 507
Urn randomization, 184, **783**
Users assistance, 17
Utrecht school of phenomenology, 470, 533–535

V

Validity, 152–154, 205–210, **783**
    construct, 216–217, 324–328, **759**
    content, 319–320, 602
    criterion, 320–324
    critical appraisal, 220, 220*b*
    cross-cultural, 328, **761**
    definition, 205
    divergent, **762**
    ecological, **762**
    external, 218, **764**
    face, 319–320
    internal, 212–216
    known-groups, **768**
    mixed methods (MM) research, 570
    qualitative research and, 551–564. *See also* Trustworthiness
    statistical conclusion, 210–212
    threats, 205
    tradeoffs and priorities in, 219–220
    types of, 205–206
Variability, 368–370, **783**
Variables, 44–45, **783**
    categorical, **757**
    characteristics of, 44
    endogenous, **763**
    extraneous, **764**
Variance, 369, **783**
Verbal portion of an entrance exam (EE-V), 408
Verification
    data entry and, 432
    qualitative research and, 563
Videoconferencing interviews, 508
Video-reflexive ethnography (VRE), 467
Video-stimulated recall interviews, 506
Vignettes, 284, **784**
Visual analog scale (VAS), 281, **784**
Vividness, qualitative research and, 556–557
Voice recognition software, 529
Volunteer sample, 488
Vulnerable groups, 142–143, **784**

W

Wait-list control group, 179
Wait-list design, **784**
Wald statistic, 421, **784**
Washout period, 187
Web-based surveys, 290, **784**
Weighted average, meta-analysis, 649
Weighting, 265, **784**
Wilcoxon signed-rank test, 391, **784**
Wild code, 430, **784**
Windshield survey, 512
Within-subjects designs, 159, **784**
Within-subjects tests, 387, 418
Wording, 76–77
Writing, 106–108

Y

Yea-sayers bias, 292, **784**

Z

Zelen design, 184
Zoom, 508
z (standard) score, 413, **784**